# Medical Microbiology

*For Churchill Livingstone*

*Publisher:* Timothy Horne
*Project Manager:* Ninette Premdas
*Copy Editor:* Rich Cutler
*Indexer:* Monica Trigg
*Project Controller:* Nancy Arnott
*Design:* Erik Bigland

# Medical Microbiology

A Guide to Microbial Infections:
Pathogenesis, Immunity, Laboratory Diagnosis and Control

Edited by

## David Greenwood BSc PhD DSc FRCPath

Professor of Antimicrobial Science, Division of
Microbiology, University of Nottingham Medical School,
Nottingham, UK; Honorary Microbiologist, Public Health
Laboratory Service

## Richard C. B. Slack MA MB BChir MRCPath DRCOG

Senior Lecturer, Division of Microbiology, University of
Nottingham Medical School, Nottingham, UK; Consultant in
Communicable Disease Control, Nottingham Health
Authority; Honorary Consultant, Public Health Laboratory
Service

## John F. Peutherer BSc MB ChB MD FRCPath FRCPE

Senior Lecturer, Department of Medical Microbiology,
University of Edinburgh Medical School; Honorary
Consultant, The Royal Infirmary of Edinburgh NHS Trust, Edinburgh, UK

FIFTEENTH EDITION

CHURCHILL
LIVINGSTONE

NEW YORK  EDINBURGH  LONDON  MADRID  MELBOURNE  SAN FRANCISCO AND TOKYO 1997

CHURCHILL LIVINGSTONE
Medical Division of Longman Group UK Limited

Distributed in the United States of America by Churchill
Livingstone Inc., 650 Avenue of the Americas, New York,
N.Y. 10011, and by associated companies, branches and
representatives throughout the world.

First edition 1925
Second edition 1928
Third edition 1931
Fourth edition 1934
Fifth edition 1938
Sixth edition 1942
Seventh edition 1945
Eighth edition 1948
Ninth edition 1953
Tenth edition 1960
Eleventh edition 1965

Twelfth edition (Vol. 1) 1973
Twelfth edition (Vol. 2) 1975
Thirteenth edition (Vol. 1) 1978
Thirteenth edition (Vol. 2) 1989
Fourteenth edition 1992
Fifteenth edition 1997

International edition of fifteenth edition published 1997

Standard edition ISBN 0443 054541
International edition ISBN 0443 055602

**British Library Cataloguing in Publication Data**
A catalogue record for this book is available from the British
Library.

**Library of Congress Cataloging in Publication Data**
A catalog record for this book is available from the Library
of Congress

Medical knowledge is constantly changing. As new
information becomes available, changes in treatment,
procedures, equipment and the use of drugs become
necessary. The editors, contributors and the publishers have,
as far as it is possible, taken care to ensure that the
information given in this text is accurate and up to date.
However, readers are strongly advised to confirm that the
information, especially with regard to drug usage, complies
with current legislation and standards of practice.

The
publisher's
policy is to use
**paper manufactured
from sustainable forests**

Produced by Longman Asia Ltd, Hong Kong
NPCC/01

# Preface

If T. J. Mackie and J. E. McCartney, the original authors of this book (first published in 1925 as *An Introduction to Practical Bacteriology as Applied to Medicine and Public Health*) were able to see the latest edition, they would be astonished at how the subject has grown. Vastly more infective agents of all kinds – bacteria, viruses, protozoa, helminths and fungi – are recognized. Spectacular advances in molecular genetics have fostered a detailed understanding of microbial physiology, mechanisms of microbial pathogenicity and the host response to microbial invasion. Antimicrobial agents and vaccines beyond the wildest dreams of workers in the 1920s are in common use. Many infectious diseases have been controlled and one scourge, smallpox, eradicated. The subject is now so large that the practical laboratory aspects, once considered essential to a proper knowledge of microbiology, have long been hived off into a companion volume: *Mackie and McCartney: Practical Medical Microbiology*, edited by J. G. Collee, A. G. Fraser, B. P. Marmion and A. Simmons.

Despite our increased understanding of microbes, and the means to control them, infection continues to flourish: one third of the population of the world is estimated to harbour the bacillus of tuberculosis; millions of infants die of bacterial, viral and protozoal infection before they reach their fifth birthday; food-borne disease, even in developed countries, is at an all time high; AIDS continues its inexorable spread; the growth of antimicrobial drug resistance is causing considerable alarm. The lesson is clear. Microbes will not be easily subdued, and medical students, indeed, all health-care professionals, need to understand the principles of infection and its control. The trouble is, that with the subject now so vast, learning is necessarily selective. Moreover, with so many other demands on students' time it is easy to consign the study of infection to a minor place in the curriculum in the mistaken belief that microbial disease has been controlled by antimicrobial drugs and vaccines. Nothing could be further from the truth, and microbiology must retain a high profile in medical schools. In this book we have tried to concentrate on essentials, while providing enough background to help the student to understand the full context of microbial disease, including the often neglected topics of the epidemiology and control of infection. The emphasis is very much on clinical microbiology, but with sufficient explanation of the laboratory aspects of the subject to allow an intelligent use of diagnostic laboratory services. Readers seeking fuller information about laboratory techniques are referred to the excellent companion volume. Rather than provide an exhaustive reference list for each chapter, a few key publications are recommended to the interested reader seeking further information.

For this new edition the text has been brought fully up to date. We are most grateful to our contributors, who have suffered our constant cajoling with equanimity and produced, mostly on time, manuscripts that required very little editorial interference. Unusually among textbooks, we have been able to encompass new developments without increase – in fact, with a modest decrease – in the size of the book. This has been achieved by attention to layout and by some rationalization of the tables, figures and text. Nothing of importance, we believe, has been sacrificed.

Once more we thank our contributing authors and the editorial staff of Churchill Livingstone, who have also endured much badgering during the genesis of this book.

David Greenwood, Richard Slack, John Peutherer
Nottingham and Edinburgh, UK, 1997

# Contributors

**R. P. Allaker** BSc PhD
Lecturer in Oral Microbiology
St Bartholomew's and the Royal London School of
Medicine and Dentistry
London, UK

**Michael R. Barer** MB BS PhD MRCPath
Reader
Department of Microbiology
University of Newcastle upon Tyne
Newcastle upon Tyne, UK

**Sheila M. Burns** MB ChB MRCPath
Consultant Virologist
The Royal Infirmary of Edinburgh NHS Trust
Director, Regional Virus Laboratory
City Hospital
Edinburgh, UK

**Evan Owen Caul** PhD FIBMS FRCPath
Deputy Director
Bristol PHL
Consultant Clinical Scientist
Bristol Public Health Laboratory
Bristol, UK

**A. Cockayne** BSc PhD
Research Fellow
Department of Microbiology
University Hospital
Nottingham, UK

**Joyce D. Coghlan** BSc PhD
Formerly Director, Leptospira Reference
Laboratory
Public Health Laboratory Service
London
Formerly Lecturer in Bacteriology
University of Edinburgh Medical School
Edinburgh, UK

**J. G. Collee** CBE MD FRCPath FRCP(Edin) FRSE
Emeritus Professor of Medical Microbiology
University of Edinburgh Medical School
Edinburgh, UK

**Heather A. Cubie** BSc MSc PhD MRCPath
Consultant Clinical Scientist
Regional Virus Laboratory
City Hospital
Edinburgh, UK

**W. David Cubitt** BTech MSc PhD MIBiol
Consultant Clinical Scientist, Honorary Senior
Lecturer
Great Ormond Street Hospital for Children
and Institute of Child Health NHS Trust
London, UK

**J. Mervyn Darville** BSc PhD FRCPath
Lecturer in Medical Virology
University of Bristol
(Honorary) Clinical Virologist
Bristol Public Health Laboratory
Bristol, UK

**Ulrich Desselberger** MD FRCPath FRCP(Glas, Lon)
Consultant Virologist and Director
Clinical Microbiology and Public Health
Laboratory
Addenbrooke's Hospital
Cambridge, UK

**E. Glyn V. Evans** BSc PhD CBiol FIBiol FRCPath
Professor of Medical Mycology
PHLS Mycology Reference Laboratory
Department of Microbiology
University of Leeds and General Infirmary
Leeds, UK

**R. J. Fallon** BSc MD FRCPath FRCP(Glas)
Formerly Consultant in Laboratory
Medicine, Ruchill Hospital
Formerly Honorary Senior Clinical
Lecturer in Bacteriology and
Infectious Diseases
University of Glasgow
Glasgow, UK

**Roger G. Finch** FRCP PRCPath FFPM
Professor of Infectious Diseases
Division of Microbiology and Infectious Diseases
The City Hospital
Nottingham, UK

**K. L. Gage** PhD
Plague Section Chief (Acting)
Division of Vector-Borne Infectious Diseases
Centers for Disease Control and Prevention
Colorado, USA

**John R. W. Govan** PhD DSc
Reader
Department of Medical Microbiology
University of Edinburgh Medical School
Edinburgh, UK

**John Grange** MD MSc
Reader in Clinical Microbiology
Imperial College School of Medicine at the
National Heart and Lung Institute
London, UK

**D. Greenwood** BSc PhD DSc FRCPath
Professor of Antimicrobial Science
Division of Microbiology
Department of Clinical Laboratory Sciences
University of Nottingham
Honorary Microbiologist
Public Health Laboratory Service, UK

**J. M. Hardie** BDS PhD DipBact FRCPath
Professor of Oral Microbiology
St Bartholomew's & the Royal London School of
Medicine and Dentistry
London, UK

**H. Humphreys** MD FRCPI MRCPath
Senior Lecturer
University of Nottingham
Honorary Consultant Microbiologist
University Hospital and Public Health Laboratory
Service
Nottingham, UK

**James Ironside** BMSc(Hons) MBChB MRCPath
Senior Lecturer in Pathology
University of Edinburgh
Honorary Consultant in Neuropathology
Western General Hospitals Trust, Edinburgh, UK

**M. J. Lewis** MD DipBact
Formerly Director
Nottingham Area Public Health Laboratory
Formerly Senior Lecturer
University of Nottingham
Nottingham, UK

**Alasdair P. MacGowan** BMedBiol(Hons) MD MRCPath
Consultant Medical Microbiologist
Regional Antimicrobial Reference Laboratory
Department of Medical Microbiology
Southmead Health Services NHS Trust
Bristol, UK

**C. R. Madeley** MD FRCPath
Professor of Clinical Virology
Department of Virology
The Medical School
University of Newcastle upon Tyne
Newcastle upon Tyne, UK

**Ruth C. Matthews** MS PhD FRCPath
Reader in Medical Microbiology
Director, Pertussis Reference Laboratory
University of Manchester, Clinical Sciences
Building
Manchester Royal Infirmary, UK

**Donald M. McLean** MD FRCP FRCPath
Professor Emeritus of Pathology
University of British Columbia
Canada

**P. Morgan-Capner** BSc MBBS FRCPath
Consultant Virologist
Public Health Laboratory Service North West
Preston, UK

**Mary Norval** BSc PhD DSc
Reader
Department of Medical Microbiology
University of Edinburgh Medical School
Edinburgh, UK

**M. M. Ogilvie** MD BSc(Hons) MRCPath
Senior Lecturer (Hon Consultant)
Department of Medical Microbiology
University of Edinburgh Medical School,
Edinburgh, UK

**J. R. Pattison** MA BSc DM FRCPath
Professor of Medical Microbiology
University College London Medical School
London, UK

**J. S. M. Peiris** MBBS FRCPath DPhil(Oxon)
Senior Lecturer
Department of Microbiology
University of Hong Kong
Hong Kong

**T. H. Pennington** MB BS PhD FRCPath
Professor of Bacteriology
University of Aberdeen
Aberdeen, UK

**J. F. Peutherer** BSc MB ChB MD FRCPath FRCPE
Senior Lecturer
Department of Medical Microbiology
University of Edinburgh Medical School
Honorary Consultant
The Royal Infirmary of Edinburgh NHS Trust
Edinburgh, UK

**T. L. Pitt** MPhil PhD
Deputy Director
Laboratory of Hospital Infection
Central Public Health Laboratory
London, UK

**Noel W. Preston** MD DpBact FRCPath LRCP LRCS LRFPS
Honorary Fellow in Microbial Immunology,
Department of Medical Microbiology
University of Manchester
WHO Expert Adviser on Bacterial Diseases
Formerly Director of Pertussis Reference
Laboratory, University of Manchester
Formerly Honorary Consultant Microbiologist,
Public Health Laboratory Service
UK

**D. Reid** DBE MD FRCP(Glas) FRCP(Edin) FFPHM DPH
Director, Scottish Centre for Infection and
Environmental Health, Ruchill Hospital, Glasgow
Honorary Professor, University of Glasgow
Visiting Professor, University of Strathclyde,
Glasgow, UK

**P. W. Ross** TD MD FRCPath FRCPE CBiol FIBiol FLS
Reader
Department of Medical Microbiology
University of Edinburgh
Honorary Consultant Bacteriologist
Royal Infirmary of Edinburgh NHS Trust
Edinburgh, UK

**R. A. Simpson** PhD MRCPath
Director of Laboratory Services
Healthcare Science Ltd, UK

**M. B. Skirrow** MB PhD FRCPath DTM&H
Honorary Emeritus Consultant Microbiologist
Public Health Laboratory Service
Gloucestershire Royal Hospital, UK

**Mary P. E. Slack** MA MB BChir FRCPath
University Lecturer, Nuffield Department of
Pathology and Bacteriology
University of Oxford
Honorary Consultant Microbiologist
Oxford Radcliffe Hospital
Honorary Consultant, Public Health Laboratory
Service
Oxford, UK

**Richard Slack** MA MB BChir MRCPath DRCOG
Senior Lecturer and Consultant in Communicable
Disease Control
University of Nottingham Medical School
Nottingham
Honorary Consultant, Public Health Laboratory
Service
UK

**Isabel W. Smith** BSc PhD
Formerly Senior Lecturer
Department of Medical Microbiology
University of Edinburgh Medical School
Edinburgh, UK

**John Stewart** BSc PhD
Lecturer
Department of Medical Microbiology
University of Edinburgh Medical School
Edinburgh, UK

**Sheena Sutherland** MBChB FRCPath
Senior Lecturer
Department of Medical Microbiology
University of Edinburgh Medical School
Honorary Consultant
The Royal Infirmary of Edinburgh NHS Trust
Edinburgh, UK

**David Taylor-Robinson** MD MRCP FRCPath
Professor of Genitourinary Microbiology and
Medicine
Imperial College School of Medicine at St Mary's
Jefferiss Research Trust Laboratories
London, UK

**K. J. Towner** BSc PhD
Consultant Clinical Scientist
Division of Microbiology and Infectious Diseases &
PHLS Laboratory
University Hospital
Queen's Medical Centre
Nottingham, UK

**David H. Walker** MD
Professor and Chairman
Department of Pathology
University of Texas Medical Branch at Galveston
Director
WHO Collaborating Center for Tropical Diseases,
UTMB
USA

**D. M. Weir** MD FRCPE
Formerly Professor of Microbial Immunology
University of Edinburgh Medical School
Edinburgh, UK

# Contents

# Part 1
## MICROBIAL BIOLOGY

# 1

# Microbiology and medicine

*D. Greenwood*

Applications of microbiology have transformed the diagnosis, prevention and cure of disease. Along with improved nutrition and living conditions, they have – at least in developed communities – revolutionized human health, doubled the average length of life and ensured the safe upbringing of most children born, where before only a minority survived.

The conquest of epidemic and fatal infections has sometimes seemed so conclusive that the main challenges in medicine are often seen to lie in other fields, such as those of the mental illnesses and degenerative diseases, but a major shift of attention away from the problems of infection could be dangerous. The relative freedom of society from fatal infections depends on the continued, informed deployment of complex countermeasures: on correct diagnosis and treatment of infections, full implementation of immunization programmes, alert epidemiological surveillance and rigorous environmental sanitation. Moreover, on a global scale, infection is far from defeated. In the developing nations of the world, an estimated 10 million young children die each year from the effects of infectious diarrhoeas, measles, malaria, tetanus, diphtheria and whooping cough alone. The tragedy is that we have the means to hand to prevent nearly all these deaths.

Even in the developed world, infection is still extremely common: at least a quarter of all illnesses for which patients consult their doctors are infective; a substantial proportion of patients acquire infection while in hospital, sometimes with multiresistant organisms. Intensive farming methods and a shift in eating habits to pre-prepared 'fast foods' have led to a sharp increase in food-related infection. In hospitals, new approaches to therapy that deplete the competence of the patient's immune system to cope with infection, as well as the increasing use of shunts, intravenous cannulae and prosthetic devices, all provide the ever-resourceful microbes with new opportunities to invade the host. Previously unsuspected links between microbes and diseases such as cancer, peptic ulcer, inflammatory bowel disease and rheumatoid arthritis have been uncovered. Surprisingly, 'new' agents of infectious disease continue to be recognized (Table 1.1). The most notorious of these is undoubtedly the human immunodeficiency virus (HIV), the causative agent of acquired immune deficiency syndrome (AIDS). The rise and spread of this condition provides a sobering reminder of the potential impact of microbial disease. It is as essential now as it ever was that health care personnel should be well trained in matters relating to infection.

**Table 1.1** Some newly recognized infectious agents, 1975–95

| Agent | Disease |
|---|---|
| *Bartonella henselae* | Cat scratch disease |
| *Borrelia burgdorferi* | Lyme disease |
| *Campylobacter jejuni* | Enteritis |
| *Chlamydia pneumoniae* | Pneumonia |
| *Clostridium difficile* | Pseudomembranous colitis |
| *Cryptosporidium parvum* | Diarrhoea |
| *Cyclospora cayetanensis* | Diarrhoea |
| *Escherichia coli* O157 | Haemolytic uraemic syndrome |
| *Helicobacter pylori* | Gastritis |
| Hepatitis C virus | Hepatitis |
| Hepatitis E virus | Hepatitis |
| Hepatitis G virus | Hepatitis |
| Human herpesvirus 6 | Exanthem subitum |
| Human herpesvirus 8 | Kaposi's sarcoma |
| Human immunodeficiency virus | Acquired immune deficiency syndrome (AIDS) |
| Human T cell lymphotropic virus | Adult T cell leukaemia; tropical spastic paraparesis |
| *Legionella pneumophila* | Legionnaires' disease |
| Microspora (various genera) | Diarrhoea |
| *Mobiluncus* spp. | Bacterial vaginosis |
| Parvovirus B19 | Fifth disease |
| 'Small round' viruses | Gastro-enteritis |
| *Tropheryma whippelii* | Whipple's disease |

## DEVELOPMENT OF MICROBIOLOGY

*Microbiology* is the study of living organisms of microscopic size. The term was introduced by the French chemist Louis Pasteur, whose demonstration that fermentation was caused by the growth of bacteria and yeasts (1857–60) provided a main impetus for the development of the science.

Micro-organisms were first seen about 1675 by the Dutchman Antony van Leeuwenhoek. His microscopes consisted of a single biconvex lens that magnified about ×200 and resolved bodies with diameters down to about 1 μm. He found many micro-organisms in materials such as water, mud, saliva and the intestinal contents of healthy subjects, and he recognized them as living creatures ('animalcules') because they swam about actively. That he saw bacteria as well as the larger microbes is known from his measurements of their size ('one-sixth the diameter of a red blood corpuscle') and his drawings of the forms we now recognize as cocci (spheres), bacilli (rods) and spirochaetes (spiral filaments).

Leeuwenhoek observed that very large numbers of bacteria appeared in watery infusions of animal or vegetable matter which were left to stand for a week or two at room temperature. He believed that these huge populations were the progeny of a few parental organisms, or seeds, that were originally present in the materials of the infusion or had entered it from the air. Other scientists suggested that the organisms arose by spontaneous generation from dead organic matter, and this began a controversy that lasted for 200 years. The prototype of the experiment that ultimately was to settle the matter was first described by the French microscopist Louis Joblot in 1718. Joblot boiled a flask of an infusion of hay for 15 min to kill any microbes originally present, covered it with a parchment cap to prevent the later entry of other microbes from the air and showed that, on subsequent standing, it remained free from microbial growth. Similar experiments, notably those of John Needham (1749), showed, by contrast, that heated, covered infusions gave a growth of organisms and so appeared to demonstrate the occurrence of spontaneous generation. It was not at first realized how exacting were the conditions needed to kill all micro-organisms, and maintain sterility. The necessary techniques were perfected only after much further work, particularly that by Lazzaro Spallanzani (1765, 1776) and Louis Pasteur (1860–64). Pasteur's flasks of infusions, sterilized by autoclaving at 115–120°C, always remained sterile despite the entry of unheated air through a dust-stopping 'swan neck' or cotton-wool stopper, and so finally proved the absence of spontaneous generation.

The controversy over spontaneous generation had the valuable outcome of establishing many of the basic techniques of bacteriology. Convenient nutrient media for preparing cultures of bacteria in the laboratory were derived from meat and vegetable infusions, and reliable methods were developed for the sterilization and maintenance of sterility of culture media and equipment. The mechanism of bacterial reproduction by asexual fission was discovered by De Saussure (1760), and the need for high temperatures for sterilization was explained by Ferdinand Cohn's (1876) discovery that certain bacteria form heat-resistant spores. Other techniques essential for the rapid progress of bacteriology were developed by the German bacteriologist Robert Koch, who in 1877 described methods for the easy microscopical examination of bacteria in dried, fixed films stained with aniline dyes, and in 1881 devised the simple method for isolating pure cultures of bacteria by plating out mixed material on a solid culture medium on which the progeny of single bacteria grow in separate colonies.

## MICRO-ORGANISMS AND DISEASE

Few of the micro-organisms that abound in nature are disease-producing, or *pathogenic*, for humans. Most are free-living in soil, water and similar habitats, and are unable to invade the living body. Some free-living micro-organisms obtain their energy from daylight or by the oxidation of inorganic matter, but the majority feed on dead organic matter, and are termed *saprophytes*. In contrast, a parasite lives in or on, and obtains its nourishment from, a living host. In medical usage, the term *parasite* is nowadays usually reserved for parasitic protozoa, helminths and arthropods. The last usually affect the outside of the body, and are termed *ectoparasites*. *Commensal* micro-organisms constitute the normal flora of the healthy body. They live on the skin and on the mucous membranes of the upper respiratory tract, intestines and vagina, and obtain nourishment from the secretions and food residues. They are generally harmless, but under certain circumstances, as when the body's defences are impaired, they may invade the tissues and cause disease, thus acting as *opportunist* pathogens. True pathogens are the micro-organisms that are adapted to overcoming the normal defences of the body and invading the tissues; their growth in the tissues, or their production of poisonous substances (*toxins*), damages the tissues and causes the manifestations of disease. The process of microbial invasion of the body is called *infection*. Those infective diseases that are readily communicable from person to person are called *infectious* or *contagious*.

The germ theory of disease was slow in gaining acceptance, though it was early recognized that epidemic diseases such as smallpox, measles, typhus and syphilis were probably spread from person to person. The Italian scholar Girolamo Fracastoro, in his book *De Contagione* (1546), distinguished three modes of transmission: (1) by direct contact, i.e. touching a patient's body; (2) by contact with clothing and household goods contaminated by a patient; and (3) at a distance through the air. He explained contagion as being due to the transmission of invisible seeds, or germs, different kinds of which were the specific causes of the different diseases. It is unclear whether he regarded the germs as living, but their ability to multiply in successive hosts would certainly be necessary for their continued spread.

Fracastoro's views were largely forgotten by the time Leeuwenhoek discovered micro-organisms, but speculations then began that these organisms might be the cause of certain diseases. The first clear demonstration of a pathogenic role was made by the Italian civil servant Agostino Bassi (1835), who showed that the calcino disease of silkworms was invariably associated with an invasion of their tissues by a fungus and that the disease could be transmitted by the inoculation of material from the tissues of an infected worm into those of a healthy one.

Despite Bassi's work, the germ theory of disease did not become firmly established until 1876, when Robert Koch, a country doctor in East Prussia, reported his observations on anthrax. Ten years earlier, C. J. Davaine had shown that the blood of sheep dying from anthrax contained numerous non-motile filaments and that its inoculation into healthy sheep caused them to develop anthrax. These findings, however, did not exclude the possibility that the filaments were inanimate products of the disease rather than its cause. Koch began his work by transmitting anthrax from infected sheep and cattle to the mouse, an unnatural but convenient laboratory host. He observed filaments in the blood and tissues of the infected mouse, and proved that they were living bacteria by watching them grow and form spores in drops of sterile ox serum or aqueous humour seeded with fragments of infected tissue. He showed that the bacteria alone were the cause of the disease by growing them in a series of eight pure cultures in aqueous humour, each seeded with a

small proportion of the preceding one, and then reproducing the disease by inoculation of the final culture into a mouse. He thus provided the evidence, now described as *Koch's postulates*, which Jacob Henle had earlier stated would be needed to prove that the particular micro-organism was the cause of a particular disease, namely: that the microbe be found in the body in all cases of the disease; that it be isolated from a case and grown in a series of pure cultures in vitro; and that it reproduce the disease on the inoculation of a late pure culture into a susceptible animal.

Koch obtained a research appointment in Berlin and there built up a successful school of bacteriology. He demonstrated the pathogenic roles of the tubercle bacillus (1882) and cholera vibrio (1883), and established the general principle that specific micro-organisms cause different kinds of disease. This principle is not absolute, and in 1883 some exceptions were demonstrated by the Scottish surgeon Alexander Ogston, who showed that *Staphylococcus aureus* and *Streptococcus pyogenes* could each cause various suppurative infections, such as abscesses and wound sepsis.

Alongside the discovery of the pathogenic role of bacteria the involvement of protozoa, helminths and fungi was soon established. Worms visible to the naked eye had, of course, been recognized in antiquity, but great strides were made in the 19th century. Among notable events were: the discovery by James Paget (while a first-year medical student at St Bartholomew's Hospital, London) of the larvae of *Trichinella spiralis* in muscle during an autopsy (1835); the observation by Alfred Donné of *Trichomonas vaginalis* in vaginal secretions (1836); the discovery of adult worms of *Schistosoma haematobium* by Theodor Bilharz in Cairo (1851); demonstration of the fungal nature of thrush by Langenbeck (1859); and the recognition of the parasites of malaria in human blood by the French Army surgeon Alphonse Laveran (1880). The complex life cycles of many of the parasitic worms and protozoa were later worked out by painstaking studies by numerous workers, of whom Patrick Manson, Ronald Ross and David Bruce are among the most celebrated.

The viruses were more difficult to demonstrate, for most were too small to be seen with the light microscope and none could be grown on an inanimate culture medium. At first they could be demonstrated only by observation of the disease they produced when infected tissue was inoculated into a susceptible animal. Thus, in studies of rabies, Pasteur and his colleagues in 1881 failed to isolate any micro-organism capable of causing the disease. They were able to reproduce the disease in dogs and rabbits by the intracerebral injection of brain tissue or saliva from a fatal case, and they suggested that the causal agent was an organism too small to be seen. Their experiments, however, did not exclude the possibility that the agent might be a bacterium, or a larger microbe which was present but undetected in the inoculum. The means of excluding such a possibility was devised by Ivanowski (1892) in experiments with the viral mosaic disease of tobacco; he transmitted the disease to healthy plants by the inoculation of juice from a diseased plant after it had been filtered through a porcelain filter fine enough to prevent the passage of bacteria. Filter-passing viruses were soon similarly demonstrated in foot-and-mouth disease of cattle by Loeffler and Frosch (1898), in yellow fever by Reed, Carroll, Agramonte and Lazear (1900), who had to test their inoculations in human volunteers, and in other diseases. Virology did not progress rapidly, however, until after the Second World War, when the availability of the electron microscope enabled viruses to be visualized and the use of living human and animal tissue cells for the in-vitro culture of viruses was developed by John Enders (1949) and others from the earlier work of pioneers such as Alexis Carrel.

## IMMUNITY AND IMMUNIZATION

It was known from ancient times that persons who had suffered from a distinctive disease, such as smallpox or measles, resisted it on subsequent exposures and rarely contracted it a second time. Such an acquired immunity is generally effective only against the same type of infection as that previously suffered.

Artificial immunization against smallpox was practised in various communities by the unsafe method of inoculating smallpox exudate through the skin (*variolation*), until, in 1796, the safer method of inoculating cowpox exudate (*vaccination*) was discovered by the Gloucestershire doctor Edward Jenner. Present-day vaccinia virus has been shown to be different from cowpox virus, and its origin is obscure. Nevertheless, it is highly effective and has been instrumental in the world eradication of natural smallpox, the last case of which occurred in Somalia in 1977. The natural existence of a safe immunizing agent such as vaccinia virus is exceptional, and we owe to Pasteur the development of immunizing strains of pathogenic microbes which are artificially *attenuated* (reduced in virulence) by prolonged or repeated culture under laboratory conditions. Pasteur derived such attenuated live *vaccines* for fowl cholera,

anthrax, swine erysipelas and rabies, and called them *vaccines* in honour of Jenner's work with cowpox, or vaccinia (Latin *vacca* = cow). In 1881 he made a convincing controlled trial of his anthrax vaccine, in which a vaccinated group of cows and sheep survived a later challenge by the inoculation of virulent anthrax bacilli, while a control group of unvaccinated animals perished from the same challenge. Today, attenuated live vaccines are used with outstanding success against such diseases as tuberculosis, poliomyelitis, measles and yellow fever.

The efficacy of vaccines consisting of killed bacteria was discovered by Salmon and Smith in 1886 in experiments on salmonellosis in pigeons, and today killed vaccines are used against, for example, typhoid fever, whooping cough and influenza. About 1900, Loewenstein in Vienna and Glenny in London discovered that bacterial toxins rendered non-poisonous by treatment with formaldehyde were effective in immunizing against diphtheria and tetanus, diseases in which the serious effects are due to the toxin. The *toxoids* are now used routinely for immunization.

The first step in elucidating the mechanisms of acquired immunity was the discovery of *antibodies* by Behring and Kitasato in 1890. They found that the injection of sublethal doses of diphtheria or tetanus toxin into guinea-pigs rendered the animals immune to the later injection of large doses of the same toxin. The immunity was associated with the appearance in the animal's blood of a substance, *antitoxin*, that specifically neutralized the toxin. These diphtheria and tetanus antitoxins were the first known antibodies, but protective antibodies which reacted directly with bacteria and viruses were soon demonstrated by other workers. Antibodies have a highly specific affinity for the microbial substances, or *antigens*, that have induced their formation, and this property is exploited in the common use of blood serum containing antibodies (*antiserum*) in laboratory tests for the precise identification of microorganisms. Discovery of the means of perpetuating the growth of single antibody-producing cells has enabled these techniques to be further refined by the use of *monoclonal antibodies* that exhibit absolute specificity for the target antigens.

## SEROTHERAPY AND CHEMOTHERAPY

The work of Behring and Kitasato led to the successful use of antisera raised in animals for the treatment of patients with diphtheria, tetanus, pneumonia and other diseases. Because, however, the antisera contained animal proteins foreign to the human body, and were given by injection, serotherapy often caused unpleasant allergic responses, called *serum sickness*. For this reason, and also because serotherapy was unsuccessful against many kinds of infection, further progress depended on the development of drugs that exhibited *selective toxicity* – the ability to inhibit or kill the microbe without harming the patient.

Although agents active against bacteria now form the most abundant group of antimicrobial drugs, the earliest therapeutic successes were achieved with antiprotozoal and anthelminthic compounds. Indeed, effective treatment for malaria (cinchona bark), amoebic dysentery (ipecacuanha root), tapeworm (male fern) and roundworm (wormseed) have been known for centuries. In contrast, effective therapy for systemic bacterial disease was unknown before the use of hexamine (methenamine) at the turn of the 20th century and Paul Ehrlich's development of the arsenical Salvarsan (arsphenamine) for spiro-chaetal disease in 1909. Even these discoveries were of limited value. The true beginning of the therapeutic revolution in infection dates from Gerhard Domagk's description of Prontosil (the forerunner of sulphona-mides) in 1935, the development of Alexander Fleming's penicillin by Howard Florey and his col-leagues in 1940, and Selman Waksman's exploitation of the potential for antibiotic production among soil micro-organisms in the 1940s. Within 25 years of these discoveries, most of the major groups of anti-microbial agents had been recognized and more recent developments have chiefly involved chemical alteration of existing molecules.

Progress in the development of antiviral, antifungal and antiparasitic compounds has been much slower and therapeutic options in non-bacterial infection consequently remain severely limited. Meanwhile, the explosion of knowledge in immunology has renewed hopes that it may be possible to manipulate immunological processes triggered by infection to the benefit of the host.

## SOURCES AND SPREAD OF INFECTION

Sources of infection are the habitats in which the pathogenic microbes ordinarily grow and from which they are disseminated to susceptible hosts. Inanimate objects may act as passive vehicles of infection, while some pathogens are derived from healthy persons, known as *carriers*, in whom infection may be un-suspected. Some infections, such as rabies, bubonic plague, brucellosis and leptospirosis, have their sources

in animals, which are the natural hosts of the patho-gen, and are called *zoonoses*. They are transmissible from animals to humans, but not ordinarily from person to person, so that prevention depends on the control of human contact with the infected animals.

As well as these kinds of *exogenous* infections from external sources, there are also many infections, termed *endogenous*, which are due to the invasion of tissues by a commensal organism that hitherto grew harmlessly elsewhere in the body, e.g. infections of the lung with pneumococci previously resident in the throat. The prevention of endogenous infections depends on the avoidance of predisposing conditions that impair the tissue defences.

Epidemiological observations may suggest the mechanism by which an infection is transmitted and so lead to the formulation of preventive measures even when the causal micro-organism is still un-known. In 1846, for instance, in a maternity clinic in Vienna, Ignaz Semmelweis deduced that puerperal fever was caused by a putrefactive agent which doctors picked up on their hands when attending patients or performing necropsies and then transferred into the birth canal when assisting women at child-birth. He reduced the number of maternal deaths from nearly 10% to about 3.5% by requiring staff to wash their hands in chloride of lime before attending the birth.

In a comparable study in London, John Snow (1849, 1854) showed that the geographical distri-bution of cholera was related to the sources of the supplies of drinking water, and concluded that the 'peculiar poison of the disease' was spread in patients' faeces, which contaminated water later drunk by other persons (*faecal–oral transmission*). Measures subsequently taken to ensure the purity of drinking water by protection, filtration and chlorination have led to the decline of cholera, typhoid fever and other water-borne infections.

The development of the techniques of antiseptic and aseptic surgery for the prevention of wound sepsis had its origin in the conception by Joseph Lister (1867) that if, as shown by Pasteur, bacteria were the cause of the fermentation and putrefaction of dead organic matter, they might well also be the cause of suppuration in living tissues. By covering operation wounds with dressings soaked in carbolic acid to kill any bacteria present in them and to exclude others from entry, and by disinfecting his hands and instru-ments, he greatly reduced the incidence of sepsis in his patients.

The discovery that blood-sucking arthropods spread certain diseases led to prevention by measures for the control of these vectors. In 1893, Theobald Smith and F. L. Kilborne first showed that Texas fever of cattle was spread by ticks that bite an infected cow and transmit its blood to another animal. Subsequently, it was shown that malaria was transmitted by anopheles mosquitoes (Ronald Ross, 1898), yellow fever by aedes mosquitoes (Walter Reed and co-workers, 1900), bubonic plague by the rat flea (W. G. Liston and co-workers, 1905) and typhus fever by lice (Charles Nicolle, 1909). Campaigns of vector control by the use of insecticides and other means have since been conducted for the prevention of these diseases.

A major group of infections that have proved largely insusceptible to control by environmental sanitation are those of the respiratory tract, e.g. common colds, sore throats, influenza, whooping cough, pneumonia, tuberculosis, measles and chickenpox. Organisms that enter and leave the body via the respiratory tract may be transmitted by a variety of means, including contact and air-borne secretion droplets. It is probably this versatility in their means of spread, as well as the frequency with which urban dwellers share and breathe indoor air polluted by others, that explains the continuing high prevalence of respiratory infections.

Although infective illness has remained common during the last 100 years, industrialized countries have seen a phenomenal decrease in the death rate from the classic infections. Since the steep decline began more than a century before preventive and curative medicine became significantly effective, the earlier reduction in deaths must have been due to improvements in nutrition and living conditions which increased the resistance of individuals to the point that they generally recovered from their many infections. Subsequently, and particularly with the introduction of immunization programmes and anti-microbial therapy in the last 50 years, medicine has made a more substantial contribution to the saving of life, but let no-one imagine that microbial disease has been conquered!

## RECOMMENDED READING

Brock T D 1961 *Milestones in Microbiology*. Prentice-Hall, Engelwood Cliffs, NJ. Reprinted 1975 by the American Society for Microbiology, Washington, DC

Bulloch W 1960 *The History of Bacteriology*. Oxford University Press, Oxford

Burnet F M 1972 *Natural History of Infectious Disease*, 4th edn. Cambridge University Press, Cambridge

Collard P 1976 *The Development of Microbiology*. Cambridge University Press, Cambridge

Foster W D 1970 *A History of Medical Bacteriology and Immunology*. Cox and Wyman, London

Grant J P 1995 *The State of the World's Children, 1995*. Oxford University Press (for UNICEF), Oxford

Grove D I 1990 *A History of Human Helminthology*. CAB International, Wallingford, Oxford.

Waterson A P, Wilkinson L 1978 *An Introduction to the History of Virology*. Cambridge University Press, Cambridge

Zinsser H 1935 *Rats, Lice and History*. Routledge, London

# 2

# Morphology and nature of micro-organisms

*D. Greenwood*

Living material is organized in units known as *cells*. Each cell consists of a body of protoplasm, the *protoplast*, enclosed by a thin semipermeable membrane, the *cytoplasmic* or *plasma membrane*, and also, in some cases, by an outer, relatively rigid *cell wall*. The protoplast is differentiated into a major part, the *cytoplasm*, and an inner body, the *nucleus*, which contains the hereditary determinants of character, the *genes*, borne on thread-like *chromosomes*.

*Micro-organisms* are generally regarded as living forms that are microscopic in size and relatively simple, usually unicellular, in structure. The diameter of the smallest body that can be resolved and seen clearly with the naked eye is about 100 μm. Nearly all bacteria are smaller than this, and a microscope is therefore necessary to see them. Viruses are even smaller, and in most cases an electron microscope is needed to visualize them.

However, when bacteria or fungi are allowed to grow on a nutritive, solid supporting medium, their numerous progeny form *colonies* that are readily visible to the naked eye. Many viruses can be grown within cultures of living cells (*tissue cultures*) in the laboratory and many cause characteristic *cytopathic effects* visible in the light microscope.

It is useful to draw a clear distinction between relatively primitive (*prokaryotic*) cells and more advanced (*eukaryotic*) cells. The bacteria and related organisms (rickettsiae, chlamydiae and mycoplasmas) are prokaryotic cells whereas the cells of fungi, protozoa, plants and animals are eukaryotic. Viruses fall into neither category; they are not cells in the accepted sense and rely on the biochemical processes of the host cell for their replication and propagation.

The main distinguishing features of the prokaryotic cell are:

1. Its nucleus appears as a simple, homogeneous body not possessing a nuclear membrane separating it from the cytoplasm, nor a nucleolus, nor a spindle, nor a number of separate non-identical chromosomes.

2. It lacks the internal membranes isolating the respiratory and photosynthetic enzyme systems in specific organelles, comparable with the membrane-bound mitochondria and chloroplasts of eukaryotic cells. Thus, the respiratory enzymes in bacteria are located mainly in the peripheral cytoplasmic membrane, and their effective functioning is dependent upon the integrity of the cell protoplast as a whole.

3. Its rigid cell wall usually contains as its main strengthening element a specific peptidoglycan substance not found in eukaryotic organisms.

The bodies of higher plants and animals including helminths are multicellular, with interdependence and specialization of function among the cells, the different kinds of cells being segregated in separate tissues. Many micro-organisms, on the other hand, are unicellular, existing as single cells, unattached to their fellows. Others grow as aggregates of cells joined together by their cell walls in clusters, chains, rods, filaments (*hyphae*) or meshworks of branching filaments (*mycelia*). Generally, these morphologically multicellular microbes are physiologically unicellular, each cell being self-sufficient and, if isolated artificially, able to nourish itself, grow and reproduce the species. Some specialization of cell function, approaching that of true multicellular organisms, is encountered in colonies of moulds and filamentous 'higher' bacteria in which certain cells form an aerial mycelium and are specialized for the formation and dissemination of spores; these cells are dependent for their nutrition on the activities of other cells comprising a vegetative mycelium.

Most fungi form an aerial mycelium, but some (*yeasts* and *yeast-like fungi*) grow by budding, or by germ-tube formation. Others (*dimorphic fungi*) can exist in the yeast or mycelial form depending on the environmental conditions (see Ch. 60). Protozoa

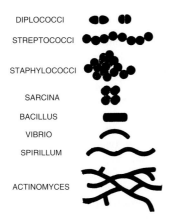

DIPLOCOCCI

STREPTOCOCCI

STAPHYLOCOCCI

SARCINA

BACILLUS

VIBRIO

SPIRILLUM

ACTINOMYCES

**Fig. 2.1** The shapes and characteristic groupings of various bacterial cells.

are all unicellular, but encompass a wide diversity of morphological forms. Some (e.g. *Entamoeba* spp. and *Giardia lamblia*) have the capacity to enter a resting phase (*cyst*) by secretion of an external wall. This enables them to survive outside the host. Other protozoa (e.g. malaria parasites) exist as very diverse morphological and metabolic types at different stages in a complex life cycle (see Ch. 61). Bacterial cells are smaller (usually between 0.4 and 1.5 μm in short diameter) than those of fungi and protozoa, and in most cases they have relatively rigid cell walls that maintain their characteristic shape; this may be spherical (*coccus*), rod-shaped (*bacillus*), comma-shaped (*vibrio*), spiral (*spirillum* and *spirochaete*) or filamentous (Fig. 2.1). They show little structural differentiation when examined by ordinary microscopical methods.

## ANATOMY OF THE BACTERIAL CELL

The principal structures of the bacterial cell are shown in Figure 2.2. The *protoplast*, i.e. the whole body of living material (*protoplasm*), is bounded peripherally by a very thin, elastic and semipermeable cytoplasmic membrane. Outside, and closely covering this, lies the rigid, supporting *cell wall*, which is porous and relatively permeable. Cell division occurs by the development, from the periphery inwards, of a transverse cytoplasmic membrane and a transverse cell wall, or *cross-wall*.

The *cytoplasm*, or main part of the protoplasm, consists of a watery sap packed with large numbers of small granules called *ribosomes* and a few convoluted membranous bodies called *mesosomes* (see below). The nuclear material, nucleus or *chromatin*, is not normally seen with the light microscope. Figure 2.3 is an electron micrograph of a thin section of a dividing bacterial cell. In addition to these essential structures, other intracellular and extracellular structures may be present in some species of bacteria; their occurrence sometimes depends upon particular conditions of growth. *Inclusion granules* of storage products such as volutin (polyphosphate), lipid (poly-β-hydroxybutyrate), glycogen or starch may occur in the cytoplasm. Outside the cell wall, there may be a protective gelatinous covering layer called a *capsule* or, when it is too thin to be resolved with the light microscope (<0.2 μm), a *microcapsule*. Soluble large-molecular material may be dispersed by the bacterium into the environment as *loose slime*. Some bacteria bear, protruding outwards from the cell wall, one or more kinds of

**Fig. 2.2** A diagram of a dividing bacterial cell with a single flagellum, four sex pili, numerous common fimbriae, a cell wall, a cytoplasmic membrane, two nuclear bodies, three mesosomes and numerous ribosomes.

**Fig. 2.3** A thin section of a dividing bacillus showing cell wall, cytoplasmic membrane, ribosomes, a developing cross-wall, and a mesosome. (By courtesy of Dr P J Highton and the editors of *Journal of Ultrastructure Research.*) ×50 000.

filamentous appendages: *flagella*, which are organs of locomotion; *fimbriae*, which appear to be organs of adhesion; and *pili*, which are involved in the transfer of genetic material. Because they are exposed to contact and interaction with the cells and humoral substances of the body of the host, the surface structures of bacteria are the structures most likely to have special roles in the processes of infection.

## Bacterial nucleus (DNA)

The genetic information of a bacterial cell is contained in a single, long molecule of double-stranded deoxyribonucleic acid (DNA) which can be extracted in the form of a closed circular thread about 1 mm long. The cell solves the problem of packaging this enormous macromolecule by condensing and looping it into a *supercoiled* state. As well as the chromosome, the bacterium may contain one or more additional fragments of DNA, known as *episomes* or *plasmids*. As the bacterial chromosome is not bound to proteins, it does not stain like a eukaryotic chromosome, and in unstained bacteria examined normally with the light microscope, or in bacteria stained by the usual methods, there is no obvious differentiation into nucleus and cytoplasm. Only a single nuclear body is present in some cells, whilst in others, as a result of nuclear division preceding cell division, two or more may be present. These can be revealed by special staining procedures. Unlike the intracellular storage granules described below, they are constantly present in all cells and under all conditions of culture. The nuclear bodies replicate by growth and simple fission, and not by mitosis; they show no outer nuclear membrane separating them from the cytoplasm, and they have no nucleolus.

## Cytoplasm of bacteria

The cytoplasm of the bacterial cell is a viscous watery solution, or soft gel, containing a variety of organic and inorganic solutes, and numerous *ribosomes*. The cytoplasm of bacteria differs from that of the higher eukaryotic organisms in not containing an endoplasmic reticulum or membrane-bearing microsomes, in not containing mitochondria and in not showing signs of internal mobility such as cytoplasmic streaming, the formation, migration and disappearance of vacuoles, and amoeboid movement.

## Ribosomes

Bacterial ribosomes are slightly smaller (10–20 nm) than those of eukaryotic cells and they have a sedimentation constant of 70S, being composed of a 30S and a 50S subunit (cf. 40S and 60S in the 80S eukaryotic counterparts). They may be seen with the electron microscope, and number tens of thousands per cell. They are strung together on strands of messenger RNA (mRNA) to form *polysomes*, and it is at this site that the code of the mRNA is translated into peptide sequences. Thus the ribosomal components link up and travel along the mRNA strand and here determine the sequence of amino acids brought to the site on transfer RNA (tRNA) molecules and built into specific polypeptides.

## Inclusion granules

In many species of bacteria, round granules are observed in the cytoplasm. These are not permanent or essential structures, and may be absent under certain conditions of growth. They appear to be aggregates of substances concerned with cell metabolism, e.g. an excess metabolite stored as a nutrient reserve. Generally, they are present in largest amount when the bacteria have access to an abundance of energy-yielding nutrients, and diminish or disappear under conditions of energy source starvation. They consist of volutin (polyphosphate), lipid, glycogen, starch or sulphur.

*Volutin granules* (syn. metachromatic granules). These granules are 0.1–1.0 μm in diameter and have an intense affinity for basic dyes. They are characteristically found in the diphtheria bacillus. With toluidine blue or methylene blue, they stain a red-violet colour, contrasting with the blue staining of the bacterial protoplasm. By special methods such as those of Neisser and Albert the granules can be demonstrated with even greater colour contrast. Their metachromatic staining is thought to be due to their content of polymerized inorganic polyphosphate, an energy-rich compound that may act as a reserve of energy and phosphate for cell metabolism or may be a by-product. Volutin granules are slightly acid-fast, resisting decoloration by 1% sulphuric acid; they are more refractile than the protoplasm and are sometimes distinguishable in unstained wet films. By electron microscopy they appear as very opaque, clearly demarcated bodies.

*Lipid granules.* These granules have an affinity for fat-soluble dyes such as Sudan black; they are then coloured black in contrast to the remaining protoplasm, which can be counterstained pink with water-soluble basic fuchsin. The granules are spherical, of varying size, highly refractile, and easily seen in unstained preparations. They appear as unstained spaces in bacteria treated with simple stains and appear to consist mainly of polymerized β-hydroxybutyric acid. The manner in which the lipid content of bacteria, e.g. in the *Bacillus* genus, varies with the conditions of culture suggests that this substance may act as a carbon and energy storage product.

*Polysaccharide granules.* These can be seen in the cytoplasm of certain bacteria when they are stained with iodine and are of either glycogen (red-brown) or starch (blue). Many other species, e.g. *Escherichia coli*, do not form granules visible with the light microscope but they can be seen with the electron microscope.

## Mesosomes

These are convoluted or multilaminated membranous bodies visible in the electron microscope. They develop by complex invagination of the cytoplasmic membrane into the cytoplasm, sometimes in relation to the nuclear body and often from the sites of cross-wall formation in Gram-positive bacteria. Similar structures have been noted in Gram-negative bacteria where they are not so common. Mesosomes are thought to be involved in mechanisms responsible for the compartmenting of DNA at cell division and at sporulation. They may also have a function analogous to the mitochondria of the eukaryotic cell – providing a membranous support for respiratory enzymes.

## Cytoplasmic membrane

The bacterial protoplast is limited externally by a thin, elastic cytoplasmic membrane, which is 5–10 nm thick, consists mainly of lipoprotein and is visible in some ultrathin sections examined with the electron microscope. *Membranes* generally appear in suitably stained electron microscope preparations as two dark lines about 2.5 nm wide separated by a lighter area of similar width. The classical model of a 'unit membrane' is shown in Figure 2.4: lipid molecules are arrayed in a double layer with their hydrophilic polar regions externally aligned and in contact with a layer of protein at each surface. The functions of membranes differ widely in nature and it is clear that this simplified model cannot account for all of the variations of function that are already known. More complex membrane architecture is gradually

**Fig. 2.4** A diagram of a unit membrane. A lipid bilayer with polar (hydrophilic) regions externally orientated towards a layer of protein at each surface has a characteristic appearance when stained and seen in cross-section in the electron microscope.

**Fig. 2.5** **a** The envelope of the Gram-positive cell wall. **b** The envelope of the Gram-negative cell wall.

being revealed by special electron microscope techniques. In bacteria, the cytoplasmic membrane lacks cholesterol, which is a normal constituent of animal cell membranes. The cytoplasmic membrane constitutes an osmotic barrier that is impermeable to many small molecular solutes and is responsible for maintaining the differences in solute content between the cytoplasm and the external environment. It permits the passive diffusion inwards and outwards of water and certain other small molecular substances, especially lipid-soluble ones, and it actively effects the selective transport of specific nutrient solutes into the cell and that of waste products out of it. In addition to the enzymes, or *permeases*, responsible for the active uptake of nutrients, the cytoplasmic membrane contains many other kinds of enzymes, notably respiratory enzymes and pigments (cytochrome system), certain enzymes of the tricarboxylic acid cycle and, probably, polymerizing enzymes that manufacture the substances of the cell wall and extracellular structures. It has little mechanical strength and is supported on the outside by the cell wall (Fig. 2.5).

## Cell wall

The cell wall encases the protoplast and lies immediately external to the cytoplasmic membrane. It is 10–25 nm thick, strong and relatively rigid, though with some elasticity, and openly porous, being freely permeable to solute molecules smaller than 10 kDa in mass and 1 nm in diameter. It supports the weak cytoplasmic membrane against the high internal osmotic pressure of the protoplasm (usually between 5 and 25 atm) and maintains the characteristic shape of the bacterium in its coccal, bacillary, filamentous or spiral form.

The integrity of the cell wall is essential to the viability of the bacterium. If the wall is weakened or ruptured, the protoplasm may swell from osmotic inflow of water and burst the weak cytoplasmic membrane. This process of lethal disintegration and dissolution is termed *lysis*.

The cell wall plays an important part in *cell division*. A transverse partition of cell wall material grows inwards, like a closing iris diaphragm, from the lateral wall at the equator of the cell and forms a complete *cross-wall* separating two daughter cells. The cell wall is not seen in conventionally stained smears examined with the light microscope. It can be demonstrated by special staining methods but most readily and clearly by electron microscopy; it is seen both in ultrathin sections and, as an empty fold surrounding the shrunken protoplast, in whole-cell preparations shadow-cast with heavy metal.

The chemical composition of the cell wall differs considerably between different bacterial species, but in all species the main strengthening component is *peptidoglycan* (syn. *mucopeptide* or *murein*). Peptidoglycan is composed of N-acetylglucosamine and N-acetylmuramic acid molecules linked alternately in a chain (Fig. 2.6). The N-acetylmuramic acid units each carry a short peptide, usually consisting of L-alanine, D-glutamic acid, either *meso*-diaminopimelic acid (in Gram-negative bacteria) or L-lysine (in Gram-positive bacteria) and D-alanyl-D-alanine. The wall is given its strength by cross-links that form between adjacent strands. These may be formed directly between the *meso*-diaminopimelic acid or L-lysine of one strand and the penultimate D-alanine of the next, or (the usual form in Gram-positive organisms) through an interpeptide bridge composed of up to five amino acids; in either case, the terminal D-alanine is lost in the cross-linking reaction (Fig. 2.7). Several antibiotics interfere with the construction of the cell wall peptidoglycan (see Ch. 5).

The walls of Gram-positive bacteria contain more peptidoglycan and are thicker and stronger (more extensively cross-linked) than those of Gram-negative bacteria. This difference is associated with a higher internal osmotic pressure in Gram-positive cells. The presence of peptidoglycan has been demonstrated in rickettsiae and chlamydiae, and this is taken to indicate that these organisms are phylogenetically related to the bacteria rather than to the viruses, in which muramic acid has not been found.

**Fig. 2.6** The basic building block of bacterial cell wall peptidoglycan. N-Acetylmuramic acid is derived from N-acetylglucosamine by the addition of a lactic acid unit. Each N-acetylmuramic acid molecule is substituted with a pentapeptide; an N-acetylglcosamine molecule is joined to the muramylpentapeptide within the cell membrane and the unit is transferred to growth points in the existing peptidoglycan, where adjacent strands are cross-linked. (See also Figs 2.7 and 5.1.)

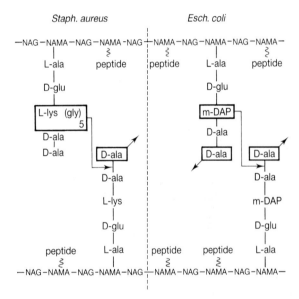

**Fig. 2.7** Schematic representation of the peptidoglycan of a representative Gram-positive organism (*Staphylococcus aureus*) and a representative Gram-negative organism (*Esch. coli*). Note that in the Gram-positive organism cross-linking occurs through a peptide bridge (pentaglycine in *Staph. aureus*) whereas direct cross-linking occurs in *Esch. coli*. In both cases the terminal D-alanine is lost. Not all peptides are engaged in cross-linking in *Esch. coli*, and carboxypeptidases remove redundant D-alanine residues.

The bacterial cell wall also contains other components whose nature and amount vary with the species. Many Gram-positive bacteria contain relatively large amounts of *teichoic acid* (a polymer of ribitol or glycerol phosphate complexed with sugar residues) interspersed with the peptidoglycan; some of this material (*lipoteichoic acid*) is linked to lipids buried in the cell membrane. Gram-negative bacteria possess a complex membrane-like structure external to the peptidoglycan layer. In *Esch. coli* this comprises lipid, polysaccharide, lipoprotein and lipopolysaccharide, and makes up over 80% of the wall weight. This outer membrane confers several important properties on Gram-negative bacteria: it protects the peptidoglycan from the effects of lysozyme and it impedes the ingress of many antibiotics that are thus rendered impotent. Components of the lipopolysaccharide, in particular the core structure, lipid A, forms *endotoxin*, which, when released in the bloodstream, may give rise to *endotoxin shock*.

Lysozyme is a natural body defence substance which lyses bacteria of many species. It cleaves the link between *N*-acetylglucosamine and *N*-acetylmuramic acid (see Fig. 2.6). Bacteriophages possess a lysozyme-like enzyme that allows their initial penetration into the bacterium and, after they have reproduced, causes lysis of the bacterium. It should be noted, moreover, that bacteria themselves possess enzymes, called *autolysins*, able to hydrolyse their own cell wall substances. Under normal conditions their action is confined to remodelling of the cell wall in the course of growth. Weakening, removal or defective formation of the cell wall is involved in the production of the various abnormal forms called *spheroplasts*, *protoplasts*, *pleomorphic involution forms*, and *L-forms* (see below).

## Capsules, microcapsules and loose slime

Many bacteria are surrounded by a discrete covering layer of a relatively firm gelatinous material that lies outside and immediately in contact with the cell wall. When this layer, in the wet state, is wide enough (0.2 µm or more) to be resolved with the light microscope, it is called a *capsule*. When it is narrower, and detectable only by indirect, serological means, or by electron microscopy, it may be termed a *microcapsule*. The capsular gel consists largely of water and has only a small content (e.g. 2%) of solids. In most species, the solid material is a complex polysaccharide, though in some species its main constituent is polypeptide or protein.

*Loose slime*, or *free slime*, is an amorphous, viscid colloidal material that is secreted extracellularly by some non-capsulate bacteria and also, outside their capsules, by many capsulate bacteria. In capsulate bacteria the slime is generally similar in chemical composition and antigenic character to the capsular substance. When slime-forming bacteria are grown on a solid culture medium, the slime remains around

**Fig. 2.8** *Bacillus megaterium*. Chain of bacilli with large capsule and pair with very small capsule. Wet film with India ink, ×3500.

the bacteria as a matrix in which they are embedded and its presence confers on the growths a watery and sticky 'mucoid' character. The slime is freely soluble in water and, when the bacteria are grown or suspended in a liquid medium, it passes away from them and disperses through the medium.

*Demonstration.* Capsules and slime are usually invisible in films stained by ordinary methods except as clear haloes surrounding the stained bacteria. Since capsules consist largely of water, they shrink greatly on drying. For this reason, dry-film methods of demonstrating capsules are unreliable; the capsules may shrink so much that they become invisible or, on the other hand, shrinkage artefacts may give the appearance of capsules on non-capsulate bacteria. The most reliable method of demonstration is by 'negative' staining in wet films with India ink; the carbon particles of the ink make a dark background in the film, but cannot penetrate the capsule, which thus appears as a clear halo around the bacterium (Fig. 2.8). When bacteria that have been grown on solid medium are being examined for capsules, it is important that they should first be washed or suspended for a sufficient time in water to ensure the removal of any loose slime which can be observed when films are made directly from the solid medium.

Microcapsules may not be seen at all, and for this reason their presence has generally to be deduced from serological evidence that the cell wall antigen (e.g. the O, or somatic, antigen in Enterobacteriaceae) is masked by a covering layer (e.g. of K, or 'capsular', antigen).

The development of capsules is often dependent on the existence of favourable environmental conditions. Thus, their size may vary with the amount of carbohydrate in the culture medium. In the later stages of growth in artificial culture (e.g. 12–24 h) they may become reduced in size due to carbon and energy starvation or they may disappear due to the accumulation in the medium of capsule-degrading enzymes (e.g. hyaluronidase in the case of *Streptococcus pyogenes*).

**Function.** It is not known with certainty what the functions of capsules and microcapsules are, but it is probable that their principal action is in protecting the cell wall against attack by various kinds of antibacterial agents, e.g. bacteriophages, colicines, complement, lysozyme and other lytic enzymes, that otherwise would more readily damage or destroy it. In the case of certain capsulate pathogenic organisms (e.g. pneumococcus, pyogenic streptococci, anthrax bacillus and plague bacillus) there is good evidence that the capsule protects the bacteria against ingestion by the phagocytes of the host. The capsule is thus an important virulence determinant, and non-capsulate mutants of these bacteria are non-virulent. In some organisms the capsule contains more than one functional component. Thus, *Str. pyogenes*, which under favourable conditions of growth may form an antiphagocytic capsule composed of hyaluronic acid, also possesses a second surface substance, M protein, which inhibits either the ingestion or the intracellular digestion of the cocci by the phagocytes; the M protein occurs in association with the hyaluronic acid capsule or, when the latter is absent, by itself in the form of a microcapsule. In *Bacillus anthracis* the capsule is a polymer of D-glutamic acid and protects the bacteria not only against phagocytosis but also, to some extent, against the action of a bactericidal basic polypeptide present in animal tissues.

The capsular substance is usually antigenic and the capsular antigens play a very important part in determining the antigenic specificity of bacteria. When capsulate pneumococci are treated with type-specific antiserum, the sharpness of outline of the capsule is greatly enhanced. This is referred to as the *capsule-swelling reaction*.

## Flagella and motility

Motile bacteria possess filamentous appendages known as *flagella*, which act as organs of locomotion. The flagellum is a long, thin filament, twisted spirally in an open, regular wave form. It is about 0.02 μm thick and is usually several times the length of the bacterial cell. It originates in the bacterial protoplasm and is extruded through the cell wall. According to the species, there may be one, or up to 20 flagella, per cell. In elongated bacteria the arrangement of the flagella may be *peritrichous*, or *lateral*, when they originate from the sides of the cell, or *polar*, when they originate from one or both ends. Where several occur on a cell, they may function coiled together as a single 'tail'. Flagella consist largely or entirely of a protein, *flagellin*, belonging to the same chemical group as myosin, the contractile protein of muscle. They are invisible in ordinary preparations by the light microscope, but may be shown by the use of special staining methods, and in special circumstances by dark-ground illumination. Because of the difficulties of these methods, the presence of flagella is commonly inferred from the observation of motility. They can be demonstrated easily and clearly with the electron microscope, usually appearing as simple fibrils without internal differentiation (Fig. 2.9). In some preparations the flagellum appears as a hollow tube formed of heli-

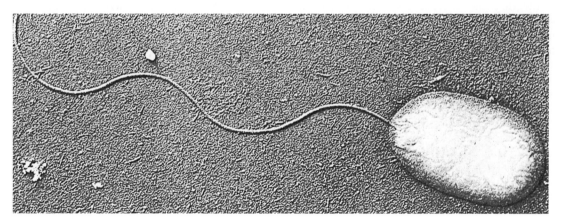

**Fig. 2.9** *Pseudomonas aeruginosa*. Bacillus with a single polar flagellum, dried and shadow-cast. Electron micrograph, ×38 000. (From Wilkinson J F, Duguid J P 1960 The influence of cultural conditions on bacterial cytology. *International Review of Cytology* 9: 1–76.)

cally twisted fibrils, and the flagella of some bacteria, e.g. vibrios, have an outer sheath. Flagella of the flagellate protozoa have the complex structure found in plants and animals, which consists of two central and nine peripheral fibrils contained in a tube-like sheath.

*Motility* may be observed microscopically or by the occurrence of spreading growth in semi-solid agar medium. By microscopy of wet films, motile bacteria are seen swimming in different directions across the field, with a darting, wriggling or tumbling movement. True motility must be distinguished from a drifting of the bacteria in a single direction due to a current in the liquid, and also from Brownian movement, which is a rapid oscillation of each bacterium within a very limited area due to bombardment by water molecules.

Among the spirochaetes, motility appears to be a function of the cell body, since flagella do not occur. The most characteristic movement is a fast spiral rotation on the long axis with slow progression in the axial line; movements of flexion and lashing movements may be observed. Some spirochaetes possess an axial filament and others a band of fibrils wound around their surface from pole to pole. It has been suggested that these structures may contribute to motility, either through being themselves contractile or by acting as stiffeners for recoil against the contractile protoplast.

*Function.* It is not known with certainty what advantage a bacterium derives from its ability to move actively. Motility may be beneficial in increasing the rate of uptake of nutrient solutes by continuously changing the environmental fluid in contact with the bacterial cell surface. Random movement and dispersion through the environment may be beneficial ensuring that at least some cells of a strain reach every locality suitable for colonization. There is, moreover, good evidence that the movement of many bacteria is *directed* by responses of the organism towards localities favourable to growth and away from unfavourable regions. Thus, bacteria tend to migrate towards regions where there is a higher concentration of nutrient solutes (a process known as *chemotaxis*) and away from regions containing higher concentrations of disinfectant substances (*negative chemotaxis*). Motile aerobic bacteria show positive *aerotaxis* and migrate towards regions where there is a higher concentration of dissolved oxygen; anaerobes migrate away from such regions.

It might be supposed that the power of active locomotion would assist pathogenic bacteria in penetrating through viscid mucous secretions and epithelial barriers, and in spreading throughout the body fluids and tissues, but it must be noted that many non-motile pathogens (e.g. meningococci and streptococci) are no less invasive than motile ones.

## Fimbriae

Certain Gram-negative bacilli, including intestinal commensal and pathogenic species, possess filamentous appendages of a different kind from the flagella. These are called *fimbriae* and they occur in non-motile, as well as in motile strains. They are far more numerous than flagella (e.g. 100–500 being borne peritrichously by each cell) and are much shorter and only about half as thick (e.g. varying from 0.1 to 1.5 μm in length and having a uniform width between 4 and 8 nm). They do not have the smoothly curved spiral form of flagella and are mostly more or less straight. They cannot be seen with the light microscope but are clearly seen with the electron microscope in preparations that have been metal-shadowed or negatively stained with phosphotungstic acid (Fig. 2.10).

Fimbriate strains of bacteria often undergo a reversible variation between a fimbriate phase and a non-fimbriate phase that is affected by the conditions of growth. Most bacilli become fimbriate, as a result of prolonged culture or serial subculture, in static liquid medium incubated aerobically. The non-fimbriate phase predominates when subcultures are made serially on a solid culture medium.

*Function.* Fimbriae probably function as organs of adhesion. The possession of fimbriae confers on bacilli the power of adhering firmly to solid surfaces of various kinds, including those of the cells of animals, plants and fungi. Comparable non-fimbriate bacilli do not adhere when they collide with such surfaces. The adhesive property may be of value to the bacteria in holding them in nutritionally favourable micro-environments. Moreover, bacteria growing in stagnant liquid medium under air are assisted by the possession of fimbriae to grow attached together in the form of a *pellicle* that floats on the surface of the medium where the growth is greatly enhanced by the free supply of atmospheric oxygen.

*Haemagglutination.* Most fimbriate bacteria bear fimbriae of a type that enables them to adhere to, among other kinds of tissue cells, the red blood cells of many animal species (e.g. to guinea-pig, fowl, horse and pig red cells very strongly, to human cells moderately strongly, to sheep cells weakly and to ox cells scarcely at all). If a drop of a concentrated suspension of fimbriate bacilli is mixed for a few minutes with a drop of a suspension of guinea-pig red cells, the adhering bacilli bind the red cells

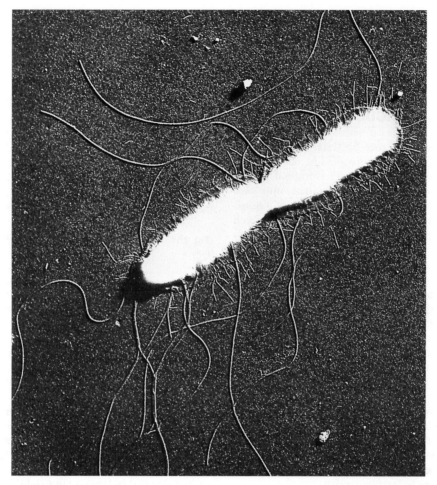

**Fig. 2.10** *Salmonella enterica* serotype Typhi Dividing bacillus from log-phase culture bears about 15 long wavy flagella and over 100 short fimbriae. Note dense (white) shrunken protoplast surrounded by an empty fold of cell wall. Whole bacillus dried and shadow-cast. Electron micrograph, ×16 000. (From Duguid J P, Wilkinson J F 1961 Environmentally induced changes in bacterial morphology. *Symposia of the Society for General Microbiology* 11: 69–99.)

together in clumps visible to the naked eye. A simple haemagglutination test can thus be used to determine whether a culture contains fimbriate bacilli.

Different types of fimbriae have different adhesive properties. The commonest kind, type 1, which occurs in escherichia, klebsiella, serratia, salmonella and shigella organisms, is about 8 nm in width, and it may be recognized by the observation that its adhesive and haemagglutinating actions are completely and specifically inhibited by the addition of a small amount (0.1–0.5%) of D-mannose to the test mixture (i.e. its activities are mannose-sensitive). A few salmonellae (e.g. *S. enterica* serotypes Gallinarum and Pullorum) possess a kind of fimbriae (type 2) apparently devoid of all haemagglutinating and adhesive properties. In addition to, or instead of, type 1 fimbriae, some *Klebsiella* and *Serratia* spp.

possess type 3 fimbriae, about 5 nm in width; these do not agglutinate red cells unless the cells are first heated or tanned, and their adhesive properties are unaffected by mannose. *Proteus* spp. possess a kind of fimbriae (type 4) which have mannose-resistant haemagglutinating activity against untreated red cells of certain species. It should be noted also that some bacteria, e.g. many strains of *Esch. coli*, possess mannose-resistant haemagglutinating factors that are not associated with fimbriae.

## Pili (sex pili)

These structures are similar to fimbriae, but are functionally different. They are longer than fimbriae and confer the ability to attach specifically to other bacteria that lack these appendages. Pili appear to be involved in the transfer of DNA during conjugation (see Ch. 6); they also act as receptor sites for certain bacteriophages described as being 'donor-specific'.

## BACTERIAL REPRODUCTION

Among the 'lower' or true bacteria, multiplication takes place by *simple binary fission*. The cell grows in size, usually elongating to twice its original length, and the protoplasm becomes divided into two approximately equal parts by the ingrowth of a transverse septum from the plasma membrane and cell wall. In some species, the cell wall septum, or cross-wall, splits in two and the daughter cells separate almost immediately. In others, the cell walls of the daughter cells remain continuous for some time after cell division and the organisms grow, adhering in pairs, clusters, chains or filaments. If cross-wall splitting is thus delayed in an organism in which the cross-walls of successive cell divisions are all formed in parallel planes, the cells will be grouped in pairs, chains, rods or filaments. If it is delayed in an organism that forms successive cross-walls in different planes, e.g. ones at right angles to each other, the cells will be grouped in pairs, forming either cubic or irregular clusters. Under favourable conditions, growth and division are repeated with great rapidity, e.g. every half hour or less, so that one individual cell may reproduce thousands of millions of new organisms in less than a day.

In the 'higher', or mycelial, bacteria, growth takes place by extension of the vegetative filaments, and multiplication by transverse division of these into shorter forms, or by the liberation of numerous conidia (see below) which later germinate and give rise to fresh mycelia.

### Bacterial spores

Some bacteria, notably those of the genera *Bacillus* and *Clostridium*, develop a highly resistant resting phase or *endospore*, whereby the organism can survive in a dormant state through a long period of starvation or other adverse environmental condition. The process does not involve multiplication: in *sporulation*, each vegetative cell forms only one spore, and in subsequent *germination* each spore gives rise to a single vegetative cell. Certain specific antigens develop in the spore that are not found in the vegetative cells.

In unstained preparations the spore is recognized within the parent cell by its greater refractility. It is

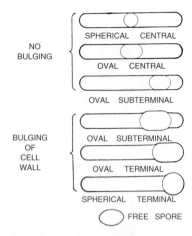

**Fig. 2.11** The shape and situation of the spore in the bacterial cell.

larger than lipid inclusion granules and is often ovoid, in contrast to the spherical shape of the lipid granules. Mature ungerminated spores are 'phase-bright' in the phase-contrast microscope; immature or germinated spores are 'phase-dark'. When mature, the spore resists coloration by simple stains, appearing as a clear space within the stained cell protoplasm. Spores are slightly acid-fast and may be stained differentially by a modification of the Ziehl–Neelsen method. The appearance of the mature spores varies according to the species, being spherical, ovoid or elongated, occupying a terminal, subterminal or central position, and being narrower than the cell, or broader and bulging it (Fig. 2.11).

*Sporulation.* Sporulation occurs as a response to starvation or, at least, the exhaustion of a limiting substance. It does not take place as long as conditions continue to favour maximal vegetative growth. In certain species, sporulation may be induced by depletion of nutrients necessary for vegetative growth, e.g. the carbon and energy source, the nitrogen source, sulphate, phosphate or iron salt; at the same time, the process requires a continued supply of other minerals (potassium, magnesium, manganese and calcium salts), and favourable conditions of moisture, temperature, pH, oxygen tension, etc. The spore is formed inside the parent vegetative cell (hence the name 'endospore'). It develops from a portion of protoplasm near one end of the cell (the 'forespore'), incorporates part of the nuclear material (equivalent to one genome) of the cell and acquires a thick covering layer, the 'cortex', and a thin, but tough, outer 'spore coat' consisting of several layers. Spores of some species have an additional, apparently rather loose covering known

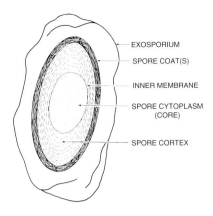

EXOSPORIUM
SPORE COAT(S)
INNER MEMBRANE
SPORE CYTOPLASM
(CORE)
SPORE CORTEX

**Fig. 2.12**  Cross-section of a bacterial spore. The core is surrounded by the inner spore membrane. The cortex, a laminated structure, is protected by a more resistant layer or multiple layers forming the spore coat. In some cases, a loose outer covering (exosporium) can be defined.

as the *exosporium* (Fig. 2.12). Finally, the remainder of the parent cell disintegrates and the spore is freed.

*Viability.*  Spores are much more resistant than the vegetative forms to exposure to disinfectants, drying and heating. Thus, application of moist heat at 100–120°C for a period of 10–20 min may be needed to kill spores, whereas heating at 60°C suffices to kill vegetative cells. In the dry state, or in moist conditions unfavourable to growth, spores may remain viable for many years. The marked resistance of spores has been attributed to several factors in which they differ from vegetative cells: the impermeability of their cortex and outer coat, their high content of calcium and dipicolinic acid, their low content of water and their very low metabolic and enzymic activity.

*Germination.*  Germination of the spore occurs when the external conditions become favourable to growth by access to moisture and nutrients. It is irreversible and involves rapid degradative changes. The spore successively loses its heat resistance and its dipicolinic acid; it loses calcium, it becomes permeable to dyes and its refractility changes. Spores that have survived exposure to severe adverse influences such as heat are much more exacting than normal spores in their requirements for germination. For this reason, specially enriched culture media are used when testing the sterility of materials, such as surgical catgut, that have been exposed to disinfecting procedures. In the process of germination, the spore swells, its cortex disintegrates, its coat is broken open and a single vegetative cell emerges.

The initiation of germination (*activation*) is incompletely understood. It is clear that the state of dormancy of spores may be altered by various treatments, e.g. transient exposure to heat at 80°C, so that germination can then proceed more rapidly in the individual cells or more completely in a spore population. Activation is distinct from germination and is reversible if germination does not proceed.

*Outgrowth.*  This term is used to denote the stage from germination up to the formation of the first vegetative cell and prior to the first cell division. The conditions required for successful outgrowth may differ markedly from those that allow germination.

## Conidia (exospores)

Some of the mycelial bacteria (*Actinomycetales*) and many filamentous fungi form *conidia*, resting spores of a kind different from endospores. The conidia are borne *externally* by abstriction from the ends of the parent cells (conidiophores), and are disseminated by the air or other means to fresh habitats. They are not specially resistant to heat and disinfectants.

## Pleomorphism and involution

During growth, bacteria of a single strain may show considerable variation in size and shape, or form a proportion of cells that are swollen, spherical, elongated or pear shaped. This pleomorphism occurs most readily in certain species (e.g. *Streptobacillus moniliformis* and *Yersinia pestis*) in ageing cultures on artificial medium and especially in the presence of antagonistic substances such as penicillin, glycine, lithium chloride, sodium chloride in high concentrations, and organic acids at low pH. The abnormal cells are generally regarded as degenerate or *involution* forms; some are non-viable, whilst others may grow and revert to the normal form when transferred to a suitable environment. In many cases the abnormal shape seems to be the result of defective cell wall synthesis; the growing protoplasm expands the weakened wall to produce a grotesquely swollen cell comparable to a spheroplast (see below) that later usually bursts and lyses.

## Spheroplasts and free protoplasts

If bacteria have their cell walls removed or weakened while they are held in a sufficiently concentrated solution such as 0.2–1.0 M sucrose with 0.01 M $Mg^{2+}$ to prevent them imbibing water by osmosis, they may escape being lysed and, instead, may become converted into viable spherical bodies. If all the cell wall material has been removed from them, the spheres are *free protoplasts*. If they remain enclosed by an intact, but weakened residual cell wall, they are called *spheroplasts*. Protoplasts, for example, are readily liberated from the Gram-positive *Bacillus megaterium* by dissolution of the cell walls with egg-white lysozyme. Spheroplasts are readily produced from Gram-negative bacilli such as *Esch. coli* by growing the organism in the presence of penicillins or other β-lactam antibiotics that specifically inhibit synthesis of the peptidoglycan component of the cell wall. A similar result may be obtained by culturing certain bacteria on media lacking a nutrient, e.g. diaminopimelic acid, lysine or a hexosamine derivative, that they require specifically for cell wall synthesis.

Protoplasts and spheroplasts are osmotically sensitive; they vary in size with the osmotic pressure of the suspending medium and, if the medium is much diluted, they swell up, burst and perish by lysis. If maintained in an osmotically protective nutrient medium, they remain viable and continue to metabolize, synthesize and grow. Protoplasts do not multiply (but see L-forms below). Spheroplasts, when kept in suitable conditions, may multiply by fission or budding and reproduce through many serial subcultures. Protoplasts cannot revert to normal bacterial morphology by re-forming their cell walls, but spheroplasts commonly revert en masse when transferred to a culture medium lacking the cell wall inhibitor.

## L-forms of bacteria

These are abnormal growth forms that may arise spontaneously (e.g. in *Streptobacillus moniliformis* and *Bacteroides* spp.) or by the inhibition of cell wall synthesis in bacteria of normal morphology. They are stable in the sense that special conditions of culture, such as the presence of penicillin, are not required to prevent their reversion to the parental bacterial forms. They continue to reproduce as L-forms through repeated subcultures in the absence of cell wall inhibitor, and give rise to revertants of normal bacterial morphology only occasionally. They differ from the parent bacteria in lacking a rigid cell wall and, in consequence, regular size and shape, but unlike protoplasts they are capable of growing and multiplying on a suitable nutrient medium. They range in size from minute bodies about 0.1 μm in diameter to large ones of 10–20 μm. The smallest viable forms are about 0.3 μm in diameter and may pass through bacteria-stopping filters.

Colonies of L-phase organisms on agar media are small and have a characteristic 'fried egg' appearance,

rather like mycoplasmas, which naturally lack peptidoglycan. Because of their fragility, microscopical examination of L-forms is best done in situ on the agar medium, a cover-slip being applied to a block of agar bearing the growth. If desired, the organisms can be stained after fixation by a fixative that is allowed to diffuse through the agar.

L-forms should probably be regarded as laboratory artefacts that do not occur or survive to any important extent in natural habitats, although it is possible that they could account for bacterial persistence during therapy with certain antibiotics. L-forms are non-pathogenic to laboratory animals.

## MORPHOLOGICAL STUDY OF MICRO-ORGANISMS

Microscopical examination is usually the first step taken in the identification of an unknown micro-organism. The morphological features of importance are the size, shape and grouping of the cells, and their possession of spores, flagella (sometimes inferred from the simple observation of motility), and other distinctive structures. The morphology of fungi, helminth eggs or larvae and some protozoa can be studied by examining them suspended in a thin film of fluid between a glass slide and cover-slip in an unstained 'wet film'. This may also be helpful in determining the general shape and motility of bacteria.

Low- or medium-power light microscopy is usually adequate for the identification of most fungi and protozoa, and the ova or larvae of helminths. Oil-immersion microscopy is needed for the identification of bacteria. Certain very slender bacteria, such as the spirochaetes, are so feebly refractile that they cannot be seen by the ordinary microscopic methods, and *dark-ground illumination* or *phase-contrast microscopy* is necessary for their demonstration. Phase-contrast microscopy may also be used to demonstrate motility, spores and intracellular granules. The electron microscope is essential for the visualization of viruses.

## Stained preparations

Bacteria and blood protozoa like malaria parasites are more readily studied when fixed and stained. Smears or films of bacterial cultures and clinical specimens are usually fixed by heat, the slide being first thoroughly dried in air and then heated gently in a flame. Vegetative bacteria are thereby killed, rendered permeable to the stain, stuck to the surface of the slide and preserved from undergoing autolytic changes. Blood films are fixed in methanol. Chemical fixatives such as formalin, mercuric chloride, and osmic acid are used for sections of infected tissue.

During staining, the coloured, positively charged cation of basic dyes such as methylene blue combines with negatively charged groups in the cell protoplasm, especially with the phosphate groups in the abundant nucleic acids. Acidic dyes, having coloured anions, do not stain bacteria strongly except at very acid pH values, and thus can be used for 'negative staining' (see below). Cells or structures that stain with basic dyes at normal pH values are described as *basophilic*, and those that stain with acidic dyes as *acidophilic*. It should be noted that the bacterial cell wall is not stained by ordinary methods, and the coloured body seen corresponds to the cell protoplasm only. This is usually much shrunken as a result of drying. Chains of stained bacteria thus show the coloured bodies separated by gaps that are the sites of unstained, connecting cell walls. Certain bacteria do not colour evenly with simple stains, perhaps due to the manner in which the protoplasm shrinks when the cell is dried and fixed. Thus, the diphtheria bacillus shows a 'beaded' appearance, with alternating dark and light bars. The plague bacillus shows 'bipolar staining', the ends being more deeply coloured than the centre.

*Negative* or *background staining* is of value as a rapid method for the simple morphological study of bacteria and yeasts. The organisms are mixed with a substance such as India ink, or nigrosin, which, after spreading as a film, yields a dark background in which the organisms stand out as bright, unstained objects. Eosin–saline can similarly be used for the negative staining of intestinal protozoa. *Silver impregnation* methods are used to stain spirochaetes, especially in tissues. The slender cells are thickened by a dark deposit of silver on their surface.

*Differential staining reactions.* For blood protozoa, polychrome dyes such as Giemsa, Leishman or other *Romanowsky stains* are used to differentially stain the characteristic morphological features of the parasites (see Ch. 61). Various stains may be helpful in the diagnosis of fungal disease, depending on the species and its location in the body (see Ch. 60).

In the case of bacteria, *Gram's stain* has the widest application, distinguishing them as 'Gram-positive' or 'Gram-negative', according to whether or not they resist decoloration with acetone, alcohol or aniline oil after staining with a triphenyl methane dye, such as methyl violet, and subsequent treatment with iodine. The Gram-positive bacteria resist decoloration

and remain stained a dark purple colour. The Gram-negative bacteria are decolorized, and are then counterstained light pink by the subsequent application of safranin, neutral red or dilute carbol fuchsin. In routine diagnostic work a Gram-stained smear is often the only preparation examined microscopically, since it shows clearly the general morphology of the bacteria as well as revealing their Gram reaction. It should be noted that characteristically Gram-positive species may sometimes appear Gram-negative under certain conditions of growth, especially in ageing cultures on nutrient agar. Gram reactivity appears to reflect a fundamental aspect of cell structure and is correlated with many other biological properties. Thus, the different species of a single genus generally show the same reaction. Gram-positive bacteria are more susceptible than Gram-negative bacteria to the antibacterial actions of penicillin, acids, iodine, basic dyes, detergents and lysozyme, and less susceptible to alkalies, azide, tellurite, proteolytic enzymes, lysis by antibody and complement, and plasmolysis in solutes of high osmotic pressure.

The mechanism of the Gram stain is not fully understood. The more acidic character of the protoplasm of Gram-positive species, which is enhanced by treatment with iodine, may partly explain their stronger retention of basic dye. Probably, however, the more important difference is in the permeability of the cell wall during the staining process. After staining with methyl violet and treatment with iodine, a dye–iodine complex or *lake* is formed within the cell; this is insoluble in water but moderately soluble and dissociable in the acetone or alcohol used as the decolorizer. Under the action of the decolorizer, the dye and iodine diffuse freely out of the Gram-negative cell, but not from the Gram-positive cell, presumably because the cell wall of the latter is less permeable. Gram-positive bacteria become Gram-negative when their cell wall is ruptured or removed.

The *acid-fast staining reaction*, as revealed by the Ziehl–Neelsen method is of value in the detection of the tubercle bacillus and some other mycobacteria. These 'acid-fast' bacteria have cell walls with a high lipid content (mycolic acids) and are relatively impermeable to simple stains, but when stained with a hot phenolic solution of basic fuchsin, or a fluorescent dye that binds to mycolic acids, such as auramine, they subsequently resist decolorization by 20% sulphuric acid. Any decoloured non-acid-fast organisms are counterstained in a contrasting colour with methylene blue or malachite green. Modifications of the Ziehl–Neelsen method are useful for the demonstration of organisms such as *Nocardia* spp. and some protozoa, notably *Cryptosporidium parvum*.

## COMPOSITION OF VIRUSES

### Structure

The basic infectious particle of a virus is known as the *virion*. In the simplest viruses this consists of nucleic acid and a surrounding coat of protein called the *capsid*. Some viruses are enclosed within an *envelope* usually derived from host cell membranes, but modified by the inclusion of viral glycoproteins. The capsid is composed of distinct morphological units or *capsomeres* which are assembled from viral proteins. Depending on the arrangement of these proteins, the capsomeres may be spherical, cylindrical or ring-like in appearance. The *nucleocapsid* is the combination of nucleic acid and capsid. The arrangement of the capsomeres around the nucleic acid determines the *symmetry* of the virion. When the capsomeres are applied directly to the helical nucleic acid this forms a coil-like structure with the appearance of a hollow tube. Viruses with this arrangement are said to have *helical symmetry*. Most helical viruses enclose the nucleocapsid within an envelope and thus do not have a rigid appearance. The other major type is shown by the viruses with *icosahedral symmetry* (Fig. 2.13) in which the capsomeres are arranged as if they lay on the faces of an icosahedron which has 20 equilateral triangular faces and 12 corners or apices (Fig. 2.14). Capsomeres on the faces and edges of this figure are called hexons as they always link with six adjacent capsomeres; those positioned at the apices are the pentons as they always join to five capsomeres. Viruses with icosahedral symmetry have a rigid structure and in the electron microscope have a characteristic hexagonal outline with triangular faces. However, if the diameter of the virion is less than about 50 nm the particle will appear spherical. Many viruses with icosahedral symmetry are enclosed by an outer envelope. The poxviruses are large and complex and do not show either type of symmetry; they are referred to as complex. The size of virions varies considerably, from 25 to 300 nm, in different families (Fig. 2.15).

### Viral nucleic acid

The commonest types of nucleic acid in viruses of humans are single-stranded RNA and double-stranded DNA. However, both double-stranded RNA and

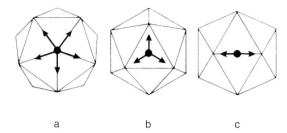

a        b        c

**Fig. 2.13**    An icosahedron viewed along its **a** five-fold, **b** three-fold and **c** two-fold axes of symmetry.

**Fig. 2.14**    A diagram of an icosahedron of an adenovirus. The core of DNA is represented by a circular mass. Some of the pentamers at the 12 vertices have been indicated with protruding fibres and terminal knobs. The remaining 240 hexamer capsids are, for the most part, shown as compressed into hollow spheres linked to each other by divalent bonds. The hexagonal shape of a few of the capsomeres is seen in the centre of the diagram.

single-stranded DNA occur in the reoviruses and parvoviruses, respectively. The genomes of RNA viruses may be present as a single strand as in paramyxoviruses, or as two copies as in the retroviruses, or exist as a specific number of fragments as in the orthomyxoviruses and reoviruses. Circular molecules of DNA are present in the virions of papovaviruses and hepadnaviruses. The amount of nucleic acid in virions is constant for a particular virus but shows considerable variation; thus the molecular weight can vary from about 1.5 million in the parvo- and hepadnaviruses to between 80 million and 240 million for the poxviruses.

### Virion enzymes

Several viruses carry essential enzymes in the virion.

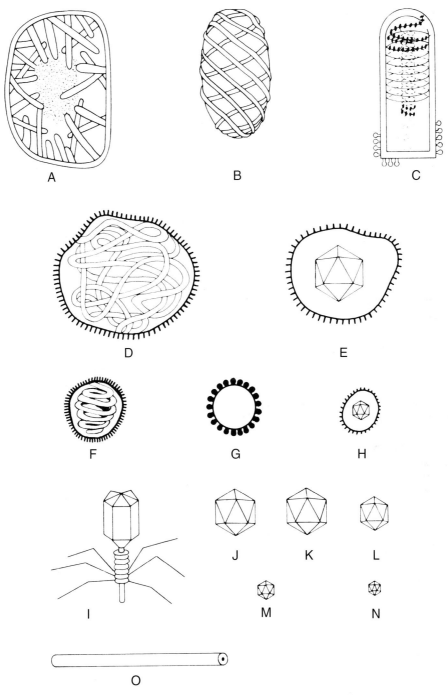

**Fig. 2.15** Morphology of viruses.

A Orthopoxvirus
B Parapoxvirus
C Rhabdovirus
D Paramyxovirus

E Herpesvirus
F Orthomyxovirus
G Coronavirus
H Togavirus

I T-even coliphage
J Adenovirus
K Reovirus
L Papovavirus

M Picornavirus
N Parvovirus
O Tobacco mosaic virus

As discussed in Chapter 9, an RNA-dependent RNA polymerase or transcriptase is an essential component of the virion in several virus families, including the negative-strand RNA viruses. Among DNA viruses only the poxviruses carry a DNA-dependent RNA polymerase. The hepadnaviruses have a virion polymerase complex that has some similarity to the reverse transcriptase complex found in the retroviruses.

## Viral proteins

Analysis of the proteins produced in a cell during viral infection shows that some are essential compo-nents of the virion; these are the structural proteins and include capsid proteins and enzymes as well as basic core proteins which may be necessary to pack-age the nucleic acid within the capsid. Other proteins such as enzymes are needed for the production of viral components but are not part of the virion; these are the non-structural proteins. The essential steps of virus attachment and penetration of the host cell are known to depend on regions of the outer capsid such as the apical fibres and knobs of adenoviruses or on parts of the envelope glycoproteins of viruses such as influenza A and B and the human immuno-deficiency virus.

## RECOMMENDED READING

Actor P, Daneo-Moore L, Higgins M L, Salton M R J, Shockman G D 1988 *Antibiotic Inhibition of Bacterial Cell Surface Assembly and Function*. American Society for Microbiology, Washington, DC

Blair D F 1995 How bacteria sense and swim. *Annual Review of Microbiology* 49: 489–522

Dawes I W, Sutherland I W 1991 *Microbial Physiology*, 2nd edn. Blackwell Scientific, Oxford

Frey D, Oldfield R J, Bridger R C 1979 *A Colour Atlas of Pathogenic Fungi*. Wolfe Medical, London

Madeley C R, Field A M 1988 *Virus Morphology*, 2nd edn.

Churchill Livingstone, Edinburgh

Mandelstam J, McQuillen K, Dawes I W 1982 *Biochemistry of Bacterial Growth*, 3rd edn. Blackwell Scientific, Oxford

Nikaido H, Vaara M 1985 Molecular basis of bacterial outer membrane permeability. *Microbiological Reviews* 49: 1–32

Olds R J 1975 *A Colour Atlas of Microbiology*. Wolfe Medical, London

Shockman G D, Barrett J F 1983 Structure, function and assembly of cell walls from Gram-positive bacteria. *Annual Review of Microbiology* 37: 501–527

# 3

# Classification and identification of micro-organisms

*T. L. Pitt*

Micro-organisms may be classified in the following large biological groups:

1. Algae
2. Protozoa
3. Slime moulds
4. Fungi
5. Bacteria
6. Archaebacteria
7. Viruses.

The algae (excluding the blue-green algae), the protozoa, slime moulds and fungi include the larger and more highly developed micro-organisms; their cells have the same general type of structure and organization, described as *eukaryotic*, as that found in higher plants and animals. The bacteria, including organisms of the mycoplasma, rickettsia and chlamydia groups, together with the related blue-green algae, comprise the smaller micro-organisms with a simpler form of cellular organization described as *prokaryotic*. The archaebacteria are a distinct phylogenetic group of prokaryotes, which bear only a remote ancestral relationship to other organisms.

The viruses are the smallest of the infective agents; they have a relatively simple structure that is not comparable with that of a cell, and their mode of reproduction is fundamentally different from cellular organisms. Even simpler are *viroids*, protein-free fragments of single-stranded circular RNA that cause disease in plants. Other types of infectious particles have been postulated: *prions* are described as infectious proteins devoid of nucleic acid, while *virinos* are said to consist of a small amount of nucleic acid complexed with protein derived from the host cell. There is considerable debate about the true status of prions and virinos and of the relationship, if any, between them.

Since the algae, slime moulds and archaebacteria are not thought to contain species of medical or veterinary importance they will not be considered further. Blue-green algae do not cause infection, but certain species produce potent peptide toxins that may affect persons or animals ingesting polluted water.

## TAXONOMY

*Taxonomy* consists of three components: *classification*, *nomenclature* and *identification*. Classification allows the orderly grouping of micro-organisms while nomenclature concerns the naming of these organisms and requires agreement so that the same name is used unambiguously by everyone. Changes in nomenclature may give rise to confusion and are subject to internationally agreed rules. In clinical practice, microbiologists are generally concerned with identification – the correct naming of isolates according to agreed systems of classification.

Protozoa, fungi and helminths are classified and named according to the standard rules of classification and nomenclature that have been developed following the pioneering work of the 18th century Swedish botanist Linnaeus (Carl von Linné). Large subdivisions (class, order, family, etc.) are finally classified into individual *species* designated by a Latin binomial, the first term of which is the *genus*, e.g. *Plasmodium* (genus) *falciparum* (species). Occasionally it is useful to recognize a biological variant with particular properties: thus, *Trypanosoma* (genus) *brucei* (species) *gambiense* (variant) differs from the variant *T. brucei brucei* in being pathogenic for humans.

Bacteria are similarly classified, but the infinite variety of microbial life and the natural capacity of bacteria for variation and adaptation make rigid classification difficult. Moreover, species of bacteria cannot be defined by the criterion of continued interbreeding used for higher plants and animals, since they reproduce asexually. At present no standard classification of bacteria is universally accepted and applied, although *Bergey's Manual of Systematic Bacteriology* is widely used as an authoritative source.

Bacterial nomenclature is governed by an international code prepared by the *International Committee on Systematic Bacteriology* and published as *Approved Lists of Bacterial Names* in the *International Journal of Systematic Bacteriology*; most new species are also first described in this journal, and since 1984 a species is only considered to be validly published if it appears on a validation list in this journal.

The *International Committee on Taxonomy of Viruses* meets regularly to classify viruses, and publishes its reports in the journal *Intervirology*. Latin names are used wherever possible for the ranks family, subfamily and genus, but at present there are no formal categories higher than family, and binomial nomenclature is not used for species. Viruses do not lend themselves easily to classification according to Linnaean principles, and vernacular names still have wide usage among medical virologists.

## METHODS OF CLASSIFICATION

In most systems of bacterial classification, the major groups are distinguished by fundamental characters, such as cell shape, Gram reaction and spore formation; genera and species are usually distinguished by properties such as fermentation reactions, nutritional requirements and pathogenicity. This system suffers from the weakness that decisions about the relative 'importance' of different characters, thus about their priority in defining the major and minor groupings, are often purely arbitrary.

## Adansonian or numerical classification

The uncertainties of arbitrary choices are avoided in the Adansonian system of taxonomy. This system determines the degrees of relationship between strains by a statistical coefficient that takes account of the widest range of characters, all of which are considered of equal weight. It is clear, of course, that some characters, e.g. cell shape or Gram reaction, represent a much wider and permanent genetic commitment than other characters which, being dependent on only one or a few genes, are relatively mutable. For this reason, the Adansonian method is most useful for the classification of strains within a larger grouping that shares major characters.

By scoring a large number of phenotypic characters it is possible to estimate a *similarity coefficient* when shared positive characters are considered, or a *matching coefficient* when both negative and positive shared characters (matches) are taken into account. The observations can be analysed by computer to indicate degrees of similarity for a group of different organisms and displayed as a *similarity matrix* (Fig. 3.1) or a dendrogram (Fig. 3.2).

## DNA composition

The hydrogen bonding between guanine and cytosine (G-C) base pairs in DNA is stronger than that between adenine and thymine (A-T). Thus, the melting or denaturation temperature of DNA (at which the two strands separate) is primarily determined by the G + C content. At the melting temperature, the separation of the strands brings about a marked

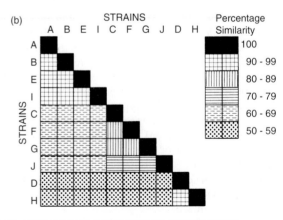

**Fig. 3.1a** A similarity matrix for 10 strains A–J arranged in alphabetical order. **b** To emphasize similarities, the matrix has been redrawn according to a process called *cluster analysis*, which shows that strains A, B, E and I are highly similar *phenons*; strains D and H form a separate group that are closely related to each other, but not to the other strains. (After Sneath P H A 1962 The construction of taxonomic groups. In: Ainsworth G C, Sneath P H A (eds) *Microbial Classification*. Cambridge University Press, Cambridge.)

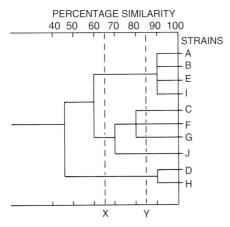

**Fig. 3.2** A hierarchic taxonomic tree (*dendrogram*) prepared from the similarity matrix data shown in Figure 3.1. The broken lines X and Y indicated levels of similarity at which separation into genera and species might be possible. (After Sneath (1962) – see Fig. 3.1 for reference.)

change in the light absorption characteristics at a wavelength of 260 nm, and this is readily detected by spectrophotometry.

There is a very wide range in the G + C component of DNA of bacteria, varying from about 25 to 80 mol% in different genera. However, for any one species, the G + C content is relatively fixed, or falls within a very narrow range, and this provides a basis for classification.

## DNA homology

Another approach to classification is to arrange individual organisms into groups on the basis of the *homology* of their DNA base sequences. This exploits the fact that double strands re-form (anneal) from separated strands during controlled cooling of a heated preparation of DNA. This process can be readily demonstrated with suitably heated homologous DNA extracted from a single species, but it can also occur with DNA from two related species, so that hybrid pairs of DNA strands are produced. These hybrid pairings occur with high frequency between complementary regions of DNA, and the degree of hybridization can be assessed if labelled DNA preparations are used. Binding studies with messenger RNA (mRNA) can also give information to complement these observations, which provide genetic evidence of relatedness among bacteria.

Organisms with different G + C ratios are very unlikely to show significant DNA homology. However, organisms with the same, or close, G + C ratios do not necessarily show homology.

## Ribosomal RNA sequencing

The structure of ribosomal RNA (rRNA) appears to have been highly conserved during the course of evolution and close similarities in nucleotide sequences reflect phylogenetic relationships. Advances in technology have made nucleotide sequencing relatively simple, so that investigation of similarities in oligonucleotides derived from rRNA is increasingly used in taxonomic studies. Far fewer full-length gene sequences are known for 23S rRNA than for 16S rRNA. A rapid and universal bacterial identification scheme is possible based on the amplification of the variable length 16S–23S rDNA spacer regions.

## CLASSIFICATION IN CLINICAL PRACTICE

The identification of micro-organisms in routine practice requires a pragmatic approach to taxonomy. Table 3.1 outlines a simple, but practical, classification scheme in which organisms are grouped according to a few shared characteristics. Within these groups, organisms may be further identified, sometimes to species level, by a few supplementary tests. Protozoa, helminths and fungi can often be definitively identified on morphological criteria alone (see appropriate chapters).

## Protozoa

These are non-photosynthetic unicellular organisms with protoplasm clearly differentiated into nucleus and cytoplasm. They are relatively large with transverse diameters mainly in the range 2–100 μm. Their surface membranes vary in complexity and rigidity from a thin, flexible membrane in amoebae, which allows major changes in cell shape and the protrusion of pseudopodia for the purposes of locomotion and ingestion, to a relatively stiff pellicle in ciliate protozoa, which preserves a characteristic cell shape. Most free-living and some parasitic species capture, ingest and digest internally solid particles of food material; many protozoa, for instance, feed on bacteria. Protozoa, therefore, are generally regarded as the lowest forms of animal life, though certain flagellate protozoa are closely related in their morphology and mode of development to photosynthetic flagellate algae in the plant kingdom. Protozoa reproduce asexually by binary fission or by multiple fission (*schizogony*), and some also by a sexual mechanism (*sporogony*). The most important

| Table 3.1 A simple classification of some micro-organisms of medical importance |
| --- |

**EUKARYOTIC GENERA**

**Protozoa**

    Sporozoa: *Plasmodium, Isospora, Toxoplasma, Cryptosporidium*
    Flagellates: *Giardia, Trichomonas, Trypanosoma, Leishmania*
    Amoebae: *Entamoeba, Naegleria, Acanthamoeba*
    Others: *Babesia, Balantidium, Pneumocystis*[a]

**Fungi**

    Mould-like: *Epidermophyton, Trichophyton, Microsporum, Aspergillus*
    Yeast-like: *Candida*
    Dimorphic: *Histoplasma, Blastomyces, Coccidioides*
    True yeast: *Cryptococcus*

**PROKARYOTIC GENERA**

**Filamentous bacteria**

    *Actinomyces, Nocardia, Streptomyces, Mycobacterium*

**'True bacteria'**

    Gram-positive bacilli:    Aerobes – *Corynebacterium, Listeria, Bacillus*
                             Anaerobes – *Clostridium, Lactobacillus, Eubacterium*
    Gram-positive cocci:    *Staphylococcus, Streptococcus, Enterococcus*
    Gram-negative cocci:    Aerobes – *Neisseria*
                             Anaerobes – *Veillonella*
    Gram-negative bacilli:    Aerobes
                              Enterobacteria – *Escherichia, Klebsiella, Proteus, Salmonella, Shigella, Yersinia*
                              Pseudomonads – *Pseudomonas, Burkholderia, Stenotrophomonas*
                              Parvobacteria – *Haemophilus, Bordetella, Brucella, Pasteurella*
                              Anaerobes – *Bacteroides, Fusobacterium*
    Gram-negative vibrios:    *Vibrio, Spirillum, Campylobacter, Helicobacter*

**Spirochaetes**

    *Borrelia, Treponema, Leptospira*

**Mycoplasmas**

    *Mycoplasma, Ureaplasma*

**Rickettsiae and chlamydiae**

    *Rickettsia, Coxiella, Chlamydia*

[a]May be a fungus.

groups of medical protozoa are the *sporozoa* (malaria parasites, etc.), amoebae and flagellates (see Ch. 61).

## Fungi

These are non-photosynthetic organisms possessing relatively rigid cell walls. They may be saprophytic or parasitic, and take in soluble nutrients by diffusion through their cell surfaces.

*Moulds* grow as branching filaments (*hyphae*), usually between 2 and 10 μm in width, which interlace to form a meshwork (*mycelium*). The hyphae are coenocytic (i.e. have a continuous multinucleate protoplasm), being either non-septate or else septate with a central pore in each cross-wall. Moulds reproduce by the formation of various kinds of sexual and asexual spores that develop from the vegetative (feeding) mycelium, or from an aerial mycelium that effects their air-borne dissemination.

*Yeasts* are ovoid or spherical cells that reproduce asexually by budding and also, in many cases, sexually, with the formation of sexual spores. They do not form a mycelium, although the intermediate *yeast-like fungi* form a pseudomycelium consisting of chains of elongated cells. The *dimorphic fungi* produce a vegetative mycelium in artificial culture, but are yeast-like in infected lesions. The higher fungi of the class *Basidiomycetes* (mushrooms), which produce large fruiting structures for aerial dissemination of spores, are not infectious for humans or animals, although some species are poisonous.

## Bacteria

The main groups of bacteria are distinguished by the microscopical observation of their morphology and staining reactions. The Gram staining procedure, which reflects fundamental differences in cell wall structure, separates most bacteria into two great divisions: *Gram-positive bacteria* and *Gram-negative bacteria* (see Ch. 2).

Details of structure provide a basis for a separate division into:

1. *Filamentous bacteria (Actinomycetes)*, most of which are capable of true branching and which may produce a type of mycelium
2. *'True' bacteria*, which multiply by simple binary fission
3. *Spirochaetes*, which divide by transverse binary fission
4. *Mycoplasmas*, which lack a rigid cell wall
5. *Rickettsiae* and *chlamydiae*, which are strict intracellular parasites.

### Filamentous bacteria

These are sometimes referred to as 'higher bacteria'. A few are of medical interest as pathogens, and some produce antibiotics.

1. *Actinomyces*. Gram-positive, non-acid-fast, tend to fragment into short coccal and bacillary forms and not to form conidia; anaerobic (e.g. *Actinomyces israelii*).
2. *Nocardia*. Similar to *Actinomyces*, but aerobic and mostly acid-fast (e.g. *Nocardia asteroides*).
3. *Streptomyces*. Vegetative mycelium does not fragment into short forms; conidia form in chains from aerial hyphae (e.g. *Streptomyces griseus*).
4. *Mycobacterium*. Acid-fast; Gram-positive, but does not readily stain by the Gram method; usually bacillary, rarely branching; aerobic (e.g. *Mycobacterium tuberculosis*).

### True bacteria

Most medically important bacteria fall into this group. They are classified on the basis of their shape:

1. Cocci – spherical, or nearly spherical cells
2. Bacilli – relatively straight, rod-shaped (cylindrical) cells
3. Vibrios and spirilla – curved or twisted rod-shaped cells.

***Cocci.*** The main groups of cocci are distinguished by their predominant mode of cell grouping and their reaction to the Gram stain. The different cocci are relatively uniform in size (usually about 1 μm in diameter). Some species are capsulate and a very few are motile.

1. *Streptococcus*. Gram-positive; cells mainly adherent in chains, due to successive cell divisions occurring in the same axis (e.g. *Streptococcus pyogenes*); sometimes predominantly diplococcal (e.g. *Streptococcus pneumoniae*).
2. *Staphylococcus* and *Micrococcus*. Gram-positive; cells mainly adherent in irregular clusters, due to successive divisions occurring irregularly in different planes (e.g. *Staphylococcus aureus*).
3. *Sarcina*. Gram-positive cells mainly adherent in cubical arrays of eight, or multiples thereof, due to division occurring successively in three planes at right angles (e.g. *Sarcinia lutea*).
4. *Neisseria*. Gram-negative; cells mainly adherent in pairs and slightly elongated at right angles to axis of pairs (e.g. *Neisseria meningitidis*).
5. *Veillonella*. Gram-negative; generally very small cocci arranged mainly in clusters and pairs; anaerobic (e.g. *Veillonella parvula*).

***Bacilli.*** The primary subdivision of the rod-shaped bacteria is made according to their staining reaction by the Gram method and the presence or absence of endospores.

1. *Gram-positive spore-forming bacilli*. Apart from some rare saprophytic varieties, the only bacteria to form endospores are those of the genera *Bacillus* (aerobic) and *Clostridium* (anaerobic). They are Gram-positive, but liable to become Gram-negative in ageing cultures. The size, shape and position of the spore may assist recognition of the species, e.g. the bulging, spherical, terminal spore ('drumstick' form) of *Clostridium tetani*.

2. *Gram-positive non-sporing bacilli*. These include several genera. *Corynebacterium* is distinguished by a tendency to slight curving, a club-shaped or ovoid swelling of the bacilli, and their arrangement in parallel or angular clusters due to the snapping mode of cell division. *Erysipelothrix* and *Lactobacillus* are distinguished by a tendency to grow in chains and filaments, and *Listeria* by flagella that confer motility.

3. *Gram-negative bacilli.* This large grouping includes numerous genera such as the pseudomonads and the family Enterobacteriaceae ('coliform bacilli') as well as small, often pleomorphic bacilli represented by *Haemophilus*, *Brucella*, etc. ('parvobacteria'), and anaerobes such as *Bacteroides*.

4. *Vibrios and spirilla.* Vibrios and the related campylobacters are recognized as short, non-flexuous, comma-shaped bacilli (e.g. *Vibrio cholerae*) and spirilla as non-flexuous spiral filaments (e.g. *Spirillum minus*). They are Gram-negative and mostly motile, having polar flagella and showing very active 'darting' motility.

## Spirochaetes

These organisms differ from the 'true' bacteria in being slender flexuous spiral filaments which, unlike the spirilla, are motile without possession of flagella. The staining reaction, when demonstrable, is Gram-negative. The different varieties are recognized by their size, shape, wave form and refractility, observed in the natural state in unstained wet films by dark-ground microscopy (Fig. 3.3).

1. *Borrelia.* Larger and more refractile than the other pathogenic spirochaetes and more readily stained by ordinary methods; coils large and open, with a wavelength of 2–3 μm; by electron microscopy a leash of 8–12 fibrils, each about 0.02 μm thick, is seen twisted round the whole length of the protoplast (e.g. *Borrelia recurrentis*).

2. *Treponema.* Thinner filaments in coils of shorter wavelength (e.g. 1.0–1.5 μm), typically presenting a regular 'corkscrew' form; feebly refractile and difficult to stain except by silver impregnation methods; by electron microscopy, a leash of four fibrils is seen wound round the protoplast within the cell wall (e.g. *Treponema pallidum*).

3. *Leptospira.* The coils are so fine and close (wavelength about 0.5 μm) that they are barely discernible by dark-ground microscopy, though clearly seen winding round two axial filaments by electron microscopy. One or both extremities of the organism are hooked, or recurved, so that it may take the shape of a walking-stick, an 'S' or a 'C' (e.g. *Leptospira interrogans*).

## Mycoplasmas

These are prokaryotes that differ from 'true' bacteria in their smaller size and their lack of a rigid cell wall, which leads to extreme pleomorphism and sensitivity to external osmotic pressure. The viable elements range from 0.15 to over 1 μm in diameter, the smallest being capable of passing through filters that retain conventional bacteria. Mycoplasmas can be cultivated on cell-free nutrient media, and are the smallest and simplest organisms capable of autonomous growth.

## Rickettsiae and chlamydiae

The rickettsiae are rod-shaped, spherical or pleomorphic Gram-negative organisms. They are generally smaller than 'true' bacteria, but are still resolvable in the light microscope. Most are strict parasites that can grow only in the living tissues of a suitable animal host, usually intracellularly (e.g. *Rickettsia prowazekii*). Chlamydiae are similar to rickettsiae, but have a more complex intracellular cycle (e.g. *Chlamydia trachomatis*).

# Viruses

Viruses usually consist of little more than a strand of DNA or RNA (never both) enclosed in a simple protein shell known as a *capsid*. Sometimes the complete nucleocapsid may be enclosed in a lipoprotein envelope largely derived from the host cell. Viruses are capable of growing only within the living cells of an appropriate animal, plant or bacterial host; none can grow in an inanimate nutrient medium. The viruses that infect and parasitize bacteria are named *bacteriophages* or *phages*.

A simple classification of the viruses that are involved in human disease is shown in Table 3.2.

# IDENTIFICATION OF MICRO-ORGANISMS

Precise identification of bacteria is time-consuming and contentious, and is best carried out in specialized reference centres. For most clinical purposes, clear, rapid guidance on the likely cause of an infection is

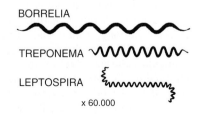

**Fig. 3.3** Morphology of spirochaetes.

**Table 3.2** Principal types of virus causing human disease

| Types of virus | Examples |
|---|---|
| **RNA viruses** | |
| Orthomyxoviruses | Influenza A, B, C viruses |
| Paramyxoviruses | Parainfluenza viruses |
| | Mumps virus |
| | Measles virus |
| | Respiratory syncytial virus |
| Rhabdoviruses | Rabies virus |
| Arenaviruses | Lassa virus |
| Filoviruses | Marburg and Ebola viruses |
| Togaviruses | Many arboviruses |
| | Rubella virus |
| Flaviviruses | Yellow fever virus |
| | Dengue virus |
| | Japanese encephalitis virus |
| Bunyaviruses | Hantaan virus |
| Coronaviruses | OC42 |
| Caliciviruses | Small round structured viruses |
| | Hepatitis E |
| Picornaviruses | Enteroviruses |
| | Poliovirus (3 types) |
| | Echovirus (31 types) |
| | Coxsackie A virus (24 types) |
| | Coxsackie B virus (6 types) |
| | Enterovirus types 68–71 |
| | Hepatitis A virus (type 72) |
| | Rhinovirus, many serotypes |
| Retroviruses | Human immunodeficiency viruses types 1 and 2 |
| | Human T-lymphotropic virus types I and II |
| Reoviruses | Rotaviruses |
| **DNA viruses** | |
| Poxviruses | Variola, vaccinia |
| | Molluscum contagiosum virus |
| | Orf |
| Herpesviruses | Herpes simplex virus types 1 and 2 |
| | Varicella–zoster virus |
| | Cytomegalovirus |
| | Epstein–Barr virus |
| | Human herpes virus type 6 |
| Adenoviruses | Many serotypes |
| Polyomaviruses | Papillomaviruses (warts) |
| | JC virus |
| Hepadnaviruses | Hepatitis B virus |
| Parvoviruses | B19 virus |

required and, consequently, microbiologists usually rely on a few simple procedures, notably microscopy and culture, backed up, when necessary, by a few supplementary tests.

Microscopy is the most rapid test of all, but culture inevitably takes at least 24 h, and sometimes longer. More rapid tests are constantly being sought, and some progress has been achieved with antigen detection methods and specific *gene probes* (see below).

Most specimens for bacteriological examination, whether from humans, animals or the environment, contain mixtures of bacteria and it is essential to obtain *pure cultures* of individual isolates before embarking on identification. Non-cultural methods, such as antigen detection or gene probes, do not have this disadvantage; however, they do have the potential limitation of being highly specific so that the investigator must know beforehand what is to be looked for.

## Microscopy

Morphology and staining reactions of individual organisms generally serve as preliminary criteria to place an unknown species in its appropriate biological group. A Gram stain smear suffices to show the Gram reaction, size, shape and grouping of the bacteria, and the arrangement of any endospores.

An unstained wet film may be examined with dark-ground illumination in the microscope to observe the morphology of delicate spirochaetes; an unstained wet film, or 'hanging-drop' preparation is examined with ordinary bright field illumination for observation of motility. To identify mycobacteria, or other acid-fast organisms, a preparation is stained by the Ziehl–Neelsen method or one of its modifications.

The microscopical characters of certain organisms in pathological specimens may be sufficient for presumptive identification, e.g. tubercle bacilli in sputum, or *T. pallidum* in exudate from a chancre. However, many bacteria share similar morphological features, and further tests must be applied to differentiate them.

## Cultural characteristics

The appearance of colonial growth on the surface of a solid medium, such as nutrient agar, is often very characteristic. Attention is paid to the diameter of the colonies, their outline (Fig. 3.4), their elevation (Fig. 3.5), their translucency (clear, translucent or opaque) and colour. Changes brought about in the medium (e.g. haemolysis in a blood agar medium) may also be significant.

The range of conditions that support growth is characteristic of particular organisms. The ability or inability of the organism to grow aerobically or anaerobically, or on media containing selective inhibitory factors (e.g. bile salt, specific antimicrobial agents, or low or high pH) may also be of diagnostic significance.

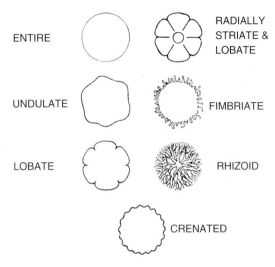

Fig. 3.4  Edges of bacterial colonies.

Fig. 3.5  Elevations of bacterial colonies.

## Biochemical reactions

Species that cannot be distinguished by morphology and cultural characters may exhibit metabolic differences that can be exploited. Is is usual to test the ability of the organism to produce acidic and gaseous end-products, when presented with individual carbohydrates (glucose, lactose, sucrose, mannitol, etc.) as the sole carbon source. Other tests determine whether the bacterium produces particular end-products (e.g. indole or hydrogen sulphide) when grown in suitable culture media, and whether it possesses certain enzyme activities, such as oxidase, catalase, urease, gelatinase or lecithinase.

Traditionally, such tests have been performed selectively and individually according to the recommendations of standard guides, such as the invalu-able *Cowan and Steel's Manual for the Identification of Medical Bacteria.* For practical reasons many workers are now turning to the commercially prepared galleries of identification tests which, though expensive, combine simplicity and accuracy. Test kits are now available for a number of different groups of organisms, including enterobacteria, staphylococci, streptococci and anaerobes.

Sometimes more elaborate procedures may be used for the analysis of metabolic products. For example, gas–liquid chromatography is widely used to recognize characteristic volatile fatty acids and alcohols produced by anaerobic bacteria.

## INDIRECT IDENTIFICATION METHODS

### Gene probes

These are cloned fragments of DNA that recognize complementary sequences within micro-organisms (see Ch. 6, p. 66). Binding is detected by tagging the DNA with a radio-active label, or with a reagent that can be developed to give a colour reaction. By selecting DNA fragments specific for features characteristic of individual organisms, gene probes can be tailored to the rapid identification of individual species in clinical material. One disadvantage of this approach is that the organism itself is not made available for subsequent tests of susceptibility to anti-microbial agents, toxin production or epidemiological investigation. However, probes able to detect genes for antibiotic resistance, toxin production or epidemiological markers are also being developed.

### Antibody reactions

Species and types of micro-organism can often be identified by specific serological reactions. These depend on the fact that the serum of an animal immunized against a micro-organism contains specific antibodies for the homologous species or type that reacts in a characteristic manner (e.g. agglutination or precipitation) with the particular micro-organism. Such simple in-vitro tests have been used for many years in microbiology, notably in the formal identification of presumptive isolates of pathogens (e.g. salmonellae) from clinical material.

The specificity and range of antibody tests have been greatly improved by the availability of highly specific *monoclonal antibodies*. These are produced by the *hybridoma* technique in which individual antibody-producing spleen cells are fused with 'immortal' tumour cells in vitro. The progeny of these hybrid cells produce only the type of antibody appropriate to the spleen cell precursor.

## Counterimmuno-electrophoresis

This technique has been widely used for the detection of pneumococcal and other capsular antigens. The specimen to be tested for the particular antigen and the homologous antibody are placed in separate wells in an agar gel and subjected to an electric current. Antigens that carry a negative charge migrate towards the anode, and the positively charged antibody towards the cathode. A line of precipitation is formed at the point at which the two meet.

## Enzyme-linked immunosorbent assay

In enzyme-linked immunosorbent assay (ELISA), a specific antibody is attached to the surface of a plastic well and material containing the test antigen is added. After washing, the presence of the antigen is detected by addition of more of the specific antibody, this time labelled with an enzyme which can initiate a colour reaction when provided with the appropriate substrate. The intensity of the colour change is related to the amount of antigen bound.

The ELISA method may also be used in the reverse manner for the quantitative detection of antibodies, by adsorbing purified antigen to the well before adding test serum; in this case the enzyme-linked system used to detect the antigen–antibody reaction is a labelled anti-human globulin.

In immunoglobulin M antibody capture ELISA (MAC-ELISA), widely used in virological diagnosis for the detection of IgM, anti-human μ chain antibody (usually raised in goats) is bound to the well. The test serum is added, and any IgM binds to the capture reagent; after washing, purified antigen (e.g. rubella antigen) is added, and this can be detected with an appropriate labelled antibody.

## Latex agglutination

By adsorbing specific antibody to inert latex particles, a visible agglutination reaction can be induced in the presence of homologous antigen. Once again, this principle can be applied in reverse to detect serum antibodies.

## Haemagglutination and haemadsorption

Certain viruses, notably the influenza viruses, have the property of attaching to specific receptors on the surface of appropriate red blood cells. In this manner the virus particles act as bridges linking the red cells in visible clumps.

In tissue culture, such haemagglutinins may appear on the surface of cells infected with a virus. If red cells are added to the tissue culture, they adhere to the surface of infected cells, a phenomenon known as *haemadsorption*.

Red blood cells can also be coated with specific antibody so that they agglutinate in the presence of the homologous virus particle in a manner similar to that described for latex agglutination above.

## Fluorescence microscopy and immunofluorescence

When certain dyes are exposed to ultraviolet light, they absorb energy and emit visible light (i.e. they fluoresce). Tissues or organisms stained with such a dye and examined with ultraviolet light in a specially adapted microscope are seen as fluorescent objects; for example, auramine can be used in this way to stain *M. tuberculosis*.

Antibody molecules can be labelled by conjugation with a fluorochrome dye such as fluorescein isothiocyanate (which fluoresces green) or rhodamine (orange-red). When fluorescent antibody is allowed to react with homologous antigen exposed at a cell surface, this *direct immunofluorescence* procedure affords a highly sensitive method for the identification of the particular antigen. For this procedure it is necessary to have a specific antibody conjugate for each antigen; however, unconjugated antibody can be used and the reaction then detected by addition of an antiglobulin conjugate which will react with any antibody from the species in which the antibody was raised.

## TYPING OF BACTERIA

A population of bacteria presumed to descend from a single bacterium as found in a natural habitat, in primary cultures from the habitat, and in subcultures from the primary cultures, is called a *strain*. Each primary culture from a natural source is called an *isolate*. The distinction between strains and isolates may be important; for example, cultures of typhoid bacilli isolated from 10 different patients should be regarded simply as 10 different *isolates* unless epidemiological or other evidence indicates that the patients have been infected from a common source with the same *strain*. Strains with demonstrable ancestral lineage have been termed *clones*, but this term should be used with caution.

The ability to discriminate between similar strains may be of great epidemiological value in tracing sources or modes of spread of infection in a community, and various typing methods have been devised.

Strains may be distinguishable only in minor characters and it is usually simpler to establish differences between isolates from a common source than unequivocally to prove their identity. Demonstration of an identical response by a single reproducible typing method is not proof that two strains are the same. However, the confidence with which similarity can be inferred is greatly increased if more than one typing method is used.

## Biotyping

Biochemical test reactions which are not universally positive or negative within a species may define *biotypes* which are efficient strain markers. Differences among strains may also be detected by variations in sensitivity to fixed concentrations of chemicals such as heavy metals, a process known as *resistotyping*.

## Serotyping

Many surface structures of bacteria (lipopolysaccharide and outer membrane, flagella, capsule etc.) are antigenic and antibodies raised against them can be used to group isolates into defined *serotypes*.

## Phage typing

Bacteria often show differential susceptibility to lysis by certain bacteriophages. The *phage type* of the culture is identified according to the pattern of susceptibility to a set of lytic phages. Phage typing is widely used to discriminate among strains of salmonellae and of staphylococci.

## Bacteriocin typing

Bacteriocins are naturally occurring antibacterial substances, elaborated by most bacterial species, that are active mainly against strains of the same genus as the producer strain. Bacteriocin typing may define the spectrum of bacteriocins produced by field strains, or the sensitivity of these strains to bacteriocins of a standard panel of strains. Patterns of production or susceptibility to bacteriocins allow the division of species into *bacteriocin types*.

## Protein typing

Bacteria manufacture thousands of proteins which can be visualized by electrophoresis in acrylamide gels in the presence of a strong detergent. The proteins separate according to molecular size and after staining with a dye the pattern of bands from each isolate can be compared. This system has been successfully used for typing many bacterial and fungal species. Investigation of microbial populations by gel electrophoresis of metabolic enzymes, which can then be detected by specific substrates, is also widely applied for clonal analysis within species.

## Restriction endonuclease typing

*Restriction endonucleases* are a family of enzymes that each cut DNA at a specific sequence recognition site, which may be rare or frequent in the DNA of the species being examined. Both plasmid and chromosomal DNA can be analysed by this means. Frequent-cutting endonucleases generate numerous small fragments which can be resolved by conventional electrophoresis in agarose gel and detected by staining with a dye. Rare cutters produce large DNA fragments that need to be separated in special electrical fields with a pulsed current (*pulsed-field gel electrophoresis*). This technique is widely used to size genomes of species and detect variations in the DNA of individual strains.

## Gene probe typing

DNA probes (see earlier) for strain typing consist of cloned specific, random or universal sequences that can detect restriction site heterogeneity in the target DNA. The detection of variation in rDNA gene loci is the basis of *ribotyping*, and this method has been universally applied to the typing of various species. Some genera such as *Mycoplasma* cannot be ribotyped as they have only a single copy of the rRNA operon. Other commonly used probes are *insertion sequences* (lengths of DNA involved in transposition; see p. 67), which may define clonal structure of populations.

## Polymerase chain reaction typing

The polymerase chain reaction (PCR) is a technique that allows specific sequences of DNA to be amplified. Multiple copies of regions of the genome defined by specific oligonucleotide primers are made by repeated cycles of polymerization under controlled conditions (see p. 68). Such methods can be used to study DNA from any source. Several variations on the PCR theme have been described, and use of these techniques continues to expand and develop.

PCR-mediated DNA fingerprinting makes use of the variable regions in DNA molecules. These may be variable numbers of tandem repeat regions or areas with restriction endonuclease recognition sequences. To do *PCR typing*, it is necessary to know the sequences of the bordering regions so that specific oligonucleotide primers can be synthesized. Primers may be specific for a known sequence or be random. Random primers are extensively used in the techniques *random applied polymorphic DNA typing* (RAPD) and *arbitrarily primed PCR* (AP-PCR).

## Miscellaneous methods

Other methods such as pyrolysis mass spectrometry of total volatile bacterial products, fatty acid profiles, and lipopolysaccharide electrophoretic profiles for Gram-negative species have been applied for strain fingerprinting.

The antimicrobial sensitivity pattern of bacteria (*antibiogram*) can sometimes be sufficiently characteristic to be useful as an epidemiological marker for tracing strains.

## Animal pathogenicity and toxigenicity

Animal pathogenicity tests were formerly much used in the diagnosis of tuberculosis and certain other diseases. They have now been almost entirely replaced by cultural methods. Similarly, animal tests for the demonstration of bacterial toxins have largely been superseded by gene probes and ELISA methodologies.

RECOMMENDED READING

Barrow G I, Feltham R K A (eds) 1993 *Cowan and Steel's Manual for the Identification of Medical Bacteria*, 3rd edn. Cambridge University Press, Cambridge

Holt J G (editor-in-chief) (1984–89) *Bergey's Manual of Systematic Bacteriology*. Williams and Wilkins, Baltimore, vols 1–4

Murphy F A, Fauquet C M, Bishop D H L et al (eds) 1995 Virus taxonomy. Classification and nomenclature of viruses. Sixth report of the International Committee on Taxonomy of Viruses. *Archives of Virology* Suppl 10: 359—67, 409–11

Murray P R, Baron, E J, Pfaller M A, Tenover F C, Yolken R H (eds) 1995 *Manual of Clinical Microbiology*, 6th edn. ASM Press, Washington, DC

Skerman V B D, McGowan V, Sneath P H A 1989 *Approved Lists of Bacterial Names*, amended edn. American Society for Microbiology, Washington, DC

Woese C R 1987 Bacterial evolution. *Microbiological Reviews* 51: 221–271

# 4

# Bacterial growth and physiology

*M. R. Barer*

Most of what we know about bacteria derives from their growth. Their ability to propagate may be seen as a supreme achievement which enables them to attain enormous populations at rates which are breathtaking from a human perspective. These properties underpin their capacity for change by mutation and the rapidity with which some infections develop.

Bacterial growth involves both an increase in the size of organisms and an increase in the number of individuals. Whatever the balance between these two processes, the net effect is an increase in the total mass (*biomass*) of the culture. Medical microbiologists have traditionally concentrated on the number of individuals in growth studies. Whether this emphasis on cell number is appropriate remains uncertain; nonetheless, it will be adopted here, since the number of individual bacteria involved is important in the course and outcome of infections and in the measurement of the effects of antibiotics.

Students of medicine may be surprised and even dismayed to hear that organisms as small as bacteria have a physiology. However, the complement of enzymes and the biochemical and biophysical processes occurring in a prokaryotic cell at any one time represent the product of genetic and biochemical control mechanisms which are every bit as sophisticated and tightly regulated as those in eukaryotic cells. Moreover, the recognition and definition of the mechanisms by which bacteria sense and adapt to nutritional and noxious stimuli in their environments have provided insights that are likely to translate into medically significant advances in the foreseeable future.

Although this chapter only discusses bacterial growth and physiology, many of the principles are also applicable to fungi. The central difference between their growth is that cell division is generally achieved in bacteria by *binary fission* to produce identical offspring which cannot be distinguished as parents and progeny, while fungi divide by budding in the case of yeast growth and hyphal septation in the mould form.

## BACTERIAL GROWTH

When placed in a suitable nutritious environment and maintained under appropriate physical and chemical conditions a bacterial cell begins to grow and, when it has manufactured approximately twice the amount of component materials that it started with, divides. The range of specific components which define 'suitable' and 'appropriate' for all known bacteria is so broad that it actually defines the global biosphere (those environments which can sustain life) and includes temperatures and pressures present at the opening of hydrothermal vents on the ocean floor to the outer reaches of the atmosphere. Although these conditions do not regularly occur in humans they serve to illustrate that no part of the body or medical device with which it may come in contact is too difficult for bacteria to colonize and that bacteria may lurk in surprising environmental niches. Conversely, the conditions required for some organisms to grow are so precise that so far we have not been able to reproduce them in artificial laboratory media. This applies to some well-known organisms such as the agents of leprosy and syphilis, but it also applies to many other potential pathogens that we are beginning to learn about through molecular methods which do not depend on growth. In fact, it is estimated that we have not yet isolated more than 1% of all the bacterial species that exist, and it is almost certain that there are many medically important organisms among the 'as yet uncultivated' micro-organisms.

As the central technique in bacteriology, growth in the laboratory has been used to serve many different purposes. From the clinical perspective, growth is used for detection and identification, and for the assessment of antibiotic effects, while scientific and industrial objectives are often served by growth in bulk to obtain sufficient biomass for detailed biochemical analysis and to produce the desirable products of the brewing and biotechnology industries.

## Types of growth

In the laboratory bacterial growth can be seen in three main forms:

1. By the development of *colonies*, the macroscopic product of 20–30 cell divisions of a single bacterium or clump of bacteria on solid media
2. By the transformation of a clear broth medium to a turbid suspension of $10^7$–$10^9$ cells per millilitre
3. In *biofilm* formation, in which growth is spread thinly (300–400 µm thick) over an inert surface and nutrition obtained from a bathing fluid.

In natural systems only biofilms, such as those that develop on the surfaces of intravascular cannulae, appear to have the same appearance and properties as growth produced in the laboratory, while colonies, the other form of *sessile* growth, rarely reach macroscopic dimensions. Turbid liquid systems due to *planktonic* growth of a single organism are also a rarity in nature. However, in spite of these unrepresentative features, growth in macroscopic colonies and growth to high cell densities in broth offer great practical advantages and remain central techniques.

## Growth phases in broth culture

Bacterial growth in broth has been studied in great detail and has provided a framework within which the growth state or growth phase of any given pure culture of a single organism can be placed; these phases are summarized in the idealized *growth curve* shown in Figure 4.1. When growth is initiated by inoculation into appropriate broth conditions, the number of cells present appears to remain constant for the *lag phase*, during which cells are thought to be preparing for growth. Increase in cell number then becomes detectable, and its rate accelerates rapidly until it is established at the maximum achievable rate for the available conditions. This is known as the *exponential phase* because the number of cells is increasing exponentially with time. In order to accommodate the astronomic changes in number, the growth curve is normally displayed on a logarithmic scale which shows a linear increase in cell number with time (hence the older term *log*

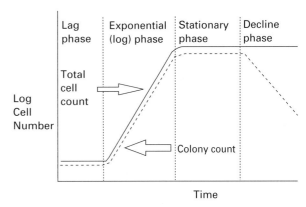

**Fig. 4.1**  Phases of growth in a broth culture.

*phase*). This log–linear relationship is sufficiently constant for a given bacterial strain under one set of conditions that it can be mathematically defined and is often quoted as the *doubling time* for that organism. Doubling times have been measured at anything between 13 min for *Vibrio cholerae* and 24 h for *Mycobacterium tuberculosis*. On this basis it is not surprising that cholera is a disease that can kill within 12 h, while tuberculosis takes months to develop. A further consequence is that when specimens are submitted to diagnostic laboratories for the detection of these organisms by culture, a result is usually available for *V. cholerae* the next day while several weeks are required for conventional culture of *M. tuberculosis*.

It is often difficult to grasp fully the scale of exponential microbial growth; the message may be strengthened by considering that the progeny of a lecture theatre containing 150 students would exceed the global population of humanity ($5 \times 10^9$) within $8\frac{1}{2}$ h if they were able to breed like *Escherichia coli*!

Exponential growth cannot be sustained indefinitely in a closed (*batch*) system with limited available nutrients. Eventually growth slows down, and the total bacterial cell number reaches a maximum and stabilizes. This is known as the *stationary* or *post-exponential phase*. At this stage it becomes important to know what method has been used to determine the growth curve. If a direct method which assesses the total number of cells present is used then the count remains constant. Such methods include counting cells in a volumetric chamber observed by microscopy, electronic particle counters and measurement of turbidity. If, however, the growth potential of the individual cells present in the culture is assessed by taking regular samples, making 10-fold dilutions of these and inoculating them onto agar, then the number of *colony forming units* (cfu) per unit volume can be determined at each sample time. Although such cfu counts closely parallel the results obtained by direct counting methods in the exponential and early stationary phases, a divergence begins to emerge towards the end of the latter; the total cell number remains constant while the colony count declines. This marks the beginning of the final, *decline phase*, in the sequence of growth states which can be observed in broth. The discrepancy between the total and cfu counts is conventionally held to represent the death of cells due to nutrient exhaustion and accumulation of detrimental metabolic end-products. However, there is some doubt concerning this interpretation (see below).

The study of bacterial growth in broth provides a valuable point of reference to which practical, experimental and routine diagnostic procedures are often related. For example, the length of the lag phase and rates of exponential growth in different circumstances are used to make predictions and contribute to safety standards for storage in the food industry. An important feature that emerges is that cultures inoculated with cells prepared at different stages in the growth curve yield different results. The exponential phase is the most reproducible and readily identified, and is therefore used most frequently. It can be extended in an open system known as *continuous culture* using a *chemostat* in which cells of a growing culture are continuously harvested and nutrients continuously replenished. Chemostat studies have provided very detailed information on the chemistry of microbial growth and the way in which different organisms convert specific substrates into biomass. The extraordinary efficiency of this process has made natural and genetically manipulated microbes a powerful resource for the biotechnology industry.

In contrast to growth in broth, far less is known about the state of the bacteria in a mature macroscopic colony on an agar plate. Such a colony presents a wide range of environments from an abundance of oxygen and nutrients at the edge to almost no oxygen or nutrients available to those cells in the centre. It is likely that all phases of growth are represented in colonies, depending on the location of a particular cell and the age of the culture. Although in practice colonies can be used reliably to inoculate routine tests of antimicrobial susceptibility in clinical laboratories, they cannot be considered a defined starting point for experimental work because they comprise such a heterogeneous population of cells. In fact, colonies are complex and dynamic communities in which cells at different locations can show startlingly different phenotypes. In spite of its complexity, the capacity for and quality of colonial growth of specific organisms on specialized media is central to the laboratory description of medically important bacteria.

## MEDIA FOR BACTERIAL GROWTH

The media used in a medical diagnostic bacteriology laboratory have their origins, for the most part, back in the 'golden age of bacteriology' in the late 19th and early 20th centuries. A vast amount of experience and knowledge has accrued from their use and, apart from better standardization and quality control in their production, little has changed in their basic design. The objectives of early medium design were to grow pathogenic bacteria, separate them from the other organisms present in samples and, ultimately, differentiate their phenotypic properties so that they could be identified. A critical development was the introduction of solidifying agents, most particularly the largely indigestible polysaccharide extract of seaweed known as agar. Alternative solidifying agents include gelatine, and egg albumen. Before the development of solid media, pure cultures could be achieved only by dilution of inocula so that only one growing cell or clump of cells was present at the initiation of growth, a very laborious and unreliable procedure. In contrast, solid media in Petri dishes provided a growth substrate onto which mixed cultures could be inoculated and, providing the population density could be made low enough to allow development of well-separated colonies, the different organisms present could be differentiated and subsequently separated into pure cultures.

### Media used for isolation and identification of pathogens

The central features of media in medical bacteriology are:

1. A source of protein or protein hydrolysate, often derived from casein or an infusion of brain, heart or liver obtained from the nearest butcher
2. Control of pH in the final product (after sterilization)
3. A defined salt content.

Early media often included blood or serum in an attempt to reproduce nutritional features present in the human body. Growth of some pathogens was found to be dependent on such supplements, and it was recognized that these relatively *fastidious* or *nutritionally exacting* organisms were dependent on *growth factors*. The identity of many of the growth factors is now known (e.g. haemin and several coenzymes) but blood often remains their most convenient source.

### Selective and indicator media

Tremendous ingenuity has gone into designing growth media that provide information relevant to patient management as early as possible. There are two main approaches, both of which depend on adding supplements to the basal medium. *Selective media* contain substances such as bile salts or antibiotics that inhibit the growth of some organisms but have little or no effect on the organisms for whose isolation they were designed. They are essential for samples containing a normal microbial flora such as faeces. The inclusion of components or specific reagents that show whether the bacteria possess a particular biochemical property characterizes an *indicator medium*. Such media are critical to the rapid presumptive identification of isolates. Combinations of selective and indicator supplements in agar media have led to formulations with some remarkably elegant differential properties which effectively colour code the colonies according to their biochemical properties and restrict growth to a desired range of organisms. Broth indicator media tend to be much simpler, since they generally require a pure inoculum of a single organism and reveal only one property per formulation. Broth media with selective properties are usually referred to as *enrichment media* as they change the balance of organisms inoculated in favour of the desired range of organisms thereby enriching them.

### Media for laboratory studies

Most of the objectives of a clinical diagnostic laboratory can be fulfilled with the range of media outlined above. However, the composition of these media is not defined, and this poses problems for some investigations including the detailed analysis of antibiotic action. Wherever possible, such investigations are based on a *defined* or *synthetic medium* where every chemical component is carefully regulated. In genetic experiments use is often made of a *minimal medium* in which every component is required for the growth of the organism under investigation, so that if one component is removed,

growth cannot occur. Minimal media also prevent the growth of mutants that have additional nutritional requirements to those of the parent strain. For some organisms, particularly those which can grow outside the human body, minimal media may comprise as little as an ammonium salt to provide nitrogen, a carbon source, which in some cases can be as simple as carbon monoxide, trace amounts of iron and other essential elements and pH adjustment to within an appropriate range. Defined and minimal media generally have to be developed for small groups of closely related organisms and should not be used for other organisms.

Relatively well-defined media are preferred, even for routine antibiotic tests, because quantitative aspects of bacterial biochemistry, growth and susceptibility to noxious stimuli can be substantially influenced by minor changes in medium composition. The use of fully defined media has underpinned almost all of what we know about bacterial physiology.

## BACTERIAL PHYSIOLOGY

The complement of processes that enable an organism to occupy and thrive in a particular environment places certain requirements on its physiology. Traditional descriptions of bacterial groups emphasize features which place a microbe in particular ecological niches. Thus we have *acidophiles* for organisms such as *Lactobacillus* spp. which grow at lower pH levels than most other organisms and *halophiles* for organisms which grow at high salt concentrations. The environments which can be colonized by a pathogen are, of course, critical in determining its reservoirs and potential modes of transmission. More recently it has been recognized that individual bacteria are not restricted to a single physiological state. Rather, they respond to environmental stimuli and undergo *adaptive responses* which confer improved capacity for survival in adverse conditions. All these properties sustain the *viability* of the organism. However, it has become apparent that our ability to measure viability by conventional means may be inadequate.

The specific means by which a particular organism obtains energy and raw materials to sustain its growth (its nutritional type) and the physical conditions it requires reflect its fundamental physiological characteristics. Placing an organism into the groups defined by these characteristics is an important step in its conventional classification.

## Nutritional types

Traditionally, all living organisms have been divided into two nutritional groups, *heterotrophs* and *autotrophs*. The former depend on the latter to produce organic molecules by fixing carbon dioxide, predominantly by photosynthesis. Bacterial metabolism is now recognized to be so diverse that it cannot be encompassed by these two terms. Three basic features are used in the present terminology, the *energy source*, the *hydrogen donors* and the *carbon source*.

Energy for adenosine triphosphate (ATP) synthesis may be obtained from light in a *phototrophic* organism and from chemical oxidations in the case of a *chemotrophic* organism. The hydrogen donor type characterizes an organism as an *organotroph* if it requires organic sources of hydrogen and as a *lithotroph* if it can use inorganic sources (e.g. ammonia or hydrogen sulphide). Finally, the terms autotroph and heterotroph are reserved for the carbon source; the former can fix carbon dioxide directly while the latter require an organic source. In general, only the energy and hydrogen donor designations are referred to routinely by combining the two terms. Hence we refer to *chemo-organotrophs* (the vast majority of currently recognized medically important organisms) and *chemolithotrophs* (e.g. some *Pseudomonas* spp.). Surprisingly, there are even some *photolithotrophs* with medical significance; the cyanobacteria are now known to produce many toxins that can affect humans.

## Physical conditions required for growth

All living organisms use oxidation to transfer energy to compounds which participate in their internal biochemical and biophysical processes. Oxidation of a molecule is equivalent to the removal of hydrogen, and requires another molecule to receive electrons in the process. In *aerobic* respiration the final electron recipient in the oxidation process is molecular oxygen (i.e. $O_2$) whilst under *anaerobic* conditions (in the absence of oxygen) most medically important organisms use an organic molecule as the final electron recipient, and the oxidative process is referred to as *fermentation*. There are also some forms of anaerobic respiration which use inorganic electron acceptors such as nitrates. Respiration in this context is generally used to denote involvement of a membrane-associated electron transport chain in the oxidation. In the early period of development of life on the earth there was no oxygen in the atmosphere, thus, at this time, all bacteria were

*anaerobes*. Subsequently, following the development of photo-autotrophic organisms, atmospheric oxygen became abundant, and organisms capable of using oxygen evolved.

Although aerobic metabolism is a more efficient means of obtaining energy than anaerobiosis, it is not without its cost. Some oxidation–reduction (redox) reactions occurring in the presence of oxygen commonly result in the formation of the reactive superoxide ($O_2^-$) and hydroxyl (OH·) radicals as well as hydrogen peroxide ($H_2O_2$), all of which are highly toxic. To cope with this, aerobic organisms or *aerobes* have developed two enzymes which detoxify these molecules. *Superoxide dismutase* converts superoxide radicals to hydrogen peroxide ($2O_2^- + 2H^+ \rightarrow H_2O_2 + O_2$) while *catalase* converts hydrogen peroxide to water and oxygen in the reaction $2H_2O_2 \rightarrow 2H_2O + O_2$. Possession or lack of these enzymes has the important consequence of defining the atmosphere necessary for growth and survival of different organisms. Moreover, when produced in large amounts, the enzymes also provide protection for pathogenic organisms against the reactive oxygen intermediates deliberately produced as a defence mechanism by phagocytic cells.

### Growth atmosphere

These oxygen-related features underpin the major practical grouping of bacteria according to their atmospheric requirements (Table 4.1). Thus, *strict* or *obligate aerobes* require oxygen, usually at ambient levels (~20%) and *strict* or *obligate anaerobes* require the complete absence of oxygen. Many organisms exhibit intermediate properties: *facultative anaerobes* generally grow better in oxygen but are still able to grow well in its absence; *micro-aerophilic* organisms require a reduced oxygen level (~5%); and *aerotolerant anaerobes* have a fermentative pattern of metabolism but can tolerate the presence of oxygen because they possess superoxide dismutase. Many medically important organisms are facultative anaerobes. There are a mixture of aerobic and anaerobic micro-environments in the human body and the capacity to replicate in both is clearly advantageous. For obvious reasons, strict anaerobes are particularly associated with infection of tissues where the blood supply has been interrupted.

Among the various physical requirements for the growth of different bacterial groups, atmosphere assumes particular importance because in practice agar cultures from most clinical specimens are set up aerobically and anaerobically. Thus, when growth is first inspected after overnight incubation the

**Table 4.1**  Key descriptive terms used to categorize bacteria according to their growth requirements

| Descriptive term | Property | Example |
|---|---|---|
| **Growth atmosphere** | | |
| Strict (obligate) aerobe | Requires atmospheric oxygen for growth | *Pseudomonas aeruginosa* |
| Strict (obligate) anaerobe | Will not tolerate oxygen | *Bacteroides fragilis* |
| Facultative anaerobe | Grows best aerobically, but can grow anaerobically | *Staphylococcus* spp.; *Esch. coli*, etc. |
| Aerotolerant anaerobe | Anaerobic, but tolerates exposure to oxygen | *Clostridium perfringens* |
| Micro-aerophilic organism | Requires or prefers reduced oxygen levels | *Campylobacter* spp.; *Helicobacter* spp. |
| Capnophilic organism | Requires or prefers increased carbon dioxide levels | *Neisseria* spp. |
| **Growth temperature** | | |
| Psychrophile | Grows best at low temperature (e.g. <10°C) | *Flavobacterium* spp. |
| Thermophile | Grows best at high temperature (e.g. >60°C) | *Bacillus stearothermophilus*[a] |
| Mesophile | Grows best between 20 and 40°C | Most bacterial pathogens |

[a]Not a pathogen; its spores are very heat-resistant and are used for testing the efficiency of heat sterilization.

isolates can readily be differentiated into strict aerobes, anaerobes and facultative anaerobes according to the conditions under which they have grown. Various atmospheric conditions can also be obtained in broth media. If the medium is unstirred, strict aerobes tend to grow on the surface, micro-aerophiles just under the surface and anaerobes in the body of the medium away from the surface. Growth of anaerobes is often improved by addition of a reducing agent such as cysteine or thioglycolate to mop up any free oxygen.

### Growth temperature

The other significant physical condition for bacterial growth from the medical perspective is temperature (see Table 4.1). Pathogens which actually replicate on or in the human body must be able to grow within the temperature range 20–40°C, and are generally referred to as *mesophiles*. Organisms which can grow outside this range are either *psychrophiles* (cold-loving) or *thermophiles* (heat-loving). The former may be capable of growth in food or pharmaceuticals stored at normal refrigeration temperatures (0–8°C) while the latter can be a source of proteins with remarkable thermotolerant properties such as taq polymerase, the key enzyme used in the polymerase chain reaction. Organisms that prefer lower growth temperatures such as the leprosy bacillus are often associated with skin and superficial infections while organisms which grow in the colon (often a few degrees warmer than normal body temperature) can grow well up to 44°C.

### Extremophiles

Some bacteria require ostensibly bizarre physical conditions for growth. For example, barophiles isolated from the ocean floor may require enormous pressures before they can replicate. Such organisms are often referred to as *extremophiles*. Their properties serve to remind us that microbes have the potential to occupy any environmental niche where energy and nutrition are available.

## Bacterial metabolism

Although some bacteria are able to obtain their resources for growth in ways that seem alien to us the core of their metabolism is essentially very similar to that of mammalian cells. The basic details of glycolysis, the tricarboxylic acid cycle, oxidative phosphorylation, ATP biosynthesis and amino acid metabolism are constant. Variations in the pathways that feed into and flow from these core processes are readily detected by what are loosely termed *biochemical tests* in medical laboratories. These detect traits such as the ability to use individual carbohydrate sources to produce acid and the possession of specific enzymes.

The common nature of central catabolic and anabolic pathways in bacteria and higher organisms reflects the economy of biology and evolution. Processes that work well cannot be out-competed and tend to be preserved in the genetic stock. Thus, many of the specific enzymes involved in bacterial metabolism show remarkable levels of conservation in their amino acid sequences across very sub-stantial distances in evolutionary terms. DNA sequencing has enabled identification of *molecular families* of proteins that have a common evolutionary origin. In addition to the metabolic enzymes, it has been recognized that many transport proteins responsible for importing and exporting specific substrates into and out of the bacterial cytoplasm are closely related in their structure and mode of function to those present in mammalian cells. Of course, because bacteria have only one cell compartment in which to operate, the location of these proteins is often different; for example, since they have no mitochondria, the cytoplasmic membrane contains the components of the electron transport chain, and the proton gradient across the inner mitochondrial membrane is generated across the cytoplasmic membrane instead. This feature actually means that bacteria can perform some energy-requiring processes at the cell surface, notably flagellar rotation (motility), by directly exploiting the proton gradient rather than consuming ATP.

Aside from its role in identification and intrinsic biological interest, bacterial metabolism has real consequences for man. In direct terms, the resident microflora have consequences in human health and disease. For example, the bacteria in dental plaque produce acid when presented with certain carbo-hydrate sources, and this acid is responsible for tooth decay; on the positive side, bacteria in the intestines deconjugate bile salts and thereby contribute to the enterohepatic circulation. It seems likely that the importance of such bioconversions will be increasingly recognized in the future. In particular, the role of bacteria in recovering nitrogen excreted into the colon in marginal human nutritional states and metabolic activity leading to the formation of carcinogens or other biologically active molecules are both areas where there is much room for further work.

Humans are also indirectly affected by microbial metabolism. At one level, the chemistry of our environment has been extensively shaped by microbes; the original development of oxygen in our atmosphere, the availability of elemental sulphur and the flow of nitrogen are all critically dependent on microbial metabolism. Exploitation of microbial metabolism in industry has, of course, given us ethanol and many of the other alcohols and acids that result from fermentation have commercial value. Finally, bacteria have been used to combat the deleterious effects of environmental pollution in the process referred to as *bioremediation*.

## Adaptive responses in bacteria

The extent to which bacteria can respond to environmental stimuli has been demonstrated by two-dimensional gel electrophoresis combined with autoradiography. This technique reveals and separates most of the several hundred proteins which are being synthesized by a pure culture at a particular time. The catalogue of different proteins detected represents those proteins that the organism requires to function in the circumstances from which the sample was drawn. Assays of this type have shown that different sets of proteins are made in the exponential and stationary phases of the growth cycle. This finding underpins the recognition of just how different the phenotype of a single organism can be in different physiological states and reinforces the need to define the inoculum used in laboratory experiments. The effects of specific sublethal but noxious stimuli on these protein profiles have also been studied. Each different stimulus leads to an adaptive *stress response*, which is to some extent specific to the stimulus applied. Heat shock (the effects of raising temperature to 45°C and above for a few minutes) has been studied most extensively. The newly synthesized proteins elicited in this response are referred to as *heat shock proteins* (HSPs). When the amino acid sequences of the principal HSPs were determined they were found to belong to a molecular family now recognized in all prokaryotic and eukaryotic cells. Apart from their role in improving the ability of bacteria to survive heat shock, HSPs, by virtue of their similarity to host cell HSP antigens, seem to be involved in initiating auto-immune damage and immune dysfunction. A very important feature of the stress response in bacteria is that many of the stimuli used are prominent aspects of the stresses applied by the human immune system to an invading pathogen. Thus, acid stress is provided by the stomach and the hostile environment of phago-lysosomes includes both oxidative and pH stress.

The information built up from studying stress responses has made it possible to identify sets of proteins which are made in response to several different stresses and those which appear exclusive to one stress. Together with other approaches, this has allowed recognition of *global regulatory systems* or *networks* within bacteria which are responsible for differential gene expression under different circumstances. The hierarchy of specific control mechanisms involved has spawned two important new terms, *stimulon* and *regulon*. A stimulon denotes all those genes whose expression is increased or decreased by a specific external stimulus while a regulon refers to all those genes under the influence of a specific regulatory protein. A regulon may affect several operons (see Ch. 6), and there may be many regulons in one stimulon.

Regulatory networks have been identified in almost every area of bacterial physiology. Thus, in addition to the stimuli cited above, osmotic stress, cold shock, nutrient limitation (separate responses for carbon, nitrogen and phosphate), anaerobic and many other stimulons are recognized. These control systems are responsible for making sure the organism only synthesizes proteins appropriate to its current circumstances. A particularly important medical example of this is the regulation of proteins concerned with an organism's progress in an infection (virulence factors). Equally important from the scientific perspective is the recognition that chemicals secreted by an organism can themselves act as regulatory stimuli to individuals of the same species in a way analogous to the pheromones released by insects.

Although it is still important to recognize that different organisms are particularly adapted to special environmental niches with descriptive terms such as mesophile, acidophile and halophile, the discovery of adaptive responses in bacteria has pushed us into an uncertain period where much of what has been established about the tolerance of micro-organisms to noxious stresses will have to be re-examined. Furthermore, since the extent to which bacteria modulate their phenotype according to their circumstances is now clear, the need for caution in concluding that any property detected in the laboratory is significant in a natural infection is unavoidably obvious.

## Bacterial viability

A central feature of the general and adaptive physiology of bacteria is its capacity to preserve the viability of a particular organism. There is, however, a persistent problem – how do we define viability in practical terms? Traditionally, the operational definition of the capacity of a cell to form a colony on an appropriate agar medium (the colony or cfu count) has been almost universally accepted. It is also often expressed as the proportion of cells within a population which are capable of forming colonies. However, it must be emphasized that viability is not a clearly measurable property. At the individual level, it expresses the expectation that, in a suitable environment, a particular cell has the capacity to grow and undergo binary fission and that its progeny will have the same potential. The key assumption is that colony counts provide an accurate measure of viability.

The central problem can be stated as follows: it is self-evident that if a bacterial cell produces a colony it must have been viable, but to what extent is it true that a cell which fails to do this is non-viable or dead? Immediately contradictions to this proposal can be identified. The bacterial pathogens such as *Mycobacterium leprae* and *Treponema pallidum* which cannot be induced to form colonies on available agar media are clearly viable. Similarly, all the 'as yet uncultivated organisms' (possibly as many as 99% of all bacterial species) are clearly able to propagate themselves. They simply have not been sporting enough to do it on our laboratory media. A further exception is the phenomenon of bacterial recovery from injury (e.g. cold or osmotic shock) in which colony counts can be shown to rise in the absence of cell division.

It is possible that some organisms which are readily cultivable may be able to switch to a physiological state in which they cannot be induced to form colonies. The current popular terminology for cells in this putative state is *viable but non-culturable* (VNC).

Epidemiological and laboratory evidence provide some support for the existence of a VNC state. In particular, the occurrence of several infectious diseases acquired from environmental sources, notably cholera, is at variance with our ability to recover the causal organisms from the implicated source. Environmental studies have demonstrated cells with immunological properties compatible with those of the cholera vibrio but failed to recover the organism in culture, and laboratory studies have indicated that the organism can persist in a non-culturable form. There is also evidence that non-culturable forms may revert to their 'normal' culturable state.

A major attraction of the VNC hypothesis is that it may resolve a number of important mysteries in medical microbiology. In general, these are situations in which we know the organism must be present but are unable to culture it. This is particularly so with diseases that have dormant phases such as tuberculosis.

The most significant problem for the VNC hypothesis is that it has not been defined in physiological or biochemical terms. On the face of it, one might expect transition to the VNC state to result from an adaptive response such as those described in the previous section. Alternatively, transition might be the result of a programme of gene expression such as that observed in spore formation or starvation. From this standpoint the stationary and decline phases in the growth cycle outlined above (when spore formation is induced in sporulating bacteria) may represent the initiation of and transition to a non-culturable phase rather than loss of viability (the traditional view). In spite of their popularity, these ideas must be presently viewed as interesting speculations for which there is circumstantial but no conclusive evidence.

Measurement of viability has been of great practical value in medical microbiology. Colony counts performed to investigate the action of antibiotics and other disruptive influences such as heat and those performed at different stages during experimental infections in animal models of human infections, have provided a wealth of valuable information. Moreover, there is no reason to doubt that this approach will continue to be extremely useful.

Nonetheless, it is necessary to maintain a clear view of the limitations of bacterial culture as a measure of the organisms present in a sample and of their viability. Studies often use the term 'viability' when in fact growth on agar or in broth was measured, and confusion would be prevented if the terms 'culturability' and 'colony counts' were used instead.

We are now entering an era in which many diagnostic and investigational techniques may be replaced by molecular detection procedures. The fact that signals based on such techniques may come from culturable, dead and potentially VNC cells should be recognized. Unravelling these three possibilities presents ample challenge for medical and non-medical microbiologists alike.

## RECOMMENDED READING

Barer M R, Gribbon L T, Harwood C R, Nwoguh C E 1993 The viable but non-culturable hypothesis and medical microbiology. *Reviews in Medical Microbiology* 4: 183–191

Moat A G, Foster J W 1995 *Microbial Physiology*, 3rd edn. Wiley-Liss, New York

Neidhardt F C, Ingraham J L, Schaechter M 1990 Physiology of the Bacterial Cell: *A Molecular Approach*. Sinauer, Sunderland, MA

Roszaak D B, Colwell R R 1987 Survival strategies of bacteria in the natural environment. *Microbiological Reviews* 51: 365–379

# 5

# Antimicrobial agents

*D. Greenwood*

The study of antimicrobial agents embraces not only antibacterial compounds, but also antiviral, antifungal, antiprotozoal and even anthelminthic agents. The treatment of individual infections is dealt with in the appropriate chapters and the general strategy of antimicrobial chemotherapy is covered in Chapter 65.

*Antibiotics* are naturally occurring microbial products; chemical compounds such as sulphonamides, quinolones, nitrofurans and imidazoles should strictly be referred to as *chemotherapeutic agents*. However, since some antibiotics can be manufactured synthetically while others are the products of chemical manipulation of naturally occurring compounds (*semi-synthetic antibiotics*) the distinction is now ill-defined. Nowadays the term *antibiotic* is generally used to describe agents (mainly, but not exclusively, antibacterial agents) that can be used to treat systemic infection. Antimicrobial substances that are too toxic to be used other than in topical therapy or for environmental decontamination are referred to as *antiseptics* or *disinfectants* (see Ch. 7).

## ANTIBACTERIAL AGENTS

The principal types of antibacterial agent are listed in Table 5.1. Because there are so many of them it

**Table 5.1** Principal types of antibacterial agent (other than agents used exclusively in mycobacterial infection)

| Agent | Site of action | Usual activity[a] against | | | | | |
|---|---|---|---|---|---|---|---|
| | | Staphylococci | Streptococci | Enterobacteria | *Pseudomonas aeruginosa* | *Mycobacterium tuberculosis* | Anaerobes |
| Penicillins | Cell wall | (+) | + | v | v | − | +[b] |
| Cephalosporins | Cell wall | + | + | + | v | − | +[b] |
| Other β-lactam agents | Cell wall | v | v | + | v | − | v |
| Glycopeptides | Cell wall | + | + | − | − | − | +[c] |
| Tetracyclines | Ribosome | (+) | (+) | (+) | − | − | (+) |
| Chloramphenicol | Ribosome | + | + | + | − | − | − |
| Aminoglycosides | Ribosome | + | − | + | v | v | − |
| Macrolides | Ribosome | + | + | − | − | − | + |
| Lincosamides | Ribosome | + | + | − | − | − | + |
| Fusidic acid | Ribosome | + | + | − | − | + | + |
| Rifamycins | RNA synthesis | + | + | + | − | + | + |
| Sulphonamides | Folate metabolism | (+) | (+) | (+) | − | − | − |
| Diaminopyrimidines | Folate metabolism | + | + | (+) | − | − | − |
| Quinolones | DNA synthesis | v | v | + | v | v | − |
| Nitrofurans | DNA synthesis | − | − | + | − | − | + |
| Nitroimidazoles | DNA synthesis | − | − | − | − | − | + |

v, variable activity among different agents of the group.
[a]Usual spectrum of intrinsic activity; parentheses indicate that resistance is common.
[b]Poor activity against anaerobes of the *Bacteroides fragilis* group.
[c]Poor activity against most Gram-negative anaerobes.

is convenient to group them according to their site of action.

## Inhibitors of bacterial cell wall synthesis

Since most bacteria possess a rigid cell wall that is lacking in mammalian cells, this structure is a prime target for agents that exhibit *selective toxicity*, the ability to inhibit or destroy the microbe without harming the host. However, the bacterial cell wall can also prevent access of agents that would otherwise be effective. Thus, the complex outer envelope of Gram-negative bacteria is impermeable to large hydrophilic molecules, which may be prevented from reaching an otherwise susceptible target.

Inhibitors of bacterial cell wall synthesis act on the formation of the peptidoglycan layer (Fig. 5.1). Bacteria that lack peptidoglycan, such as mycoplasmas, are resistant to these agents.

### β-Lactam agents

Penicillins, cephalosporins and other compounds that feature a β-lactam ring in their structure fall into this group (Fig. 5.2). All these compounds bind to proteins situated at the cell wall–cell membrane interface. These *penicillin-binding proteins* are involved in cell wall construction, including the cross-linking of the peptidoglycan strands that gives the wall its strength. Opening of the β-lactam ring by hydrolytic enzymes, collectively called *β-lactamases*, abolishes antibacterial activity. Many such enzymes are found in bacteria. Those elaborated by Gram-negative enteric bacilli are particularly diverse in their activity and properties. Most prevalent are the so-called *TEM β-lactamases* (TEM-1, TEM-2, etc.)

*Penicillins.* Benzylpenicillin (penicillin G) exhibits unrivalled activity against staphylococci, streptococci, neisseriae, spirochaetes and certain other organisms. However, resistance, normally due to the production of β-lactamase (penicillinase), has undermined its activity against staphylococci and, to a lesser extent, gonococci. Strains of pneumococci that exhibit reduced susceptibility to penicillin by a non-enzymic mechanism are also increasingly encountered. Benzylpenicillin revolutionized the treatment of infection caused by some of the most virulent bacterial pathogens, but it also suffered from a number of shortcomings:

1. Breakdown by gastric acidity when given orally
2. Very rapid excretion by the kidney
3. Susceptibility to penicillinase (β-lactamase)
4. A restricted spectrum of activity.

Further development of the penicillin family has been directed towards improving these properties. Crucial to this was the discovery that removal of the phenylacetic acid side-chain left intact the core structure, 6-aminopenicillanic acid, the starting point for the numerous semi-synthetic penicillins that have been produced (Fig. 5.3). Among the most important penicillins are: procaine penicillin, the long-acting

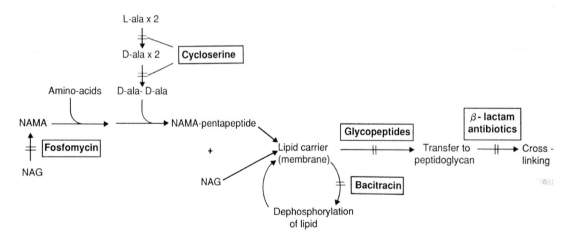

NAG = *N*-acetylglucosamine

NAMA = *N*-acetylmuramic acid

**Fig. 5.1**   Sites of action of inhibitors of bacterial cell wall synthesis.

**Fig. 5.2** Examples of different types of molecular structure among β-lactam antibiotics.

salt of benzylpenicillin; flucloxacillin, an anti-staphylococcal compound; ampicillin and amoxycillin, which have activity against some enterobacteria; and the antipseudomonal agents, ticarcillin, azlocillin and piperacillin. None of these compounds, with the exception of flucloxacillin and other antistaphylococcal penicillins, exhibits stability to staphylococcal β-lactamase. So-called *methicillin-resistant Staphylococcus aureus* (MRSA), and other staphylococci that owe their resistance to alterations in the target penicillin-binding proteins, are resistant not only to all penicillins but to all other β-lactam antibiotics.

**Cephalosporins.** Cephalosporins are close cousins of the penicillins, but the β-lactam ring is fused to a six-membered dihydrothiazine ring rather than the five-membered thiazolidine ring of penicillins. The additional carbon offers the possibility of additional substitutions that may alter the pharmacological

behaviour of the molecule, and sometimes its anti-bacterial activity. Some cephalosporins (e.g. cephalothin and cefotaxime) carry an acetoxymethyl group on the extra carbon. This can be de-acetylated by hepatic enzymes in the body to produce a less active derivative, but it is doubtful whether this has any therapeutic significance. Other cephalosporins (e.g. cephamandole, cefoperazone, cefotetan and the oxa-cephem latamoxef) possess a methyltetrazole substituent. Use of compounds with this feature has been associated with hypoprothrombinaemia and bleeding in some patients.

Cephalosporins have some apparent advantages over penicillins in that they are generally stable to staphylococcal penicillinase (though they are differentially susceptible to hydrolysis by the various types of enterobacterial β-lactamase); they normally exhibit a broader spectrum; and they are less prone

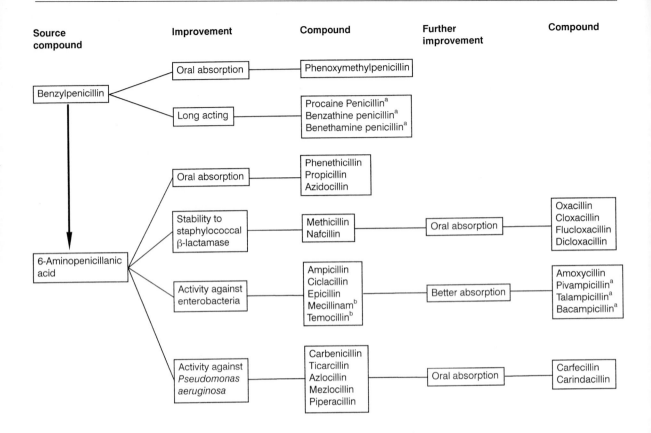

| Source compound | Improvement | Compound | Further improvement | Compound |
|---|---|---|---|---|

Benzylpenicillin
- Oral absorption → Phenoxymethylpenicillin
- Long acting → Procaine Penicillin[a], Benzathine penicillin[a], Benethamine penicillin[a]

6-Aminopenicillanic acid
- Oral absorption → Phenethicillin, Propicillin, Azidocillin
- Stability to staphylococcal β-lactamase → Methicillin, Nafcillin → Oral absorption → Oxacillin, Cloxacillin, Flucloxacillin, Dicloxacillin
- Activity against enterobacteria → Ampicillin, Ciclacillin, Epicillin, Mecillinam[b], Temocillin[b] → Better absorption → Amoxycillin, Pivampicillin[a], Talampicillin[a], Bacampicillin[a]
- Activity against *Pseudomonas aeruginosa* → Carbenicillin, Ticarcillin, Azlocillin, Mezlocillin, Piperacillin → Oral absorption → Carfecillin, Carindacillin

[a] Pro-drugs that release active penicillins
[b] Inactive against Gram-positive bacteria

**Fig. 5.3** Development of penicillins. 'Improvement' means a qualitative improvement, and is not intended to indicate that compounds listed together are necessarily equivalent.

to cause hypersensitivity reactions. On the other hand, the more active compounds can only be administered parenterally, and the group lacks activity against enterococci. Among the most important cephalosporin derivatives are: the oral agents cephalexin and cefaclor; the β-lactamase-stable compounds, cefuroxime and cefoxitin; and the expanded-spectrum compounds, cefotaxime, ceftriaxone and ceftazidime (Fig. 5.4).

***Other β-lactam agents.*** Various agents with diverse properties share the structural feature of a β-lactam ring with penicillins and cephalosporins (Table 5.2). Latamoxef (moxalactam) is an *oxa-cephem* with properties similar to those of broad-spectrum, β-lactamase-stable cephalosporins. Aztreonam is a monocyclic β-lactam antibiotic (*monobactam*) with a spectrum that is restricted to aerobic Gram-negative bacteria. In contrast, the *carbapenems* imipenem and meropenem have an unusually broad spectrum of

activity embracing most Gram-positive and Gram-negative aerobic and anaerobic bacteria. Imipenem is inactivated by a dehydropeptidase in the human kidney, and is co-administered with a dehydro-peptidase inhibitor, cilastatin. The clavam, clavulanic acid, and the sulphones, sulbactam and tazobactam, exhibit poor antibacterial activity, but have proved useful as β-lactamase inhibitors when used in combination with β-lactamase-susceptible compounds (e.g. co-amoxiclav, the combination of amoxycillin and clavulanic acid).

### Glycopeptides

Vancomycin and teicoplanin are large molecules that are unable to penetrate the outer membrane of Gram-negative bacteria, and the spectrum is consequently restricted to Gram-positive organisms. Their chief importance resides in their action

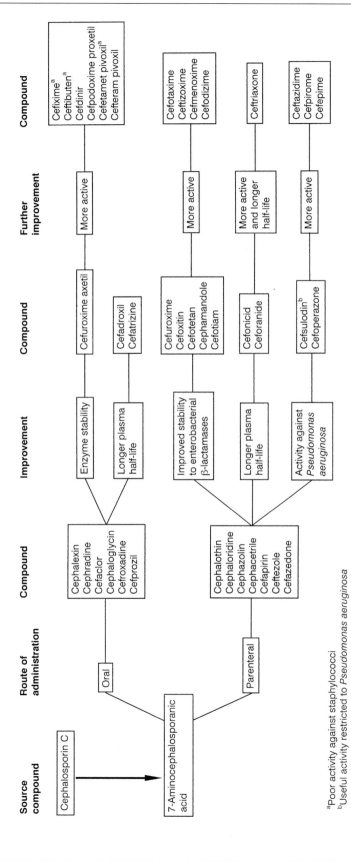

[a]Poor activity against staphylococci
[b]Useful activity restricted to *Pseudomonas aeruginosa*

**Fig. 5.4** Development of cephalosporins. 'Improvement' means a qualitative improvement, and is not intended to indicate that compounds listed together are necessarily equivalent.

**Table 5.2** Clinically useful β-lactam compounds other than penicillins and cephalosporins

| Compound | Structure[a] | Chief properties |
|---|---|---|
| Aztreonam | Monobactam | Narrow spectrum |
| Imipenem | Carbapenem | Very broad spectrum |
| Meropenem | Carbapenem | Very broad spectrum |
| Latamoxef | Oxa-cephem | Broad spectrum |
| Clavulanic acid | Clavam | β-Lactamase inhibitor |
| Sulbactam | Sulphone | β-Lactamase inhibitor |
| Tazobactam | Sulphone | β-Lactamase inhibitor |

[a]See Figure 5.2.

against organisms with multiple resistance to other drugs. Resistance among enterococci and coagulase-negative staphylococci, which was once rare, is being reported more frequently, but *Staph. aureus* strains, including MRSA, presently remain fully susceptible.

### Other inhibitors of bacterial cell wall synthesis

Fosfomycin is a naturally occurring antibiotic with a simple epoxypropylphosphonic acid structure. It exhibits a fairly broad spectrum, notably against Gram-negative bacilli, and is mainly used for the treatment of urinary tract infection. Resistance arises readily in vitro. Bacitracin is active against Gram-positive bacteria, but is too toxic for systemic use. It is found in many topical preparations, and is also used in the laboratory in the presumptive identification of haemolytic streptococci of Lancefield group A. Cycloserine is an analogue of D-alanine formerly used as an antituberculous agent (see below). Isoniazid and some other compounds used in tuberculosis probably act by interfering with formation of the mycolic acids of the mycobacterial cell wall.

## Inhibitors of bacterial protein synthesis

Bacterial ribosomes are sufficiently different from those of mammalian cells to allow selective inhibition of protein synthesis. Most of these agents are true antibiotics (or derivatives thereof) produced by *Streptomyces* species or other soil organisms.

### Tetracyclines

These are broad-spectrum agents with important activity against chlamydiae, rickettsiae and mycoplasmas as well as most conventional Gram-positive and Gram-negative bacteria. They prevent binding of amino-acyl transfer RNA (tRNA) to the ribosome. The various members of the tetracycline group are closely related and differ more in their pharmacological behaviour than in antibacterial activity. Doxycycline and minocycline are the tetracyclines in most common use. Resistance has limited the value of tetracyclines against many Gram-positive and Gram-negative bacteria, but not so far against rickettsiae, chlamydiae and mycoplasmas.

### Chloramphenicol

This compound and the related thiamphenicol also possess a very broad antibacterial spectrum. They act by blocking the growth of the peptide chain. Use of chloramphenicol has been limited to typhoid fever, meningitis and a few other clinical indications, because of the occurrence of a rare but fatal side-effect, aplastic anaemia. Thiamphenicol is said to lack this disadvantage, but is more likely to cause a reversible type of bone marrow toxicity.

### Aminoglycosides

Streptomycin, the first antibiotic to be discovered by random screening of soil organisms, is predominantly active against enterobacteria and *Mycobacterium tuberculosis*. Like all members of the aminoglycoside family it has no useful activity against streptococci, anaerobes or intracellular bacteria. The group also has in common a tendency to damage the eighth cranial nerve (ototoxicity) and the kidney (nephrotoxicity). The chief properties of aminoglycosides are shown in Table 5.3. They inhibit formation of the ribosomal initiation complex and also cause misreading of messenger RNA (mRNA). They are bactericidal compounds, and some, notably gentamicin and tobramycin, exhibit good activity against *Pseudomonas aeruginosa*. Such compounds have been widely used, often in combination with β-lactam antibiotics, with which they interact synergically, in the 'blind' treatment of sepsis in immunocompromised patients. Resistance may arise from ribosomal changes (streptomycin), or alterations in drug uptake. However, it is more often caused by bacterial enzymes that phosphorylate, acetylate or adenylate exposed amino or hydroxyl groups. Enzymic resistance consequently affects the various aminoglycosides differentially depending on the possession of exposed groups that can be attacked by the enzyme involved. Amikacin is resistant to most of the common enzymes.

**Table 5.3** Summary of the important differential properties of aminoglycoside antibiotics

| Aminoglycoside | Activity against | | Susceptibility to inactivation by bacterial enzymes | Relative degrees of | |
|---|---|---|---|---|---|
| | *Pseudomonas aeruginosa* | *Mycobacterium tuberculosis* | | Ototoxicity | Nephrotoxicity |
| Amikacin | + | + | ± | ++ | + |
| Gentamicin | + | − | ++ | ++ | ++ |
| Kanamycin | − | + | ++ | ++ | ++ |
| Neomycin | − | ± | ++ | +++ | ++ |
| Netilmicin | + | − | + | + | + |
| Sissomicin | + | − | ++ | ++ | ++ |
| Streptomycin | − | + | ++ | +++ | ± |
| Tobramycin | + | − | ++ | ++ | ++ |

## Macrolides

Macrolides act by interfering with the translocation of mRNA on the bacterial ribosome. The first macrolide, erythromycin, established itself as a useful antistaphylococcal and antistreptococcal agent, chiefly for use in patients allergic to penicillins. More recently it has found extended use in Legionnaires' disease and in those cases of campylobacter enteritis that require antimicrobial therapy. Erythromycin and other macrolides have no useful activity against enteric Gram-negative bacilli. Erythromycin is usually administered orally as the stearate salt or as esterified *pro-drugs* (pharmacological preparations that improve absorption and deliver the active drug into the circulation). Salts suitable for intravenous administration are also available.

Other macrolides include spiramycin, which is generally less active than erythromycin against Grampositive cocci, but has some useful activity against the protozoan parasite *Toxoplasma gondii*. Oleandomycin and josamycin exhibit properties similar to those of erythromycin. Some newer macrolides, such as azithromycin (in which the macrolide ring has been expanded by inclusion of a nitrogen atom to form an *azalide*), clarithromycin, dirithromycin and roxithromycin offer improved pharmacological properties.

## Lincosamides

The original lincosamide antibiotic, lincomycin, has been superseded by the 7-deoxy-7-chloro derivative, clindamycin, which is better absorbed after oral administration and is more active against the organisms within its spectrum. These include staphylococci, streptococci and most anaerobic bacteria, against which clindamycin exhibits outstanding activity. Enthusiasm for the use of clindamycin has been tempered by an association with the occasional development of severe diarrhoea which sometimes progresses to a life-threatening pseudomembranous colitis (see *Clostridium difficile*, Ch. 23).

Lincosamides bind to the 50S ribosomal subunit at a site closely related to that at which macrolides act. Inducible resistance to macrolides caused by enzymic modification of the ribosomal binding site also renders the cells resistant to lincosamides (and sreptogramins; see below), but only in the presence of macrolides, which alone are able to act as inducers.

## Fusidic acid

The structure of fusidic acid is related to that of steroids, but the antibiotic is devoid of steroid-like activity. It blocks factor G, which is involved in peptide elongation. Fusidic acid has an unusual spectrum of activity that includes corynebacteria, nocardia and *M. tuberculosis*, but the antibiotic is usually regarded simply as an antistaphylococcal agent. It penetrates well into bone and has been widely used (generally in combination with a β-lactam antibiotic to prevent the selection of resistant variants) in the treatment of staphylococcal osteomyelitis.

## Streptogramins

This is a family of naturally occurring antibiotics, each member of which consists of two synergic components, a peptolide and a depsipeptide. The best known member of the group, pristinamycin, is predominantly an antistaphylococcal agent. Use has been limited by poor solubility, but water soluble derivatives suitable for parenteral administration are under development.

## Mupirocin

This is an antibiotic, produced by *Pseudomonas fluorescens*, which blocks incorporation of isoleucine into proteins. Its useful activity is restricted to staphylococci and streptococci, and, since it is inactivated when given systemically, it is used only in topical preparations.

## Inhibitors of nucleic acid synthesis

Nucleic acids are ubiquitous in living cells, and it is perhaps surprising that a number of important antibacterial agents act directly or indirectly on DNA or RNA synthesis.

### Sulphonamides and diaminopyrimidines

These agents act indirectly on DNA synthesis because of their effect on folic acid metabolism. Folic acid is used in many one-carbon transfers in living cells, including the conversion of deoxyuridine to thymidine. During this process the active form of the vitamin, tetrahydrofolate, is oxidized to dihydrofolate, and this must be reduced before it can function in further reactions. Sulphonamides are analogues of p-aminobenzoic acid, and prevent the condensation of this compound with dihydropteridine during the formation of folic acid. Diaminopyrimidines, which include the broad-spectrum antibacterial agent trimethoprim and the antimalarial compounds pyrimethamine and cycloguanil (the metabolic product of proguanil), prevent the reduction of dihydrofolate to tetrahydrofolate. Sulphonamides and diaminopyrimidines thus act at sequential stages of the same metabolic pathway and interact synergically, but in bacterial infections trimethoprim is generally sufficiently effective, and less toxic, when used alone.

Sulphonamides are broad-spectrum antibacterial agents, but resistance is common and the group also suffers from problems of toxicity. They are now little used alone, but the combination of sulphamethoxazole with trimethoprim (co-trimoxazole) is still widely used, notably in the prophylaxis and treatment of *Pneumocystis carinii* pneumonia. Sulfadoxine or sulphadiazine combined with pyrimethamine are used in malaria and toxoplasmosis, respectively. The numerous sulphonamides exhibit similar, but not identical, antibacterial activity, but differ widely in their pharmacokinetic behaviour.

### Quinolones

These drugs act on the α subunit of DNA gyrase. Two groups are presently available (Table 5.4). Nalidixic acid and its early congeners are narrow-spectrum agents active only against Gram-negative

**Table 5.4** Types of quinolone antibacterial agent

| Older, narrow-spectrum quinolones | Newer, broad-spectrum quinolones |
|---|---|
| Acrosoxacin | Ciprofloxacin |
| Cinoxacin | Enoxacin |
| Flumequine | Lomefloxacin |
| Nalidixic acid | Norfloxacin |
| Oxolinic acid | Ofloxacin |
| Pipemidic acid | Pefloxacin |
| Piromidic acid | Sparfloxacin |

bacteria. Their use is virtually restricted to urinary tract infection, although they have also been used in enteric infections and, in the case of acrosoxacin, in gonorrhoea. Newer fluoroquinolones, such as ciprofloxacin and ofloxacin, display much enhanced activity and a broader spectrum, although activity against some Gram-positive cocci, notably *Streptococcus pneumoniae* is unreliable.

Quinolones are quite well absorbed when given orally and are widely distributed throughout the body. Extensive metabolization may occur, particularly with nalidixic acid and the older derivatives. Ciprofloxacin and the newer fluoroquinolones have been successfully used in a wide variety of infections, but resistance is becoming more prevalent.

### Nitroimidazoles

Azole derivatives feature prominently among antifungal, antiprotozoal and anthelminthic agents. Those that exhibit antibacterial activity are 5-nitroimidazoles that, at the low redox ($E_h$) values produced intracellularly in anaerobic organisms, are reduced to a short-lived intermediate which causes strand breakage in DNA. Because of the requirement for low $E_h$ values, 5-nitroimidazoles are active only against anaerobic (and certain micro-aerophilic) bacteria and anaerobic protozoa. The representative of the group most commonly used clinically is metronidazole, but similar derivatives include tinidazole, ornidazole and nimorazole.

### Nitrofurans

The most familiar nitrofuran derivative is nitrofurantoin, an agent used exclusively in urinary tract infection. Other nitrofurans, including furazolidone, which is used in enteric infections, are in use for a variety of purposes in some parts of the world. The mode of action of nitrofurans has not been elucidated, but it is probable that a reduced metabolite acts on DNA in a manner analogous to that of the nitroimidazoles.

### Novobiocin

This compound acts on the β subunit of DNA gyrase (cf. quinolones). It was once widely used as a reserve antistaphylococcal agent, but is no longer favoured because of problems of resistance and toxicity.

### Rifamycins

This group of antibiotics is characterized by excellent activity against mycobacteria, although other bacteria are also susceptible; staphylococci in particular are exquisitely sensitive. These compounds act by inhibiting transcription of RNA from DNA. Rifampicin, the best known member of the group, is used in tuberculosis and leprosy. Wider use has been discouraged on the grounds that it might inadvertently foster the emergence of resistance in mycobacteria. Rifapentine has similar properties, but exhibits a longer plasma half-life. Rifabutin (ansamycin) is used in infections caused by atypical mycobacteria of the avium-intracellulare group (see Ch. 20).

## Miscellaneous antibacterial agents

### Polymyxins

Two members of this family are in use: polymyxin B and colistin (polymyxin E). They act like cationic detergents to disrupt the cell membrane. Polymyxins exhibit potent antipseudomonal activity, but toxicity has limited their usefulness except in topical preparations. If systemic use is contemplated, a sulphomethylated derivative, colistin sulphomethate, is preferred.

### Antimycobacterial agents

As well as streptomycin and rifampicin (see above), a number of other agents are used exclusively for the treatment of mycobacterial infection. These include isoniazid, ethambutol and pyrazinamide, which are commonly found in antituberculosis regimens, and diaminodiphenylsulphone (dapsone) and clofazimine, which are used in leprosy. Cycloserine and *p*-aminosalicylic acid (PAS), which were formerly used in tuberculosis, have now been largely abandoned except for drug-resistant tu-

berculosis. Some fluoroquinolones and macrolides exhibit activity against certain mycobacteria, and may have a role in treatment.

## ANTIFUNGAL AGENTS

Although fungi cause a wide variety of infections (see Ch. 60), relatively few agents are available for treatment, especially for the systemic therapy of serious mycoses. Superficial fungal infections of the skin and mucous membranes can often be treated with topical agents, including *polyenes*, such as nystatin, or *azole* derivatives, of which many (clotrimazole, miconazole, econazole, etc.) are marketed as vaginal pessaries. For dermatophyte infections of the nails, oral therapy with griseofulvin or the allylamine derivative terbinafine is peculiarly suitable, since these agents are deposited in newly formed keratin. Serious systemic disease caused by yeasts and other fungi is often treated with the polyene, amphotericin B, which is extremely toxic. Newer formulations of the drug, in which it is complexed with liposomes or lipids, are better tolerated. The pyrimidine analogue 5-fluorocytosine is active against many yeasts, and is sometimes used in combination with amphotericin B in severe systemic yeast infections.

Azole derivatives exhibit the broadest spectrum of activity, embracing yeasts, filamentous fungi and dimorphic fungi, but few are suitable for systemic use. Those that are include the 2-nitroimidazole ketoconazole, and the triazoles itraconazole and fluconazole. Itraconazole is unique in exhibiting useful activity against *Aspergillus fumigatus*; fluconazole is particularly well distributed after oral administration, and has been used successfully in systemic yeast infections, including cryptococcal meningitis.

The spectrum of activity of the common antifungal compounds is shown in Table 5.5. Most act by interfering with the integrity of the fungal cell membrane, either by binding to membrane sterols (polyenes), or by preventing the synthesis of ergosterol (azoles and allylamines). Their use in individual fungal diseases is considered in Chapter 60.

## ANTIVIRAL AGENTS

Relatively few agents are available for the treatment of viral infection (Table 5.6). Most of those presently

**Table 5.5** Summary of the spectrum of activity of antifungal agents

| Agent | Candida albicans | Cryptococcus neoformans | Dermatophytes | Aspergillus fumigatus | Dimorphic fungi |
|---|---|---|---|---|---|
| Amphotericin B | + | + | − | + | + |
| Flucytosine | + | + | − | − | − |
| Griseofulvin | − | − | + | − | − |
| Nitroimidazoles | + | + | + | − | + |
| Nystatin[a] | + | − | + | − | − |
| Terbinafine | − | − | + | +[b] | +[b] |
| Triazoles | + | + | + | (+)[c] | + |

[a]For topical use only.
[b]Clinical efficacy not yet established.
[c]Itraconazole is active against *A. fumigatus*, but fluconazole is not.

**Table 5.6** Antiviral agents in clinical use

| Compound | Mode of action | Indication |
|---|---|---|
| Acyclovir[a] | Nucleoside analogue | Herpes simplex |
| Amantadine (and rimantadine) | Viral uncoating and assembly | Influenza A |
| Dideoxynucleosides | Nucleoside analogues | HIV |
| Foscarnet | Inhibition of polymerase | Cytomegalovirus retinitis |
| Ganciclovir | Nucleoside analogue | Cytomegalovirus |
| Idoxuridine (and trifluridine) | Nucleoside analogue | Herpes simplex (topical) |
| Interferon-α | Immunomodulator | Hepatitis B and C |
| Penciclovir[a] | Nucleosiode analogue | Herpes simplex |
| Ritonavir | Protease inhibitor | HIV |
| Saquinavir | Protease inhibitor | HIV |
| Tribavirin[b] | Nucleoside analogue | Respiratory syncytial virus |
| Zidovudine | Nucleoside analogue | HIV |

HIV, human immunodeficiency virus.
[a]Available in pro-drug formulations.
[b]Also known as ribavirin.

available are nucleoside analogues, which are phosphorylated within cells and inhibit DNA replication. The most widely used antiviral agent, acyclovir (aciclovir), and the related penciclovir, are phosphorylated by a thymidine kinase produced by the herpes simplex virus. Since the drugs are activated only in cells infected with the virus, they exhibit true selective toxicity. Valaciclovir and famciclovir are oral pro-drug formulations of acyclovir

and penciclovir, respectively. Ganciclovir, which exhibits preferential activity against cytomegalovirus is phosphorylated by cellular enzymes, and is much more toxic. Another nucleoside analogue, tribavirin (ribavirin), has no useful antiherpes activity, but is used in the treatment of respiratory syncytial virus infection (see p. 438) and Lassa fever (see p. 508).

*Interferons*, naturally occurring antiviral compounds produced by mammalian cells in response to viral infection, are now manufactured by genetic recombination. Interferon-α is in clinical use to cure carriage of hepatitis B and C viruses. Interferon-β may have some effect in reducing exacerbations of disease in multiple sclerosis.

The acquired immune deficiency syndrome (AIDS) pandemic has generated an enormous interest in potential antiviral agents. Several *nucleoside analogues*, including zidovudine (azidothymidine) and the dideoxynucleosides, didanosine (dideoxyinosine), zalcitabine (dideoxycytidine), stavudine (didehydrodeoxythymidine) and lamivudine (deoxythiacytidine) are now in use. A number of other compounds, including some *HIV protease inhibitors*, which act at a later stage in the viral cycle by interfering with the cleavage of essential polyprotein precursors, are showing promise. Saquinavir and ritonavir are examples of such compounds that are in limited clinical use, principally in combination with zidovudine or zalcitabine.

## ANTIPARASITIC AGENTS

Progress in the development of new agents for the treatment of protozoal and helminthic infections has been slow, and the choice remains extremely limited. Part of the problem is that protozoa and helminths are very varied, reflecting diverse solutions to the problems of their specialized parasitic existence. Consequently, there are few 'broad-spectrum' antiprotozoal or anthelminthic agents, although some compounds exhibit a surprising range of activity. Thus the antiprotozoal nitroimidazoles, such as metronidazole, are active against *Entamoeba histolytica*, *Trichomonas vaginalis* and *Giardia lamblia* (see Ch. 61); benzimidazoles, like mebendazole and albendazole, act against most intestinal nematodes; praziquantel not only exhibits good activity against all human schistosomes but also includes other trematodes and tapeworms in its spectrum (see Ch. 62). Most remarkably of all, ivermectin is active not only against many filarial worms and some intestinal roundworms but also against ectoparasites such as the scabies mite.

Antimicrobial agents commonly used against patho-genic protozoa and helminths are shown in Tables 5.7 and 5.8.

**Table 5.8** Spectrum of activity of the principal anthelminthic agents

| Agent | Active against |
| --- | --- |
| Benzimidazoles[a] | Intestinal nematodes |
| Diethylcarbamazine | Filariae |
| Ivermectin | *Onchocerca volvulus* |
| | Other filariae |
| Niclosamide | Tapeworms |
| Metriphonate | *Schistosoma haematobium* |
| Oxamniquine | *Schistosoma mansoni* |
| Piperazine | *Ascaris lumbricoides* |
| | *Enterobius vermicularis* |
| Praziquantel | *Schistosoma* spp. |
| | Other trematodes |
| | Tapeworms |
| Pyrantel pamoate | Intestinal nematodes |
| Tetrachloroethylene | *Necator americanus* |
| Trivalent antimonials | *Schistosoma* spp. |

[a]Includes mebendazole, thiabendazole and albendazole.

**Table 5.7** Principal agents used against the major protozoan parasites of man

| Species | Agent |
| --- | --- |
| *Cryptosporidium parvum* | None |
| *Entamoeba histolytica* | Metronidazole |
| | Emetine |
| | Diloxanide furoate |
| *Giardia lamblia* | Metronidazole |
| | Mepacrine |
| *Leishmania* spp. | Sodium stibogluconate |
| | Amphotericin B |
| *Plasmodium* spp. | Chloroquine |
| | Quinine |
| | Pyrimethamine |
| | Proguanil |
| | Mefloquine |
| | Halofantrine |
| | Artemisinin |
| *Pneumocystis carinii*[a] | Co-trimoxazole |
| | Pentamidine |
| | Trimetrexate |
| | Atovaquone |
| *Toxoplasma gondii* | Pyrimethamine + sulphadiazine |
| *Trichomonas vaginalis* | Metronidazole |
| *Trypanosoma brucei* | Melarsoprol |
| spp. *rhodesiense* | Suramin |
| and *T. brucei gambiense* | Pentamidine |
| | Eflornithine[b] |
| *Trypanosoma cruzi* | Nifurtimox |

[a]Taxonomy uncertain; may be a fungus.
[b]Not active against *T. brucei rhodesiense*.

## ANTIBIOTIC SENSITIVITY TESTS

To establish the activity of an antimicrobial agent, micro-organisms are tested for their ability to grow in the presence of different concentrations of the drug. In the case of antibacterial agents, dilutions are made in an appropriate nutrient broth or incorporated into agar during the preparation of agar plates. In the latter case, many different isolates can be tested at the same time by spot inoculation of the plate. The *minimum inhibitory concentration* (MIC) is the lowest concentration of the antimicrobial agent that prevents the development of visible growth during overnight incubation. By semi-quantitative subculture of dilutions of the antibiotic in which inhibition has occurred, the *minimum bactericidal concentration* (MBC) can additionally be estimated. This is usually taken as the lowest concentration able to reduce the original inoculum by a factor of a thousand, e.g. from $10^5$ colony-forming units (cfu)/ml to $10^2$ cfu/ml or below. To establish the rate of killing, the number of viable organisms in broth cultures is measured at timed intervals after addition of appropriate concentrations of the antibiotic.

Antibiotic titrations are too laborious for the routine assessment of antibiotic activity in clinical practice, although a truncated form of the method, in which isolates are tested at agreed *break points* of sensitivity or resistance, is sometimes used. A common alternative method is the *disc diffusion test*. The culture to be examined is seeded confluently, or semiconfluently, over the surface of an agar plate, and paper discs individually impregnated with different antibiotics are spaced evenly over the inoculated plate. Antibiotic diffuses outwards from each disc into the surrounding agar and produces a diminishing gradient of concentration. On incubation, the bacteria grow on areas of the plate except those around the drugs to which they are sensitive. The width of the *zone of inhibition* is a rough measure of the degree of sensitivity to the drug.

Characteristics of the growth medium (such as pH or the presence of antagonizing substances), the size of the bacterial inoculum and the conditions of the test may influence the results of sensitivity tests. In disc methods, the size of the inhibition zone is additionally affected by the diffusion characteristics of the antibiotic. It is therefore important that suitable control organisms are tested in parallel in all tests of antibiotic susceptibility. In *Stokes's comparative disc method*, control is achieved by placing antibiotic discs at the interface between inocula of the test and control bacteria on the same plate. In this way the zone of inhibition obtained with the test organism can be directly compared with that of a known control, and variations in the cultural conditions or in disc content can be avoided.

Tests of antibiotic sensitivity are routinely carried out only on rapidly growing bacteria, although tests of mycobacteria, fungi and some other organisms are available in certain laboratories and reference centres.

## ANTIBIOTIC ASSAY

In most clinical circumstances in which antimicrobial agents are used it is not usually necessary to measure the concentrations achieved in blood or other body fluids (see Ch. 65). Such measurements are needed, however, during the development of new agents in order to establish the pharmacokinetic behaviour of the drug.

Various techniques are available, including microbiological methods in which the antibiotic-containing material and known dilutions of the drug are titrated in parallel against a susceptible indicator organism. Chemical methods, or analytical techniques such as high-pressure liquid chromatography, may also be used. In the few cases in which clinical assays are needed, notably during treatment with aminoglycosides, immunochemical methods are often used with commercially available instrumentation.

### RECOMMENDED READING

Franklin T J, Snow G A 1989 *Biochemistry of Antimicrobial Action*, 4th edn. Chapman and Hall, London
Greenwood D (ed) 1995 *Antimicrobial Chemotherapy*, 3rd edn. Oxford University Press, Oxford
Greenwood D, O'Grady F 1985 *The Scientific Basis of Antimicrobial Chemotherapy*. Cambridge University Press, Cambridge
Kucers A, Bennett N McK 1987 *The Use of Antibiotics*, 4th edn.

Heinemann, London
Lambert H P, O'Grady F W, Finch R G, Greenwood D 1997 *Antibiotic and Chemotherapy*, 7th edn. Churchill Livingstone, Edinburgh
Pratt W B, Fekety R 1986 *The Antimicrobial Drugs*. Oxford University Press, Oxford
Russell A D, Chopra I 1996 *Understanding Antibacterial Action and Resistance*, 2nd edn. Ellis Horwood, Chichester

# 6

# Bacterial genetics

*K. J. Towner*

## GENETIC ORGANIZATION AND REGULATION OF THE BACTERIAL CELL

All properties of a bacterial cell, including those of medical importance such as virulence, pathogenicity and antibiotic resistance, are determined ultimately by the genetic information contained within the cell *genome*. This information is normally encoded by the specific sequence of nucleotide bases comprising the deoxyribonucleic acid (DNA) of the cell. There are four common nucleotide bases in DNA: adenine, guanine, cytosine and thymine; it is the linear order in which these bases are arranged that determines the properties of the cell. In virtually all bacteria so far studied, most of the genetic information required by the cell is arranged in the form of a single circular double-stranded chromosome. In *Escherichia coli* the chromosome is about 1300 μm long and occurs in an irregular coiled bundle lying free in the cytoplasm. The DNA is not associated with protein or histone molecules as it is in eukaryotic cell chromosomes.

In addition to the single main chromosome, bacterial cells may also carry one or more small circular extrachromosomal elements. These were originally called episomes, but are now termed *plasmids*. Plasmids replicate independently of the main chromosome in the cell. Although dispensable, they often carry supplementary genetic information coding for beneficial properties (e.g. resistance to antibiotics) that enable the host cell to survive under a particular set of environmental conditions.

A third source of genetic information in a bacterial cell can be provided by the presence of certain types of bacterial viruses, *bacteriophages*. Bacteriophages consist essentially of just a protein coat enclosing the virus genome and, since they are unable to multiply in the absence of their bacterial host, generally they are lethal to their host cell. In some instances, they can enter a potentially long-term state of controlled replication, *lysogeny*, within the bacterial cell without

causing lysis. In such a state the bacteriophage genome effectively becomes a temporary part of the total genetic information available to the cell and may consequently bestow additional properties on the cell.

Not all genetic material consists of double-stranded DNA. Some bacteriophages contain single-stranded molecules of either DNA or RNA which can be either circular or linear in configuration. Within the prokaryotic kingdom, and including bacteriophages, genome size varies over more than three orders of magnitude from about 3 to 5000 kilobases (kb) (Table 6.1).

## Processes leading to protein synthesis

The character of a bacterial cell is determined essentially by the specific polypeptides that comprise its enzymes and other proteins. The DNA acts as a template for the *transcription* of RNA by RNA polymerase for subsequent protein production within the cell. In the transcription process the specific sequence of nucleotides in the DNA determines the corresponding sequence of nucleotides in the

**Table 6.1** Examples of prokaryotic genetic elements

| Genetic element | Type | Configuration | Size (kb) |
|---|---|---|---|
| Bacterial chromosome | | | |
| *Escherichia coli* | DNA | ds circular | $3.8 \times 10^3$ |
| *Bacillus subtilis* | DNA | ds circular | $2.0 \times 10^3$ |
| Plasmids | | | |
| R300B | DNA | ds circular | 9.0 |
| RK2 | DNA | ds circular | 60.0 |
| Bacteriophages | | | |
| MS2 | RNA | ss linear | 3.6 |
| Φ174 | DNA | ss circular | 5.4 |
| T7 | DNA | ds linear | 40.4 |

Abbreviations: ss, single-stranded; ds, double-stranded.

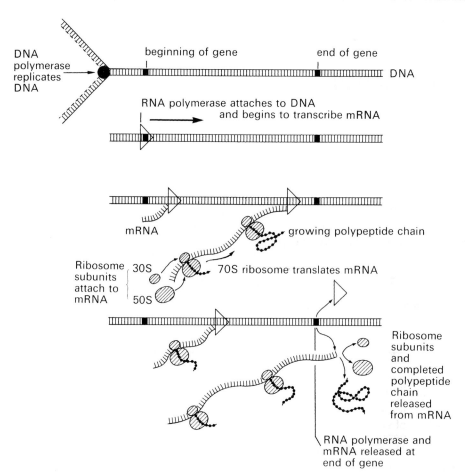

**Fig. 6.1** The central dogma of molecular biology.

messenger RNA (mRNA). This, in turn, is then *translated* into the appropriate sequence of amino acids by ribosomes. Finally, the sequence of amino acids in the resulting polypeptide chain determines the configuration into which the polypeptide chain folds itself, which in many cases determines the enzymic properties of the completed protein. A segment of DNA that specifies the production of a particular polypeptide chain is called a *gene*, while the processes of transcription and translation leading to protein synthesis are collectively termed the *central dogma* of molecular biology. These processes are illustrated schematically in Figure 6.1.

## Gene regulation

Most bacteria contain enough DNA to code for the production of between 1000 and 3000 different polypeptide chains, i.e. 1000–3000 different genes. However, during normal bacterial life, some polypeptides will be required only at particular stages, while others will be needed only when the cell is provided with a new or unusual growth substrate. Protein production is an energy-intensive process, and therefore the expression of many genes is controlled actively within the cell to prevent wasteful energy consumption.

In prokaryotic bacteria the process of gene expression is regulated mainly at the transcriptional level, thereby conserving the energy supply and the transcription–translation apparatus. This is achieved by means of regulatory elements that either inhibit or enhance the rate of RNA chain initiation and termination for a particular gene. Numerous complex regulatory chain mechanisms are involved in coordinating the many biochemical reactions that proceed inside a cell, but related genes involved in a common regulatory system are often clustered on the bacterial chromosome. Such functional clusters are known as *operons* (Fig. 6.2).

**Fig. 6.2** The *lac* operon of *Esch. coli.*
**1** The *lac* repressor is produced from the *i* gene
**2** Binding of the repressor to the operator site (*o*) prevents transcription of the genes *z* (β-galactosidase), *y* (galactoside permease) and *a* (transacetylase)
**3** The inducer (lactose, or a closely related derivative) can bind specifically to the repressor
**4** The repressor molecule is thereby altered at its operator-binding site and the repressor–inducer complex is released from the DNA
**5** RNA polymerase can now attach to the promoter site (*p*) and transcribe the structural genes of the *lac* operon.

For transcription to occur as the first stage in protein synthesis, RNA polymerase has to attach to DNA at a specific *promoter* region and transcribe the DNA in a fixed direction. This process can be switched off by the attachment of a *repressor* molecule to a specific region of the DNA, known as the *operator*, which lies between the promoter and the structural gene(s) being transcribed; the repressor then blocks the movement of the RNA polymerase molecule so that the following genes are not transcribed.

The repressor is often an allosteric molecule with two active sites. One recognizes the operator region so that the repressor can bind to it to prevent transcription. The other recognizes an *inducer* molecule. When the inducer is present it binds to the repressor and alters simultaneously the binding specificity at the other site, so that the repressor no longer binds to the operator and transcription can resume.

There are many different variations on this basic regulatory system. For example, a repressor may be normally inactive, but activated by the end-product of a biosynthetic pathway; thus only when the end-product is present in adequate concentration will the repressor combine with the operator and switch off transcription of the operon. Alternatively, regulation of certain operons involves proteins that bind to the DNA and assist RNA polymerase to initiate transcription. These are just a few examples, and other regulatory systems display both minor and major differences. Finally, it should be stressed that prokaryotic gene regulation frequently involves interwoven regulatory circuits that respond to a variety of different stimuli.

## MUTATION

As bacteria reproduce by asexual binary fission, the genome is normally identical in all the progeny. The DNA replication process is therefore very accurate, but occasional rare inaccuracies produce a slightly altered nucleotide sequence in one of the progeny cells. Such a mutation is heritable and will be passed on stably to subsequent generations. One of the fundamental requirements for evolution is that, although gene replication must normally be completely accurate to ensure stability, there must also be occasional variation to produce new or altered characters that could prove to be of selective value to the organism. Mutations may not produce any observable effect on the structure or function of the corresponding protein, but in a small proportion of cases an enzyme with altered specificity for substrates, inhibitors or regulatory molecules may be produced. This is the kind of mutation that is most likely to be of evolutionary value to an organism; indeed, many examples of acquired antibiotic resistance have been shown to be of this type (see p. 66). Other mutations may alter a gene so that a non-functional protein is formed; if this protein is essential to the cell then the mutation will be lethal.

Since mutation may occur in any of the several thousand genes of the cell, and different mutations in the same gene may produce different effects in the cell, the number of possible mutations is very large. Particular mutations occur at fairly constant rates, normally between once per $10^4$ and once per $10^{10}$ cell divisions. As a large bacterial colony contains at least $10^9$ cells, even a 'pure' bacterial culture will contain many thousands of different mutations affecting many of the genes in the cell. Some of these mutations will be viable and could be selected by particular environmental conditions during subculture. For the same reason, in an infected patient, a variety of mutants will appear spontaneously in the population that grows from the few bacteria originally entering the body. Such mutations may enhance the ability of an organism to grow in the body, e.g. by conferring antibiotic resistance, enhanced virulence, or altered surface antigens. In such a situation, cells with the mutation will rapidly outgrow cells without the mutation, so that selection of the mutant cells occurs and they soon become the predominant type.

## Phenotypic variation

The properties of a bacterial cell at a particular time are referred to as the *phenotype* of the cell. These properties are determined not only by its genome (*genotype*), but also by its environment. *Phenotypic variation* occurs when the *expression* of genes is changed in response to the environment, e.g. by the induction or repression of synthesis of particular enzymes. The distinction is important: genotypic mutation is heritable and maintained through changes in environmental conditions, whereas phenotypic variation is reversible, being dependent on environmental conditions and altering when these change. Phenotypic variation is therefore not a form of mutation.

## Types of mutation

Mutations can be divided conveniently into *multisite mutations*, involving extensive chromosomal rearrangements such as inversions, duplications and deletions, and *point mutations*, which are defined as only affecting one, or very few, nucleotides. The structure of DNA is such that point mutations can be divided into one of three basic types: the substitution of one nucleotide for another, the deletion of one or more nucleotides, and the insertion of one or more nucleotides (Fig. 6.3).

Mutations occur spontaneously during replication of DNA, but most are corrected immediately by the editing apparatus of the cell. The frequency of stable spontaneous mutation is often too low for convenient experimentation, and *mutagens* are therefore used to increase the frequency of mutants in cultures. Common mutagens include irradiation (X-rays or ultraviolet light) and chemicals (5-bromouracil, 2-aminopurine, nitrous acid or hydroxylamine) that interfere with DNA replication either by acting as base analogues or by altering DNA bases in situ.

Mutations are normally inherited stably by the progeny, but secondary mutations can occasionally restore the original nucleotide sequence. It is important to distinguish this relatively rare event of *back-mutation* from the separate process of *phase variation*, which is readily reversible and occurs with relatively high frequency in either direction, e.g. once per $10^3$ cell divisions. The variation of certain Gram-negative bacteria between a fimbriate and a non-fimbriate phase, and the variation of flagellar antigens in *Salmonella* species are examples of phase variation. These seem to involve special genetic regions that are specifically inverted to yield alternative gene products and different phenotypes. In some cases

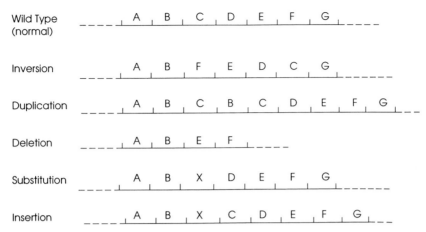

**Fig. 6.3** Examples of types of mutations. The top sequence represents a portion of the wild-type chromosome from which the different mutational rearrangements shown below are derived.

it is known that promoters initiate RNA transcription in different directions to give a flip–flop type of action. The number of such switching systems is probably quite limited, but they have value to the organism in providing a mechanism to switch to a reversible alternative, as opposed to an irreversible change.

## Isolation of mutants

Until the invention of the polymerase chain reaction (see p. 68), the study of bacterial genetics was dependent largely upon the isolation and characterization of mutants in particular genes. Mutations may occur in any gene, but many individual mutations are lethal. Other mutations affect gene products that are essential only under particular cultural conditions. Considerable ingenuity may be required to devise laboratory conditions that promote growth of mutants defective in a particular function and that allow selection of small numbers of these mutants from the large numbers of normal (wild-type) cells in the culture. A few general principles are described below.

### Drug-resistant mutants

Mutations can be found that produce increased resistance to almost any antimicrobial agent, and these can be isolated readily in the laboratory since resistant mutants grow in the presence of drug concentrations that inhibit the growth of drug-sensitive cells. Study of such mutants is an essential step in understanding the modes of action of antibiotic agents and mechanisms of resistance to them.

### Auxotrophic mutants

Many organisms can grow in simple defined culture media because they have the ability to synthesize all of their own essential metabolites; such cells are termed *prototrophic*. Mutants that have lost the ability to make a particular essential metabolite, such as an amino acid, are called auxotrophic mutants (*auxotrophs*). To select an auxotrophic mutant from a prototrophic population, colonies resulting from a large number of cells growing on a complex medium must be tested for the ability to grow on media with and without the specific metabolite of interest. A common short cut is to use the technique of *replica plating* to test simultaneously all the colonies from one plate. This is done with a circular pad of sterile velvet that is first pushed against the master plate of colonies. The velvet picks up an imprint of the original colonies, which can then be used to inoculate several replica plates containing combinations of different metabolites. The ability of the original colonies to grow on the different sets of media can then be compared directly. Studies of auxotrophs with mutations affecting different enzymes in a biosynthetic pathway are very valuable in the elucidation of such pathways.

### Metabolic mutants

Other commonly studied mutations affect enzymes involved in the fermentation of sugars and the breakdown of a variety of other substances in the bacterial environment. Mutations in some of these genes can be detected by growing the cells on special media that produce a distinctive colour in or around colonies producing the enzyme. For example, the production of β-galactosidase can be demonstrated on media containing lactose as the only sugar and an indicator such as neutral red. Colonies producing β-galactosidase turn red following the production of acid, whereas colonies of mutants unable to ferment lactose remain colourless.

The detailed function and regulation of processes in the bacterial cell can be analysed only by searching systematically for mutations that affect each separate step in a process. Many different types of regulation occur in the co-ordination of all the biochemical reactions that proceed inside a cell and the isolation of specific mutants is fundamental to their understanding.

## GENE TRANSFER

A change in the genome of a bacterial cell may be caused either by a mutation in the DNA of the cell or result from the acquisition of additional DNA from an external source. DNA may be transferred between bacteria by three mechanisms: *transformation*, *conjugation* and *transduction*. Each of these mechanisms probably occurs at a low frequency in nature and has therefore probably been of value in bacterial evolution. It should, however, be noted that the acquisition by bacteria of new properties following gene transfer is significant, as with mutation, only if the new genetic end-product is subject to favourable selection by the conditions under which the bacteria are growing.

## Transformation

Most species of bacteria are unable to take up exogenous DNA from the environment; indeed, most bacteria produce nucleases that recognize and break down foreign DNA. However, bacteria in some genera, notably pneumococci, *Haemophilus influenzae* and certain *Bacillus* species, have been shown to be capable of taking up DNA either extracted artificially or released by lysis from cells of another strain. Cells are *competent* for transformation only under certain conditions of growth, usually in late log phase or, in *Bacillus* species, during sporulation. However, bacterial geneticists have also developed treatments by means of which organisms can be made artificially competent. In the case of *Esch. coli* the treatment involves incubation at a low temperature (4°C) in the presence of calcium ions, followed by a short exposure to a temperature of 42°C. Several other factors, including other metal ions, also stimulate

the process. The absolute requirement for calcium ions in producing competent cells of *Esch. coli* indicates that structural alterations in the cell wall, sufficient to allow the passage of DNA molecules, are probably taking place.

Once a piece of DNA has entered the cell by transformation, it has to become incorporated into the existing chromosome of the cell by a process of *recombination* in order to survive. This is a complex molecular process for which the transformed DNA must have been derived from a closely related strain, since pieces of DNA can normally recombine with the chromosome only when there is a high degree of nucleic acid similarity (*homology*).

Any gene may be transferred by transformation, as any fragment of a donor chromosome may be taken up by the recipient cells. However, a piece of DNA introduced into a cell by transformation will normally be relatively short, and will only contain a very small number of genes. For this reason, transformation is only of limited use for studying the organization of genes in relation to one another (*genetic mapping* – see later).

## Conjugation

Conjugation is a process in which one cell, the *donor* or male cell, makes contact with another, the *recipient* or female cell, and DNA is transferred directly from the donor into the recipient. Certain types of plasmids, known as *transfer factors* or *sex factors*, carry the genetic information necessary for conjugation to occur. Only cells that contain such a plasmid can act as donors; those lacking a sex factor act as recipients.

Transfer of DNA between cells by conjugation requires direct contact between the donor and recipient cells. Plasmids capable of mediating conjugation carry genes coding for the production of a 1–2 μm-long protein appendage, termed a *pilus*, on the surface of the donor cell. The tip of the pilus attaches to the surface of a recipient cell and holds the two cells together so that DNA can then pass into the recipient cell. It is probable, but not absolutely certain, that transfer actually occurs through the pilus; alternatively, the pilus could act simply as a mechanism by which the donor and female cells are drawn together. Different types of pilus are specified by different types of plasmid and can therefore be used as an aid to plasmid classification.

In the vast majority of cases, the only DNA transferred during the conjugation process is the sex factor (plasmid) that mediates the process. It is thought that one strand of the circular DNA of the sex factor is nicked open at a specific site and the free end is passed into the recipient cell. The DNA is replicated during transfer so that each cell receives a copy. As donor ability is dependent upon having a copy of the sex factor, the recipient strain becomes converted into a donor, able to conjugate with further recipients and convert them in turn! In this way a sex factor may spread rapidly through a whole population of recipient cells; this process is sometimes described as infectious spread of a plasmid.

### Mobilization of chromosomal genes by conjugation

Many plasmids have the ability to act as sex factors and transfer themselves. Some plasmids also have the ability to mobilize the chromosomal genes of bacteria. The prototype plasmid of this type is the 'F factor' (fertility factor) of *Esch. coli*. The F factor is a sex factor that contains the basic genetic information for extrachromosomal existence and for self-transfer. Cells that contain the F plasmid free in the cytoplasm (F$^+$ cells) have no unusual characteristics apart from the ability to produce F pili and to transfer the F plasmid to *F$^-$ cells* by conjugation. In a very small proportion of F$^+$ cells, the F plasmid becomes inserted into the bacterial chromosome. Once inserted, the entire chromosome behaves like an enormous F plasmid, and hence chromosomal genes can be transferred in the normal sex factor manner to a recipient cell at a relatively high frequency. Cultures of cells in which the F plasmid has inserted into the chromosome are consequently termed *high-frequency recombination* (Hfr) strains. One important difference is that the chromosome tends to break randomly during the longer time period required for complete transfer. Only the very rare recipient cell that receives the whole chromosome, complete with the entire integrated F plasmid, will also become F$^+$.

There is an additional mechanism by which chromosomal genes may be mobilized by conjugation to a recipient cell. In any culture of Hfr cells there are a few in which the F plasmid has excised itself from the chromosome and reverted to the free state. The F plasmid is not always excised accurately, and occasionally an F plasmid is excised together with some of the neighbouring chromosomal genes. An F plasmid that has picked up a small portion of the chromosome in this way is known as an *F-prime* (F'). A well-known example is the F-*lac* plasmid, which is an F' carrying the genes of the *Esch. coli* lactose operon. When an F' transfers itself into a recipient cell, its associated genes function normally on the plasmid in the new host. Thus non-lactose-fermenting organisms become lactose fer-

menters when they receive F-*lac*. When F-*lac* is transferred into *Esch. coli*, the cells become diploid for the *lac* genes. The particular value of this partial diploidy is that it allows the study of interactions between different *lac* operon mutations within the same cell.

It is important to emphasize that the F plasmid system is confined to *Esch. coli* and other closely related enteric bacteria. Many other plasmids are capable of mediating conjugation, and sometimes chromosome mobilization, not only in *Esch. coli* but also in other bacteria. For example, plasmid RP4 and its relatives have been used to mediate conjugation in a wide range of Gram-negative bacteria, and there have been reports of conjugation systems in Gram-positive bacteria, such as *Enterococcus faecalis*, and several *Streptomyces* species.

## Transduction

The third known mechanism of gene transfer in bacteria involves the transfer of DNA between cells by bacteriophages. Most bacteriophages carry their genetic information (the phage genome) as a length of double-stranded DNA coiled up inside a protein coat. Other phages are known in which the phage genome consists of single-stranded DNA or RNA but, as far as is known, transducing phages all contain double-stranded DNA. Two major types of transduction are known to occur in bacteria: *generalized* transduction and *specialized* transduction.

### Generalized transduction

When bacteriophages multiply inside an infected bacterial cell, each phage head is normally filled with a copy of the replicated phage genome. However, with certain types of phage a new phage particle is formed, at a frequency of about 1 in 10$^6$, which accidentally contains a length of bacterial chromosome DNA instead of phage DNA. When such a phage particle subsequently infects a second bacterial cell, the DNA that enters the cell is a short segment of chromosome from the original host. Bacterial genes have been *transduced* by the phage into the second cell. Since phages of this type pick up any portion of the bacterial chromosome at random, they can transduce any chromosomal gene at approximately the same frequency, and are termed *generalized transducing phages*. Genes can be transduced only between fairly closely related strains as particular phages usually attack only a limited range of bacteria. As well as chromosomal genes, generalized transducing bacteriophages may also pick up and transfer plasmid DNA. As an example, the penicillinase gene in staphylococci is usually located on a plasmid, and it may be transferred into other staphylococcal strains by transduction.

### Specialized transduction

Bacteriophages that lyse the host cell are known as *virulent* phages, and are said to produce a lytic cycle of infection. In contrast, *temperate* phages are able to infect a cell without necessarily causing immediate cell lysis and death. The surviving bacterial cell (carrying a copy of the bacteriophage genome) is termed a *lysogen*. The cells are said to be *lysogenic*, and the latent phage is called a *prophage*. In such cases the phage DNA is often inserted into the host cell DNA and is replicated stably as part of the host cell chromosome. This is a symbiotic relationship in which the integrated phage DNA imparts *immunity* to the lysogenized cell against superinfection by genetically related phages, as well as certain unrelated phages.

The lysogenic state is stable but not permanent. The prophage may become excised from the chromosome, followed by the replication of phage DNA and lysis of the cell in the normal way. This process of phage induction occurs spontaneously at low frequency ($10^{-2}$–$10^{-5}$ per cell per generation), but the frequency can be increased artificially, e.g. with ultraviolet light.

Following induction, excision of prophage is usually exact. However, occasionally the prophage picks up DNA adjacent to the phage integration site. Since the phage protein coat can contain only a fixed amount of DNA, a transducing phage that contains a few bacterial genes at one end of its DNA often lacks a few phage genes at the other end. When the defective phage genome is transduced into a second cell, the phage can still integrate into its normal site on the chromosome, but is unable to replicate normally and lyse the cell. The result is that the added piece of bacterial DNA is transduced to the chromosome of the new host cell by the defective phage DNA. Since a temperate phage normally has a specific insertion site on the chromosome, it can pick up and transduce only a short length of DNA containing a few genes on either side of this site. The process is therefore termed *specialized* or *restricted transduction*.

### Lysogenic conversion

The presence of prophage DNA constitutes a genetic alteration to the host cell. Usually only the phage repressor gene is expressed, but in certain cases it can be demonstrated that other genes are also expressed by the host cell. For example, *Corynebacterium diphtheriae* only produces diphtheria toxin when it is lysogenized by β phage; the toxin is specified by one of the phage genes. This process is termed *lysogenic conversion*. It is probable that the production of many toxins by staphylococci, streptococci and clostridia is also dependent upon lysogenic conversion by specific bacteriophages. In such cases, lysogenic conversion not only gives the cell superinfection immunity, but also actively influences the virulence of the bacterium for humans.

## PLASMIDS

### Properties encoded by plasmids

As described earlier, plasmids are circular extrachromosomal genetic elements that may encode a variety of supplementary genetic information, including the information for self-transfer to other cells by conjugation. Not all plasmids can transfer themselves: the *non-conjugative* class of plasmids encodes neither donor pili nor transfer. They can, however, be *mobilized* by other conjugative plasmids present in the same donor cell. Apart from this optional transfer ability, all bacterial plasmids contain the basic genetic information necessary for self-replication and segregation into daughter cells at cell division. Plasmids seem to be ubiquitous in bacteria; many encode genetic information for such properties as resistance to antibiotics, bacteriocin production, resistance to toxic metal ions, enterotoxin production, enhanced pathogenicity, reduced sensitivity to mutagens, or the ability to degrade complex organic molecules.

### Plasmid classification

Because of the vast range of plasmids, it is necessary to have a means of classification so that their distribution and epidemiology can be studied.

Plasmids can be grouped initially according to the properties which they encode, but other methods are needed in order to study their spread and distribution. These methods can be subdivided conveniently into physical and genetic methods.

### Physical methods

Since all plasmids are relatively small structures that are normally separate from the bacterial cell chromo-

**Fig. 6.4** Examples of plasmid fingerprints. Plasmids in tracks 4, 5 and 6 are closely related to each other. Similarly, plasmids in tracks 9 and 10 are closely related. Plasmids in the other tracks appear to be unrelated.

the enteric bacteria to the *Pseudomonas* family, while others can be transferred between almost any Gram-negative bacteria. Similar host range relationships exist amongst plasmids of Gram-positive bacteria.

Once the host range of a plasmid has been determined, plasmids may be classified by *incompatibility testing*. This method relies on the fact that closely related plasmids are unable to coexist stably in the same bacterial cell. Plasmids which are sufficiently closely related to interfere with each other's replication in this manner are said to be *incompatible* and to belong to the same *incompatibility group*. In contrast, unrelated plasmids can coexist stably and are therefore said to belong to different incompatibility groups.

If the introduction of an unknown plasmid into a host that contains a plasmid of known incompatibility group results in the elimination of the resident plasmid, this is evidence that they are incompatible; the unknown plasmid belongs to the same group as the known plasmid. However, for reproducible results, plasmids must be classified by incompatibility in one chosen host since incompatibility relationships may differ in different hosts.

A final method for plasmid classification involves the use of specific virulent bacteriophages. All members of the same plasmid incompatibility group produce the same type of pilus for conjugation. For some incompatibility groups, specific virulent bacteriophages have been isolated that will adhere only to the type of pilus produced by that particular group of plasmids. Lysis by such a phage shows that a particular type of pilus is being produced, which in turn allows the identification of the group to which the plasmid contained in the cell belongs.

## Plasmid epidemiology and distribution

Some plasmid groups have been identified in many different countries of the world, while others have so far been found only in a single bacterial species isolated from a solitary ecological niche. There seem to be two major ways in which plasmids spread: (1) by direct transfer from one bacterium to another in a particular micro-environment; (2) by being carried in a particular host from one environment, e.g. a hospital, to another. The epidemiological tracing of these pathways requires identification not just of the plasmids involved but also of their host bacterial strains.

## GENETIC MAPPING

The location of genes with reference to each other

some, it is possible to isolate them from the chromosome by physical techniques. Centrifugation and electrophoresis techniques allow the sizes of different plasmids to be compared directly. Plasmids of similar size that confer identical phenotypes on the host cells may, however, be totally unrelated from a molecular viewpoint. Such relationships can be examined by generating *restriction endonuclease fingerprints* from purified plasmid DNA. A restriction endonuclease is an enzyme that cuts the DNA molecule at, or near to, a specific nucleotide sequence to produce discrete DNA fragments which can be separated by gel electrophoresis. The pattern ('fingerprint') of fragments produced is dependent on the distribution of the specific DNA sequences recognized by the enzyme. Closely related plasmids will produce the same, or very similar, fingerprints, while unrelated plasmids will produce different fingerprints (Fig. 6.4). Restriction endonucleases of different specificities may be needed to generate distinctive fingerprints.

### Genetic methods

An initial genetic test will distinguish groups of plasmids which are self-transmissible from those that are not. Linked with the question of transferability is the question of host range: for example, some groups can be transferred only between members of the enterobacteria, others can be transferred from and to their respective control regions by mapping techniques is an essential part of genetic analysis. Historically this required the transfer of genetic material between different mutants, initially by conjugation to locate the approximate position of an unknown gene on the chromosome or a plasmid, followed by fine structure mapping with generalized transduction. By far the most extensive genetic map available is that of the *Esch. coli* strain K12 chromosome. It is now a relatively simple matter to map an 'unknown' gene on the chromosome of *Esch. coli* K12, but is much more difficult for less intensively studied genera.

A more modern approach that can be used for all bacterial genera makes use of molecular techniques allowing the isolation, cloning and nucleotide sequencing of individual genes. Once a particular gene or sequence of DNA has been selected and analysed, it is then possible to label it and use the gene as a *probe* in hybridization experiments. Alternatively, it is possible to synthesize a small stretch of nucleotides, termed an *oligonucleotide*, from within the overall gene sequence for use as a probe. *Hybridization* is a process in which two single strands of nucleic acid come together to form a stable double-stranded molecule. As long as the sequence of bases is complementary on each strand, the two strands will bind together by the formation of hydrogen bonds. Oligonucleotide probes are normally only 10–40 bases in length, and can be synthesized and chemically labelled by automated instruments designed specifically for this purpose. The labelled probe can then be used in hybridization experiments with relatively large fragments ('fingerprints') generated from the entire bacterial chromosome with rare-cutting restriction endonucleases. The probe will hybridize only to the chromosomal DNA fragment containing the original gene from which the probe was derived, and will therefore indicate the precise physical location of the original gene in relation to other known genes and control regions. It is therefore now possible to elucidate the relationship between gene structure and function in the cell at the most fundamental molecular level.

## THE GENETIC BASIS OF ANTIBIOTIC RESISTANCE

All of the properties of a micro-organism are determined ultimately by genes located either on the chromosome or on plasmids or on lysogenic bacteriophages. With regard to antibiotic resistance it is important to distinguish between *intrinsic* and *acquired* resistance. Intrinsic resistance is dependent upon the natural insusceptibility of an organism. In contrast, acquired resistance involves changes in the DNA content of a cell, such that the cell acquires a phenotype (i.e. antibiotic resistance) which is not inherent in that particular species.

### Intrinsic resistance

Organisms that are naturally insensitive to a particular drug will always exist. The most obvious determinant of bacterial response to an antibiotic is the presence or absence of the target for the action of the drug. Thus, polyene antibiotics such as amphotericin B kill fungi by binding tightly to the sterols in the fungal cell membrane and altering the permeability of the fungal cell. Since bacterial membranes do not contain sterols they are intrinsically resistant to this class of antibiotics. Similarly, the presence of a permeability barrier provided by the cell envelopes of Gram-negative bacteria is important in determining sensitivity patterns to many antibiotics. Intrinsic resistance is usually predictable in a clinical situation and should not pose problems provided that an informed and judicious choice is made of appropriate antimicrobial therapy.

### Acquired resistance

A problem of chemotherapy has been the appearance of resistance to particular drugs in a normally sensitive microbial population. An organism may lose its sensitivity to an antibiotic during a course of treatment. In some cases the loss of sensitivity may be slight, but often organisms become resistant to clinically achievable concentrations of a drug. Once resistance has appeared, the continuing presence of an antibiotic exerts a *selective pressure* in favour of the resistant organisms. Three main factors affect the frequency of acquired resistance: the amount of antibiotic which is being used; the frequency with which bacteria can undergo spontaneous mutations to resistance; and the prevalence of plasmids able to transfer resistance from one bacterium to another.

#### Chromosomal mutations

Random spontaneous mutations occur continuously at a low frequency in all bacterial populations, and some mutations may confer resistance to a particular antibiotic. The rate at which these mutations occur is not influenced by the antibiotic, but in the presence of the drug the resistant mutant can survive, grow and eventually become the predominant, or only, member of the population. The degree of resistance conferred by chromosomal mutation depends upon the biological consequences of the mutation. With *single large-step mutations* the drug target is altered by mutation so that it is totally unable to bind a drug, although it can still carry out its normal biological functions sufficiently well to permit the continued survival of the cell. This type of mutation occurs with streptomycin, but is otherwise not very common clinically. More commonly, the target is altered so that it can no longer bind a drug as efficiently, although it still has some residual affinity. In such a case a higher concentration of antibiotic would be required to produce the same antimicrobial effect: the *minimum inhibitory concentration* (MIC) of the antibiotic for the organism would be increased. Once a slightly resistant organism has been produced, additional mutational events – each conferring an additional small degree of resistance – can eventually lead to the production of organisms that are highly resistant. This is called the *multistep pattern of resistance*. Spontaneous chromosomal mutation is of clinical importance in tuberculosis in which mutants resistant to any single drug, e.g. streptomycin, rifampicin or isoniazid, are likely to be present in the patient before the start of treatment. If only one drug is given to the patient, the few resistant mutant bacteria will multiply and eventually cause a relapse of the disease. Combined therapy with several drugs to which the organism is sensitive is used in the treatment of tuberculosis, so that each drug kills the few mutants that are resistant to the other. The frequency with which double or triple mutations occur spontaneously in the same cell is so low as to be clinically insignificant.

There are many other examples of chromosomal mutations to antibiotic resistance which have assumed clinical importance. Bacterial enzymes called β-lactamases are commonly responsible for resistance to penicillins, cephalosporins and related antibiotics that contain a β-lactam ring (see p. 46). Mutations in the genes controlling the production of chromosomally encoded β-lactamases in Gram-negative bacteria can result in overproduction of these enzymes and consequent resistance to the cephalosporin antibiotics normally regarded as stable to β-lactamase.

Chromosomal mutations leading to antibiotic resistance are in many cases just as important clinically as the types of transferable resistance described in the next section.

### Transferable antibiotic resistance

Of the three modes of gene transfer in bacteria, it is plasmid-mediated conjugation that is of greatest significance in terms of drug resistance. Plasmids conferring resistance to one or more unrelated groups of antibiotics (*R plasmids*) can be transferred rapidly by conjugation throughout the population.

R plasmids were first demonstrated in Japan in 1959, when it was shown that resistance to several antibiotics could be transferred by conjugation between strains of *Shigella* and *Esch. coli*. Many surveys since then in all parts of the world have shown that R plasmids are common and widespread.

The way in which R plasmids are built up in vivo probably varies from case to case, but it is clear that simple transfer factors can pick up resistance genes and combine with non-transmissible resistance plasmids to produce complex transmissible R plasmids that encode resistance to as many as eight or more different antimicrobial drugs. This process of plasmid evolution is accelerated considerably by genetic elements termed *transposons*. These are linear pieces of DNA, often including genes for antibiotic resistance, that can migrate between unrelated plasmids and/or the bacterial chromosome independently of the normal bacterial recombination processes. R plasmids can transfer themselves into a wide range of commensal and pathogenic bacteria. Once resistance to an antibiotic appears in any one of these species, the process of *transposition* assists the dissemination of the responsible gene between different R plasmids and subsequent distribution to other bacterial species.

As the prevalence of multiple-resistance R plasmids continues to increase, infections caused by a wide range of pathogens become more difficult to treat. In addition, R plasmids can also carry genes, e.g. for toxin production, that confer increased virulence on a bacterial cell. Thus, use of antibiotics may select for bacteria carrying plasmids that confer not only multiple drug resistance but also increased pathogenicity.

## Control of antibiotic resistance

The major cause of the spread of genes conferring antibiotic resistance is the selection pressure brought about by the increased, and often indiscriminate, use of antibiotics in humans and animals. Plasmid-encoded drug resistance is increased by the widespread use of antibiotics in animal husbandry, where antibiotics are used as animal feed supplements and whole animal populations may be treated, rather than an individual patient as occurs in medical practice. When R plasmids are present, the mass use of antibiotics fails to prevent the spread of resistance and selects R plasmids in the gut flora of the whole population of animals. Such R plasmids, evolved in farm animals, can spread to human commensal *Esch. coli*, followed by transfer to more important human pathogens.

It is important to minimize the use of antibiotics as much as possible and to reduce the chance of cross-infection. Rational use of antibiotics and sensible restriction of their availability in humans and animals could prevent further spread of R plasmids and perhaps reduce their incidence. Some R plasmids are unstable and tend to lose resistance genes when the selection pressure is removed. R plasmids are also lost spontaneously from a small proportion of cells in a culture since plasmid replication and segregation are not always precisely synchronous with chromosome replication and segregation. Cells that lose an R plasmid may have a slight metabolic advantage and may slowly outgrow drug-resistant organisms. Moreover, R plasmids that evolve in one species may be unstable in another or may transfer themselves to other organisms much less efficiently. Similarly, organisms that are adapted to the gut of a calf, pig or chicken may not establish readily in humans. Such factors may help to contain the spread of R plasmids.

## APPLICATIONS OF MOLECULAR GENETICS

### Specific gene probes

Every properly classified species must, by definition, have somewhere on its chromosome a unique DNA sequence that distinguishes it from every other species. If this sequence can be identified, a specific labelled DNA probe (see earlier) can be used in a hybridization reaction to recognize pathogen-specific DNA released from clinical samples. Initial isolation of the infecting pathogen is not necessary and, consequently, DNA probes can be used to detect pathogens that cannot be cultured easily in vitro.

DNA probes have already been used successfully to identify a wide variety of pathogens, from simple viruses to pathogenic bacteria and parasites. Probes have also been developed which can recognize specific antibiotic resistance genes, so that antimicrobial susceptibility of an infecting organism can be determined directly without primary isolation and growth. Commercial kits incorporating DNA probes are now available to detect a range of bacteria and viruses.

### Polymerase chain reaction

In the *polymerase chain reaction* (PCR) a thermostable DNA polymerase and two specific oligonucleotide

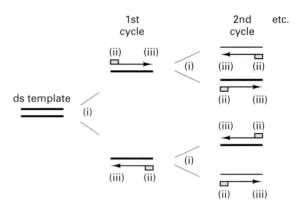

**Fig. 6.5** Schematic outline of PCR. Each cycle in the exponential reaction consists of three steps: (i) heat denaturation, typically at 94°C, to dissociate double-stranded (ds) DNA; (ii) annealing of primers ( □ ) at a temperature determined empirically for each individual PCR; (iii) elongation at an optimal temperature for thermostable polymerase activity, typically 72°C for *Taq* polymerase.

primers are used to produce multiple copies of specific nucleic acid regions quickly and exponentially (Fig. 6.5). The specificity of the reaction is controlled by the oligonucleotide primers that direct replication of the intervening 'target' region. In an exponential reaction, the target sequence is amplified a million-fold or more within a few hours. Once the reaction has occurred, a variety of methods are available to detect the amplified product, of which the simplest is to identify the product by size following electrophoresis and migration on an agarose gel. For many diagnostic applications, the simple visualization of a PCR product of characteristic size is a significant result since it indicates the presence of the target DNA sequence in the original sample.

PCR offers an exquisitely sensitive approach to the detection and identification of specific microorganisms in a variety of sample types. Potentially, a characteristic DNA sequence from a single virus particle or bacterial cell can be amplified to detectable levels within a very short period of time. The method has received particular attention for detecting the presence of low numbers of bacteria or virus particles in clinical and environmental specimens. For example, while a diagnostic antibody response may take up to 8 weeks to develop in an individual infected with human immunodeficiency virus (HIV), specific HIV sequences can be detected in a few hours by PCR, even if present at only 1 part per 100 000 human genome equivalents.

## Molecular typing of micro-organisms

Typing of micro-organisms is increasingly important for studying cross-infection and epidemiological relationships, particularly during outbreaks of nosocomial infection (see p. 33–4). The DNA-based molecular techniques described above offer the possibility of a unified approach to microbial typing that can be applied immediately to a new epidemiological problem, with no prior knowledge of the organisms being investigated, and can be used to study any organism from which DNA can be prepared.

### RECOMMENDED READING

Broda P 1979 *Plasmids*. Freeman, San Francisco

Bryan L E (ed) 1984 *Antimicrobial Drug Resistance*. Academic Press, New York

Erlich H A 1989 *PCR Technology – Principles and Applications of DNA Amplification*. Stockton Press, New York

Glass R E 1982 *Gene Function*: E. coli *and its Heritable Elements*. Croom Helm, London

Innis M A, Gelfand D H, Sninsky J J, White T 1990 *PCR Protocols – A Guide to Methods and Applications*. Academic Press, San Diego

Schleif R 1986 *Genetics and Molecular Biology*. Addison Wesley, Reading, MA

Tenover F C 1988 Diagnostic deoxyribonucleic acid probes for infectious diseases. *Clinical Microbiology Reviews* 1: 82–101

Towner K J, Cockayne A 1993 *Molecular Methods for Microbial Identification and Typing*. Chapman and Hall, London

# 7

# Sterilization and disinfection

*R. A. Simpson*

Procedures that kill micro-organisms have important applications in practical microbiology and in the practice of medicine and surgery. Laboratory work with pure cultures requires the use of apparatus and culture media that have been rendered sterile, while the need to avoid infecting the patient requires the use of equipment, instruments, dressings and parenteral drugs that are free from all living micro-organisms, or at least from those which may give rise to infection.

## General definitions

Several terms are used to describe processes for the killing or removal of micro-organisms, and it is important to recognize the difference in meaning.

*Sterilization* is a process used to achieve sterility, an absolute term meaning the absence of all viable micro-organisms.

*Disinfection* is a process which reduces the number of contaminating micro-organisms, particularly those liable to cause infection, to a level which is deemed no longer harmful to health. The term *sanitization* is also used, particularly in the USA, to describe disinfection, generally in conjunction with catering and food equipment.

*Antisepsis* is used to describe disinfection applied to living tissue such as a wound.

*Cleaning* is a soil-removing process which removes many micro-organisms. The reduction in contamination by cleaning processes is difficult to quantify other than visually. However, they have wide application in the hospital environment and as the necessary prerequisite to sterilization and disinfection.

*Decontamination* is a general term for the treatment used to make equipment safe to handle, and includes microbiological, chemical, radio-active and other contamination.

## STERILIZATION

Sterilization means the freeing of an article from all living organisms, including viruses, bacteria and their spores, and fungi and their spores. In practice, all processes of sterilization have a finite probability of failure. An article may be regarded as sterile if it can be demonstrated that there is a probability of less than 1 in a million of there being viable micro-organisms on it.

### Uses

Sterilization is required for instruments and materials used in procedures that involve penetration into normally sterile parts of the body, e.g. in surgical operations, intravenous infusions, hypodermic injections and diagnostic aspirations. It is also required for media, reagents and equipment used in laboratory practice.

### Methods

Five main methods are used for sterilization.

*Heat*. The only method of sterilization that is both reliable and widely applicable is by heating under carefully controlled conditions at temperatures above 100°C to ensure that bacterial spores are killed.

*Ionizing irradiation*. Both β (electrons) irradiation and γ (photons) irradiation are employed industrially for the sterilization of single-use disposable items such as needles and syringes, latex catheters and surgical gloves.

*Filtration*. Filters are used to remove bacteria and all larger micro-organisms from liquids that are liable to be spoiled by heating, e.g. blood serum and antibiotic solutions in which contamination with filter-passing viruses is improbable or unimportant.

*Sterilant gases*. Ethylene oxide is used mainly by industry for the sterilization of plastics and other thermolabile material that cannot withstand heating. Formaldehyde in combination with subatmospheric steam is more commonly used in hospitals for reprocessing thermolabile equipment. Both processes carry toxic and other hazards for the user and the patient.

*Sterilant liquids.* Use of liquids such as glutaraldehyde is generally the least effective and the most unreliable method. Such methods should be regarded as 'high-grade disinfection' only, to be applied when no other sterilization method is available.

## DISINFECTION

Disinfection, the freeing of an article from some or all of its burden of contaminating micro-organisms, is a relative term embracing a wide range of efficacy against particular viruses, vegetative bacteria and fungi, but not usually including bacterial spores.

### Uses

Disinfection is applied in circumstances in which sterility is unnecessary or sterilizing procedures are impracticable. Thus, in the absence of demonstrable clinical need, it is uneconomic to sterilize bed-pans, eating utensils, bed linen and other items of everyday living which may spread infection within hospitals. Moreover, the pathogens likely to be present on these articles rarely include those that form spores.

Similarly, it is a valuable precaution to treat the skin around the site of an invasive procedure, such as an injection or surgical operation, with an antiseptic that will kill many of the vegetative micro-organisms and reduce the chance of some of them being carried into the wound.

### Methods

Disinfection is achieved by means of processes similar to, although less severe than, those used for sterilization.

*Heat.* Various methods are available using steam or water; some incorporate a cleaning stage within an automatic controlled process.

*Ultraviolet radiation.* This has limited application for the disinfection of surfaces and some piped-water supplies, but lacks penetrative power for more widespread application.

*Gases.* Formaldehyde is used as a fumigant in laboratory environments, e.g. before changing a filter in a safety cabinet or in the event of a gross spillage.

*Filtration.* Air supplied to operating theatres and other critical environments is filtered to remove potentially hazardous micro-organisms.

*Chemical.* Various chemicals with antimicrobial properties are used as disinfectants. They are all liable to be inactivated by excessive dilution and contact with organic materials such as dirt or blood, or a variety of other materials. Nevertheless, they may provide a convenient method for environmental disinfection and other specific applications.

## CHOICE OF METHOD

The choice of method of sterilization or disinfection depends on the nature of the item to be treated, the likely microbial contamination, and the risk of transmitting infection to patients or staff in contact with the item. Choice is based on an assessment of risk according to different categories of patient (e.g. immunocompromised), the equipment involved and its application (Table 7.1). The selection of sterilization, disinfection or simple cleaning processes for individual items of equipment and the environment should be agreed as part of the infection control policy of a hospital (see Ch. 67). The preferred option wherever possible, for both sterilization and disinfection, is heat rather than chemicals. This relates not only to the antimicrobial efficacy but to safety considerations, which are more difficult to control in some chemical processes. Wherever chemicals are to be used for disinfection and sterilization, the safety of persons involved directly or indirectly in the procedure must be considered. It should be remembered that all sterilizing and disinfecting agents have some action on human cells. No method should be assumed to be safe unless appropriate precautions are taken.

## MEASUREMENT OF MICROBIAL DEATH

Every method used must be validated to demonstrate the required degree of microbial kill. With heat sterilization and irradiation, a biological test may not be required if the physical conditions are sufficiently well defined and controlled. For practical purposes

| Table 7.1    Risks to patients from equipment and the environment | | |
| --- | --- | --- |
| Risk group | Examples | Choice of process |
| **1. High risk (critical)** | | |
| Direct contact with a break in skin or mucous membrane or entering a sterile body area | Surgical instruments; needles, syringes; parenteral fluids; arthroscopes | Must be sterile: heat sterilization, irradiation |
| **2. Intermediate risk (semi-critical)** | | |
| Direct contact with mucous membrane but tissue is intact | Endotracheal tubes; aspirators; gastroscopes | Need not be sterile: disinfection acceptable; thorough cleaning with liquid chemicals |
| **3. Low risk (non-critical)** | | |
| No direct contact with the patient other than via unbroken skin | Bed-pans, urinals; furniture; sinks, drains; walls, floors | Thorough cleaning (with disinfection as necessary) by washer or disinfector with detergents |

a micro-organism may be regarded as 'dead' when it has lost the ability to reproduce.

When micro-organisms are subjected to a lethal process, the number of viable cells decreases exponentially in relationship to the extent of exposure. If the logarithm of the number of survivors is plotted against the lethal dose received (e.g. time of heating at a particular temperature) the resulting curve is described as the *survivor curve*. This is independent of the size of the original population and is approximately linear. The linear survivor curve is an idealized concept and, in practice, minor variations, such as an initial shoulder or final tail, occur (Fig. 7.1).

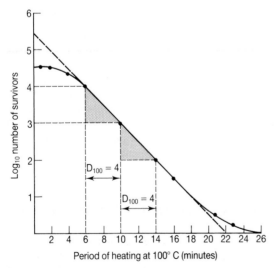

**Fig. 7.1** The rate of inactivation of an inoculum of bacterial spores showing the decimal reduction time (*D* value) at 100°C and the non-linear 'shoulder and tail' effects.

D **value.** The *D value* or *decimal reduction value* is the dose required to inactivate 90% of the initial population. From Figure 7.1, it can be seen that the time (dose) required to reduce the population from 1 000 000 to 100 000 is the same as the time (dose) required to reduce the population from 100 000 to 10 000, i.e. the *D* value remains constant over the full range of the survivor curve. Extending the treatment beyond the point where there is one surviving cell does not give rise to fractions of a surviving cell but rather to a statement of the probability of finding one survivor. Thus by extrapolation from the experimental data it is possible to determine the lethal dose required to give a probability of less than $10^{-6}$ which is required to meet the pharmacopoeial definition of 'sterile'.

## FACTORS INFLUENCING RESISTANCE

Many common factors affect the ability of micro-organisms to withstand the lethal effects of sterilization or disinfection processes. Factors specific to individual processes are considered in the description of those processes.

### Species or strain of micro-organism

In general, vegetative bacteria and viruses are more susceptible, and bacterial spores the most resistant, to sterilizing and disinfecting agents. However, within different species and strains of species there may be wide variation in intrinsic resistance. For example, within the Enterobacteriaceae, *D* values at 60°C range from a few minutes (*Escherichia coli*) to 1 h (*Salmonella senftenberg*). The typical *D* value for *Staphylococcus aureus* at 70°C is less than 1 min compared with 3 min for *Staph. epidermidis*. However, an unusual strain of *Staph. aureus* has been isolated with a *D* value of 14 min at 70°C. Such variations may be attributed to morphological or physiological changes such as alterations in cell proteins or specific targets in the cell envelope affecting permeability.

Inactivation data obtained for one micro-organism should not be extrapolated to another; thus it should not be assumed that bactericidal disinfectants are also potent against viruses. The inactivation data for scrapie, bovine spongiform encephalopathy and Creutzfeldt–Jakob disease suggest a highly resistant agent requiring six times the normal heat sterilization cycle (134°C for 18 min).

## Physiological state

The conditions under which the micro-organisms were grown before exposure to the lethal process have a marked effect on their resistance. Organisms grown under nutrient-limiting conditions are typically more resistant than those grown under nutrient-rich conditions. Resistance usually increases through the late logarithmic phase of growth of vegetative cells and declines erratically during the stationary phase.

## Ability to form spores

Bacterial endospores, formed principally by *Bacillus* and *Clostridium* species, are relatively resistant to most processes. Similarly, fungal spores are more resistant than the vegetative mycelium, although they are not usually as resistant as bacterial spores. Bacterial spores were used to define the sterilization processes in current use, and preparations of bacterial spores (biological indicators) are used to monitor the efficacy of ethylene oxide sterilization, in which physical monitoring is inadequate. In general, disinfection processes have little or no activity against bacterial spores.

## Suspending menstruum

The micro-environment of the organism during exposure to the lethal process has a profound effect on its resistance. Thus, micro-organisms occluded in salt have greatly enhanced resistance to ethylene oxide; the presence of blood or other organic material will reduce the effectiveness of hypochlorite solution.

## Number of micro-organisms

The higher the initial 'bioburden', the more extensive must be the process to achieve the same assurance of sterility.

## STERILIZATION BY HEAT

Moist heat is much more effective than dry heat because it kills micro-organisms by coagulating and denaturing their enzymes and structural proteins, a process in which water participates. It is therefore necessary for all parts of the load to be sterilized to be in direct contact with water molecules or steam. Sterilization requires exposure to moist heat at 121°C for 15 min.

Dry heat is believed to kill micro-organisms by causing a destructive oxidation of essential cell constituents. Killing of the most resistant spores by dry heat requires a temperature of 160°C for 2 h. This high temperature causes slight charring of paper, cotton and other organic materials.

## Factors influencing sterilization by heat

The factors to be considered include:

1. The temperature
2. The time of exposure
3. The number of vegetative micro-organisms and spores present
4. The species
5. The strain and spore-forming ability of the micro-organisms
6. The nature of the contaminated material.

*Temperature and time.* These are inversely related, shorter times sufficing at higher temperatures. The recommended combinations of temperature and holding time are listed in Table 7.2. These do not include time for heating up or cooling the load

| Table 7.2 Minimum recommended hold times for heat sterilization | | |
|---|---|---|
| Process | Temperature (°C) | Hold time (min) |
| Dry heat | 160 | 120 |
| | 170 | 60 |
| | 180 | 30 |
| Moist heat | 121 | 15 |
| | 126 | 10 |
| | 134 | 3 |

for safe handling. Thus the total cycle time for processing a sterilized article will be much longer.

**Microbial load.**    The number of micro-organisms and spores affects the rapidity of sterilization. The number of survivors falls exponentially with the duration of heating (see Fig. 7.1) and the time of complete sterilization increases in relation to the numbers initially present. In practice it is usual to minimize the number of contaminating bacteria by prior cleaning. If this is not possible, e.g. contaminated laboratory cultures, an extended period of heating to achieve the required temperature will be needed.

## Sterilization by moist heat

Moist heat sterilization requires temperatures above that of boiling water. Such conditions are attained under controlled conditions by raising the pressure of steam in a pressure vessel (*autoclave*). At sea-level, boiling water at atmospheric pressure (1 bar) will produce steam at 98–100°C, whereas raising the pressure to 2.4 bar increases the temperature to 125°C, and at 3.0 bar to 134°C. Conversely, at subatmospheric pressures, including those at higher altitude, water will boil at lower temperatures.

### The quality of steam for sterilization

Steam is non-toxic and non-corrosive, but for effective sterilization it must be *saturated*, which means that it holds all the water it can in the form of a transparent vapour. It must also be *dry*, which means that it does not contain water droplets.

Saturated steam is more efficient than dry heat, partly because of the greater lethal action of moist heat but also because it is quicker in heating up the article to be sterilized. When dry saturated steam meets a cooler surface it condenses into a small volume of water and liberates the latent heat of vaporization. The energy available from this latent heat is considerable, e.g. 6 litres of steam at a temperature of 134°C (and a corresponding pressure of 3 bar absolute) will condense into 10 ml of water and liberate 2162 J of heat energy. By comparison, less than 100 J of heat energy is released to an article by the sensible heat from air at 134°C.

Steam at a higher temperature than the corresponding pressure would allow is referred to as *superheated steam*, and behaves in a similar manner to hot air. Conversely, steam which contains suspended droplets of water at the same temperature is referred to as *wet steam* and is less efficient. The presence of air in steam affects the sterilizing efficiency by changing the pressure–temperature relationship.

### Types of steam sterilizer

**Sterilizers for porous loads.**    These are intended to deal with dressings, textiles, wrapped instruments and wrapped utensils. Such loads are liable to trap air within the fabric, packaging or within narrow lumen instruments. This type of sterilizer must have a vacuum-assisted air removal stage to ensure that adequate air is removed from the load before admission of steam. The vacuum pulsing of air also ensures that the load is dry on completion of the cycle.

**Sterilizers for fluids in sealed containers.** Sterilizers for pharmaceutical fluids and laboratory media in sealed containers and ampoules must have a safety feature to ensure that the door cannot be opened until the contents of the glass containers have fallen below 80°C. Otherwise the thermal stress of cold air on opening the door may cause the bottles to explode under pressure, causing serious injury.

**Sterilizers for unwrapped instruments and utensils.**    These simple machines should not be used for wrapped articles. They are recommended for use in dental clinics and in general practice.

**Laboratory sterilizers.**    These are needed for several different types of load, such as culture media in containers, laboratory glassware and equipment.

### Monitoring of steam sterilizers

Physical measurements of temperature, pressure and time with thermometers and pressure gauges are recorded for every load, and periodic detailed tests are undertaken with temperature-sensitive probes (thermocouples) inserted into standard test packs. Biological indicators comprising dried spore suspensions of a reference heat-resistant bacterium, *Bacillus stearothermophilus*, are no longer considered appropriate for routine testing, although spore indicators are essential for low-temperature gaseous processes in which the physical measurements are not reliable.

Sterilizers incorporating a vacuum-assisted air removal cycle are fitted with an air detector. In addition, the *Bowie–Dick test* monitors penetration of steam into a wrapped pack and will detect uneven steam penetration by a 'bubble' of residual air in the pack. In the original test, an adhesive indicator tape, in the shape of a cross, was stuck onto a sheet of paper which was placed at the centre of a stack of towels (the test pack). The indicator shows a colour change from colourless to black, which should be even along the entire cross of the tape.

# Sterilization by dry heat

## Incineration

This is an efficient method for the sterilization and disposal of contaminated materials at a high temperature. It has a particular application for pathological waste materials, surgical dressings, sharp needles and other clinical waste.

## Red heat

Inoculating wires, loops and points of forceps are sterilized by holding them in the flame of a Bunsen burner until they are red hot.

## Flaming

Exposure of scalpels and the necks of flasks to a flame for a few seconds is of uncertain efficacy. Inoculating loops and needles are sometimes treated by immersing them in methylated spirit and burning off the alcohol, but this does not produce a sufficiently high temperature for sterilization, and care must be taken to avoid the flammable risk of alcohol.

## Hot air sterilizer

Hot air sterilizers are used to process materials which can withstand high temperatures for the length of time needed for sterilization by dry heat (see Table 7.2), but which are likely to be affected by contact with steam. Examples include oils, powders, carbon steel microsurgical instruments and empty laboratory glassware. The overall cycle of heating up and cooling may take several hours.

## Microwave ovens

The heating effect in microwave ovens is not uniform and no reliable sterilization process using microwaves is presently available.

# STERILIZATION BY IRRADIATION

Ionizing radiations, including $\gamma$ rays, X-rays and accelerated electrons, are lethal to all cells. Bacterial species differ in their sensitivity to ionizing radiations, although the degree of resistance varies during the growth cycle and bacterial spores are generally more resistant than vegetative cells. Sterilization is achieved by the use of high-speed electrons from a machine such as a linear accelerator or by an isotope source such as cobalt-60; a dose of 255 kGy is generally adequate, which makes this a large-scale industrial process. It is used to sterilize large amounts of prepacked single-use items such as plastic syringes and catheters.

# STERILIZATION BY GASEOUS PROCESSES

## Ethylene oxide

This is a highly penetrative, non-corrosive and microbicidal gas which is used in industry for the sterilization of single-use, heat-sensitive medical devices such as prosthetic heart valves and plastic catheters. Ethylene oxide sterilization is usually carried out at temperatures below 60°C in conditions of high relative humidity. To ensure sterility, material should be exposed to a gas concentration of 700–1000 mg/l at 45–60°C and a relative humidity above 70% for about 2 h. Care must be taken because of toxicity to personnel, flammability and explosion risk. The sterilized product must be aerated to remove residual ethylene oxide before it can be safely used on the patient, and the turn-round time is consequently slow.

## Low-temperature steam and formaldehyde

This combines the thermal effects of steam generated at subatmospheric pressure (73–80°C) and a gaseous agent, formaldehyde, to give an effective sporicidal process. This method is appropriate for the reprocessing of heat-sensitive instruments and items of hospital equipment which can withstand temperatures up to 80°C only. Again, safely requirements make the process inappropriate for routine hospital use.

# STERILIZATION BY FILTRATION

Fluids, including bacterial cultures, can be rendered free of bacteria by passage through filters with a pore size of less than 0.45 µm. The method is used in the separation of toxins and other soluble products of bacterial growth, and in the preparation of thermolabile parenteral fluids such as antibiotic solutions, radiopharmaceuticals and blood products which would not withstand the preferred option of sterilization by heat. The efficiency of microbial retention is dependent on many factors, including the initial number of micro-organisms, their type and the composition and pore size of the filter. Most viruses, and certain bacteria such as mycoplasmas, can pass through filters with a pore size as low as 0.22 μm.

Early filter types, including unglazed ceramic *Chamberland* filters, asbestos *Seitz* filters and *sintered glass* filters, have been largely superseded by *membrane* filters made of cellulose esters or other polymers.

## DISINFECTION

The efficacy of disinfection depends on the severity of the treatment (temperature and/or chemical concentration) and the process time. There are no methods that are instantaneously effective or that will 'kill all known (household) germs'.

### Cleaning

Thorough cleaning is a prerequisite for successful disinfection, and it is also a valuable method for disinfection in its own right. Any process used to kill micro-organisms has a limited capacity and, for both disinfection and sterilization, it is essential that the lowest possible number of organisms are present at the start of the process. Removal of debris dried on instruments or other items that are difficult to clean may be enhanced by the use of *ultrasonic baths*. The detergents used in cleaning have some disinfection properties, and the dilution effect of thorough rinsing further reduces the microbial load.

### Disinfection by moist heat

This is the method of first choice. It can be precisely controlled, leaves no toxic residues and does not promote the development of resistant strains. Washing or rinsing laundry or eating utensils in water at 70–80°C for a few minutes will kill most non-sporing micro-organisms present. Similarly, steam maintained at subatmospheric pressure at 73°C is used in *low-temperature steam* disinfectors in hospitals to disinfect thermolabile reusable equipment.

Exposure to boiling water for 20 min achieves highly effective disinfection; although this is not a sterilization process it can be useful in emergencies if no sterilizer is available.

### Disinfection by ultraviolet radiation

Ultraviolet radiation is a low-energy, non-ionizing radiation with poor penetrating power that is lethal to micro-organisms under optimum conditions. The shortest ultraviolet rays that reach the earth's surface in quantity have a wavelength of about 290 nm, but even more effective radiation of 240–280 nm is produced by mercury lamps. It is used in the treatment of air, water, thin films and surfaces such as laboratory safety cabinets.

### Disinfection by gases

Traditionally, formaldehyde gas was used to disinfect rooms previously occupied by patients with contagious diseases such as smallpox. It is still used for disinfection of complex heat-sensitive equipment including anaesthetic machines and baby incubators, and for periodic decontamination of laboratory safety cabinets.

### Disinfection by filtration

This method is used to remove micro-organisms from air supplied to critical sites such as operating theatres, pharmaceutical clean rooms, ultraclean laminar airflow ventilation systems and for the treatment of extracted air from laboratories handling dangerous pathogens.. A properly installed *high-efficiency particulate air* (HEPA) filter achieves 99.997% or better arrestance to particles of 0.5 μm, and can produce sterile air at the filter face.

### Disinfection by chemicals

Chemicals used in the environment or on the skin (*disinfectants* or *antiseptics*) cannot be relied on to kill or inhibit all pathogenic micro-organisms. The distinction between disinfectants and antiseptics is not clear cut: an antiseptic can be regarded as a special kind of disinfectant which is sufficiently free from injurious effects to be applied to the surface of the body, though not suitable for systemic administration. Some would restrict the term *antiseptic* to preparations applied to open wounds or abraded tissue and would prefer the term *skin disinfection* for the removal of organisms from the hands and intact skin surfaces.

#### Factors influencing the performance of chemical disinfectants

These include:

1. The concentration of the disinfectant
2. The number, type and location of micro-organisms

3. The temperature and pH
4. The presence of organic or other interfering substances.

In general, the rate of inactivation of a susceptible microbial population in the presence of an anti-microbial chemical is dependent on the relative concentration of the two reactants, the micro-organism and the chemical. The optimum concentration required to produce a standardized microbial effect in practice is described as the *in-use* concentration. Care must always be taken in preparing an accurate in-use dilution of concentrated product. Accidental or arbitrary overdilution may result in failure of disinfection.

The velocity of the reaction depends upon the number and type of organisms present. In general, Gram-positive bacteria are more sensitive to disinfectants than Gram-negative bacteria; mycobacteria and fungal spores are relatively resistant and bacterial spores are highly resistant. Enveloped or lipophilic viruses are relatively sensitive, whereas hydrophilic viruses such as poliovirus and other enteroviruses are less susceptible. Although difficult to test in vitro, there is evidence that the hepatitis B virus is more resistant than other viruses (including the human immunodeficiency virus) and most vegetative bacteria to the action of chemical disinfectants and heat.

Glutaraldehyde is highly active against bacteria, viruses and spores. Other disinfectants such as hexachlorophane have a relatively narrow range of activity, predominantly against Gram-positive cocci. Some disinfectants are more active or stable at a particular pH value; although glutaraldehyde is more stable under acidic conditions, use at a higher pH value (8.0) improves the antimicrobial effect.

Disinfectants may be inactivated by hard tapwater, cork, plastics, blood, urine, soaps and detergents, or another disinfectant. Information should be sought from the manufacturer or from reference authorities to confirm that the disinfectant will remain active in the circumstances of use.

## Alcohols

Isopropanol, ethanol and industrial methylated spirits have optimal bactericidal activity in aqueous solution at concentrations of 70–90% and have little bactericidal effect outside this range. They have limited activity against mycobacteria and are not sporicidal. Action against viruses is generally good. Because they are volatile, alcohols have been widely recommended as rapidly drying disinfectants for skin and surfaces.

However, they may not achieve adequate penetration and kill, particularly if organic matter such as blood or other protein-based contamination is present. Alcohols are suitable for physically clean surfaces such as washed thermometers or trolley tops but not for dirty surfaces. Care must be taken when used on the skin in conjunction with diathermy and other instances of flammable risk. Alcohols or alcohol-based formulations with chlorhexidine or povidone iodine are good choices for hand disinfection; they are applied to dry skin, often with added emollient to counteract the drying effect.

## Aldehydes

Most aldehyde disinfectants are based on glutaraldehyde or formaldehyde formulations, alone or in combination. *Glutaraldehyde* has a broad-spectrum action against vegetative bacteria, fungi and viruses, but acts more slowly against spores. It is often used for equipment such as endoscopes that cannot be sterilized or disinfected by heat. It is an irritant to the eyes, skin and respiratory mucosa, and must be used with adequate protection of staff and ventilation of the working environment. It must be thoroughly rinsed from treated equipment with sterile water to avoid carry-over of toxic residues and recontamination. The alkaline buffered solution is claimed to remain active for several days, but this will vary depending on the 'in-use' situation, including the amount of organic material.

## Biguanides

**Chlorhexidine.** This is commonly used for disinfection of the skin and mucous membranes. It is less active against Gram-negative bacteria such as *Pseudomonas* and *Proteus* species, and in aqueous solution has limited virucidal, tuberculocidal and negligible sporicidal activity. It is often combined with a compatible detergent for handwashing or with alcohol as a handrub. Chlorhexidine has low irritancy and toxicity, and is effective even on exposed healing surfaces. It is inactivated by organic matter, soap, anionic detergents, hard water and some natural materials such as the cork liners of bottle closures.

## Halogens

**Hypochlorites.** These broad-spectrum, inexpensive chlorine-releasing disinfectants are the disinfectants of choice against viruses, including hepatitis B virus. For circumstances of heavy soilage such as blood spillage, a concentration of 10 000 ppm of available chlorine is recommended.

They are inactivated by organic matter and corrode metals, so that contact with metallic instruments and equipment should be avoided. The bleaching action of hypochlorites may have a detrimental effect on fabrics, e.g. in treating a spillage on a carpet.

Chlorine-releasing disinfectants are relatively stable in concentrated form as liquid bleach or as tablets (sodium dichloroisocyanurates) but should be stored in well-sealed containers in a cool, dark place. On dilution to the required concentration for use, activity is rapidly lost.

Hypochlorites have widespread application as laboratory disinfectants on bench surfaces and in discard pots. Care should be taken to remove all chlorine-releasing agents from laboratory areas before the use of formaldehyde fumigation to avoid the production of carcinogenic reaction products.

*Iodine*. Like chlorine, iodine is inactivated by organic matter and has the additional disadvantages of staining and hypersensitivity. The *iodophors*, which contain iodine complexed with an anionic detergent, or *povidone iodine*, a water-soluble complex of iodine and polyvinyl pyrrolidone, are less irritant and cause less staining. Aqueous and alcohol-based povidone iodine preparations are widely used in skin disinfection, including pre-operative preparation of the skin.

## Phenolics

These have been widely used as general-purpose environmental disinfectants in hospital and laboratory practice. They exhibit broad-spectrum activity and are relatively cheap. Clear soluble phenolics have been used to disinfect environmental surfaces and spillages if organic soil and transmissible pathogens may have been present. As hospital disinfection policies are rationalized, phenolics are being replaced by detergents for cleaning, and by hypochlorites for disinfection of contaminated sources. Most phenolics are stable and not readily inactivated by organic matter, with the exception of the chloroxylenols ('Dettol'), which are also inactivated by hard water and are not recommended for hospital use. Phenolics are incompatible with cationic detergents. Contact should be avoided with rubber and plastics, such as mattress covers, since they are absorbed and may increase the permeability of the material to body fluids. The slow release of phenol fumes in closed environments and the need to avoid skin contact are other reasons for care in use of phenolics.

The bis-phenol *hexachlorophane* has particular activity against Gram-positive cocci, and has been used in powder or emulsion formulations as a skin disinfectant, notably for prophylaxis against staphylococcal infection in nurseries. There has been some concern about the possible toxic effect of absorption across the neonatal skin barrier on repeated exposure. An alternative, which has been used in the control of methicillin-resistant *Staph. aureus* (MRSA) outbreaks is *triclosan*.

## Oxidizing agents and hydrogen peroxide

Various agents, including chlorine dioxide, peracetic acid and hydrogen peroxide, have good antimicrobial properties but are corrosive to skin and metals. Hydrogen peroxide is highly reactive and has limited application for the treatment of wounds.

## Surface-active agents

Anionic, cationic, non-ionic and amphoteric *detergents* are generally used as cleaning agents. The cationic (*quaternary ammonium compounds*) and amphoteric agents have limited antimicrobial activity against vegetative bacteria and some viruses but not mycobacteria or bacterial spores. Quaternary ammonium compounds disrupt the membrane of the microorganisms, leading to cell lysis. Care must be taken to avoid overgrowth by Gram-negative contaminants and inactivation by mixing cationic and anionic agents. Disinfection may be enhanced by the appropriate combination of a surface-active agent with disinfectant to improve contact spread and cleansing properties.

## Disinfectant testing

A wide range of testing methods have been developed for different products and different applications in the medical, food and veterinary areas. Standardization of test methods within Europe is currently in progress, and will include:

1. Simple screening tests of the rate of kill
2. Laboratory tests simulating in-use conditions (skin disinfection tests and inanimate surface tests)
3. In-use tests on equipment and solutions.

The purpose of the 'in-use' test is to monitor not only the performance of a particular disinfectant but also how it is being used. Samples of the disinfectant dilutions in use around the hospital are taken to determine the survival and multiplication of contaminating pathogens in a stale or over-diluted formulation.

# STERILIZATION AND DISINFECTION POLICY

Each hospital, through the infection control team, should agree a policy to ensure that staff responsible for sterilization and disinfection are familiar with the agents to be used and the procedures involved. The policy should consider:

1. The sources (equipment, skin and environment) for which a choice of process is required.

2. The processes and products available for sterilization and disinfection. An effective policy may include a limited number of process options; restrictions on the range of chemical disinfectants will eliminate unnecessary costs, confusion and chemical hazards.

3. The category of process required for each item: sterilization for surgical instruments and needles; heat disinfection for laundry, crockery, bed-pans; cleaning for floors, walls and furniture.

4. The specific products and method to be used for each item of equipment, the site of use and the staff responsible for the procedure.

Effective implementation of the policy requires liaison and training of staff and updating the policy. Safety considerations for staff and patients require a careful assessment of specific procedures to minimize risks, e.g. to avoid skin contact and fumes from disinfectants by the use of protective clothing and local ventilation.

## RECOMMENDED READING

Ayliffe G A J, Coates D, Hoffman P N 1993 *Chemical Disinfection in Hospitals*, 2nd edn. Public Health Laboratory Service, London

Block S S (eds) 1991 *Disinfection, Sterilization and Preservation*, 4th edn. Lea and Febiger, Philadelphia

Gardner J F, Peel M M 1991 *Introduction to Sterilization and Disinfection*, 2nd edn. Churchill Livingstone, Edinburgh

Maurer I M 1985 *Hospital Hygiene*, 3rd edn. Edward Arnold, London

Medical Devices Agency 1996 *Sterilization, Disinfection and Cleaning of Medical Equipment. Guidance on Decontamination from the Microbiology Advisory Committee to the Department of Health*. Medical Devices Agency, London

Russell A D, Hugo W B, Ayliffe G A J (eds) 1992 *Principles and Practice of Disinfection, Preservation and Sterilisation*, 2nd edn. Blackwell Scientific, Oxford

# 8

# Bacterial pathogenicity

*A. Cockayne*

Pathogenicity, or the capacity to initiate disease, is a relatively rare quality among microbes. It requires the attributes of *transmissibility* or communicability from one host or reservoir to a fresh host, *infectivity* or the ability to breach the new host's defences, and *virulence*, a variable that is multifactorial and denotes the capacity of a pathogen to harm the host. Virulence in the clinical sense is a manifestation of a complex parasite–host relationship in which the capacity of the organism to cause disease is considered in relation to the resistance of the host.

## TYPES OF BACTERIAL PATHOGEN

Bacterial pathogens can be classified into two broad groups, *opportunists* and *primary pathogens*.

## Opportunistic pathogens

These rarely cause disease in individuals with intact immunological and anatomical defences. Only when such defences are impaired or compromised, as a result of congenital or acquired disease or by the use of immunosuppressive therapy or surgical techniques, are these bacteria able to cause disease. Many opportunistic pathogens, e.g. coagulase-negative staphylococci and *Escherichia coli*, are part of the normal human flora and are carried on the skin or mucosal surfaces where they cause no harm and may actually have a beneficial effect by preventing colonization by other potential pathogens. However, introduction of these organisms into anatomical sites in which they are not normally found, or removal of competing bacteria by the use of broad-spectrum antibiotics, may allow their localized multiplication and subsequent development of disease.

## Primary pathogens

These are capable of establishing infection and causing disease in previously healthy individuals with intact immunological defences. However, these bacteria may more readily cause disease in individuals with impaired defences.

## VIRULENCE DETERMINANTS

Both opportunistic and primary pathogens possess *virulence determinants* or *aggressins* that facilitate pathogenesis. Possession of a single virulence determinant is rarely sufficient to allow the initiation of infection and production of pathology. Many bacteria possess several virulence determinants, all of which play some part at various stages of the disease process. In addition, not all strains of a particular bacterial species are equally pathogenic. For example, although six separate serotypes of encapsulated *Haemophilus influenzae* are recognized, serious infection is almost exclusively associated with isolates of serotype b. Moreover, even within serotype b isolates, 80% of serious infections are caused by six out of over 100 clonal types.

Different strains of a pathogenic species may cause distinct types of infection, each associated with possession of a particular complement of virulence determinants. Different strains of *Esch. coli*, for example, cause several distinct gastro-intestinal diseases, urinary tract infections, septicaemia, meningitis and a range of other minor infections (see Ch. 27).

## Expression and analysis of virulence determinants

Many pathogens produce an impressive armoury of virulence determinants in vitro. However, relatively early in the study of pathogenesis, it was appreciated that a knowledge of the behaviour of the pathogen in vivo is crucial to an understanding of virulence.

Animal models have been used to compare the virulence of naturally occurring variants differing in the expression of a particular determinant, and have provided much useful information, but the possibility that observed differences in virulence may be due to additional cryptic phenotypic or genotypic variations cannot always be excluded. More recently, molecular techniques have been used to construct *isogenic* mutants of bacteria that differ only in the particular determinant of interest, and these constructs have allowed more detailed analysis of the role of such components in pathogenesis.

Most studies of bacterial virulence determinants are by necessity performed in model systems in vitro. However, growth conditions in vitro differ significantly from those found in tissues, and since the expression of many virulence determinants is influenced by environmental factors, it is essential that such studies use cultural conditions that mimic as closely as possible those found in the host.

Genetic studies have shown that expression of several different virulence determinants in a single bacterium are sometimes regulated in a co-ordinated fashion. Iron limitation, the situation encountered in host tissues, is one environmental stimulus which co-ordinately increases production of many bacterial proteins including virulence determinants such as haemolysin of *Esch. coli* and diphtheria toxin from *Corynebacterium diphtheriae*. In other bacteria, e.g. *Staphylococcus aureus* and *Pseudomonas aeruginosa*, some virulence determinants are expressed exclusively or maximally during the stationary phase of growth. Expression of these factors is associated with production of inducer molecules or pheromones in the bacterial culture which accumulate as the bacteria grow until a threshold level is reached and gene expression is triggered – a process known as *quorum sensing*. The ability to regulate production of virulence determinants may save energy in situations in which expression is not required, e.g. in the environment, and quorum sensing may be important in establishing a sufficiently large population of bacteria in tissue to guarantee survival of the infecting organism.

Molecular studies have also allowed mechanisms of transmission of virulence determinants to be investigated. Virulence determinants encoded by genomic DNA sequences, plasmids, bacteriophage and transposons have been reported.

## Establishment of infection

Potential pathogens may enter the body by various routes, including the respiratory, gastro-intestinal, urinary or genital tracts. Alternatively, they may directly enter tissues through insect bites or by accidental or surgical trauma to the skin. Many opportunistic pathogens are carried as part of the normal human flora, and this acts as a ready source of infection in the compromised host. For many primary pathogens, however, transmission to a new host and establishment of infection are more complex processes. Transmission of respiratory pathogens, such as *Bordetella pertussis*, may require direct contact with infectious material since the organism cannot survive for any length of time in the environment. Sexually transmitted pathogens such as *Neisseria gonorrhoeae* and *Treponema pallidum* have evolved further along this route, and require direct person-to-person mucosal contact for transmission. Man is the only natural host for these pathogens, which die rapidly in the environment. The source of infection may be individuals with clinical disease or subclinically infected *carriers*, in whom symptoms may be absent or relatively mild either because the disease process is at an early stage or because of partial immunity to the pathogen.

In contrast, for many gastro-intestinal pathogens such as *Salmonella*, *Shigella* and *Campylobacter* species the primary source is environmental, and infection follows ingestion of contaminated food or water. Many of these organisms also infect other animals, often without harmful effect, and these act as a *reservoir of infection* and source of environmental contamination.

## Colonization

For many pathogenic bacteria, the initial interaction with host tissues occurs at a mucosal surface and colonization – the establishment of a stable population of bacteria in the host – normally requires *adhesion* to the mucosal cell surface. This allows the establishment of a focus of infection that may remain localized or may subsequently spread to other tissues. Adhesion is necessary to avoid innate host defence mechanisms such as peristalsis in the gut and the flushing action of mucus, saliva and urine which remove non-adherent bacteria. For invasive bacteria, adhesion is an essential preliminary to penetration through tissues. Successful colonization also requires that bacteria are able to acquire essential nutrients – in particular iron – for growth.

## Adhesion

Adhesion involves surface interactions between specific *receptors* on the mammalian cell membrane (usually carbohydrates) and *ligands* (usually proteins) on the bacterial surface. The presence or absence of specific receptors on mammalian cells contributes significantly to tissue specificity of infection. Non-specific surface properties of the bacterium, including surface charge and hydrophobicity, also contribute to the initial stages of the adhesion process. Several different mechanisms of bacterial adherence have evolved, all utilizing specialized cell surface organelles or macromolecules, that help to overcome the natural forces of repulsion that exist between the pathogen and its target cell.

## Fimbrial adhesins

Electron microscopy of the surface of many Gram-negative and some Gram-positive bacteria reveals the presence of numerous thin, rigid rod-like structures called *fimbriae* that are easily distinguishable from the much thicker bacterial flagella (see Ch. 2). Fimbriae are involved in mediating attachment of some bacteria to mammalian cell surfaces. Different strains or species of bacteria may produce different types of fimbriae which can be identified on the basis of antigenic composition, morphology and receptor specificity (Table 8.1). A broad division can be made between those fimbriae in which adherence in vitro is inhibited by D-mannose (*mannose-sensitive fimbriae*) and those unaffected by this treatment (*mannose-insensitive fimbriae*).

The antigenic composition of fimbriae can be complex. For instance, two fimbrial antigens called colonization factor antigens (CFA) I and II have been detected in enteropathogenic *Esch. coli* strains. CFA II consists of three distinct fimbrial antigens designated as coli surface (CS) antigens 1, 2 and 3. Another *Esch. coli* strain, E8775, has been found to produce three other CS antigens, CS4, CS5 and CS6. Pyelonephritogenic *Esch. coli* isolates produce a group of adhesins called X-adhesins; two fimbrial types designated S and M on the basis of receptor specificity have been identified in this group.

The evolutionary significance of such heterogeneity may be that the ability of an individual bacterium to express several different types of fimbriae allows different target receptors to be used at different anatomical sites of the infected host. In vitro, production of fimbriae is influenced by cultural conditions such as incubation temperature and medium composition, which may switch off production of fimbriae or induce a phase change from one fimbrial type to another.

For some fimbriae the association with infection is clear. Thus the K88 fimbrial antigen is clearly associated with the ability of *Esch. coli* K88 to cause diarrhoea in pigs; pigs lacking the appropriate intestinal receptors are spared the enterotoxigenic effects of *Esch. coli* strains of this type. In many other instances the association between production of fimbriae and infection remains putative at present. Production of fimbriae is controlled by either chromosomal or plasmid genes (see Table 8.1). The structure of one of these fimbrial types – *type 1* or

| Table 8.1 | Examples of fimbriae produced by Gram-negative pathogens | |
|---|---|---|
| Designation | Bacterium | Gene location |
| Common (type 1)[a] | Enterobacteriaceae<br>Uropathogenic *Escherichia coli* | Chromosome |
| CFA I, CFA II (CS1, CS2, CS3)<br>E8775 (CS4, CS5, CS6) | Enterotoxigenic *Esch. coli* from humans | Plasmid<br>Unknown |
| K88<br>K99<br>F41 | Enterotoxigenic *Esch. coli* from animals | Plasmid<br>Plasmid<br>Unknown |
| Pap-G, Prs-G | Uropathogenic *Esch. coli* | Unknown |
| P fimbriae<br>X-adhesins (S, M) | Pyelonephritogenic *Esch. coli* | Chromosome<br>Unknown |
| *N*-Methylphenylalanine fimbriae | *Pseudomonas, Neisseria, Moraxella,*<br>*Bacteroides, Vibrio* species | Chromosome |

See text for abbreviations and explanation.
[a]Mannose-sensitive fimbriae.

*common fimbriae* – has been studied in detail. These consist of aggregates of a structural protein subunit called *fimbrillin* arranged in a regular helical array to produce a rigid rod-like structure of 7 nm diameter, with a central hole running along its length. A highly conserved minor protein, located at both the tip and at intervals along the length of the fimbriae, mediates specific adhesion. Type 1 fimbriae bind specifically to D-mannose residues. Their role in vivo remains controversial; however, they may be involved in the pathogenesis of urinary tract infections.

Other Gram-negative bacteria, including those of the genera *Pseudomonas*, *Neisseria*, *Bacteroides* and *Vibrio*, produce fimbriae that share some homology, especially in the amino-terminal region of the fimbrillin subunits (the so-called *N-methylphenylalanine fimbriae*). These fimbriae have been shown to act as virulence determinants for *Ps. aeruginosa* and *N. gonorrhoeae*.

## Non-fimbrial adhesins

Non-fimbrial adhesins include the filamentous haemagglutinin of *Bord. pertussis*, a mannose-resistant haemagglutinin from *Salmonella* serotype Typhimurium and a fibrillar haemagglutinin from *Helicobacter pylori*. Outer membrane proteins are involved in the adherence of *N. gonorrhoeae* and enteropathogenic *Esch. coli* to cell surfaces.

Exopolysaccharides present on the surface of some Gram-positive bacteria are also involved in adhesion. For example, *Streptococcus mutans*, which is involved in the pathogenesis of dental caries, synthesizes a homopolymer of glucose which anchors the bacterium to the tooth surface and contributes to the matrix of dental plaque. *Actinomyces* may adhere to other oral bacteria – a process called *co-aggregation*. Teichoic acid and surface proteins of coagulase-negative staphylococci mediate adherence of the bacterium to prosthetic devices and catheters, contributing to increasing numbers of hospital-acquired infections. Continued growth following attachment to these biomaterials may result in formation of a *biofilm* which may hinder succesful antibiotic treatment by restricting access of drugs to the bacterium.

Flagella act as adhesins in *Vibrio cholerae* and *Campylobacter jejuni*. Bacterial motility is also thought to be important in chemotaxis of these organisms and *H. pylori* towards intestinal cells and in penetration of these bacteria through the mucous layer during colonization.

## Binding to fibronectin

Fibronectin is a complex multifunctional glycoprotein found in plasma and associated with mucosal cell surfaces, where it promotes numerous adhesion functions. Many pathogenic bacteria bind fibronectin at the bacterial surface, and for some organisms fibronectin has been shown to act as the cell surface receptor for bacterial adhesion. In *Streptococcus pyogenes*, lipoteichoic acid mediates attachment of the bacterium to the amino terminus of the fibronectin molecule. Attachment of *Staph. aureus* to cell surfaces also involves the amino terminus of fibronectin, but the bacterial ligand appears to be protein in this instance. *T. pallidum* also binds fibronectin. The significance of the interaction with fibronectin in the pathogenesis of syphilis and many other bacterial diseases needs further clarification. Binding of bacterial pathogens to a number of other connective tissue proteins including collagen, laminin and vitronectin have also been described.

## Consequences of adhesion

In addition to preventing loss of the pathogen from the host, adhesion induces structural and functional changes in mucosal cells, and these may contribute to disease. For example, adherance of enteropathogenic *Esch. coli* (EPEC) to epithelial cells induces rearrangements of the cell cytoskeleton causing loss of microvilli and localized accumulation of actin. In contrast, adherance of *H. pylori* to gastric epithelial cells causes enhanced production of the pro-inflammatory chemokine interleukin-8 (IL-8), which contributes to gastric pathology. In both cases, these changes involve induction of intracellular signalling pathways triggered following binding of the bacteria to specific receptors on the epithelial cell surface. Adhesion of bacteria to mammalian cells may also induce changes in bacterial protein synthesis.

## Invasion

Once attached to a mucosal surface, some bacteria exert their pathogenic effects without penetrating the tissues of the host: toxins, other aggressins and induction of intracellular signalling pathways mediate tissue damage at local or distant sites. For a number of pathogenic bacteria, however, adherence to the mucosal surface represents but the first stage of the invasion of tissues. Examples of organisms that are able to invade and survive within host cells include mycobacteria and those of the genera *Salmonella*, *Shigella*, *Escherichia*, *Yersinia*, *Legionella*, *Listeria*,

*Campylobacter* and *Neisseria*. Cell invasion confers the ability to avoid humoral host defence mechanisms and potentially provides a niche rich in nutrients and devoid of competition from other bacteria. However, survival of bacteria in professional phagocytes, such as macrophages or polymorphonuclear leucocytes, depends on subverting intracellular killing mechanisms that would normally result in microbial destruction (see below). For some bacteria, e.g. *Neisseria meningitidis*, penetration through or between epithelial cells allows dissemination from the initial site of entry to other body sites.

### Uptake into host cells

The initial phase of cellular invasion involves penetration of the mammalian cell membrane and many intracellular pathogens use normal phagocytic entry mechanisms to gain access.

Shigellae invade colonic mucosal cells but rarely penetrate deeper into the host tissues. Inside the cell, they are surrounded by a membrane-bound vesicle derived from the host cell. Soon after entry, this vesicle is lysed by the action of the plasmid-encoded haemolysin, and the bacteria are released into the cell cytoplasm. *Listeria monocytogenes* produces a heat shock protein with a similar function termed *listeriolysin*. Once free in the cell cytoplasm, shigellae multiply rapidly with subsequent inhibition of host cell protein synthesis. Several hours later the host cell dies, and bacteria spread to adjacent cells where the process of invasion is repeated.

In contrast to shigellae, most salmonellae proceed through the superficial layers of the gut and invade deeper tissues, in particular cells of the reticulo-endothelial system such as macrophages. Salmonellae also occupy a host-derived vesicle, but this does not lyse. Instead, several vesicles coalesce to form large intracellular vacuoles. These vacuoles traverse the cytoplasm to reach the opposite side of the cell and initiate spread to adjacent cells and deeper tissues. For both *Salmonella* and *Shigella* species, bacterial protein and RNA synthesis are required for invasion.

### Role of cell receptors

The availability of specific receptors defines the type of host cells that are involved. As a result some pathogens can invade a wide range of cell types whilst others have a much more restricted invasive potential. The receptors for some of the invasive pathogens have been identified. For example, *Legionella pneumophila* and *Mycobacterium tuberculosis* adhere to complement receptors on the surface of phagocytic cells. The receptor for *Yersinia pseudotuberculosis* belongs to a family of proteins termed *integrins* that form a network on the surface of host cells to which host proteins such as fibronectin can bind. Mimicry of the amino acid sequence (Arg-Gly-Asp) of fibronectin that mediates attachment to the integrins may represent a common mechanism of effecting intracellular entry.

The ability to utilize integrins may not be restricted to intracellular bacteria. The filamentous haemagglutinin of *Bord. pertussis* may use the fibronectin integrin to mediate attachment in the respiratory tract.

## Avoidance of host defence mechanisms

Colonization by bacterial pathogens results in the induction of specific and non-specific humoral and cell-mediated immune responses designed to eradicate the organism from the site of infection. Products of the organism may be chemotactic for phagocytic cells which are attracted to the site. Moreover, complement components may directly damage the bacterium and release peptides chemotactic for phagocytic cells. Other humoral antibacterial factors include lysozyme and the iron chelators transferrin and lactoferrin. Lysozyme is active primarily against Gram-positive bacteria but potentiates the activity of complement against Gram-negative organisms. Transferrin and lactoferrin chelate iron in body fluids, and reduce the amount of free iron to levels below that necessary for bacterial growth.

Pathogenic bacteria have evolved ways of avoiding or neutralizing these highly efficient clearance systems. Since most of the interactions between the bacterium and the immune effectors involve the bacterial surface, resistance to these effects is related to the molecular architecture of the bacterial surface layers.

### Capsules

Many bacterial pathogens need to avoid phagocytosis, and production of an extracellular capsule is the most common mechanism by which this is achieved. Virtually all the pathogens associated with meningitis and pneumonia, including *H. influenzae*, *N. meningitidis*, *Esch. coli* and *Str. pneumoniae*, have capsules, and non-capsulate variants usually exhibit much reduced virulence. Most capsules are polysaccharides composed of sugar monomers that vary among different bacteria. Polysaccharide capsules reduce the efficiency of phagocytosis in a number of ways:

1. In the absence of specific antibody to the bacterium, the hydrophilic nature of the capsule may hinder uptake by phagocytes, a process which occurs more readily at hydrophobic surfaces. This may be overcome if the phagocyte is able to trap the bacterium against a surface – a process referred to as *surface phagocytosis*.

2. Capsules prevent efficient opsonization of the bacterium by complement or specific antibody, events that promote interaction with phagocytic cells. Capsules may either prevent complement deposition completely or cause complement to be deposited at a distance from the bacterial membrane where it is unable to damage the organism.

3. Capsules tend to be weakly immunogenic and may mask more immunogenic surface components and reduce interactions with both complement and antibody.

### Streptococcal M protein

The M protein present on the surface of *Str. pyogenes* is not a capsule but functions in a similar manner to prevent complement deposition at the bacterial surface. The M protein binds both fibrinogen and fibrin, and deposition of this material on the streptococcal surface hinders the access of complement activated by the alternative pathway.

### Resistance to killing by phagocytic cells

Some pathogens not only survive within macrophages and other phagocytes, but may actually multiply intracellularly. The normal sequence of events following phagocytosis involves fusion of the *phagosome* in which the bacterium is contained with *lysosomal granules* present in the cell cytoplasm. These granules contain enzymes and cationic peptides involved in oxygen-dependent and oxygen-independent bacterial killing mechanisms (see Ch. 11).

Different organisms use different strategies for survival (Table 8.2). *M. tuberculosis* is thought to resist intracellular killing by preventing phagosome–lysosome fusion; other bacteria are able to resist the action of such lysosomal components following fusion. Some organisms stimulate a normal respiratory burst but are intrinsically resistant to the effects of the potentially toxic oxygen radicals produced. Production of catalase by *Staph. aureus* and *N. gonorrhoeae* is thought to protect these organisms from such toxic products. The smooth lipopolysaccharide of many bacterial pathogens is also thought to contribute to their resistance to the

**Table 8.2** Some strategies adopted by bacteria to avoid intracellular killing

| Species | Method |
|---|---|
| *Mycobacterium tuberculosis* | May prevent phagosomelysosome fusion |
| *Salmonella* serotype Typhi | Fails to stimulate $O_2$-dependent killing |
| *Staphylococcus aureus* *Neisseria gonorrhoeae* | Produce catalase to negate effect of toxic $O_2$ radicals |
| *Legionella pneumophila* | Inhibits phagolysosome acidification |

effects of bactericidal cationic peptides present in the phagolysosome.

### Antigenic variation

Variation in surface antigen composition during the course of infection provides a mechanism of avoidance of specific immune responses directed at those antigens. This strategy is most highly developed in blood-borne parasitic protozoa, such as trypanosomes, but is also exhibited by bacteria. *N. gonorrhoeae* shows antigenic variation in an outer-membrane protein known as PII and in its fimbriae. Expression of individual PII proteins is controlled by frame shifts in the nucleotide sequence encoding the protein leader sequence, which varies as a result of recombination or mutation during DNA replication. Individual PII genes appear to be independently regulated such that there are many possible combinations of these proteins on a single organism.

Variation in the fimbriae is controlled by a different mechanism in *N. gonorrhoeae*. Usually only one complete fimbrillin gene is expressed, though several incomplete 'silent' gene sequences are present on the chromosome. Movement of the incomplete gene sequences to an expression locus results in synthesis of a protein that may differ antigenically from that previously expressed. Alternatively, variant fimbrillin gene DNA may be acquired from other gonococci by transformation to allow new genes to be constructed by recombination at the expression site.

The borreliae that cause relapsing fever use a similar strategy to generate antigenic variation in their outer surface proteins. Other bacteria show strain-specific antigenic variability, for example group A streptococci produce up to 75 antigenically distinct serotypes of M protein.

The capacity for variation in surface antigens means that antibody produced in response to infection by one strain of a pathogen may not protect against subsequent challenge with a different strain of that bacterium. This makes development of vaccines based on inhibition of attachment or generation of opsonic antibody particularly difficult for these organisms.

## Immunoglobulin A proteases

Several species of pathogenic bacteria that cause disease on mucosal surfaces produce a protease that specifically cleaves immunoglobulin A (IgA), the principal antibody type produced at these sites. These proteases are specific for human IgA isotype I. Nearly all the pathogens causing meningitis possess an IgA protease and a polysaccharide capsule enabling them to persist on the mucosal surface and resist phagocytosis during the invasive phase of the disease.

## Serum resistance

To survive in the bloodstream, bacteria must be able to resist lysis as a result of deposition of complement on the bacterial surface. In the Enterobacteriaceae, resistance is primarily due to the composition of the lipopolysaccharide (LPS) present in the bacterial outer membrane. *Smooth* colonial variants which possess polysaccharide 'O' side-chains in their LPS are more resistant than *rough* colonial variants that lack such side-chains (see below). The side-chains sterically hinder deposition of complement components on the bacterial surface. Conversely, however, some O chain polysaccharides activate complement by an alternate pathway leading to lysis of the bacterial cell. In *N. meningitidis* group B and *Esch. coli* K1, sialic acid capsules prevent efficient complement activation and, in *N. gonorrhoeae*, complement binds but forms an aberrant configuration in the bacterial outer membrane so that it is unable to effect lysis.

## Iron acquisition

The concentration of free iron in bodily secretions is below that required for bacterial growth because it is chelated by high-affinity mammalian iron-binding proteins such as transferrin and lactoferrin. In order to multiply in body fluids or on mucous membranes, bacteria must therefore obtain iron, and many bacterial pathogens have evolved very efficient mechanisms for scavenging iron from mammalian iron-binding proteins. Bacteria such as *Esch. coli*, *Klebsiella pneumoniae* and some staphylococci produce extracellular iron chelators called *siderophores* for this purpose. Others including *N. meningitidis*, *Haemophilus parainfluenzae*, *H. influenzae* type b, *Staphylococcus epidermidis* and *Staph. aureus* have specific receptors for transferrin or lactoferrin, or both, on their surfaces, and are able to bind these proteins and their chelated iron directly from body fluids. Production of siderophores, their cell surface receptors and receptors for transferrin, lactoferrin and other mammalian iron-binding proteins is iron regulated and only occurs under conditions of iron restriction.

Two other mechanisms of iron acquisition from mammalian iron chelators have been described. Some *Bacteroides* species remove iron by proteolytic cleavage of the chelator. In *Listeria monocytogenes*, reduction of the $Fe^{3+}$ ion to $Fe^{2+}$ reduces the affinity for the chelator sufficiently for it to be removed by the bacterium.

## Toxins

In many bacterial infections the characteristic pathology of the disease is caused by toxins. Toxins may exert their pathogenic effects directly on a target cell or may interact with cells of the immune system resulting in the release of immunological mediators (cytokines) that cause pathophysiological effects. Such effects may not always lead to the death of the target cell but may selectively impair specific functions. Substances that have toxic physiological effects on target cells in vitro do not necessarily exert the same effects in vivo, but a number of toxins have been shown to be responsible for the typical clinical features of bacterial disease.

Two major types of toxin have been described: *endotoxin*, which is a component of the outer membrane of Gram-negative bacteria, and *exotoxins*, which are produced extracellularly by both Gram-negative and Gram-positive bacteria.

## Endotoxin

Endotoxin, also called LPS, is a component of the outer membrane of Gram-negative bacteria, and is released from the bacterial surface following natural lysis of the bacterium or by disintegration of the organism in vitro. LPS is anchored into the bacterial outer membrane through a unique molecule termed *lipid A* (Fig. 8.1). Covalently linked to lipid A is an eight-carbon sugar, ketodeoxyoctonate (KDO), in

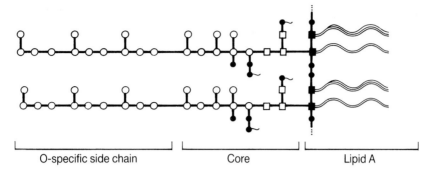

O-specific side chain          Core          Lipid A

○ = various sugar residues

□ = ketodeoxyoctonate (KDO)

■ = glucosamine

●～ = phosphoethanolamine

～ = fatty acid residues

**Fig. 8.1**  Diagrammatic representation of the structure of bacterial lipopolysaccharide. (After Reitschel E T, Galanos C, Lüderlitz O 1975 Structure, endotoxicity and immunogenicity of the lipid A component of bacterial lipopolysaccharide. In: Schlessinger D (ed) *Microbiology – 1975*. American Society for Microbiology, Washington, DC, pp 307–314.)

turn linked to the oligosaccharides which form the highly variable O antigen structures of Gram-negative bacteria. Bacteria carrying LPS containing O antigen form *smooth* colonies on bacteriological media in contrast to those lacking the O antigen, which form *rough* colonies.

The term *endotoxin* was originally introduced to describe the component of Gram-negative bacteria responsible for the pathophysiology of *endotoxic shock*, a syndrome with high mortality, particularly in immunocompromised or otherwise debilitated individuals. LPS activates complement via the alternative pathway, but most of the biological activity of LPS is attributable to lipid A. Both LPS and lipid A are potent activators of macrophages, resulting in the induction of a range of cytokines which are involved in the regulation of immune and inflammatory responses (see Ch. 11).

## Exotoxins

*Exotoxins*, in contrast to endotoxin, are diffusable proteins secreted into the external medium by the pathogen. Some exotoxins can be partially denatured (e.g. by formaldehyde treatment) to generate toxoids which lack toxic activity but still induce protective immunity when used as vaccines. The molecular structure and mechanism of action of many exotoxins have now been determined. Exotoxins can be classified by their mode of action on animal cells: type I

toxins bind surface receptors and stimulate transmembrane signals; type II toxins act directly on membranes, forming pores or disrupting lipid bilayers; type III toxins translocate an active enzymatic component into the cell which modifies an intracellular target molecule. Examples of exotoxins and their effects on target cells are shown in Table 8.3.

*Enterotoxins* cause symptoms of gastro-intestinal disease, including diarrhoea, dysentery or vomiting. In some cases the disease is caused by ingestion of preformed toxin in food, but in most cases colonization of the intestine is required before toxin is made.

Cholera toxin and heat-labile toxins of enterotoxigenic *Esch. coli* do not induce inflammatory changes in the intestinal mucosa, but perturb the processes that regulate ion and water exchange across the intestinal epithelium (see Chs 27 and 31). In contrast, the enterotoxins of *Clostridium difficile, C. perfringens* type A and *Bacillus cereus* cause structural damage to epithelial cells resulting in inflammation. Other gastro-intestinal pathogens such as enteropathogenic *Esch. coli* mediate damage by ill-defined mechanisms, following close contact between the bacterium and the cell surface.

## Toxins in respiratory infections

The involvement of exotoxins in the pathogenesis of bacterial respiratory infections is unclear, but for

**Table 8.3** Some effects of bacterial exotoxins

| Toxic effect | Examples |
|---|---|
| **Lethal action** | |
| Effect on neuromuscular junction | *Clostridium botulinum* toxin A |
| Effect on voluntary muscle | Tetanus toxin |
| Damage to heart, lungs, kidneys, etc. | Diphtheria toxin |
| **Pyrogenic effect** | |
| Increase in body temperature | Exotoxins of *Staphylococcus aureus* and *Streptococcus pyogenes* |
| | Staphylococcal toxic shock syndrome toxin 1 |
| **Action on gastro-intestinal tract** | |
| Secretion of water and electrolytes | Cholera and *Escherichia coli* enterotoxins |
| Pseudomembranous colitis | *Clostridium difficile* toxins A and B |
| Bacillary dysentery | Shigella toxin |
| Vomiting | *Staph. aureus* enterotoxins A–E |
| **Action on skin** | |
| Necrosis | Clostridial toxins; staphylococcal α-toxin |
| Erythema | Diphtheria toxin; streptococcal erythrogenic toxin |
| Permeability of skin capillaries | Cholera enterotoxin; *Esch. coli* heat-labile toxin |
| Nikolsky sign[a] | *Staph. aureus* epidermolytic toxin |
| **Cytolytic effects** | |
| Lysis of blood cells | *Staph. aureus* α-, β- and δ-lysins, leucocidin |
| | Streptolysin O and S |
| | *Clostridium perfringens* α and θ toxins |
| **Inhibition of metabolic activity** | |
| Protein synthesis | Diphtheria toxin; shiga toxin |

[a]Separation of epidermis from dermis.

*Bord. pertussis*, the causative agent of whooping cough, the role of toxins is more clear cut. This organism produces various extracellular products, including a tracheal cytotoxin which inhibits the beating of cilia on tracheal epithelial cells, pertussis toxin, which exhibits several systemic effects, and an adenylate cyclase that interferes with phagocyte function (see Ch. 33).

## Toxins acting on subepithelial tissues

Another group of toxins causes damage to subepithelial tissues following penetration and multiplication of the pathogen at the site of infection. Many of these toxins also inhibit or interfere with components of the host immune system. Membrane-damaging toxins such as staphylococcal α and β toxins, streptolysin O and streptolysin S and *C. perfringens* α and θ toxins inhibit leucocyte chemotaxis at subcytolytic concentrations, but cause necrosis and tissue damage at higher concentrations.

## Systemic effects of toxins

Some toxins cause damage to internal organs following absorption from the focus of infection. Included in this category are the toxins causing diphtheria, tetanus and botulism and those associated with streptococcal scarlet fever and staphylococcal toxic shock syndrome. The diphtheria toxin, the gene for which is bacteriophage-encoded, inhibits protein synthesis in mammalian cells. Tetanus toxin, in contrast, exerts its effect by preventing the release of inhibitory neurotransmitters whose function is to prevent overstimulation of motor neurones in the central nervous system, resulting in the convulsive muscle spasm characteristic of tetanus. Diphtheria and tetanus toxins represent the sole determinant of disease and are neutralized by specific antitoxin antibody. As a result, vaccination with diphtheria and tetanus toxoids is highly effective.

Botulism results from the ingestion of preformed toxin produced by *Clostridium botulinum* in food contaminated with this bacterium, and is not a true infectious disease. The toxic activity is due to a family of serologically distinct polypeptide neurotoxins that prevent release of acetylcholine at neuromuscular junctions, resulting in the symptoms of flaccid paralysis. These toxins have been used clinically in treating squints and muscle spasm.

Other toxins cause disseminated multisystem organ damage. Such pathology is seen in staphylococcal *toxic shock syndrome* caused by certain strains of *Staph. aureus* that produce a toxin designated *toxic shock syndrome toxin 1* (TSST-1). This toxin belongs to a group of functionally related proteins collectively referred to as *superantigens*, which includes the staphylococcal enterotoxins, staphylococcal exfoliative toxin and streptococcal pyrogenic exotoxin A. These molecules are potent T cell mitogens whose reactivity with lymphocytes induces cytokine release, and may initiate tissue damage by mechanisms similar to those postulated to account for Gramnegative endotoxic shock (see Ch. 14).

## Other extracellular aggressins

Many bacteria secrete a range of enzymes that may be involved in the pathogenic processes.

*Proteus* spp. and some other bacteria that cause urinary tract infections produce *ureases* that break down urea in the urine, and the release of ammonia may contribute to the pathology. The urease produced by the gastric and duodenal pathogen *H. pylori* is similarly implicated in the virulence of the organism. *L. pneumophila* produces a metalloprotease thought to contribute to the characteristic pathology seen in legionella pneumonia.

Many other degradative enzymes, including *mucinases, phospholipases, collagenases* and *hyaluronidases*, are produced by pathogenic bacteria. Many non-pathogenic bacteria also produce such enzymes, and their role in pathogenesis requires further clarification.

Understanding of the basic mechanisms of pathogenesis is important for the design of new or improved vaccines and appropriate therapies. Such knowledge is also invaluable in the analysis of 'new' bacterial pathogens that are recognized from time to time. However, for some bacterial diseases, e.g. syphilis, such approaches have still not defined the mechanisms of pathogenesis or the virulence determinants involved, and new strategies employed by such successful pathogens may yet be discovered.

### RECOMMENDED READING

Hormaeche C E, Penn C W, Smyth C J (eds) 1992 *Molecular Biology of Bacterial Infection: Current Status and Future Perspectives. Society for General Microbiology Symposium 49*. Cambridge University Press, Cambridge

Inglewski B H, Clark L V (eds) 1990 *The Bacteria. Molecular Basis of Bacterial Pathogenesis*. Academic Press, London, vol XI

Litwin C M, Calderwood S B 1993 Role of iron in regulation of virulence genes. *Clinical Microbiology Reviews* 6: 137–149

Ofek I, Doyle R J 1994 *Bacterial Adhesion to Cells and Tissues*. Chapman and Hall, London

Patrick S, Larkin M J 1995 *Immunological and Molecular Aspects of Bacterial Virulence*. Wiley, Chichester

Salmond G P C, Bycroft B W, Stewart G S A B, Williams P 1995 The bacterial enigma: cracking the code of cell – cell communication. *Molecular Microbiology* 16: 615–624

# 9

# Virus–cell interactions: antiviral agents

*M. Norval*

Viruses are totally dependent on the cells they infect to provide the energy, metabolic intermediates and most, in some cases all, of the enzymes required for their replication. With advances in the techniques of molecular virology and modelling together with the classical methods of electron microscopy, titration and biochemical assay, it has become possible to study virus–cell interactions to a sophisticated level. The picture that has emerged, and is still emerging, is a fascinating one, as viruses are found to associate with, and affect, cells in a wide variety of ways. The range of possible interactions is indicated in Table 9.1. It is possible to divide these into three broad categories which show considerable overlap:

1. Viruses which infect and replicate within cells causing the cells to lyse when the progeny virions are released. This is called a *cytolytic cycle*, the infection is *productive* and the cell culture shows *cytopathic effects*, which are often characteristic of the infecting virus. The host cells are termed *permissive*. In some instances viruses are produced from the infected cells but the cells are not killed by the process, i.e. the infection is *productive* but *non-cytolytic*, and may become *persistent*.

2. Viruses which infect cells but which do not complete the replication cycle. Thus the infection is called *abortive* or *non-productive*. Abortive infections can be due to a mutation in the virus so that some essential function is lost, or to the production of defective interfering particles, or to the action of interferons. It may be possible to manipulate the conditions in vitro to obtain a *steady state* or *persistent infection* in which infected and uninfected cells coexist and there is some, generally limited, virus production.

3. Viruses which enter cells but are not produced by the infected cell. The virus is maintained within the cell in the form of DNA which replicates in association with the host cell DNA. The host cell is termed *non-permissive* and the infection is *non-productive*. Occasionally this type of interaction induces cell *transformation*. In other cases a *latent infection* may result in which very little or no viral gene expression occurs and the cell retains its normal properties.

## THE LYTIC OR CYTOCIDAL GROWTH CYCLE

While there are large differences in the details of the lytic growth cycle depending on the virus studied and to some extent on the host cell, certain features are common, and a simplified description will be given first. The quantitative aspects of virion production were determined initially using bacteriophages but have now been ascertained for many animal viruses growing in vitro in cell culture. A one-step growth curve is obtained when samples are removed from an infected cell culture at intervals and assayed for the total content of infectious virus after artificial lysis of the cells (Fig. 9.1).

In the early part of the cycle, virus particles come into contact with the cells, and may then *attach* or *adsorb* to them. This marks the start of the *eclipse phase*. The virion then *penetrates* into the host cell and is partially *uncoated* to reveal the viral genome. *Macromolecular synthesis* of viral components follows. Often this can be divided into *early* and *late phases*

| Table 9.1 The range of virus–cell interactions | |
|---|---|
| Type of infection/effect on cells | Comment |
| Cytolytic | Virus produced |
| Non-cytolytic (persistent) | Virus produced |
| Abortive | Virus not produced |
| Abortive (persistent) | Virus produced |
| Latency (persistent) | Viral nucleic acid present |
| Transformation (persistent) | Viral nucleic acid present |

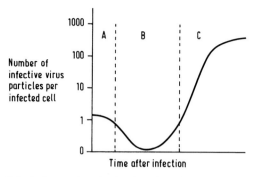

**Fig. 9.1** Lytic growth cycle of a virus. Samples are removed from the infected culture at intervals and assayed for the total content of virus. Phase A, adsorption; phase B, eclipse; phase C, assembly and release.

separated by the replication of the viral nucleic acid. Early messenger RNA (mRNA) is first transcribed and translated into proteins. These are frequently non-structural proteins and enzymes required to undertake nucleic acid synthesis and the later stages of replication. Viral nucleic acid is then produced, followed by late mRNA transcription and translation. Most proteins made at this stage are structural ones, and will make up part of the final virion. The eclipse phase ends with the *assembly* and *release* of newly formed virus particles. The cycle is shown in diagrammatic form in Figure 9.2, and can vary from as little as 8 h for some picornaviruses to more than 40 h for cytomegalovirus, a human herpesvirus.

## Attachment (adsorption)

The initial interaction is by random collision, and depends on the relative concentrations of virus particles and cells. The ionic composition of the culture medium is an important factor as both viruses and cells are negatively charged at neutral pH and would tend to repel each other. The presence of cations, such as $Mg^{2+}$, therefore helps to promote close contact. Adsorption then takes place through a *specific binding site* on the virus and a *receptor* on the plasma membrane of the cell. It is largely temperature- and energy-independent.

Viruses vary widely in the range of cells to which they can adsorb, depending on the nature of the site to which they attach and how widespread it is amongst cells of different types, tissues and species. Rabies virus binds to the acetylcholine receptor found on neurones. Orthomyxo- and paramyxo-viruses have envelope glycoproteins protruding from the surface of the virion, which have specific binding sites for the oligosaccharide side-chains of glycoproteins or glycolipids terminating in *N*-acetylneuraminic acid (sialic acid). These are found on the membranes of most cells. The haemagglutinin consists of trimers of two polypeptides, $HA_1$ and $HA_2$, and the binding site for sialic acid is located on the globular part of $HA_1$, which is furthest from the envelope of the virus. Poliovirus, a picornavirus, infects only primate cells, and only those of the central nervous system or the intestine. The receptor in this case is a member of the immunoglobulin gene superfamily coded by a gene on the human chromosome 19. It has been estimated that there are up to $3 \times 10^3$ such receptor sites per cell. The attachment is through an arrangement of the structural proteins VP1, VP2 and VP3 of the virus. Another picornavirus, rhinovirus, also uses a member of the immunoglobulin gene superfamily as a receptor; in this case intercellular adhesion molecule-1

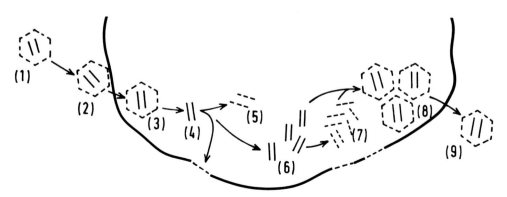

**Fig. 9.2** A simplified viral replication cycle showing a hypothetical virus particle (1), attaching to the surface of a susceptible cell (2), penetrating into the cell (3), being uncoated (4), undergoing early transcription and translation (5), then replication of the viral nucleic acid (6), late transcription and translation (7), and, finally, assembly of new virus particles (8) and release from the cell (9).

(ICAM-1), a ligand important in the adhesion of leucocytes. Epstein–Barr virus infects human B lymphocytes, and is largely selective for them due to the expression in mature B cells of a receptor for one of the complement cleavage fragments to which the virus binds. The attachment of human immunodeficiency virus (HIV) to cells is mediated by the interaction between a glycoprotein, gp120, in the viral envelope and CD4 antigen expressed on T helper cells, monocytes and some dendritic cells.

Most cellular receptors are glycoproteins, and the number expressed on different cell types and tissues is an important factor in determining susceptibility, i.e. the capacity of a cell or animal to become infected with a particular virus. The number per cell is generally several thousand. The expression of the receptors may change if the cells are cultured in vitro. Thus, monkey kidney cells are commonly used for the growth of poliovirus in vitro although this virus does not infect the kidney in vivo in infected monkeys. With some viruses, the requirement for specific receptors on the cell membrane can be bypassed, experimentally at least, by infection with extracted viral nucleic acid. Cells which are normally resistant can therefore become infected. For example, chick fibroblasts, resistant to infection with poliovirus, can be infected for one cycle by poliovirus RNA; the virions produced are not infectious for other chick fibroblasts as they still do not possess an appropriate binding site for chick cells.

## Penetration (uptake)

Penetration occurs immediately after adsorption and, unlike adsorption, requires energy and does not proceed at 0°C. Despite much study, it is still not clear how many viruses enter cells, particularly in vivo, and, furthermore, which route of entry leads to a successful infection. There are probably two main mechanisms.

### 1. Receptor-mediated endocytosis

This method is used by both enveloped and non-enveloped viruses, and is essentially the same as the normal uptake of macromolecules bound to cell surface receptors. Receptors with adsorbed virus particles move together (patch) to pits coated with clathrin, before moving into the cytosol to form small uncoated vesicles which then fuse together as endosomes. A proton pump in the endosome lowers the pH to about 5. For enveloped viruses, this change causes a rearrangement of the hydrophobic components of selected viral polypeptides leading to their fusion with the endosome membrane. Thus the viral nucleocapsid is released into the cytosol. The endosomes combine with lysosomes, which

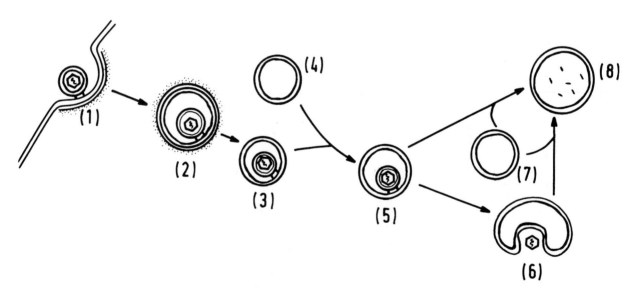

**Fig. 9.3** Receptor-mediated endocytosis of an enveloped virus. The virus attaches to specific receptors on the cell membrane (1), which patch at coated pits before being pinched off to form vesicles (2). These lose their coat (3) and fuse with other vesicles (4) to form endosomes (5). At the acid pH of endosomes, fusion of the viral envelope and the endosome membrane occurs releasing the virus into the cytosol (6). (7) Fusion of the endosome with lysosomes leads to the final degradation of viral components and their return to the surface (8).

eventually cause degradation of any viral components contained within. This process is outlined in Figure 9.3. In the case of influenza virus, a part of the haemagglutinin (the hydrophobic amino ($N$)-terminal of $HA_2$) is responsible for the fusion, the fusion sequence being activated by the low pH of the endosome. There is also a contribution from $M_2$, another membrane glycoprotein of the virus, which forms an ion channel at low pH and allows the liberation of the ribonucleoproteins from the virions into the cytoplasm. Non-enveloped viruses also enter by receptor-mediated endocytosis, but the end-point is not fusion and is ill-defined, as yet. In adenoviruses, a viral protein may be activated at low pH, capable of lysing the endosomal membrane. In other viruses, proteolytic cleavage of the capsid may occur, thus activating a viral component which may then lyse or permeabilize the endosomal membrane.

## 2. Fusion with the plasma membrane

This mechanism is used only by certain enveloped viruses including paramyxoviruses, retroviruses and herpesviruses. It requires the presence of a specific viral protein in the envelope which facilitates the fusion between the envelope and the plasma membrane at physiological pH. Subsequently there is release of the nucleocapsid into the cytosol. An example of such a protein is the F (fusion) protein of paramyxoviruses which is activated following attachment of the virus to the cell membrane via the haemagglutinin–neuraminidase glycoprotein.

## Uncoating

Uncoating can take place at several stages and sites in the cell. Some viruses, such as poliovirus, undergo conformational changes on attachment which result in the integrity of the particle being lost as it is transported into the cell. Those enveloped viruses entering by receptor-mediated endocytosis may be affected by the low pH and the action of lysosomal enzymes. Uncoating can also be found in the cytosol and, in the case of some DNA viruses such as herpes simplex virus, this stage occurs at the nuclear pore, allowing the viral DNA to enter the nucleus thereafter. Reoviruses never fully uncoat, the viral genome remaining within a recognizable capsid structure. Poxviruses become uncoated in two stages. In the first, the outer layers and lateral bodies are removed within endosomal vesicles using host enzymes, and the core lies in the cytosol. Poxviruses carry their own DNA-dependent RNA polymerase, and this enzyme is used in the second stage to transcribe mRNA, which is translated into a special

uncoating protein; this enables the final release of viral DNA from the core.

Following uncoating, it is necessary for the viral nucleic acid with, in some instances, viral enzymes or proteins from the capsid to proceed to the correct site in the cell to commence synthesis of the macromolecules which will comprise the new virions. In some cases this happens entirely in the cytosol, e.g. poliovirus, others replicate in the nucleus, e.g. herpesviruses, while a third category has nuclear and cytoplasmic stages, e.g. influenza viruses. In most instances it is not known how the transport is controlled although an important role for the cytoskeleton has been proposed.

## Synthesis of viral components

The nucleic acid in viruses is either single or double stranded, circular or linear, in one piece or segmented. In addition, viruses vary enormously in their complexity, ranging from ones with nucleic acid sufficient to code for only a few proteins, such as the papovaviruses, up to ones coding for several hundred proteins, such as the poxviruses. Although every virus has a unique method of replicating and has a strict temporal control on the synthesis of components, each must present functional mRNA to the cell, so that new virally encoded polypeptides and nucleic acid can be synthesized using the normal cellular processes. Thus, only viruses which contain DNA and replicate in the nucleus can use solely cellular enzymes for transcription and translation. All other viruses require to synthesize their mRNA by processes other than those found in uninfected cells. Six different classes, first described by Baltimore in 1970, can be distinguished (Fig.

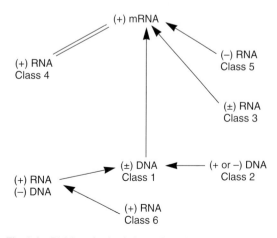

**Fig. 9.4** Division of animal viruses into six classes, based on mechanisms of transcription.

9.4). Conventionally in the scheme, nucleic acid of the same polarity or sense as mRNA is called 'positive' (+), while that of the opposite polarity or anti-sense is called 'negative' (−). Rather than be exhaustive, one or two illustrative examples from each class will now be described.

## Class 1. Double-stranded DNA viruses

This comprises a very large group of viruses which contain double-stranded DNA in a linear, e.g. herpesviruses, adenoviruses and poxviruses, or a circular form, e.g. papovaviruses. In all cases, apart from the poxviruses, transcription of the viral genome occurs in the nucleus. Herpes simplex virus is used as an example (Fig. 9.5). On uncoating at the nuclear pore, the viral nucleic acid enters the nucleus and, using the normal host cell mechanisms of transcription and translation, three groups of viral polypeptides are synthesized in a strict temporal fashion. They are called immediate early (α), early (β) and late (γ). A component in the virus particle (α-TIF, a γ protein), acting as a trans-activator, induces the transcription of the first set of mRNAs. A second component of the viral tegument called VHS inhibits host cell macromolecular synthesis, and all the metabolic energy of the cell is turned towards the production of new virus particles. The genes coding for the α, β and γ proteins have been mapped on the genome and, while the β and γ genes tend to be scattered, the α genes are located together. Amongst the early gene products are thymidine kinase and a virus-specific DNA polymerase. Most of the late proteins are structural proteins, and they inhibit the synthesis of the α and β proteins. Between β and γ protein synthesis, new viral DNA begins to be made, probably by circularization using a rolling circle model.

The replication of hepadnaviruses is unique amongst the double-stranded DNA viruses. Here the first stage, taking place in the nucleus, is the synthesis of single-stranded positive-sense RNA using the cellular DNA-dependent RNA polymerase. The RNA is transported into the cytoplasm and the core protein is translated which encapsidates the RNA, together with newly synthesized viral RNA-dependent DNA polmerase (reverse transcriptase – see below). Then, using this enzyme, a complementary negative strand of DNA is made, while the RNA is degraded. The DNA is next transcribed into positive-sense DNA, and is found as partially double-stranded DNA in the new virus particles.

## Class 2. Single-stranded DNA viruses

Parvoviruses comprise the sole family in this group. They are small, with DNA of molecular weight about $2 \times 10^6$. Some parvoviruses contain DNA of '−' polarity, and grow only in rapidly dividing cells; others contain either '+' or '−' DNA, and depend on co-infection with a helper virus for their replication. Parvoviruses use the cellular DNA polymerases to make the viral genome double stranded, called the replicative form. Priming is by the viral nucleic acid itself forming a loop at the 3′ terminus. This is followed by displacement of the parental DNA strand and synthesis of more DNA complementary to the template strand. Messenger RNAs are made using the appropriate DNA strand as the template, and are translated into viral proteins (Fig. 9.6).

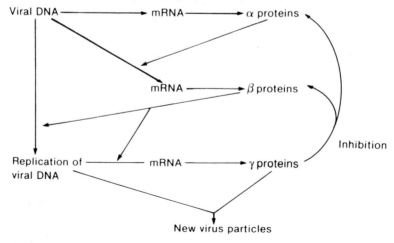

**Fig. 9.5** Diagram of macromolecular synthesis during the replication of herpes simplex virus.

**Fig. 9.6**   Diagram of parvovirus replication.

## Class 3. Double-stranded RNA viruses

In this group are found the reoviruses and rota-viruses. All members have segmented genomes, and each RNA segment codes for a single polypeptide. Replication of viral nucleic acid, transcription and translation occur solely in the cytoplasm without nuclear involvement at any stage. The virus carries its own RNA-dependent RNA polymerase, an enzyme unique to some RNA viruses and not found in uninfected cells. It enables the transcription of one strand (–) into mRNAs, subsequently translated into viral proteins. The transcription is thus asymmetric and conservative, i.e. only mRNAs are formed, and the parental duplex is not broken apart. Each mRNA is later encapsidated and copied once to form double-stranded molecules (Fig. 9.7). Several hours pass between the '+' and '–' strands of the new virus particles being synthesized. Thus the replication of the double-stranded DNA and RNA viruses is very different.

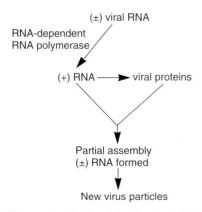

**Fig. 9.7**   Diagram of replication of double-stranded RNA virus.

## Class 4. '+' single-stranded RNA viruses

This class comprises a large group of viruses containing RNA of the same polarity as mRNA. Because they code for all the proteins they require during replication, the viral RNA extracted from the virions is infectious by itself. Poliovirus falls into this category, and is used as an example (Fig. 9.8). Macromolecular synthesis of viral components occurs entirely in the cytoplasm. Following entry of poliovirus into the cell, the viral RNA binds to ribosomes, acts as mRNA and is translated in its entirety into one large polypeptide. This is then proteolytically cleaved to give as products RNA polymerase and protease enzymes and new capsid proteins. Using the polymerase enzyme, '–'-strand RNA is synthesized with the genomic RNA as the template, and a temporary double-stranded RNA is formed, called the replicative intermediate. The replicative intermediate consists of complete '+' RNA and numerous partially completed '–' strands. When the '–' strands are ready, they can be used as templates to make more '+'-strand RNA. This is required as genomic RNA for assembly into new virus particles and for transcription into more viral proteins. At the same time as viral replication, host cell protein synthesis and RNA synthesis are inhibited. Initiation of translation of cellular mRNA requires the participation of a cap-binding protein at the 5′ end. Poliovirus induces the cleavage of this protein, and thus halts the synthesis of cellular proteins. The RNA genome of poliovirus does not have such a cap. Instead it has a small protein, called VPg, at the 5′ end which is required to initiate replication of the '+' or '–' form of RNA. VPg is not found on viral mRNA, implying that the translation machinery of the cell is modified to cope with translating this molecule without a cap. The capsid of poliovirus consists of 60 copies of each of four proteins, VP1, VP2, VP3 and VP4, forming the icosahedron. One of the first cleavages of the polyprotein produces VP1, which is then broken into VP0, VP3 and VP1. Finally, on assembly, VP0 is cleaved into VP4 and VP2, a process catalysed by VP0 itself.

## Class 5. '–' single-stranded RNA viruses

Viruses of this group have single-stranded RNA of '–' polarity, and all must carry their own RNA transcriptase complex to be infectious, as the normal cellular enzymes are unable to replicate RNA. Influenza virus is an example (Fig. 9.9). It contains eight segments of '–'-strand RNA, plus the

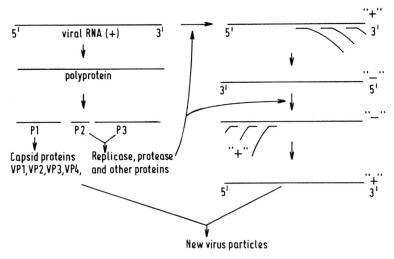

**Fig. 9.8** Diagram of poliovirus replication.

RNA transcriptase complex within each virus particle. After entry into the cell by receptor-mediated endocytosis, transcription to viral mRNA occurs in the nucleus. Influenza virus is the only '−'-strand RNA virus to replicate in the nucleus. To initiate transcription, a nucleotide sequence of about 10–13 bases, found at the 5′ end of the cellular mRNAs and already capped, is used. This is cleaved from cellular mRNAs by an endonuclease activity of the viral RNA transcriptase complex. Thus all the viral mRNAs have a 5′-terminal segment of the host cell mRNA. Once the mRNAs have been generated, they are translated into poly-peptides. Each genomic segment produces one mRNA, translated into one polypeptide except in two instances where, by RNA splicing of the original transcript, more than one mRNA is produced and therefore more than one protein. Unlike the transcription of mRNAs, the production of '+'-strand RNAs, required as intermediates to make the progeny '−'-strand RNAs, proceeds without the need for primers. There is much trafficking of viral polypeptides in the cell; the haemagglutinin, neuraminidase and $M_2$ protein are inserted in the plasma membrane, and the $M_1$ protein below this point on the membrane, while the nucleocapsid assembles around the viral RNAs in the nucleus.

## Class 6. Retroviruses

Viruses of this group are unique as they contain single-stranded RNA (in the form of two identical subunits), yet they replicate via an integrated double-stranded DNA stage. Retroviruses are the only such family and the virus particles contain a reverse transcriptase complex, with RNA-dependent DNA polymerase activity, from which the name 'retrovirus' is derived. This enzyme is not found in normal cells. Following entry, synthesis of DNA complementary to the viral RNA occurs using the

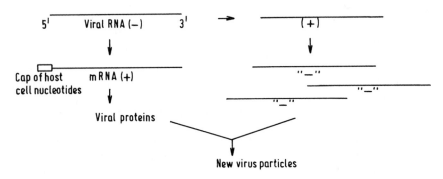

**Fig. 9.9** Diagram of influenza virus replication.

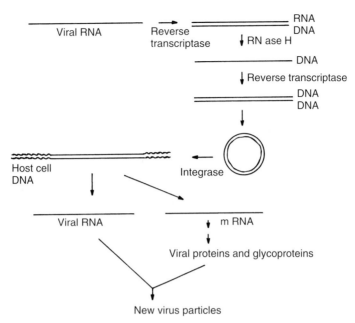

**Fig. 9.10**   Diagram of retrovirus replication.

reverse transcriptase, originating at a primer binding site near the 5′ end of the viral genome. The primer is a specific transfer RNA (tRNA); for example tRNA$^{lys}$ in human immunodeficiency virus. Transcription proceeds towards the 5′ end, and is probably continued by a jump across to the 3′ end of the same molecule. In addition to RNA-dependent DNA polymerase activity, the reverse transcriptase complex has ribonuclease (RNAase) H activity, i.e. it is able to digest RNA from a DNA–RNA hybrid (Fig. 9.10). The resulting single-stranded DNA is then made double stranded, using the reverse transcriptase as enzyme and starting from a purine-rich sequence. Thus, a linear double-stranded DNA form is produced, first found in the cytoplasm. The viral RNA has a short sequence of about 12–235 bases repeated at each end. During replication there is generation of a longer repeat sequence, from 250 to 1000 nucleotides, at both ends of the DNA molecule. This is called the long terminal repeat; it contains the enhancer and promoter sequences controlling the expression of the viral genome as well as the sequence for the initiation of transcription. The linear double-stranded DNA is able to circularize, and is found in this form in the nucleus. The next step is integration of the circular DNA into the host cell DNA. This is catalysed by an integrase carried by the virion. It is thought that the circular viral DNA is cleaved leaving staggered ends, and the cellular DNA similarly, to allow insertion of the viral DNA into the cellular DNA; the viral DNA is now called a provirus. The site of insertion is not thought to be specific. The provirus is colinear with the original viral genome, and is always flanked by a 4–6 base pair direct repeat of the host DNA: this repeat is also found flanking transposons. The integrated state is a stable one and, as the DNA of the cell is replicated during cell growth, so the viral DNA is also replicated. Integration can result, on occasion, in cell transformation (see below). The replication cycle is completed using the normal cellular RNA polymerase II to synthesize viral RNA and viral mRNAs, which are translated into polyproteins and processed into the final proteins found in the virus particle. A viral protease is responsible for many of these cleavages. The control of this stage is complex.

## Assembly and release

Following synthesis of viral proteins and viral nucleic acid, there is a stage of assembly called *morphogenesis*, followed by *release* of virus particles, the productive phase of the infection. The release is either through *cell lysis* or through *budding* without cell death in many instances. The former method is used by non-enveloped icosahedral viruses and the latter by enveloped viruses. There is also some recent evidence for active release without cell lysis for some non-enveloped viruses. Generally the com-

**Fig. 9.11** Budding of retroviruses. ×70 000.

ponents which will constitute the new virions are produced in high quantities, and the assembly process is probably rather inefficient.

Viruses which are released by killing the cell depend on the cell disintegrating to let them out. There is no specific mechanism for their egress. For this type of virus, morphogenesis may occur spontaneously once the capsid proteins have been made, the specificity depending on the amino acid sequence of the proteins. Thus the structural proteins of the viruses can form capsomeres by themselves which then aggregate to form the procapsid, a structure without nucleic acid. Often there is proteolytic cleavage of a capsid protein to form the final virus particle, as has been described for poliovirus. The precise nature of the interaction beween the nucleic acid and the structural proteins which make up the capsid is not known, despite extensive study. It is possible that the viral nucleic acid is inserted into the procapsid through a pore, or it might cause a structural re-orientation of the procapsid thereby becoming internalized. Alternatively the capsomeres may accumulate around a condensed core of nucleic acid as the nucleic acid is being synthesized.

The second method of assembly and release is by budding. This can take place through the plasma membrane, thus releasing the virions from the cell e.g. orthomyxoviruses and retroviruses (Fig. 9.11), or through internal membranes, such as the inner nuclear membrane in the case of the herpesviruses (Fig. 9.12b), followed by fusion of the vesicles con-

taining the viruses with the plasma membrane. Envelope glycoproteins specified by the virus are synthesized by essentially the same mechanism as cellular membrane glycoproteins. The viral proteins destined to become envelope proteins contain a sequence of 15–30 hydrophobic amino acids known as the signal sequence. This sequence binds the growing polypeptide chain to a receptor on the cytoplasmic side of the rough endoplasmic reticulum and enables its passage through the membrane. Glycosylation occurs in the lumen of the rough endo-plasmic reticulum, and the proteins are transported to the Golgi apparatus. There they are further glycosylated and acylated before transport to the plasma membrane, the direction probably deter-mined by a sorting signal in the polypeptide sequence. In some cases, the signal directs the viral glycoprotein to one surface of the cell only, e.g. orthomyxoviruses bud only from the outer (apical) surface of epithelial cells, while rhabdoviruses bud only from the inner (basal) surface. The viral glyco-proteins are very important in terms of antigenicity as the hydrophilic domains protrude from the surface of the cell, with the N terminus being furthest away, and change its surface structure significantly. They remain anchored in the membrane via a hydro-phobic domain near the carboxyl (C) terminus. After insertion into the membrane, the viral glycoproteins accumulate together to form oligomers; at the same time the host cell glycoproteins move away. At the C terminus there is frequently a short hydrophilic

**Fig. 9.12**  Effects of viruses on cells. **a** Light microscopy of a skin lesion due to herpesvirus to show cell fusion and intranuclear inclusions (Cowdry type A). ×60. **b** Electron micrograph of a cell infected with herpes simplex virus. Assembly of capsids within nucleus – enveloped virus between layers of nuclear membrane. ×9000. **c** Type A (accumulation of viral protein) and type B (virus factory) inclusions (identified as A and B, respectively) in the cytoplasm of a poxvirus-infected cell. V, virus; N, the cell nucleus. ×700.

sequence which remains inside the cell and is assumed to interact with the internal components of the virus during assembly. The nucleocapsid becomes engulfed by the membrane, forming a bud which matures and eventually pinches off. In some cases, a final cleavage of the glycoprotein is required to make the virus infectious. For example, the haemagglutinin $H_0$ of influenza virus is cleaved into two peptides, $HA_1$ and $HA_2$, linked by disulphide bridges.

Several thousand virus particles can be produced per infected cell, although this number varies considerably with virus type and host cell type. The budding viruses tend to be released slowly over several hours, while the lytic ones are released together. Only a few of the newly formed virus particles are infectious, as indicated by a high ratio of particles to infectious virions. Presumably most do not have the correct complement of proteins, enzymes or viral nucleic acid, or have been assembled incorrectly.

## Microscopy of infected cells

It is possible to observe effects on the host cell microscopically. In the first place there may be morphological changes called *inclusion bodies* in the infected cell, seen by altered staining behaviour. The inclusion bodies are nuclear or cytoplasmic and vary in their composition. They can consist of viral factories where morphogenesis occurs, crystalline arrays of virus particles ready for release, overproduction of a particular viral protein or proteins, or some aberrant cellular structure, such as clumped chromatin. Some inclusion bodies are shown in Figure 9.12. Secondly the cells may be killed by the viral infection. There are several possible reasons for this. It is likely that the accumulation of viral structural proteins is toxic for the cells in some cases. In addition, some viruses, such as herpes simplex virus and the poxviruses, inhibit host cell macromolecular synthesis from an early stage in the

**Fig. 9.13** Cytopathic effects: **a** uninfected fibroblast cells; **b** cell rounding due to herpes simplex virus; **c** syncytium formation or cell fusion due to respiratory syncytial virus. All unstained. ×65.

replication cycle which leads to structural and functional damage. Plasma membrane function and permeability change, and lysosomal membranes begin to break down, allowing leakage of the contents with degradative activity into the cytoplasm. There may also be marked effects on the cytoskeleton. These changes lead to a *cytopathic effect*, clearly seen in cell culture. It can take several forms, one of the commonest being *cell rounding* and subsequent detachment from the solid surface (Fig. 9.13b). Another is the formation of a *syncytium*, where the membranes of adjacent infected cells fuse and a giant cell is formed containing many nuclei (Fig. 9.13c). Also in some cases the nuclei fuse to make hybrid cells, a property which used to be exploited in monoclonal antibody production.

## NON-CYTOCIDAL PRODUCTIVE INFECTIONS

Some viruses are able to infect cells productively but the cells are not killed by the replication process. Viruses which are released by budding frequently come into this category. The cell type used for the infection is critical, and, presumably, any inhibitory effect of the virus on the cellular metabolism does not take place. This type of interaction may lead to a *persistent infection* in which infected cells and viruses coexist over a long period of time. There will, however, be antigenic changes in the infected cells, often the insertion of viral glycoproteins in the plasma membrane. This can be exploited for the detection of a virus; e.g. if influenza virus is cultured in monkey kidney cells, virus is produced from the cells but there is no immediate cytopathic effect. However, there is insertion of viral haemagglutinin into the plasma

membrane during replication. Thus if red blood cells of certain species are added to the infected cells, they adhere to the haemagglutinin and can be seen microscopically. This phenomenon is called *haemadsorption*.

## ABORTIVE (NON-PRODUCTIVE) INFECTIONS

Some viruses are unable to infect cells because they cannot adsorb to them; the cells are therefore called *resistant*. In other cases viruses are able to infect cells but are not produced from them; the infection is therefore called *non-productive* or *abortive*, and the cells are *non-permissive*. Often there is a block on one stage of the replication cycle due to the absence of a cellular function essential for viral replication. The same interaction can also occur in a permissive cell if the viral genome itself is *defective* in some way, so that the replication cannot be completed. This can happen in two ways. First the virus is too small to code for all the proteins required in replication. An example is provided by the adeno-associated viruses, belonging to the Parvoviridae family. They are unable to replicate on their own but depend on a second 'helper' virus infecting the same cell and providing the essential function which they lack. Adenoviruses act as the helper viruses and are thought to activate transcription of the parvovirus genome in the infected cell. Secondly, abortive infections can arise due to viral mutation. In fact only a few animo acid substitutions in selected proteins of the virus can change the nature of a lytic infection. In some cases the non-productive infection can be converted into a persistent one where new virus particles are synthesized: three examples follow.

## Temperature-sensitive mutants

Here the wild-type virus has mutated to produce a variant – a temperature-sensitive (ts) mutant – lacking an essential gene function at the *non-permissive temperature*, normally above 38°C. This is thought to be due to the thermal instability of the secondary or tertiary structure of a particular protein. The temperature can be lowered, generally to below 35°C, to a level called *permissive* where the defect is no longer functional and the infection becomes productive. However, ts mutants tend to be less cytopathic than the wild type, even at permissive temperatures, probably because they synthesize less mRNA and protein. Thus, within a cell culture, a persistent infection can result with a balance between infected and uninfected cells together with virus production. Ts mutants have been used to identify the gene responsible for a particular replication step and to map where functions lie on the viral genome. It is possible to place ts mutants into complementation groups where, at the non-permissive temperature, the defect in one ts mutant is compensated for by a second ts mutant with a defect in a different gene.

## Defective interfering particles

It has been known for many years that, if cells are infected at high multiplicity, then, amongst the progeny, there will be a number of virus particles with genomes shorter than normal, containing at least one deletion – so-called defective interfering particles (DIPs). Thus these particles are not able to replicate themselves although they are able to infect new cells. However, they can replicate in the presence of helper virus, often the parental virus, which compensates for the lack of a particular gene or gene cluster in the DIPs. The DIPs retain an origin of replication and the ability to form capsids. One of their important properties is that they *interfere* with the replication of normal parental viruses because, firstly, it requires less time and energy to replicate the defective genome compared with the full-length genome and, secondly, the transcriptase complex has a greater affinity for the defective genome than the full-length one. Hence DIPs, as their numbers increase, have a greater and greater effect on the replication of parental virus. It is possible to obtain an in-vitro cell culture in which infected and uninfected cells together with infectious virus and DIPs are in balance over a prolonged period of time. Thus a steady state exists and the infection is persistent.

## Abortive infections maintained by interferons

The final example of abortive infections arises due to the action of *interferons* in infected cell cultures. Interferons are produced from virally infected cells and can protect other cells from attack by viruses. These molecules, of α or β types, inhibit various stages of the viral replication cycle, especially polypeptide synthesis (see Ch. 12 for details). In cell culture, persistent infections can be obtained where the antiviral effects of interferons protect sufficient cells from the cytolytic effects of viral replication to allow cells and viruses to coexist.

## LATENCY

Latency represents a type of persistence where the virus is present in the form of its genome only and there is limited expression of viral genes, occasionally as mRNA only and not at the level of protein. The genome is found either integrated into the host cell chromosome or as a circular non-integrated episome. It is maintained throughout cell division when the host cell replicates. Latent infections are more common with DNA viruses than RNA viruses, perhaps because no mechanisms exist to maintain RNA for long periods of time intracellularly. One example of latency is provided by Epstein–Barr virus, which persists in B lymphocytes as episomal viral DNA with limited transcription of viral genes, probably around 11 protein products being expressed. In some cases specific stimuli trigger the *reactivation* of the virus from the latent state, and the infection becomes productive.

## TRANSFORMATION

In this type of virus–cell interaction, the virus infects the cell non-productively, and is found in the form of viral DNA, either integrated in the host cell DNA, or non-integrated, or in both states. The properties of the cells are changed dramatically, a process called *transformation*. Transformed cells have similar properties to tumour cells, and a detailed study of the mechanism of viral transformation has led to some understanding of the molecular basis of cancer. Only members of some virus families are able to tranform cells. These include herpesviruses, adenoviruses, hepadnaviruses, papovaviruses and poxviruses, of the DNA viruses, and, of the RNA viruses, only retroviruses. The type of cell infected and the species are also important. It should be noted that transformation is a rare event: at most only 1 in $10^5$ cells infected by a particular virus will become transformed.

Some of the main properties of transformed cells which distinguish them from normal cells are listed below:

1. Loss of contact inhibition of growth
2. High saturation density
3. Less requirement for serum factors
4. Indefinite number of cell divisions
5. Viral antigens expressed
6. Fibronectin absent
7. Fetal antigens often found
8. Changes in agglutinability by plant lectins
9. Induction of tumours in experimental animals.

One of the most striking changes is the loss of contact inhibition of growth, so that cells which normally grow in an ordered fashion beside their neighbours and stop dividing when they touch each other, now grow on top of each other and lose their orientation with respect to each other (Fig. 9.14). As a result they reach much higher densities. They have less requirements for serum factors in the medium and can be cultured in suspension without being attached to a solid surface (anchorage-independent). Normal cells have a limited number of cell divisions, called the Hayflick limit, which they can undergo in vitro before apoptosis, e.g. for cells taken from a human fetus it is around 60. Transformed cells no longer have this limit and thus can grow and divide indefinitely. There are many changes in the surface properties of transformed cells. Often viral-specific antigens are found, particularly ones synthesized early in the replication cycle. Fibronectin, a surface glycoprotein thought to be important in keeping cells together in a tissue or organ, is no longer found. Commonly fetal antigens are expressed and the agglutinability of cells by plant lectins changes, demonstrating alterations in the distribution of membrane glycoproteins. Finally, some transformed cells form tumours when injected into susceptible animals. Often these animals have to be immunocompromised in some way before tumours are produced, or the cells inserted into an immunologically protected site, such as the cheek pouch of the hamster. In addition, it is important to appreciate that by no means all transformed cells will form tumours. It is thought that there are degrees of transformation and that several stages have to be completed before the cells are fully transformed and equivalent to malignant tumour cells. Viral transformation may represent only the first step or a single step in such a pathway. There are no in-vitro markers which determine the degree of transformation; thus the potential ability of the transformed cell to produce

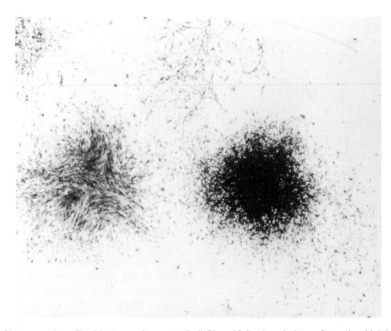

**Fig. 9.14** Colonies of human embryo fibroblasts growing normally (left) and following viral transformation (right).

tumours in experimental animals cannot be predicted, as yet.

All the viruses which cause transformation in vitro have a similar interaction with the host cell (Fig. 9.15). The initial stages are exactly as for the productive infections described earlier in this chapter. There is adsorption, penetration, uncoating and, in most but not all cases, selected viral genes are expressed as proteins, giving the cell new antigenic properties. At this stage the viral nucleic acid becomes integrated in the host cell DNA, probably not at a specific site, or it circularizes and is maintained in a non-integrated episomal form in the nucleus. The association is a stable one, so that when the host cell DNA is replicated, the viral nucleic acid is also replicated and the number of viral genome copies per cell remains constant over many cell generations. Thus, transformation is a heritable alteration. With some viruses, such as Epstein–Barr virus and the papovaviruses, the whole viral genome is normally integrated, while with others, such as herpes simplex virus and adenoviruses, only part is integrated, and the remainder is lost.

Recent work in this area has concentrated on the molecular events surrounding transformation and in analysing the functions of the viral proteins found in transformed cells. Two examples of transforming viruses, one RNA and the other DNA, are briefly described now to illustrate the approaches taken. Both are associated with human tumours.

The first is human T lymphotropic or T cell leukaemia virus type I (HTLV-I), a retrovirus, which is found in CD4$^+$ T cells of patients with adult T cell leukaemia. It is able to transform CD4$^+$ lymphocytes in vitro with integration of the DNA provirus. Genetic analysis has revealed that the viral genome can code for several non-structural proteins including one of special interest called Tax, of molecular weight 40 kDa. This protein, which has no cellular homologue, is able to activate transcription in the long terminal repeat of the integrated virus. It may also activate transcription of cellular genes at more distant sites, including the genes for interleukin-2 and the interleukin-2 receptor. Interleukin-2 is an important cytokine, and increasing its expression, plus that of its receptor, may have profound implications for the control of T cell activation.

The second example is human papillomavirus type 16 (HPV-16), found as integrated DNA in many cases of carcinoma of the cervix. In vitro this virus is able to transform most types of human epithelial cells including keratinocytes. The viral genes responsible for transformation are the products of two genes, E6 and E7: E6 protein interacts with p53, and E7 with retinoblastoma protein, thereby inactivating them. As both p53 and retinoblastoma protein act as cellular growth-suppressing proteins, loss of their functions is likely to lead to transformation. In addition, integration of the viral genome normally involves the disruption of the E2 gene, the product of which is required to stop transcription of the E6 and E7 promoter.

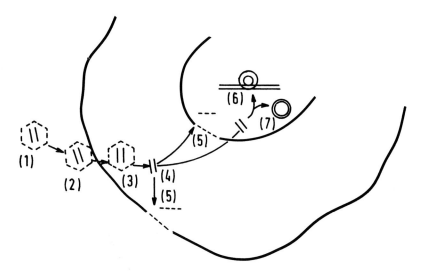

**Fig. 9.15** A simplified diagram showing the events of viral transformation. The hypothetical virus (1) adsorbs (2), penetrates (3), is uncoated (4), and usually some early viral proteins are synthesized (5) followed by integration of the viral genome in the host cell DNA (6) or formation of a circular non-integrated genomic DNA (7).

**Table 9.2** Site of action of available and potential antiviral agents

| Stage of replication | Potential antiviral target | Example |
|---|---|---|
| Attachment | Block virion attachment<br>Down-regulation of cellular receptor | Antibody to virion binding site<br>Antibody to cell receptor |
| Penetration/uncoating | Stabilize viral capsid in endosome<br>Inhibit uncoating | Amantadine<br>WIN compounds (disoxaril, arildone, rhodanine) |
| Viral nucleic acid synthesis | RNA and DNA polymerase inhibitors and chain terminators | Nucleoside analogues (acyclovir, vidarabine, zidovudine, famciclovir, tribavirin), foscarnet |
| Transcription/RNA genomes | Anti-sense oligonucleotides<br>Anti-gene oligonucleotides<br>Decoy RNA (corresponding to regulatory region)<br>Ribozymes | |
| Translation/protein processing | Capping inhibitors<br>Translation inhibitors<br>Inhibitors of glycosylation and myristylation<br>Proteolytic cleavage inhibitors | Interferons<br>Castanospermine, myristic acid analogues<br>Saquinavir, ritonavir |
| Virion assembly | Nucleocapsid assembly<br>Budding | Transdominant mutant proteins<br>Amantadine |

**Fig. 9.16** Structures of some antiviral agents: **a** amantadine, **b** disoxaril, **c** vidarabine, **d** acyclovir, **e** zidovudine, **f** tribavirin, **g** phosphonoformic acid (foscarnet).

# AGENTS WHICH INTERFERE WITH THE REPLICATION OF VIRUSES

While one of the major advances in medicine this century has been the development of antibiotics to combat bacterial infections, the same cannot be said of antiviral agents. Since viruses are totally dependent on their host cells, it has proved difficult to obtain inhibitory agents which will not also adversely affect the normal functions of the cells. However, selected stages of the replication cycle are potentially vulnerable to inhibition by suitable agents (Table 9.2), and a few effective compounds are in clinical use (see Ch. 5, pp 53–4). One major impetus to the development of novel antiviral agents has been the HIV pandemic, and, in addition, there is increasing awareness of the importance of persistent viral infections in human health. Thus, many approaches are being evaluated currently and rapid progress is anticipated. Table 9.2 indicates the different stages of the growth cycle that may be blocked and lists those compounds effective at each stage. The chemical structures of some of them are illustrated in Figure 9.16.

## RECOMMENDED READING

Ansardi D, Porter D C, Anderson M J, Morrow C D 1996 Poliovirus assembly and encapsidation of genomic RNA. *Advances in Virus Research* 46: 1–68

Bangham C R, Kirkwood T B 1993 Defective interfering particles and virus evolution. *Trends in Microbiology* 1: 260–264

Dalgleish A G 1991 Viruses and cancer. *British Medical Bulletin* 47: 21–46

de la Torre J C, Oldstone M B A 1996 Anatomy of viral persistence: mechanisms of persistence and associated diseases. *Advances in Virus Research* 46: 311–343

Fields D N, Knipe D M, Howley P M (eds) 1996 *Virology*, 3rd edn. Lippencott-Raven, Philadelphia

Gaudin Y, Ringrok R W H, Brunner J 1995 Low-pH induced conformational changes in viral fusion proteins: implications for the fusion mechanism. *Journal of General Virology* 76: 1541–1556

Greber U F, Singh I, Helenius A 1994 Mechanism of virus uncoating. *Trends in Microbiology* 2: 52056

Harper D R 1994 *Molecular Virology*. BIOS Scientific, Oxford

Hay J, Ruyechan W T 1992 Regulation of herpes simplex virus type 1 gene expression. *Current Topics in Microbiology and Immunology* 179: 1–14

Haywood A M 1994 Virus receptors: binding, adhesion strengthening, and changes in viral structure. *Journal of Virology* 68: 1–5

Hobman T C 1993 Targeting of viral glycoproteins to the Golgi complex. *Trends in Microbiology* 1: 124–130

Nomoto A, Kioke S, Aoki J 1994 Tissue tropism and species specificity of poliovirus infection. *Trends in Microbiology* 2: 47–51

zur Hausen H, de Villiers E-M 1994 Human papillomaviruses. *Annual Review of Microbiology* 45: 927–433

# Part 2
## INFECTION AND IMMUNITY

# 10

# Antigens

*J. Stewart and D. M. Weir*

An antigen is any substance capable of provoking the lymphoid tissues of an animal to respond by generating an immune reaction specifically directed at the inducing substance and not at other unrelated substances. The response is not to the entire molecule but to individual chemical groups that will have a specific three-dimensional shape. The specificity of the response to these *antigenic determinants* or *epitopes* is an important characteristic of immune responses. The reaction of an animal to contact with antigen, called the *acquired immune response*, takes two forms, (1) the *humoral* or *circulating antibody response* and (2) the *cell-mediated response*, and their characteristics are described in Chapter 11. Most of the information available on the specificity of the immune response comes from studies of the interaction of circulating antibody with antigen. An antibody directed against an epitope of a particular molecule will react only with this determinant or other very similar structures. Even minor chemical changes in the conformation of the epitope will markedly reduce the ability of the original antibody to react with the altered material.

The term 'antigen', referring to substances either acting as stimulants of the immune response or reacting with antibody, is used rather loosely by immunologists. Use is made of the functional classification of antigens into (1) substances that are able to generate an immune response by themselves, which are termed *immunogens*, and (2) molecules that are able to react with antibodies but are unable to stimulate their production directly. The latter substances are often low molecular weight chemicals, termed *haptens*, that will react with preformed antibodies but only become immunogenic when attached to large molecules, called *carriers*. The hapten forms an epitope on the carrier molecule that is recognized by the immune system and stimulates the production of antibody. In other words, the ability of a chemical grouping to interact with an antibody is not enough to stimulate an immune response. As we will see later, when discussing the sites on molecules recognized by cells of the immune system, all antigens can be considered to be composed of haptens on larger carrier structures.

## GENERAL PROPERTIES OF ANTIGENS

A substance that acts as an antigen in one species of animal may not do so in another if it is represented in the tissues or fluids of the second species. This underlines the requirement that an antigen must be a foreign substance to elicit an immune response. For example, egg albumin, whilst an excellent antigen in rabbit, fails to induce an antibody response in fowl. The more foreign and evolutionarily distant a substance is to a particular species, the more likely it is to be a powerful antigen.

A widely recognized requirement for a substance to be antigenic in its own right, without having to be attached to a carrier molecule, is that it should have a molecular weight in excess of 5000. It is, however, possible to induce an immune response to substances of lower molecular weight. For example, glucagon (molecular weight of 3800) can stimulate antibody production but only if special measures are taken such as the use of an *adjuvant* which gives an additional stimulus to the immune system. Very large proteins, such as the crustacean respiratory pigment haemocyanin, are very powerful antigens and are widely used in experimental immunology. Polysaccharides vary in antigenicity, e.g. dextran with a molecular weight of 600 000 is a good antigen, whereas dextran with a molecular weight of 100 000 is not.

Some low molecular weight chemical substances appear to contradict the requirement that an antigen be large. Among these are picryl chloride, formaldehyde and drugs such as aspirin, penicillin and sulphonamides. These substances are highly antigenic, particularly if applied to the skin. The reason for this appears to be that such materials form complexes by means of covalent bonds with tissue proteins. The complex of such a substance, acting as a hapten, with a tissue protein acting as a carrier, forms a complete antigen. This phenomenon has important implications in the development of certain types of hypersensitivity (see Ch. 11).

## ANTIGENIC DETERMINANTS

The immune system does not recognize an infectious agent or foreign molecule as a whole but reacts to structurally distinct areas – antigenic determinants or epitopes. Thus, exposure to a micro-organism will generate an immune response to many different epitopes. The antiserum produced will contain different antibodies reactive with each determinant. This will ensure that an individual will be protected from the micro-organism by producing a response to at least a few of the possible determinants. If the host only reacted to the organism as a whole then failure to react to this one site would have dire consequences, i.e. it would not be able to eliminate the pathogen. Certain antibodies may react with an epitope composed of residues that can also be part of two other epitopes recognized by different antibodies (Fig. 10.1).

A response to antigen involves the specific interaction of components of the immune system, antibodies and lymphocytes, with epitopes on the antigen. The lymphocytes have receptors on their surface that function as the recognition units – on B lymphocytes surface-bound immunoglobulin is the receptor and on T lymphocytes the recognition unit is known as the T cell receptor. The interaction between an antibody (or cell-bound receptor) and antigen is governed by the complementarity of the electron cloud surrounding the determinants. The overall configuration of the outer electrons, not the chemical nature of the constituent residues, determines the shape of the epitope and its complementary *paratope* (the part of the antibody or T cell

receptor that interacts with the epitope). The better the fit between the epitope and the paratope the stronger the non-covalent bonds formed and consequently the higher the affinity of the interaction.

Antigenic determinants have to be topographical, i.e. composed of structures on the surface of molecules, and can be constructed in two ways. They may be contained within a single segment of primary sequence or assembled from residues far apart in the primary sequence but brought together on the surface by the folding of the molecule into its native conformation. The former are known as *sequential* epitopes, and those formed from distant residues are *conformational* epitopes. The antigenic structures seen by antibody depend on the tertiary configuration of the immunogen (conformational), while epitopes seen by T cells are defined by the primary structure (sequential).

## ANTIGENIC SPECIFICITY

Foreignness of a substance to an animal can depend on the presence of chemical groupings that are not normally found in the animal's body. Arsenic acid, for example, can be chemically introduced into a protein molecule and, as a hapten, acts as a determinant of antigenic specificity of the molecule. There are many other examples where antibodies are able to distinguish subtle chemical differences between molecules. Thus, antisera can distinguish between glucose and galactose, which differ only by the interchange of a hydrogen atom and a hydroxyl group on one carbon atom.

The ability of antibody (or T cell receptors) to form a high-affinity interaction with an antigen depends on intermolecular forces which act strongly only when the two molecules come together in a very precise manner. The better the fit, the stronger the bond. An antibody molecule directed against a particularly shaped antigenic determinant might be able to react with another similar but not quite identical determinant, as shown in Figure 10.2. This type of cross-reaction does occur but the

**Fig. 10.1** Overlapping epitopes. Two epitopes (1 and 2) on an antigen induce the formation of three antibodies (A, B and C).

**Fig. 10.2** Specificity and cross-reactions. Antibody produced in response to an antigen that contains epitope 1 will also combine with epitope 2.

strength of the bond between the two molecules will be diminished in the case of the less well-fitting determinant.

A common source of confusion concerning the specificity of antibodies arises when an antibody to a particular antigen is found to be capable of combining with an apparently unrelated antigen. For example, glucose residues are present in many different types of molecule, and an antibody that binds to a glucose determinant in antigen X–glucose would be likely to react with the glucose group in antigen Y–glucose provided the two determinants are equally accessible. The antibody directed against the glucose determinant is not a non-specific type of antibody but is simply reacting with an identical chemical determinant in another antigen molecule.

In laboratory practice, cross-reactivity is often found between antisera to certain bacterial antigens and antigens present on cells such as erythrocytes. Antigens shared in this way are known as *heterophile antigens*. The best known of the heterophile antigens is the Forssman antigen, which is present on the red cells of many species as well as in bacteria such as pneumococci and salmonellae. Another heterophile antigen is found in *Escherichia coli* and human red cells of blood group B individuals. These cross-reactivities are probably responsible for the generation of antibodies found in individuals of a certain blood group that bind to the red blood cells of individuals of a different blood group. These antibodies are known as *isohaemagglutinins* because they are able to bind the red blood cells and clump them together, i.e. cause agglutination.

## IMMUNOGLOBULINS

Towards the end of the 19th century, von Behring and Kitasato in Berlin found that the blood serum of an appropriately immunized animal contained specific neutralizing substances or antitoxins. This was the first demonstration of the activity of what are now known as *antibodies* or *immunoglobulins*. Antibodies are glycoproteins, present in the serum and body tissues, that are induced when immunogenic molecules are introduced into the host's lymphoid system. They bind specifically to the antigen that induced their formation.

The liquid collected from blood that has been allowed to clot is known as *serum*. It contains a number of molecules but no cells or clotting factors. If serum is prepared from an animal that has been

**Fig. 10.3** Separation of serum proteins by electrophoresis.

exposed to an antigen then it is known as an *antiserum* since it will contain antibodies reactive to the inducing antigen. When the components of serum are separated electrophoretically then the heterogeneity of immunoglobulins can be seen, i.e. they appear as broad bands (Fig. 10.3). This technique separates serum components into various fractions, labelled α, β and γ. Most of the antibody molecules are present within the γ fraction, and they are sometimes referred to as γ-globulins.

There are five distinct *classes* or *isotypes* of immunoglobulins, namely IgG, IgA, IgM, IgD and IgE. They differ from each other in size, charge, carbohydrate content and, of course, amino acid composition (Table 10.1). Within certain classes there are subclasses that vary slightly in structure and function. These classes and subclasses can be separated from each other serologically, i.e. using antibody. If injected into the correct species they will induce the formation of antibodies that can be used to differentiate between the different isotypes.

### Antibody structure

All antibody molecules have the same basic four-chain structure composed of two light chains and two heavy chains (Fig. 10.4). The light chains (molecular weight of 25 000) are one of two types designated κ and λ and only one type is found in one antibody. The heavy chains vary in molecular weight from 50 000 to 70 000, and it is these chains that determine the isotype. They are designated α, δ, ε, γ and μ for the respective classes of immunoglobulin (Table 10.1). The individual chains are held together by disulphide bridges and non-covalent interactions.

**Table 10.1** Physicochemical properties of human immunoglobulins. The immunoglobulin serotype is determined by the type of heavy chain present. The different characteristics observed are also controlled by the heavy chain. Variation within a class gives rise to subclasses

| Characteristic | Immunoglobulin isotype | | | | |
| --- | --- | --- | --- | --- | --- |
| | IgA[a] | IgD | IgE | IgG | IgM[b] |
| Mean serum concentration (mg/dl) | 300 | 5 | 0.005 | 1400 | 150 |
| Mass (kDa) | 160 | 184 | 188 | 160 | 970 |
| Carbohydrate (%) | 7–11 | 9–14 | 12 | 2–3 | 12 |
| Half-life (days) | 6 | 3 | 2 | 21 | 5 |
| Heavy chain | $\alpha$ | $\delta$ | $\varepsilon$ | $\gamma$ | $\mu$ |

[a]IgA is also found as a dimer, and in secretions IgA is present in dimeric form associated with a protein known as secretory component.
[b]Data for IgM as a pentamer.

**Fig. 10.4** Basic structure of an immunoglobulin molecule. See text for details.

When individual light chains are studied it is found that they are composed of two distinct areas or *domains* of approximately 110 amino acids. One end of the chain is identical in all members of the same isotype, and is termed the constant region of the light chain, $C_L$. The other end shows considerable sequence variation, and is known as the variable region, $V_L$. The heavy chains are also split into domains of approximately the same size, the number varying between the five types of heavy chain. One of these domains will show considerable sequence variation ($V_H$) while the others ($C_H$) are similar for the same isotype. The tertiary structure generated by the combination of the $V_L$ and $V_H$ regions determines the shape of the antigen-combining site or paratope. Since the two light and

two heavy chains are identical, each antibody unit will have two identical paratopes situated at the amino (*N*)-terminal end of the molecule that recognize the antigen. The carboxyl (C)-terminal end of the antibody will be the same for all members of the same class or subclass, and is involved in the biological activities of the molecule. The area of the heavy chains between the $C_H1$ and $C_H2$ domains contains a varying number of interchain disulphide bonds and is known as the *hinge region*. A number of enzymes cleave immunoglobulins at distinct points to generate different peptide fragments. Using these enzymes, antibodies can be divided into a Fab region ('fragment antigen binding') containing the paratope and an Fc region ('fragment crystallizable') that is similar for all antibodies of the same isotype.

Despite the differences between the various isotypes, as shown in Table 10.1, all antibody molecules are composed of the same basic unit structure, with the Fab portion containing the antigen-recognizing paratope and the Fc region carrying out the activities that protect the host, i.e. effector functions. The differences seen in the Fc region between the various heavy chains are responsible for the different biological activities of the antibody isotypes.

## IgG

This is the major immunoglobulin of serum, making up 75% of the total and having a molecular weight of 150 000 in humans. Four subclasses are found in humans – IgG1, IgG2, IgG3 and IgG4 – that differ in their relative concentrations, amino acid composition, number and position of interchain disulphide bonds and biological function. IgG is the major antibody of the secondary response (see Ch. 11) and is found in both the serum and tissue fluids.

## IgA

In man, most of the serum IgA occurs as a monomer, but in many other mammals it is mostly found as a dimer. The dimer is held together by a J chain, which is produced by the antibody-producing plasma cells. IgA is the predominant antibody class in seromucous secretions such as saliva, tears, colostrum and respiratory, gastro-intestinal and genito-urinary secretions. This secretory IgA (sIgA) is always in the dimeric form and is composed of two basic four-chain units (two light chains and two heavy chains), a J chain and the secretory component. The secretory component is part of the molecule that transports the dimer produced by a submucosal plasma cell to the mucosal surface (Fig. 10.5). It not only facilitates passage through the epithelial cells but protects the secreted molecule from proteolytic digestion. There are two subclasses of IgA – IgA1 and IgA2.

## IgM

IgM is a pentamer of the basic unit with μ heavy chains and a single J chain. Because of its large size this isotype is mainly confined to the intravascular

pool, and is the first antibody type to be produced during an immune response.

## IgD

Many circulating B cells have IgD present on their surface, but it accounts for less than 1% of the circulating antibody. It is composed of the basic unit with δ heavy chains. The protein is very susceptible to proteolytic attack and therefore has a very short half-life in serum.

## IgE

The IgE is present in extremely low levels in the serum. However, it is found on the surface of mast cells and basophils, which possess a receptor specific for the Fc part of this molecule.

## Antigen binding

The variability in amino acid sequence in the variable domains of light and heavy chains is not found over their entire length but is restricted to short segments. These segments show considerable variation, and are termed *hypervariable regions*. Hypervariable regions are now known to contain the residues that make direct contact with the antigen, and are referred to as *complementarity determining regions* (CDRs). Although the remaining *framework* residues do not come into direct contact with the antigen, they are essential for the formation of the correct tertiary structure of the variable domain and maintenance of the integrity of the binding site. In both light and heavy chains there are three CDRs which, in combination, form the paratope.

The antigen and antibody are held together by various individually weak non-covalent inter-actions. However, the formation of a large number of hydrogen bonds and electrostatic, van der Waals and hydrophobic interactions leads to a consider-able binding energy. These attractive forces are only active over extremely short distances and therefore the epitope and paratope must have complementary structures to enable them to combine. If the electron clouds overlap or residues of similar charge are brought together then repulsive forces will come into play. The balance of attraction against repulsion will dictate the strength of the interaction between an antibody and a particular antigen, i.e. the affinity of the antibody for the antigen.

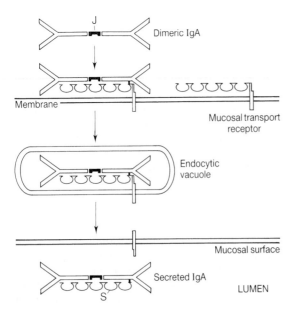

**Fig. 10.5** Transport of secretory IgA. J, J chain; S, secretory component.

## Antibody diversity

It is now known that an antigen selects from the available antibodies those that can combine with its epitopes. It therefore follows that an individual must have an extremely large number of different antibodies to cope with the vast array of different antigens present in the environment.

### Immunoglobulin variability

The paratope is produced by the CDRs of the light and heavy chains generating a specific three-dimensional shape. Any light chain can join with any heavy chain to produce a different paratope. Thus, theoretically, with $10^4$ different light chains and $10^4$ different heavy chains, $10^8$ different specificities could be generated.

The germ-line DNA is the structure of the gene as it is inherited. All cells in the body contain all the inherited genes but different genes become active in different cells at different times. Within B lymphocytes, the cells that differentiate to antibody-producing plasma cells, the functional immunoglobulin genes are formed by gene rearrangements and recombinations. These events give rise to the production of different variable domains in each B lymphocyte. Once a functional gene has been constructed no other rearrangements are allowed to take place within this cell. This dictates that one particular cell will produce antibodies with an identical antigen-combining site and is known as *allelic exclusion*. There is evidence that the gene segments for the variable region of immunoglobulins are particularly susceptible to mutations. This can lead to subtle changes in specificity and/or affinity that are important as an immune response develops (see Ch. 11).

When a B lymphocyte is first stimulated by antigen it will produce IgM. As the immune response develops, the class of antibody changes. However, the immunoglobulin produced will have the same variable domain and therefore bind to the same antigen. All that is altered, or *switched*, is the heavy chain constant region. Thus the progeny of a single B cell will produce different immunoglobulin isotypes as the response to a particular antigen develops, but each will have the same paratope.

## Secreted and membrane immunoglobulins

At different stages in its development a B cell will produce immunoglobulins that have to be inserted into the membrane or secreted. The membrane-bound immunoglobulin will be used as the antigen receptor of the B cell and a cell that binds antigen through this molecule will then secrete immunoglobulin of the same specificity. The only difference between the two types of antibody is to be found at the C terminus, where the membrane form has an additional part, the transmembrane portion.

## Antibody function

Knowledge gained from the structural studies discussed above has gone some way towards an understanding of the biological activities of the immunoglobulin molecule.

The primary function of an antibody is to bind the antigen that induced its formation. Apart from cases where this results in direct neutralization (e.g. inhibition of toxin activity or of microbial attachment) other effector functions must be generated. The binding of antigen is mediated by the Fab portion, and the Fc region controls the biological defence mechanisms. For every antibody the paratope will be different, and it will therefore recognize different epitopes. However, for every antibody of the same

**Table 10.2** Biological properties of human immunoglobulins. These activities are determined by the Fc portion of the molecules

| Function | Immunoglobulin isotype | | | | | | | |
|---|---|---|---|---|---|---|---|---|
| | IgA | IgD | IgE | IgG1 | IgG2 | IgG3 | IgG4 | IgM |
| Complement fixation | ±[a] | − | − | ++ | + | +++ | − | +++ |
| Placental transfer | − | − | − | + | ± | + | + | − |
| Binding to phagocytes | ±[b] | − | − | +++ | ± | +++ | + | − |
| Binding to mast cells | − | − | +++ | − | − | − | + | − |

[a]IgA will activate the alternative pathway.
[b]Receptors for the Fc portion of IgA have been found on neutrophils and alveolar macrophages.

isotype the heavy chain constant domains will be the same, and they will therefore all perform the same functions (Table 10.2).

## Neutralization

The fact that antibodies are at least divalent means that they can form a complex with multivalent antigen. Depending on the physical nature of the antigen these *immune complexes* exist in various forms (Fig. 10.6). If the antibody is directed against surface antigens of particulate material such as micro-organisms or erythrocytes then *agglutination* will occur. This is a clump or aggregate that will isolate the potential pathogen, stop its dissemination and stimulate its removal by other mechanisms. If the antigen is soluble then the size of the complex will determine its physical state. Small complexes will remain soluble while large complexes will form *precipitates*.

As might be expected from knowledge of the structure of IgM, its 10 combining sites make it a very efficient agglutinating antibody molecule. Rabbit IgM has been shown to be more than 20 times as active as IgG in bringing about bacterial agglutination. Because of its size, IgM is largely

(a)   (b)

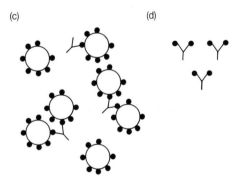

(c)   (d)

**Fig. 10.6**   Immune complex formation: **a** antibody excess; **b** equivalence; **c** antigen excess; **d** monovalent antigen.

confined to the bloodstream and probably plays an important role in protecting against blood invasion by micro-organisms. Certain sites on micro-organisms are critical to the establishment of an infection. Antibody bound to these sites will interfere with attachment processes and could, therefore, stop infection by the microbe. The binding of an antibody to functionally important residues in a toxin will neutralize their harmful effects.

## Complement activation

The activation of the complement system is one of the most important antibody effector mechanisms. The complement cascade is a complex group of serum proteins that mediate inflammatory reactions and cell lysis. It is discussed more fully in Chapter 11. The Fc portion of certain isotypes (Table 10.2), once antigen has been bound, will activate complement; this requires that C1q, a subunit of the first complement component, cross-links two antibody Fc portions. For this to happen the two regions must be in close proximity. It has been calculated that a single IgM molecule is 1000 times more efficient than IgG. This is because two IgG molecules must be close together for complement activation. A large number of IgG molecules would be required for this to occur if the epitopes are spread. Not all isotypes activate complement, presumably because they do not have the required amino acid sequence, and therefore tertiary structure, in the Fc portion. C1q binds to residues in the $C_H3$ domain of IgM and the $C_H2$ domain of IgG. Some isotypes when interacting with antigen can activate the alternative pathway of complement that does not use C1 but gives rise to the same biological activities.

## Cell binding and opsonization

The Fc portion of certain immunoglobulin isotypes is able to interact with various cell types (Table 10.2). Antibodies specific for particular antigens, such as bacteria, play a valuable role by binding to the surface and making the antigen more susceptible to phagocytosis and subsequent elimination. This process is known as *opsonization*, and is again mediated by the Fc portion of the antibody. A specific conformation on the Fc region of certain isotypes is recognized by *Fc receptors* on the surface of the phagocyte. The important residues are in the $C_H2$ domain near the hinge region. Individually, the interactions are not strong enough to signal the uptake of the antibody molecule; therefore, free immunoglobulin is not internalized. However, when an antigen is coated by many antibody molecules then summation of all the interactions stimulates phagocytosis or other effector mechanisms.

Certain phagocytic cells have receptors for activated complement components, *complement receptors*. If the binding of antibody to the antigen can activate the complement cascade then various complement components will be deposited on the antigen–antibody complex. Phagocytic cells that have receptors for these complement components will then ingest the complexes.

The above-mentioned processes require that the antibody is first complexed with antigen. However, certain cell types will bind free antibody. Mast cells and basophils have Fc receptors that are specific for IgE. These cells perform a protective function but are also involved in hypersensitivity reactions described in Chapter 11. In humans, IgG has the ability to cross the placenta and reach the fetal circulation. This is a passive process involving specific Fc receptors. This route is limited to primates whereas, in ruminants, immunoglobulin from colostrum is absorbed through the intestinal epithelium. Another Fc-mediated mechanism, already described, is the selective transport of IgA into mucosal secretions.

## ANTIGEN RECOGNITION

The immune system has evolved to protect us from potentially harmful material but it must not respond to self molecules. Two separate recognition systems are present: humoral immunity and cell-mediated immunity. Antibody is the recognition molecule of humoral immunity. This glycoprotein is produced by plasma cells and circulates in the blood and other body fluids. Antibody is also present on the surface of B lymphocytes. The interaction of this surface immunoglobulin with its specific antigen is responsible for the differentiation of these cells into plasma cells. Antibody molecules, whether free or on the surface of a B cell, will recognize free native antigen. This contrasts dramatically with the situation in cell-mediated immunity; the T lymphocyte antigen receptor will only bind to fragments of antigen that are associated with products of the *major histocompatibility complex* (MHC). T cell recognition of antigen is said to be *MHC restricted*. These MHC products are present on the surface of cells, therefore T cells only recognize cell-associated antigens. This MHC-restricted recognition mechanism has evolved because of the functions carried out by T lymphocytes. Some T cells produce immuno-regulatory molecules, *lymphokines*, some of which influence the activities of host cells and others that directly kill infected or foreign cells. Therefore, it would be inefficient or dangerous to produce these effects in response to either free antigen or antigen sitting idly on some cell membrane. The joint recognition of MHC molecules and antigen ensures that the T cell makes contact with antigen on the surface of the appropriate target cell.

## B cell receptor

Antibody is found free in body fluids and as a transmembrane protein on the surface of B lymphocytes, i.e. surface immunoglobulin, where it acts as the B cell antigen receptor. The antibody present on the surface of the B cell is exactly the same molecule as will be secreted when the cell develops into a plasma cell except for the extreme C-terminal end as described above. It should be noted that the molecules present on the cell surface are present as monomers even though they are secreted in a polymeric form.

## T cell receptor

The complex on T lymphocytes that is involved in antigen recognition is composed of a number of glycoprotein structures. Some of these molecules have been systematically named by CD (cluster of differentiation) nomenclature using antibodies. These generic names will be used in preference to other symbols sometimes found in the literature.

The T cell antigen receptor is a heterodimer composed of an $\alpha$ and a $\beta$ or a $\gamma$ and a $\delta$ chain. Each chain contains a variable and constant domain, transmembrane portion and cytoplasmic tail. The variable domain folds to form a paratope that will interact with antigenic peptides that are associated with MHC molecules on a cell surface. The majority of T cells use the $\alpha/\beta$ heterodimer in antigen recognition. The role of cells that possess the $\gamma/\delta$ molecules is unknown but they may be involved in the immune response to particular types of antigens at specific anatomical sites. The T cell receptor is the molecule that is responsible for the recognition of specific MHC–antigen complexes and will be different for every T cell. Genetic rearrangements of germ-line genes, similar to those seen in B cells, produce functional T cell receptors.

CD3 is present on all T cells and is non-covalently linked to the T cell receptor. The CD3 complex is thought to be involved in signal transduction, leading to cell activation, when a ligand binds to the T cell receptor.

CD4 and CD8 are mutually exclusive molecules. They are present on T cells that are restricted in their recognition of antigen by MHC class II and class I molecules, respectively. Due to their almost exclusive correlation with a specific MHC class it is thought that these molecules bind to non-polymorphic determinants on the MHC molecules. This interaction could stabilize the binding of the T cell receptor to the MHC–antigen complex or it may in fact have a co-receptor function. In the former case the CD4 or CD8 molecule could interact with the same MHC molecule as the T cell receptor or with a different one and this interaction does not generate a stimulatory signal, i.e. it solely stabilizes the specific interaction (T cell receptor with antigen–MHC). In the latter case the T cell receptor and CD4 or CD8 bind to the same MHC molecule but at different sites, and the joint signal that is generated leads to the stimulation of the T cell.

## MAJOR HISTOCOMPATIBILITY COMPLEX

The MHC is part of the genome that codes for molecules that are important in immune recognition – including interactions between lymphoid cells and other cell types. It is also involved in the rejection of allografts. The MHCs of a number of species have been studied but most is known about those of the mouse and humans.

The gene complex contains a large number of individual genes that can be grouped into three classes on the basis of structure and function of their products. The products of the genes are sometimes referred to as *MHC antigens* because they were first defined by serological analysis, i.e. using antibodies.

The MHC of humans is known as *human leucocyte group A* (HLA), and in mice it is referred to as *histocompatibility-2* (H-2).

## Gene organization

The genes that code for the HLA antigens are found on the short arm of chromosome 6. They are arranged over a region of between 2000 and 4000 kilobases in size containing enough DNA for over 200 genes. The MHC genes are contained within regions known as A, B, C and D (Fig. 10.7). MHC class I molecules consist of two non-covalently associated polypeptide chains. A single gene that codes for the larger chain is present in the A, B and C regions while the lighter chain, known as $\beta_2$-microglobulin, is coded for elsewhere in the genome. The class II molecules are composed of two chains, both of which are coded for within the D region. There are three class II molecules, DP, DQ and DR. The class III genes are grouped together in a region between D and B. These genes code for a number of complement components but most have nothing to do with the immune system.

## MHC antigen structure and distribution

The MHC class I molecule is a dimer composed of a glycosylated transmembrane peptide, of molecular weight 45 000, coded for within the MHC, linked to a peptide, $\beta_2$-microglobulin (Fig. 10.8a). The globular protein formed by these two peptides is present on the surface of all nucleated cells in humans, except neurones. $\beta_2$-Microglobulin is required for the processing and expression of MHC-encoded molecules on the cell membrane. The MHC-encoded class I glycoprotein folds into three globular domains ($\alpha_1$, $\alpha_2$ and $\alpha_3$) held in place by disulphide bonds and non-covalent interactions. These globular domains are found on the outer surface of the cell. There is a short cytoplasmic tail

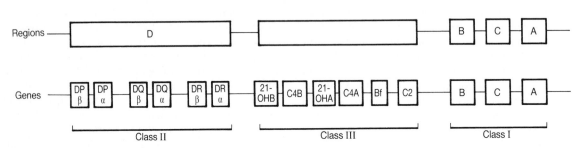

**Fig. 10.7**    MHC gene map of humans.

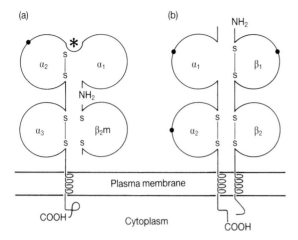

**Fig. 10.8** Structure of MHC class I and class II molecules. Schematic representation of **a** class I and **b** class II molecules as found in the plasma membrane $\beta_2$m, $\beta_2$-microglobulin •, carbohydrate moieties; *, antigen-binding cleft.

and a transmembrane portion. $\beta_2$-Microglobulin is non-covalently associated with the $\alpha_3$ domain.

The MHC class II molecules consist of two polypeptide chains ($\alpha$ and $\beta$) held together by non-covalent interactions (Fig. 10.8b). They have a much more limited cellular distribution being limited to the surface of certain cells of the immune system. In humans, they are normally found on B lymphocytes, macrophages, monocytes and activated T lymphocytes. The MHC class II molecule

consists of two non-covalently associated peptides, $\alpha$ and $\beta$. Each chain is composed of two extracellular domains, a transmembrane portion and a cytoplasmic tail.

These two types of molecule are folded into domains of a similar overall structure to immunoglobulin and, along with other molecules of the immune system involved in recognition processes, are thought to have evolved from a common ancestral molecule. A number of members of this *immunoglobulin supergene family* are depicted in Figure 10.9. MHC class II molecules, some interleukin receptors and Fc receptors are also included in the family.

The MHC antigens of each class have a similar basic structure. However, fine structural differences can be detected in the $\alpha_1$ and $\alpha_2$ domains of class I molecules and in $\alpha_1$ and $\beta_1$ domains of class II molecules. These domains form a cleft on the outermost part of the molecules in which antigen fragments are found. The variations found are due to differences in the amino acid sequence and can be detected serologically. The variable residues will give rise to different three-dimensional shapes on the MHC molecules. This will in turn influence the way in which antigen fragments can bind to the MHC molecule.

There are, therefore, many different forms of these molecules that can be identified in a population – they are highly *polymorphic*. Thus, it is highly unlikely that two individuals will have exactly

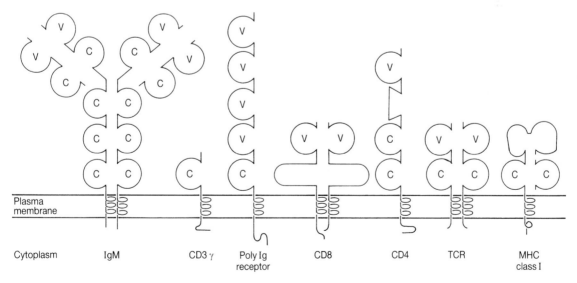

**Fig. 10.9** The immunoglobulin supergene family. A number of molecules involved in the immune system display striking similarities in overall structure. Regions similar to immunoglobulin domains are shown as circles; those related to variable and constant domains are designated V and C, respectively.

the same MHC antigens. The MHC molecules of a particular individual, his or her *haplotype*, can be given a designation using tissue-typing reagents. So, on each chromosome of an individual will be the genes that code for an A, B, C, DP, DQ and DR molecule. As the MHC genes are co-dominant, the products of both alleles are expressed on the cell surface. All the nucleated cells in the body will therefore express multiple copies of two HLA-A, two HLA-B and two HLA-C molecules. On certain cell types there will also be HLA-DP, -DQ and -DR molecules that were inherited from both parents.

## Function

The MHC class I and class II molecules are essential for immune recognition by T lymphocytes, which are only able to bind to antigens when they are associated with these molecules. The different classes of molecule are involved in antigen recognition by different T cell types or subsets. T lymphocytes that have CD4 molecules on their surface recognize antigen in association with MHC class II molecules, while those that have CD8 molecules are restricted by MHC class I molecules.

The T lymphocyte subsets perform different functions, but the division is not absolute. The one thing that they have in common is that they recognize, through their T cell receptor complex (CD3, CD4 or CD8, TCR), antigen fragments in association with MHC molecules (Fig. 10.10). In general terms, CD4-positive (CD4[+]) cells produce molecules, lymphokines, that stimulate and support the production of immune system cells while the CD8[+] fraction is involved in the destruction of virally infected cells.

Viruses replicate within host cells. During this process fragments of viral proteins become associ-

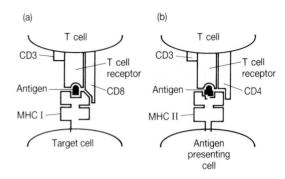

**Fig. 10.10** Molecules involved in T cell recognition. **a** Antigen fragments that associate with class I molecules are recognized by T cells that have the CD8 molecule. **b** Antigen fragments that associate with MHC class II are recognized by T cells that have the CD4 molecule on their surface.

ated with MHC class I molecules, and these complexes are then transported to the surface of the infected cell. The CD8 T cell recognizes this complex and destroys the infected cell before it can release progeny virus. Thus, MHC-restricted recognition of peptide fragments is responsible for directing the effector cells onto infected targets. These cytotoxic cells are also capable of destroying tissue grafts from MHC-incompatible donors.

The CD4[+] cells produce molecules that stimulate growth and differentiation of cells. These molecules are most effective over short distances since they will be more concentrated. This will happen when the two cells involved are actually joined together or in close proximity. The stimulation of CD4[+] T cells by antigen fragments on the surface of a responsive cell, or on a cell in the vicinity of a responsive cell, will greatly increase the effectiveness of the messenger molecules produced by the T cell.

RECOMMENDED READING

Abbas A K, Lichtman A H, Pober J S 1994 *Cellular and Molecular Immunology*, 2nd edn. W B Saunders, Philadelphia
Janeway C A 1993 How the immune system recognizes

invaders. *Scientific American* Sept: 41–47
Weir D M, Stewart J 1997 *Immunology*, 8th edn. Churchill Livingstone, Edinburgh

# 11

# Innate and acquired immunity

*J. Stewart and D. M. Weir*

The environment contains a vast number of potentially infectious organisms – viruses, bacteria, fungi, protozoa and worms. Any of these can cause damage if they multiply unchecked, and many could kill the host. However, the majority of infections in the normal individual are of limited duration and leave very little permanent damage. This fortunate outcome is due largely to the *immune system.*

The immune system is split into two functional divisions. *Innate immunity* is the first line of defence against infectious agents, and most potential pathogens are checked before they establish an overt infection. If these defences are breached, the acquired immune system is called into play. *Acquired immunity* produces a specific response to each infectious agent, and the effector mechanisms generated normally eradicate the offending material. Furthermore, the adaptive immune system remembers the particular infectious agent and can prevent it causing disease later.

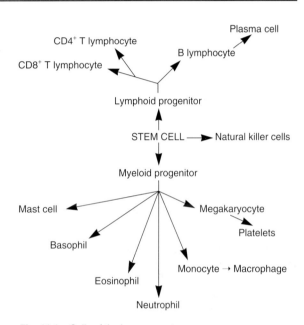

**Fig. 11.1** Cells of the immune system.

## THE IMMUNE SYSTEM

The immune system consists of a number of organs and several different cell types. All the cells of the immune system, tissue cells and white blood cells or *leucocytes*, develop from pluripotent stem cells in the bone marrow. These haemopoietic stem cells also give rise to the red blood cells or *erythrocytes*. The production of leucocytes is through two main pathways of differentiation (Fig. 11.1). The *lymphoid* lineage produces T lymphocytes and B lymphocytes. Natural killer (NK) cells, also known as large granular lymphocytes, develop along an unknown pathway. The *myeloid* pathway gives rise to mononuclear phagocytes, monocytes and macrophages, and granulocytes, basophils, eosinophils and neutrophils, as well as platelets and mast cells. Platelets are involved in blood clotting and inflammation while

mast cells are similar to basophils but are found in tissues.

## Lymphoid cells

Lymphocytes make up about 20% of the white blood cells present in the adult circulation. Mature lymphoid cells are long lived and may survive for many years as memory cells. These mononuclear cells are heterogeneous in size and morphology. The typical small lymphocytes are agranular and comprise the T and B cell populations. The larger cells are referred to as large granular lymphocytes because they contain cytoplasmic granules. Cells within this population are able to kill certain tumour and virally infected cells (natural killing) and destroy cells coated with immunoglobulin (antibody-dependent cell-mediated cytotoxicity).

**Table 11.1** Major T lymphocyte markers

| Marker | Distribution | Proposed function |
|--------|-------------|-------------------|
| CD2 | All T cells | Adherence to target cell |
| CD3 | All T cells | Part of T cell antigen receptor complex |
| CD4 | Helper subset ($T_H$) | MHC class II-restricted recognition |
| CD7 | All T cells | Unknown |
| CD8 | Cytotoxic subset ($T_C$) | MHC class I-restricted recognition |

MHC, major histocompatibility complex.

Morphologically it is quite difficult to distinguish between the different lymphoid cells and impossible to differentiate the subclasses of T cell. Since these cells carry out different processes they possess molecules on their surface unique to that functional requirement. These molecules, referred to as markers, can be used to distinguish between different cell types and also identify cells at different stages of differentiation. The different cell surface molecules have been systematically named by the CD (cluster of differentiation) system, and some of those expressed by different T cell populations are shown in Table 11.1. These CD markers are identified using specific monoclonal antibodies (see p. 135). The presence of these specific antibodies on the cell surface is then visualized using labelled antibodies that recognize the first antibody.

## Myeloid cells

The second pathway of development gives rise to a variety of cell types of different morphology and function.

### Mononuclear phagocytes

The common myeloid progenitor in the bone marrow gives rise to *monocytes* that circulate in the blood and migrate into organs and tissues to become *macrophages*. The human blood monocyte is larger than a lymphocyte and usually has a kidney-shaped nucleus. This actively phagocytic cell has a ruffled membrane and many cytoplasmic granules. These *lysosomes* contain enzymes and molecules that are involved in the killing of micro-organisms. Mononuclear phagocytes adhere strongly to surfaces and have various cell membrane receptors to aid the binding and ingestion of foreign material. Their activities can be enhanced by molecules produced by T lymphocytes, called *lymphokines*. Macrophages and monocytes are capable of producing various complement components, prostaglandins, interferons and *monokines* such as interleukin-1 and tumour necrosis factor. Lymphokines and monokines are collectively known as *cytokines*.

### Polymorphonuclear leucocytes

These cells are sometimes referred to as *granulocytes* and are short-lived cells (2–3 days) compared to macrophages which may survive for months or years. They constitute 60–70% of the leucocytes, but also migrate into tissues in response to injury or infection. The mature forms have a multilobed nucleus and many granules. They are classified as *neutrophils*, *eosinophils* and *basophils* on the basis of their histochemical staining.

**Neutrophils.** These are the most abundant circulating granulocyte. Their granules contain numerous microbicidal molecules and the cells enter the tissues when a chemotactic factor is produced, as the result of infection or injury.

**Eosinophils.** Eosinophils are also phagocytic cells, although they appear to be less efficient than neutrophils. They are present in low numbers in a healthy, normal individual (1–2% of leucocytes), but their numbers rise in certain allergic conditions. The granule contents can be released by the appropriate signal, and the cytotoxic molecules can then kill parasites that are too large to be phagocytosed.

**Basophils.** These cells are found in extremely small numbers in the circulation (<0.2%) and have certain characteristics in common with tissue *mast cells*. Both cell types have receptors on their surface for the Fc portion of IgE, and cross-linking of this immunoglobulin by antigen leads to the release of various pharmacological mediators. These molecules stimulate an inflammatory response. There are two types of mast cell: one is found in connective tissue and the other is mucosa associated. Mast cells and basophils are both bone marrow derived, but their developmental relationship is not clear.

### Platelets

Platelets are also derived from myeloid progenitors. In addition to their role in clotting they are involved in inflammation.

**Table 11.2** Characteristics and determinants of innate and acquired immunity

| Innate immunity | Acquired immunity |
| --- | --- |
| Non-specfic | Specific |
| No change with repeat exposure | Memory |
| Mechanical barriers<br>Bactericidal substances<br>Natural flora | |
| **Humoral** | |
| Acute phase proteins | Antibody |
| Interferons | |
| Lysozyme | |
| Complement | |
| **Cell mediated** | |
| Natural killer cells | T lymphocytes |
| Phagocytes | |

# INNATE IMMUNITY

The healthy individual is protected from potentially harmful micro-organisms in the environment by a number of very effective mechanisms, present from birth, that do not depend upon prior exposure to any particular micro-organism. The innate defence mechanisms are non-specific in the sense that they are effective against a wide range of potentially infectious agents. The characteristics and constituents of innate and acquired immunity are shown in Table 11.2.

## Determinants of innate immunity

### Species and strains

Marked differences exist in the susceptibility of different species to infective agents. The rat is strikingly resistant to diphtheria whilst the guinea-pig and humans are highly susceptible. The rabbit is particularly susceptible to myxomatosis, and humans to syphilis, leprosy and meningococcal meningitis. Susceptibility to an infection does not always imply a lack of resistance to disease caused by the micro-organism. For example, although humans are highly susceptible to the common cold, the infection is overcome within a few days. In some diseases, it may be difficult to initiate the infection, but once established the disease can progress rapidly – inferring a lack of resistance. For example, rabies occurs in both humans and dogs but is not readily established as the virus does not ordinarily penetrate healthy skin. Once infected, however, both species are unable to overcome the disease. Marked variations in resistance to infection have been noted between different strains of mice, and it is possible to breed, by selection, rabbits of low, intermediate and high resistance to experimental tuberculosis.

### Individual differences and influence of age

The role of heredity in determining resistance to infection is well illustrated by studies on tuberculosis in twins. If one homozygous twin develops tuberculosis, the other twin has a 3 to 1 chance of developing the disease compared with a 1 in 3 chance if the twins are heterozygous. Sometimes genetically controlled abnormalities are an advantage to the individual in resisting infection as, for example, in a hereditary abnormality of the red blood cells (sickling). These red blood cells cannot be parasitized by *Plasmodium falciparum*, thus conferring a degree of resistance to malaria in the affected individuals.

Infectious diseases are often more severe in early childhood and in young animals; this higher susceptibility of the young appears to be associated with immaturity of the immunological mechanisms affecting the ability of the lymphoid system to deal with and react to foreign antigens. This is also the time when infectious agents are encountered for the first time (primary exposure), and a memory-acquired immune response cannot be called upon to aid elimination. In certain viral infections, e.g. polio and chickenpox, the clinical illness is more severe in adults than in children. This may be due to a more active immune response producing greater tissue damage. In the elderly, besides a general waning of the activities of the immune system, physical abnormalities (e.g. prostatic enlargement leading to stasis of urine) or long-term exposure to environmental factors (e.g. smoking) are common causes of increased susceptibility to infection.

### Hormonal influences and sex

There is decreased resistance to infection in diseases such as diabetes mellitus, hypothyroidism and adrenal dysfunction. The reasons for this decrease have not yet been clarified but may be related to enzyme or hormone activities. It is known that glucocorticoids are anti-inflammatory agents, decreasing the ability of phagocytes to ingest material. They also have beneficial effects by interfering in some way with the toxic effects of bacterial products such as endo-toxins.

There are no marked differences in susceptibility to infections between the sexes. Although the over-all incidence and death rate from infectious disease are greater in the male than in the female, both infectious hepatitis and whooping cough have a higher morbidity and mortality in females.

### Nutritional factors

The adverse effects of poor nutrition on susceptibility to certain infectious agents are not now seriously questioned. Experimental evidence in animals has shown repeatedly that inadequate diet may be correlated with increased susceptibility to a variety of bacterial diseases, associated with decreased phagocytic activity and leucopenia. In the case of viruses which are intracellular parasites, malnutri-tion might have an effect on virus production, but the usual outcome is enhanced disease due to impair-ed immune responses, especially the cytotoxic responses.

## Mechanisms of innate immunity

### Mechanical barriers and surface secretions

The intact skin and mucous membranes of the body afford a high degree of protection against pathogens. In conditions where the skin is damaged, such as in burns patients and after traumatic injury or surgery, infections can be a serious problem. The skin is a resistant barrier because of its outer horny layer consisting mainly of keratin, which is indigestible by most micro-organisms, and thus shields the living cells of the epidermis from micro-organisms and their toxins. The relatively dry condition of the skin and the high concentration of salt in drying sweat are inhibitory or lethal to many micro-organisms.

The sebaceous secretions and sweat of the skin contain bactericidal and fungicidal fatty acids, and these constitute an effective protective mechanism against many potential pathogens. The protective ability of these secretions varies at different stages of life, and some fungal 'ringworm' infections of children disappear at puberty with the marked increase of sebaceous secretions.

The sticky mucus covering the respiratory tract acts as a trapping mechanism for inhaled particles. The action of cilia sweeps the secretions, containing the foreign material, towards the oropharynx so that it is swallowed; in the stomach the acidic secretions destroy most of the micro-organisms present. Nasal secretions and saliva contain mucopolysaccharides capable of blocking some viruses and the tears and the mucous secretions of the respiratory, alimentary and genito-urinary tracts contain lysozyme that is particularly active against some Gram-positive bacteria.

The washing action of tears and flushing of urine are effective in stopping invasion by micro-organisms. The commensal micro-organisms that make up the natural bacterial flora covering epithelial surfaces are protective in a number of ways: (1) their very presence uses up a niche that cannot be used by a pathogen; (2) they compete for nutrients and also produce by-products that can inhibit the growth of other organisms. It is important not to disturb the relationship between the host and its indigenous flora.

Commensal organisms from the gut or bacteria normally present on the skin can cause problems if they gain access to an area that they do not nor-mally populate. An example of this is urinary tract infections resulting from the introduction of *Esche-richia coli*, a gut commensal, by means of a urinary catheter. Commensal organisms that are provided with the circumstances by which to cause infections are called *opportunistic pathogens*. Infections with these opportunists are quite widespread, often appear-ing as a result of medical or surgical treatment which breaches the innate defences or reduces the host's ability to respond.

### Humoral defence mechanisms

A number of microbicidal substances are present in the tissue and body fluids. Some of these molecules are produced constitutively, e.g. lysozyme, and others are produced in response to infection, e.g. acute-phase proteins and interferon. These molecules all show the characteristics of innate immunity – there is no specific recognition of the micro-organism and the response is not enhanced on re-exposure to the same antigen.

***Lysozyme.*** This is a basic protein of low mole-cular weight found in relatively high concentrations in neutrophils as well as in most tissue fluids, except cerebrospinal fluid, sweat and urine. It functions as a mucolytic enzyme, splitting sugars off the struc-tural peptidoglycan of the cell wall of many Gram-positive bacteria and thus causing their lysis. It seems likely that lysozyme may also play a role in the intracellular destruction of some Gram-negative bacteria. In many pathogenic bacteria the peptido-glycan of the cell wall appears to be protected from the access of lysozyme by other wall components, e.g. lipopolysaccharide. The action of other enzymes from phagocytes or of complement may be needed to remove this protection and expose the peptidoglycan to the action of lysozyme.

**Basic polypeptides.** A variety of basic proteins, derived from tissues and blood cells, have some antibacterial properties. This group includes the basic proteins called spermine and spermidine, which can kill tubercle bacilli and some staphylococci. Other toxic compounds are the arginine- and lysine-containing proteins protamine and histone. The bactericidal activity of basic polypeptides probably depends on their ability to react non-specifically with acid polysaccharides at the bacterial cell surface.

**Acute-phase proteins.** The concentration of acute-phase proteins rises dramatically during an infection. Microbial products such as endotoxin can stimulate macrophages to release interleukin-1, which stimulates the liver to produce increased amounts of various acute-phase proteins, the concentrations of which can rise over 1000-fold. One of the best-characterized acute-phase proteins is *C-reactive protein*, which binds to phosphorylcholine residues in the cell wall of certain micro-organisms. This complex is very effective at activating the classical complement pathway. Also included in this group of molecules are $\alpha_1$-antitrypsin, $\alpha_2$-macroglobulin, fibrinogen and serum amyloid A protein, all of which act to limit the spread of the infectious agent or stimulate the host response.

**Interferon.** The observation that cell cultures infected with one virus resist infection by a second virus, i.e. viral interference, led to the identification of the family of antiviral agents known as *interferons*. A number of molecules have been identified; $\alpha$- and $\beta$-interferons are part of innate immunity, and $\gamma$-interferon is produced by T cells as part of the acquired immune response (see Ch. 12).

## Complement

The existence of a heat-labile serum component with the ability to lyse red blood cells and destroy Gram-negative bacteria has been known since the 1930s. The chemical complexity of the phenomenon was not appreciated by early workers, who ascribed the activity to a single component, called complement. Complement is in fact an extremely complex group of serum proteins present in low concentration in normal serum. These molecules are present in an inactive form but can be activated to form an enzyme cascade, i.e. the product of the first reaction

is the catalyst of the next and so on. Complement comprises nine functional components denoted C1 to C9, of which there are further subdivisions.

There are about 20 proteins involved in the complement system, some of which are enzymes, some are control molecules and others are structural proteins with no enzymic activity. A number of the molecules involved are split into two components (a and b fragments) by the product of the previous step. There are two pathways of complement activation, the alternative and classical, that lead to the same physiological consequences – opsonization, cellular activation and lysis – but use different initiation processes. Component C3 forms the connection between the two pathways, and the binding of this molecule to a surface is the key process in complement activation.

**Classical pathway.** The classical pathway of activation leading to the cleavage of C3 is initiated by the binding of two or more of the globular domains of the C1q component of C1 to its ligand: immune complexes containing IgG or IgM and certain micro-organisms and their products. This causes a conformational change in the C1 complex that leads to the auto-activation of C1r. The enzyme C1r then converts C1s into an active serine esterase that acts on the thioester-containing molecule C4 to produce C4a and a reactive C4b (Fig. 11.2). C4a is released and some of the C4b becomes attached to a surface. The rest is inactivated by reacting with water. C2 binds to the surface-bound C4b, becomes a substrate for the activated C1 complex and is split into C2a and C2b. The C2b is released, leaving C4b2a – the classical pathway C3 convertase. This active enzyme then generates C3a and the unstable C3b from C3. A small amount of the C3b generated will bind to the activating surface and act as a focus for further complement activation. The activation of the classical pathway is regulated by C1 inhibitor and by a number of molecules that limit the production of the 'C3 convertase'.

**Alternative pathway.** Intrinsically, C3 undergoes a low level of hydrolysis of an internal thioester bond to generate C3b. This molecule complexes, in the presence of $Mg^{2+}$ ions, with factor B, which is then acted on by factor D to produce C3bBb. This is a 'C3 convertase' that is capable of splitting more C3 to C3b, some of which will become membrane bound.

The initial binding of C3b generated by either the classical or alternative pathway leads to an amplification loop that results in the binding of many more C3b molecules to the same surface. Factor B binds to the surface-bound C3b to form C3bB, the

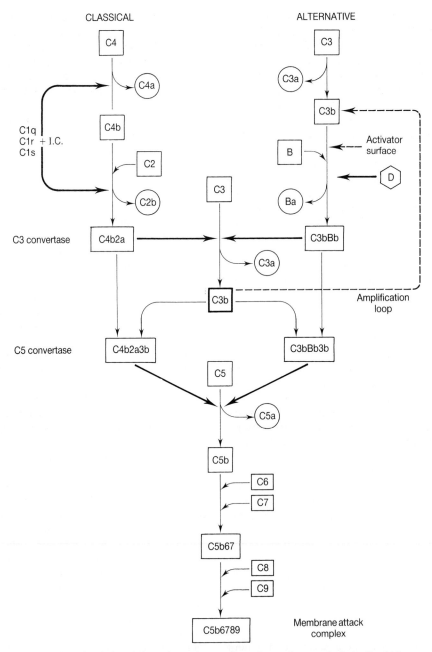

**Fig. 11.2** Complement activation: classical and alternative pathways. Enzymic reactions are indicated by thick arrows. I.C., immune complex.

substrate for factor D – a serine esterase – that is present in very low concentrations in an already active form. The cleavage of factor B results in the formation of the C3 convertase, C3bBb, which dissociates rapidly unless it is stabilized by the binding of properdin (P) – forming the complex C3bBbP. This convertase can cleave many more C3 mole-

cules, some of which become surface bound. This amplification loop is a positive-feedback system that will cycle until all the C3 is used up unless it is regulated carefully.

***Regulation.*** The nature of the surface to which the C3b is bound regulates the outcome. Self cell membranes contain a number of regulatory molecules that promote the binding of factor H rather than factor B to C3b. This results in the inhibition of the activation process. On non-self structures the C3b is protected since regulatory proteins are not present, and factor B has a higher affinity for C3b than factor H at these sites.

Thus the surface of many micro-organisms can stabilize the C3bBb by protecting it from factor H. In addition, another molecule, properdin, stabilizes the complex. The deposition of a few molecules of C3b onto these surfaces is followed by the formation of the relatively stable C3bBbP complex. This C3 convertase will lead to more C3b deposition. Immune complexes composed of certain immunoglobulins, e.g. IgA and IgE, also function as protected sites for C3b and activate complement by the alternative pathway. Poor activation surfaces will be made more susceptible to deposition by the presence of antibody that generates C3b by the classical pathway.

***Membrane attack complex.*** The next step after the formation of C3b is the cleavage of C5 (Fig. 11.3). The 'C5 convertases' are generated from C4b2a of the classical pathway and C3bBb of the alternative pathway by the addition of another C3b molecule. These membrane-bound trimolecular complexes selectively bind C5 and cleave it to give fluid phase C5a and membrane-bound C5b. The formation of the rest of the membrane attack complex is non-enzymic. C6 binds to C5b, and this joint complex is released from the C5 convertase. The formation of C5b67 generates a hydrophobic complex that inserts into the lipid bilayer in the vicinity of the initial activation site. Usually this will be on the same cell surface as the initial trigger, but occasionally other cells may be involved. Therefore,

'bystander' lysis can take place, giving rise to damage to surrounding tissue. There are a number of proteins present in body fluids to limit this potentially dangerous process by binding to fluid phase C5b67. C8 and C9 bind to the membrane-inserted complex in sequence, resulting in the formation of a lytic polymeric complex containing up to 20 C9 monomers. A small amount of lysis can occur when C8 binds to C5b67, but it is the polymerized C9 that causes the most damage.

***Functions.*** The activation of complement by either pathway gives rise to C3b and the generation of a number of factors that can aid in the elimination of foreign material.

The complete insertion of the membrane attack complex into a cell will lead to membrane damage and lysis, probably by osmotic swelling. Some thin-walled pathogens, such as trypanosomes and malaria parasites, are killed by complement-mediated lysis. Some Gram-negative bacteria can be killed by complement in conjunction with lysozyme. However, complement-mediated lysis is of limited importance as a bactericidal mechanism when compared to phagocyte destruction of bacteria. Inherited deficiencies of the terminal components are associated with infection by gonococci and meningococci which can survive inside neutrophils and for which complement-mediated killing is important.

Phagocytic cells have receptors for C3b and iC3b that facilitate the adherence of complement-coated particles. Therefore, complement is an *opsonin*, and in certain circumstances this attachment may lead to phagocytosis.

Two of the molecules released during the complement cascade, C3a and C5a, have potent biological activities. These molecules, known as *anaphylatoxins*,

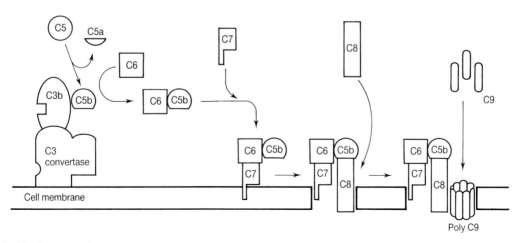

**Fig. 11.3** Membrane attack complex.

trigger mast cells and basophils to release mediators of inflammation (see below). They also stimulate neutrophils to produce reactive oxygen intermediates, while C5a on its own is a chemoattractant and acts directly on vascular endothelium to cause vasodilation and increased vascular permeability.

## Cells

***Phagocytes.***   Micro-organisms entering the tissue fluids or bloodstream are very rapidly engulfed by *neutrophils* and *mononuclear phagocytes*. In the blood the latter are known as *monocytes* while in the tissues they differentiate into *macrophages*. In connective tissue they are known as *histiocytes*, in kidney as *mesangial cells*, in bone as *osteoclasts*, in brain as *microglia* and in the spleen, lymph node and thymus as the *sinus-lining macrophages*.

The essential features of these cells are that they: (1) are actively phagocytic; (2) contain digestive enzymes to degrade ingested material; and (3), mononuclear phagocytes are an important link between the innate and acquired immune mechanisms. Part of their role in regard to acquired immunity is that they can process and present antigens and produce molecules that stimulate lymphocyte differentiation into effector cells.

The role of the phagocyte in innate immunity is to engulf particles (phagocytosis) or soluble material (pinocytosis), and digest them intracellularly within specialized vacuoles. The macrophages present in the walls of capillaries and vascular sinuses in spleen, liver, lungs and bone marrow serve a very important role in clearing the bloodstream of foreign particulate material such as bacteria. So efficient is this process that the finding of a few micro-organisms in the bloodstream usually indicates that there is a continuing release of micro-organisms from an active focus such as an abscess or the heart valve vegetations found in bacterial endocarditis.

The ability of macrophages to ingest and destroy micro-organisms can be impaired or enhanced by depression or stimulation of the phagocyte system. Some micro-organisms such as mycobacteria and brucellae can resist intracellular digestion by normal macrophages, though they may be digested by 'activated' ones.

***Chemotaxis.***   For phagocytic cells to be effective they must be attracted to the site of infection. Once they have passed through the capillary walls they move through the tissues in response to a concentration gradient of molecules that have been produced at the site of damage. These chemotactic factors include products of injured tissue, factors from the blood (C5a), substances produced by neutrophils and mast cells (leukotrienes and histamine) and bacterial products (formyl-methionine peptides). Neutrophils respond first and move faster than monocytes.

***Phagocytosis.***   Phagocytosis involves (1) recognition and binding, (2) ingestion and (3) digestion. It may occur in the absence of antibody, especially on surfaces such as those of the lung alveoli and when inert particles are involved. Cell membranes carry a net negative charge that keeps them apart and stops autophagocytosis. The hydrophilic nature of certain bacterial cell wall components stops them passing through the hydrophobic membrane. To overcome these difficulties the phagocytes have receptors on their surface that mediate the attachment of particles that have been coated with the correct ligand. Phagocytes have receptors for the Fc portion of certain immunoglobulin isotypes and for some components of the complement cascade. The presence of these molecules or *opsonins* on the particle surface markedly enhances the ingestion process and, in some cases, digestion. Whether mediated by specific receptors or not, the foreign particle is surrounded by the cell membrane, which then invaginates and produces an *endosome* or *phagosome* within the cell (Fig. 11.4).

The microbicidal machinery of the phagocyte is contained within organelles known as *lysosomes*. This compartmentalization of potentially toxic molecules is necessary to protect the cell from self-destruction and produce an environment where the molecules

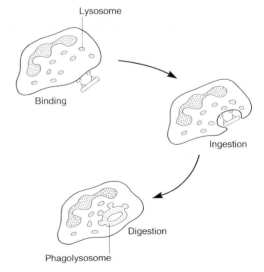

**Fig. 11.4**  Stages in phagocytosis.

can function efficiently. The phagosome and lysosome fuse to form a *phagolysosome* in which the ingested material is killed and digested by various enzyme systems.

Ingestion is accompanied by enhanced glycolysis and an increase in the synthesis of proteins and membrane phospholipids. After phagocytosis there is a respiratory burst consisting of a steep rise in oxygen consumption. This is accompanied by an increase in the activity of a number of enzymes and leads to the reduction of molecular oxygen to various highly reactive intermediates, e.g. the superoxide anion ($O_2^-$), hydrogen peroxide ($H_2O_2$), singlet oxygen ($O\cdot$) and the hydroxyl radical ($OH\cdot$). All these chemical species have microbicidal activity and are termed oxygen-dependent killing mechanisms. The superoxide anion is a free radical produced by the one-electron reduction of molecular oxygen; it is very reactive and highly damaging to animal cells, as well as to micro-organisms. It is also the substrate for superoxide dismutase that generates hydrogen peroxide for subsequent use in microbial killing. Myeloperoxidase uses hydrogen peroxide and halide ions, such as iodide or chloride, to produce at least two bactericidal systems. In one, halogenation (incorporation of iodine or chlorine) of the bacterial cell wall leads to death of the organism. In the second mechanism, myeloperoxidase and hydrogen peroxide damage the cell wall by converting amino acids into aldehydes that have antimicrobial activity.

A number of oxygen-independent mechanisms are also present within phagocytes that are capable of destroying ingested material. Some of these enzymes can damage membranes. For example, *lysozyme* and *elastase* attack peptidoglycan of the bacterial cell wall, and then hydrolases are responsible for the complete digestion of the killed organism. The cationic proteins of lysosomes bind to and damage bacterial cell walls and enveloped viruses, such as herpes simplex virus. The iron-binding protein *lactoferrin* has antimicrobial properties. It complexes with iron, rendering it unavailable to bacteria that require iron for growth. The high acidity within phagolysosomes (pH 3.5–4.0) may have bactericidal effects: it probably results from lactic acid production in glycolysis. In addition, many lysosomal enzymes, such as acid hydrolases, have acid pH optima. There are significant differences between macrophages and neutrophils in the killing of micro-organisms. Although macrophage lysosomes contain a variety of enzymes, including lysozyme, they lack cationic proteins and lactoferrin. Tissue macrophages do not have myeloperoxidase but probably use catalase to generate the

hydrogen peroxide system. Normal macrophages are less efficient killers of certain pathogens, such as fungi, than neutrophils. The microbicidal activity of macrophages can, however, be greatly improved after contact with products of lymphocytes, known as lymphokines.

Once killed, most micro-organisms are digested and solubilized by lysosomal enzymes. The degradation products are then released to the exterior.

***Natural killer cells.*** NK cells recognize changes on virus-infected cells and destroy them by an extracellular killing mechanism. After binding to the target cell, by an as yet undefined mechanism, the NK cell produces molecules that damage the membrane of the infected cell, leading to its destruction.

Natural killing can be performed by a number of different cell types. This activity has been shown to be carried out by cells described as large granular lymphocytes and also by cells with T cell markers, macrophage markers and others that do not have the characteristics of any of the main cells of the immune system. Natural killing is present without prior exposure to the infectious agent and shows all the characteristics of an innate defence mechanism. NK cells have also been implicated in host defence against cancers. They are thought to recognize changes in the cell membranes of transformed cells in a mechanism similar to that used to combat virus infection. Natural killing is enhanced by interferons which appear to stimulate the production of NK cells and also increase the rate at which they kill the target cells.

***Eosinophils.*** Eosinophils are polymorphonuclear leucocytes with a characteristic bilobed nucleus and cytoplasmic granules. They are present in the blood of normal individuals at very low levels (<1%), but their numbers increase in patients with parasitic infections and allergies. They are not efficient phagocytic cells but their granules contain molecules that are toxic to parasites. Large parasites such as helminths cannot be internalized by phagocytes and therefore must be killed extracellularly. Eosinophil granules contain an array of enzymes and toxic molecules that are active against parasitic worms. The release of these molecules must be controlled so that tissue damage is avoided. The eosinophils have specific receptors, including Fc and complement receptors, that bind the labelled target, i.e. antibody or complement-coated parasites. The granule contents are then released into the space between the cell and the parasite, thus targeting the toxic molecules onto the parasite membrane.

## Temperature

The temperature dependence of many micro-organisms is well known, and it is therefore apparent that temperature is an important factor in determining the innate immunity of an animal to some infectious agents. It seems likely that the pyrexia that follows so many different types of infection can function as a protective response against the infecting micro-organism. The febrile response in many cases is controlled by interleukin-1 produced by macrophages as part of the immune response.

## Inflammation

A number of the above factors are responsible for the process of *inflammation*. This is the reaction of the body to injury, such as invasion by an infectious agent, exposure to a noxious chemical or physical trauma. The signs of inflammation are redness, heat, swelling, pain and loss of function. The molecular and cellular events that occur during an inflammatory reaction are (1) vasodilation, (2) increased vascular permeability and (3) cellular infiltration. These changes are brought about mainly by chemical mediators (Table 11.3) that are widely distributed in a sequestered or inactive form throughout the body and are released or activated locally at the site of inflammation. After release they tend to be rapidly inactivated to ensure control of the inflammatory process.

There is increased blood supply to the affected area due to the action of vaso-active amines such as histamine and 5-hydroxytryptamine and other mediators stored within mast cells. These molecules are released (1) as a consequence of the production of the anaphylatoxins (C3a and C5a) that trigger specific receptors on mast cells and (2) following interaction of antigen with IgE on the surface of mast cells or (3) by direct physical damage to the cells. Other mediators, such as bradykinins and prostaglandins, are produced locally or released by platelets. The vasodilation causes increased blood supply to the area, giving rise to redness and heat. The result is an increase in the supply of the molecules and cells that can combat the agent responsible for the initial trigger.

The same molecules, vaso-active amines, prostaglandins and kinins, increase vascular permeability allowing plasma and plasma proteins to traverse the endothelial lining. The plasma proteins will include immunoglobulins and molecules of the clotting and complement cascades. This leaking of fluid will cause swelling (oedema) that will in turn lead to increased tissue tension and pain. Some of the molecules themselves, e.g. prostaglandins and histamine, stimulate the pain responses directly. The inflammatory exudate has several important functions. Bacteria often produce tissue-damaging toxins that will be diluted by the exudate. Clotting factors present result in the deposition of fibrin, creating a physical obstruction to the spread of bacteria. The

---

**Table 11.3**  Mediators of inflammation

| Mediator | Main source | Function |
|---|---|---|
| Histamine[a] | Mast cells, basophils | Vasodilation, increased vascular permeability, contraction of smooth muscle |
| Kinins (e.g. bradykinin) | Plasma | Vasodilation, increased vascular permeability, contraction of smooth muscle, pain |
| Prostaglandins | Neutrophils, eosinophils, monocytes, platelets | Vasodilation, increased vascular permeability, pain |
| Leukotrienes | Neutrophils, mast cells, basophils | Vasodilation, increased vascular permeability, contraction of smooth muscle, induce cell adherence and chemotaxis |
| Complement components (e.g. C3a, C5a) | Plasma | Cause mast cells to release mediator C5a is chemotactic factor |
| Plasmin | Plasma | Breaks down fibrin, kinin formation |
| Cytokines | Lymphocytes, macrophages | Chemotactic factors, colony stimulation factors, macrophage activation |

[a]In rodents, 5-hydroxytryptamine (serotonin) is present in mast cells and basophils.

exudate is continuously drained off by the lymphatic vessels, and antigens, such as bacteria and their toxins, are carried to the draining lymph node where immune responses can be generated.

Chemotactic factors produced, including C5a, histamine, leukotrienes and molecules specific for certain cell types, will attract phagocytic cells to the site. The increased vascular permeability will allow easier access for neutrophils and monocytes and the vasodilation means that more cells are in the vicinity. The neutrophils will arrive first and begin to destroy or remove the offending agent. Most will be successful but a few will die, releasing their tissue-damaging contents to increase the inflammatory process. Mononuclear phagocytes will arrive on the scene to finish off the removal of the residual debris and stimulate tissue repair.

When the swelling is severe there may be loss of function to the affected area. If the offending agent is quickly removed then the tissue will soon be repaired. The inflammatory process continues until the conditions responsible for its initiation are resolved. In most circumstances this occurs fairly rapidly with an acute inflammatory reaction lasting a matter of hours or days. If, however, the causative agent is not easily removed or is reintroduced continuously then chronic inflammation will ensue with the possibility of tissue destruction and complete loss of function.

## ACQUIRED IMMUNITY

Micro-organisms that overcome or circumvent the innate non-specific defence mechanisms or are administered deliberately, i.e. active immunization, come up against the host's second line of defence – *acquired immunity*. To give expression to this acquired form of immunity it is necessary that the antigens of the invading micro-organism should come into contact with cells of the immune system (macrophages and lymphocytes) and so initiate an immune response specific for the foreign material. The cells that respond are precommitted, because of their surface receptors, to respond to a particular epitope on the antigen. This response takes two forms, *humoral* and *cell mediated*, which usually develop in parallel. The part played by each will depend on a number of factors, including the nature of the antigen, the route of entry and the individual who is infected.

Humoral immunity depends on the appearance in the blood of antibodies produced by plasma cells.

The term 'cell-mediated immunity' was orginally coined to describe localized reactions to organisms mediated by T lymphocytes and phagocytes rather than by antibody. It is now used to describe any response in which antibody plays a subordinate role. Cell-mediated immunity depends mainly on the development of T cells that are specifically responsive to the inducing agent and is generally active against intracellular organisms.

Specific immunity may be acquired in two main ways. (1) It may be induced by overt clinical infection, inapparent clinical infection or deliberate artificial immunization. This is *active acquired immunity*, and contrasts with (2) *passive acquired immunity*, which is the transfer of preformed antibodies to a non-immune individual by means of blood, serum components or lymphoid cells.

Actively acquired immunity is long-lasting although it may be circumvented by antigenic change in the infecting micro-organism. Passively acquired immunity provides only temporary protection. Passive immunity may be transferred to the fetus by the passage of maternal antibodies across the placenta.

## Tissues involved in immune reactions

For the generation of an immune response, antigen must interact with and activate a number of different cells. In addition, these cells must interact with each other. The cells involved in immune responses are organized into tissues and organs in order that these complex cellular interactions can occur most effectively. These structures are collectively referred to as the *lymphoid system*, which comprises lymphocytes, epithelial and stromal cells arranged into discrete capsulated organs or accumulations of diffuse lymphoid tissue. Lymphoid organs contain lymphocytes at various stages of development and are classified into primary and secondary lymphoid organs.

The primary lymphoid organs are the major sites of lymphopoiesis. Here, lymphoid progenitor cells develop into mature lymphocytes by a process of proliferation and differentiation. In mammals, T lymphocytes develop in the thymus, and B lymphocytes in the bone marrow and fetal liver. It is within the primary lymphoid organs that the lymphocytes acquire their repertoire of specific antigen receptors in order to cope with the antigenic challenges that the individual receives during its life. The ability to differentiate between self and non-self is also acquired in these tissues.

The secondary lymphoid organs create the environment in which lymphocytes can interact with each other and with antigen and then disseminate the effector cells and molecules generated. Secondary lymphoid organs include lymph nodes, spleen and mucosal-associated lymphoid tissue, e.g. tonsils and Peyer's patches of the gut. These organs have a characteristic structure which relates to the function they carry out, with areas composed mainly of B cells or T cells.

## Development of the immune system

In humans, lymphoid tissue appears first in the thymus at about 8 weeks of gestation. Peyer's patches are distinguishable by the 5th month, and immuno-globulin-secreting cells appear in the spleen and lymph nodes at about 20 weeks. From this period onwards, IgM and IgD are synthesized by the fetus (Fig. 11.5). At birth the infant has a blood concentration of IgG comparable to that of the maternal circulation, having received IgG but not IgM via the placenta. The rate of synthesis of IgM in the infant increases rapidly within the first few days of life but does not reach adult levels until about a year. Serum IgG does not reach adult levels until after the second year, and IgA takes even longer. There is an actual drop in the level of IgG from birth due to the decay of maternal antibody, with the lowest levels of total IgG at around 3 months of age. This corresponds to an age of marked susceptibility to a number of infections. Cell-mediated immunity can be stimulated at birth, but these reactions may not be as powerful as in the adult.

## Lymphocyte trafficking

Lymphocytes differentiate and mature in the primary lymphoid organs and then enter the blood lympho-cyte pool. B cells are produced in the bone marrow and mature there before proceeding via the circulation to the secondary lymphoid organs. T cell pre-cursors leave the bone marrow and mature in the thymus before migrating to the secondary lymphoid organs. Once in the secondary lymphoid tissues the lymphocytes do not remain there but move from one lymphoid organ to another through the blood and lymphatics (Fig. 11.6). One of the main advan-tages of this *lymphocyte recirculation* is that during the course of a natural infection the continual trafficking of lymphocytes enables very many dif-ferent lymphocytes to have access to the antigen.

Only a very small number of the lymphocytes will recognize a particular antigen. Pathogens can enter the body by many routes but must be carried from the site of infection to the secondary lymphoid tissues where they are localized and concentrated on the dendritic processes of macrophages or on the sur-face of antigen-presenting cells. If the infection is in

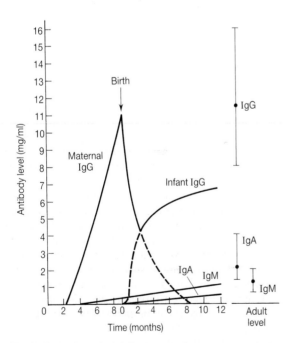

**Fig. 11.5** Immunoglobulin levels in the fetus and neonate. The adult levels of the major isotypes are shown as normal ranges with mean serum levels (●).

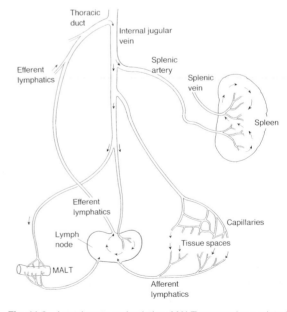

**Fig. 11.6** Lymphocyte recirculation. MALT, mucosal-associated lymphoid tissue.

the tissues, antigen is carried in the lymphatics to the draining lymph node. Under normal conditions there is a continuous active flow of lymphocytes through lymph nodes, but when antigen and antigen-reactive cells enter there is a temporary shutdown of the exit. Thus, antigen-specific cells are preferentially retained in the node draining the source of the antigen. This is partly responsible for the swollen glands (lymph nodes) that can sometimes be found during an infection. Antigens that enter through a mucosal surface are collected into the mucosal-associated lymphoid tissues such as the tonsils and Peyer's patches. Blood-borne antigens are trapped in the spleen. The passage of lymphocytes through an area where antigen has been localized facilitates the induction of an immune response. Lymphocytes with appropriate receptors bind to the antigen and become activated. Once activated the lymphocytes mature into effector cells. In the case of B lymphocytes they become plasma cells and secrete antibody. T lymphocytes will leave the secondary lymphoid tissue and return to the site of infection to destroy the infectious agent.

There is now evidence for non-random migration of lymphocytes to particular lymphoid compartments. For example, lymphocytes that home to the gut are selectively transported across endothelial cells of venules in the intestine. It appears that lymphocytes have specific molecules on their surface that preferentially interact with endothelial cells in different anatomical sites. A lymphocyte that was initially stimulated by antigen in a Peyer's patch will migrate to the draining lymph node, respond, and memory cells will be produced. It is important that these memory cells migrate back to the area where the same pathogen might be encountered again. Therefore, they are found preferentially in the mucosal-associated lymphoid tissue.

## Clonal selection

During their development in the primary lymphoid tissues both T and B lymphocytes acquire specific cell surface receptors that commit them to a single antigenic specificity. For T cells this receptor will remain the same for its life, but the surface immunoglobulin on B cells can be modified due to somatic mutations. In the B cell this is mirrored in the modification of the antibody the cell produces on exposure to its specific antigen. The cell is activated when it binds its specific antigen, the lymphocytes then proliferate, differentiate and mature into effector cells.

Each lymphocyte produced has a unique receptor capable of recognizing a particularly shaped epitope. Since the immune system can specifically recognize a very large number of antigens this means that the lymphocytes reactive to any particular antigen are only a small proportion of the total pool. Therefore, antigen binds to the small number of cells that can recognize it and *selects* them to proliferate and mature so that sufficient cells are formed to mount an adequate immune response. A cell that responds to an antigenic trigger and proliferates will give rise to cells with a genetically identical make-up, i.e. *clones*. Therefore, this phenomenon is known as *clonal selection*.

Lymphocyte receptors appear to be created in a random fashion, so there is no reason why they should not recognize 'self' molecules. It is obviously an important attribute of the immune system that it is able to discriminate between 'self' and 'non-self'.

## Cellular activation

When an individual is exposed to foreign material, those cells with receptors that recognize antigenic determinants are selected to respond. B lymphocytes proliferate and differentiate into antibody-producing plasma cells and memory cells. T lymphocytes are stimulated to become effector cells that can directly eliminate the foreign material or produce molecules that help other cells destroy the pathogen. The type (immunity or tolerance) and magnitude of the response, if generated, will depend on a number of factors, including the nature, dose and route of entry of the antigen and the individual's genetic make-up and previous exposure to the antigen.

The first stage in the production of effector cells and molecules is the activation of the resting cells. This involves various cellular interactions with maturation of the response, leading to a co-ordinated, efficient production of effector T cells, immunoglobulin and memory cells.

Cross-linking of the B cell antigen receptor, surface immunoglobulin, is the initial trigger for activation. When this happens, a number of biochemical changes are instigated. These changes probably act through protein kinases that cause the synthesis of RNA and ultimately immunoglobulin production. In a number of cases this is all that is required to stimulate antibody production. However, for the majority of antigens this initial cross-linking is not enough, and molecules produced by T cells are also required.

***Thymus-independent antigens.*** A number of antigens will stimulate specific immunoglobulin production directly. These T-independent antigens are of two types: *mitogens* and certain large molecules.

**Mitogens** are substances that cause cells, particularly lymphocytes, to undergo cell division, i.e. proliferation. Certain glycoproteins, called lectins, have mitogenic activity. These molecules have specificity for sugars and bind to the cell surface and will activate all responsive cells. The response to the mitogens will therefore be polyclonal since lymphocytes of many different specificities will be activated. However, at low concentrations these mitogens do not cause polyclonal activation but can lead to the stimulation of specific B cells. Lipopolysaccharide is an example of a B cell mitogen.

Some large molecules with regularly repeating epitopes, e.g. polymers of D-amino acids and simple sugars such as pneumococcal polysaccharide and dextran, can interact directly with the B cell surface immunoglobulin. They may also be held on the surface of specialized macrophages in secondary lymphoid tissues and the B cells interact with them there. The multiple repeats of the epitope interact with a large number of surface immunoglobulin molecules and the signal that is generated is sufficient to stimulate antibody production.

The immune response generated to these antigens tends to be similar on each exposure, i.e. IgM is the main antibody, and the response shows little memory. This suggests that class switch and memory production require additional factors, i.e. products of T lymphocytes.

***Thymus-dependent antigens.*** Many antigens do not stimulate antibody production without the help of T lymphocytes. These antigens first bind to the B cell, which must then be exposed to T cell-derived lymphokines, i.e. helper factors, before antibody can be produced. For the second activation signal, i.e. help, to be effectively targeted at the B cell the T and B cells must be in direct contact. For this to happen the B and T cell epitopes must be physically linked. However, T cells only recognize antigen that has been processed and is presented in association with products of the major histocompatibility complex (MHC), so it is impossible for native antigen to form a bridge between surface immunoglobulin and the T cell receptor. The B cell binds to its epitope on free antigen, but there is no site on this molecule that the T cell can bind to since it requires antigen associated with MHC products. The answer to this problem can be seen when the requirements for antigen presentation in T cell recognition are considered.

## Antigen processing and presentation

The development of an antibody response to a T-dependent antigen requires that the antigen becomes associated with MHC class II molecules, i.e. *processed*, and expressed on the cell surface, i.e. *presented*, in a form that helper T cells can recognize.

All cells express MHC class I molecules, but class II molecules are confined to cells of the immune system – the antigen-presenting cells. These cells present antigen to MHC class II-restricted T cells (the CD4-positive (CD4$^+$) population) and therefore play a key role in the induction and development of immune responses. Within lymph nodes, different antigen-presenting cells are found in each of the main areas (Table 11.4).

There are a large number of antigen-presenting cells in the body (Table 11.5), most of which constitutively express MHC class II molecules. Other cells, such as T lymphocytes and endothelium, can be induced to express MHC class II molecules by suitable stimuli such as lymphokines. The relative importance of each type depends on whether a primary or secondary response is being stimulated and on the location. The most studied antigen-presenting cells are the macrophages and dendritic cells. However, it is now apparent that in certain situations B cells may be important antigen-presenting cells. The relative importance of B cells becomes greatest during secondary responses, especially if the antigen concentration is low. Here the B cells can specifically engulf antigen via their surface immunoglobulin. In a primary response, specific B

**Table 11.4**  Antigen-presenting cells in the lymph nodes

| Area | Antigen-presenting cell | Antigen |
|---|---|---|
| Subcapsular marginal sinus | Marginal zone macrophage | T-independent antigens |
| Follicles and B cell areas | Follicular dendritic cells | Antigen–antibody complexes |
| Medulla | Classical macrophages | Most antigens |
| T cell areas | Interdigitating dendritic cells | Most antigens |

**Table 11.5**   Antigen-presenting cells

| Group | Type | Location | MHC class II expression |
|---|---|---|---|
| Phagocytic cells | Monocytes | Blood | |
| | Macrophages | Tissues | + |
| | Marginal zone macrophages | Spleen and lymph node | |
| | Kupffer's cells | Liver | |
| | | | ++++ |
| | Microglia | Brain | |
| Lymphocytes | B cells | Lymphoid tissue and site of | + → +++ |
| | T cells | immune responses | 0 → ++ |
| Non-phagocytic constitutive | Langerhans' cells | Skin | ++ |
| presenters | Interdigitating cells | Lymphoid tissue | ++ |
| | Follicular dendritic cells | Lymphoid tissue | 0 |
| Facultative presenters | Astrocytes | Brain | |
| | Follicular cells | Thyroid | 0 |
| | Endothelium | Vascular and lymphoid tissue | |
| | Fibroblasts | Connective tissue | ++ |

Level of MHC class II expression is indicated by the number of + signs: 0, none present. Arrow indicates that MHC class II is inducible.

cells are at a low frequency and their receptors are of low affinity; in this situation macrophages and dendritic cells are probably most important.

The key feature of all antigen-presenting cells is that they can ingest antigen, degrade it and present it, in the context of MHC class II molecules, to T cells. The antigen is taken into the antigen-presenting cells and enters the endocytic pathway. Before it is completely destroyed, peptide fragments are taken to a structure called the compartment for peptide loading (CPL). MHC class II molecules are synthesized within the endoplasmic reticulum and are also transported to the CPL, where they associate with the processed antigen. The MHC class II molecule with the bound peptide is then transported to the cell surface.

## T cell activation

The activation of resting $CD4^+$ T cells requires two signals. The first is antigen in association with MHC class II molecules and the second is the co-stimulatory signal. The generation of the first of these signals has just been discussed, i.e. antigen presentation. The second signal is delivered by the same antigen-presenting cell which gave the first signal. The co-stimulatory signal is mediated by the inter-action of a molecule on the antigen-presenting cell engaging with its receptor on the T cell. The best characterized pairing is B7 on the antigen-presenting cell, and CD28 on the T cell.

When both these signals are generated, biochemical changes occur within the T cell, leading to RNA and protein synthesis. The responsive cells progress through the cell cycle from the $G_0$ to the $G_1$ phase. The cells start to express interleukin-2 receptors and produce interleukin-2. Interleukin-2 is a T cell growth factor and causes the expansion of the responsive T cell population. Interleukin-2 was originally thought to be the only T cell growth factor, but it is now known that interleukin-4 and interleukin-1 will support T cell growth although they are not as potent. After about 2 days, interleukin-2 synthesis stops, while interleukin-2 receptors remain for up to a week if the cell is not reactivated. Therefore, there is a built-in limitation on T cell growth and clonal expansion. When stimulated, T cells secrete interleukin-2, which interacts with interleukin-2 receptors to mediate growth. This can be in an 'autocrine' fashion if the same cell that released the interleukin-2 is stimulated. If the responding cell is in the vicinity of the producer then the stimulation is in a 'paracrine' manner. Interleukin-2 is not present at detectable levels in the blood, therefore there is no '*endocrine*' activity involved, i.e. action at a distant site. The end result is the production of a large number of activated CD4+ T lymphocytes.

The other main type of T lymphocyte is the CD8+ T cell. Antigen recognition by these cells is restricted by MHC class I molecules. Again, these cells require two signals to be activated – antigen fragment in association with MHC class I is the first signal, and the co-stimulatory signal the second signal. A cell that 'sees' both these signals responds by clonal expansion and differentiation into a fully active effector T cell.

### B cell activation

Mitogens and T-independent antigens have an inherent ability to drive B cells into division and differentiation. T-dependent responses rely on T cells and their products to control the antibody class, affinity and memory. The first cells to be activated are CD4+ T cells that recognize the antigen in association with MHC class II molecules (see above). These cells respond to the signal of the antigen fragment–MHC complex, and produce a variety of lymphokines that act on B cells.

As far as B cell development is concerned, the antigen-stimulated cells develop under the influence of interleukin-4 (previously known as B cell stimulation factor) that is produced by closely adherent T cells. Interleukin-5 and interleukin-6 then bring the cells to a state of full activation with terminal differentiation into an immunoglobulin-producing plasma cell. All this will happen within a germinal centre of a lymph node secondary follicle which has evolved to facilitate the necessary cellular and molecular interactions.

Therefore, for both B and T cell activation two stimuli are required. The recognition of antigen makes sure that only those cells that will be effective against the foreign material are recruited. The provision of the co-stimulatory signal has evolved to control the process and aid discrimination of 'self' and 'non-self'.

## Humoral immunity

### Synthesis of antibody

On exposure to antigen, antibody production follows a characteristic pattern (Fig. 11.7). There is a lag phase during which antibody cannot be detected. This is the time taken for the interactions described above to take place and antibody to reach a level that can be measured. Then there is an exponential

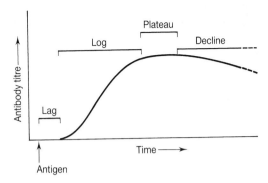

**Fig. 11.7**   Pattern of antibody production following antigen exposure.

rise in the antibody level or titre. This log phase is followed by a plateau with a constant level of antibody where the amount produced equals the amount removed. The amount of antibody then declines due to the clearing of antigen–antibody complexes and the natural catabolism of the immunoglobulin.

If the response is to a T-dependent antigen then the B cells can switch to the production of another isotype, e.g. in a primary response IgM gives way to IgG production. This process is under the control of T cells, since the class of antibody produced will depend on signals from the T cell. At some point, again under the control of T cells, a proportion of the antigen-reactive cells will develop into memory cells. These cells will react if the epitope is encountered again.

There are a number of differences in the reaction profile on second and subsequent exposures to an antigen compared to the primary response (Fig. 11.8). There is a shortened lag and an extended plateau and decline. The level and affinity of antibody produced are much increased, and it is mostly of

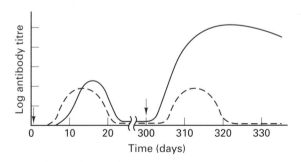

**Fig. 11.8**   Primary and secondary antibody response. The level of serum IgM (- - -) and IgG (—) detected with time after primary immunization (day 0) and challenge (day 300) with the same antigen.

the IgG isotype. Some IgM will be generated, but it will follow the same pattern as in the primary response.

When first introduced the antigen selects the cells that can react with it. However, before antibody is produced the B cell must differentiate into a plasma cell, involving the interactions already described. The B cells that are stimulated in the primary response synthesize IgM. With time, class switch will occur in some of the B cells, leading to the production of other isotypes. Somatic mutations will occur, giving rise to *affinity maturation* through selection of cells bearing high-affinity receptors as the amount of antigen in the system falls. Memory cells will also be produced. An equilibrium is reached where there is a balance between the amount of antibody synthesized and the amount used. Then various mechanisms come into play to turn off the response when it is no longer needed (see below). The simplest is the removal of the stimulant, i.e. antigen. So the production of antibody is stopped and there is a natural decline in antibody levels.

On subsequent exposure the responding cells, i.e. memory cells, are at a different level of activation and present at an increased frequency. Therefore, there is a shorter lag before antibody can be detected: the main isotype is IgG. The level of antibody produced is 10 or more times greater than during the primary response. The antibody is present for an extended period and has a higher affinity for antigen due to affinity maturation. As is seen in Figure 11.8 some IgM is also produced during a secondary response. This immunoglobulin is produced by the activation of B cells that were not present in the lymphocyte pool on the previous exposure but have developed since. The development of these cells follows the characteristics of a primary response, and they will give rise to a secondary response if the antigen is encountered again.

## Monoclonal antibodies

When an antigen is introduced into the lymphoid system of a mouse, all the B cells that recognize epitopes on the antigen will be stimulated to produce antibody. The serum of the immunized animal is known as a polyclonal antiserum since it is the product of many clonally derived B cells. Even if highly purified antigen is used, the antiserum produced will contain a number of antibodies that react to the antigen and others that interact with antigens that the animal encountered naturally during this time. It is extremely difficult to purify the antibodies of interest from this complex mixture, but it is possible to fuse single plasma cells with a myeloma (a tumour) cell line to form a hybridoma which will grow in tissue culture. These cells will all be identical and therefore secrete the same antibody, a *monoclonal antibody.*

Human monoclonal antibodies are potentially of value in patient treatment. As starting material, peripheral blood or secondary lymphoid tissue such as tonsils have been used. It is impossible for ethical reasons to expose human subjects to most of the antigenic material that would be required to induce useful antibodies. Therefore, cells are only available from patients with certain diseases, such as tumours, infections and auto-immune diseases, or from individuals who have received vaccinations.

All the molecules in a monoclonal antibody preparation will have the same isotype, specificity and affinity, in contrast to the polyclonal antiserum produced by the inoculation of antigen into an experimental animal. In addition, the same polyclonal antiserum can never be reproduced, not even when using the same animal. However, monoclonal antibodies are defined reagents that can be produced indefinitely and on a large scale. They provide a standard material that can be used in studies ranging from the identification and enumeration of different cell types to blood typing and diagnosis of disease.

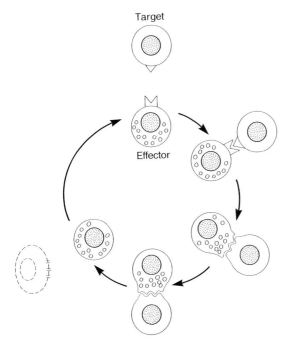

Target

Effector

**Fig. 11.9** Mechanism of cell-mediated cytotoxicity. The effector cell has a receptor that is able to bind to a target cell that possesses the appropriate ligand (△).

They are also increasingly used in attempts to treat and prevent disease.

## Cell-mediated immunity

Specific cell-mediated responses are mediated by two different types of T lymphocyte. T cells that have the CD8 molecule on their surface recognize antigen fragments in association with MHC class I molecules on a target cell and cause cell lysis. MHC class II-restricted recognition is seen with T cells that have the CD4 marker. These cells secrete lymphokines when stimulated by the antigen–MHC class II complex. CD4$^+$ T cells are involved in two main activities: (1) cell-mediated reactions, as the lymphokines can aid in the elimination of foreign material by recruiting and activating other leucocytes and promoting an inflammatory response; and (2) the generation and control of an immune response, as some of the lymphokines produced are growth and differentiation factors for T and B cells.

The other cell types, NK cells and phagocytes, which can participate in cell-mediated defence mechanisms have been described.

### Cell-mediated cytotoxicity

Certain subpopulations of lymphoid and myeloid cells can destroy target cells to which they are closely bound. The stages and processes involved are similar for the different cell types although the molecules that mediate the recognition of the target by the effector differ.

*Cytotoxic T lymphocytes.* Cytotoxic T cells (T$_C$ cells) are small T lymphocytes that are derived from stem cells in the bone marrow. These cells mature in the thymus. Most cells that mediate MHC-restricted cytotoxicity are CD8$^+$ and, therefore, recognize antigen in association with MHC class I antigens. Some are CD4$^+$ and, therefore, MHC class II restricted.

*MHC-unrestricted cytotoxic cells.* A number of partially overlapping cell populations are able to carry out MHC-unrestricted killing. These include NK cells, lymphokine-activated killer (LAK) cells and killer (K) cells.

Most cells that have the capacity to perform natural killing have the morphology of large granular lymphocytes and have a broad target range. The receptor on the NK cell and the structures that they recognize on the target have not been identified. NK cells have been shown to produce a number of cytokines, including γ-interferon.

Several types of cells are able to destroy foreign material by antibody-dependent cell-mediated cytotoxicity. The cells that carry out this activity have a receptor for the Fc portion of immunoglobulin and are, therefore, able to bind to antibody-coated targets.

*Lytic mechanism.* Three distinct phases have been described in cell-mediated cytotoxicity: (1) binding to target; (2) rearrangement of cytoplasmic granules and the release of their contents; and (3) target cell death (Fig. 11.9).

Once the effector–target conjugate is formed the cytoplasmic granules appear to become rearranged and concentrated at the side of the cell adjacent to the target. The granule contents are then released into the space between the two cells. There are at least three different types of molecule stored within the granules that can cause cell death. T cells and NK cells contain perforin, which is a monomeric protein related to the complement component C9. In the presence of Ca$^{2+}$ ions the monomers bind to the target cell membrane and polymerize to form a transmembrane pore. This upsets the osmotic balance of the cell and leads to cell death. The granules also contain at least two serine esterases that may play a role in destroying the target cell. A number of other toxic molecules are also produced by cytotoxic cells, including tumour necrosis factor (TNFα), lymphotoxin (TNFβ), γ-interferon and NK cytotoxic factor. The process is unidirectional with only the target cell being destroyed. The effector cell can then move on and eliminate another target cell.

### Lymphokine production

The other arm of cell-mediated immunity is dependent on the production of lymphokines from antigen-activated T lymphocytes. These molecules produced in an antigen-specific fashion can act in an antigen non-specific manner to recruit, activate and regulate effector cells with the potential to combat infectious agents.

The first documented reference to the production of lymphokines is credited to Robert Koch in 1880. Injection of purified antigen (tuberculin) into the skin of immune individuals produced a reaction that peaked within 24–72 h. The response was characterized by reddening and swelling and was accompanied by the accumulation of lymphocytes, monocytes and basophils. Because of the time course of the reaction this response has become known as *delayed-type hypersensitivity* (DTH) and the cells responsible were called delayed-type hypersensitivity T lymphocytes (T$_{DTH}$ or T$_D$ cells). These cells are identical to the helper T ($T_H$) cell subset as far as antigen recognition is concerned. CD4$^+$ T cells, usually still referred to as $T_H$ cells, are therefore capable of mediating both helper activities and so-called delayed hypersensitivity reactions by producing lymphokines. Although the term 'delayed hypersensitivity' suggests a disease process, the production of lymphokines has a physiological function, and only in some situations do pathological consequences occur.

Cytokines are biologically active molecules released by specific cells that elicit a particular response from other cells on which they act. A number of these regulatory molecules produced by lymphocytes (lymphokines) and monocytes (monokines) are shown in Table 11.6. The responses caused by these substances are varied and interrelated. In general, cytokines control growth, mobility and differentiation of lymphocytes, but they also exert a similar effect on other leucocytes and some non-immune cells.

The exact signals and mechanisms controlling the activation of T cells and the release of lymphokines are not known. The balance between the different lymphokines produced will determine the response generated. CD4$^+$ T cells can be divided into two main types depending on the profile of lymphokines they secrete. The $T_H2$ subset produces interleukin-4 and interleukin-5, which act on responsive B cells giving antibody production as the main feature of the response. The $T_H1$ subset secretes mainly interleukin-2 and $\gamma$-interferon. The production of

**Table 11.6** Cytokines of importance in the immune system. Many of the molecules detailed below act synergistically to produce their biological effects

| Cytokine | Immune system source | Other source | Target | Effect |
|---|---|---|---|---|
| IL-1 | Macrophages | Epithelial cells | T lymphocytes<br>B lymphocytes<br>Tissue cells | Fever<br>Inflammation<br>T cell activation<br>Macrophage activation |
| TNF$\alpha$ | Macrophages<br>NK cells | | Macrophages<br>Endothelial cells | Cell activation<br>Local inflammation<br>Cachexia |
| TNF$\beta$ | T lymphocytes | | Granulocytes<br>Endothelial cells<br>NK cells | Killing<br>Cell activation<br>Increased adherence of leucocytes to endothelium |
| IFN-$\alpha$ | Leucocytes | | Tissue cells | Antiviral effect<br>Induction of MHC class I |
| IFN-$\beta$ | Fibroblast | | Tissue cells | Antiviral effect<br>Induction of MHC class I |
| IFN-$\gamma$ | T lymphocytes<br>NK cells | | Leucocytes and tissue cells | Macrophage activation<br>Induction of MHC class I and II |
| Macrophage (M–) CSF | Monocytes | Endothelium<br>Fibroblasts | Stem cells | Stimulate division and differentiation |
| Granulocyte (G–) CSF | Macrophages | Fibroblasts | Stem cells | Stimulate division and differentiation |
| GM–CSF | T lymphocytes<br>Macrophage | Endothelium<br>Fibroblasts | Stem cells | Stimulate division and differentiation |
| Migration inhibition factor (MIF) | T lymphocytes | | Macrophages | Migration inhibition |
| Chemotactic factors | Lymphocytes<br>Macrophages<br>Granulocytes | Tissue cells | Leucocytes | Attract to site of infection or tissue damage |

IL, interleukin; TNF, tumour necrosis factor; IFN, interferon; CSF colony-stimulating factor.

interleukin-2 stimulates T cell growth while γ-interferon will have multiple effects, including macrophage activation.

## Role of macrophages

Macrophages are able to carry out a remarkable array of different functions (Fig. 11.10). They play a key role in several aspects of cell-mediated immunity, being involved at the initiation of the response, as antigen-presenting cells, and as effector cells having microbicidal and tumoricidal activities. They also produce a number of cytokines (or more precisely monokines) that function as regulatory molecules. These monokines contribute to inflammation and fever and affect the functioning of other cells. Macrophages can also produce various enzymes and factors that are involved in reorganization and repair following tissue damage. However, since they contain many important biological molecules they themselves can cause damage if these enzymes and factors are released inappropriately.

Many of these activities are enhanced in macrophages that have been 'activated' by exposure to lymphokines, such as γ-interferon produced by T cells. Macrophage activation is a complex process which probably occurs in stages with different effector functions being expressed at different stages. Macrophages from different sites in the body show different characteristics, i.e. they are very heterogeneous, and will have different activation requirements.

γ-Interferon is a powerful macrophage-activating molecule which increases the uptake of antigens by an enhanced expression of Fc and complement receptors; the activities of intracellular enzymes involved in killing are also elevated. Since γ-interferon causes an increase in MHC class II expression there will be an enhanced presentation of antigen to CD4$^+$ T cells. This will lead to the production of more lymphokines and more effective elimination of the offending material.

The lymphokines that activate macrophages are secreted by CD4$^+$ T cells. Therefore, the presentation of antigen by an antigen-presenting cell will lead to the production of lymphokines by $T_H1$ cells *specific* for the antigen involved. The lymphokines produced will then activate *any* responsive macrophage in the vicinity of the responding cells. The activation process appears to depend on the presence of a number of lymphokines that act synergistically to induce activation. For example, pure interleukin-2, interleukin-4 or γ-interferon is unable to induce resistance to infection, but if γ-interferon is combined with any of the others then resistance is observed.

Macrophages and monocytes themselves are capable of producing a number of important cytokines. These monokines include interleukin-1, interleukin-6, various colony-stimulating factors and tumour necrosis factor. Tumour necrosis factor and interleukin-1 acting independently and together have effects on many leucocytes and tissues. Tumour necrosis factor is responsible for the tumoricidal activity of macrophages but is also implicated in the elimination of certain bacteria and parasites. It has a synergistic effect with γ-interferon on resistance to a number of viral infections.

## Generation of immune responses

As discussed previously, the generation of humoral and cell-mediated responses requires the recogni-

**Fig. 11.10** The central role of macrophages.

tion of antigen, by the responding cell, as the first signal and a co-stimulation second signal. $T_H$ cells, as has been emphasized, only recognize antigen fragments in association with MHC class II molecules. The distribution of MHC class II molecules is limited, in normal situations, to certain cells of the immune system – the antigen-presenting cells. In certain circumstances non-lymphoid cells can present antigens if they are induced to express MHC class II molecules. In order to stimulate a $T_H$ cell the antigen must be taken into the cell and re-expressed on the surface in association with MHC class II molecules. Since the T cell antigen receptor recognizes antigen fragments bound to the MHC molecules, the antigen-presenting cell must also be able to process the antigen. MHC class I- and class II-restricted recognition by $CD8^+$ and $CD4^+$ T cells requires antigen processing. The pathways that lead to association of an antigen fragment with a particular restriction element are not fully understood.

Immune responses are generated in secondary lymphoid tissues, such as lymph nodes. Since a number of cells and molecules must all interact, the architecture of the secondary lymphoid tissue has evolved for the efficient induction of an immune response. In a secondary immune response the cells involved are at a different stage of activation, i.e. they are memory cells having already been exposed to antigen. Therefore, the growth factor signals may not be so critical but antigen in association with MHC class II molecules is still required. In this situation B cells are important as antigen-presenting cells.

$CD8^+$ T cells, as we have seen, recognize antigen fragments associated with MHC class I molecules. All cells have MHC class I molecules on their surface and would therefore be expected to be capable of presenting antigen fragments to cytotoxic T cells that are in the most part MHC class I restricted. The antigen fragments derived from endogenously synthesized molecules, e.g. from a virus, are produced at a site distinct from the endocytic vesicles where exogenous antigens are processed.

At or around the site of protein synthesis, endogenously produced antigen fragments become associated with the newly produced MHC class I molecules. The MHC class II molecule picks up internalized antigen within a structure, known as the compartment for peptide loading (CPL), as it moves to the cell surface. In this compartment, antigen fragments cannot bind to the MHC class I molecules because these molecules have already associated with endogenously produced antigenic fragments within the endoplasmic reticulum and never go to CPL. Thus the site where the antigen is processed

determines whether it will associate with MHC class I or class II molecules. This separation of processing pathways explains why $CD4^+$ and $CD8^+$ T cells are involved in the destruction of exogenous and endogenous antigens, respectively.

If a particular antigen does not become associated with either MHC class I or II molecules then no T-dependent immune response will be directed against that antigen. Since MHC class II molecules are involved in the initiation of immune responses by presenting antigen fragments to $T_H$ cells, they can control whether a response takes place or not. It has been clearly shown that the level of an immune response to a particular antigen is controlled by the MHC class II molecules. The genes that code for these molecules, i.e. MHC class II genes, have therefore been referred to as *immune response genes* (*Ir* genes).

It should be obvious that if an antigen cannot associate with the MHC class II molecules of an individual then no immune response will be generated. Since the MHC molecules are polymorphic, the cells of some individuals will present, and therefore respond to, certain antigen fragments while cells from other individuals will not. Fortunately, more than one antigenic fragment can be generated from each pathogen, otherwise individuals who did not respond to the particular sequence would be vulnerable to that micro-organism. In addition, individuals can have six different MHC class II genes and therefore an increased chance that some fragments will bind to at least one of their MHC class II molecules. Variations in the levels and specificity of response will occur in individuals who have different MHC class II molecules and have therefore produced different MHC–antigen complexes on their cells.

*Ir* gene effects can also be controlled at the level of the T cell receptor. If an individual does not have a T cell with a receptor that recognizes a particular antigen–MHC complex then no response will be generated. The T cell receptor repertoire is generated in the thymus where the genes of the immature T cells are rearranged to give rise to a functioning receptor. T cells that cross-react too strongly with self molecules are deleted, as are cells whose receptors do not interact with self MHC molecules. Therefore, T cells that interact weakly with MHC molecules are selected to mature and leave the thymus. When these cells later come across an antigen–MHC complex the presence of antigen strengthens the weak T cell receptor–MHC interaction, leading to a stimulatory signal being transmitted to the T cell. If for some reason T cells that respond to a particular MHC–antigen configuration have been deleted, suppressed or not formed then no immune response will be generated to that antigen. There is what is known as a 'hole' in the T cell repertoire.

## Control of immune responses

An antigen can induce two types of response, immunity or tolerance. Tolerance is the acquisition of non-reactivity towards a particular antigen. The generation of immunity or tolerance depends largely on the way the immune system first encounters the antigen. Once the immune system has been stimulated the cells involved proliferate and produce a response that will eliminate the offending agent. It is then important to dampen down the reacting cells and various feedback mechanisms operate to bring this about.

### Role of antigen

The primary regulator of an immune response is the antigen itself. This makes sense since it is important to initiate a response when antigen enters the host and once it has been eliminated it is wasteful and in some cases dangerous to continue to produce effector mechanisms.

### Role of antibody

Many biological systems are controlled by the product inhibiting the reaction once a certain level is reached. This type of negative feedback is seen with antibody which may act by blocking the epitopes on the antigen so that it can no longer stimulate the cell through its receptor.

As antibody levels rise there is competition between free antibody and the B cell receptor. Consequently, only those B cells that have a receptor with a high affinity for antigen will be stimulated and therefore produce high-affinity antibody. For this reason antibody feedback is thought to be an important driving force in affinity maturation.

### Regulatory T cells

$T_H$ cells control the generation of effector cells by producing helper factors. However, the factors that stimulate the expansion of B and T cell numbers do not work indefinitely. Maturation factors are also produced that control terminal differentiation into effector cells. Under the influence of these latter lymphokines the action of the proliferation factors is inhibited mainly by making the effector cell unresponsive to its effects.

Other T lymphocytes have been described that provide negative signals to the immune system. Suppressor T cells ($T_S$ cells) limit the development of antibody-producing cells and effector T cells. The activity of suppressor cells can involve both the production of soluble factors and direct cell–cell interactions.

## Tolerance

Two forms of tolerance can be identified – *natural* tolerance and *acquired* tolerance. The non-response to self molecules is due to natural tolerance. If this tolerance breaks down and the body responds to self molecules then an auto-immune disease will develop. Natural tolerance appears during fetal development when the immune system is being formed. In experimental animals the introduction of foreign material at the time of birth leads to tolerance. Acquired tolerance arises when a potential immunogen induces a state of unresponsiveness to itself. This has consequences for host defences since the presence of a tolerogenic epitope on a pathogen may compromise the ability of the body to resist infection.

An antigen can induce different effects on the two arms of the immune system. During an infection the host will be exposed to a variety of antigenic determinants on a micro-organism. These epitopes will be present at differing concentrations and possibly at different times during the infection. The epitopes can act as either immunogens or tolerogens. Therefore, it is possible that the antibody response to a particular antigen may be quite pronounced while the cell-mediated response might be lacking, or vice versa. Alternatively, both arms of the immune response may be stimulated or tolerized.

Generally, high doses of antigen tolerize B cells, while minute doses given repeatedly tolerize T cells. For acquired tolerance to be maintained the tolerogen must persist or be repeatedly administered. This is probably necessary because of the continuous production of new T and B cells that must be made tolerant.

Several mechanisms play a role in the selective lack of response to specific antigens. Since each lymphocyte has a receptor with a single specificity the elimination of a specific cell will render the individual tolerant to the epitope it recognizes and leave the rest of the repertoire untouched. This mechanism relies on self molecules interacting with the receptor and causing their elimination. It is proposed that during lymphocyte development the cell goes through a phase in which contact with antigen leads to death or permanant inactivation.

Immature B cells encountering antigen for the first time are particularly susceptible to tolerization in the presence of low doses of antigen. The requirement for two signals in the stimulation of B cells and the generation of effector T cells can give rise to tolerance. Both cell types require stimulation via the antigen receptor and 'help' from a specific T cell. If the helper factors are not produced then the responding cells will be functionally deleted. Therefore, the elimination of self-reactive T cells in the thymus during T cell maturation is an important step in maintaining a state of tolerance. Tolerance can also be induced by active suppression. Some T cells are capable of inducing unresponsiveness by acting directly on B cells or other T cells. These $T_S$ cells can be antigen-specific and probably produce signals that actively suppress cells capable of responding to a particular antigen.

Tolerance to self tissues is fundamental to the functioning of the immune system. It was originally thought that unresponsiveness to self was controlled by the elimination of all self-reactive cells before they matured. This cannot be true since self-reactive B cells are found in normal adult animals. It is thought that these B cells are controlled by a lack of T cell help, i.e. $T_H$ cells have been eliminated. It is thought that $T_S$ cells play a subordinate role acting as a back-up mechanism.

## Immunodeficiency

The immunologically competent cells of the lymphoid tissues derived from, renewed by and influenced by the activities of the thymus, bone marrow and other lymphoid tissues can be the subject of disease processes. The deficiency states seen are due either to defects in one of the components of the system itself, or are secondary to some other disease process affecting the normal functioning of some part of the lymphoid tissues. Deficiency of one or more of the defence mechanisms can be inherited, developmental or acquired. The types of infections and diseases seen in patients with immunodeficiencies relate to the role the affected component plays in the normal situation. An individual whose immune system has been depressed in any of these ways is said to be immunocompromised. The *compromised host* is prone to infectious diseases that the normal individual would easily eradicate or not succumb to in the first place. Some examples of predisposing factors are given in Table 11.7.

### Defective innate defence mechanisms

Defects in phagocyte function take two forms: (1) where there is a quantitative deficiency of neutrophils which may be congenital (e.g. infantile agranulocytosis) or acquired as a result of replacement of bone marrow by tumour cells or the toxic effects of drugs or chemicals; (2) where there is a qualitative deficiency in the functioning of neutrophils which, while ingesting bacteria normally, fail, because of an enzymic defect, to digest them. Characteristic of these diseases is a susceptibility to bacterial and fungal, but not viral or protozoan, infections. Among the enzyme deficiency disorders are *chronic granulomatous disease* and the *Chédiak–Higashi syndrome*.

| Table 11.7 The compromised host | | |
|---|---|---|
| Predisposing factor | Effect on immune system | Type of infection |
| Immunosuppression for transplant or cancer | Diminished cell-mediated and humoral immunity | Lung infections, bacteraemia, fungal infections, urinary tract infections |
| Viral immunosuppression, e.g. measles, human immunodeficiency virus, Epstein–Barr virus | Impaired function of infected cells | Secondary bacterial infections, opportunistic pathogens |
| Tumour of immune cells | Replacement of cells of the immune system | Bacteraemia, pneumonia, urinary tract infections |
| Malnutrition | Lymphoid hypoplasia Decreased lymphocytes and phagocyte activity | Measles, tuberculosis, respiratory infections, gastro-intestinal infections |
| Breakdown of tissue barriers, e.g. surgery, burns, catheterization | Breach innate defence mechanisms | Bacterial infections Opportunistic pathogens |
| Inhalation of particles due to employment or smoking | Damage to cilia, destruction of alveolar macrophages | Chronic respiratory infections, hypersensitivity reactions |

The complement system can also suffer from certain defects in function leading to increased susceptibility to infection. The most severe abnormalities of host defences occur, as would be expected, if there is a defect in the functioning of C3. Severe deficiency or absence of C3 is associated with increased susceptibility to infection, particularly septicaemia, pneumonia, meningitis, otitis and pharyngitis.

## Defective acquired immune defence mechanisms

**Primary immunodeficiencies.** Primary deficiencies in immunological function can arise through failure of any of the developmental processes from stem cell to functional end cell. A complete lack of all leucocytes is seen in *reticular dysgenesis* due to a defect in the development of bone marrow stem cells in the fetus. A baby born with this defect usually dies within the first year of life from recurrent, intractable infections. Defects in the development of the common lymphoid stem cell give rise to severe combined immunodeficiency. Both T and B lymphocytes fail to develop but functional phagocytes are present.

There are several types of B cell defect that give rise to hypogammaglobulinaemias, i.e. low levels of γ-globulins (antibodies) in the blood. Deficiency of immunoglobulin synthesis is almost complete in X-linked infantile hypogammaglobulinaemia (*Bruton's disease*). Male infants suffer from severe, chronic bacterial infections after maternal antibody has disappeared. There is an absence, or deficiency, of all five classes of serum immunoglobulins. Therefore, the defect is thought to be caused by the absence of B cell precursors or their arrest at a pre-B cell stage. In these patients cell-mediated immune mechanisms function normally and they seem to be able to handle viral infections relatively well.

Partial defects in immunoglobulin synthesis have been described affecting one or more of the immunoglobulin classes. In the *Wiskott–Aldrich syndrome* that is inherited as an X-linked recessive character there are low IgM levels but IgA and IgE levels are elevated. Patients are susceptible to pyogenic infections, along with recurrent bleeding and eczema. The bleeding is due to reduced platelet production (thrombocytopenia), and the allergy-related eczema is linked to the elevated IgE levels. In patients with *dysgammaglobulinaemia* there is a deficiency in only one antibody class. Some patients have reduced levels of IgA whereas the other isotypes are normal. These patients have an increased incidence of infec-tions in the upper and lower respiratory tracts where IgA is normally protective.

Individuals with T cell defects tend to have more severe and persistent infections than those with antibody deficiencies. A lack of T lymphocytes is often associated with abnormal antibody levels since $T_H$ cells are involved in the generation and control of humoral immunity. Patients with T cell defects suffer from viral, intracellular bacterial, fungal and protozoan infections rather than acute bacterial infections. In the *DiGeorge syndrome* (congenital thymic aplasia) the patient is born with little or no thymus. Individuals who survive develop recurrent and chronic infections, including pneumonia, diarrhoea and yeast infections once passive maternal immunity wanes.

**Secondary immunodeficiencies.** Acquired deficiencies can occur secondarily to a number of disease states or after exposure to drugs and chemicals.

Deficiency of immunoglobulins can be brought about by excessive loss of protein through diseased kidneys or via the intestine in protein-losing enteropathy. Malnutrition and iron deficiency can lead to depressed immune responsiveness, particularly in cell-mediated immunity. Medical and surgical treatments such as irradiation, cytotoxic drugs and steroids often have undesirable effects on the immune system. Viral infections are often immunosuppressive. For example, measles, human immunodeficiency and other viruses infect cells of the immune system.

In contrast to the deficiency states just described, raised immunoglobulin levels are found in certain disorders of plasma cells due to malignant proliferation of a particular clone or group of plasma cells. In these conditions, such as chronic lymphocytic leukaemia and multiple myeloma, malignant clones will each produce one particular type of antibody. There is usually a decreased synthesis of normal immunoglobulins and an associated deficiency in the immune response to acute bacterial infections. These B-lymphoproliferative disorders contrast with the situation in *Hodgkin's disease*, a reticular cell neoplasm, where the patients show defective cell-mediated immunity and are susceptible to viruses and intracellular bacteria.

## Hypersensitivity

Immunity was first recognized as a resistant state that followed infection. However, some forms of immune reaction, rather than providing exemption or safety, can produce severe and occasionally fatal results. These are known as *hypersensitivity reactions* and result from an excessive or inappropriate response to an antigenic stimulus. The mechanisms underlying these deleterious reactions are those that normally eradicate foreign material but for various reasons the response leads to a disease state. When considering each of the four hypersensitivity states it is important to remember this fact and consider the underlying defence mechanism and how it has given rise to the observed immunopathology.

Various classifications of hypersensitivity reactions have been proposed, and probably the most widely accepted is that of Coombs and Gell. This recognizes four types of hypersensitivity that will be considered in turn.

## Type I: anaphylactic

If a guinea-pig is injected with a small dose of an antigen such as egg albumin, no adverse effects are noted. If a second injection of the same antigen is given intravenously after an interval of about 2 weeks a condition known as *anaphylactic shock* is likely to develop. The animal becomes restless, starts chewing and rubbing its nose, begins to wheeze and may develop convulsions and die. The initial injection of antigen is termed the sensitizing dose while the second injection causes anaphylactic shock. Such a reaction is seen in humans after a bee sting or injection of penicillin in sensitized individuals. Localized reactions are seen in patients with hay fever and asthma. In all these situations the host responds to the first injection by producing IgE, and it is the level of IgE produced to a particular antigen that will determine whether an anaphylactic reaction will occur on re-exposure to the same antigen. Asthma results from a similar response in the respiratory tract.

The biologically active molecules that are responsible for the manifestations of type I hypersensitivity are stored within mast cell and basophil granules or are synthesized after cell triggering. The signal for the release or production of these molecules is the cross-linking of surface-bound IgE by antigen. The release of these molecules, vaso-active amines and chemotactic factors, is responsible for the symptoms of type I hypersensitivity. IgE has been implicated in the control of parasitic worms, and the importance of this is discussed in Chapter 13.

## Type II: cytotoxic

Type II reactions are initiated by the binding of an antibody to an antigenic component on a cell surface. The antibody is directed against an epitope that can be a self molecule or a drug or microbial product passively adsorbed onto a cell surface. The cell that is covered with antibody is then destroyed by the immune system. A variety of infectious diseases due to salmonella organisms and mycobacteria are associated with haemolytic anaemia. There is evidence, particularly in studies on salmonella infections, that the haemolysis is due to an immune reaction against a lipopolysaccharide bacterial endotoxin that becomes coated onto the erythrocytes of the patient.

## Type III: immune complex

As discussed previously, when a soluble antigen combines with antibody the size and physical form of the immune complex formed will depend on the relative proportions of the participating molecules and will be affected by the class of antibody. Monocytes and macrophages are very efficient at binding and removing large complexes. These same cell types can also eliminate the smaller complexes made in antibody excess but are relatively inefficient at removing those formed in antigen excess. Type III hypersensitivity reactions appear if there is a defect in the systems, involving phagocytes and complement, that remove immune complexes or if the system is overloaded and the complexes are deposited in tissues. This latter situation occurs when antigens are never completely eliminated, as with persistent infection with an organism, autoimmunity and repeated contact with environmental factors.

The tissue damage that results from the deposition of immune complexes is caused by the activation of complement, platelets and phagocytes, in essence an acute inflammatory response. In general, the degree and site of damage depends on the ratio of antigen to antibody. At equivalence or slight excess of either component the complexes precipitate at the site of antigen injection or production and a mild, local type III hypersensitivity reaction occurs, e.g. the *Arthus reaction*. In contrast, the complexes formed in large antigen excess become soluble and circulate, causing more serious systemic reactions, i.e. *serum sickness*, or eventually deposit in organs, such as skin, kidneys and joints. The type of disease and its time course will depend on the immune status of the individual.

The local release of antigens from an infectious organism can cause a type III reaction. A number of parasitic worms, although undesirable, cause little or no damage. However, if the worm is killed it can become lodged in the lymphatics, and the inflammatory response initiated by antigen–antibody complexes causes a blockage of lymph flow. This leads to the condition of elephantiasis in which enormous swellings can occur. In some cases of tuberculosis, sarcoidosis, leprosy and streptococcal infections, vascular inflammatory lesions are seen mainly in the legs. These are variously referred to as *erythema nodosum*, *nodular vasculitis* and *erythema induratum*, and may be due to the deposition of immune complexes and the development of an Arthus reaction.

In systemic disease the clinical manifestations depend upon where the immune complexes form or lodge – skin, joints, kidney and heart being particularly affected.

Drugs such as penicillin and sulphonamides can cause type III reactions. The most susceptible patients will develop rashes (urticarial, morbilliform or scarlatiniform), pyrexia, arthralgia, lymphadenopathy and perhaps nephritis some 8–12 days after being given the drug. It is likely that similar events occur in many bacterial and viral infections (see Chs 14 and 12, respectively).

### Type IV: cell-mediated or delayed

This form of hypersensitivity can be defined as a specifically provoked, slowly evolving (24–48 h), mixed cellular reaction involving lymphocytes and macrophages. The reaction is not brought about by circulating antibody but by sensitized lymphoid cells. This type of response is seen in a number of allergic reactions to bacteria, viruses and fungi, in contact dermatitis and in graft rejection. The classical example of this type of reaction is the tuberculin response that is seen following an intradermal injection of a purified protein derivative (PPD) from tubercle bacilli in immune individuals. An indurated inflammatory reaction in the skin appears about 24 h later and persists for a few weeks. In humans the injection site is infiltrated with large numbers of mononuclear cells, mainly lymphocytes, with about 10–20% macrophages. Most of these cells are in or around small blood vessels. The type IV hypersensitivity state arises when an inappropriate or exaggerated cell-mediated response occurs.

Cell-mediated hypersensitivity reactions are seen in a number of chronic infectious diseases due to mycobacteria, protozoa and fungi. Because the host is unable to eliminate the micro-organism the antigens persist and give rise to a chronic antigenic stimulus. Thus, continual release of lymphokines from sensitized T cells results in the accumulation of large numbers of activated macrophages that can become epithelioid cells. These cells can fuse together to form giant cells. Macrophages will express antigen fragments on their surface in association with MHC class I and II molecules and will therefore be the targets of $T_C$ cells and stimulate more lymphokine production. This whole process leads to tissue damage with the formation of a chronic granuloma and resultant cell death.

Penicillin sensitization is a common clinical complication following the topical application of the antibiotic in ointments or creams. This and other substances that cause contact sensitivity are not themselves antigenic and only become so in combination with proteins in the skin. The Langerhans's cells of the epidermis are efficient antigen-presenting cells favouring the development of a T cell response. These cells pick up the newly formed antigen in the skin and transport it to the draining lymph node where a T cell response is stimulated. Here, the specific T cells will be stimulated to mature and will then return to the site of entry of the offending material and release their lymphokines. In a normal situation these would help to eliminate a pathogen but in this case the continual or subsequent exposure to the foreign material leads to an inappropriate response. The reaction site is characterized by a mononuclear cell infiltrate peaking at 48 h. The clinical symptoms in these contact dermatitis lesions include redness, swelling, vesicles, scaling and exudation of fluid, i.e. eczema.

## Auto-immunity

A fundamental characteristic of the immune system of an animal is that it does not, under normal circumstances, react against its own body constituents. Mechanisms, as we have seen, exist that allow the immune system to tolerate self and destroy non-self. Occasionally these mechanisms break down and auto-antibodies are produced.

Genetic factors appear to play a role in the development of auto-immune diseases and there is a strong association between several auto-immune diseases and particular HLA (human leucocyte group A) specificities, suggesting that *Ir* gene effects may be involved.

There are a number of examples where potential auto-antigenic determinants are present in exogenous material. These preparations may provide a new carrier, i.e. a T cell-stimulating determinant that provokes auto-antibody formation. The encephalitis sometimes seen after rabies vaccination with the older vaccines is thought to result from a response directed against the brain that is stimulated by heterologous brain tissues present in the vaccine.

Micro-organisms are a source of cross-reacting antigens sharing antigenic determinants with tissue components. These may provide an important way of inducing auto-immunity. The group A streptococci, which are closely associated with rheumatic fever, share an antigen with the human heart. Heart lesions are a common finding in rheumatic fever, and anti-heart antibody is found in just over 50% of patients with this condition. Nephritogenic strains of type 12 group A streptococci carry surface antigens similar to those found in human glomeruli, and infection by these organisms has been associated with the development of acute nephritis. Some of the immunopathology seen in Chagas' disease has been attributed to a cross-reaction between *Trypanosoma cruzi* and cardiac muscle.

Auto-immunity can be induced by bypassing T cells. Self-reactive cells can be directly stimulated by polyclonal activators that directly activate B cells. A number of micro-organisms or their products are potent polyclonal activators; however, the response that is generated tends to be IgM and to wane when the pathogen is eliminated. Bacterial endotoxin, the lipopolysaccharide of Gram-negative bacteria, provides a non-specific inductive signal to B cells, bypassing the need for T cell help. A variety of antibodies are present in infectious mononucleosis, including auto-antibodies, that are caused by the polyclonal activation of B cells by Epstein–Barr virus.

---

## RECOMMENDED READING

Abbas A K, Lichtman A H, Pober J S 1994 *Cellular and Molecular Immunology*, 2nd edn. W B Saunders, Philadelphia

Engelhard V H 1994 How cells process antigens. *Scientific American* Aug: 44–51

Germain R N 1994 MHC-dependent antigen processing and peptide presentation: providing ligands for T lymphocyte activation. *Cell* 76: 287–299

Janeway C A, Travers P 1994 *Immunobiology*. Current Biology, London

Weir D M, Stewart J 1997 *Immunology*, 8th edn. Churchill Livingstone, Edinburgh

# 12

# Immunity in viral infections

*J. Stewart and D. M. Weir*

The host response to an invading virus will depend upon the characteristics of the infectious agent and where it is encountered. In many cases viral infections are subclinical, i.e. symptomless, but exposure gives rise to protection on re-exposure later in life. A vast array of host defence mechanisms work in a concerted way to protect the individual from viruses and to eliminate them if an infection occurs. In several instances, virus-induced immune responses may have immunopathological consequences.

## THE RESPONSE TO VIRAL INFECTIONS

### Interferons

At the time of their discovery in 1957 the term *interferon* identified a factor produced by cells in response to viral infection that protected other cells of the same species from attack by a wide range of viruses. It is now clear that this activity is mediated by members of a family of regulatory proteins.

In humans, as in a number of other species, there are three types of interferon; α-interferon (IFN-α) and β-interferon (IFN-β), produced by peripheral blood mononuclear cells and fibroblasts, respectively, and γ-interferon (IFN-γ), a lymphokine produced in response to a specific antigenic signal. There is only one gene for IFN-β and one for IFN-γ but there are at least 23 different IFN-α genes coding for 15 functional proteins. All the IFN-α genes are closely related and clustered on chromosome 9, close to the IFN-β gene; the IFN-γ gene is on chromosome 12. The production of interferons is under strict inductional control. IFN-α and IFN-β are produced in response to the presence of viruses and certain intracellular bacteria. Double-stranded RNA may be the important inducer. IFN-γ, which has an extensive role in the control of immune responses, is produced by antigen-activated T lymphocytes and natural killer (NK) cells (see pp. 136–8).

To exert their biological effects these molecules must interact with cell surface receptors. IFN-α and IFN-β share a common receptor while IFN-γ binds to its own specific receptor. After binding to the cell surface receptors, interferons act by rapidly and transiently inducing or up-regulating some cellular genes and down-regulating others. The overall effect is to inhibit viral replication and activate host defence mechanisms.

The antiviral activity is mediated by the interferon released from a virus-infected cell binding to a neighbouring cell and inducing the synthesis of antiviral proteins (Fig. 12.1). Interferons are extremely potent in this function, acting at femtomolar ($10^{-15}$ M) concentrations. They can inhibit many stages of the virus life cycle – attachment and uncoating, early viral transcription, viral translation, protein synthesis and budding. Many new proteins can be detected in cells exposed to interferon, but major roles have been proposed for two enzymes that inhibit protein synthesis: 2',5'-oligoadenylate synthetase (2,5-A synthetase) and a protein kinase. The activity of both these enzymes is dependent on double-stranded RNA provided by viral intermediates in the cell. The protein kinase is responsible for phosphorylation of histones and the protein synthesis initiation factor $eIF_2$. This leads to the inhibition of protein synthesis within interferon-stimulated cells due to inhibition of ribosome assembly. The 2,5-A synthetase is strongly induced in human cells by all three types of interferon and forms 2',5'-linked oligonucleotides of adenosine from ATP. These oligonucleotides activate a latent cellular endonuclease that degrades both messenger and ribosomal RNA with a resultant inhibition of protein synthesis. The requirement for the presence of double-stranded RNA for the full expression of these effects will safeguard uninfected cells from the damaging effects of these enzymes. Apart from these well-characterized changes, many other changes occur in cells treated with interferons. Some viral proteins can inhibit the interferon response.

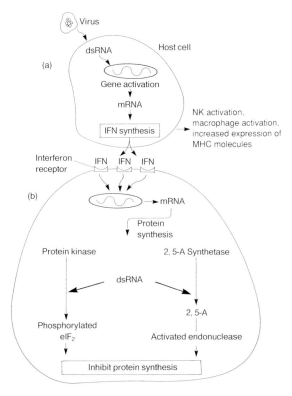

**Fig. 12.1** Proposed mechanisms of **a** induction of synthesis of INF-α and INF-β and **b** production of resistance to virus infection. dsRNA, double-stranded RNA; mRNA, messenger RNA; 2,5-A, 2',5'-oligoadenylate; MHC, major histocompatibility complex; NK natural killer cells.

Some effects of interferon are viral-specific. The Mx protein induced in mice by IFN-α/β is specifically involved in the resistance to influenza virus infection. There is a related protein in human cells, and it is possible that some of the other interferon-induced proteins may confer resistance to specific virus types. Resistance of IFN-γ-treated cells to the parasite *Toxoplasma gondii* is associated with induction of the enzyme indolamine dioxygenase, which catabolizes the essential amino acid tryptophan. However, interferons have effects on host cell growth and differentiation. Interferons, particularly IFN-α and IFN-β, are potent inhibitors of normal and malignant cell growth. A number of clinical trials have shown that IFN-α is active against some human cancers, especially those of haemopoietic origin.

Interferons are able to modify immune responses by (1) altering expression of cell surface molecules, (2) altering the production and secretion of cellular proteins and (3) enhancing or inhibiting effector cell functions. One of the main ways in which

interferons control immune responses is by the induction or enhancement of major histocompatibility complex (MHC)-encoded molecules. Class I MHC genes are up-regulated by all types of interferon, as is the production of $\beta_2$-microglobulin. IFN-γ induces and increases the expression of MHC class II antigens. In addition, interferons can induce or enhance the expression of Fc receptors and receptors for a number of cytokines. These activities will increase the efficiency of antigen recognition and lead to a more effective immune response.

Interferons have also been implicated in the control of B cell responses. When added in vitro or in vivo they can suppress or enhance primary or secondary antibody responses, depending on the dose and time of addition. The regulatory effects seem to be on the B cells themselves, on increased antigen presentation and through an effect on regulatory T cells.

A number of immune effector cells act by killing infected target cells. The cytotoxicity of macrophages, neutrophils, T cells and NK cells is enhanced by interferons. IFN-γ produced by T lymphocytes is capable of activating macrophages to kill intracellular bacteria. This lymphokine has all the activities of the molecule that used to be known as macrophage-activating factor (MAF). NK cells are able to destroy a range of syngeneic, allogeneic and xenogeneic cells in an MHC-unrestricted fashion (see below). The interaction of NK cells with their target generates the release of IFN-α and IFN-β. All three types of interferon increase NK cell activity in vitro and in vivo, not only by recruiting pre-NK cells to become actively lytic but also by increasing the spectrum of cells lysed. The mechanisms by which interferons make cells cytotoxic are not clear but it is of interest that interferons can stimulate the production of cytotoxins such as tumour necrosis factor.

Tumour necrosis factor has also been reported to have several antiviral activities similar to IFN-γ, but working through a different pathway. However, if both tumour necrosis factor and IFN-γ are added together then a synergistic effect is seen. If tumour necrosis factor is added to cells after viral infection, it can lead to their destruction even though the cells are normally resistant to tumour necrosis factor. This effect is also synergistic with IFN-γ. Certain viruses have been shown to trigger the release of tumour necrosis factor from mononuclear cells, and it seems likely that this cytokine is an important host response to viral infections.

Certain cell-mediated reactions are also part of the innate defences against viral infections. In natural killing the structures recognized by the effector cells, the NK cells, are not known, but changes in the level of expression of a number of surface molecules on the infected cells may be important. The formation of a close conjugate between the NK cell and the target induces the effector cell to produce toxic molecules that lead to the death of the infected cell. Antibodies that recognize NK cells have been used to deplete these cells in mice. It was found that these treated mice were more susceptible to murine cytomegalovirus than were normal mice. Therefore, natural killing may form a first-line defence against viral attack before the acquired immune response is generated. Natural killing is increased by interferons, both the number of effector cells and their killing potential, and, therefore, these two innate defence mechanisms appear to work together to protect the host from viral infections.

## Acquired immunity

The response to viral antigens is almost entirely T cell-dependent. Immunodeficiencies involving T cells are always characterized by markedly enhanced susceptibility to viral infections. However, this tells us little about the effector mechanisms involved as T cells are required for both antibody production and cytotoxic reactions.

The viral epitopes that the immune system responds to have been studied to give an insight into the mechanisms involved in the host response to these pathogens and also to aid in the development of better vaccines. The recognition of viral antigens is similar to that for all foreign material. B cells and immuno-globulin are able to combine with exposed epitopes while processed viral fragments presented in the context of MHC molecules are recognized by T cells. The B cell will recognize a conformationally deter-mined epitope while the T cell epitope is a sequential epitope.

Antigen-specific B cells can act as antigen-presenting cells and therefore support the generation of an immune response by presenting viral antigens in association with MHC class II molecules to helper T ($T_H$) cells. B cells will present antigen to T cells and in return will be stimulated by growth and differentiation molecules. Intramolecular help may explain hapten–carrier effects. For virus particles the uptake of an intact virion will mean that the B cell will be able to present peptides derived from internal proteins to T cells (Fig. 12.2). Thus, a B cell specific for a surface antigen can receive help from a T cell specific for another molecule as long as it is present within the same particle, i.e. intrastructural help.

In most cases, exogenous virus proteins, i.e. those derived from an extracellular virus and taken into a

**Fig. 12.2** Intrastructural T cell help. A B cell that is specific for a surface component of a virus binds the virus through its receptor, surface immunoglobulin. The virus contains three potential T cell epitopes (a, b and c) within its nucleocapsid. The entire virus can be internalized, and all viral polypeptides will be processed and fragments will be re-expressed in association with MHC class II molecules (presentation) on the B cell surface.

cell, will be presented in the context of MHC class II molecules and stimulate $T_H$ cells. Cells that are supporting viral replication express virus-derived peptides in association with MHC class I molecules, i.e. the endogenous pathway. The fact that some endogenous viral proteins are presented in the context of MHC class II molecules suggests that the cellular compartment in which they are found is not transected by the MHC class I pathway.

### Humoral immunity

There are several ways in which antibody against viral components can protect the host. Antibodies cannot enter cells, and therefore are ineffective against latent viruses and those that spread directly from cell to cell. They will, however, bind to extra-cellular viral epitopes. These epitopes can be on intact virions or on the surface of infected cells. The binding of antibody to free virus can inhibit a number of processes essential to virus replication. Antibodies can block binding to the host cell membrane, and will thus stop attachment and penetration. The immunoglobulins IgG and IgM have this important function in serum and body fluids, and IgA can neutralize viruses by a similar mechanism on mucosal surfaces. Antibody can also work at stages after penetration. Uncoating with its release of viral nucleic acid into the cytoplasm can be inhibited if the virion is covered by antibody.

Antibody can also cause aggregation of virus particles, thus limiting the spread of the infectious particles and forming a complex that is readily phagocytosed. Complement can aid in the neutralization process by opsonizing the virus or directly lysing enveloped viruses. In certain cases complement alone can inactivate viruses. Some retroviruses have a protein that can act as a receptor for C1q, and other viruses have been reported to activate the alternative pathway. In some infections, viral proteins remain on the surface of the cell after entry or become associated with the cell membrane during replication. Antibodies against these molecules can cause cell lysis by the classical pathway but an intact alternative pathway is necessary to amplify the initial triggering by the antibody-dependent pathway. In certain situations antibody-mediated reactions are not always of benefit (see below). Antibodies are also capable of modulating or stripping viral antigens from the cell surface, allowing the infected cell to avoid destruction by other effector mechanisms.

Viral infections, particularly those caused by enteroviruses, are frequent and severe when humoral immunity is impaired, as in certain inherited immunodeficiency states. In Bruton-type deficiencies, poliomyelitis may develop after vaccination with the live virus vaccine; meningoencephalitis caused by echovirus and coxsackievirus may also be seen. In many situations, viruses seem to be able to escape the humoral defence mechanisms. Some viruses become latent, e.g. herpesviruses, and are reactivated despite the presence of circulating antibody, as they can pass directly from cell to cell. Other escape mechanisms include antigenic variation in which the antigenic structure of the virus is altered so that antibodies formed to the previous strain are no longer effective.

In viral infections the efficiency of antibody depends largely on whether the virus passes through the bloodstream outside host cells in order to reach its target organ. Poliovirus crosses the intestinal wall, enters the bloodstream to cause a cell-free viraemia and passes to the spinal cord and brain where it replicates. Small amounts of antibody in the blood can neutralize the virus before it reaches its target cells in the nervous system.

In comparison, in viral diseases such as influenza and the common cold, the viruses do not pass through the bloodstream. These infections have a short incubation period, their target organ being at the site of entry into the body, namely the respiratory mucous membranes. In this type of infection a high level of antibody in the blood will be relatively ineffective in comparison with its effect on blood-borne viruses. In this case the antibody must be present in the mucous secretions at the time of infection. There are very low levels of IgG or IgM in secretions but IgA has been shown to be responsible for most of the neutralizing activity present in nasal secretions against rhinoviruses and other respiratory tract viruses.

One consequence of this is that conventional immunization methods using killed virus or viral subunits which produce high levels of circulating antibody are unlikely to be effective against viruses which attack the mucous membranes. Some considerable effort is being directed at developing methods for stimulating local production of IgA in the mucous membranes themselves. Live virus vaccines are effective in this respect, and the intranasal administration of a live attenuated influenza virus vaccine is an attempt to overcome this problem. The high degree of immunity provided by the oral polio vaccine is due in part to locally produced antibody in the gut neutralizing the virus before it attaches to cell receptors to cause infection. The presence of IgA against polio has been demonstrated in faeces, in duodenal fluid and in saliva. Recent evidence suggests that parenteral administration of a killed virus may give rise to a secretory IgA response if the individual has been previously exposed to the virus or has received an oral attenuated vaccine. So there appears to be a link between the systemic immune system and local mucosal immunity.

Humoral immunity does play a major protective role in polio and a number of other viral infections, and is probably the predominant form of immunity responsible for protection from reinfection. Passively administered antibody can protect humans against several infections, including measles, hepatitis A and B and chickenpox, if given before or very soon after exposure. Immunity to many viral infections is life-long. This may occur because antibodies are boosted by occasional re-exposure to the virus.

### Cell-mediated immunity

The destruction of virus-infected cells is an important mechanism in the eradication of virus from the host. Antibody can neutralize free virions but once these agents get into cells other strategies are employed. The destruction of an infected cell before progeny particles are released is an effective way of terminating a viral infection. For this process to occur the immune system must recognize the infected cell and various types of effector cell have evolved to mediate these processes.

As viral proteins are synthesized within the cell some of these molecules are processed into small peptides. These endogenously produced antigen fragments become associated with MHC class I molecules, and this complex is then transported to the cell surface where it acts as the recognition unit for cytotoxic T ($T_C$) lymphocytes. Most $T_C$ cells have a receptor that binds to fragments of the virus sitting in the cleft of an MHC class I molecule. This T cell will also have the CD8 molecule on its surface. Some $T_C$ cells are restricted in their recognition of antigen by MHC class II molecules and therefore have the CD4 molecule.

Many viruses, such as poliovirus and papillomavirus, replicate and produce fully infectious particles inside the cell. These viruses are liberated from the infected cell as it disintegrates. Other viruses do not wait for the cell to die but are released by a process of budding through the cell membrane. During the replicative process virus-encoded molecules, i.e. viral antigens, are inserted into the host cell membrane, and the nucleocapsid becomes associated with these molecules. The virus particle finally acquires an envelope as it is released. Such viruses include herpesviruses, alphaviruses, flaviviruses, retroviruses, hepadnaviruses and ortho- and paramyxoviruses. Viral antigens often appear on the cell surface very early in the replicative cycle, many hours before progeny virus is liberated. In cells infected with herpes simplex virus as many as five different viral glycoproteins appear on the cell surface. In other virus infections such as those caused by poxviruses and papovaviruses, the viral particles are not released by budding, but viral antigens appear on the cell surface. These molecules, including those which are not incorporated into the released virion, can therefore act as signals indicating the presence of virus within a cell.

Antibody-dependent cell-mediated cytotoxicity is carried out by a number of different cell types, all of which have Fc receptors. These killer cells recognize the Fc portion of immunoglobulin bound to viral antigens present on the infected cell surface. This interaction brings the two cells close together, and toxic molecules are released onto the target cell membrane causing cell death.

$CD4^+$ and $CD8^+$ T cells can produce various lymphokines when stimulated by antigen. These will include molecules that are active in the elimination of virus, e.g. IFN-$\gamma$ and tumour necrosis factor and others that generally increase the effectiveness of the immune system by attracting cells to the site of infection, stimulating the production of more cells and supporting their growth. Macrophages will be activated, and this will lead to enhanced microbicidal activities and the production of monokines.

## Induction of an immune response

The precise nature of the acquired immune reactions that are generated in response to infection will depend to a great extent on the site of infection, type of virus, previous exposure to the agent and the genetic make-up of the host. Both humoral and cell-mediated responses will be produced to all infections. The importance of genetic factors is illustrated by the severe *X-linked recessive lymphoproliferative syndrome* in which fatal infectious mononucleosis results from the unrestricted replication of Epstein–Barr virus as affected males have reduced numbers of normal lymphocytes.

The virus or viral components entering the peripheral tissues or being produced there will be carried to the draining lymph node. Once in the secondary lymphoid tissues the virus is processed by an antigen-presenting cell, and viral peptides associate with MHC class II molecules and are transported to the cell surface. When antigen enters the lymph node the outlet is closed so that the antigen-specific cells that enter have a chance to interact with the peptide–MHC complex on the antigen-presenting cells, and the effector cells can respond to the helper factors that will be produced in the node. A $T_H$ cell will bind to the peptide–MHC class II complex, and in the presence of co-stimulatory signals expand clonally and produce helper factors for the growth and differentiation of T and B cells. The proportions of the different lymphokines produced will determine the type and level of the response generated. B cells will enter the node, and those that bind antigen through their surface immunoglobulin, or enter the node already having interacted with antigen, will be responsive to the growth factors produced by the $T_H$ cells and will be stimulated into antibody production. Other T cells will enter the lymph node. If these cells have a receptor that interacts with an antigen fragment–MHC class I complex then they will respond to the growth factors present in the node and proliferate and mature into effector T cells. After a time the valve on the efferent lymphatic will open, and the products of the immune response will leave to circulate round the body and localise at the site of infection. As the response progresses the pathogen will be eliminated, the tissue repaired and memory cells generated. Finally, when all the antigen is eliminated the immune response will be terminated. In some instances virus-induced immune responses may have immunopathological consequences.

## IMMUNOPATHOLOGY

Viruses have evolved a multitude of mechanisms for exploiting weaknesses in the host immune system and avoiding, and sometimes actually subverting, immune mechanisms. Some viruses are so successful in avoiding host defences that they persist in the host indefinitely, sometimes in a latent form without producing disease.

One of the most important strategies developed by viruses is to infect cells of the immune system itself. The effect of this is often to disable the normal functioning of the cell type that has been infected. Many common human viruses including rubella, mumps, measles and herpesviruses infect cells of the immune system, as does the human immunodeficiency virus (HIV). The consequences of viral infection of cells of the immune system have been categorized in two ways:

1. Infections that cause temporary immune deficiency to unrelated antigens and sometimes to the antigens of the infecting virus. It is known that infection with influenza, rubella, measles and cytomegalovirus predisposes to bacterial and other infections. This is sometimes associated with depressed immunoglobulin synthesis and interference with the antimicrobial functions of phagocytes.

2. Permanent depression of immunity to unrelated antigens and occasionally to antigens of the infecting virus. The acquired immune deficiency syndrome is an example of such a disease where the patient becomes susceptible to otherwise harmless protozoa, bacteria, viruses and fungi.

Viruses have also developed other mechanisms to avoid the immune system. These include antigenic variation, release of antigens and the production of antigens at sites that are inaccessible to the immune system.

Viruses that cannot enter and replicate within phagocytic cells will be destroyed if they are engulfed by a neutrophil or macrophage. Since neutrophils are short-lived cells they do not usually give rise to progeny virus. On the other hand, monocytes and macrophages are long-lived cells and can be responsible for disseminating a virus throughout the body. Viruses that do replicate within macrophages must escape from the phagosome very rapidly before it fuses with the lysosome. Reovirus infection of macrophages is actually helped by the lysosomal enzymes which initiate 'uncoating' of the virus and therefore enhance viral replication.

A virus will remain relatively safe from immune destruction if it remains within the cell and allows only very low or no viral antigen expression on the infected cell membrane. This is what happens in latent infections where herpes simplex or varicella–zoster virus is present in the dorsal root ganglion.

Antibody can actually remove viral antigens from cell membranes, as cross-linking of antigens on the cell surface can lead to their internalization by capping. Here the antigens complexed with the antibody are drawn to one pole of the cell and are internalized or shed into the surrounding tissue. Capping occurs on brain cells infected with measles virus in subacute sclerosing panencephalitis. Viruses that move from cell to cell without entering the extracellular fluids will also escape the action of antibodies as will those passed from cell to cell by cell division.

A number of infections continually shed virus into external secretions, such as saliva, milk or urine. As long as the infected cell only forms virus on the luminal surface of the mucosa then cells of the immune system and antibody will be unable to destroy the infected cell. IgA present in the secretions may neutralize the virus, but this class of antibody does not activate complement efficiently so the cell will not be lysed. A similar situation applies to epidermal infections with wart virus. The infected cell is keratinized and about to be released from the surface of the body before any virus or viral antigens are produced. The infected cell is therefore isolated from the host's immune cells.

During the course of an infection various antibodies will be formed against different epitopes on a virus. These antibodies will be of differing affinities and also stimulate different effector functions. Antibodies against some of the epitopes will neutralize the virus, but other antibodies will be against unimportant epitopes or be of an ineffective isotype, which may fail to neutralize the virus and may actually aid in its infectivity by allowing uptake of virus–antibody complexes via Fc receptors or cause tissue damage through immune complex disease. Soluble antigens liberated from infected cells could 'mop- up' free antibody so that it can no longer interact and destroy extracellular virus. Whether the small particles present in the serum of patients and carriers with hepatitis B virus infections function in this way is not known, although patients in the prodromal phase may suffer from rash, myalgia and arthralgia. Polyarteritis nodosa and glomerulonephritis can also occur, all suggestive of immune complex formation.

Susceptibility to infection is generally greater in the very young and very old because of a weaker immune response. However, the immunopathology tends to be less severe. In the very young, infections can spread rapidly and prove fatal without the clinical and pathological changes seen in adults. Latent infections are kept under control by the immune system, and in older people the infections show an increased incidence of activation, e.g. zoster or shingles. Immunological immaturity makes the neonate highly susceptible to many viral infections. Maternal-derived antibody provides passive protection for about 3–6 months, after which time the infant is at risk of infection: respiratory and alimentary tract infections are frequent.

Physical and physiological differences may also contribute to age-related disease susceptibility. Respiratory infections in old age are probably a bigger problem than in young adults because of weaker respiratory muscles and a poorer cough reflex. In the young the airways are narrower and more easily blocked by secretions and exudate. Infants, because of their low body weight, show signs of distress from loss of fluid and electrolytes, so that fever, vomiting and diarrhoea tend to be very serious at this time of life. Often the reasons for the differences between infants and adults are not known. Respiratory syncytial virus causes severe illness in the early months of life with croup, bronchiolitis and bronchopneumonia, despite the presence of maternal IgG. In adults the virus usually causes a mild upper respiratory tract infection.

Certain viral infections produce a milder disease in children than in adults, e.g. varicella, mumps, polio-myelitis and Epstein–Barr virus infections. Varicella often causes pneumonia in adults, and mumps may involve the testes and ovaries after puberty, giving rise to orchitis and oophoritis. Epstein–Barr virus is excreted in saliva, and in developing countries most individuals are infected early in life, usually asymp-tomatically. In developed countries where the childhood infection is less common, first infection can be delayed to adolescence or early adulthood, when salivary exposure occurs during kissing. In this age group, Epstein–Barr virus infection gives rise to glandular fever. It is not clear why these infections are more severe in adults, but it may be linked to the more powerful immune defences giving rise to immunopathological sequelae in adults.

There are also age-related differences in the incidence of infections. It is not surprising that most infections are commonest in childhood when the individual will be exposed to the micro-organisms for the first time.

## Antigenic variation

A micro-organism can avoid the acquired immune response by periodically changing the structure of molecules that are recognized by the host immune system. The immune system will select the variants by not being able to mount an immune response against them before they are shed. The micro-organism will only be able to change a component in a way that does not alter the functioning of the molecule. The molecules involved can be either active enzymes, recognition molecules or structural proteins. HIV shows considerable variation in parts of the envelope glycoprotein within a given individual.

The significance of antigenic variation is well illustrated by influenza viruses. Here changes in the surface glycoproteins are linked to the occurrence of epidemics of infection (see Ch. 50).

With influenza virus the infection is localized to the respiratory tract where the principal protection against reinfection will be secretory IgA. The amount of this antibody produced tends to be low compared to the level of humoral immunity developed against viraemic infections such as poliovirus and measles. The virus-specific IgA still present at the mucosal surface a few years after infection can protect against the original infecting virus but may be insufficient to deal with an antigenic variant despite antigenic overlap. Thus, in effect, IgA levels become a selective pressure which will allow infection by the mutant, and antigenic drift occurs. The very short incubation period (1–3 days) is more rapid than the secondary antibody response so that the IgA levels cannot be boosted to abort infection.

Antigenic variation is likely to be an important viral adaptation for overcoming host immunity in long-lived species such as humans where there is a need for multiple reinfection of the same individual if the virus is to survive and the virus is unable to become latent. In shorter-lived animals such as mice and rabbits a susceptible population appears quickly enough to maintain the infectious cycle.

## Persistence of virus

Certain viruses give rise to a persistent infection which is held in check as long as the immune system remains intact.

Chickenpox is a persistent infection characterized by latency in that there is apparent recovery from the original infection but the virus can reappear later in life when a localized eruption, shingles, results. Other herpesviruses, cytomegalovirus and Epstein–Barr virus also persist after infection. If the carrier's immune system remains intact, there will be no evidence of disease. However, cytomegalovirus causes many problems in immunosuppressed patients. The polyomavirus, JC, usually causes asymptomatic infections, but, in the immunosuppressed, it has been found in areas of destruction in the central nervous system: the disease is progressive multifocal leucoencephalopathy.

In other persistent infections, the immune system contributes to the pathology of the disease, often over a period of years. Thus, in subacute sclerosing panencephalitis, persistence of measles virus in neurones triggers their destruction by the host's immune system. Similarly the chronic active hepatitis seen in those carriers of hepatitis B who continue to produce virions appears to be triggered by a $T_C$ cell response to viral antigens present in the hepatocyte membrane. In both examples, several years may elapse before symptoms appear.

## VACCINES

Natural infection with a virus is an extremely effective means of giving life-long immunity from the disease. In most cases, where there is one virus type, this means that second attacks are extremely rare. The memory of the immune system ensures that for these infections a secondary response can be generated before the virus has time to cause the disease. The level of immunity needed to protect an individual will depend on the incubation period of the virus and its life cycle. For viruses with very short incubation periods a high level of protective immunity must be present before exposure to the infective agent. In the case of a virus with a long incubation period (10–20 days) then the immune system has time to generate a protective response.

It is also important to consider the type of immune response that will be protective against different viruses. If antibody gives protection then steps must be taken to ensure that the material to be used for immunization contains the correct epitopes. A denatured antigen will not generate antibodies that can combine with the native virus. Sometimes the chemical treatment of the antigen may destroy important components. Thus the original killed measles virus vaccine did not contain the fusion protein. As a result, vaccinees suffered enhanced disease when exposed to the virus as viral replication and spread could occur in the presence of antibody to the other viral proteins. If T cell immunity is important then the vaccine must be in a form that will give rise to peptides in the correct compartment of the cell to produce antigen fragments in association with MHC-encoded products. It will have to associate with the MHC class II molecules to generate help and MHC class I molecules to stimulate effector cell formation. For antibody production, T cell help will also be required. Therefore, for an antibody response, a killed vaccine may be sufficient but, when T cell immunity is required, a live attenuated vaccine will be needed.

Vaccination has been responsible for the elimination of smallpox and reducing the incidence of other viral diseases. It should be possible to control many viral diseases but with some the problem is more difficult. New technologies and a better understanding of the immune system are helping with this task.

## RECOMMENDED READING

Mims C, Dimmock N, Nash A, Stephen J 1995 *Mims' Pathogenesis of Infectious Disease*, 4th edn. Academic Press, London

Taussig M J 1984 *Processes in Pathology and Microbiology*, 2nd edn. Blackwell Scientific, Oxford

# 13

# Parasitic infections: pathogenesis and immunity

*J. Stewart and D. M. Weir*

By convention the term 'parasitic diseases' refers to those caused by protozoa, worms (helminths) and arthropods (insects and arachnids). Such parasites affect many hundreds of millions of people in tropical parts of the world and are responsible for many severe and debilitating diseases (see Chs 61 and 62).

These infections are associated with a broad spectrum of effects. Some are due to the parasites themselves and others are a consequence of the host response to the invader. The nature and extent of the pathological effects are dependent upon the site and mode of infection and also on the level of the parasite burden.

Development of protective immunity to such parasites is more complicated than to bacteria and viruses because of the complicated life cycles of the parasites involved.

## PATHOGENIC MECHANISMS

As with other infectious agents the site occupied by a parasite is important. A host will survive with a large number of lung flukes, *Paragonimus* spp., in their usual site in the lungs, but infection in the brain may cause far more serious effects. The severity of disease depends not only on the degree of infestation but also on the physiological state of the host. A lowering of general health, due to malnutrition for example, will predispose to more serious consequences following infection by parasites.

### Mechanical tissue damage

Physical obstruction of anatomical sites leading to loss of function can be a major component of the diseases caused by parasites. The intestinal lumen can be blocked by worms such as *Ascaris* spp. or tapeworms, and filarial parasites (*Wuchereria* and *Brugia* spp.) can obstruct the flow of lymph through lymphatics.

Within tissues the site of a parasite infection can give rise to serious consequences. Intestinal infection with the tapeworm *Taenia solium* is usually of little consequence, but the eggs may develop into larvae (cysticerci) in humans, causing cysticercosis. The cysticerci can be found in muscle, liver, eye or, most dangerously, in the brain. Hydatid cysts, the larval stage of the dog tapeworm (*Echinococcus granulosus*) in humans, may reach volumes of 1–2 litres, and such masses can cause severe damage to any infected organ.

### Physiological effects

Large numbers of *Giardia* spp. covering the walls of the small intestine can lead to malabsorption, especially of fats. Competition by parasites for essential nutrients leads to host deprivation. Thus, depletion of vitamin $B_{12}$ by the tapeworm *Diphyllobothrium latum* sometimes leads to pernicious anaemia. Other forms of anaemia result from blood loss, especially in hookworm infection and from red blood cell destruction in malaria.

Some parasites produce metabolites that may have profound effects on the host. *Trypanosoma cruzi* secretes a neurotoxin that affects the autonomic nervous system. Malaria parasites are thought to produce a metabolite with vasoconstrictor activity.

### Tissue damage

The presence of parasites can result in the release of proteolytic enzymes that damage host tissues. Ulceration of the intestinal wall occurs in amoebic dysentery, and trophozoites (the active, motile forms of a protozoan parasite) can penetrate deep into the wall of the intestine to reach the blood and hence the liver, lungs and brain where secondary amoebic abscesses may occur. The skin damage caused by skin-penetrating helminths, such as *Strongyloides* spp. and hookworms, can also permit entry of other infectious agents.

The host reaction to parasites and their products can evoke immunological reactions that may lead to secondary damage to host tissues. This is seen in schistosomiasis where the host response to parasite eggs in tissues leads to the formation of a granuloma with subsequent tissue destruction through fibrosis. Other types of hypersensitivity reactions can be generated in various parasite infections (see below).

## IMMUNE DEFENCE MECHANISMS

The large size of parasites means that they will display more antigens than bacteria or viruses to the immune system. When the parasite has a complicated life cycle some of these antigens may be specific to a particular stage of development. Parasites have evolved to be closely adapted to the host, and most parasitic infections are chronic and show a degree of host specificity. For example the malaria parasites of humans, birds and rodents are confined to their own particular species. An exception to this is *Trichinella spiralis*, which is able to infect many animal species.

In the natural host there is no one defence mechanism that acts in isolation against a particular parasite. In turn the parasite will have evolved a number of strategies to evade elimination. In general terms, cell-mediated immune mechanisms are more effective against intracellular protozoa while antibody, with the aid of certain effector cells, is involved in the destruction of extracellular targets. Again due to the life cycles of some parasites, either cell-mediated or humoral immunity may be of greater importance at different stages of their development.

### Innate defences

Several of the innate or natural defence mechanisms that are active against bacteria and viruses are also effective against parasitic infections. The physical barrier of the skin protects against many parasites but it is ineffective against those that are transmitted by a blood-feeding insect. In addition, other parasites, such as schistosomes, have evolved mechanisms for actively penetrating intact skin. Certain individuals are genetically less susceptible to certain parasites. Thus, individuals with the sickle cell trait have a genetic defect in their haemoglobin that causes a mechanical distortion in their erythrocytes. This somehow leads to the destruction of intracellular malaria parasites. The Duffy blood group antigen is the attachment site for one of the plasmodium parasites. Individuals

who lack this determinant are therefore protected from malaria caused by *Plasmodium vivax*.

A variety of other non-specific host defence mechanisms are involved in the control of parasitic infections. These include direct cellular responses by monocytes, macrophages and granulocytes, and by natural killer cells. The antiparasitic activity of these cells will be enhanced by products of acquired immune reactions. For example, certain protozoan parasites infect macrophages. In particular, *Leishmania* spp. are obligate parasites of mononuclear phagocytes, and are completely dependent upon macrophages, where they survive in the phagolysosome. The parasite appears to be able to survive within non-stimulated resident macrophages whereas they are destroyed in activated macrophages.

Complement, through activation by the alternative pathway, is active against a number of parasites including adult worms and active larvae of *T. spiralis* and schistosomula of *Schistosoma mansoni*. The spleen is thought to be active in the elimination of intracellular parasites as its filtering of infected erythrocytes is thought to remove intracellular plasmodium.

### Acquired immunity

An individual with a parasitic infection will mount a specific response against the invading parasite. These immune reactions will generate antibody and effector T cells directed against specific parasite antigens. Memory B and T cells will also be produced. For a number of reasons described later, much of acquired immunity is ineffective in protecting the host against recurrent infection. However, in certain cases, such as amoebiasis and toxoplasmosis, immunity to reinfection is fairly complete. In schistosomiasis, the presence of surviving adult forms protects against further infections. However, this is probably an effect of the parasite and not of the host.

#### Antibody

The specific immune response to parasites leads to the production of antibody. Infection by protozoan parasites is associated with the production of the immunoglobulins IgG and IgM. With helminths there is in addition the synthesis of substantial amounts of IgE. IgA is produced in response to intestinal protozoa, such as *Entamoeba* and *Giardia* spp.

In addition to these specific T-dependent responses a non-specific hypergammaglobulinaemia is present in many parasitic infections. Much of this non-specific antibody is the result of polyclonal B cell activation by released parasite antigens acting as mitogens. This

**Table 13.1**   Humoral defence mechanisms against parasite infections

| Mechanism | Effect | Parasite |
|---|---|---|
| Neutralization | Blocks attachment to host cell | Protozoa |
| | Acts to inhibit evasion mechanisms of intracellular organisms | Protozoa |
| | Binding to toxins or enzymes | Protozoa and worms |
| Physical interference | Obstructs orifices of parasite | Worms |
| | Agglutination | Protozoa |
| Opsonization | Increases clearance by phagocytes | Protozoa |
| Cytotoxicity | Complement-mediated lysis | Protozoa and worms |
| | Antibody-dependent cell-mediated cytotoxicity | Protozoa and worms |

response is ineffective at counteracting the parasite and can enhance the pathogenicity by causing the production of auto-antibodies, and may actually lead to a diminished specific response due to B cell exhaustion. It has also been reported that some parasite molecules are T cell mitogens. This could lead to the generation of autoreactive T cells or activation of suppressor responses.

There are a number of mechanisms by which specific antibody can provide protection against and control parasitic infections (Table 13.1). As with viral infections, antibody is only effective against extracellular parasites and where parasite antigens are displayed on the surface of infected cells. Antibody can neutralize parasites by combining with various surface molecules, blocking or interfering with their proper functioning. The binding of antibody to an attachment site will stop infection of a new host cell. The agglutination of blood parasites by IgM may occur, leading to the prevention of spread, as in the acute phase of infection with *Tryp. cruzi*. Toxins and enzymes produced by certain parasites add to their pathogenicity and antibodies that inhibit these molecules will protect the host from damage and also affect the infection process directly. Intracellular parasites have evolved a number of mechanisms to allow them to survive in this environment. Antibodies against the molecules that aid the parasite in these activities, e.g. to escape from endosomes or inhibit lysosomal fusion, will lead to removal of the intruder by the phagocyte. Parasitic worms are multicellular organisms with defined anatomical features that are responsible for functions such as feeding and reproduction. Antibodies that block particular orifices, e.g. oral and genital, will interfere with critical physiological functions and could cause starvation or curtail reproduction.

Antibodies can bind to the surface of parasites and cause direct damage, or by interacting with comple-

ment lead to cell lysis. Antibody also acts as an opsonin and hence increases uptake by phagocytic cells. In this context, complement activation will lead to enhanced ingestion due to complement receptors. Macrophage activation leads to the expression of increased Fc and complement receptors, so phagocytosis will be enhanced in the presence of macrophage-activating factors. Phagocytes play an important role in the control of infections by *Plasmodium* spp. and *Trypanosoma brucei*.

Antibody-dependent cell-mediated cytotoxicity has been shown to play a part in infections caused by a number of parasites, including *Tryp. cruzi*, *T. spiralis*, *S. mansoni* and filarial worms. The effector cells, macrophages, monocytes, neutrophils and eosinophils, bind to the antibody-coated parasites by their Fc and complement receptors. Close apposition of the effector cell and the target are necessary because the toxic molecules produced are non-specific and could damage host cells. Major basic protein from eosinophils damages the tegument of schistosomes and other worms, causing their death. It appears that different cell types and immunoglobulin isotypes are active against different developmental stages of parasites. Eosinophils are more effective at killing newborn larvae of *T. spiralis* than other cells, whereas macrophages are very effective against microfilariae.

## T cells

The importance of T cells in counteracting protozoan infections has been shown using nude (athymic) or T cell-depleted mice, which have a reduced capacity to control trypanosomal and malaria infections. The transfer of spleen cells, especially T cells, from immune animals gives protection against most parasitic infections. The type of T cell that is effective depends on the parasite. CD4+ T cells transfer protection against *Leishmania major* and *L. tropica*, and may be necessary for the elimination of other parasites. The intracellular parasite of cattle, *Theileria parvum*, is destroyed by cytotoxic T ($T_C$) cells.

CD4$^+$ T cells may act by providing help in antibody production, but they also secrete various lymphokines that interact with other effector cells. CD8$^+$ cells may be cytotoxic in certain situations, but these cells also produce a variety of lymphokines. Interleukin-2 is an important lymphokine that has been shown to be deficient during parasitic infections, such as malaria and trypanosomiasis. Administration of interleukin-2 to mice infected with *Tryp. cruzi* reduces parasitaemia and increases survival.

Colony-stimulating factors, e.g. interleukin-3 and granulocyte/monocyte colony-stimulating factor, are also produced by activated T cells. These molecules act on myeloid progenitors in the bone marrow, causing increased production of neutrophils, eosinophils and monocytes. They also increase the activity of these cells; the monocytosis and splenomegaly in malaria are caused by these T cell-derived molecules. The accumulation of macrophages in the liver as granulomata in schistosomiasis and the eosinophilia that is characteristic of worm infestations are also T cell-dependent phenomena.

In certain cases the production of lymphokines may have adverse effects. Leishmania infect macrophages and the release of molecules that stimulate the production of more host cells may potentiate the infection.

γ-Interferon does not appear directly to inhibit or kill parasites, although multiplication of the liver stages of the malaria parasite is inhibited by γ-interferon, possibly through interaction with its receptor on the surface of hepatocytes. γ-Interferon is a potent macrophage activation factor and is probably involved in the resistance and elimination of intracellular parasites, such as *Toxoplasma gondii* and *Leishmania* spp. Activated macrophages are more effective killers and can destroy intracellular parasites before they establish themselves within the cell.

## Macrophages

Macrophages play an important role in the elimination and control of parasitic protozoa and worms. They secrete monokines, such as interleukin-1, tumour necrosis factor and colony-stimulating factors that affect not only T cells and antibody production but also granulocytes. However, other monokines, e.g. prostaglandins, are immunosuppressive. Macrophages are also phagocytic cells and function as such in the elimination of parasites. In the same way as in the eradication of other infectious agents, opsonins will greatly enhance this process. Once internalized, the parasite will be killed, by oxygen-dependent and oxygen-independent mechanisms, and digested. Many of the molecules produced by macrophages are cytotoxic, and when produced in close proximity to a parasite will kill it. Specific antibody, IgG and IgE, can mediate the attachment of the macrophage to the surface of parasites that are too large to internalize but are vulnerable to antibody-dependent cell-mediated cytotoxicity. Acting as antigen-presenting cells, they can aid elimination by helping in the initiation of an immune response.

In addition to lymphokines some products of parasites themselves, such as those produced by *Tryp. brucei* and the malaria parasite, can cause macrophage activation. These may be direct effects or result from the production of monokines such as tumour necrosis factor.

In some parasitic infections the immune system is unable to eradicate the offending organism. The body reacts by trying to isolate the parasite within a granuloma. In this situation there is chronic stimulation of those T cells specific for antigens on the parasite. The continual release of lymphokines leads to macrophage accumulation, release of fibrogenic factors, stimulation of granuloma formation and, ultimately, fibrosis. Granuloma formation around schistosome eggs can occur in the liver, and this response is thought to benefit the host by isolating host cells from the toxic substances produced by the eggs. It can, however, lead to pathological consequences if the damage to the liver leads to loss of liver function.

## Granulocytes

Neutrophils and eosinophils are thought to play a role in the elimination of protozoa and worms. The smaller parasites can be phagocytosed and destroyed by both oxygen-dependent and -independent processes. The phagocytic capacity of neutrophils is superior to that of eosinophils. Both cell types possess receptors for the Fc portion of immunoglobulin and for various complement components, so the presence of opsonins increases phagocytosis. Extracellular destruction of large parasites can occur by antibody-dependent cell-mediated cytotoxicity.

Neutrophils are attracted to sites of inflammation and will clear the offending parasite. They have been reported to be more effective than eosinophils at eliminating several species of nematode, including *T. spiralis*, although the relative importance of the two cell types may depend on the class of antibody present.

Eosinophilia and high levels of IgE are characteristics of many parasitic worm infections. It has been suggested that eosinophils are especially active against helminths, and IgE-dependent degranulation of mast cells has evolved to attract these cells to the site where the parasite is localized. The eosinophilia is T cell-dependent and the lymphokines that induce the production of the cells also cause an increase in their activation state. These effector cells are attracted to the site by chemotactic factors produced by mast cells (see below). Once at the site they degranulate in response to perturbation of their cell membrane induced by antibodies and complement bound to the surface of the parasite. The toxic molecules are therefore released onto the surface of the target and cause its destruction.

## Mast cells

The mediators stored and produced by mast cells play an important role in eliminating worm infections. Parasite antigens cause the release of mediators from mast cells; these molecules induce a local inflammatory response. Chemotactic factors are produced and attract eosinophils and neutrophils. Thus the IgE-dependent release of mast cell products helps in the expulsion of the worm. The number of mucosal mast cells rises during a parasitic worm infestation due to a T cell-dependent process.

## Platelets

Platelet activation results in the release of molecules that are toxic to various parasites, including schisto-somula, *Tox. gondii* and *Tryp. cruzi*. The release process does not require antibody, although IgE-dependent cytotoxicity is possible, but seems to involve acute-phase proteins. The cytotoxic potential of platelets is enhanced by various cytokines, including γ-interferon and tumour necrosis factor.

# EVASION MECHANISMS

All animal pathogens, including parasitic protozoa and worms, have evolved effective mechanisms to avoid elimination by the host defence systems (Table 13.2).

## Seclusion

Many parasites inhabit cells or anatomical sites that are inaccessible to host defence mechanisms. Those that attempt to survive within cells avoid the effects of antibody but must possess mechanisms to avoid destruction if the cell involved is capable of destroying them. *Plasmodium* spp. inhabit erythrocytes while toxoplasmas are less selective and will infect non-phagocytic cells as well as phagocytes. A number of different ways of avoiding destruction in macrophages have evolved. *Leishmania donovani* amastigotes are able to survive and metabolize in the acidic environment (pH 4–5) found in phagolysosomes while *Tox. gondii* is able to inhibit the fusion of lysosomes with the parasite-containing phagosome.

| Table 13.2    Parasite escape mechanisms | |
| --- | --- |
| Intracellular habitat | Malaria parasites, trypanosomes and *Leishmania* spp. |
| Encystment | *Toxoplasma gondii* and *Trypanosoma cruzi* |
| Resistance to microbicidal products of phagocytes | *Leishmania donovani* |
| Masking of antigens | Schistosomes |
| Variation of antigen | Trypanosomes and malaria parasites |
| Suppression of immune response | Most parasites, e.g. malaria parasites, *Trichinella spiralis* and *Schistosoma mansoni* |
| Interference by antigens Polyclonal activation | Trypanosomes |
| Sharing of antigens between parasite and host – molecular mimicry | Schistosomes |
| Continuous turnover and release of surface antigens of parasite | Schistosomes |

*L. major* has a similar escape mechanism by attaching to a phagocyte complement receptor (CR1) that does not trigger the respiratory burst. The activation of the complement system by protozoan parasites seems to be a common mechanism to achieve attachment to target cells. *Tryp. cruzi* trypomastigotes can infect T cells of both the CD4 and CD8 subsets, and may be similar to retroviruses in using receptor molecules on the T cell surface for penetration.

The effectiveness of macrophages in the elimination of *Tryp. cruzi* depends upon the stage of development of the parasite. Trypomastigotes are able to escape from the phagocytic vacuole and survive in the cytoplasm whereas epimastigotes do not escape and are killed. Macrophages are also the preferred habitat of *Leishmania* spp., which multiply in the phagolysosome where they are resistant to digestion.

In an immune host these evasion mechanisms are less effective because of the presence of antibody and lymphokines. The ability to resist complement destruction also appears to be important. For example, *L. tropica* is easily killed by complement and causes only a localized self-healing lesion in the skin whereas a disseminating, often fatal, disease is seen with *L. donovani*, which is 10 times more resistant to complement killing. Large parasites such as helminths cannot infect individual cells; however, they can still achieve anatomical seclusion. *T. spiralis* larvae avoid the immune system by encysting in muscle; intestinal nematodes live in the lumen of the intestine.

## Evasion

Parasites may avoid recognition by antigenic variation and by acquiring host-derived molecules. African trypanosomes have the capacity to express more than 100 different surface glycoproteins. By producing novel antigens throughout their lives, these parasites continuously evade the immune system. By the time the host has mounted a response against each new antigen the parasite has changed again. Plasmodia pass through several discrete developmental stages, each with its own particular antigens. A similar situation is seen in certain helminths such as *T. spiralis*. As a result, each new stage of the life cycle will be seen by the host as a 'new' infective challenge.

A number of parasites are known to adsorb host-derived molecules onto their surface. This is thought to mask their own antigens and enable them to evade immunological attack.

Parasitic protozoa and worms also use devices to avoid immune destruction. Certain parasites retain a surface coat, or glycocalyx, that blocks direct exposure of its surface antigens.

## Immunosuppression

Parasites are not always able to evade detection and many have evolved mechanisms to suppress or divert immune reactions. Some parasites produce or generate molecules that act against cells of the immune system. Thus, the larvae of *T. spiralis* produce a molecule that is cytotoxic towards lymphocytes, and schistosomes can cleave a peptide from IgG, thereby decreasing its effectiveness. During many parasitic infections a large amount of antigenic material is released into the body fluids, and this may inhibit the response to or divert the response away from the parasite. High antigen concentrations can lead to tolerance by clonal exhaustion or clonal deletion. The immune complexes formed can also inhibit antibody production by negative feedback via Fc receptors on plasma cells. Many of these released molecules are polyclonal activators of T and B cells. This leads to the production of non-specific antibody, impairment of B cell function and immunosuppression. It has also been proposed that many parasites can cause unresponsiveness by activating immune suppressor mechanisms.

In many cases the immunosuppression has been attributed to macrophage dysfunction associated with antigen overload or the presence of intracellular parasites. In addition to the non-specific immunosuppression there can be parasite-specific effects. Mice infected by *Leishmania* spp. show antigen-specific depression of lymphokine production. Since this genus inhabits macrophages and is partly controlled by activation of these cells by lymphokines the effect is a diminished response against the pathogen.

Schistosomes have a receptor for part of the antibody molecule. They also release several proteases that cleave antibody molecules and release products that prevent macrophage activation. A schistosome-derived inhibitory factor suppresses T cell activity and is believed to allow other parasites to survive the effects of T cells and may explain the inefficiency of cytotoxic T cells in damaging the parasite.

When tested in a lymphocyte proliferation assay, peripheral blood lymphocytes of patients infected with *Plasmodium falciparum* are unresponsive to antigen prepared from the parasite, and in nearly 40% of the patients this persists for more than 4 weeks. Patients infected with *P. falciparum* show a suppression of lymphocyte reactivity which is not related to the degree of parasitaemia or severity of the clinical illness. The depressed lymphocyte reactivity is associated with a loss of both $CD4^+$ and $CD8^+$ lymphocytes from the peripheral blood. Once the parasite is cleared the response returns to normal. An even more sophisticated strategy has been evolved by *Leishmania mexicana* and *L. donovani*, which use interleukin-2 to stimulate their own growth. Mammalian epidermal growth factor has also been shown to stimulate the growth of certain trypanosomes in vitro.

## IMMUNOPATHOLOGY

The immune response to parasites is aimed at eliminating the organisms, but many of the host reactions have pathological effects.

The IgE produced in parasitic worm infections can have severe effects on the host if it stimulates excessive mast cell degranulation, i.e. type I hypersensitivity. Anaphylactic shock can occur if a cyst ruptures and releases vast amounts of antigenic material into the circulation of a sensitized individual. Asthma-like symptoms occur in *Toxocara canis* infections when larvae of worms migrate through the lungs.

The polyclonal B cell activation seen with many parasitic infections can give rise to auto-antibodies. In trypanosomiasis and malaria antibodies against red blood cells, lymphocytes and DNA have been detected. Host antigens incorporated into the parasite, as an immune evasion mechanism, may stimulate auto-antibody production by giving rise to T cell help and overcoming tolerance. In Chagas' disease about 20% of individuals develop progressive cardio-myopathy and neuropathy of the digestive tract that is believed to be auto-immune in nature. These effects are thought to result from cross-reactivity between antibody or T cells responsive to *Tryp. cruzi* and nerve ganglia.

Immune complex-mediated disease occurs in malaria, trypanosomiasis, schistosomiasis and oncho-cerciasis. The deposition of immune complexes in the kidney is responsible for the nephrotic syndrome of quartan malaria.

Enlargement of the spleen and liver in malaria, trypanosomiasis and visceral leishmaniasis is associated with increases in the number of macrophages and lymphocytes in these organs. The liver, renal and cardiopulmonary pathology of schistosomiasis is related to cell-mediated responses to the worm eggs. Symptoms similar to those seen in endotoxaemia induced by Gram-negative bacteria are found in the acute stages of malaria.

The non-specific immunosuppression discussed above may explain why individuals with parasite infections are especially susceptible to bacterial and viral infections.

## VACCINATION

No effective vaccine, for humans, has so far been developed against parasitic protozoa and worms, mainly due to the complex parasite life cycles and their sophisticated adaptive responses. Since protection in many cases depends on both antibody and cell-mediated reactions a vaccine must induce long-lived B and T cell immunity. In addition, since the recognition by T cells is genetically restricted, the vaccine preparation must stimulate T cells from most haplotypes and preferably be without suppressor epitopes. Due to the immunopathology seen in many parasite infections, antigens that induce a potentially damaging response must be avoided.

A much better understanding of the biological mechanisms underlying the natural history of parasitic diseases is required before it will be possible to control these globally important diseases.

---

RECOMMENDED READING

Mims C, Dimmock N, Nash A, Stephen J 1995 *Mims' Pathogenesis of Infectious Disease*, 4th edn. Academic Press, London
Taussig M J 1984 *Processes in Pathology and Microbiology*, 2nd edn. Blackwell Scientific, Oxford

Wakelin D 1996 *Immunity to Parasites*, 2nd edn. Cambridge University Press, Cambridge
Wyler D J 1990 *Modern Parasite Biology*. W H Freeman, New York

# 14

# Immunity in bacterial infections

*J. Stewart and D. M. Weir*

Modern medical science has managed to subdue many of the classical infectious diseases, but has helped to create new ones which result from interference with normal host defence mechanisms, consequent upon medical and surgical procedures such as chemotherapy, catheterization, immunosuppression and irradiation. Infections that develop in this way are known as *iatrogenic* (physician-induced) diseases.

It is important to differentiate infection from disease. A host may be infected with a particular micro-organism and be unaware of its presence. If the microbe reproduces itself to such an extent that toxic products or sheer numbers of organisms begin to harm the host then a disease process has developed. Potentially pathogenic bacteria such as pneumococci, streptococci and salmonellae are found in the nose, throat or bowel; this is known as the carrier state and is a source of infection to other individuals. These bacteria may also cause disease in the carrier if they enter a vulnerable tissue.

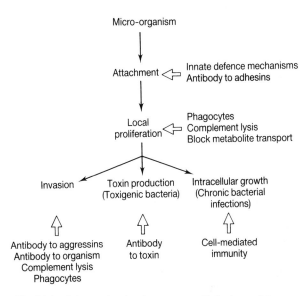

**Fig. 14.1** Scheme showing the progress of infection and the immunological defence mechanisms.

## HOST DEFENCES

Very few organisms can penetrate intact skin, and the various other innate defence mechanisms are extremely efficient at keeping bacteria at bay. When bacteria do gain access to the tissues the ability of the host to limit damage and eliminate the microbe will depend on the generation of an effective immune response against microbial antigens. In most cases the host defences will be directed against external components and secreted molecules. Bacteria are surrounded by a cytoplasmic membrane and a peptidoglycan cell wall. Associated with these basic structures there can be a variety of other components such as proteins, capsules, lipopolysaccharide or teichoic acids. There are also structures involved in motility or adherence to the cells of the host (see

Chs 2 and 8). These are some of the components to which the immune system directs its response. In general, peptidoglycan is attacked by lysosomal enzymes, and the outer lipid layer of Gram-negative bacteria by cationic proteins and complement. Specific antibodies can bind to flagella or fimbriae, affecting their ability to function properly and can inactivate various bacterial enzymes and toxins. Antibodies therefore interfere with many important bacterial processes but, ultimately, phagocytes are needed to destroy and remove the bacteria (Fig. 14.1). In some situations cell-mediated responses are required.

### Inflammation

Having successfully avoided the innate immune mechanisms that protect the individual (mechanical barriers, antibacterial substances and phagocytosis; described in Ch. 11), a bacterium starts to proliferate in the tissues, and its toxic products trigger an inflammatory reaction. The resulting increase in vascular permeability leads to an exudation of serum proteins, including complement components, antibodies and clotting factors, as well as phagocytic cells. The phagocytes are attracted to the site of inflammation by chemotactic factors. Anaphylatoxins generated by complement activation further increase vascular permeability and encourage exudation of fluid and cells at the site of inflammation. Many of these mediators also cause vasodilation, thereby increasing blood flow to the area.

Many types of micro-organisms, e.g. staphylococci and streptococci, are effectively dealt with by the phagocytes. The intensity and duration of the inflammatory process that is stimulated depends on the degree of success with which the micro-organism initially establishes itself. This, in turn, depends on the extent of the injury, the amount of associated tissue damage and the number and type of micro-organisms introduced. A localized abscess may arise at the site of infection.

If bacteria are not eliminated at the site of entry and continue to proliferate, they will pass via the tissue fluids and lymphatics to the draining lymph node, where a specific acquired immune response will be generated. The antibody and effector cells generated will leave the node to return to the area of infection to eliminate the bacteria. Some capsulate micro-organisms, such as pneumococci, are able to resist phagocytosis and are not dealt with effectively until large amounts of antibody are made. These 'mop up' the released capsular polysaccharide, and phagocytosis occurs. Other micro-organisms produce exotoxins, and effective immunity to exotoxins requires the development of specific antibodies against the toxin, i.e. antitoxin.

The types of infection described above are usually referred to as acute infections, and contrast with the protracted or chronic infections that are usually induced by bacteria which are adapted to survive within the cells of the host. Included amongst these are tuberculosis and leprosy, brucella infections and listeriosis. In these infections, cell-mediated immunity plays a predominant part in the final elimination of the micro-organism.

## Humoral immunity

The attachment of a micro-organism to an epithelial surface is a prerequisite for the development of an infectious process (see Ch. 8). A first line of attack by antibody could be to inhibit colonization by stopping attachment.

The immunoglobulin IgA can be detected in many mucous secretions in higher concentrations than those found in serum. This secretory IgA can stop colonization of the mucosal surface if it interferes with the attachment molecules (adhesins) present on the bacterial surface. IgA does not activate complement very efficiently; therefore, an inflammatory reaction is not stimulated. Damage to the gut wall during an inflammatory reaction would allow the entry of many potential pathogens into vulnerable tissues.

Many micro-organisms owe their pathogenic abilities to the production of exotoxins. Amongst diseases dependent on this type of mechanism are diphtheria, cholera, tetanus and botulism. Antibodies acquired by either immunization or previous infection or given passively as antiserum are able to neutralize bacterial toxins.

Many bacterial exotoxins are enzymes, and protective antibody is able to interfere with the ability of the enzyme to interact with its substrate. The antibody can bind directly to the active site of the enzyme or to adjacent residues and inhibit by steric hindrance. They may also act by stopping activation of a zymogen into an active enzyme, interfere with the interaction between the toxin and its target cell or bind to a site on the molecule, causing a conformational change that destroys the enzymic activity.

The direct binding of antibody to a bacterium can interfere with its normal functioning in numerous ways. Antibody can kill bacteria on its own or in conjunction with host factors and cells. To survive and multiply, bacteria must ingest nutrients and ions mainly by specific transport systems. Antibodies that affect the activity of specific transport systems will deprive the bacteria of its energy supply and other essential chemicals. A number of bacteria are invasive, moving into the tissues aided by enzymes that they produce. Invasion can also be inhibited by antibody that attaches to the flagella of the micro-organism in such a way as to affect their motility. Antibodies can agglutinate bacteria, and formation of the aggregate will impede the spread of the organism. In addition, the formation of an immune complex of bacteria and antibody will stimulate phagocytosis and complement activation.

When a particle is coated with antibody a large number of Fc portions are exposed to the outside. This increases the chance that the particle will be held in contact with the phagocyte long enough to stimulate phagocytosis. The interaction of multiple ligands will increase the overall affinity of the binding and if antibody and complement components are present on the same particle the binding will be even stronger.

The bacteria are internalized and attacked by the oxygen-dependent and oxygen-independent killing mechanisms within the phagocyte. Phagocytes are also responsible for the removal and digestion of bacteria that have been killed extracellularly. Bacteria are susceptible to the lytic action of complement, which may be activated by bacterial components. The presence of antibody on the bacterial cell surface will further stimulate the activation of complement. In certain circumstances, antibodies in conjunction with other bactericidal molecules lead to more efficient bacterial destruction. Gram-negative organisms are normally resistant to the action of lysozyme, probably due to the lipopolysaccharide component of the cell. The action of antibody and complement is thought to expose the underlying cell wall, which is then attacked by the lysozyme.

## Cell-mediated immunity

Ultimately, all bacteria will be engulfed by a phagocyte, either to be killed or removed after extracellular killing. The host defence mechanisms of macrophages and monocytes can be enhanced by various activating stimuli, including such microbial products as muramyl dipeptide and trehalose dimycolate. The chemotactic formyl-methionyl peptides have been shown to increase the activities of various macrophage functions. The linkage of chemotaxis to activation has the advantage that the cell that is being attracted to the site of tissue injury will be better equipped to deal with the insult. Endotoxin present in the cell wall of Gram-negative bacteria and various carbohydrate polymers, such as β-glucans, are also potent macrophage activators.

The immune system is also active in the production of macrophage-activating factors. In particular, lymphokines, produced by T lymphocytes, are often required to potentiate bacterial clearance both by attracting phagocytes to the site of infection and by activating them. The most important activator is γ-interferon, although tumour necrosis factor and colony-stimulating factors have also been implicated (see Ch. 11). All T lymphocytes produce some lymphokines when stimulated, and the balance of the different factors produced dictates the effect on surrounding cells. The overall effect of the lymphokines is to increase the effectiveness of host defence mechanisms, but if these molecules are produced in excess or to an inappropriate signal then a type IV hypersensitivity reaction can occur.

## EVASION

Once a micro-organism becomes established in the tissues, having escaped the innate defence mechanisms, it can often make use of a number of evasion strategies that protect it from the immune reactions of the host. Pathogenic bacteria produce a rather ill-defined group of bacterial products called *aggressins* and *impedins*, possession of which is associated with virulence (see Ch. 8). If antibody to such substances is present, the pathogenicity of the micro-organism is likely to be reduced.

## Intracellular bacteria

Bacteria that can survive and replicate within phagocytic cells are at an advantage as they are protected from host defence mechanisms. Some micro-organisms reside intracellularly only transiently while others spend most, if not all, their life inside cells. An intracellular lifestyle demands potent evasion mechanisms to survive this hostile environment. Some bacteria, such as *Mycobacterium leprae*, have become so accustomed to their intracellular environment that they can no longer live in the extracellular space.

*Listeria monocytogenes*, the causative agent of listeriosis, can survive and multiply in normal macrophages; but it is killed within macrophages activated by lymphokines released from T lymphocytes. Listeriosis is most commonly seen in immuno-compromised patients, pregnant women and neonates in whom a lack of adequate T cell-derived macrophage-activating factors is probably the critical factor. *Salmonella* spp. and *Brucella* spp. can also survive intracellularly. Unlike *L. monocytogenes* they owe their resistance to a glycolipid capsule that is resistant to destruction.

Mycobacteria have a waxy cell wall that is very hydrophobic. This external surface is very resistant to lysosomal enzymes and persists for a long time even when the bacteria have been killed. In addition, these micro-organisms have evolved other strategies to evade destruction. *Mycobacterium tuberculosis* secretes molecules that inhibit lysosome/phagosome fusion, while *M. leprae* can escape from the phagosome and grow in the cytoplasm. The cell wall of both these bacteria contains lipoarabinomannan that blocks the effects of γ-interferon on macrophages.

T lymphocytes represent the major host defence against intracellular pathogens. In many cases the bacteria themselves do not directly harm the host but the pathogenesis is caused by the immune response.

After invasion of the host, intracellular bacteria will be taken up by macrophages, evade intracellular killing and multiply. During intracellular replication some microbial molecules will be processed and presented on the surface of the infected cell in association with major histocompatibility complex (MHC) gene products. The exact nature of the microbial molecules and the processing mechanism are not known. The processing appears to produce mainly antigen fragments in association with MHC class II molecules. This complex on the cell surface will be recognized by specific CD4$^+$ T cells, which will be stimulated to release lymphokines. These molecules will in turn activate the macrophage so that the intracellular bacteria are killed.

It has also been proposed that peptides derived from the bacteria can become associated with MHC class I molecules. This complex will lead to the destruction of the infected cell by CD8$^+$ T cells. These cells also produce lymphokines that can aid in the elimination of the infection. The lymphokines produced will attract blood monocytes to the site and activate them. If these newly recruited cells take up the released mycobacteria they will be more likely to destroy them since they will be in an activated state. The accumulation of macrophages will also cause the formation of a granuloma, which will prevent dissemination of the bacteria to other sites in the body. As conditions for the survival of the pathogens become less suitable they stop replicating and die. Some intracellular bacteria infect cells that are unable to destroy them. In this situation a more aggressive immune response may be needed to remove the pathogen and this can cause pathogenic damage unless kept under control (see below).

## IMMUNOPATHOLOGY

The immune response to an organism will lead to some tissue damage through inflammation, lymph node swelling and cell infiltration. Sometimes the damage caused by the immune system is very severe, leading to serious disease and death. Rheumatic fever can follow group A streptococcal infections of the throat and is believed to be due to antibodies formed against a streptococcal cell wall component cross-reacting with cardiac muscle or heart valve. Myocarditis develops a few weeks after the throat infection and can be restimulated if the patient is reinfected with different streptococci.

Immune complex disease (type III hypersensitivity) is frequently associated with bacterial infections.

Infective endocarditis due to staphylococci and streptococci is associated with circulating complexes of antibody and bacterial antigen. Detection of these complexes can be helpful in diagnosis, but they can lead to joint and kidney lesions, vasculitis and skin rashes. Immune complexes may play a role in the pathogenesis of leprosy, typhoid fever and gonorrhoea.

## Effects of endotoxin

Endotoxin interacts with cells and molecules of inflammation, immunity and haemostasis. Fever is induced by interleukin-1, produced by the liver in response to endotoxin, acting on the temperature-regulating hypothalamus. The action of lipopolysaccharide on platelets and activation of Hageman's factor causes disseminated intravascular coagulation with ensuing ischaemic tissue damage to various organs. Septic shock occurs during severe infections with Gram-negative organisms when bacteria or lipopolysaccharide enter the bloodstream. Endotoxin acts on neutrophils, platelets and complement to produce, both directly and through mast cell degranulation, vaso-active amines that cause hypotension. The mortality is very high.

Endotoxin causes macrophages to produce large quantities of potent cytokines such as interleukin-1, tumour necrosis factor and colony-stimulating factors. It also causes polyclonal activation of B cells and can stimulate natural killer cells and other cell types to produce γ-interferon. A substantial part of the pathogenesis of endotoxic shock is probably due to the production of these molecules by cells of the immune system. In small amounts, endotoxin may actually be beneficial to the host but when present in excess the results can be disastrous.

## Mycobacterial disease

Activated macrophages secrete a variety of biologically active molecules, including proteases, tumour necrosis factor and reactive oxygen intermediates that are harmful to the surrounding tissue. Hence tissue destruction will be an inevitable side-effect of this important mechanism of resistance. In the acute phase of a response this is likely to be tolerated; but, in the case of resistant organisms such as mycobacteria the process may become chronic and the tissue destruction extensive. Mycobacterial components are still able to stimulate a response after the bacterium has been killed since they persist for a long time, adding to the tissue damage.

Recent evidence suggests that lysis of infected cells may also occur. At first sight this may appear beneficial. Such a direct effect may be particularly relevant in the case of obligate intracellular pathogens like *M. leprae*. Release into the hypoxic centre of a productive granuloma may also be fatal for *M. tuberculosis*, which is highly sensitive to low oxygen pressures. The same cytolytic event may also result in microbial discharge from the granuloma into surrounding capillaries or alveoli and hence facilitate dissemination to other parts of the body or to other individuals. Lysis of infected cells causes tissue destruction, the severity of the effects depending on the importance of the tissue involved. *M. leprae* infects a particularly essential cell, the Schwann cell, that is an irreplaceable component of the peripheral nervous system. Although the presence of *M. leprae* does not appear to affect the host cell to any extent,

the presence of activated macrophages releasing toxic molecules or direct lysis by cytotoxic cells constitutes a major pathological mechanism in leprosy.

If the leprosy bacillus is released from a lysed non-phagocytic cell to be engulfed by an activated macrophage then the bacterium will be eliminated. Therefore, macrophage activation and target cell lysis can be beneficial as well as detrimental to the host.

The cell-mediated response that has the potential to eliminate these infections will give rise to type IV hypersensitivity reactions if the antigen is not efficiently removed. Chronic production of lymphokines will cause granuloma formation that with time can lead to fibrosis and loss of organ function. This type of response is particularly prevalent in patients with tuberculosis.

## RECOMMENDED READING

Mims C, Dimmock N, Nash A, Stephen J 1995 *Mims' Pathogenesis of Infectious Disease*, 4th edn. Academic Press, London

Patrick S, Larkin M J 1995 *Immunological and Molecular Aspects of Bacterial Virulence*. Wiley, Chichester

Taussig M J 1984 *Processes in Pathology and Microbiology*, 2nd edn. Blackwell Scientific, Oxford

# Part 3
## BACTERIAL PATHOGENS AND ASSOCIATED DISEASES

# 15

# Staphylococcus

Skin infections; osteomyelitis; food poisoning; foreign body infections

*H. Humphreys*

Sir Alexander Ogston, a Scottish surgeon, first showed in 1880 that a number of pyogenic diseases in humans were associated with a cluster-forming micro-organism. He introduced the name 'staphylococcus' (Greek: *staphyle* = bunch of grapes; *kokkos* = grain or berry) now used as the genus name for a group of facultatively anaerobic, catalase-positive, Gram-positive cocci. The major pathogen within the genus, *Staphylococcus aureus*, causes a wide range of major and minor infections in humans and animals (Table 15.1) and is characterized by its ability to clot blood plasma by action of the enzyme *coagulase*. There are about 30 other species of staphylococci which all lack this enzyme. The coagulase-negative staphylococci are skin commensals that can cause opportunistic infections associated with prostheses or foreign bodies, catheters and implants (usually *Staph. epidermidis*), and urinary tract infections (*Staph. saprophyticus*). It is not usually necessary to identify coagulase-negative staphylococci to the species level.

Staphylococci are hardy, being resistant to dry conditions and high salt concentrations, and are well suited to their ecological niche, which is the skin surface of humans and animals. Staphylococci are also commonly present on other animals; mastitis caused by *Staph. aureus* is a common and costly complication of milking. Contamination of food can occur from human or animal sources and result in staphylococcal food poisoning.

## STAPHYLOCOCCUS AUREUS

### Description

*Staph. aureus* is a Gram-positive coccus about 1 µm in diameter. The cocci are mainly arranged in grape-like clusters (Fig. 15.1); but some, especially when

**Table 15.1** Infections caused by staphylococci

| *Staph. aureus* | | Coagulase-negative staphylococci |
|---|---|---|
| Pyogenic infections | Toxin-mediated infections | |
| Boils, carbuncles | Scalded skin | Infected prostheses |
| Wound infection | syndrome | Infected implants |
| Abscesses | Pemphigus | Infected intra- |
| Impetigo | neonatorum | vascular lines |
| Mastitis | Toxic shock | Ventriculitis[a] |
| Bacteraemia | syndrome | Peritonitis (CAPD) |
| Osteomyelitis | Food poisoning | Bacteraemia |
| Pneumonia | | Endocarditis |
| | | Urinary tract |
| | | infection |

CAPD, continuous ambulatory peritoneal dialysis.
[a]Shunt associated.

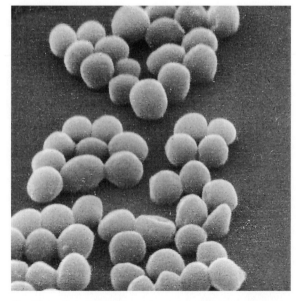

**Fig. 15.1** Scanning electron micrograph of *Staph. aureus*.

examined in pathological specimens, occur as single cells or pairs of cells. The organisms are non-sporing, non-motile and usually non-capsulate. When grown on nutrient agar, milk agar or blood agar for 24 h at 37°C, individual colonies are circular, 2–3 mm in diameter with a smooth, shiny surface; colonies appear opaque and are often pigmented (golden-yellow, fawn or cream), though a few strains are unpigmented. Staphylococci are salt-tolerant and can be selectively isolated from materials such as faeces and food by use of media containing 7–10% sodium chloride. The main distinctive diagnostic features of *Staph. aureus* are:

1. Production of an extracellular enzyme, coagulase, that converts fibrinogen in citrated human or rabbit plasma into fibrin, aided by an activator present in plasma. This test is done by adding a drop of fresh young broth culture into a tube containing 0.5 ml of citrated plasma diluted 1 in 10. A positive result is seen within a few hours as a distinct clot.

2. Production of thermostable *nucleases* that break down DNA. This activity is detected by the ability of a boiled broth culture to degrade DNA in an agar diffusion test.

3. Production of a surface-associated protein known as *clumping factor* or *bound coagulase* that reacts with fibrinogen. Clumping factor is easily detected within a few seconds by adding undiluted plasma to a saline suspension of the organism on a microscope slide.

Various commercial systems are available that rapidly identify coagulase-positive and coagulase-negative species. They are particularly useful for screening large numbers of strains obtained from environmental and food samples.

## Pathogenesis

*Staph. aureus* is present in the nose of 30% of healthy people and may be found on the skin. It causes infection most commonly at sites of lowered host resistance, e.g. damaged skin or mucous membranes.

### Virulence factors

*Staph. aureus* strains possess a large number of cell-associated and extracellular factors, some of which contribute to the ability of the organism to overcome the body's defences and to invade, survive in and colonize the tissues (Table 15.2). Though the role of each individual factor is not fully understood, it is likely that they are responsible for the establishment of infection, enabling the organism to bind to connective tissue, opposing destruction by the bactericidal

**Table 15.2** Virulence factors of *Staph. aureus*

| Virulence factor | Activity |
| --- | --- |
| **Cell wall polymers** | |
| Peptidoglycan | Inhibits inflammatory response; endotoxin-like activity |
| Teichoic acid | Phage adsorption; reservoir of bound divalent cations |
| **Cell surface proteins** | |
| Protein A | Reacts with Fc region of IgG |
| Clumping factor | Binds to fibrinogen |
| Fibronectin-binding protein | Binds to fibronectin |
| Collagen-binding protein | Binds to collagen |
| **Exoproteins** | |
| α-Lysin | Impairment of membrane permeability; cytotoxic effects on phagocytic and tissue cells |
| β-Lysin | |
| γ-Lysin | |
| δ-Lysin | |
| Panton–Valentine leucocidin | |
| Epidermolytic toxins | Cause blistering of skin |
| Toxic shock syndrome toxin | Induces multisystem effects; superantigen effects |
| Enterotoxins | Induce vomiting and diarrhoea; superantigen effects |
| Coagulase | Converts fibrinogen to fibrin in plasma |
| Hyaluronidase | Degrades hyaluronic acid in connective tissue |
| Staphylokinase | Degrades fibrin |
| Lipase | Degrades lipid |
| Phospholipases | Degrade phospholipids |
| Deoxyribonuclease | Degrades DNA |
| Proteases | Cause proteolysis |

activities of humoral factors such as complement and overcoming uptake and intracellular killing by phagocytes.

Animal experiments, with mutants defective in individual virulence factors, support the view that no single virulence factor is pre-eminent in overcoming host resistance and establishing a focus of staphylococcal infection. However, particular exotoxins are responsible for the symptoms of certain syndromes.

### Staphylococcal toxins

***Enterotoxins.*** Five types of enterotoxin (types A–E) are commonly produced by up to 65% of strains of *Staph. aureus*, sometimes singly and sometimes in combination. These toxic proteins are heat-stable, withstanding exposure to 100°C for several minutes. When ingested as preformed toxins in contaminated food, microgram amounts of toxin can induce within a few hours the symptoms of staphylococcal food poisoning: nausea, vomiting and diarrhoea. The serotypes A–E can be detected by various sensitive serological tests, such as latex agglutination.

***Toxic shock syndrome toxin (TSST-1).*** This was discovered in the early 1980s as a result of epidemiological and microbiological investigations in the USA of an apparently new multisystem disease named *toxic shock syndrome* due to staphylococcal TSST-1 or enterotoxin, or both. The disease reached public notice when large numbers of cases were reported in healthy young menstruating women. A link was established with the use of highly absorbent tampons, although non-menstrual cases are now as common. The absence of circulating antibodies to TSST-1 is a factor in the pathogenesis of this syndrome.

TSST-1 and the enterotoxins are now recognized as *superantigens*, i.e. they are potent activators of T lymphocytes resulting in the liberation of cytokines such as tumour necrosis factor, and they bind with high affinity to mononuclear cells. These characteristics partly explain the florid and multisystem nature of the clinical conditions associated with these toxins.

***Epidermolytic toxins.*** Two kinds of epidermolytic toxin (types A and B) are commonly produced by strains, mainly belonging to phage group II (see below), that cause blistering diseases. These toxins induce intra-epidermal blisters at the granular cell layer. Such blisters range in severity from the trivial to the distended blisters of *pemphigus neonatorum*. Outbreaks of blistering disease are not uncommon in busy nursing units where careful observation of hygiene practice is essential if skin sepsis is to be avoided.

The most dramatic manifestation of epidermolytic toxin is the *scalded skin syndrome* in which toxin spreads systemically in individuals who lack neutralizing antitoxin: extensive areas of skin are affected, which, after the development of a painful rash, slough off; the skin surface resembles scalding. Such blistering lesions are seen mainly, but not exclusively, in small children.

## Epidemiology

### Sources of infection

***Infected lesions.*** Large numbers of staphylococci are disseminated in pus and dried exudate discharged from large infected wounds, burns, secondarily infected skin lesions, and in sputum coughed from the lung of a patient with bronchopneumonia. Direct contact is the most important mode of spread, but air-borne dissemination may also occur. Small discharging lesions, on the hands of doctors and nurses, are a special danger to their patients. Cross-infection is an important method of spread of staphylococcal disease, particularly in hospitals, and scrupulous handwashing is essential in preventing spread. Food handlers may similarly introduce enterotoxin-producing food poisoning strains into food.

***Healthy carriers.*** *Staph. aureus* grows harmlessly on the moist skin of the nostrils in many healthy persons, and the perineum is also commonly colonized. Organisms are spread from these sites into the environment by the hands, handkerchiefs, clothing, and dust consisting of skin squames and cloth fibres. Some carriers, called *shedders*, disseminate exceptionally large numbers of cocci, comparable to the numbers disseminated by patients with large superficial lesions or lower respiratory tract infections.

During the first day or two of life most babies become colonized in the nose and skin by staphylococci acquired from their mother, nurse or environment. Nasal carriage in babies, as in older persons, is usually long-lasting. Transmission from babies to nursing mothers, who then develop mastitis, is well described.

***Animals.*** Domesticated and some wild species may disseminate *Staph. aureus* from infected lesions or carriage sites and so cause infections in humans, e.g. a dairy cow with staphylococcal infection of the udder may give infected milk which can cause staphylococcal food poisoning.

### Modes of infection

The mode of acquisition of an infection may be either *exogenous* (from an external source), or *endogenous* (from a carriage site, or minor lesion, elsewhere in the patient's own body). Staphylococci do not grow outside the body except occasionally in moist nutrient materials such as meat, milk and dirty water, and it is important to remember that the body surfaces of humans and animals are the main reservoir. Although not spore-forming, they may remain alive in a dormant state for several months when dried in pus, sputum, bed clothes or dust. They are fairly readily killed by heat (e.g. by moist heat at 65°C for 30 min), by exposure to light and by common disinfectants.

## Laboratory diagnosis

One or more of the following specimens should be collected to confirm a diagnosis:

1. *Pus* from abscesses, wounds, burns, etc., is much preferred to swabs
2. *Sputum* from cases of lower respiratory tract infections, e.g. postinfluenzal or ventilator-associated pneumonia
3. *Faeces* or *vomit* from patients with suspected food poisoning or the *remains of foods* implicated
4. *Blood* from patients with suspected bacteraemia, e.g. septic shock, osteomyelitis or endocarditis
5. *Mid-stream urine* from patients with suspected cystitis or pyelonephritis
6. *Anterior nasal* and *perineal swabs* (moistened in saline or sterile water) from suspected carriers; nasal swabs should be rubbed in turn over the anterior walls of both nostrils.

The characteristic Gram-positive cocci arranged in clusters can often be demonstrated by microscopy, and the organisms can be cultured readily on blood agar and most other media. The tube or slide coagulase test is performed to distinguish *Staph. aureus* from coagulase-negative species.

## *Typing*

Most staphylococcal infections are sporadic, but outbreaks do occur, especially in hospitals. The identification of an outbreak strain by determining whether all the isolates are of the same type is an important aspect in the investigation of a source, e.g. a heavy shedder in the operating theatre. For many years, strains of *Staph. aureus* have been differentiated into different *phage types* by observation of their pattern of susceptibility to lysis by a standard set of 23 different *Staph. aureus* bacteriophages. Virulent phages cause lysis of staphylococci that they can infect, and thus produce a clearing in the lawn of growth (Fig. 15.2). Phage types are designated according to the phages able to cause this effect, and there is international agreement on the interpretation of results. Thus, a strain of type 3B/3C/55 is one that is lysed by phage 3B, phage 3C and phage 55 but not by any of the other phages. Strains isolated from patients, carriers and fomites may be precisely identified ('fingerprinted') by this means and their source and pattern of spread in an outbreak discovered. Strains of *Staph. aureus* can be allocated to three main phage groups, I, II and III, according to their susceptibility to three groups of related phages,

**Fig. 15.2** Phage-typing plate showing lysis produced by the International Standard set of 23 different bacteriophages in a lawn of *Staph. aureus*. More than 50 plaques, irrespective of size, in the area surrounding the phage inoculum is scored as a positive result. The *Staph. aureus* strain shown belongs to lytic group III (6/47/53/54/75/83a/85). (By courtesy of George Sharp and Carol Webster.)

e.g. group I contains many hospital epidemic strains such as types 80 and 52A/79.

Strains resistant to the typing phages have become common, even after incorporating additional phages into the typing set. There has therefore been considerable interest in molecular techniques to overcome the problem of strains untypable with phages. Pulsed field gel electrophoresis, ribotyping and polymerase chain reaction-based techniques (see Ch 3) have been used, methods that do not rely on phenotypic characteristics which may alter with time. There are presently no standardized techniques or agreed criteria for the interpretation of results as is the case with phage typing. Nonetheless, it seems likely that these typing methods will become accepted as they become more widely available.

## Treatment

### Sensitivity to antibiotics

*Staph. aureus* and other staphylococci are inherently sensitive to many antimicrobial agents (Table 15.3). Among the most active is benzylpenicillin, but about 90% of those found in hospitals are now resistant. Resistance to penicillin depends on production of the enzyme penicillinase, a β-lactamase that opens the β-lactam ring. Penicillinase also inactivates most of the other penicillins, but a few compounds, including methicillin, cloxacillin and flucloxacillin have been developed that exhibit stability to the enzyme. Cephalosporins and β-lactamase inhibitors are also stable to penicillinase (see Ch. 5).

Antibiotic resistance can arise by various mechanisms (Table 15.4). Methicillin-resistant *Staph. aureus* (MRSA) is an increasing infection control problem and therapeutic challenge. These strains, which are resistant to all β-lactam agents, and often to other agents such as the aminoglycosides and fluoroquinolones, commonly colonize broken skin but can cause the full range of minor and systemic staphylococcal infections. These strains have probably arisen by a succession of mutations and the acquisition of resistance plasmids. The resistance gene *mecA* codes for a unique penicillin-binding protein and is transmitted chromosomally. Although predominantly a hospital pathogen in debilitated patients, MRSA is becoming more common in the community, especially in long-stay institutions. Eradication of colonized sites such as the nose or skin with topical agents, such as mupirocin or chlorhexidine, is often indicated to reduce the risks of cross-infection in hospital. Glycopeptides (vancomycin or teicoplanin) are the agents of choice in the treatment of systemic infection, but

**Table 15.3** Antibiotics and staphylococci

| Active agents | Agents lacking useful activity |
| --- | --- |
| Penicillins[a] | Mecillinam |
| Cephalosporins | Temocillin |
| Aminoglycosides | Aztreonam |
| Tetracyclines | Polymyxins |
| Macrolides | Nitroimidazoles |
| Lincosamides | Quinolones[b] |
| Glycopeptides | |
| Fluoroquinolones[c] | |
| Rifampicin | |
| Fusidic acid | |
| Trimethoprim | |
| Chloramphenicol | |
| Carbapenems | |

[a]Resistance common (see text).
[b]Nalidixic acid, etc.
[c]Ciprofloxacin, etc.

**Table 15.4** Common mechanisms of resistance to antistaphylococcal agents

| Agent | Mechanism of resistance | Usual genetic location |
| --- | --- | --- |
| Penicillins[a] | β-Lactamase | Plasmid |
| Methicillin[b] | Altered binding protein | Chromosome |
| Chloramphenicol | Acetyltranferase | Plasmid |
| Tetracyclines | Reduced accumulation | Plasmid |
| Erythromycin | Methylation of ribosome | Plasmid |
| Streptomycin | Altered ribosomal protein | Chromosome |
| Other aminoglycosides | Enzymic modification | Plasmid |
| Fusidic acid | Altered factor G | Chromosome |
| Rifampicin | Altered RNA polymerase | Chromosome |

[a]Except methicillin, nafcillin and isoxazolylpenicillins.
[b]And other β-lactam agents, including isoxazolylpenicillins, cephalosporins and carbapenems.

these agents are expensive and may be toxic. Resistance to the glycopeptides in *Staph. aureus* has yet to be described in vivo.

### Choice of antibiotic for therapy

Since strains of *Staph. aureus* vary in sensitivity to different antibiotics, treatment should be based on the results of sensitivity tests made on a culture of the strain isolated from the patient. Pending receipt of the results, the treatment of severe infections suspected of being due to *Staph. aureus* should be begun with flucloxacillin unless MRSA is endemic locally, in which case a glycopeptide is indicated. If tests show that the infecting organism is penicillin-sensitive, the drug of choice for further treatment is benzylpenicillin, which is narrow-spectrum and bactericidal. If the patient is hypersensitive to penicillin, erythromycin, clindamycin or vancomycin is used. Fusidic acid and rifampicin are not usually used alone in serious infections since mutation to resistance arises readily.

Collections of pus may require surgical drainage, and infected prostheses (e.g. hip joint) or intravascular lines (e.g. Hickmann catheter) usually require removal if antibiotic treatment is to be successful. Life-threatening toxin-mediated disease, such as toxic shock syndrome, requires major medical support such as intravenous fluids to prevent multi-organ failure, often best provided in an intensive care unit.

# COAGULASE-NEGATIVE STAPHYLOCOCCI

Coagulase-negative staphylococci comprise a large group of related species which are commonly found on the surface of healthy persons in whom they are rarely the cause of infection. More than 30 species are recognized, but only a few are commonly incriminated in human infection. *Staph. epidermidis* accounts for about 75% of all clinical isolates, probably reflecting its preponderance in the normal skin flora. The emergence of coagulase-negative staphylococci as major pathogens reflects the increased use of implants such as cerebrospinal fluid shunts, intravascular lines and cannulae, cardiac valves, pacemakers, artificial joints, vascular grafts and urinary catheters, and the increasing numbers of severely debilitated patients in hospitals.

## Description

Coagulase-negative staphylococci are morphologically similar to *Staph. aureus*, and the methods for isolation are the same. Colonies are usually non-pigmented (white), and they can be distinguished from *Staph. aureus* by their failure to coagulate plasma and by their lack of clumping factor and deoxyribonuclease. Because *Staph. epidermidis*, which accounts for the majority of isolates, may contaminate clinical specimens, care has to be exercised in assessing its significance, especially from superficial sites. When isolated from sites such as blood or cerebrospinal fluid, further specimens should be obtained to confirm their clinical significance.

Coagulase-negative staphylococci are opportunistic pathogens that cause infection in debilitated or compromised patients such as premature neonates and oncology patients, often by colonizing plastic devices. The organisms cause particular problems after cardiac surgery (prosthetic valve endocarditis); in patients fitted with cerebrospinal fluid shunts (meningitis); in continuous ambulatory peritoneal dialysis (peritonitis); and in immunocompromised patients (e.g. bacteraemia). One species, *Staph. saprophyticus*, is a common cause of urinary tract infection in women during the reproductive years but is rarely implicated in other infections.

## Pathogenesis

Unlike *Staph. aureus*, coagulase-negative staphylococci produce few, if any, toxins, and their pathogenicity is believed to be related to their ability to adhere to biomaterials consisting of synthetic polymers and production of extracellular 'slime'. Adherence is mediated by polysaccharides and is enhanced by the presence of fibrinogen. 'Slime', which largely consists of teichoic acid, inhibits the proliferation of human peripheral mononuclear cells, and may be partly responsible for the failure of treatment with antimicrobial agents because of difficulties in drug penetration. Biomaterials vary in their ability to aggregate platelets, tissue components and bacteria. Current developments include the production of materials less likely to facilitate colonization and the impregnation of implantable devices with antibacterial substances. Little is known about the virulence factors of *Staph. saprophyticus* causing urinary tract infection, but 'slime' and urease production are believed to be implicated.

## Treatment

Antibiotic treatment of coagulase-negative staphylococcal infections is complicated because susceptibility is generally unpredictable. Strains resistant to penicillin, methicillin, gentamicin, erythromycin and chloramphenicol are common. If a strain is the cause of systemic infection, then vancomyin or teicoplanin should be used. Rifampicin in combination with a glycopepetide is occasionally useful in treating central nervous system infections. Vancomycin resistance is rare, but one species, *Staph. haemolyticus*, is often resistant to teicoplanin. Uncomplicated urinary tract infection caused by *Staph. saprophyticus* usually responds to trimethoprim or one of the fluoroquinolones such as norfloxacin.

## RECOMMENDED READING

Cafferkey M T 1992 *Methicillin-Resistant* Staphylococcus aureus. *Clinical Management and Laboratory Aspects*. Marcel Dekker, New York

Easmon C S F, Adlam C 1983 *Staphylococci and Staphylococcal Infections*. Academic Press, London, vols 1 and 2

Elek S D 1959 Staphylococcus pyogenes *and its Relation to Disease*. Livingstone, Edinburgh

Jones D, Board R G, Sussman M 1990 *Staphylococci. Society for Applied Microbiology Symposium Series*, No. 19. Blackwell Scientific, Oxford

Kloos W E, Bannerman T L 1994 Update on clinical significance of coagulase-negative staphylococci. *Clinical Microbiology Reviews* 7: 117–140

Macdonald A, Smith G 1981 *The Staphylococci*. Aberdeen University Press, Aberdeen

# 16

# Streptococcus and enterococcus

Sore throat; scarlet fever; impetigo; rheumatic fever; glomerulonephritis; bacterial endocarditis

*P. W. Ross*

Streptococci form part of the normal flora of man and animals. They inhabit various sites, notably the upper respiratory tract, and usually live harmlessly as commensals. Some species, of which *Streptococcus pyogenes* is the most important, may adopt a more aggressive role. This organism can cause a wide spectrum of diseases, including tonsillitis, erysipelas, impetigo, scarlet fever and septicaemia, which range in severity from the trivial to the life-threatening. *Str. pyogenes* is also involved in the aetiology of rheumatic fever and acute glomerulonephritis. Other pathogenic species include *Str. agalactiae*, an important cause of neonatal infection, and *Str. pneumoniae* (see Ch. 17). Related organisms include: *Peptostreptococcus* spp., which are strictly anaerobic; enterococci, of which *Enterococcus faecalis* is the most important; and certain species that are rarely incriminated in infection, including *Pediococcus* spp. and *Leuconostoc* spp.

| Table 16.1 | Streptococci of importance in human infection | |
|---|---|---|
| Species | Lancefield group | Type of haemolysis on horse blood agar |
| *Str. pyogenes* | A | β |
| *Str. agalactiae* | B | β |
| *Str. equisimilis* | C | β |
| *Str. zooepidemicus* | C | β |
| *Str. bovis* | D | α or none |
| *Str. equinus* | D | α or none |
| *Str. milleri*[a] | A, C, G or F | α, β or none |
| *Str. pneumoniae* | None | α |
| *Str. sanguis* | None | α |
| *Str. mitior*[b] | None | α |
| *Str. mutans* | None | None |

[a] Includes strains designated *Str. intermedius, Str. constellatus* and *Str. anginosus*.
[b] Includes strains known as *Str. mitis* and *Str. oralis*.

## CLASSIFICATION OF STREPTOCOCCI

Streptococci that are most commonly encountered in medical laboratory practice are shown in Table 16.1. They are Gram-positive bacteria arranged in chains of varying length (Fig. 16.1); each cell is approximately 1.0 μm in diameter, non-motile, non-sporing and may be capsulate. Most are facultative anaerobes, but there are species that are strictly anaerobic. All have an anaerobic type of metabolism and are catalase-negative.

Classification depends traditionally on the type of haemolysis seen on blood agar. Some strains have soluble haemolysins (streptolysins O and S), which produce a clear zone of haemolysis on fresh blood agar media. This is known as β-haemolysis, a phenomenon associated with the majority of streptococcal species that cause primary infections in man and animals. These haemolytic streptococci can be

**Fig. 16.1** Scanning electron micrograph of *Str. pyogenes* showing typical chain formation.

further subdivided serologically into a number of broad groups exploiting differences in the group-specific polysaccharide antigens contained in the cell wall. Lancefield thus identified a number of different groups lettered sequentially A–H and K–V.

*Str. pyogenes* belongs to Lancefield group A. These strains may be further subdivided by specific sera into Griffith types according to their surface protein antigens (M, T and R). The M protein is the antigen of most importance, and it exists in approximately 60 different antigenic forms, each of which is present in a different serotype of *Str. pyogenes* (type 1, type 2, etc.). The determination of the serotype of strains of *Str. pyogenes* isolated from patients and carriers plays a valuable part in the epidemiological investigation of outbreaks of infection in a way comparable to the use of phage typing in the study of *Staphylococcus aureus* infection.

Streptococci that do not possess soluble haemolysins are divided into two categories: (1) those that cause a narrow zone of partial clearing and green coloration and are called α-haemolytic streptococci, or viridans streptococci; (2) those that produce no obvious changes around colonies on blood agar and are called non-haemolytic. These are sometimes called γ-haemolytic, but this term may be misleading in terms of classification and should not be used.

## STREPTOCOCCUS PYOGENES (GROUP A β-HAEMOLYTIC STREPTOCOCCI)

### Pathogenesis

The most common route of entry of *Str. pyogenes* is the upper respiratory tract, where the primary infection is established, usually in the throat, but only a proportion of infected individuals develop tonsillitis or pharyngitis. The others may have mild atypical infections or become symptomless carriers. In tropical climates the skin is a common site of entry.

### Structural components

The virulence of *Str. pyogenes* is closely related to a surface antigen, the M protein, which is the main antiphagocytic factor. M-associated protein antigen, which is not type-specific, is found in M-positive variants. Two other surface proteins, T and R, do not play any part in virulence but are useful in

identification of the infecting serotype. Antibodies to M protein are mainly responsible for immunity; they counteract the antiphagocytic action of the M protein and are effective only against the homologous serotype. Fimbriae on the surface of streptococci enable attachment to epithelial cells and consist of M protein. Hyaluronic acid capsules are produced by streptococci in the early stages of artificial culture and also when spreading in the blood and tissues, but they have only a weak antiphagocytic effect.

### Extracellular products

β-Haemolytic streptococci, notably *Str. pyogenes*, possess a formidable battery of diffusible products, but it is not yet possible to link definitively any individual toxin or enzyme, or combination, with any particular syndrome or infection. Not all of these substances are produced by any one strain but most strains can form the majority of them, depending on environmental conditions. These products can also be isolated from some other β-haemolytic streptococci.

***Erythrogenic agents.*** There are three distinct toxins, erythrogenic toxins A, B and C (streptococcal pyrogenic exotoxins; SPE A, SPE B and SPE C). Type A toxin is encoded by bacteriophage gene *speA*, type B toxin by chromosomal gene *speB* and toxin C by bacteriophage gene *speC*. These exotoxins are superantigens, T cell mitogens that induce lymphocytes to synthesize and release cytokines such as tumour necrosis factor, interleukin-1β and interleukin-6, with the subsequent production of fever, shock and tissue damage.

***Streptolysin O.*** Most group A streptococci and some group C and G streptococci produce this haemolysin. Other bacteria also form streptolysin O-like products. Streptolysin O lyses red blood cells by linking to bound cholesterol in the cell membrane, causing holes to form in this structure; it is also cytotoxic for other cells, including neutrophils, platelets and cardiac tissue. It is inactivated by oxygen.

***Streptolysin S.*** This haemolysin is not inactivated by oxygen and is responsible for the haemolysis produced on the surface of an aerobic blood agar plate. As well as its haemolytic properties it also has a leucocidal action.

***Streptokinase (fibrinolysin).*** Streptokinase, produced by group A, C and G streptococci, is protein in nature and is antigenic.

The role of streptokinase in streptococcal infections is not clear but because of its action in preventing the formation of an effective fibrin barrier it may well influence the character of the lesions by interfering with the localization of the infection. This property is used therapeutically in the early treatment of coronary thrombosis.

*Deoxyribonucleases (DNAases).* There are at least four of these enzymes, designated A, B, C and D. As with other extracellular products of streptococci, they are found in group C and G as well as in group A streptococci; they are antigenic. DNAase B is the most common form in *Str. pyogenes*. They hydrolyse nucleic acids and nucleo-proteins, and since the products can be used by streptococci they may have an important nutritional role. Nucleases have been used clinically to liquefy viscous exudates, e.g. empyema.

*Hyaluronidase.* This antigenic substance is produced by strains of group A, B, C and G streptococci. A characteristic feature of streptococcal infections, whether the portal of entry is the throat, the skin or the genital tract, is the ability of the organisms to spread through the tissues. Cellulitis and erysipelas are classical examples of the spread-ing lesion, and this may be related to the production of hyaluronidase; however, *Staph. aureus* also produces hyaluronidase, but rarely causes spreading infections in the skin.

*Nicotinamide adenine dinucleotidase (NADase).* This is produced by strains of group A, C and G streptococci and is antigenic. There is a close connection between the ability of a streptococcal strain to produce NADase and its leucotoxic effect.

*Serum opacity factor (lipoproteinase).* The ability to produce opacity in horse serum is a characteristic of certain M types of group A streptococci. The opacity factor is closely associated with the M protein and is loosely bound to the cell. It is antigenically specific, the specificity corres-ponding to that of the M antigen.

Other extracellular products that have been isolated from streptococci include bacteriocines, amylase, esterase, proteinase, lipase and β-glucuronidase.

## Laboratory diagnosis

Identification of β-haemolytic streptococci that have been isolated from the patient and examination of patients' sera for a rising titre of antibodies to one or more streptococcal antigens are the means of diagnosis.

Swabs are taken from patients or from suspected carriers. Microscopy is of little help in the diagnosis of streptococcal pharyngitis, though it may reveal other pathogens such as Vincent's organisms. If there is likely to be a delay of more than a few hours before the swab can be despatched to the laboratory or processed, it should be refrigerated. In a search for carriers, as in an institutional outbreak of sore throat or scarlet fever, nasal as well as throat swabs must be taken. Saliva can yield positive results when the throat swab is negative.

Swabs are cultured on blood agar and incubated for 24 h. Anaerobic as well as aerobic incubation should be carried out because group A strains that form only haemolysin O fail to show haemolysis on aerobic culture.

It is unhelpful for a service laboratory to report to the clinician growth of β-haemolytic streptococci from a specimen without grouping the organisms. Grouping of all β-haemolytic streptococci is mandatory for the following reasons: (1) to facilitate epidemiological surveillance of streptococcal infec-tions in hospital and in the wider community; (2) to monitor drug resistance patterns effectively; and (3) because various Lancefield groups are associated with characteristic infections.

For the presumptive identification of β-haemolytic streptococci belonging to group A, bacitracin sen-sitivity may be tested. Group A organisms are much more sensitive than other groups to bacitracin but the test is not totally reliable as some non-group A strains may also be sensitive. For accurate identifi-cation of streptococci, Lancefield's serogrouping must be performed. Commercial kits are used increasingly for streptococcal grouping, and are convenient, quick and reliable.

Tests for streptococcal serum antibodies may also be performed, but such tests do not give the clini-cian an immediate answer during the initial phase of an acute infection. They may be used to identify or confirm primary infections but are more commonly used for the diagnosis of the non-suppurative sequelae of group A streptococcal infection such as rheumatic fever or glomerulonephritis. Single titres are difficult to evaluate as they do not differentiate between past and current infections; a second serum sample must always be tested about 10 days after the first to detect a rise in antibody titre. If the results are equivocal, a further sample must be analysed.

The antistreptolysin O (ASO) test is most com-monly performed, and the anti-DNAase B test may also be useful.

## Epidemiology

The severity of streptococcal infections has become steadily and markedly reduced in many countries in the past century. The strongest evidence in support of this statement comes from the mortality rates for scarlet fever, which is a notifiable disease in the UK. Death rates in the UK from this once dreaded disease have fallen from about 1000 per million of the population in the decade 1860–69 to virtually zero at the present time. The remarkable reduction in the severity of scarlet fever was accompanied by a decline in the incidence and mortality of other severe streptococcal infections such as septicaemia, puerperal sepsis, acute endocarditis and rheumatic fever, and was apparent before the advent of antibiotics. This general amelioration was probably related to a steady improvement in nutrition and in social and environmental conditions compared with the abject poverty and gross overcrowding of earlier decades when the rapid transfer of *Str. pyogenes* in a highly susceptible population led to an exaltation in the virulence of the pathogen. However, since the late 1980s there has been a marked change in the epidemiology of infections caused by *Str. pyogenes*. Several cases of rheumatic fever have occurred, particularly in the USA, and the incidence of invasive infections with bacteraemia and toxaemia has increased significantly. Notable among these are necrotizing fasciitis and the streptococcal toxic shock syndrome, produced by M types 1 and 3 but also by M types 12 and 28.

The capsules of types 1 and 3 contain substantial amounts of hyaluronic acid which has an anti-phagocytic action, but the reason for the increase in incidence and severity of streptococcal infections during the last decade is due more probably to factors relating to the organisms and the individuals affected. For example, some M strains, particularly type 1, represent a virulent clone of bacteria with new genetic information, carrying genes for the production of specific exotoxins. These include erythrogenic toxins A, B and C (see above).

Besides the acute case of sore throat and the nasal or saliva carrier, other dangerous sources of infection are patients with streptococcal otitis media, vulvovaginitis or infected skin lesions. Although the nasal carrier is important in initiating streptococcal infections, carriage in the throat or saliva is more common. At least 10% of children will be throat carriers at any one time and this proportion increases sharply at times of greater prevalence of clinical infection.

## Chemotherapy

*Str. pyogenes* is highly sensitive to a wide range of antibacterial drugs, including penicillin and erythro-mycin, but strains resistant to sulphonamides and tetracyclines are common. Benzylpenicillin (penicillin G) or oral phenoxymethylpenicillin (penicillin V) are the drugs of choice. Penicillin-resistant strains of *Str. pyogenes* are presently unknown, so that antibiotic sensitivity tests are unnecessary if *Str. pyogenes* is identified as the infecting organism and penicillin is to be used.

Treatment for 3–5 days will limit the effect of severe attacks of streptococcal infection and prevent suppurative complications such as otitis media, but studies have shown that only if treatment is continued for 10 days will the streptococci be eliminated from the infected area.

If the use of any other antimicrobial agent is contemplated, as in cases of hypersensitivity to penicillin, antimicrobial sensitivity testing must be done because of dangers of resistance to the drug.

## Clinical infections

The most common and typical infection caused by *Str. pyogenes* is an acute sore throat. If the infecting streptococcus is capable of producing an erythrogenic toxin and the host has not developed antibodies to this toxin, the sore throat may be accompanied by a generalized punctate erythema or rash. This syndrome is called *scarlet fever*. Local extension of the infection from the throat may result rarely in such complications as peritonsillar abscess (quinsy), sinusitis, otitis media or mastoiditis. Bronchopneumonia may develop as a complication of viral infections of the respiratory tract such as measles and influenza.

Puerperal sepsis or child-bed fever is traditionally associated with infection by *Str. pyogenes*, although other bacteria are now more commonly involved. Besides local inflammation of uterine tissues, infection may spread to the adnexa (pelvic cellulitis or peritonitis). Wounds, burns and chronic skin lesions (eczema, psoriasis) may become infected with *Str. pyogenes*; these superficial infections may extend in the local tissues (cellulitis) or be carried by lymphatics to regional lymph glands (lymphadenitis) or get into the bloodstream and become generalized (septicaemia).

*Str. pyogenes* can cause two types of primary skin infection, erysipelas and impetigo.

### Sore throat

Sore throat – acute tonsillitis and/or pharyngitis – may be caused by non-infective agents such as tobacco smoke and be associated with blood diseases such as leukaemia, but it is caused most commonly by infective agents. It is a feature of the common cold and influenza and with the prodromal stages of infectious diseases such as chickenpox and measles. It accompanies local throat infections such as infectious mononucleosis, candida infection, Vincent's infection and – very rarely now in Western societies – diphtheria. Sore throat is one of the most common ailments seen by family doctors, especially in the winter months. It is uncommon in infants and in the elderly. Boys and girls are equally affected, and its peak incidence is in young schoolchildren who succumb to the cross-infection hazards of the classroom because of a poorly developed level and range of antibodies. It is less common in the older schoolchild, adolescent and young adult.

Acute pharyngitis and acute tonsillitis are caused by both bacteria and viruses. The bacteria are almost exclusively *Str. pyogenes*. Group C and G streptococci may also be involved, but other bacteria such as staphylococci and *Haemophilus* spp. are rarely implicated. For all practical purposes a bacterial sore throat means a streptococcal sore throat. Specific antibodies to the M protein, the virulence antigen of the infecting streptococcus, develop slowly after sore throat or other streptococcal illness but persist for a long time. Consequently, attacks by the same streptococcal serotype are unlikely though specific antibody does not protect against infection with other serotypes. Only 30–40% of cases of sore throat are caused by streptococci. Most of the rest are caused by viruses or, occasionally, *Mycoplasma pneumoniae*. It is not possible to diagnose the aetiology of sore throat on clinical grounds because streptococci and viruses both cause pain on swallowing, tender, enlarged tonsillar lymph nodes, pyrexia, headache and malaise. An exudate over the back of the throat can be produced by both streptococci and viruses. The throat must be swabbed if an accurate diagnosis of the cause of infection is to be established.

***Throat swabbing***. The technique of swabbing is all important. As large an area of the soft palate as possible should be covered, and rotation of the swab-head is also recommended so that as many bacteria as possible will be gathered onto the swab. A sample of saliva may also be useful as streptococci may be shed into the saliva.

## Cellulitis

*Str. pyogenes* predominates in causing cellulitis and highly invasive soft tissue infections, but group C and G β-haemolytic streptococci also play a role, in addition to *Staph. aureus* and *Clostridium perfringens*. Commonly there is no obvious portal of entry for the bacteria, although a breach of the skin or mucosa is the most likely. Streptococcal cellulitis is a spreading infection that may become bacteraemic.

## Bacteraemia

Streptococcal bacteraemia, an indicator of invasive streptococcal disease, is reported with increasing frequency. Organisms have been isolated from sites normally sterile, such as blood, cerebrospinal fluid, brain, lung, kidney, bone marrow and the uterus. Sources of infection are unclear but intravenous drug abuse is a well-recognized factor.

## Impetigo

Although *Str. pyogenes* is the predominant infecting agent, impetigo may also be caused by group C and G streptococci and by *Staph. aureus*; the primary skin lesion may be bullous rather than vesicular (bullous impetigo or pemphigus neonatorum).

## Erysipelas

This acute spreading skin lesion is rarer than impetigo. The infected area of the skin shows marked oedema and erythema.

## Scarlet fever

This disease comprises a streptococcal sore throat and a generalized erythema, although occasionally the rash may accompany a streptococcal wound infection (surgical scarlet fever). The incidence and severity of scarlet fever decreased dramatically in the 20th century, but severe cases are still seen sporadically. Many strains of group A and some strains of group G streptococci produce scarlet fever. The incubation period is 2–3 days, and the disease occurs most often in children under the age of 10 years. The characteristic rash, consisting of a widespread erythema with punctate spots, varies considerably depending on the severity of the infection.

Although chemotherapy has completely altered the clinical course of the disease by shortening the acute stage and by virtually eliminating suppurative complications, the natural course of the rash is not altered in any way by antibiotics.

## Necrotizing fasciitis

This infection progresses very rapidly, destroying fat and fascia. Although *Str. pyogenes* gains entry to these tissues through the skin after trauma, often of a minor nature, the skin itself may show only minimal signs of infection and may indeed be spared. Systemic shock and general deterioration occur very quickly. The disease affects the fit, young person with no obvious underlying pathology, as well as the immunocompromised.

Diagnosis clinically may be difficult because *Staph. aureus* and anaerobes, e.g. *Cl. perfringens* can produce a similar clinical picture. Streptococci can be isolated from the blood, blister fluid and from cultures of the infected area. Types M1 and 3 are implicated most often; they possess the *speA* gene with variants *speA*2 in type 1 and *speA*3 in type 3.

Antibiotic penetration of the infected area is poor, and surgery is essential to remove damaged tissue. Clindamycin is preferred to penicillin because it inhibits protein synthesis including production of exotoxin.

## Streptococcal toxic shock syndrome

A striking feature of this acute fulminating disease is severe pain at the site of infection, usually the soft tissues. There is bacteraemia and toxaemia, accompanied by fever and shock. There may be organ damage, acute respiratory distress and renal failure. Although the age group affected is relatively young, mortality is between 20 and 30%. As in necrotizing fasciitis, types M1 and 3, possessing the *speA* gene, are the most common, but types 12 and 28 are also involved. Antibiotics that inhibit protein synthesis, such as clindamycin, are useful.

A crucial factor in necrotizing fasciitis and streptococcal toxic shock syndrome is the immune status of the individual. Invasion of a non-immune host by a particular M type will produce disease; if the M type additionally possesses SPE A or SPE B to which the person has no immunity, fever and shock with or without organ damage will follow. Effective immunity prevents these conditions.

## Streptococcal myositis

This rare infection mimics necrotizing fasciitis clinically, although at operation they look quite different. As a breach of the skin or soft tissue damage is unusual, the source is considered to be the throat, with bacteraemic spread to the muscle. The infection may be precipitated by trauma or muscle strain.

## Non-suppurative complications

### Rheumatic fever

An attack of rheumatic fever is related to antecedent streptococcal throat infection occurring 1–5 weeks earlier. Support for this association is based on clinical, bacteriological, epidemiological, serological and chemoprophylactic evidence.

***Epidemiology.*** Altitude, humidity and other physical factors were thought to have a role in rheumatic fever, but it now appears that it can occur anywhere in the world. In general, there is an increased incidence when the streptococcal carriage rate increases, and in the UK the age group with the highest incidence (7–9 years) is also that which has the highest incidence of streptococcal sore throat. Social factors such as overcrowding, poor nutrition and clothing are all important. In the USA since the late 1980s clusters of cases of rheumatic fever have been identified in various geographical areas such as Pennsylvania, Ohio and Utah. Young adults in military populations in Missouri and California have also contracted the disease.

***Diagnosis.*** Rheumatic fever may be difficult to diagnose and, since throat swabs may or may not yield growth of *Str. pyogenes*, the most important investigations are serological. Two samples of serum must be assayed to check for a rising titre of antibody to *Str. pyogenes*. Titres become detectable in the 2nd week after the onset of infection, are maximal by the 6th week and thereafter decrease.

Many serotypes of *Str. pyogenes* are involved, but it does not occur in the absence of immunological evidence of streptococcal infection.

***Chemoprophylaxis.*** Penicillin prophylaxis after a primary attack of rheumatic fever will reduce substantially the risk of a second attack by preventing further streptococcal infection of the throat. However, prevention of primary attacks is virtually impossible, and penicillin treatment of streptococcal sore throat plays little or no part. Moreover, only a few persons with streptococcal throat infection are treated, either because infection is subclinical or because those with a sore throat do not consult their doctor.

***Aetiology.*** There is conclusive evidence of an association with an antecedent streptococcal throat infection, but not with primary streptococcal infections of other tissues. The streptococci are not present in the lesions in the heart and joints. No particular streptococcal serotypes are incriminated, as happens with glomerulonephritis, and it is for this reason that throat infections with different serotypes can cause relapses of rheumatic fever.

An immunological relationship exists between a streptococcal antigen and human myocardial tissue. The antigen responsible for the cross-reactivity is localized in the cell wall and is associated with the M protein. It is probable that several cross-reactive antigen–antibody systems occur between the streptococcus, heart valves and heart muscle. Group-specific polysaccharide antigen of *Str. pyogenes* cross-reacts with the structural glycoprotein of both human and bovine valves.

Specific host factors have not been excluded in the pathogenesis of this disease. Some individuals seem prone to develop the rheumatic syndrome and such individuals are particularly liable to recurrent attacks after further streptococcal sore throats. However, the significance of hereditary predisposition is very difficult to disentangle from predisposing environmental factors, such as overcrowding in families or in communities.

### Acute glomerulonephritis

Post-streptococcal glomerulonephritis is a common type of acute nephritis. It is almost always produced by group A streptococci but group C streptococci may also be involved. In comparison with rheumatic fever, which can be caused by a wide range of serotypes of *Str. pyogenes*, acute glomerulonephritis is produced by a much narrower range. Also, whereas the *Str. pyogenes* strains associated with rheumatic fever are isolated from the upper respiratory tract only, those involved in acute glomerulonephritis may be isolated from the upper respiratory tract or from skin lesions such as impetigo (Table 16.2).

The role of skin and throat infections in the development of acute glomerulonephritis is now firmly established, although there are clear differences in the epidemiology: acute glomerulonephritis following streptococcal throat infection occurs at the colder times of the year and mostly in children or young adults. Outbreaks in institutions can occur and there may be epidemic waves in the community. Following infected skin lesions it occurs in all age groups in hot humid weather, notably in parts of the USA and in the West Indies, where flies of the genus *Hippelates* are important vectors of streptococci. Recurrences of acute glomerulonephritis are rare.

Post-streptococcal glomerulonephritis arises because components of the glomerular basement membrane are immunologically similar to the cell membranes of nephritogenic β-haemolytic streptococci.

***Laboratory diagnosis.*** β-Haemolytic streptococci may be isolated from the throat and skin but serological tests are generally more helpful in establishing the diagnosis. Immune responses vary depending on whether the source of infection is the throat or skin. For example, the ASO estimation is reliable in the throat-associated form but unreliable in pyoderma-associated acute glomerulonephritis, whereas the anti-DNAase B titre is raised more frequently and to a greater degree in pyoderma-associated disease.

## OTHER STREPTOCOCCI

### Group B streptococci

Group B streptococci (*Str. agalactiae*) were known at the end of the last century as a cause of bovine mastitis but it was not until the 1930s that their association with human disease was recognized. Such infections have been reported with increasing frequency, and group B streptococci have now replaced group A streptococci, the scourge of the pre-1940s, as the major streptococcal pathogens in neonates and young infants.

A real change in the incidence and epidemiology of infections has occurred. Improvements in laboratory methods and techniques and a greater awareness of group B infections cannot account solely for the dramatic increase in the last two decades.

### Infections in the neonate

These represent a wide spectrum of clinical disease, some minor, some major.

'Early-onset' infection occurs soon after birth, and the 'late-onset' form occurs several days to several weeks after birth. Although these terms are in common use they do not have clear-cut clinical

| Table 16.2 M protein types of *Str. pyogenes* associated with acute glomerulonephritis | |
|---|---|
| Antecedent infection | Common M protein types |
| Throat infection | 12, 1, 25, 4 and 3 |
| Pyoderma | 49, 52, 53–55 and 57–61 |

significance, since there is no universally accepted line of demarcation between them.

*Early-onset infection.* This is a particularly devastating neonatal septicaemic disease. Neonates may be ill at birth or develop acute and fulminating illness a few hours, or a day or two, later. Neonates may be lethargic, cyanosed and apnoeic, and when septicaemia progresses, shock ensues and death will occur if treatment is not quickly instituted. Meningitis and pulmonary infection may be associated.

Early rupture of the membranes, prolonged labour, prematurity, low birth weight and heavy colonization of the mother's genital tract by group B streptococci lead to infection. Group B streptococci may be isolated from many sites in the neonate but diagnosis is sometimes made only after death.

Group B colonization of neonates, with or without infection, is via the mother's genital tract; in almost every case the serotype of group B isolated from the neonate (the anterior nares, external auditory meatus, umbilicus and rectum are the sites from which organisms are most commonly isolated) is similar to that isolated from the cervicovaginal canal, urethra or rectum of the mother. Group B streptococci can be isolated from infants delivered by caesarian section, implying that the organisms can spread directly into the uterus from the genital tract of the mother.

*Late-onset infection.* Purulent meningitis is the most common group B infection after the immediate newborn period. Signs and symptoms of meningitis relate to the degree of maturity of the infant. There is usually no history of obstetric complications and seldom does the mother have genital tract colonization by group B streptococci. Infection is probably nosocomial, since some studies have shown that a substantial number of ward staff can be group B carriers. Transfer of the organisms to the baby takes place during nursing procedures. Baby-to-baby spread also occurs.

*Prevention of group B neonatal infection.* Whereas late-onset infection may be prevented or decreased by standard aseptic nursing procedures, early onset infection is more difficult to prevent. Swabbing the mother's genital tract during pregnancy is not helpful because carriage can be intermittent, and isolation of the organism during pregnancy does not indicate that it will be present during labour. Moreover, administration of antibiotics to women who are positive during pregnancy has little effect on the carriage of group B streptococci.

Group B streptococci can produce other infections in infants, including septic arthritis, osteomyelitis, conjunctivitis, sinusitis, otitis media, endocarditis, peritonitis and omphalitis.

Localized infections are seen more commonly in older infants.

### Infections in the adult

Infections in adults have a bimodal distribution:

1. Abortion, chorioamnionitis, postpartum sepsis (endometritis) and other infections (e.g. pneumonia) in the postpartum period may occur in young, previously healthy women.

2. Meningitis, otitis media, endocarditis, pneumonia, empyema, arthritis, abscesses, infections of wounds and burns, urinary tract infection and osteomyelitis may occur in the elderly and in immunocompromised individuals.

## Group C streptococci

These organisms comprise four species, *Str. equi*, *Str. equisimilis*, *Str. dysgalactiae* and *Str. zooepidemicus*. They resemble group A streptococci, although they do not cause as many infections.

Group C streptococci are notably animal pathogens but certain species such as *Str. zooepidemicus* and *Str. equisimilis* can produce disease in humans. They can cause epidemic sore throat, especially in communities such as schools, nurseries and institutions, often associated with unpasteurized milk. Some group C strains have been related to acute glomerulonephritis and other infections such as postpartum sepsis, septicaemia, meningitis, pneumonia and skin and wound infections.

## Group G streptococci

Although antigenically quite distinct, these streptococci resemble those of groups A and C in their pathogenic properties and in the types of infections produced. They can cause sore throat, sometimes after ingestion of contaminated food, and pneumonia. They are isolated from 3 to 4% of cases of septicaemia and are sometimes associated with underlying malignancy in the patient. Erysipelas and cellulitis may be caused as well as bone and joint infection.

## Group D streptococci and enterococci

Whereas group A, C and G streptococci are commonly linked together because of a number of shared features, group D is a separate entity in terms of its biochemical, serological and pathogenic profiles. Many group D strains are much less sensitive to penicillin than other streptococci, and as they are genetically unrelated these strains have been reclassified as *Enterococcus* species. The enterococcal species most commonly associated with human disease are *E. faecalis* and *E. faecium* but infections caused by others, such as *E. durans* and *E. avium*, also occur.

*E. faecalis* and *E. faecium* are important causes of nosocomial infection and may cause sporadic outbreaks. Bacteraemia carries a poor prognosis and is often present in patients with major underlying pathology and in those who are immunocompromised. Resistance to the commonly used antibiotics, including vancomycin, is on the increase.

The non-enterococcal group D strains which include *Str. bovis* and *Str. equinus* remain sensitive to penicillin. *Str. bovis* bacteraemia is associated with endocarditis and carcinoma of the bowel. The normal habitats of enterococci and group D streptococci are the intestine and vagina, and the diseases with which they are associated are: urinary tract infection; infective endocarditis; biliary tract infections; suppurative abdominal lesions; and peritonitis.

## Group R streptococci

Rarely do streptococci of groups other than A, B, C, D, F and G cause human infections, but *Str. suis*, serotype 2, known also as group R streptococcus, a well-established cause of septicaemia and meningitis in pigs, can infect people in contact with contaminated pork or infected pigs, causing septicaemia, meningitis and respiratory tract infections. Abattoir workers, butchers and, to a lesser extent, housewives are at risk.

## Viridans streptococci

Sometimes known as the oral streptococci, they characteristically produce partial (α) haemolysis when grown on blood agar, but some are nonhaemolytic and produce no change in blood. An important difference between these organisms and the pyogenic β-haemolytic streptococci is that, because of cross-reactions and lack of definite antigens in many species, serological tests are of little use in their identification. Instead, biochemical and cultural tests are used, but these can give equivocal results.

Viridans streptococci are important in clinical medicine and dentistry. The normal habitat of most species is the mouth but they are not evenly distributed there; each species has its own characteristic ecological niche. They are involved in dental

caries and in more serious non-oral conditions such as infective endocarditis, septicaemia and deep-seated abscesses, e.g. in the brain and liver. These are the result of bacteraemic spread from caries, periodontal disease, periodontal abscess and periapical abscess.

A substantial obstacle to understanding the pathogenic potential of this heterogeneous group of bacteria has been related to confused nomenclature, but advances in taxonomy have clarified this, and intimate associations between particular species and specific infections have been established. At present, viridans streptococci are classified thus:

1. *Str. mutans*, now collectively known as 'mutans streptococci', is divided into seven species, the two most prominent of which are *Str. mutans* and *Str. sobrinus*.

2. The *Str. sanguis* group, now divided into *Str. sanguis* and *Str. gordonii*, includes the related species *Str. parasanguis* and *Str. crista*.

3. *Str. milleri* has been superseded by the identification of three separate species within this group, *Str. constellatus*, *Str. intermedius* and *Str. anginosus*. *Str. mitior* has been subdivided into *Str. mitis* and *Str. oralis*.

Viridans streptococci associated with infective endocarditis are predominantly *Str. sanguis*, *Str. oralis* and *Str. gordonii*; those with septicaemia, *Str. oralis* and *Str. mitis*; and those with deep abscesses, *Str. intermedius*.

### Dental caries

Bacteria, a susceptible host and a cariogenic diet are the three essentials for the production of caries. Viridans streptococci, chiefly *Str. mutans*, are involved in the production of caries. Other acidogenic bacteria, including *Actinomyces* and *Lactobacillus* spp., may contribute to the progression of the disease but are less important.

***Dental plaque.*** This soft but adherent deposit covers the fissures and pits of the teeth adjacent to the gingivae. It consists initially of glycoprotein, which by the action of enzymes precipitates and is adsorbed onto the enamel surfaces. Bacteria instantly become associated with this glycoprotein pellicle. Plaque is a dynamic entity and whereas the bacterial composition of early plaque consists of mainly aerobic or facultatively anaerobic organisms, it later becomes colonized by strict anaerobes. Supragingival plaque plays an essential role in the causation of dental caries and subgingival plaque in periodontal disease.

*Prevention of caries.* Dietary sucrose is an important contributor to caries production and restriction of this reduces the substrate for the activities of the plaque bacteria. The form in which sucrose is taken is important, as sticky sweet foods can remain in the mouth for some time and are more completely metabolized to form acid than drinks containing sucrose, which are soon swallowed.

Plaque control, involving regular tooth-brushing and the use of toothpicks and dental floss, is mandatory. Also, the addition of 1 ppm of fluoride to drinking water has proved very effective in reducing caries.

The possibility of using a vaccine against *Str. mutans*, serotype C, has been rejected because too many inherent problems exist, not the least being a cross-reactivity with human heart muscle.

### Infective endocarditis

*Aetiology.* Viridans streptococci account for about 40% of cases of infective endocarditis; *Str. sanguis* and *Str. mitis* are most commonly incriminated, followed by *Str. mutans* and *Str. milleri*. Most other cases are caused by other Gram-positive cocci, notably enterococci (especially *E. faecalis*), *Staph. aureus* and coagulase-negative staphylococci. *Coxiella burneti* and fungi are sometimes involved; hence the term *infective* endocarditis, rather than *bacterial* endocarditis.

*Pathogenesis.* Various factors predispose to endocarditis (Table 16.3). Minute platelet thrombi adhere to the roughened epithelium and organisms may grow in the thrombi and produce fragile vegetations from which emboli can break off. Infected vegetations consist of bacteria enmeshed in fibrin and platelets. Fibrosis can occur in the valve and this surrounds and further protects the bacteria.

*Epidemiology.* Acute and subacute forms occur; pyogenic organisms are more common in the acute form. Endocarditis associated with rheumatic fever has decreased dramatically in developed countries, but with the increasing age of the population, more older persons with cardiac pathology are now infected. Formerly, the age group involved was about 30 years of age. Other factors influencing

**Table 16.3** Factors predisposing to infective endocarditis

| Cardiac factors | Non-cardiac factors |
|---|---|
| Rheumatic heart disease | Dental manipulations |
| Atherosclerotic heart disease | Endoscopy |
| Congenital heart disease | Intravenous drug abuse |
| Cardiac surgery | Intravenous cannulae and shunts |
| Prosthetic heart valves | Sepsis |

the changing pattern include the increased use of prosthetic valves and drug abuse.

*Laboratory diagnosis.* Blood culture should be performed as soon as infective endocarditis is suspected, before antibiotic therapy is started.

Some patients with infective endocarditis have negative blood cultures. This can be explained by administration of antibiotics before taking blood for culture, by intermittent bacteraemia or by the presence of organisms that will only grow in cell culture such as *Cox. burneti* (Q fever endocarditis), *Chlamydia psittaci* and *C. trachomatis*. Fungi (usually *Candida albicans*) may also be responsible.

*Treatment.* In most cases, initial therapy is blind and should start as soon as blood has been taken for culture. A combination of benzylpenicillin and gentamicin is generally used and if staphylococci are thought to be involved flucloxacillin should be added. Subsequent therapy will depend on the results of blood culture.

## *Leuconostoc* and *Pediococcus* spp.

Leuconostoc and pediococci are catalase-negative Gram-positive cocci of uncertain taxonomic affinity. They are occasionally encountered as opportunist pathogens. Like the lactobacilli (to which leuconostocs are related) they are unusual among Gram-positive organisms in being resistant to the glycopeptide antibiotics, vancomycin and teicoplanin.

## Anaerobic streptococci

Streptococci that can only grow as obligate aerobes are dealt with in Chapter 37.

RECOMMENDED READING

Beighton D, Hardie J M, Whiley R A 1991 A scheme for the identification of viridans streptococci. *Journal of Medical Microbiology* 35: 367–372

Douglas C W I, Heath J, Hampton K K, Preston F E 1993 Identity of viridans streptococci isolated from cases of infective endocarditis. *Journal of Medical Microbiology* 39: 179–182

Marsh P D, Martin M W 1992 *Oral Microbiology*, 3rd edn. Chapman and Hall, London

Ross P W 1984 Group B streptococcus – profile of an organism. *Journal of Medical Microbiology* 18: 139–166

Schwartz B, Facklam R R, Breiman R F 1990 Changing epidemiology of group A streptococcal infection in the USA. *Lancet* 336: 1167–1171

Stevens D L 1992 Invasive group A streptococcus infections. *Clinical Infectious Diseases* 14: 2–11

# 17

# Pneumococcus

**Respiratory infections; meningitis**

*R. G. Finch*

---

*Streptococcus pneumoniae*, commonly called the pneumococcus, was first identified in sputum in 1881 by Louis Pasteur in France and G. M. Sternberg in the USA. It is a member of the normal oropharyngeal flora of most people, and an important human pathogen. It primarily causes disease of the middle ear, paranasal sinuses, mastoids and the lung parenchyma but may spread to other sites, such as the joints, peritoneum, endocardium and biliary tract and, in particular, the meninges. It is thus responsible for a major burden of ill health with its attendant economic consequences.

Among the pyogenic cocci the pneumococcus is probably second only to *Staphylococcus aureus* as a cause of community bacterial infections but, unlike *Staph. aureus*, until recently it has largely remained sensitive to penicillin. The major virulence factors are pneumolysin and the polysaccharide capsule, which is antigenic, allowing serotype discrimination and the development of a polyvalent vaccine for use in individuals at either increased risk or severity of pneumococcal disease.

## DESCRIPTION

*Str. pneumoniae* (formerly called *Diplococcus pneumoniae*) is a member of the family Lactobacillaceae. It is a Gram-positive, non-motile, encapsulated ovoid or lanceolate coccus approximately 1 μm in diameter, with a tendency to occur in pairs with the broader ends opposed (Fig. 17.1). Most strains are facultatively anaerobic, although occasional isolates are strict anaerobes. Their complex nutritional requirements are satisfied by enriched media, especially when supplemented with whole or defibrinated blood. Growth is enhanced by 0.1% glucose and an atmosphere of 5–10% carbon dioxide.

Overnight growth on blood agar produces 1 mm colonies which are round, domed and surrounded

**Fig. 17.1** Scanning electron micrograph of pneumococci. (By courtesy of A. P. Shelton.)

by a zone of α-haemolysis. With more prolonged incubation, autolysis results in subsidence of the centre of the colony to create the typical 'draughtsman' appearance (Fig. 17.2). Some strains such as those belonging to serotypes 3 and 7 produce mucoid

**Fig. 17.2** Culture of *Str. pneumoniae* on blood agar, showing the typical 'draughtsman' colonies.

colonies on blood agar from excessive capsular polysaccharide production.

In broth, *Str. pneumoniae* occurs as short chains or isolated cocci. In common with other streptococci, lactic acid formation on prolonged incubation causes a fall in pH which is inhibitory to growth. Pneumococci survive with difficulty outside the pH range 7–7.8; buffering agents are therefore added to enrichment media such as Todd–Hewitt broth.

*Str. pneumoniae* lacks a cytochrome system, which reflects its relationship to anaerobic bacteria. Oxygen is utilized through a flavoprotein enzyme system with the formation of hydrogen peroxide, which is also inhibitory to growth. Pneumococci, like other streptococci, lack catalase, which is necessary for the breakdown of hydrogen peroxide. The red blood cells in blood media provide a source of catalase and hence encourage growth in vitro.

The pneumococcus is soluble in bile, and this distinguishes it from other α-haemolytic streptococci (viridans streptococci); alternatively, *optochin* (ethylhydrocuprein hydrochloride), an alkaloid related to quinine, may be added to laboratory media; a zone of inhibition around an optochin-impregnated disc on blood agar serves to differentiate pneumococci from viridans streptococci, which are optochin-resistant.

## PATHOGENESIS

*Str. pneumoniae* is a member of the normal resident oropharyngeal flora of 5–70% of the population, with the highest isolation rate in winter months. Its presence is of significance in relation to the pathogenesis of pneumococcal infections of the respiratory tract. Contiguous spread can result in otitis media, mastoiditis and paranasal sinusitis, which are infections largely of childhood and early adult life. In these situations pneumococcal infection may occur as a primary problem, although it is often secondary to an acute upper respiratory tract viral infection.

### Predisposing factors

Within the lower respiratory tract *Str. pneumoniae* is the commonest pathogen to cause pneumonia. Although occasional clusterings of pneumococcal infections are recognized, person-to-person spread is uncommon, and infection usually results from aspiration of pneumococci within upper airway secretion into the lower respiratory tract. Aspiration occurs under a variety of circumstances, usually when the normal mechanisms of mucous entrapment and expulsion by an intact glottic reflex and mucociliary escalator are impaired. This situation may arise when consciousness is disturbed in association with general anaesthesia, convulsions, cerebrovascular accidents, epilepsy or head trauma. However, aspiration of small quantities of oropharyngeal secretions can also be demonstrated in the healthy during sleep. Antecedent and pre-existing respiratory diseases such as acute lower respiratory tract viral infections, chronic bronchitis and other forms of chronic bronchial sepsis are well known to predispose to secondary bacterial infection, including pneumococcal disease.

Other predisposing disease states include valvular and ischaemic heart disease, chronic renal failure, diabetes mellitus, bronchogenic and metastatic malignancy as well as advancing age. Pneumococcal pneumonia may be the terminal event in these conditions and this has given rise to the description of the disease as 'the old man's friend'.

Other specific deficiencies in host defence which predispose to pneumococcal infection include hypogammaglobulinaemia, asplenia or hyposplenism, and malignancies such as multiple myeloma. In these conditions there is either a relative or absolute deficiency of opsonic antibody activity or an inability to manufacture sufficient type-specific antibody. Tuftsin is a naturally occurring tetrapeptide secreted by the spleen which also plays a role in combating pneumococcal sepsis; those deficient in splenic activity as a result of congenital absence, traumatic removal, or functional impairment as occurs with selected haemoglobinopathies (homozygous sickle cell disease), are particularly at risk.

Human immunodeficiency virus (HIV) infection, whilst largely predisposing to parasitic and fungal disease, also carries an increased risk of bacterial infections, including those caused by the pneumococcus. This is even more marked in children with HIV infection.

## Pneumococcal bacteraemia

Bacteraemia may complicate pneumococcal pneumonia in up to 15% of patients. This usually arises from pulmonary lymphatic spread and can result in metastatic involvement of the meninges, joints and, rarely, the endocardium. However, bloodstream access may presumably occur from the pharynx.

## Pneumococcal pneumonia

Pneumococcal pneumonia follows aspiration with subsequent migration through the bronchial mucosa to involve the peribronchial lymphatics. The inflammatory reaction is primarily focused within the alveolus of a single lobule or lobe, although multilobar disease can also occur. The initial red blood cell diapedesis is followed by a primarily polymorphonuclear inflammatory reaction with a marked proteinaceous exudate, resulting in stiff, congested, consolidated lungs. This sequence of events gives rise to the classical descriptions of 'red and grey hepatization'. Blood is shunted through these areas of consolidation without oxygenation; hypoxaemia is therefore a frequent and variably severe accompaniment of pneumococcal pneumonia. Contiguous spread commonly results in inflammatory involvement of the pleura. This may progress to empyema. Pericarditis is another uncommon but well-recognized complication. Occasionally, lung necrosis and intrapulmonary abscess formation occur with the more virulent pneumococcal serotypes. Mortality from pneumococcal pneumonia in those admitted to hospital in the UK is approximately 15%. This is increased by age, underlying disease, bloodstream involvement, metastatic infection and certain types of pneumococci such as serotypes 3 and 7.

## Meningitis

In primary pneumococcal meningitis it is assumed that invasion arises from the pharynx to the meninges via the bloodstream since bacteraemia usually coexists. Meningitis may occasionally complicate pneumococcal infection at other sites, e.g. the lung.

The incidence of pneumococcal meningitis is bimodal and affects children less than 3 years of age and adults of 45 years and above. Pneumococcal meningitis is the most virulent of the major bacterial meningitides with a mortality of approximately 20%.

## Capsular polysaccharides

Approximately 90% of cases of bacteraemic pneumococcal pneumonia and meningitis are caused by some 23 serotypes. The capsular polysaccharide is the major pneumococcal virulence factor which is both antigenic and type-specific. The capsule is antiphagocytic, inhibiting entrapment and phagocytosis where type-specific opsonic antibody is absent. Non-capsulate mutants are avirulent in experimental animals such as the mouse and rabbit, where they are readily removed by phagocytosis.

The surface composition of the capsular polysaccharide has been established for a few serotypes. For example, serotype 3 has repeating units of cellobiuronic acid. Virulence is also proportional to the degree of capsular polysaccharide, thus explaining the demonstrably greater virulence of serotypes 3 and 7. Repeated subculturing in the presence of specific anticapsular antibody results in non-encapsulated strains which can be recognized by their colonial appearances on blood agar; the non-capsulate form produces rough (R) colonies compared with the smooth (S) colonies of the encapsulated form.

The pneumococcal capsule is demonstrable by several techniques. Mixing with type-specific antisera increases its thickness, and is the basis of the *quellung reaction* or *capsular swelling test*. Similarly, the addition of India ink to a suspension of pneumococci will demonstrate the presence of the capsule as a clear halo around the organisms.

## Pneumolysin

*Str. pneumoniae* elaborates a membrane-damaging toxin known as pneumolysin. In experimental models it induces the features of lobar pneumonia and contributes to the mortality of this disease. Pneumolysin is immunogenic, and the possibility that it might be suitable for a new pneumococcal vaccine is under investigation.

## LABORATORY DIAGNOSIS

The diagnosis of pneumococcal infection is established by demonstrating the presence of the pathogen in pathological specimens. The choice of specimen varies according to the site of infection. *Str. pneumoniae* is the commonest cause of community-acquired pneumonia, yet sputum culture is only positive in approximately 20% of cases for several reasons:

1. There may be difficulty in obtaining an expectorated specimen, although postural drainage or inhaled aerosolized saline can encourage its production. A more invasive technique that is occasionally employed is the induction of expectoration by transtracheal saline injection. Sputum may also be obtained by bronchoscopy in patients who are ventilated.

2. Previous antibiotic treatment substantially reduces the chance of isolating the pneumococcus from the sputum.

The adequacy of the sputum sample should be confirmed by microscopy, which should show a predominance of pus cells rather than squamous epithelial cells of buccal origin. The specimen is then homogenized with an agent such as *N*-acetylcysteine which permits semi-quantitative culture. The pneumococcus is readily isolated on 5% blood agar, and the majority of isolates will grow in air although occasional isolates are strict anaerobes.

Colonial morphology on blood agar is characteristic (see above), and further identification of the pneumococcus is usually restricted to demonstrating its susceptibility to optochin to distinguish the organism from other α-haemolytic streptococci. Serotyping pneumococci is no longer routinely carried out, but is available in reference laboratories. Methods available include the capsule swelling test (quellung reaction) and the latex agglutination test. Monospecific antisera are used for both these tests.

In the case of pneumococcal meningitis the cerebrospinal fluid is often macroscopically cloudy. The cell count is usually markedly increased and shows a predominance of polymorphonuclear leucocytes. Typical Gram-positive diplococci can commonly be demonstrated, sometimes in enormous numbers, by Gram-stain examination of a cerebrospinal fluid deposit. The appearance is often typical, and a presumptive diagnosis can be made to allow appropriate therapy to be started before the identity of the organism is confirmed by culture.

Blood cultures are of value in patients with pneumococcal pneumonia, particularly when this is severe, since up to 15% of patients will be bacteraemic. Blood cultures may also be positive in those with pneumococcal meningitis.

Other body sites which may merit investigation

according to the clinical presentation include joint and peritoneal fluids. Tympanocentesis provides the possibility of establishing the microbial cause of otitis media, but since most of these infections settle spontaneously, or with the assistance of a few days' antibiotic treatment, tympanocentesis is not usually necessary.

## TREATMENT

*Str. pneumoniae* is sensitive to a wide range of antimicrobial agents. These include the penicillins, cephalosporins, erythromycin, tetracycline, clindamycin, vancomycin, teicoplanin, chloramphenicol and the sulphonamides. Penicillin has had a major impact on the morbidity and mortality of pneumococcal infections. However, mortality rates for those hospitalized with pneumonia remain at approximately 15% while for pneumococcal meningitis the rate is higher at 20% despite the use of penicillin.

The dose of penicillin necessary to treat pneumococcal infection is largely determined by pharmacological factors at the site of infection. For example, pneumococcal pneumonia will respond to doses of penicillin as low as 0.3 g (0.5 mega-unit) twice daily, although it is customary to prescribe higher doses; pneumococcal meningitis requires much higher doses, of the order of 7.2 g per day in divided doses. The use of even higher doses is of unproven advantage and runs the risk of inducing convulsions.

Aminopenicillins can also be used to treat pneumococcal infection in the community, and amoxycillin is most widely prescribed. This is well absorbed following oral administration, and is used to treat many community-acquired infections of the lung, middle ear and the sinuses. In patients unable to tolerate penicillin, erythromycin is the most widely used alternative agent for respiratory pneumococcal infections.

Resistance of pneumococci to antibiotics varies geographically. Resistance to erythromycin, tetracycline and chloramphenicol is not uncommon, and is often linked to, and reflects the widespread use of, one or more of these agents. For example, erythromycin resistance in the UK occurs in approximately 5–10% of isolates while in France, where erythromycin and other macrolide antibiotics are much more widely used, it can be as high as 30%.

Resistance to penicillin has rapidly emerged as a problem world-wide. Strains with reduced susceptibility (minimum inhibitory concentration (MIC)

>0.1 mg benzylpenicillin/l) were first recognized in 1967 in Papua New Guinea. The first strains with reduced susceptibility in the UK were reported in 1976. Although this increase in MIC was a cause of concern it was rarely associated with failure to respond to penicillin. However, high-level penicillin resistance was recognized in 1977 in South Africa, where it was responsible for an epidemic of pneumococcal meningitis unresponsive to penicillin. The MIC of penicillin for these isolates was above 2 mg/l. The strains were also resistant to several other antibiotics, with the exception of vancomycin and extended-spectrum cephalosporins, such as cefotaxime. Since 1977 there has been a world-wide increase in resistance to penicillin in pneumococci, and this is quite variable geographically. The reported incidence exceeds 10% in Spain, South Africa, the southern USA, Alaska and Iceland. In the UK, about 5% of isolates show reduced susceptibility (MIC = 0.1–1 mg/l), while fully resistant strains (MIC >1 mg/l) are less common. While penicillin resistance is clearly linked to treatment failures in pneumococcal meningitis and otitis media in childhood, most other forms of pneumococcal infection remain susceptible, although the possibility that higher doses may be necessary in the future is under review.

## EPIDEMIOLOGY

*Str. pneumoniae* is second only to *Haemophilus influenzae* as a respiratory tract pathogen. The estimated annual incidence of pneumococcal pneumonia is 68–260 per 100 000 of the population in the USA with a 5% case fatality rate. Comparable data for bacteraemia and meningitis are 7–25 and 1.2–2.8 per 100 000 of the population with fatality rates of 20 and 30%, respectively. The annual incidence of pneumococcal pneumonia in the UK is estimated to be between 1 and 3 per 1000 of the population. Otitis media affects approximately half of all children between the ages of 6 months and 3 years; approximately one-third of cases are caused by *Str. pneumoniae*. Apart from the acute morbidity of otitis media, other complications include mastoiditis and, occasionally, temporal lobe abscess. These complications are reduced significantly by early antibiotic treatment of middle ear disease and are now more common in developing countries.

Mortality from pneumococcal infection is related to age, pre-existing disease and serotype. The highest mortality rates occur in those over 65 years of age

with underlying disease and in whom bacteraemia complicates infection. Infections caused by serotype 3 are among the most virulent, and bacteraemic pneumococcal pneumonia with this serotype has a mortality rate of up to 50% in the elderly.

## IMMUNOPROPHYLAXIS

Before the widespread availability of effective antimicrobial drugs the treatment of pneumococcal infections was based on the use of type-specific antiserum. This reduced mortality in bacteraemic pneumococcal pneumonia, but not to the same extent that penicillin was subsequently shown to achieve. However, it indicated that type-specific antibody had a role in the control of pneumococcal disease, and led to a variety of prototype vaccines. The vaccine that is currently licensed for use contains a mixture of 23 polysaccharide serotypes chosen according to the prevalence of serotypes responsible for bacteraemic pneumococcal infection. It offers protection against 90% of isolates. Unfortunately, the immunogenicity of this vaccine is inadequate in those below 2 years of age and in those immunosuppressed as a result of malignancy, steroid therapy or other chronic disease. The recommended indications for vaccine use in the UK are shown in Table 17.1. In the USA, where the vaccine has been used most widely, it is also recommended for those over 65 years of age, with or without previous ill health, although there have been difficulties in establishing scientifically the efficacy in this group.

Immunization is particularly recommended for those with either functional or anatomical asplenia in whom pneumococcal infection can be fulminant. Such patients include those with

| Table 17.1 Recommended indications for the use of pneumococcal vaccine in the UK |
| --- |
| Asplenia or severe dysfunction of the spleen[a] |
| Homozygous sickle cell disease and coeliac disease[a] |
| Chronic renal disease or nephrotic syndrome[a] |
| Immunodeficiency or immunosuppression due to disease or treatment, including HIV infection at all stages |
| Chronic heart disease |
| Chronic lung disease |
| Chronic liver disease including cirrhosis |
| Diabetes mellitus |
| [a]Licensed for use in children. |

congenital or surgical asplenia and those with hereditary haemoglobinopathies such as sickle cell disease. Vaccine efficacy is not complete and many clinicians also prescribe oral phenoxymethylpenicillin as long-term chemoprophylaxis in this high-risk group.

## RECOMMENDED READING

Anon 1989 Pneumococcal polysaccharide vaccine. *Morbidity and Mortality Weekly Report* 38: 64–68, 73–76

Applebaum P C 1987 World-wide development of antibiotic resistance in pneumococci. *European Journal of Clinical Microbiology* 6: 367

Fine M J, Smith M A, Carson C A et al, 1994 Efficacy of pneumococcal vaccination in adults. A meta-analysis of randomized controlled trials. *Archives of Internal Medicine* 154: 2666–2677

Gransden W R, Eykyn S J, Phillips I 1985 Pneumococcal bacteraemia: 325 episodes diagnosed at St Thomas's Hospital. *British Medical Journal* 290: 505–508

Johnson A P, Speller D C E, George R C et al 1996 Prevalence of antibiotic resistance and serotypes in pneumococci in England and Wales: results of observational surveys in 1990 and 1995. *British Medical Journal* 312: 1454–1456

Paton J C, Andrew P W, Boulnois G J, Mitchell T J 1994. Molecular analysis of the pathogenicity of *Streptococcus pneumoniae*: the role of pneumococcal proteins. *Annual Review of Microbiology* 47: 89–115

# 18

# Coryneform bacteria, listeria and erysipelothrix

Diphtheria; listeriosis; erysipeloid

*A. P. MacGowan*

In the medical laboratory, '*diphtheroids*' or '*coryneforms*' are defined as pleomorphic Gram-positive rods which stain irregularly, are arranged in V forms or palisades, are non-motile, catalase-positive, non-acid-fast, non-branching and form acid but not gas from carbohydrates. The group includes the diphtheria bacillus but also encompasses many commensals and pathogens of humans and animals as well as environmental bacteria.

## *CORYNEBACTERIUM DIPHTHERIAE*

*Corynebacterium diphtheriae* is the causative organism of diphtheria, a localized inflammation of the throat with greyish white adherent exudate (*pseudo-membrane*) and a generalized toxaemia due to the secretion and dissemination of a highly potent toxin.

### Description

*C. diphtheriae* has a characteristic appearance in films from growth on suitable culture media. When dividing, the bacilli snap and bend abruptly and appear as angled pairs or parallel rows (*palisades*), resembling 'Chinese lettering'; the average size is $3.0 \times 0.3\,\mu m$, but there is considerable pleomorphism with club-shaped, oval and globular forms appearing in older cultures. The rods are Gram-positive, but are easily decolorized. When stained with Neisser or Albert stains the volutin (metachromatic) granules stain dark purple in contrast to the brown or green counterstain, giving the rods a beaded appearance.

*C. diphtheriae* is aerobic and facultatively anaerobic, growing best at 37°C on a blood- or serum-containing medium. It is non-motile, non-sporing and non-

capsulate. Loeffler's serum slopes allow quick growth and provide characteristic morphology for stained films. On blood or serum tellurite media the bacilli grow more slowly as greyish to black colonies. The shape, size and colour of these colonies enable them to be differentiated into the three main biotypes, called *gravis*, *intermedius* and *mitis* because of a relationship with the clinical severity of the infection (severe, intermediate and mild, respectively). Biochemical tests are important in differentiating *C. diphtheriae* from other coryneforms (Table 18.1).

The demonstration of toxin production is essential to differentiate toxigenic from commensal corynebacteria. Isolates identified as *gravis* or *intermedius* types are usually toxigenic but 10–20% of *mitis* strains isolated from 'sore throats' are non-toxigenic. Toxigenicity is demonstrated by the agar gel precipitation (Elek) test or by the polymerase chain reaction (PCR). There is almost complete concordance between the two tests, but PCR is quicker and may occasionally produce a positive result with a non-toxigenic strain.

### Epidemiology

#### Incidence

Diphtheria is rare in most developed countries but remains prevalent in many Third World countries and in the former Soviet Union. Twenty-five cases were reported in the UK between 1990 and 1994; most were imported from the Indian subcontinent, Africa or Asia. There was one death in the UK in 1994, but no secondary case has occurred since 1985. In contrast there has been a large outbreak of diphtheria in the countries of the former Soviet Union, with almost 50 000 cases and 1750 deaths in 1994.

Infection is confined to humans and usually spreads directly from person to person via nasopharyngeal secretions. Spread is facilitated by intimate contact. Children are susceptible after the age of 3–6 months, when passive immunity derived from maternal antibodies has disappeared. Incidence is highest among young children, but outbreaks also occur among teenagers and young adults. In the course of immunization programmes directed at preschool children and schoolchildren there may be a shift in distribution of cases to older age groups.

In some tropical countries cutaneous infections with *C. diphtheriae* occur, and latent skin infections play an important part in the natural acquisition of immunity.

## Transmission

In endemic areas there may be up to 100 healthy carriers for every clinical case. Most clinical infections are probably contracted from carriers rather than symptomatic patients. Nasal carriers are particularly dangerous because they shed large numbers of bacilli. The bacillus may survive for many weeks in dust and on dry fomites contaminated with nasal, oral or pharyngeal secretions. Dust in hospitals and institutions may become heavily infected with dried secretions, and may be a source of infection.

## Pathogenesis

Diphtheria bacilli elicit an inflammatory exudate and cause necrosis of the cells of the faucial mucosa. Infection may spread to the postnasal cavity or the larynx, causing respiratory obstruction. The serocellular exudate clots and remains adherent to the fauces, and attempts to remove the pseudo-membrane leave a raw, bleeding surface. The bacilli do not as a rule penetrate deeply in the underlying tissues, or the blood, but they produce a very powerful exotoxin which is spread by the bloodstream and has a special affinity for certain tissues, notably heart muscle, nerve endings and the adrenal glands. Diphtheria toxin is a heat-stable polypeptide which is composed of two fragments, denoted A and B. Fragment B is required for transport of fragment A into the cell, where it inhibits polypeptide chain elongation at the ribosome. Inhibition of protein synthesis is probably responsible for both the necrotic and neurotoxic effects of the toxin. Death from laryngeal diphtheria may be due to asphyxia because, in the confined space within the larynx, even a small patch of membrane can cause a fatal obstruction. In pharyngeal infections most deaths are related to toxin-mediated cardiac damage and heart failure.

Diphtheria toxin is produced most actively in vitro when the iron concentration is decreased, although other factors such as osmolality, amino acid concentrations and pH have a role. Factors affecting toxin production in vivo are, by contrast, poorly understood.

## Schick test

A simple screening test to separate susceptible from immune individuals is the injection intradermally of a suitably diluted stabilized diphtheria toxin (*Schick test*). A localized erythema (with some oedema), reaching its maximum size (1–3 cm) and intensity in 2–4 days, indicates that there is little or no neutralizing antitoxin in the tissue, and that the individual is susceptible to diphtheria. Absence of a reaction indicates immunity. The Schick test serves only as a rough guide to the amount of antitoxin in the blood and is no longer used in the UK.

## Clinical aspects of infection

The incubation period is 2–6 days. Patients present with malaise, fatigue, fever and sore throat, though this is not a major feature. Anterior nasal diphtheria presents with a thick nasal discharge and intoxication is rare. Tonsillar infection presents with a thick, adherent green pseudomembrane on one or both tonsils. Intoxication is common. In pharyngeal infection the pseudomembrane may involve the soft palate, uvula, pharyngeal wall and nasal mucosa. Oedema, heat and tenderness may occur in the anterior tissues of the neck (bull neck) and there is local lymphadenopathy. Laryngeal and bronchial diphtheria usually result from extension of the membrane down the respiratory tract.

Intoxication takes the form of myocarditis and peripheral neuritis, and may be associated with thrombocytopenia. Electrocardiogram abnormalities are common in the first week of the illness. Visual disturbance, difficulty in swallowing and paralysis of the arms and legs also occur but usually resolve spontaneously.

## Treatment

Therapy involves isolation of the patient, bed rest, appropriate antibiotics and early administration of antitoxin. Supportive therapy may be required such as intubation and ventilation for airway obstruction. *C. diphtheriae* is sensitive to penicillin, tetracycline, rifampicin and clindamycin. Erythromycin may be preferred to penicillin for elimination of the bacilli from the throat, particularly in treatment of persistent carriers. Erythromycin- and tetracycline-resistant strains have been described. Antibiotics have no effect on preformed toxin, which rapidly diffuses from the local lesion and, unless neutralized by antitoxin, soon becomes irreversibly bound to tissue cells.

Treatment should not await laboratory confirmation if there is a strong clinical suspicion, as the fatality rate is directly related to the period of delay before giving antitoxin, rising from zero to 20% between the onset of disease and day 5 of the infection; the average case fatality rate is 5–7%.

## Prophylactic immunization

The evidence in favour of immunization for the control of diphtheria in communities where it is endemic is overwhelming. In England and Wales, where large-scale immunization was begun in 1941, the incidence of diphtheria fell from about 55 000 cases annually with 2780 deaths, to an average of less than 10 cases between 1984 and 1991, with no deaths. Immunization schedules are dealt with in Chapter 68.

The control of outbreaks of diphtheria requires close collaboration between public health doctors and medical microbiologists. All home and close school contacts must have swabs taken from both the nose and throat or any other possible focus (discharging ear, skin lesion), preferably on two separate occasions; cases and carriers should be isolated in hospital and given antibiotic therapy and antitoxin if clinically indicated. The immunization histories of all home and school contacts should be ascertained and a primary course of immunization or a booster should be given if necessary. Unimmunized close contacts require urgent protection by immunization and prophylactic antibiotics. The routine use of antitoxin is no longer recommended due to hypersensitivity reactions.

## OTHER MEDICALLY IMPORTANT CORYNEFORMS

The non-diphtheria corynebacteria are diverse and include *Actinomyces pyogenes* (formerly *C. pyogenes*) and *Arcanobacterium haemolyticum* (formerly *C. haemolyticum*). Many isolates from humans, animals or the environment cannot be fitted into any species.

On the basis of the infections they produce, they can be classified into those which cause infection in immunocompetent patients: *C. ulcerans*, *A. haemolyticum*, *C. pseudotuberculosis* (*C. ovis*) and *C. minutissimum*; and those which cause opportunistic infection: *C. jeikeium*, *C. xerosis*, *C. pseudodiphtheriticum* (*C. hofmanni*), *Rhodococcus equi*, *C. urealyticum* and CDC groups A-4 and G-2. The differential characteristics of the most important species and the main clinical syndromes associated with infection are shown in Tables 18.1 and 18.2.

### Corynebacterium ulcerans

*C. ulcerans* causes bovine mastitis and sporadic infections, with outbreaks occurring in rural communities exposed to infected animals or milk. Human-to-human transmission has not been reported. Almost all infections are pharyngeal, though occasional soft tissue infections occur. A toxin identical to that of *C. diphtheriae* is produced by some strains which produce a diphtheria-like ill-

| Table 18.1 | Biochemical reactions of some medically significant coryneform bacteria | | | | | | | |
|---|---|---|---|---|---|---|---|---|
| Organism | Catalase | β-haemolysis on blood agar | Urease | Nitrate reduction | Acid production from | | | |
| | | | | | Glucose | Maltose | Sucrose | Xylose |
| C. diphtheriae | + | v | − | + | + | + | − | − |
| C. ulcerans | + | + | + | − | + | + | − | − |
| C. pseudotuberculosis | + | + | + | v | + | + | − | − |
| C. minutissimum | + | − | − | − | + | + | v | − |
| C. xerosis | + | − | − | + | + | + | + | − |
| C. pseudodiphtheriticum | + | − | + | + | − | − | − | − |
| C. jeikeium | + | − | + | − | + | v | − | − |
| C. urealyticum | + | − | + | − | − | − | − | − |
| A. haemolyticum | − | + | − | − | + | + | v | + |

+, 90% or more positive in 4 days; −, 90% or more negative; v, more than 10% but less than 90% positive.

**Table 18.2** Clinical syndromes associated with non-diphtheria coryneform bacteria

| Syndrome | Species |
|---|---|
| Acute pharyngitis | C. ulcerans<br>A. haemolyticum |
| Cutaneous infections | C. minutissimum<br>C. jeikeium |
| Granulomatous lymphadenitis<br>Infective endocarditis | C. pseudotuberculosis<br>C. jeikeium<br>C. xerosis<br>C. pseudodiphtheriticum<br>C. bovis |
| Line, shunt or cannula<br>infections | C. jeikeium<br>C. xerosis<br>C. bovis<br>Others unclassified |
| Necrotizing pneumonia | R. equi |
| Urinary infections associated<br>with renal tract abnormality<br>and stones | C. urealyticum |

ness. Infection usually takes the form of acute pharyngitis; pseudomembranes may form, and cardiac or neurological complications can occur. These infections merit treatment with antitoxin, though its efficacy is not proven. Erythromycin is the antibiotic of choice but *C. ulcerans* is sensitive to several other agents in vitro.

## Arcanobacterium haemolyticum

The main clinical infections are acute pharyngitis, which is usually sporadic, and chronic skin ulcers. Most patients are young adults who present with sore throat; some have cervical lymphadenopathy and many develop a scarlatiniform rash. A few patients may develop peritonsillar abscesses or systemic features resembling group A streptococcal infection. *A. haemolyticum* has occasionally been isolated from cellulitis, osteomyelitis and brain abscess.

Erythromycin is effective, but mild pharyngitis settles in a few days without therapy. *A. haemolyticum* is also sensitive to penicillin, but clinical failures have occurred.

## Corynebacterium pseudotuberculosis

*C. pseudotuberculosis* causes a caseous lymphadenitis in sheep. Infection has been described among those with prolonged exposure to sheep, mainly in Australia. Infection presents as a subacute or chronic

lymphadenitis involving the axillary or cervical nodes, often with systemic symptoms. Long courses of erythromycin, tetracycline or penicillin have been used; however, surgical drainage or excision may be necessary.

## Corynebacterium minutissimum

*C. minutissimum* is associated with the skin condition *erythrasma*, a localized infection of the stratum corneum which produces red scaly patches in the toewebs, groins and axillae. The lesions fluoresce 'coral red' in Wood's light. The organism can be cultured from pulped stratum corneum, but this is rarely necessary.

## Corynebacterium jeikeium

Numerically, *C. jeikeium* is now the most important pathogenic coryneform in North America and Europe. The organism is found on mucosal surfaces and the skin of a few healthy individuals. Hospital patients, particularly neutropenic patients and those receiving antibiotics, are commonly colonized. It has been isolated from blood, tissue and cerebrospinal fluid (CSF), in patients with neutropenia and after cardiac surgery. The largest infected group are patients with haematological malignancy receiving cytotoxic chemotherapy. Infection in this group is usually related to long-term intravenous cannulae, and infections may involve exit sites, subcutaneous tunnels or intraluminal infection. Bone marrow biopsy sites and perianal fissures may also become infected and give rise to bacteraemia. After a bacteraemic episode, secondary soft tissue infection and abscesses can occur.

*C. jeikeium* may infect prosthetic and porcine heterograft valves, usually presenting 1–2 months after insertion. Other infections such as peritonitis in patients on peritoneal dialysis and central nervous system (CNS) infection in those with ventriculoperitoneal or atrial shunts for hydrocephalus are an increasing problem. Myocardial abscesses and pyelonephritis have been reported in immunocompromised patients.

*C. jeikeium* is usually resistant to penicillins, cephalosporins and aminoglycosides but sensitive to glycopeptides. Vancomycin and teicoplanin are effective in treating line-associated infection in neutropenic patients. Combinations of penicillin or vancomycin with gentamicin are synergic in vitro and have been used to treat infective endocarditis. Peritonitis secondary to peritoneal dialysis and meningitis related to shunts can be treated with intraperitoneal or intrathecal vancomycin, respectively. In CSF infection, systemic gentamicin, rifampicin or trimethoprim can also be administered.

## Other coryneform bacteria

*C. xerosis* is a commensal of the nasopharynx and rarely causes infection. Infective endocarditis on prosthetic valves and infections of CSF shunts have been described, as have infections in patients with malignancy and respiratory or renal failure. Isolates are resistant to aminoglycosides and clindamycin but usually susceptible to penicillins, cephalosporins and glycopeptides.

*C. pseudodiphtheriticum* (*C. hoffmanni*) is also a commensal of the nasopharynx, and almost all human infections have been infective endocarditis, usually on prosthetic valves.

*Rhodococcus equi* causes infections in horses or swine, and most human infections have taken the form of pulmonary infection in patients with the acquired immune deficiency syndrome, neoplasia, or after renal transplantation. Many patients were receiving steroids. The course is subacute or relapsing and may be difficult to distinguish from mycobacterial infection. The diagnosis is usually established from bronchoscopy specimens or blood cultures. Isolates are sensitive to penicillin, tetracycline, erythromycin and lincomycin in vitro and prolonged therapy with erythromycin in combination with rifampicin has been successful.

*C. bovis* is a commensal of the cow's udder which may cause bovine mastitis and also infection of prosthetic human heart valves and CNS infection. Infections secondary to trauma are also described. Sensitivity to penicillin is variable, and erythromycin and rifampicin are probably the antibiotics of choice.

*C. urealyticum* is a commensal of healthy human skin. It has been associated with urinary tract infection and stone formation, perhaps related to its strong urease production. Acute pyelonephritis, bacteraemia and pneumonia have also occurred.

Various other species of coryneform bacteria have been rarely associated with human infection.

## LISTERIA

Organisms of the genus *Listeria* are non-sporing Gram-positive bacilli. The main pathogenic species is *Listeria monocytogenes*, which chiefly affects pregnant women, their babies and immunosuppressed adults, especially the elderly.

## Description

*Listeria* species are short rods measuring $0.4–0.5 \times 0.5–2.0$ μm. They grow well on a wide variety of laboratory media; some species are β-haemolytic and others non-haemolytic. The bacilli are feebly motile at 37°C, but exhibit characteristic 'tumbling' motility when tested at 25°C.

Species can be differentiated by a few biochemical tests (Table 18.3). The CAMP test with *R. equi* and *Staphylococcus aureus* and fermentation of D-xylose are the major means of discriminating between species; fermentation of L-rhamnose and α-methyl D-mannoside provide secondary characteristics. By serotyping with antisera raised in rabbits, 13 serovars of *L. monocytogenes* can be recognized. Other typing methods used include bacteriophage typing, plasmid profiling, multilocus enzyme electrophoresis and random amplified polymorphic DNA analysis.

**Table 18.3** Differential characteristics of *Listeria* species

| Species | Haemolysis | CAMP test | | Acid from | | |
| | | *Staphylococcus aureus* | *Rhodococcus equi* | L-Rhamnose | D-Xylose | α-Methyl D-mannoside |
| --- | --- | --- | --- | --- | --- | --- |
| *L. monocytogenes* | + | + | − | + | − | + |
| *L. ivanovii* | ++ | − | + | − | + | − |
| *L. innocua* | − | − | − | ± | − | + |
| *L. welshimeri* | − | − | − | ± | + | + |
| *L. seeligeri* | + | + | − | − | + | ± |

CAMP refers to a test originally devised by Christie R, Atkins N E, Munch-Petersen E 1944 *Australian Journal of Experimental Biology and Medical Science* 22: 197–200. A positive test is indicated by enhanced haemolysis in the presence of toxigenic strains of *Staph. aureus* or *R. equi*.

Pathogenicity varies widely in humans and experimental animals. *L. monocytogenes* of serovar 4 is most commonly isolated from human infection, and serovar 1/2 is the second commonest in the UK; other serovars are rarely incriminated in human disease. The other *Listeria* species are generally non-pathogenic for humans, although rare infection with *L. ivanovii* has been described.

## Epidemiology

### Incidence

There are few good studies of the incidence of listeriosis. The most recent figures for Western countries indicate infection rates of between 0.1 and 1.0 cases per 100 000 of the population per year. In the UK the number of reported cases rose sharply in the mid-1980s and then declined again; from 1990 to 1993 the incidence was 0.22 cases per 1 million of the population per year.

Most cases are sporadic and in only a few is any source found. In contrast, epidemics involving several hundred cases have occurred, some of which have been traced to contaminated foodstuffs. Hospital-associated outbreaks have been reported.

Clinical listeriosis falls into two groups: pregnancy and neonatal infection; and infection in non-pregnant adults. Pregnancy and neonatal disease account for 30–45% of cases. In pregnancy-related infection, abortion and stillbirth account for 15–25% of infections, while about 70% are neonatal infections. In about 5% of maternal infections the fetus is not affected.

The incidence of infection increases with age so that with adult infections the mean age is over 55 years. Men are more commonly infected than women over the age of 40 years, and since women are infected in the child-bearing years the overall sex distribution is more or less equal. Most patients with listeriosis live in urban areas and usually have no exposure to animals, although occasional infections occur as a result of direct animal contact, usually in vets or farmers. Immunosuppression is a major risk factor for both the epidemic and sporadic forms of listeriosis, and probably accounts for the increasing incidence with age. Human immuno-deficiency virus disease is also a major pre-disposing factor to infection in some geographical areas. The peak incidence of human disease occurs in July, August or September.

Asymptomatic carriage of listeria in human populations is common; up to 5% of healthy adults are carriers at any one time. The duration of faecal carriage is often short but may exceed a year. About 50% of faecal isolates are *L. monocytogenes*, and the remainder are non-pathogenic species. The high incidence of carriage among humans may reflect the consumption of contaminated foods.

Over 75% of raw meat and poultry and about 90% of raw sausages contain listeria, but less than 5% of most pâtés and soft cheeses now contain the organism. Poultry tends to have the highest counts per gram of meat. Epidemiological studies suggest that pasteurized milk can be a source of listeriosis, and listeria can survive some forms of pasteurization within phagocytes. Cook–chill foods may be contaminated before reheating, but microwave ovens are effective in reducing the number of viable bacteria in heavily contaminated food by a factor of 1 million per gram, provided the recommended standing time is observed to ensure even distribution of heat throughout the food.

Although many food products are contaminated with listeria, the number of organisms required to produce infection and the incubation period is unknown, so it is difficult to evaluate the importance of different foods as a source of infection.

### Transmission

Various routes of infection have been proposed, but the number of infections in which any route can be directly implicated is very small. There is little evidence to support dust or insect spread, but in hospitals neonatal infections have been associated with the contamination of resuscitation equipment in obstetric theatres and also with direct spread between patients. A small number of pregnancy-associated infections and cases of adult meningitis have been related to consumption of contaminated chickens or cheeses, indicating that food spread is of importance in sporadic infection.

Epidemics of listeriosis usually occur in the community but hospital-associated outbreaks have occurred in renal transplant and in neonatal units. In well-documented community outbreaks in North America, coleslaw, milk and Mexican-style cheese have been implicated.

## Pathogenesis

The virulence of listeria has not been studied in as much depth as the host response to infection, but the different species within the genus have varying virulence in experimental animals and in humans. All strains that are pathogenic to mice produce a haemolysin, listeriolysin O, which is antigenically similar to streptolysin O, suggesting that it may have a potential role in virulence. Listeriolysin O is important for bacterial survival after phagocytosis, and its production is regulated by extracellular iron concentrations. Several other toxins are produced: a factor which promotes bacterial entry into the cells, a cytolysin and enzymes which protect the bacteria from the harmful effects of reactive oxygen radicals such as superoxide dismutase and catalase.

Oral administration of bacteria to germ-free animals causes gut wall infection and occasional spread to the liver and spleen, but colonization of the bowel is inhibited by the normal gastro-intestinal flora. In humans, gastro-intestinal disease, causing low gastric pH, disrupted bowel flora (perhaps related to antibiotic use) or damaged bowel tissues, may help to establish listeria in the bowel.

Non-specific mechanisms of resistance are important as first lines of defence once the mucous membranes are breached. Lysozyme can lyse some strains of listeria, and human neutrophils and non-activated macrophages can phagocytose and kill the bacteria. In experimental rodent listeriosis, protective immunity depends on T lymphocytes, antibodies playing little or no role. T cells confer protection by attracting monocytes to infectious foci and activating them, producing a listeriocidal action which destroys the intracellular bacteria. Granulomata are formed, and the listeria are eliminated. It is thought that immunity in humans is similar, although there is little direct evidence.

## Clinical aspects of infection

### Infection in pregnancy and the neonate

Listeriosis in pregnancy is classified by fetal gestation at onset, as this correlates best with the clinical features, microbiology and prognosis. Neonatal infection is divided into early (<2 days old), intermediate (3–5 days old) and late (>5 days old).

Maternal listeriosis before 20 weeks of pregnancy is rare. The mother is usually previously well and having a normal pregnancy. Pregnant women often have very mild symptoms and may be asymptomatic until the delivery of an infected infant. Chills, fever, back pain, sore throat and headache are cardinal features of infection, but conjunctivitis, drowsiness and other symptoms are sometimes present. Symptomatic women may have positive blood cultures. High vaginal swabs (HVSs), stool cultures and midstream urine samples are generally of little help in antepartum diagnosis. With the onset of fever, fetal movements are reduced, and premature labour

occurs within about 1 week. There may be a transient fever during labour, and the amniotic fluid is often discoloured or meconium stained. Culture of the amniotic fluid, placenta or HVS post delivery usually yields *L. monocytogenes*. Fever resolves soon after birth, and the HVS is usually culture-negative after about 1 month. While the outcome of infection for the mother is usually benign, the outcome for the infant is more variable. Abortion, stillbirth and early-onset neonatal disease are common, depending on the gestation at infection. However, maternal infection without infection of the offspring can occur and even progress to placental infection without ill effects for the fetus.

Repeated pregnancy-associated infections are exceedingly rare, and an association between listeria carriage and habitual abortion has not been substantiated.

Early neonatal listeriosis is predominantly a septicaemic illness, contracted in utero. In contrast, late neonatal infection is predominantly meningitic and may be associated with hospital cross-infection. The main characteristics of these two forms are summarized in Table 18.4. Early disease represents a spectrum of mild to severe infection, which can be correlated with the microbiological findings. Those neonates who die of infection usually do so within a few days of birth and have pneumonia, hepato-splenomegaly, petechiae, abscesses in the liver or brain, peritonitis and enterocolitis.

Late-onset disease is the third commonest form of meningitis in neonates. The CSF protein content is almost always raised and the glucose level reduced. The total number of white cells is increased but the counts are variable; neutrophils usually predominate, but lymphocytes or monocytes may be the main cell type. In about 50% of Gram films, bacteria are seen which may resemble rods or cocci.

### Adult and juvenile infection

Listeriosis in children older than 1 month is very rare, except in children with underlying disease. In adults the main syndromes are CNS infection, septicaemia and endocarditis. Most cases occur in immunosuppressed patients receiving steroid or cytotoxic therapy. However, about one-third of patients with meningitis and around 10% with primary bacteraemia have no predisposing factors.

### Meningitis

The clinical presentation is the same in all groups, but progression is more rapid in immuno-

**Table 18.4** Characteristics of neonatal infection with *L. monocytogenes*

| | Type of infection | |
| --- | --- | --- |
| | Early | Late |
| Onset after delivery | <2 days | >5 days |
| Maternal factors[a] | Common | Rare |
| Source of infection | Maternal | Hospital acquired and (?) maternally acquired |
| Signs/symptoms | Disseminated infection<br>Cardiopulmonary distress<br>CNS signs<br>Vomiting and diarrhoea<br>Hepatosplenomegaly<br>Skin rash | Meningitis<br>Irritability<br>Poor appetite<br>Fever |
| Laboratory findings | Leucocytosis or leucopenia<br>Thrombocytopenia<br>Mottling on chest radiograph<br>Increased fibrinogen | Leucocytosis; occasional radiographic changes<br>CSF: total protein and white cell count raised; glucose level lowered |
| Sites of isolation | Blood, superficial sites and amniotic fluid; less commonly gastric aspirate, CSF and HVS | Commonly CSF; rarely blood |
| Mortality | 30–60% | 10–12% |

[a]Obstetric problems; low birth weight; maternal fever; abnormal amniotic fluid.

compromised subjects. A peripheral blood leucocytosis occurs, and the CSF white blood cell count is raised. The CSF glucose level is low and the protein level is raised; a very high protein concentration may be a poor prognostic indicator. Gram stains of the CSF are often negative, and the clinical features of infection are such that it is not possible to tell listeria meningitis from meningococcal or pneumococcal infection. However, listeria are isolated from blood cultures in most cases.

In the rare cases of encephalitis, cerebritis or abscesses of the CNS the CSF may be normal, but often the white blood cell count is mildly raised and the protein level slightly elevated with a low glucose concentration. The Gram film and culture are usually negative. Blood cultures are the main source of isolation in many of these patients.

### Bacteraemia and endocarditis

Primary bacteraemia is more common in men than in women, and occurs most often in patients with haematological malignancy or renal transplants. A few patients develop CNS infection, which has a poor prognosis.

Infective endocarditis is twice as common in men as in women. The main predisposing factors are prosthetic valves or damaged natural valves, but some patients belong to other risk groups.

### Other infections

Rare manifestations of listeriosis include arthritis, hepatitis, endophthalmitis and CAPD (continuous ambulatory peritoneal dialysis) – associated peritonitis. Pneumonia occurs in renal transplant recipients and other groups of patients.

### Treatment

*L. monocytogenes* is susceptible to a wide range of antibiotics in vitro, including ampicillin, penicillin, vancomycin, tetracyclines, chloramphenicol, aminoglycosides and co-trimoxazole. There is little agreement as to what is the best treatment, but many patients have been successfully treated with ampicillin or penicillin with or without an aminoglycoside.

Ampicillin and penicillin are probably equivalent agents for the treatment of meningitis. Co-trimoxazole is an excellent alternative. Aminoglycosides interact synergistically with penicillin or ampicillin in vitro and improve mortality rates in experimental animals, but no such evidence exists for human infection. Chloramphenicol was formerly used in listeria meningitis but, when used alone, it is less effective than penicillin or ampicillin and results in relapses. The combination of chloramphenicol with penicillin or ampicillin has resulted in increased mortality. Cephalosporins are ineffective.

The combination of ampicillin and an aminoglycoside is used most commonly in other forms of neonatal and adult listeriosis. Vancomycin is a useful alternative in bacteraemia.

## Prognosis

The mortality rate in late neonatal disease is about 10%. In contrast, mortality in early disease is 30–60%, and about 20–40% of survivors develop sequelae such as lung disease, hydrocephalus or other neurological defects. Early use of appropriate antibiotics in infected mothers may improve neonatal survival.

The mortality in adult infection is about 20–50% in CNS infection; 5–20% in primary bacteraemias; and 50% in infective endocarditis. About 25–75% of patients surviving CNS infection suffer sequelae such as hemiplegias and other neurological defects.

## ERYSIPELOTHRIX

*Erysipelothrix* is a small, possibly monospecific, genus comprising aerobic, non-sporing Gram-positive bacilli of uncertain taxonomic status. The bacilli are short (1–2 μm), but may produce long filamentous forms resembling lactobacilli. Growth on blood agar, or in glucose broth is improved by incubation in 5–10% carbon dioxide. The species *E. rhusiopathiae* causes economically important disease in domestic animals, notably pigs. Human infections are rare, but include a form of cellulitis (*erysipeloid*), which occasionally becomes diffuse, septicaemia and endocarditis. Infection is most often associated with close animal contact.

Penicillin and other β-lactam antibiotics are effective. Erythromycin and clindamycin offer suitable alternatives, but *E. rhusiopathiae* is resistant to vancomycin.

## RECOMMENDED READING

Christie A B 1987 Diphtheria. *Infectious Diseases*, 4th edn. Churchill Livingstone, Edinburgh, vol 2, pp 1183–1209

Jones E M, MacGowan A P 1995 Antimicrobial chemotherapy of human infection due to *Listeria monocytogenes. European Journal of Clinical Microbiology and Infectious Diseases* 14: 165–175

Lipsky B A, Goldberger A C, Tompkins L S, Plorde J J 1982 Infections caused by nondiphtheria corynebacteria. *Reviews of Infectious Diseases* 4: 1220–1235

MacGowan A P 1994 *Listeria* spp and listeriosis – 25 years on. *Journal of Medical Microbiology* 41: 160–163

Mitchell R G 1996 Listeria, Erysipelothrix. In: Collee J G, Fraser A G, Marmion B P, Simmons A (eds) *Mackie and MacCartney. Practical Medical Microbiology*, 14th edn. Churchill Livingstone, Edinburgh, pp 309–315

Reboli A C, Farrar W E 1989 *Erysipelothrix rhusiopathiae*: an occupational pathogen. *Clinical Microbiology Reviews 2*: 354–359

Schuchat A, Swaminathan B, Broome C V 1991 Epidemiology of human listeriosis. *Clinical Microbiology Reviews* 4: 169–183

Wilson A P R 1995 Treatment of infection caused by toxigenic and non-toxigenic strains of *Corynebacterium diphtheriae. Journal of Antimicrobial Chemotherapy* 35: 717–720

Zamiri I 1996 Corynebacterium. In: Collee J G, Fraser A G, Marmion B P, Simmons A (eds) *Mackie and MacCartney. Practical Medical Microbiology*, 14th edn. Churchill Livingstone, Edinburgh, pp 299–308

# 19

# Mycobacterium

**Tuberculosis; leprosy**

*J. M. Grange*

The mycobacteria, or acid-fast bacilli, are responsible for tuberculosis and leprosy, and a number of saprophytic species occasionally cause opportunist disease (see Ch. 20). The name of the genus, *Mycobacterium* (fungus-bacterium), is an allusion to the mould-like pellicles formed when members of this genus are grown in liquid media. This hydrophobic property is due to their possession of thick, complex, lipid-rich, waxy cell walls. A further important characteristic of mycobacteria, also due to their waxy cell walls, is their *acid-fastness*, or resistance to decolorization by a dilute mineral acid (or alcohol) after staining with hot carbol fuchsin or other arylmethane dyes.

There are about 60 species of mycobacteria, which are divisible into two major groups, the slow and rapid growers, although the growth rate of the latter is slow relative to that of most other bacteria. The leprosy bacillus has never convincingly been grown in vitro.

## MYCOBACTERIUM TUBERCULOSIS

Tuberculosis is a chronic granulomatous disease affecting humans and many other mammals. It is caused by four very closely related species: *Mycobacterium tuberculosis* (the human tubercle bacillus), *M. bovis* (the bovine tubercle bacillus), *M. microti* (the vole tubercle bacillus) and *M. africanum*.

Most human tuberculosis is caused by *M. tuberculosis*, but some cases are due to *M. bovis*, which is the principal cause of tuberculosis in cattle and many other mammals. The name *M. africanum* is given to tubercle bacilli with rather variable properties and which appear to be intermediate in form between the human and bovine types. It causes human tuberculosis and is mainly found in Equatorial Africa. *M. microti*, which is very rarely, if ever, encountered nowadays, is a pathogen of voles and other small mammals but not of humans.

## Description

Tubercle bacilli are non-motile, non-sporing, non-capsulate straight or slightly curved rods about $3 \times 0.3$ μm in size. In sputum and other clinical specimens they may occur singly or in small clumps, and in liquid cultures human tubercle bacilli often grow as twisted rope-like colonies termed *serpentine cords* (Fig. 19.1).

Tubercle bacilli are able to grow on a wide range of enriched culture media, but Löwenstein–Jensen (LJ) medium is the most widely used in clinical practice. This consists of whole eggs, glycerol, asparagine and some mineral salts, and is solidified

**Fig. 19.1** Microcolony of *M. tuberculosis* showing 'serpentine cord' formation.

by heating (inspissation). Malachite green dye is added to the medium to inhibit the growth of some contaminating bacteria and to provide a contrasting colour against which colonies of mycobacteria are easily seen. Agar-based media or broths enriched with bovine serum albumin are also used.

Human tubercle bacilli produce visible growth on LJ medium in about 2 weeks, although on primary isolation from clinical material colonies may take up to 8 weeks to appear. Colonies are of an off-white (buff) colour and often have a dry breadcrumb-like appearance. Growth is characteristically heaped up and luxuriant or 'eugonic' in contrast to the small, flat 'dysgonic' colonies of bovine tubercle bacilli on this medium. The growth of the latter is much better on media containing sodium pyruvate in place of glycerol, e.g. Stonebrink's medium.

Tubercle bacilli have a rather limited temperature range of growth: their optimal growth temperature is 35–37°C but they fail to grow at 25 or 41°C. Most other mycobacteria grow at one or other, or both, of these temperatures.

Like all mycobacteria, the tubercle bacilli are obligate aerobes, but *M. bovis* grows better in conditions of reduced oxygen tension. Thus, when incorporated in soft agar media, *M. tuberculosis* grows on the surface while *M. bovis* grows as a band a few millimetres below the surface. This provides a useful differentiating test. The human tubercle bacillus also differs from the bovine type in its ability to reduce nitrates to nitrites; its production of large amounts of niacin; its sensitivity to pyrazinamide; and, usually, in its resistance to thiophen-2-carboxylic acid hydrazide (TCH), a substance related to the antituberculosis drug isoniazid (Table 19.1).

The tubercle bacilli are obligate pathogens, but they survive in milk and in other organic materials and on pasture-land so long as they are not exposed to ultraviolet light, to which they are very sensitive. They are also heat-sensitive, and are destroyed in the process of pasteurization. Mycobacteria are susceptible to alcohol, formaldehyde and glutaraldehyde and, to a lesser extent, to hypochlorites and phenolic disinfectants. They are considerably more resistant than other bacteria to acids, alkalis and quaternary ammonium compounds.

## Pathogenesis

The tubercle bacillus owes its virulence to its ability to survive within the macrophage rather than to the production of a toxic substance. The immune response to the bacillus is of the cell-mediated type which, depending on the type of T helper cells involved, may either lead to protective immunity and resolution of the disease or to tissue-destroying hypersensitivity reactions and progression of the disease process. The nature of the immune responses following infection changes with time so that human tuberculosis is divisible into primary and post-primary forms with quite different pathological features.

### Primary tuberculosis

The site of the initial infection is usually the lung, following the inhalation of bacilli. These bacilli are engulfed by alveolar macrophages in which they replicate to form the initial lesion or *Ghon focus*. Some bacilli are carried in phagocytic cells to the hilar lymph nodes where additional foci of infection develop. The Ghon focus together with the enlarged hilar lymph nodes form the *primary complex*. In addition, bacilli are seeded by further lymphatic and haematogenous dissemination in many organs and tissues, including other parts of the lung. When the bacilli enter the mouth, as in milk-borne bovine tuberculosis, the primary complexes involve the tonsil and cervical nodes (*scrofula*; Fig. 19.2) or the intestine, often the ileocaecal region, and the mesenteric lymph nodes. Likewise, the primary focus may be in the skin with involvement of the regional lymph nodes. This form of tuberculosis was an occupational disease of anatomists and pathologists and was termed *prosector's wart*.

**Table 19.1** Some differential characteristics of tubercle bacilli causing human disease

| Species | Atmospheric preference | Nitratase | TCH | Pyrazinamide |
|---|---|---|---|---|
| M. tuberculosis | Aerobic | Positive | Resistant[a] | Sensitive |
| M. bovis | Micro-aerophilic | Negative | Sensitive | Resistant |
| M. africanum | Micro-aerophilic | Variable | Sensitive | Sensitive |

[a]Strains from south India may be sensitive to TCH.

**Fig. 19.2** Tuberculous cervical lymphadenitis (scrofula) with sinus formation in an Indonesian woman.

Within about 10 days of infection, clones of antigen-specific T lymphocytes are produced. These release lymphokines which activate macrophages and cause them to form a compact cluster, or granuloma, around the foci of infection. These activated macrophages are termed *epithelioid cells* from their microscopical resemblance to epithelial cells. Some of them fuse to form multinucleate giant cells. The centre of the granuloma contains a mixture of necrotic tissue and dead macrophages which, from its cheese-like appearance and consistency, is referred to as *caseation*.

Activated human macrophages inhibit the replication of the tubercle bacilli, but there is no clear experimental evidence that they can actually kill them. Being metabolically very active, the macrophages in the granuloma consume oxygen and the resulting anoxia and acidosis in the centre of the lesion probably kills most of the tubercle bacilli. Granuloma formation is usually sufficient to limit the primary infection: the lesions become quiescent and surrounding fibroblasts produce dense scar tissue which may become calcified. Not all bacilli

are destroyed: some remain in a poorly understood dormant form which, when reactivated, cause post-primary disease.

In a minority of cases one of the infective foci progresses and gives rise to the serious manifestations of primary disease, including progressive primary lesions (particularly in infants; Fig. 19.3), meningitis, pleurisy and disease of the kidneys, spine (*Pott's disease*) and other bones and joints. If a focus ruptures into a blood vessel, bacilli are disseminated throughout the body with the formation of numerous granulomata (Fig. 19.3). This, from the millet seed-like appearance of the lesions, is known as *miliary tuberculosis*. The 'timetable' of events in primary tuberculosis is shown in Table 19.2.

### Tuberculin reactivity

About 6 or 8 weeks after the initial infection, the phenomenon of tuberculin conversion occurs. This altered reactivity was discovered by Robert Koch whilst attempting to develop a remedy for tuberculosis. When tuberculous guinea-pigs were injected intradermally with living tubercle bacilli, the skin around the injection site became necrotic within a day or two and was sloughed off, together with the bacilli. Koch then found that the same reaction occurred when he injected *old tuberculin*, which was a heat-concentrated filtrate of a broth in which tubercle bacilli had been grown. This reaction became known as the *Koch phenomenon*, and its characteristic feature is extensive tissue necrosis.

Injection of tuberculin into the skin causes an inflammatory reaction with a huge increase in the cellularity of the skin and a compensatory increase in local capillary blood flow. In the large, indurated reactions, the blood flow is reduced, causing anoxia, acidosis, ischaemia and necrosis. This appears to be the result of mediators, including tumour necrosis factor, which are released from lymphocytes and macrophages. This necrotic reaction is largely responsible for the characteristic features of post-primary tuberculosis. Smaller, non-indurated tuberculin reactions are, by contrast, associated with protective immunity.

### Post-primary tuberculosis

In many individuals, the primary complex resolves and the only evidence of infection is a conversion to tuberculin reactivity. After an interval of months, years or decades, reactivation of dormant foci of tubercle bacilli or exogenous reinfection may lead to post-primary tuberculosis, which differs in several

**Fig. 19.3** Progressive primary tuberculous lesion in the right upper lobe of the lung and numerous miliary lesions in other parts of the lung in a child aged 6 months.

**Table 19.2** Stages of primary tuberculosis in childhood

| Stage | Time (from onset) | Characteristics |
|---|---|---|
| 1 | 3–8 weeks | Primary complex develops and tuberculin conversion occurs |
| 2 | 2–6 months | Progressive healing of primary complex Possibility of pleural effusion |
| 3 | 6–12 months | Possibility of miliary or meningeal tuberculosis |
| 4 | 1–3 years | Possibility of bone or joint tuberculosis |
| 5 | 3–5 years or more | Possibility of genito-urinary or chronic skin tuberculosis |

Adapted from Miller F J W 1982 *Tuberculosis in Children*. Churchill Livingstone, Edinburgh.

**Table 19.3** Main differences between primary and post-primary tuberculosis in non-immunocompromised patients

| Characteristics | Primary | Post-primary |
|---|---|---|
| Local lesion | Small | Large |
| Lymphatic involvement | Yes | Minimal |
| Cavity formation | Rare | Frequent |
| Tuberculin reactivity | Negative (initially) | Positive |
| Infectivity (pulmonary cases) | Uncommon | Usual |
| Site | Any part of lung | Apical region |
| Local spread | Uncommon | Frequent |

respects from primary disease (Table 19.3). Reactivation may occur spontaneously or after an intercurrent illness or other condition that lowers the host's immune responsiveness (see below). For unknown reasons reactivation or reinfection tuberculosis often occurs in the upper lobes of the lungs. The same process of granuloma formation occurs, but the necrotic element of the reaction causes tissue destruction and the formation of large areas of caseation termed *tuberculomata*. Proteases liberated by activated macrophages cause softening and liquefaction of the caseous material and an excess of tumour necrosis factor (cachectin) and other immunological mediators cause the wasting and fevers characteristic of the disease.

The interior of the tuberculoma is acidic and anoxic and contains few viable tubercle bacilli. Eventually, however, the expanding lesion erodes through the wall of a bronchus, the liquefied contents are discharged and a well-aerated cavity is formed (Fig. 19.4). The atmosphere of the lung, with a high carbon dioxide level, is ideal for supporting the growth of the bacilli, and huge numbers of these are found in the cavity walls. For this reason, closure of the cavities by collapsing the lung, either by artificial pneumothorax or by excising large portions of the chest wall, was a standard treatment for tuberculosis in the pre-chemotherapeutic era.

Once the cavity is formed, large numbers of bacilli gain access to the sputum, and the patient becomes an open or infectious case. This is a good example of the transmissibility of a pathogen being depen-

**Fig. 19.4** Large tuberculous cavity in the lung of a man aged 24 years. Other parts of the lung show secondary lesions due to endobronchial spread of disease.

dent upon the host's response to infection. Surprisingly, about 20% of cases of open cavitating tuberculosis resolve without treatment.

In post-primary tuberculosis, dissemination of bacilli to lymph nodes and other organs is unusual. Instead, spread of infection occurs through the bronchial tree so that secondary lesions develop in the lower lobes of the lung (Fig. 19.4). Likewise, secondary lesions may occur in the trachea, larynx and mouth, and swallowed bacilli cause intestinal lesions; secondary lesions may also develop in the bladder and epididymis in cases of renal tuberculosis. Post-primary cutaneous tuberculosis (*lupus vulgaris*) usually affects the face and neck. Untreated, it is a very chronic condition leading to gross scarring and deformity. Some cases are secondary to sinus formation between tuberculous lymph nodes and the skin (*scrofuloderma*).

## Tuberculosis in immunocompromised individuals

Reactivation tuberculosis is particularly likely to occur in immunocompromised individuals, including the elderly, transplant recipients and those who are human immunodeficiency virus (HIV)-positive. In the latter, tuberculosis is usually diagnosed before the other features of the acquired immune deficiency syndrome (AIDS) are apparent. Cavity formation is unusual in the more profoundly immunocompromised patients, emphasizing the importance of the immune response in this pathological process. Instead, diffuse infiltrates develop in any part of the lung, and non-pulmonary lesions due to lymphatic and haematogenous dissemination are common. Sometimes there are numerous minute lesions teeming with tubercle bacilli throughout the body – a rapidly fatal condition termed *cryptic disseminated tuberculosis*.

## The tuberculin test

Although Robert Koch's attempts to use old tuberculin as a remedy for tuberculosis failed, an Austrian physician, Clemens von Pirquet, used the Koch phenomenon in humans as an indication of bacterial 'allergy' resulting from previous infection. Individuals with active tuberculosis were usually tuberculin-positive, but many of those with disseminated and rapidly progressive disease were negative. This led to the widespread but erroneous belief that tuberculin reactivity is an indicator of immunity to tuberculosis.

Old tuberculin caused non-specific reactions, and it has been replaced by *purified protein derivative*

(PPD). This is given by intracutaneous injection (*Mantoux* method) or by means of a spring-loaded gun which fires six prongs into the skin through a drop of PPD (*Heaf* method). In addition, disposable devices with PPD dried onto prongs are available for single tests (*tine tests*).

The biological activity of tuberculins is compared with international standards and their activities are expressed in international units (IU). In the UK, solutions of PPD for Mantoux testing are supplied as dilutions of 1 in 10 000, 1 in 1000 and 1 in 100, which correspond to 1, 10 and 100 IU in the injected dose of 0.1 ml. The standard test dose is 10 IU but those suspected of having tuberculosis, and therefore likely to react strongly, may first be tested with 1 IU. Undiluted PPD is supplied for use with the Heaf gun.

The tuberculin test is widely used as a diagnostic test, although its usefulness is limited by its failure to distinguish active disease from quiescent infections and past BCG (bacille Calmette–Guérin; see later) vaccination. In addition, exposure to various mycobacteria in the environment may induce low levels of tuberculin reactivity. In the USA, more diagnostic reliance is placed on the tuberculin test as BCG is not used in that country. The test is used in epidemiological studies as outlined below.

## Laboratory diagnosis

The definitive diagnosis of tuberculosis is based on the detection of acid-fast bacilli in clinical specimens by microscopy, cultural techniques or by polymerase chain reaction (PCR). Numerous attempts have been made to develop serological tests for the disease with little success.

### Specimens

The most usual specimen for diagnosis of pulmonary tuberculosis is sputum but, if none is produced, bronchial washings, brushings or biopsies, laryngeal swabs and early-morning gastric aspirates (to harvest any bacilli swallowed overnight) may be examined. Tissue biopsies are homogenized by grinding in Griffith's tubes for microscopy and culture. Cerebrospinal fluid, pleural fluid, urine and other fluids are centrifuged and the deposits are examined.

### Microscopy

Use is made of the acid-fast property of mycobacteria to detect them in sputum and other clinical material. In the Ziehl–Neelsen (ZN) staining technique, heat-fixed smears of the specimens are flooded with a solution of carbol fuchsin (a mixture of basic fuchsin and phenol) and heated until steam rises. After washing with water, the slide is flooded with a dilute mineral acid (e.g. 3% hydrochloric acid) and, after further washing, a green or blue counterstain is applied. Red bacilli are seen against the contrasting background colour. In some methods, the acid is diluted in 95% ethanol rather than water. This gives a cleaner background but, contrary to a common belief, it does not enable tubercle bacilli to be distinguished from other mycobacteria. Fluorescent dyes are also used, and there are modifications of the staining techniques for use with tissue sections.

### Cultural methods

As sputum and certain other specimens frequently contain many bacteria and fungi that would rapidly overgrow any mycobacteria on the culture media, these must be destroyed. *Decontamination* methods make use of the relatively high resistance of myco-bacteria to acids, alkalis and certain disinfectants. In the widely used *Petroff method*, sputum is mixed well with 4% sodium hydroxide for 15–30 min, neutralized with potassium dihydrogen orthophosphate and centrifuged. The deposit is used to inoculate LJ or similar media. Specimens such as cerebrospinal fluid and tissue biopsies which are unlikely to be contaminated do not require such treatment before inoculation onto culture media.

Inoculated media are incubated at 35–37°C and inspected weekly for at least 8 weeks. Cultures of material from skin lesions should also be incubated at 33°C. Any bacterial growth is stained by the ZN method and, if acid-fast, it is subcultured for further identification. A more rapid bacteriological diagnosis is achieved by the radiometric detection of $^{14}CO_2$ released from liquid media containing $^{14}C$-labelled palmitic acid or by systems based on activation of fluorescent dyes by released $CO_2$.

The first step in identification is to determine whether an isolate is a tubercle bacillus (*M. tuberculosis*, *M. bovis* or *M. africanum*) or one of the other species. Tubercle bacilli grow slowly, do not produce yellow pigment and fail to grow at 25 and 41°C and on egg media containing *p*-nitrobenzoic acid (500 mg/l). Strains differing in any of these properties belong to other species.

### Nucleic acid technology

Nucleic acid probes for the identification of the *M. tuberculosis* complex and, specifically, *M. tuberculosis*

are commercially available. These are not sensitive enough to detect mycobacteria in clinical specimens, which thus require cultivation by conventional techniques. Amplification of specific nucleic acid sequences in specimens is achievable by PCR. Various primers and techniques have been described, and some are commercially available. Problems of low sensitivity, 'false'-positive reactions and cross-contamination have reduced the useful-ness of conventional PCR techniques but these have, to a great extent, been overcome by the introduction of closed-system, isothermal amplifi-cation techniques for detection of species-specific amplification of 16S ribosomal RNA. Most mem-bers of the *M. tuberculosis* complex contain from 1 to 20 copies of the insertion sequence IS6110 which has been used to develop restriction fragment length polymorphism analysis (DNA 'fingerprinting') for epidemiological purposes.

### Drug susceptibility testing

Several methods have been described. In the UK there is a preference for the resistance-ratio method in which test strains and a number of known susceptible control strains are inoculated on LJ medium containing doubling dilutions of drug. The results are expressed as the ratio of the drug con-centration inhibiting the test strain to that inhibiting the control strains. Susceptible strains have ratios of 1 or 2, while higher ratios indicate resistance (Table 19.4). More rapid susceptibility testing is achieved by the use of radiometry. Nucleic acid technology offers even more rapid approaches: mutations conferring rifampicin resistance have been detected in the *rpoB* gene by a modified PCR suitable for routine use.

## Treatment

The antituberculosis drugs are divisible into three groups: bactericidal drugs that effectively sterilize tuberculous lesions, bactericidal drugs that only kill tubercle bacilli in certain situations and bacteristatic drugs (Table 19.5). Streptomycin is ineffective against bacilli within macrophages and acidic inflammatory tissue, and isoniazid kills bacilli only if they are replicating. Bacteristatic drugs are of limited usefulness and are not included in modern regimens.

Mutation to drug resistance occurs at a rate of about one mutation every $10^8$ cell divisions. Success-ful therapy requires the prevention of the emergence of drug-resistant strains by the simultaneous use of at least two drugs to which the organism is sensitive.

**Table 19.4** Examples of the interpretation of drug sensitivity testing by the resistance ratio method

| Strain | Increasing drug concentration (mg/l) | | | | | | Resistance ratio | Result |
|---|---|---|---|---|---|---|---|---|
| | 1 | 2 | 4 | 8 | 16 | 32 | | |
| Controls | + | + | – | – | – | – | — | — |
| Test 1 | + | (+) | – | – | – | – | 1 | Sensitive |
| Test 2 | + | + | – | – | – | – | 1 | Sensitive |
| Test 3 | + | + | + | – | – | – | 2 | Sensitive |
| Test 4 | + | + | + | + | (+) | – | 4 | Resistant |
| Test 5 | + | + | + | + | + | – | 8 | Resistant |
| Test 6 | + | + | + | + | + | + | >8 | Resistant |

+, confluent growth or innumerable discrete colonies; (+), 20–100 colonies; –, less than 20 colonies.

**Table 19.5** Antituberculosis drugs (in vivo)

| Sterilizing | Bactericidal | Bacteristatic |
|---|---|---|
| Rifampicin | Isoniazid | Ethionamide |
| Pyrazinamide | Streptomycin | Prothionamide |
| | Ethambutol[a] | Thiacetazone |
| | | p-Aminosalicylic acid |
| | | Cycloserine |

[a]In early stages of therapy.

The once widely used 2 year regimen of streptomycin, isoniazid and p-aminosalicylic acid has been replaced by much more acceptable orally administered short-course regimens (Table 19.6). These are mostly based on an intensive phase of rifampicin, isoniazid and pyrazinamide for 2 months followed by the first two drugs for a total of 6 months. A fourth drug, usually ethambutol, is given in the intensive phase in regions where resistance to one of the former drugs is common. In some regimens,

drugs are given daily throughout, in others they are given daily during the intensive phase and then twice or thrice weekly, while in some they are given intermittently throughout. Experience has shown that it is essential to supervise the administration of the drugs to ensure compliance and, when this proves difficult, the intermittent regimens are particularly useful. The early intensive phase ensures that a significant proportion of patients are rapidly cured, thereby reducing the relapse rate in early defaulters.

The response to therapy is divisible into three phases. During the first week or two, the large numbers of actively replicating bacilli in cavity walls are killed, principally by isoniazid but also by rifampicin and ethambutol. As a result the patient rapidly ceases to be infectious, and hospitalization with barrier nursing is now rarely necessary. In the following few weeks the less active bacilli within macrophages, caseous material and dense, acidic, inflammatory lesions are killed by rifampicin and pyrazinamide. In the continuation phase any remaining dormant bacilli are killed by rifampicin

**Table 19.6** Some examples of short-course chemotherapy recommended by the International Union Against Tuberculosis and Lung Disease

| Initial phase | | Continuation phase | | |
|---|---|---|---|---|
| Drugs | Duration (months) | Drugs | Duration (months) | Notes |
| HRZ | 2 | HR | 4 | Standard regimen |
| HRZ | 2 | $H_3R_3$ | 4 | Intermittent regimens for use when |
| HRZ | 2 | $H_2R_2$ | 4 | supervision is indicated |
| $H_3R_3Z_3E_3$ | 2 | $H_3R_3$ | 4 | |
| HRZE | 2 | HR | 4 | Regimens for use when there is a high |
| HRZS | 2 | HR | 4 | incidence of initial drug resistance |

H, isoniazid; R, rifampicin; Z, pyrazinamide; E, ethambutol; S, streptomycin.
The subscript numerals 2 and 3 indicate twice- and thrice-weekly doses, respectively.

during their short bursts of metabolic activity. Any rifampicin-resistant mutants that start to replicate are killed by isoniazid.

The emergence of drug-resistant strains (acquired resistance) during adequately supervised short-course chemotherapy is uncommon – most relapses are due to drug-sensitive bacilli. Multidrug-resistant strains (resistant to isoniazid and rifampicin and sometimes to additional drugs) pose serious problems and, even if sensitive in vitro to newer fluoroquinolones and macrolides, the mortality approaches 50%, or 85% in HIV-positive patients, within 2 years.

Short-course regimens are usually well tolerated by the patient. Isoniazid, rifampicin and pyrazinamide are all potentially hepatotoxic, and rifampicin may cause an influenza-like syndrome which, paradoxically, is more likely to occur when the drug is given intermittently. Rifampicin antagonizes the action of oral contraceptives – an important point to be considered when treating young women. Isoniazid may cause mild psychiatric disturbances and peripheral neuropathy, particularly in alcoholics, but these usually respond to treatment with pyridoxine (vitamin $B_6$). Ethambutol is toxic for the eye and, although this is rare with standard dosages, care is required and the patient should be informed of this possibility.

Owing to the serious problems of non-compliance and the emergence of multidrug resistance, immunotherapeutic approaches are being considered, and one agent, heat-killed *M. vaccae*, is currently undergoing extensive clinical trials.

## Epidemiology

Human tuberculosis is principally transmitted by inhalation of bacilli in moist droplets coughed out by individuals with open pulmonary tuberculosis. Dried bacilli in dust appear to be less of a health hazard. As a general rule, only sputum smear-positive individuals are infectious: 1 ml of sputum from these individuals contains at least 5000 tubercle bacilli. Most transmission of the disease occurs within households or other environments where individuals are close together for long periods.

For epidemiological purposes, the incidence of infection by the tubercle bacillus in a community is calculated from the number of tuberculin-positive individuals in different age groups, provided that they have not received BCG vaccination. The annual infection rate gives an indirect measure of the number of open or infectious individuals in the community. Thus, a 1% annual infection rate indicates that there are around 50 infectious cases in every 100 000 members of the community. The prevalence of tuberculosis in a region is not the same as the annual infection rate because only a minority of infected individuals develop overt disease and they often become ill several years after their initial infection. Determinations of the incidence of tuberculosis world-wide are notoriously difficult but, according to World Health Organization (WHO) estimates, one-third of the world's population has been infected, about 100 million individuals are infected annually, between 8 million and 10 million develop overt disease, from 4 million to 5 million become open or infectious and around 3 million die.

In the industrially developed nations, tuberculosis is uncommon, with an annual infection rate of 0.3–0.1% or less, but the previous decline has halted and in several countries there has been an increase in notifications since around 1990. In the developing countries the annual infection rates are usually between 2 and 5% and there is little or no decline. The impact of AIDS on the epidemiology of tuberculosis and predictions of future trends are very worrying. In 1995, 8% of all cases of tuberculosis were HIV related, rising to 20% in Africa. A person infected by the tubercle bacillus and HIV has an 8% chance of developing active tuberculosis annually and, even if the tuberculosis is treated, the mortality rate is very high. The interval between infection and overt disease is considerably shortened, resulting in explosive mini-epidemics in institutions where HIV-positive persons congregate. Some such mini-epidemics have involved multidrug-resistant strains, notably in the USA.

Bovine tuberculosis is spread from animal to animal, and sometimes to human attendants, in moist cough spray. About 1% of infected cows develop lesions in the udder, and bacilli are excreted in the milk which can then infect people who drink it. Thus, primary human tuberculosis due to *M. bovis* usually involves the cervical or mesenteric lymph nodes. Heat treatment, or pasteurization, prevents such milk-borne disease. In many countries, bovine tuberculosis has been drastically reduced by regular tuberculin testing of herds and the slaughter of reactors. In such countries, human disease due to *M. bovis* is very rare and is usually the result of reactivation of old lesions: person-to-person spread of *M. bovis* leading to active disease is very uncommon. The total eradication of bovine tuberculosis has been prevented by infection of cattle from wild animals, notably badgers, and also from farm workers with open tuberculosis due to *M. bovis*.

## Control

Human tuberculosis is preventable by the early detection and effective therapy of the open or infectious individuals in a community, by lowering the chance of infection by reducing overcrowding and, to a limited extent, by vaccination.

Active case finding involves a deliberate search, often on a house-to-house basis or in workplaces, for suspects with a chronic cough of a month or more in duration. Merely waiting for patients with symptoms to seek medical attention is much less effective, even when supported by education programmes. Regular chest examination by mass miniature radiography never detected more than 15% of individuals with tuberculosis and is no longer used routinely except in certain high-risk situations.

The most important factors affecting the incidence of tuberculosis are socio-economic ones, particularly those leading to a reduction of overcrowding in homes and workplaces. In the developing countries it is estimated that each patient with open tuberculosis infects about 20 contacts annually, while in Europe the corresponding figure is two or three.

### Vaccination

Bacille Calmette-Guérin (BCG) is a living attenuated vaccine derived from a strain of *M. bovis* by repeated subculture between the years 1908 and 1920. This species was selected rather than *M. tuberculosis* on the false assumption that it was of limited virulence in humans. The vaccine was originally given orally to neonates but it is now given by intracutaneous injection.

The protective efficacy of BCG has been determined in a number of studies, and varies enormously from country to country. In the UK, administration of BCG to schoolchildren affords 78% protection, but in a major trial in south India involving individuals of all ages no protection was demonstrated (Table 19.7). This difference in protection appears to be the result of prior exposure of the population to environmental mycobacteria which, in some regions, confer some protection, but in others induce inappropriate immune reactions. For this reason, neonatal vaccination is now gaining popularity.

When BCG vaccination is introduced into a region it has an immediate impact on the incidence of the serious but non-infectious forms of childhood tuberculosis such as meningitis but it has little impact on the annual infection rate in the com-

**Table 19.7** Variations in the protective efficacy of BCG vaccinations in nine major trials

| Country or population | Age range of vaccinees (years) | Protection (%) |
|---|---|---|
| North American Indian | 0–20 | 80 |
| UK | 14–15 | 78 |
| Chicago, USA | Neonates | 75 |
| Puerto Rico | 1–18 | 31 |
| South India (Bangalore) | All ages | 30 |
| Georgia and Alabama, USA | >5 | 14 |
| Georgia, USA | 6–17 | 0 |
| Illinois, USA | Young adults | 0 |
| South India (Chingleput) | All ages | 0[a] |

[a]Some protection demonstrated in those vaccinated neonatally on 15 year follow-up.

munity as the smear-positive source cases arise mostly from amongst the older, unvaccinated, tuberculin-positive members of the community. Vaccination has therefore not proved to be an effective control measure.

### Prophylactic chemotherapy

In true prophylactic chemotherapy, drugs are administered to uninfected individuals who are in unavoidable contact with a patient with open tuberculosis. The main example is a baby born to a mother with the disease. More usually, it refers to therapy, principally with isoniazid alone, given to individuals who have been infected but show no signs of active disease. In the UK, such therapy may be given to unvaccinated children who have converted to tuberculin-positivity after exposure to a source case. The use of prophylactic chemotherapy in older tuberculin reactors is controversial and virtually restricted to countries, such as the USA, where BCG vaccination is no longer given. In principle, prophylactic chemotherapy is beneficial in those infected with both the tubercle bacillus and HIV, but the identification of such dually infected persons poses serious difficulties.

## MYCOBACTERIUM LEPRAE

Leprosy is a particularly tragic affliction as the nature of the infection often causes severe disfigurement and deformity which, throughout history, have led to the social ostracism or total banishment of its victims. Unfortunately, such attitudes towards the disease are still prevalent in many parts of the world. Despite effective chemotherapy, there were about 5.5 million registered patients in 1995, but there are probably many more who are not registered. About 600 000 new cases are detected annually, with little sign of a decreasing incidence, and 2 million to 3 million patients have been bacteriologically cured but have significant residual deformities requiring life-long care.

Leprosy is often cited as a disease of great antiquity but, in fact, literary and skeletal evidence of this very characteristic disease go back no further than 500 BC. Biblical leprosy was almost certainly not the same as the disease that now bears this name.

Potentially, leprosy is of world-wide distribution although it is now mainly confined to developing nations in the tropics. The disease was long endemic in the British Isles, and Robert the Bruce of Scotland was one of its victims. The last British leprosy patient to acquire the disease in this country died in the Shetland islands in 1798. In Norway the disease persisted into the 20th century, and the causative organism was first described in that country by Armauer Hansen in 1874.

## Description

*M. leprae* has never convincingly been cultivated in vitro, and this has been a major limiting factor in the study of leprosy. Limited replication occurs in the mouse footpad, and this has been used for testing the sensitivity of bacilli to antileprosy drugs.

A major breakthrough occurred in the 1970s when it was found that armadillos infected with *M. leprae* often developed extensive disease with up to $10^{10}$ bacilli in each gram of diseased tissue. This animal has therefore provided sufficient bacilli for a number of studies and for the production of a skin test reagent, leprosin-A.

Leprosy bacilli resemble tubercle bacilli in their general morphology, but they are not so strongly acid-fast. In clinical material from lepromatous patients they are typically found within macrophages in dense clumps.

Studies of the metabolism, biochemical properties and antigenic composition of *M. leprae* are difficult. However, a genomic library has been prepared from this bacillus, thereby providing a potentially un-limited source of recombinant protein antigens for immunological studies. A characteristic surface lipid, peptidoglycolipid I (PGL-I), has been extracted from *M. leprae*, and its unique carbohydrate antigenic determinant has been synthesized and used to develop serodiagnostic tests for leprosy. *M. leprae* may be detected in tissues and nasal secretions by PCR.

## Pathogenesis

The principal target cell for the leprosy bacillus is the Schwann cell, and the resulting nerve damage is responsible for the main clinical features of leprosy, which are anaesthesia and muscle paralysis. Repeated injury to, and infections of, the anaesthetic extremities leads to their gradual destruction (Fig. 19.5). Infil-tration of the skin and cutaneous nerves by bacilli leads to the formation of visible lesions, often with pigmentary changes. The first sign of leprosy is a non-specific or indeterminate skin lesion which often heals spontaneously. If the disease progresses, its clinical manifestation is determined by the specific immune responsiveness of the patient to the bacillus, and there is a distinct immunological spec-trum with hyper-reactive *tuberculoid* (TT) leprosy at one pole and anergic *lepromatous* (LL) leprosy at the other (Table 19.8). At the TT pole there are small numbers of localized skin lesions containing so few bacilli that they are hardly ever seen microscopically

**Fig. 19.5** Borderline tuberculoid leprosy. Trophic changes in the hands secondary to nerve damage and anaesthesia. Compare the normal face with Figure 19.6.

**Table 19.8** Characteristics of the five points on the spectrum of leprosy

|  | TT | BT | BB | BL | LL |
|---|---|---|---|---|---|
| Bacilli seen in skin | − | +/− | + | ++ | +++ |
| Bacilli in nasal secretions | − | − | − | + | +++ |
| Granuloma formation | +++ | ++ | + | − | − |
| Reaction to lepromin | +++ | + | +/− | − | − |
| Antibodies to *M. leprae* | +/− | +/− | + | ++ | +++ |
| Main phagocytic cell | Mature epithelioid | Immature epithelioid | Immature epithelioid | Macrophage | Macrophage |
| In-vitro correlates of CMI | +++ | ++ | + | +/− | − |
| Type 1 reactions | − | + | + | + | − |
| Type 2 reactions | − | − | − | +/− | ++ |

CMI, cell-mediated immunity; see text for other abbreviations.

(*paucibacillary disease*) and an inappropriately intense granulomatous response that often damages major nerve trunks. At the LL pole the skin lesions are very numerous or confluent and contain huge numbers of bacilli (*multibacillary disease*), usually seen as clusters or globi within monocytes, but there is no histological evidence of an immune response. Cooler parts of the body, such as the ear lobes, are particularly heavily infiltrated by bacilli (Fig. 19.6). Many patients occupy an intermediate position on the spectrum, and may be classified as *borderline tuberculoid* (BT), *mid-borderline* (BB) or *borderline lepromatous* (BL).

The nasal bones are also involved in leprosy, and their destruction may lead to collapse of the nose (Fig. 19.7). In addition, large numbers of leprosy bacilli are discharged in nasal secretions in multibacillary disease. The eye is frequently damaged by direct bacillary invasion, uveitis or corneal infection secondary to paralysis of the eyelids. Blindness is a common and tragic complication of untreated leprosy.

Additional tissue damage in leprosy is caused by immune reactions which are due to delayed hypersensitivity (Jopling type 1 reactions) or to a vasculitis associated with the deposition of antigen–antibody complexes (Jopling type 2 reactions, *erythema nodosum leprosum*) (Table 19.9). The former, which occurs in borderline cases (BT, BB and BL), may rapidly cause severe and permanent nerve damage, and requires urgent treatment with anti-inflammatory agents and, sometimes, surgical decompression of a greatly swollen nerve.

## Laboratory diagnosis

The clinical diagnosis of leprosy may be confirmed by histological examination of skin biopsies and by the detection of acid-fast bacilli in nasal discharges, scrapings from the nasal mucosa and *slit-skin smears*. The latter are prepared by making superficial incisions in the skin, scraping out some tissue fluid and cells and making smears on glass slides. Smears

**Fig. 19.6** Lepromatous leprosy. Nodular swelling of face, enlargement of ear lobes and loss of eyebrows.

**Fig. 19.7** Treated lepromatous leprosy. The nodularity of the skin has resolved on treatment but the absence of eyebrows and the nasal collapse remain.

| 1+ | 1–10 bacilli per 100 fields |
| 2+ | 1–10 bacilli per 10 fields |
| 3+ | 1–10 bacilli per field |
| 4+ | 10–100 bacilli per field |
| 5+ | 100–1000 bacilli per field |
| 6+ | >1000 bacilli per field. |

It is widely assumed, but unproven, that leprosy bacilli that stain strongly and evenly are viable while those that stain weakly and irregularly are dead. The percentage of the former gives the *morphological index* (MI), which declines during chemotherapy. An increase in the MI is a useful indication of non-compliance of the patient and the emergence of drug resistance. The polymerase chain reaction has also been used to detect *M. leprae* in clinical specimens.

## Treatment

Until 1982, dapsone (4,4′-diaminodiphenyl sulphone; DDS) monotherapy was the standard treatment for all forms of leprosy. Unfortunately, the increasing incidence of leprosy due to dapsone-resistant bacilli made it necessary to introduce multidrug therapy based on dapsone, rifampicin and clofazimine (Table 19.10).

Clofazimine has the unfortunate property of causing skin discoloration, particularly in fair-skinned people. If this causes the patient to refuse the drug, prothionamide, ofloxacin or minocycline may be used instead.

The treatment of leprosy demands far more than the administration of antimicrobial agents. It is often necessary to correct deformities, prevent blindness and further damage to anaesthetic extremities, treat reactions with anti-inflammatory drugs and to attend to the patient's social, psychological and spiritual welfare.

are obtained from obvious lesions, the ear lobes and apparently unaffected skin. Secretions and skin smears are stained by the ZN method, and the number of bacilli seen in each high-power field is recorded as the *bacillary index* (BI):

| Table 19.9 | Main characteristics of the reactions in leprosy | |
|---|---|---|
| Characteristics | Type 1 (reversal reaction) | Type 2 (erythema nodosum leprosum) |
| Immunological basis | Cell mediated | Vasculitis with antigen–antibody complex deposition |
| Type of patient | BT, BB, BL | BL, LL |
| Systemic disturbance | No (or mild) | Yes |
| Haematological changes | No | Yes |
| Proteinuria | No | Frequently |
| Relation to therapy | Usually within first 6 months | Rare during first 6 months |
| See text for explanation of abbreviations. | | |

**Table 19.10** WHO recommendations for multidrug therapy

| Type of leprosy | Drug | Dose | Frequency | Total duration |
|---|---|---|---|---|
| Paucibacillary | Rifampicin | 600 mg | Monthly, supervised | 6 months |
| | Dapsone | 100 mg | Daily, unsupervised | |
| Multibacillary | Rifampicin | 600 mg | Monthly, supervised | 2 years or more |
| | Dapsone | 100 mg | Daily, unsupervised | |
| | Clofazimine ⎰ | 300 mg | Monthly, supervised | |
| | ⎱ | +50 mg | Daily, unsupervised | |

## Epidemiology

Until recently, leprosy was thought to be restricted to humans but the disease has been reported in chimpanzees and sooty mangabey monkeys in Africa and in free-living armadillos in Louisiana, USA. It was also thought that leprosy was transmitted by skin-to-skin contact but it now appears more likely that the bacilli are disseminated from the nasal secretions of patients with lepromatous leprosy. In addition, the blood of patients with lepromatous leprosy contains enough bacilli to render transmission by blood-sucking insects a definite, though unproven, possibility.

The infectivity of leprosy has been the subject of much misunderstanding. In olden days this disease was regarded as being highly contagious but more recently it gained a place in the *Guinness Book of Records* as the least infectious of the communicable diseases. The truth lies somewhere in between: as in the case of tuberculosis, transmission of bacilli from multibacillary patients to their contacts occurs readily, but only a minority of those infected develop overt disease. Leprosy often commences during childhood or early adult life but, as the incubation period is long, usually 3–5 years, it is rare in children aged less than 5 years.

Epidemiological studies on the prevalence and transmission of leprosy have been aided by skin test reagents, of which there are two types: *lepromins*, which are prepared from boiled bacilli-rich lepromatous lesions, and *leprosins*, which are ultrasonicates of tissue-free bacilli extracted from lesions (the suffixes -H and -A are used to denote human and armadillo origins, respectively). These reagents elicit two types of reaction. The *Fernandez reaction* is analogous to tuberculin reactivity and appears in sensitized subjects 48 h after skin testing. It is best seen with leprosins. The *Mitsuda reaction* is a granulomatous swelling which appears about 3 weeks after testing with lepromin. This reaction is indicative of the host's ability to give a granulomatous response to antigens of *M. leprae*, and is positive at or near the TT pole. Skin testing is of limited diagnostic value, but it is useful in epidemiological studies to establish the extent of infection in contacts and in the community, and in classifying patients according to the immunological spectrum.

## Control

The most effective control measure in leprosy, as in tuberculosis, is the detection and treatment of infectious cases. This requires that patients should attend for therapy as soon as signs of the disease appear. Unfortunately, owing to the stigma associated with the disease, many patients delay seeking treatment until they have infected many contacts and have developed irreversible disfigurement and handicap.

No living attenuated vaccines have been prepared for *M. leprae*, but BCG vaccine seems to protect against leprosy in those regions where it protects against tuberculosis, strongly suggesting that protection is induced by common mycobacterial antigens.

## RECOMMENDED READING

Collins C H, Grange J M, Yates M D 1997 *Tuberculosis Bacteriology: Organization and Practice*, 2nd edn. Butterworth-Heinemann, London

Davies P D O (ed) 1994 *Clinical Tuberculosis*. Chapman and Hall, London

Davies P D O, Girling D J, Grange J M 1995 Tuberculosis. In: Weatherall D J, Ledingham J G G, Warrell D A (eds) *Oxford Textbook of Medicine*, 3rd edn. Oxford University Press, Oxford, pp 638–661

Grange J M 1996 *Mycobacteria and Human Disease*, 2nd edn. Arnold, London

Heifets L B (ed) 1991 *Drug Susceptibility in the Chemotherapy of Mycobacterial Infections*. CRC Press, Boca Raton

Porter J D H, McAdam K P W J (eds) 1994 *Tuberculosis: Back to the Future*. Wiley, Chichester

Ridley D S 1988 *Pathogenesis of Leprosy and Related Diseases*. Wright, London

Waters M F R 1995 Leprosy (Hansen's disease, hanseniasis) In: Weatherall D J, Ledingham J G G, Warrell D A (eds) *Oxford Textbook of Medicine*, 3rd edn. Oxford University Press, Oxford, pp 667–679

# 20

# Environmental mycobacteria

## Opportunist disease

### J. M. Grange

In addition to the tubercle and leprosy bacilli there are many species of mycobacteria that normally exist as saprophytes of soil and water. Termed environmental mycobacteria, some species occasionally cause opportunist disease in animals and humans. Although such opportunist pathogens were described towards the end of the 19th century, their classification remained in a state of chaos for over 50 years and they were often called *anonymous mycobacteria*. Order began to replace chaos in 1959 when a botanist, Ernest Runyon, described four groups of mycobacteria associated with human disease according to their production of yellow or orange pigment and their rate of growth:

| | | |
|---|---|---|
| Group I | *Photochromogens* | – pigmentation on exposure to light |
| Group II | *Scotochromogens* | – pigmentation formed in the dark |
| Group III | *Non-chromogens* – no pigmentation | |
| Group IV | *Rapid growers*. | |

All strains in groups I, II and III grow slowly. The photochromogens are colourless when incubated in the dark, but if young cultures are exposed to a light source for an hour or more and then re-incubated they develop a bright yellow or orange coloration. The caps of the culture bottles must be loosened during exposure to light as oxygen is essential for pigment formation. Rapid growers, which may be photo-, scoto- or non-chromogens, produce visible growth on Löwenstein–Jensen medium within 1 week on subculture; the appearance of growth on primary culture of clinical material often takes considerably longer.

In 1980, 41 species of mycobacteria were included in the Approved Lists of Bacterial Names, and about 20 more have since been described. Identification is usually undertaken by specialist reference laboratories. There is no universally recognized identification scheme for mycobacteria, although reliance is usually placed on cultural characteristics (rate and tempera-

ture of growth and pigmentation), various biochemical reactions and resistance to antimicrobial agents. Some centres also use thin-layer chromatography of cell wall lipids or detection of specific antigens by sero-agglutination or immunodiffusion techniques. Nucleic acid probes are available commercially for the identification of some of the more commonly encountered species.

## CLINICAL IMPORTANCE

The principal species that cause human disease are shown in Table 20.1.

### Photochromogens

This group contains three species, *Mycobacterium*

**Table 20.1** The principal environmental mycobacteria causing human disease

| Runyon group | Species |
|---|---|
| I (photochromogens) | M. kansasii |
| | M. marinum |
| | M. simiae |
| II (scotochromogens) | M. scrofulaceum |
| | M. gordonae |
| | M. szulgai |
| III (non-chromogens) | M. avium[a] |
| | M. intracellulare[a] |
| | M. malmoense |
| | M. xenopi |
| | M. ulcerans |
| | M. terrae group[b] |
| IV (rapid growers) | M. chelonae[c] |
| | M. fortuitum |

[a]Usually grouped together as the *M. avium* complex (MAC) or as *M. avium-intracellulare*.
[b]Includes *M. nonchromogenicum* and *M. triviale*.
[c]Previously spelt *M. chelonei*.

215

*kansasii*, *M. simiae* and *M. marinum*. The first two grow well at 37°C, and are principally isolated from cases of pulmonary disease. *M. marinum*, previously termed the fish tubercle bacillus, is the cause of a warty skin infection known as swimming pool granuloma. It grows poorly or not at all at 37°C, and cultures from skin lesions should therefore be incubated at 33°C. On microscopy, *M. kansasii* and *M. marinum* are often elongated with a distinct beaded appearance.

## Scotochromogens

The principal pathogen in this group is *M. scrofulaceum* which, as the name suggests, is associated with scrofula or cervical lymphadenitis, although it also causes pulmonary disease. *M. szulgai*, an uncommon cause of pulmonary disease and bursitis, is a scotochromogen when incubated at 37°C but a photochromogen at 25°C. *M. gordonae* (formerly *M. aquae*) is a rare cause of pulmonary disease but is frequently found in water and is a common contaminant of clinical material.

## Non-chromogens

The most prevalent and important opportunistic pathogens of humans are the avian tubercle bacillus, *M. avium*, and the closely related *M. intracellulare*, formerly known as the Battey bacillus. These two species are usually grouped together as the *M. avium* complex (MAC) or *M. avium-intracellulare*. Most clinical isolates are smooth and easily emulsifiable, and 28 serotypes are delineated by agglutination by specific antisera, although untypable strains are not uncommon. In humans, this complex is responsible for lymphadenitis, pulmonary lesions and disseminated disease, notably in patients with the acquired immune deficiency syndrome (AIDS). *M. avium* causes tuberculosis in birds and lymphadenitis in pigs as well as occasional disease in various other wild and domestic animals. The *M. avium* complex is closely related to three animal pathogens: *M. paratuberculosis*, the cause of chronic hypertrophic enteritis or Johne's disease of cattle, *M. sylvaticum*, the cause of tuberculosis in wood pigeons, and *M. lepraemurium*, the cause of a leprosy-like disease of rats, mice and cats. *M. paratuberculosis* and *M. sylvaticum* produce little or no mycobactin, a lipid-soluble iron-binding compound essential for growth. Mycobactin must therefore be added to media used for the cultivation of these species.

*M. xenopi*, first isolated from a xenopus toad, is a thermophile and grows well at 45°C. It is principally responsible for pulmonary lesions, and is of limited geographical distribution. Most reported cases have been from London and south-east England and northern France. Two phenetically similar species, *M. celatum* and *M. branderi*, have been recently described.

*M. malmoense* is a cause of pulmonary disease and lymphadenitis. It grows very slowly, often taking as long as 10 weeks to appear on primary culture, and is therefore likely to be missed if cultures are not maintained for this length of time. For unknown reasons, isolations of this pathogen are increasing in number in several European countries. In some regions, notably northern England, it has become one of the most frequently isolated of the environmental mycobacteria from cases of pulmonary disease.

*M. ulcerans*, the cause of *Buruli ulcer*, is a very slowly growing species which will only grow in vitro between 31 and 34°C. Colonies are non-pigmented or a pale lemon-yellow colour. Unlike other mycobacterial pathogens, *M. ulcerans* produces a toxin which causes tissue necrosis and is involved in the pathogenesis of disease. Inoculation of *M. ulcerans* into the mouse footpad leads to progressive disease with swelling and eventual ulceration or auto-amputation. For unknown reasons, some infected mice develop generalized oedema – the 'fat mouse syndrome'.

Other rare pathogens in this group include *M. terrae* (the radish bacillus), *M. nonchromogenicum* and *M. triviale*, which are sometimes grouped as the *M. terrae* complex. *M. haemophilum*, characterized by its growth requirement for haem or other sources of iron, is a rare cause of granulomatous or ulcerative skin lesions in xenograft recipients and other immunocompromised individuals.

## Rapid growers

Only two of the rapidly growing species, *M. chelonae* and *M. fortuitum*, are well-recognized pathogens of humans. These two species were originally identified as the turtle and frog tubercle bacilli, respectively. They occasionally cause pulmonary or disseminated disease but are principally responsible for post-injection abscesses and wound infections including corneal ulcers. Both species are non-chromogenic. Some workers divide *M. chelonae* into two species, *M. chelonae* and *M. abscessus*, and likewise divide *M. fortuitum* into *M. fortuitum* and *M. peregrinum*, but this subdivision is of little clinical usefulness.

There are many other rapidly growing species of mycobacteria, most of which are pigmented. Disease due to them is exceedingly rare but they frequently contaminate clinical specimens. They are found on the genitalia, and gain access to urine samples, although, contrary to a common belief, the species *M. smegmatis* is rarely found in this site. One species, *M. vaccae*, is a powerful immunomodulator, able to down-regulate the tissue-destroying hypersensitivity reactions in tuberculosis and enhance granuloma-forming protective immunity. Extensive clinical trials of the therapeutic efficacy of an injectable heat-killed suspension of this mycobacterium as an adjunct to chemotherapy of tuberculosis are being conducted.

## Non-cultivable or very poorly growing species

A few species, mostly isolated from the blood of patients with AIDS are either non-cultivable, or grow very poorly in certain liquid media. These have been classified according to unique base sequences in their 16S ribosomal RNA, and include *M. genavense*, *M. confluentis*, *M. intermedium* and *M. interjectum*.

## ECOLOGY AND EPIDEMIOLOGY

Mycobacteria are widely distributed in the environment and are particularly abundant in wet soil, marshland, streams, rivers and estuaries. Some species, such as *M. terrae*, are found in soil while others, including *M. marinum* and *M. gordonae*, prefer free water. Some potential pathogens, notably *M. avium*, *M. kansasii* and *M. xenopi*, are able to colonize piped-water supplies. Human beings are therefore regularly exposed to mycobacteria as a result of drinking, washing, showering and inhalation of natural aerosols. Such repeated subclinical infection may induce sensitization to tuberculin and other mycobacterial skin-testing reagents. There is also evidence that contact with environmental mycobacteria profoundly affects the subsequent ability of BCG (bacille Calmette–Guérin) vaccine to induce protective immunity, thereby explaining the great regional differences in the efficacy of this vaccine.

Compared with tubercle bacilli, environmental mycobacteria are of low virulence and, although humans are frequently infected by them, overt disease is very uncommon except in those who are profoundly immunodeficient. The incidence and type of disease in any region are determined by the species and numbers of mycobacteria in the environment and the opportunities for their transmission to humans.

Unlike tuberculosis, person-to-person transmission of opportunist mycobacterial disease rarely, if ever, occurs. Thus the incidence of such disease is independent of that of tuberculosis and unaffected by public health measures designed to control the latter. In countries where tuberculosis is uncommon, the opportunist mycobacterial infections are relatively common. In south-east England, about 5% of mycobacterial disease is due to environmental species; the proportion is much higher in some parts of the USA. In addition, the absolute incidence is increasing as a result of the growing number of immunocompromised individuals, notably patients with AIDS.

A number of 'epidemics' of falsely diagnosed mycobacterial pulmonary disease and urinary tract infection have resulted from the collection of sputum and urine specimens in containers rinsed out with water from taps colonized by mycobacteria. Inadequate cleaning of endoscopes has also led to mycobacterial contamination of clinical specimens and diagnostic confusion. Likewise, false-positive sputum smear examinations for acid-fast bacilli have occurred when staining reagents were prepared from contaminated water.

## DISEASE DUE TO ENVIRONMENTAL MYCOBACTERIA

Four main types of opportunist mycobacterial disease of humans have been described: skin lesions

**Table 20.2** Principal types of opportunist mycobacterial disease in man and the usual causative agents

| Disease | Usual causative agent |
| --- | --- |
| Lymphadenopathy | *M. avium* complex |
| | *M. scrofulaceum* |
| Skin lesions | |
| Post-trauma abscesses | *M. chelonae* |
| | *M. fortuitum* |
| | *M. terrae* |
| Swimming pool granuloma | *M. marinum* |
| Buruli ulcer | *M. ulcerans* |
| Pulmonary disease | *M. avium* complex |
| | *M. kansasii* |
| | *M. xenopi* |
| | *M. malmoense* |
| Disseminated disease | |
| AIDS related | *M. avium* complex |
| | *M. genevense* |
| Non-AIDS related | *M. avium* complex |
| | *M. chelonae* |

following traumatic inoculation of bacteria, localized lymphadenitis, tuberculosis-like pulmonary lesions and disseminated disease (Table 20.2).

## Lymphadenitis

This is caused by a number of different species which vary in relative frequency from region to region. In the USA, *M. scrofulaceum* is common while in the UK the *M. avium complex* is the predominant cause. In most cases a single node, usually a tonsillar node, is involved, and the majority of patients are children aged less than 5 years. Excision of the node, usually performed for diagnostic purposes, is almost always curative. The incidence of this disease has increased in England since 1990, but it is not clear whether this is a real increase or merely due to a greater diagnostic awareness of mycobacterial disease. Lymphadenitis occasionally occurs as part of a more disseminated infection, particularly in individuals with AIDS.

## Skin lesions

Three main types have been described: post-injection (and post-traumatic) abscesses, swimming pool granuloma and Buruli ulcer.

## Post-injection abscesses

These are usually caused by the rapidly growing pathogens *M. chelonae* and *M. fortuitum*. Abscesses occur sporadically, particularly in the tropics, or in small epidemics when batches of injectable materials are contaminated by these bacteria. Abscesses develop within a week or so or up to a year or more after the injection. They are painful and may become quite large – up to 8 or 10 cm in diameter – and may persist for many months. Treatment is by drainage with curettage or total excision. Chemotherapy is not required unless there is local spread of disease or multiple abscesses, as may occur in insulin-dependent diabetics.

More serious lesions, also usually due to *M. chelonae* and *M. fortuitum*, have followed surgery, usually those procedures involving insertion of prostheses such as heart valves, and corneal infections have followed ocular injuries. Infections by *M. terrae* have occurred in farmers and others who have been injured while working with soil.

## Swimming pool granuloma

This is also known as *fish tank granuloma* and *fish fancier's finger*, and is caused by *M. marinum*. As suggested by the names, most of those affected are users of swimming pools, keepers of tropical fish and others involved in aquatic hobbies. The bacilli enter scratches and abrasions and cause warty lesions similar to those seen in skin tuberculosis. The lesions, which usually occur on the knees and elbows of swimmers and on the hands of aquarium keepers, are usually localized but secondary lesions sometimes appear along the line of the dermal lymphatics. This is termed *sporotrichoid spread* as a similar phenomenon occurs in the fungus infection sporotrichosis. The disease is usually self-limiting although chemotherapy with minocycline, co-trimoxazole or rifampicin with ethambutol hastens its resolution.

## Buruli ulcer

This disease, caused by *M. ulcerans*, was first described in Australia, but the name is derived from the Buruli district of Uganda where a large outbreak of the disease was extensively investigated. Buruli ulcer occurs in several tropical countries, notably Nigeria, Ghana, Zaire, Mexico, Malaysia and Papua New Guinea, and is limited to certain localities which, characteristically, are low-lying marshy areas subject to periodic flooding. Although never isolated from the environment, there is strong evidence that *M. ulcerans* is a free-living species that is introduced into the human dermis by minor injuries, particularly by spiky grasses.

The first manifestation of the disease is a hard cutaneous nodule which is often itchy. This enlarges and develops central softening and fluctuation due to necrosis of the underlying adipose subcutaneous tissues caused by a toxin. The overlying skin becomes anoxic and breaks down, the liquefied necrotic contents of the lesion are discharged and one or more ulcers with deeply undermined edges are thereby formed (Fig. 20.1). At this stage the lesion is teeming with acid-fast bacilli, there is no histological evidence of an active cell-mediated immune response and the patient does not react to burulin, a skin test reagent prepared from *M. ulcerans*. During this anergic stage the lesion may progressively extend to an enormous size, sometimes involving an entire limb or a major part of the trunk.

For unknown reasons, the anergic phase eventually gives way to an immunoreactive phase when a granulomatous response develops in the lesion, the acid-fast bacilli disappear and the patient reacts to burulin. Healing then occurs but the patient is often left with considerable disfigurement and disability due to extensive scarring and contractures.

**Fig. 20.1** Buruli ulcer. Undermined ulcer overlying the biceps and swelling of the surrounding tissues. (By courtesy of Dr Alan Knell, Wellcome Tropical Institute.)

The early, pre-ulcerative, lesions are easily treatable by excision and primary closure by suture. Ulcerated lesions require excision and skin grafting. In the anergic phase, the excision must be extensive enough to remove all disease in order to avoid recurrences. Therapy with rifampicin and clofazimine has been attempted but with unconvincing results.

## Pulmonary disease

This is most frequently seen in middle-aged or elderly men with lung damage due to smoking or exposure to industrial dusts. It also occurs in individuals with congenital or acquired immune deficiencies, malignant disease and cystic fibrosis, but a substantial minority of cases occur in persons with no apparent underlying localized or generalized disorder. The disease may be caused by many species, but the most frequent are the *M. avium* complex and *M. kansasii*. There are no clinical or radiological characteristics that reliably differentiate opportunist mycobacterial disease from tuberculosis, and the diagnosis is therefore made by isolation and identification of the pathogen. Great care must, however, be taken to differentiate true disease from transient colonization or superinfection. As a general rule, a diagnosis of opportunist mycobacterial disease may be made when a heavy growth of the pathogen is repeatedly isolated from the sputum of a patient with compatible clinical and radiological features and in whom other causes of these features have been carefully excluded.

## Disseminated disease

Up to a half of all individuals dying of AIDS in the USA have disseminated mycobacterial disease, almost always due to the *M. avium* complex. Such disease also occurs in Europe but is uncommon in Africa. The source of the causative organisms is uncertain: some workers consider that disease is due to reactivation of dormant foci of infection acquired in childhood whereas others argue that they result from recent infection from the environment, but these explanations are not mutually exclusive. For unknown reasons, the serotypes of the *M. avium* complex causing human immunodeficiency virus (HIV)-related disease are more restricted than those causing non HIV-related disease and are those corresponding to *M. avium* rather than *M. intracellulare*. Acid-fast bacilli are readily isolated from bone marrow aspirates, intestinal biopsies, blood and faeces. Such disease occurs in those who are profoundly immunosuppressed and who survive, on average, only 7 months from the time of diagnosis. Although treatment is unlikely to prolong life and to completely eradicate the disease, it certainly increases the quality of life. A few cases of AIDS-related

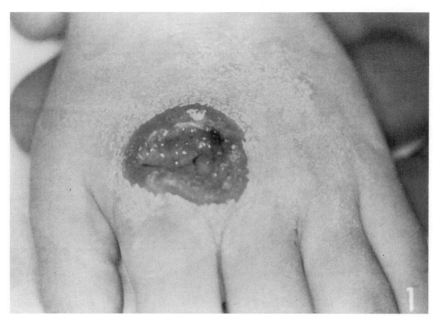

**Fig. 20.2** Skin ulcer on the dorsum of the hand due to disseminated *M. chelonae* in an immunocompromised child. (By courtesy of Dr Kurt Schopfer.)

disseminated disease have been caused by other species, including *M. genavense*.

Disseminated disease occasionally occurs in individuals with other congenital or acquired causes of immunosuppression, including renal transplantation. Again, the *M. avium* complex is the usual cause, but disseminated *M. chelonae* infections have occurred in recipients of renal transplants and in other immunocompromised patients (Fig. 20.2).

Chronic, localized non-pulmonary lesions, usually in the kidney or bone, caused by various species and with no evident predisposing cause have been described but they are extremely uncommon.

## TREATMENT

Most environmental mycobacteria are resistant to many antituberculosis drugs in vitro although infections often respond to various combinations of these drugs. Regimens containing five or six antituberculosis drugs have been used for pulmonary disease due to the *M. avium* complex, *M. kansasii*, *M. xenopi* and *M. malmoense*, but equal success has been obtained with standard triple therapy –

rifampicin, isoniazid and ethambutol – provided that all three drugs are given for up to 18 months. Treatment is, however, unsuccessful in a substantial minority of cases, and localized lesions are surgically excised when possible. Limited experience indicates that the newer macrolides may be efficacious.

Based on the results of in-vitro susceptibility tests, pulmonary and non-pulmonary disease due to the rapidly growing species *M. chelonae* and *M. fortuitum* have been treated successfully by various regimens based on one or more of the following drugs: erythromycin, sulphonamides, trimethoprim, amikacin, gentamicin, imipenem, cephalosporins and fluoroquinolones. Despite in-vitro susceptibility to antibacterial agents, some infections, notably keratitis due to *M. chelonae*, frequently relapse and require surgical intervention.

Various multidrug regimens for AIDS-associated disease due to the *M. avium* complex have been described. All regimens should include clarithromycin or azithromycin with at least two other drugs, selected, when possible on the basis of in-vitro susceptibility tests, from rifabutin, clofazimine, fluoroquinolones and ethambutol. Amikacin is added if oral regimens are ineffective.

## RECOMMENDED READING

Collins C H, Grange J M, Noble W C, Yates M D 1985 *Mycobacterium marinum* infections in man. *Journal of Hygiene* 94: 135–149

Grange J M 1996 *Mycobacteria and Human Disease*, 2nd edn. Arnold, London

Pitchenik A E, Fertel D 1992 Medical management of AIDS patients: tuberculosis and nontuberculous mycobacterial disease. *Medical Clinics of North America* 76: 121–171

Ratledge C, Stanford J L, Grange J M (eds) 1989 *The Biology of the Mycobacteria, Clinical Aspects of Mycobacterial Disease.* Academic Press, London, vol 3, chs 3, 10 and 11

Salfinger M, Pfyffer G E 1994 The new diagnostic mycobacteriology laboratory. *European Journal of Clinical Microbiology and Infectious Diseases* 13: 961–979

# 21

# Actinomyces and nocardia

Actinomycosis; nocardiasis

*J. M. Grange*

Gram-positive bacteria with branching filaments that sometimes develop into mycelia are included in the rather loosely defined order Actinomycetales. Although mostly soil saprophytes, four genera, *Actinomyces*, *Nocardia*, *Propionibacterium* and *Bifidobacterium* occasionally cause chronic granulomatous infections in animals and humans. Another genus, *Streptomyces*, is an extremely rare cause of disease but is the source of several antibiotics. In addition, repeated inhalation of thermophilic actinomycetes, notably *Faenia rectivirgula* and *Thermoactinomyces* species, causes *extrinsic allergic alveolitis (farmer's lung, mushroom worker's lung, bagassosis)* in those who are occupationally exposed to mouldy vegetable matter.

## ACTINOMYCES

## DESCRIPTION

Actinomyces are branching Gram-positive bacilli. They are facultative anaerobes but they often fail to grow aerobically on primary culture. They grow best under anaerobic or micro-aerophilic conditions with the addition of 5–10% carbon dioxide. Almost all species are commensals of the mouth and have a narrow temperature range of growth around 35–37°C. They are responsible for the disease known as *actinomycosis*, which, in humans, is usually caused by *Actinomyces israelii* and *A. gerencseriae*. A further four species, *A. meyeri*, *A. naeslundii*, *A. odontolyticus* and *A. viscosus*, are very rare causes of human actinomycosis, and the last (the usual cause of actinomycotic disease in dogs) has been isolated from cases of deep caries. *A. meyeri* is sometimes encountered as part of the mixed bacterial flora of brain abscesses. *A. bovis* causes cervicofacial infections in cattle (*lumpy jaw*). Similar human disease is occasionally caused by members of the closely related

genus *Propionibacterium*, notably *P. propionicum*, and also by *Bifidobacterium dentium*.

Concomitant bacteria, notably a small Gram-negative rod, *Actinobacillus actinomycetemcomitans*, but also *Haemophilus* species, fusiforms and anaerobic streptococci, are sometimes found in actinomycotic lesions, but their contribution to the pathogenesis of the disease, if any, is unknown. *Act. actinomycetemcomitans* is a rare cause of endocarditis.

## PATHOGENESIS

Actinomycosis is a very chronic disease characterized by multiple abscesses and granulomata, tissue destruction, extensive fibrosis and the formation of sinuses. Within diseased tissues the actinomycetes form large masses of mycelia embedded in an amorphous protein–polysaccharide matrix and surrounded by a zone of Gram-negative, weakly acid-fast, club-like structures (Fig. 21.1). These clubs were once thought to consist, at least in part, of material derived from host tissue, but it now appears that they are formed entirely from the bacteria. The mycelial masses may be large enough to be visible to the naked eye and, as they are often light yellow in colour, they are called *sulphur granules*. In older lesions the sulphur granules may be dark brown and very hard due to the deposition of calcium phosphate in the matrix.

In man, the great majority of cases of actinomycosis occur in the cervicofacial region, and the jaw is often involved. The disease is endogenous in origin: dental caries is a predisposing factor, and infection may follow tooth extractions or other dental procedures. Males are affected more frequently than females, and in some regions the disease is more common in rural agricultural workers than in town dwellers, probably due to lower standards of dental care in the former.

**Fig. 21.1** Actinomycotic granule in tissue. (By courtesy of Professor R. J. Hay.)

which reveal the Gram-positive mycelia and the zone of radiating acid-fast clubs. Sulphur granules and mycelia in tissue sections are identifiable by use of fluoroscein-conjugated specific antisera. Granules for culture are washed thoroughly in saline in a tube or Petri dish, crushed in a drop of saline with a glass rod and used to inoculate brain–heart infusion agar, blood agar and either glucose broth, enriched thioglycollate broth or commercially available actinomyces broth. Cultures are incubated, both aerobically and anaerobically, with the addition of 5% carbon dioxide for up to 10 days. After incubation for several days, *A. israelii* may form so-called *spider colonies* which resemble molar teeth, and its identity may be confirmed by means of biochemical tests, staining with specific fluorescent antisera or preferably, when the equipment is available, by gas chromatography of metabolic products of carbohydrate fermentation.

Thoracic actinomycosis commences in the lung, probably as a result of aspiration of actinomyces from the mouth. Sinuses often appear on the chest wall, and the ribs and spine may be eroded. Abdominal cases commence in the appendix or, less frequently, in colonic diverticula. Pelvic actinomycosis occasionally occurs in women fitted with plastic intra-uterine contraceptive devices. 'Punch actinomycosis' is a rare infection of the hand acquired by injury of the knuckles on an adversary's teeth.

The lymphatics are not usually involved in actinomycosis but haematogenous spread to the liver, brain and other internal organs occasionally occurs. Involvement of bone is much less common in humans than in animals and is usually the result of direct extension of adjacent soft tissue lesions.

## LABORATORY DIAGNOSIS

Specimens should be obtained directly from lesions by open biopsy, needle aspiration or, in the case of pulmonary lesions, by fibre-optic bronchoscopy. Examination of sputum is of no value as it frequently contains oral actinomycetes. Material from suspected cases is shaken with sterile water in a tube. Sulphur granules settle to the bottom and may be removed with a Pasteur pipette. Granules crushed between two glass slides are used to prepare Gram- and Ziehl–Neelsen-stained films (the latter modified by using 1% sulphuric acid for decolorization),

## TREATMENT

Actinomyces are sensitive to many antibiotics, but the penetration of drugs into the densely fibrotic diseased tissue is poor. Thus, large doses are required for prolonged periods, and recurrence of disease is not uncommon. Surgical debridement reduces scarring and deformity, hastens healing and lowers the incidence of recurrences. Penicillins are frequently used: the most active being the aminopenicillins. As lesions are often concomitantly infected with β-lactamase-producing bacteria, the preferred treatment for cervicofacial disease is amoxycillin plus clavulanic acid, 2.2 g thrice daily for 1 week and 1.1 g thrice daily for a further week. Thoracic disease requires treatment for up to 4 weeks and, in severe cases, the addition of 2 g of ampicillin thrice daily. Tetracyclines are used if the patient is allergic to penicillin. Additional drugs including aminoglycosides, clindamycin and metronidazole may be required if concomitant organisms are present.

## NOCARDIA

## DESCRIPTION

The nocardiae are branched, strictly aerobic, Gram-positive bacteria which are closely related to the rapidly growing mycobacteria. Like the latter, but

**Table 21.1**  Differences between the genera *Actinomyces* and *Nocardia*

| *Actinomyces* spp. | *Nocardia* spp. |
| --- | --- |
| Facultative anaerobes | Strict aerobes |
| Grow at 35–37°C | Wide temperature range of growth |
| Oral commensals | Environmental saprophytes |
| Non-acid-fast mycelia | Usually weakly acid-fast |
| Endogenous cause of disease | Exogenous cause of disease |

unlike actinomyces, they are environmental saprophytes with a broad temperature range of growth. The properties of nocardiae and actinomycetes are compared in Table 21.1. Most species are acid-fast when decolorized with 1% sulphuric acid, but a few are not acid-fast, and some bacteriologists prefer to place these in the separate genus *Actinomadura*.

Many species of nocardiae are found in the environment, notably in soil, but opportunist disease in humans is almost always caused by *Nocardia asteroides*, so named because of its star-shaped colonies, *N. brasiliensis* and *N. caviae* (*N. otitidis-caviarum*).

*Bovine farcy*, a lymphocutaneous disease of cattle in Africa, was thought to be nocardial, but the causative agents are now known to be mycobacteria, namely *Mycobacterium farcinogenes* and *M. senegalense*.

## PATHOGENESIS

Nocardiae, principally *N. asteroides*, are uncommon causes of opportunist pulmonary disease that usually, but not always, occurs in immunocompromised individuals including those receiving corticosteroid therapy and post-transplant immunosuppressive therapy and those with the acquired immune deficiency syndrome (AIDS). Pre-existing lung disease, notably alveolar proteinosis, also predisposes to nocardial disease. The infection is exogenous, resulting from inhalation of the bacilli. The clinical and radiological features are very variable and non-specific and diagnosis is not easy. In most cases there are multiple confluent abscesses with little or no surrounding fibrous reaction and local spread may result in empyema. In some cases the disease is very chronic while in others it spreads rapidly through the lungs. Secondary abscesses in the brain and, less frequently, in other organs occur in about one-third of patients with pulmonary

**Fig. 21.2**  Actinomycotic mycetoma of the thigh, showing multiple fungating nodules and sinuses. (By courtesy of Mr R. D. Rosin.)

nocardiasis. Acute dissemination with involvement of many organs occurs in profoundly immuno-suppressed persons, notably those with AIDS.

Nocardiae, notably *N. asteroides*, also cause primary post-traumatic or post-inoculation cutaneous infections with involvement of the lymphatics. In the USA and the southern hemisphere but rarely in Europe, cutaneous infections may result in fungating tumour-like masses termed *mycetomata* (Fig. 21.2), and the causative agent is *N. brasiliensis* or, less frequently, *N. caviae*.

*Madura foot* is a chronic granulomatous infection of the bones and soft tissues of the foot resulting in mycetoma formation and gross deformity. It occurs in Sudan, north Africa and the west coast of India, principally amongst those who walk barefoot and are therefore prone to contamination of foot injuries by soil-derived organisms. A common causative organism is *Actinomadura (Nocardia) madurae*, but it is also caused by other actinomycetes including *Streptomyces somaliensis* and by fungi (see Ch. 60).

## LABORATORY DIAGNOSIS

A presumptive diagnosis of pulmonary nocardiasis may be made by a microscopical examination of sputum. In many cases the sputum contains numerous lymphocytes and macrophages, some of which contain pleomorphic Gram-positive and weakly acid-fast bacilli, and occasionally extracellular branching filaments. Nocardiae are not so easily seen in tissue biopsies stained by the Gram or modified Ziehl–Neelsen methods but they may be seen in preparations stained by the Gomori methenamine silver method.

Nocardiae grow on most standard bacteriological media in 2 days to 1 month. Suitable media include Löwenstein–Jensen medium, brain–heart infusion agar and trypticase–soy agar enriched with blood. In addition, the technique of *paraffin baiting* may be used: a paraffin wax-coated glass rod is placed in inoculated carbon-free broth. Nocardiae grow on the rod at the air/liquid interface and may be subcultured onto agar media.

Colonies of nocardiae are cream, orange or pink coloured; their surfaces may develop a dry, chalky appearance and they adhere firmly to the medium. Identification of species is not easy and is usually undertaken by reference laboratories.

## TREATMENT

The therapy of choice for all types of nocardial infections is a sulphonamide, with or without trimethoprim, for an extended period, often 3 months or more. Alternative useful agents are minocycline, amikacin and imipenem, particularly for the treatment of AIDS patients who are unable to tolerate the standard drugs. Mycetomata due to nocardiae are much easier to treat than those due to fungi. Even long-standing cases with extensive mycetoma formation respond well to chemotherapy.

## TROPHERYMA WHIPPELII

*Whipple's disease* is a multisystem disease with symptoms including diarrhoea and malabsorption, often with arthralgia and fever. Gene amplification techniques indicate that an uncultivable Gram-positive bacillus seen histologically in gut tissue is likely to be an actinomycete. The organism has been tentatively named *Tropheryma whippelii*. Empirical treatment with penicillin (with or without an aminoglycoside) and long-term doxycycline or co-trimoxazole brings clinical improvement, but the condition may relapse.

## RECOMMENDED READING

Collins C H, Yates M D, Uttley A H C 1988 Presumptive identification of nocardias in a clinical laboratory. *Journal of Applied Bacteriology* 65: 55–59

Curry W A 1980 Human nocardosis – a clinical review with selected case reports. *Archives of Internal Medicine* 140: 818–826

Gyles C L 1995 Nocardia; actinomyces; dermatophilus. In: Gyles C L, Thoen C O (eds) *Pathogenesis of Bacterial Infections in Animals.* Iowa State University Press, Ames, pp 124–132

Hay R J 1995 Nocardiosis. In: Weatherall D J, Ledingham J G G, Warrell D A (eds) *Oxford Textbook of*

*Medicine*, 3rd edn. Oxford University Press, Oxford, pp 686–687

Roberts I F, Karim Q N, Rosin R D 1988 Actinomycotic mycetoma of the thigh. *Journal of the Royal Society of Medicine* 82: 552–553

Schaal K P, Lee H-J 1995 Actinomycete infections in humans – a review. *Gene* 115: 201–211

Schaal K P 1995 Actinomycoses. In: Weatherall D J, Ledingham J G G, Warrell D A (eds) *Oxford Textbook of Medicine*, 3rd edn. Oxford University Press, Oxford, pp 680–686

Wilson K H, Wilson J A P 1995 Whipple's disease. *Current Opinion in Infectious Diseases* 8: 380–383

# 22

# Bacillus

**Anthrax; food poisoning**

*R. C. B. Slack*

Anthrax is an example of a zoonotic disease, primarily recognized in large domesticated animals, which infects man accidentally through contact with infected products. *Bacillus anthracis*, the causative organism, is of world-wide distribution and, although rare in the industrialized nations, the very name *anthrax* strikes terror in the public, evoking horrors of 'germ warfare'. It is an important and interesting disease for a number of reasons. It holds a crucial place in the history of medical microbiology because of the work of Robert Koch, who first showed that a causative organism could be isolated from the blood of infected animals, artificially grown in pure culture and then used to reproduce the disease in animals. Koch's work on anthrax led to the development of the present-day methods of isolation and identification of bacteria and to the formulation of *Koch's postulates* (see Ch. 1). Pasteur showed that animals could be actively immunized by infecting them with cultures of *B. anthracis* that had been attenuated by growth at 43°C. Anthrax is a disease in which the infection is transmitted by the spores of the bacillus, which are shed in large numbers in the terminal stages of infection. The disease is therefore unusual in that the infection is spread only from a dying or dead host and that the causative organism may survive for a long time in the environment. More recent work has elucidated the mechanism of virulence of *B. anthracis* and improved protective vaccines.

The genus *Bacillus* originally included all rod-shaped bacteria but now comprises only large, spore-forming Gram-positive bacilli which form chains and will usually grow both aerobically and anaerobically. They are common environmental organisms and are frequently isolated in laboratories as contaminants of media or specimens. *B. anthracis* is the most important pathogen of the group. *B. cereus* may contaminate food, especially rice, in large numbers and has been implicated in many episodes of food poisoning. Other species of *Bacillus* are less often incriminated as pathogens, usually in the immunocompromised.

## *BACILLUS ANTHRACIS*

### Description

*B. anthracis* is a non-motile straight, sporing bacillus, rectangular in shape and 4–8 by 1–1.5 μm in dimensions, i.e. just smaller in length than the diameter of a red blood corpuscle. The spore is oval, refractile, central in position and of the same diameter as the bacillus. The organism is a strongly Gram-positive aerobe and facultative anaerobe with a temperature range for growth of 12–45°C (optimum, 35°C); it grows on all ordinary media as typical colonies with a wavy margin and small projections, the so-called

**Table 22.1** Distinguishing properties of some important *Bacillus* species

| Property | B. anthracis | B. cereus | B. subtilis | B. stearothermophilus |
|---|---|---|---|---|
| Cell size (μm) | Large (6 × 1.5) | Large | Small (3 × 0.6) | Small |
| Motility | – | + | + | + |
| Capsule | + | – | – | – |
| Mouse pathogenicity | +++ | + | – | – |
| Anaerobic growth | + | + | – | +/– |
| Temperature for optimal growth (°C) | 35 | 30 | 37 | 55 |

*medusa head* appearance. Table 22.1 lists some of the differences between *B. anthracis* and other important members of the genus *Bacillus*.

Spores are never found in the tissues but appear when the organism is shed or grown on artificial media; they stain only with special spore-staining procedures. The spores are resistant to chemical disinfectants and heat; the spores of many strains will resist dry heat at 140°C for 1–3 h and boiling or steam at 100°C for 5–10 min. However, autoclaving at 121°C (15 lb/in² or 1 bar) destroys them in 15 min. The spores are relatively resistant to chemical agents.

## Pathogenesis

### Clinical infection

Man is relatively resistant to infection with *B. anthracis* and anthrax most commonly arises by inoculation through the skin of material from infected animals or their products. The resulting lesion of cutaneous anthrax is often described as a *malignant pustule* because of its characteristic appearance (Fig. 22.1). Coagulation necrosis of the centre of the pustule results in the formation of a dark-coloured *eschar*, which is later surrounded by a ring of vesicles containing serous fluid and an area of oedema and induration which may become extensive. In patients with severe toxic signs and widespread oedema the prognosis is poor.

Inhalation of spores in dust or wool fibres may result in respiratory anthrax: *wool-sorter's disease*. This condition carries a high mortality due to the intense inflammation, haemorrhage and septicaemia which result from the multiplication of organisms in bronchi and spread to the lungs, lymphatics and bloodstream. The production of toxins and the considerable bacterial load which rapidly occurs in the terminal septicaemic phase produce increased vascular permeability and hypotension similar to endotoxic shock.

The intestinal form of anthrax occurs among pastoralists who may be forced through poverty to eat infected animals which have been found dead. An individual may suffer after a day or so from haemorrhagic diarrhoea, and dies rapidly from septicaemia. Often these episodes occur as small outbreaks in a family or village. Because some individuals may only suffer cutaneous lesions the recognition of the microbial cause of the outbreak is easily made clinically.

### Animal infection

All mammals are suceptible, though to a varying

**Fig. 22.1** A malignant pustule in a Kenyan farmer. (By courtesy of Professor I. A. Wamola, University of Nairobi Medical School.)

degree. Guinea-pigs and mice are highly susceptible to experimental inoculation. If a guinea-pig is injected subcutaneously with pathological material containing the bacilli, or with pure cultures, the animal dies, usually within 2–3 days, showing a marked inflammatory lesion at the site of inoculation and extensive gelatinous oedema in the subcutaneous tissues. Large numbers of the bacilli are present in the local lesion, and are also profusely present in the heart blood and in the capillaries of the internal organs. They are specially numerous in the spleen (Fig. 22.2), which is enlarged and soft, giving rise to the description *splenic fever* in the ox and the German name for the organism – *Milzbrandbazillus* (spleen-destroying bacillus).

The production of anthrax in monkeys and guinea-pigs by inhalation of contaminated aerosols has also been studied experimentally. Spores deposited on the alveolar walls are taken up by phagocytes and carried to the tracheobronchial glands, which

**Fig. 22.2**    Guinea-pig spleen imprint showing typical anthrax bacilli.

become inflamed and enlarged. Infection spreads via the lymphatics to the general circulation. About 20 000 organisms can produce lethal infection if the particle size of the aerosols is less than 5 μm. The smaller particles are more likely to penetrate in the air-stream to the alveolar walls, but the lethal dose is much higher if the particles are larger. Much of the work on the aerobiology of infection has been conducted in military establishments, and many of the results have not been released in the public domain under the mistaken view that anthrax could be an effective biological weapon.

In natural conditions both wild herbivores and domesticated animals are susceptible. The condition is usually septicaemic following ingestion of contaminated pasture. The spores are ingested with coarse vegetation, which probably predisposes to trauma of the intestinal tract. Infection also occurs by inhalation of dust into the respiratory tract and, as in human disease, through skin abrasions leading to malignant pustules.

The spores germinate and the vegetative cells produce toxin, leading to the formation of gelatinous oedema and haemorrhage. In susceptible animals the bacilli resist phagocytosis and reach the lymphatics and the bloodstream. Before death the bacilli multiply freely in the blood and tissues. In resistant animals there is a more profuse leucocyte response with phagocytosis and decapsulation of the organism.

## Virulence determinants

The pathogenicity of *B. anthracis* depends on two properties not found in a saprophytic *Bacillus* spp. The most easily demonstrated is the capsule, which is unusual in being a polypeptide, of D-glutamic acid, which inhibits opsonophagocytosis. The other determinant is the plasmid-encoded toxin complex comprising three proteins, all of which are required for pathogenicity: the *protective antigen* binds the complex to receptors on the macrophage surface; after proteolysis, *oedema factor* and *lethal factor* are released and, after endocytosis, work inside the cell by blocking the adenyl cyclase pathway. The main effect of this toxin complex is to increase vascular permeability, which leads to shock. Knowledge of the biochemistry of these determinants has led to the development of protective antigen vaccines to replace the original non-encapsulated avirulent strains.

## Laboratory diagnosis

### Clinical specimens

The fully developed malignant pustule may be difficult to swab and the central necrotic area gives a poor yield. Fluid aspirated from the surrounding vesicles, when present, is more likely to yield anthrax bacilli. Specimens should be taken before antibiotic therapy has been instituted.

In laboratories unfamiliar with the disease, additional precautions for staff safety need to be organized. However, the relative ease of clinical diagnosis, given the characteristic appearance and occupational exposure, often makes laboratory confirmation superfluous.

Gram's stain may show typical large Gram-positive bacilli, and culture on blood agar yields the large, flat, greyish colonies with a characterisic swirl (the *medusa head*). Staining of films from these colonies will show long chains of Gram-positive bacilli, some containing spores. Serological diagnosis by enzyme-linked immunosorbent assay (ELISA) may be of value retrospectively, but is seldom used diagnostically.

### Confirmatory tests

Animal inoculation was used in the past to confirm that the organism was *B. anthracis*. Guinea-pigs may be inoculated subcutaneously with a suspension of bacilli. Death usually ensues within 2–3 days, and post mortem reveals numerous bacteria on cardiac puncture or impression of splenic cells (Fig. 22.2). These specimens when stained with polychrome methylene blue show large, blue bacilli surrounded by a red granular-stained capsule (*McFadyean's reaction*). This appearance is given only by *B. anthracis*.

Confirmation in vitro is also made by simple biochemical and physiological reactions (Table 22.1). Demonstration of non-motility, gelatin liquefaction, growth in straight chains and enhanced growth aerobically, as seen in the characteristic *inverted fir tree* appearance in a gelatin stab, will generally identify *B. anthracis* completely. Toxin production can be demonstrated by immunological or gene probe methods in reference laboratories.

## Environmental samples

It is occasionally necessary to isolate *B. anthracis* from potentially contaminated material such as animal hair, hides or soil. This task is particularly difficult because of the large number of non-pathogenic *Bacillus* spp. found in the environment.

## Treatment

*B. anthracis* is susceptible in vitro to a wide range of antimicrobial agents and many have been used successfully in the treatment of anthrax in man. Penicillin remains the drug of choice as β-lactamase-producing strains are rare. In contrast, penicillin resistance is common in other *Bacillus* species. This may be partly due to the fact that *B. anthracis* generally is found in remote areas where antibiotic pressures for selection of resistance is less. Most strains tested have also been found to be sensitive to macrolides, aminoglycosides, tetracyclines and chloramphenicol.

The choice of antimicrobial agent is not a limiting factor in the treatment of anthrax; a delay in initiating therapy is the main reason for failure. This is due to late presentation for medical care or, in the case of intestinal or respiratory infection, lack of specific symptoms to establish the diagnosis before an overwhelming septicaemia. In the later stages of disease, general principles applied to the management of any patient in shock are more important than antimicrobial therapy.

It has been common practice to isolate patients with anthrax because of its highly infectious reputation. In fact, human-to-human spread is extremely uncommon and appropriate antibiotics render the patient free from bacilli. In addition, actively multiplying bacteria are not as infectious as spores, which are only found in dead or dying animals.

The use of specific antiserum is not recommended presently although, in the future, immunotherapy may play an important role in the treatment of septicaemic individuals.

## Epidemiology and control

### Agricultural anthrax

Anthrax is a *zoonosis*: a disease of animals transmissible secondarily to man. The exact incidence of anthrax in humans and animals is unknown, but many countries in Africa and Asia regularly report cases to the World Health Organization. When the disease is established in livestock and pasture becomes heavily contaminated in a country, an *enzootic* focus is created. Occasionally the disease may erupt into large numbers of domestic animals with associated human cases. In this situation anthrax is *epizootic*. This occurred in the 1980s in Zimbabwe where over 9000 human cases were recorded and countless cattle died. Areas where anthrax used to be enzootic, such as much of Europe, have been able to control the disease by control of livestock, animal feeds (especially bone meal) and strict regulations on importation of animal hides.

In the UK, the disease is occasionally found in livestock, chiefly cattle, but there were only two confirmed human cases between 1991 and 1995. Sudden death in any herbivore should be treated with suspicion, and a veterinary officer summoned to examine the carcass without a post mortem. A blood slide should be taken for Gram or methylene blue staining. Under the Anthrax Order the animal must remain on the farm and be incinerated on site if found to be positive. Deep burial in quicklime was the alternative method of disposal, but the spores remain viable for many years and may subsequently contaminate pasture and infect grazing animals. Very large numbers of bacilli are present in the terminal stages of disease in animals so that widespread dissemination may occur on death. These highly infectious animals serve as a source of anthrax both by direct spread to another beast and by contamination of the environment.

When anthrax becomes established in livestock in an area, a relatively permanent enzootic focus of infection is created. Heavy contamination of soil exists in many parts of the world, and spores may be recovered many years after the last known case. Artificial contamination of an uninhabited small island (Gruinard) off the north-west coast of Scotland occurred in 1942–43 as a result of tests of a biological warfare bomb containing live anthrax spores. Subsequent sampling showed wide areas to be contaminated with spores and even by 1979 spores could still be detected in a 3 ha area of the island. It was calculated that, even if left untouched, it would not be safe to graze sheep on Gruinard for another 70 years. In the 1980s the area was decontaminated by burning the vegetation and spraying with 5% formaldehyde in sea water. By 1987 the ground was declared anthrax-free and, after reseeding, sheep were able to graze safely.

In enzootic areas, disinfection of soil is not a practical control measure, but pastures known to be heavily contaminated should not be used for grazing animals. The organism multiplies when the soil pH is greater than 6 and when early rain has been followed by a long dry spell. Control in animals depends on early diagnosis, isolation and incineration and the use of vaccines.

### Industrial anthrax

In countries where the disease is relatively rare in animals, industrial anthrax from contamination with imported materials is the commonest form of infection in man. In general, the infectivity of *B. anthracis* for man is not of a high order, and when a case occurs in a factory spores are often widely distributed in large numbers in the dust and air. Anthrax is a recognized industrial hazard which, in the UK, is notifiable to Consultants in Communicable Disease Control and to the Health and Safety Executive. There is control on the importation of animal hides and hair, which are disinfected if considered infected. Workers at risk of exposure in the leather or wool industries and veterinarians may be offered immunization routinely and antibiotic prophylaxis if exposed to a known risk.

### Immunization

Live attenuated bacilli were first used by Louis Pasteur in May 1881. In spite of great scepticism from professionals about the effectiveness of vaccination outside the laboratory, Pasteur volunteered to make a public demonstration in an area where the disease was common. The Society of Agriculture of Seine-et-Marne took up the challenge, and the experiment took place on a farm in Pouilly-le-Fort. The 25 sheep which were vaccinated with heat-attenuated live bacilli and then inoculated with virulent anthrax material resisted infection whereas 22 of 25 sheep acting as controls succumbed within 48 h. During the next few summer months, thousands of sheep, cattle and horses were vaccinated, and the mortality among domesticated animals fell dramatically. This

discovery lead to international acclaim for Pasteur and the highest award of the Légion d'Honneur.

Subsequently, the *Sterne strain* of live spore vaccine has been used for animal immunization. Live bacterial vaccines are not considered safe for man. *Alum-precipitated toxoid* has been used to immunize workers at risk of exposure. Frequent booster doses are necessary as immunity, measured by toxin antibodies, declines rapidly. New recombinant protective antigen preparations may give better immunity.

## BACILLUS CEREUS

### Description

*B. cereus* is a large Gram-positive bacillus resembling *B. anthracis*, except that it is motile and lacks the glutamic acid capsule. Like other members of the genus it is a saprophyte and frequents soil, water and vegetation. *B. cereus* closely resembles *B. anthracis* in culture, forming large, grey, irregular colonies described as *anthracoid*. Large inocula injected into laboratory animals may cause death but without the haemorrhagic appearance of anthrax and blood smears do not show the characteristic pink capsule with McFadyean's stain.

### Pathogenesis

Spores of *B. cereus* are particularly heat-resistant and most strains produce toxins. The organism is widespread in the environment and found in most raw foods, especially cereals such as rice. Most episodes of food poisoning caused by *B. cereus* are due to preformed toxin, often found in lightly cooked Chinese dishes. In such cases vomiting is the main symptom, occurring within 6 h of ingestion. Strains associated with this emetic syndrome are low molecular weight peptides which are heat- and acid-stable and can withstand intestinal proteolytic enzymes. *B. cereus* strains may also produce an enterotoxin, which is heat-labile and formed in the intestine. This causes a diarrhoeal form of food poisoning which is similar to enteritis caused by *Escherichia coli* or *Salmonella* spp. In both situations enormous numbers of organisms (up to $10^{10}$ per gram) are found in contaminated food.

### Laboratory diagnosis

If food is available for testing, and this is often not the case in investigations of gastro-enteritis, the laboratory confirmation is easy. High numbers of *B. cereus*, often $10^8$ or more per gram, in the absence of other food poisoning bacteria are sufficient to make the diagnosis. Large facultatively anaerobic Gram-positive bacilli which produce anthracoid colonies on blood agar after overnight incubation at 37°C are almost certain to be *B. cereus*. Food reference laboratories are able to confirm identification and type if necessary.

## Management and control

Both the emetic and diarrhoeal syndromes are short-lived clinical entities. Most sufferers, even those with underlying conditions, seldom come to any harm. Acute symptoms last less than 24 h and recovery on a reduced diet and fluids is rapid. There is no specific treatment and the disease may be easily prevented by proper cooling and storage of food. Ideally, all dishes should be freshly prepared and eaten. Rice, in particular, should not be stored for long periods above 10°C.

## OTHER *BACILLUS* SPECIES

*B. subtilis*, *B. pumilis* and *B. licheniformis* have been implicated in causing food poisoning similar to that due to *B. cereus*. They do not appear to form toxins, but some strains produce antibacterial peptides, like the antibiotic bacitracin, which may facilitate growth in the intestinal tract. *B. polymyxa* is the source of the antibiotic polymyxin.

*B. cereus*, *B. subtilis* and, rarely, other members of the genus may be found in wounds and tissues of immunocompromised or burned patients. These opportunist pathogens are also common contaminants of specimens and laboratory media so that the interpretation of significance is sometimes difficult. When found in numbers in otherwise sterile sites, such as blood or cerebrospinal fluid, these otherwise insignificant pathogens require specific treatment. Most strains produce abundant β-lactamase that differs from the enzyme found in staphylococci.

## Sterilization test bacilli

*B. stearothermophilus* was, until the discovery of archaebacteria in hot springs, the most heat-resistant organism known. Spores withstand 121°C for up to 12 min, and this has made the organism ideal for testing autoclaves which run on a time–temperature cycle designed to ensure the destruction of spores. Strips containing *B. stearothermophilus* are included with the material being autoclaved, and are subsequently examined by culture for surviving spores. The organism grows only at raised temperatures, typically between 50 and 60°C; there is hardly any growth below 40°C.

*B. globigi*, a red-pigmented variant of *B. subtilis*, has been used to test ethylene oxide sterilizers, and *B. pumilis* has been used to test the efficacy of ionizing radiation.

RECOMMENDED READING

Drobniewski F A 1993 *Bacillus cereus* and related species. *Clinical Microbiology Reviews* 6: 324–338
Farrar W E 1994 Anthrax: Virulence and vaccines. *Annals of Internal Medicine* 121: 379–380
Granum P E 1994 *Bacillus cereus* and its toxins. *Journal of Applied Bacteriology Symposium Supplement* 23: 61S–66S
International Workshop on Anthrax 1990 *Salisbury Medical Bulletin* 68 (Suppl)

LaForce F M 1994 Anthrax. *Clinical Infectious Diseases* 19: 1009–1014
Parry J M, Turnbull P C B, Gibson J R 1983 *A Colour Atlas of Bacillus Species*. Wolfe Medical, London
Turnbull P C B 1996 Proceedings of the International Workshop on Anthrax *Salisbury Medical Bulletin* No. 87

# 23

# Clostridium

Gas gangrene; tetanus; food poisoning; pseudomembranous colitis

*J. G. Collee*

The clostridia are Gram-positive spore-bearing anaerobic bacilli. Most of the species are saprophytes that normally occur in soil, water and decomposing plant and animal matter; they play an important part in natural processes of putrefaction. Some, such as *Clostridium perfringens* and *C. sporogenes*, are commensals of the animal and human gut. On the death of the host, these organisms and other members of the intestinal flora rapidly invade the blood and tissues, and initiate the decomposition of the corpse. A few species are opportunistic pathogens and can produce disease, among which are: *C. perfringens*, *C. septicum* and *C. novyi*, the causes of gas gangrene and other infections; *C. tetani*, the cause of tetanus; *C. botulinum*, the cause of botulism; and *C. difficile*, the cause of pseudomembranous colitis.

A subgroup of *C. perfringens* produces particularly heat-resistant spores and is associated with a form of food poisoning, but classic strains of this species which are not particularly heat-resistant can also cause food poisoning.

## GENERAL DESCRIPTION

The clostridia are typically large, straight or slightly curved rods with slightly rounded ends. Pleomorphism is common and various forms may be seen in stained smears from cultures or wounds. These include filaments or elongated cells, spindle-shaped forms (*clostridium* is Latin for 'little spindle'), and club forms. They are often Gram-variable and may appear to be Gram-negative. All produce spores and these enable the organisms to survive in adverse conditions, e.g. in soil and dust and on skin.

A few species grow in the presence of trace amounts of air and some actually grow slowly under normal atmospheric conditions, but most of the species are obligate anaerobes. Their spores do not germinate,

and growth does not normally proceed unless a suitably low redox potential ($E_h$) exists.

These organisms are biochemically active, frequently possessing both saccharolytic and proteolytic properties, though in varying degrees.

The toxins produced by the organisms of tetanus and botulism attack nervous pathways and are referred to as neurotoxins. The organisms associated with gas gangrene attack soft tissues by producing toxins and aggressins and they are referred to as histotoxic.

## CLOSTRIDIUM PERFRINGENS

This species (formerly called *C. welchii*) is commonly implicated in gas gangrene and certain types of food poisoning.

## Description

The organism is a relatively large Gram-positive bacillus (about $4$–$6 \times 1$ μm) with stubby round ends. It is capsulate and non-motile.

*C. perfringens* can be grown quickly on selective media and can be identified by the *Nagler reaction*, which exploits the action of its phospholipase on egg yolk medium; colonies are surrounded by zones of turbidity, and the effect is specifically inhibited if *C. perfringens* antiserum containing α antitoxin is present on the medium. Typical food poisoning strains produce heat-resistant spores which can survive boiling for several hours, whereas the spores of the type A strains that cause gas gangrene are inactivated within a few minutes by boiling.

## Gas gangrene

*C. perfringens* is the commonest cause of gas gangrene, although various other species of clostridia may be

**Table 23.1** Clostridia that may be associated with gas gangrene

*C. perfringens* type A
*C. septicum*
*C. novyi* type A
*C. histolyticum*
*C. sordellii*

Note: These organisms may occur alone or in combination. Gas gangrene is almost always a polymicrobial infection involving anaerobes and facultative organisms.
*C. perfringens* is most commonly involved; other clostridia not listed here are occasionally associated with gas gangrene.

implicated (Table 23.1). The disease is characterized by rapidly spreading oedema, myositis, necrosis of tissues, gas production and profound toxaemia occurring as a complication of wound infection.

The main source of the organisms is animal and human excreta, and the spores of the causative clostridia occur widely. The infection usually results from contamination of a wound with soil, particularly that of manured and cultivated land. However, it may be indirectly derived from dirty clothing, street dust, and even the air of an operating theatre if the ventilating system is poorly designed or improperly maintained. The skin often bears spores of *C. perfringens*, especially in areas of the body that may be contaminated with intestinal organisms.

## Pathogenesis of gas gangrene

Impairment of the normal blood supply of tissue with a consequent reduction in oxygen tension may allow an anaerobic focus to develop. The patient's condition may deteriorate rapidly with the development of severe shock (Fig. 23.1).

Crushing of tissue and the severing of arteries in accidental injuries; rough handling of tissue and over-zealous clamping during surgery; or shock waves from gunshot injuries may compromise the microcirculation in an extensive area of tissue and prejudice tissue perfusion. The presence of devitalized or dead tissue, blood clot, extravasated fluid, foreign bodies and coincident pyogenic infection are all factors that promote the occurrence of gas gangrene in a wound. The spores of the clostridia and their vegetative bacilli cannot readily initiate infection in healthy tissues, presumably because the $E_h$ is too high and the organisms and spores are unable to avoid destruction and clearance by phagocytosis. Predisposing host factors include debility, old age and diabetes.

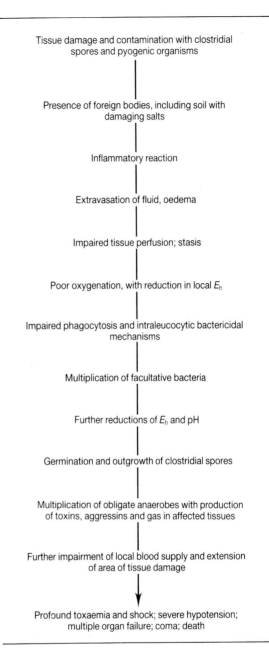

Tissue damage and contamination with clostridial spores and pyogenic organisms

↓

Presence of foreign bodies, including soil with damaging salts

↓

Inflammatory reaction

↓

Extravasation of fluid, oedema

↓

Impaired tissue perfusion; stasis

↓

Poor oxygenation, with reduction in local $E_h$

↓

Impaired phagocytosis and intraleucocytic bactericidal mechanisms

↓

Multiplication of facultative bacteria

↓

Further reductions of $E_h$ and pH

↓

Germination and outgrowth of clostridial spores

↓

Multiplication of obligate anaerobes with production of toxins, aggressins and gas in affected tissues

↓

Further impairment of local blood supply and extension of area of tissue damage

↓

Profound toxaemia and shock; severe hypotension; multiple organ failure; coma; death

**Fig. 23.1** Circumstances and events that may lead to gas gangrene.

When clostridial infection has been initiated in a focus of devitalized anaerobic tissue, the organisms multiply and produce a range of toxins and aggressins. These damage tissue by various necrotizing effects, and some have demonstrable lethal effects. They spread into adjacent viable tissue, particularly muscle, kill it and render it anaerobic and vulnerable to further colonization, with the production of more toxins and aggressins. Hyaluronidase produced by *C. perfringens* breaks down intercellular cement substance and promotes the spread of the infection along tissue planes; collagenase and other proteinases break down tissues and virtually liquefy muscles. The whole of a muscle group or segment of a limb may be affected. The principal toxin of *C. perfringens* is the α toxin, which is a phospholipase C (lecithinase). It is generally considered to be the main cause of the toxaemia associated with gas gangrene, though other clostridial species can produce similar manifestations.

In puerperal infections or in cases of septic abortion, the organisms may gain access from faeces-contaminated perineal skin or contaminated instruments to necrotic or devitalized tissues in the uterus or adnexa. Here they set up a dangerous and often fulminating pelvic infection, possibly with prompt invasion of the bloodstream. There may be intravascular haemolysis and anuria.

*C. perfringens* may also participate in peritoneal infections occurring as a result of extension of pathogens from the alimentary tract, as in cases of gangrenous appendicitis or intestinal obstruction or mesenteric thrombosis.

If a preparation of adrenalin used for injection is contaminated with clostridial spores, the combination of an infective inoculum with the local ischaemia that follows the injection may be catastrophic. Gas gangrene may be a complication of surgical operations on the lower limb or hip of a patient whose blood supply is inadequate to maintain oxygenation in the postoperative period.

It is important to appreciate that clostridia may be associated with other less severe forms of infection without the toxaemia and aggression of gas gangrene. Moreover, potentially pathogenic anaerobes may be cultivated from a wound that never shows any sign of gas gangrene, and sometimes the laboratory isolation may be attributed to the germination of a few contaminating spores when the specimen is processed. Thus, the onus is on the clinician to relate a laboratory report to the patient's circumstances.

Clinical clues include *crepitus* in the adjacent tissues; this is the sponge-cake consistency caused by small bubbles of gas. In the early stages, the patient has an anxious, frightened appearance. Local pain is increased, and there is swelling of the affected tissues. Toxaemia and shock supervene and the patient's conscious state drifts to drowsiness and into coma. Prompt diagnosis and intensive surgical and antimicrobial treatment greatly influence the patient's chance of survival and may avoid the loss

of the affected limb, but all devitalized tissue must be excised (see below).

## Laboratory diagnosis

If there are sloughs of necrotic tissue in the wound, small pieces should be transferred aseptically into a sterile screw-capped bottle and used immediately for microscopical examination and culture. Specimens of exudate should be taken from the deeper areas of the wound where the infection seems to be most pronounced. Gram smears are prepared. If gas gangrene exists, typical Gram-positive bacilli may predominate, often with other bacteria present in a mixed infection. Initiation of treatment should not await a full laboratory report, but early discussion with the bacteriologist is crucial. A direct smear of a wound exudate is often of great help in providing the evidence of the relative numbers of different bacteria that may be participating in a mixed infection or may merely be present as contaminants, but the distinction is not invariably easy and joint discussions are important.

## Treatment

Prompt and adequate surgical attention to the wound is of the utmost importance. Sutures are removed, necrotic and devitalized tissue is excised with careful debridement; fascial compartments are incised to release tension; any foreign body is found and removed. The wound is not resutured but is left open after thorough cleansing and loosely packed.

Antibiotic therapy is started immediately in very high doses. This must take account of the clostridial element and the likely coexistence of coliform organisms, Gram-positive cocci and faecal anaerobes. Accordingly, penicillin, metronidazole and an aminoglycoside may be given in combination. Alternatively, clindamycin, or a broad-spectrum β-lactam antibiotic such as cefotaxime or imipenem, may be considered. Much intensive supportive therapy is needed.

Enthusiastic claims have been made for the efficacy of hyperbaric oxygen therapy in gas gangrene. Patients are placed in a special pressurized chamber where they breathe oxygen at 2–3 atm pressure for periods of 1–2 h twice daily on several successive days. This may limit the amount of radical surgery needed, but the practice is not universally adopted.

A polyvalent antiserum used to be available in the UK for the treatment of gas gangrene; it contained *C. perfringens*, *C. septicum* and *C. novyi* antitoxins and was given intravenously. Intensive antimicrobial therapy has now replaced antitoxic therapy, and the polyvalent serum is not now recommended.

## Prophylaxis

**Surgical wounds.** C. perfringens is normally present in large numbers in human faeces, and its spores occur regularly on the skin, especially of the buttocks and thighs. As clostridial spores are very resistant to most disinfectants, they are likely to survive normal pre-operative skin preparation and spores may persist in the area of the planned incision. The numbers can be reduced by more prolonged skin preparation with the sustained action of an antiseptic such as povidone–iodine for a day or two, and this procedure has a place in orthopaedic surgery.

When inevitable skin contamination is combined with circumstances that predispose to devitalization of tissue and reduced oxygen tension, a patient may be vulnerable to the development of postoperative gas gangrene. These circumstances arise if an elderly patient or a patient with some vascular insufficiency receives major surgery to the hip or lower limb. Peri-operative antimicrobial prophylaxis with penicillin is justified in such cases.

**Accidental wounds.** The prevention of gas gangrene in accidentally sustained wounds must take account of the endogenous factors noted above and the exogenous sources of clostridial spores and vegetative forms in soil, on contaminated clothing, etc. In addition, there is an increased risk of anaerobic infection developing when foreign bodies such as soil, clothing, metal (nails, wire, bullets, shrapnel) and skin are driven into devitalized tissues. Road accidents and gunshot injuries feature in these considerations. Prompt and adequate surgical attention is of paramount importance but prophylactic administration of benzylpenicillin for patients presenting with serious contaminated wounds is also worthwhile. Many workers prefer to avoid such prophylaxis, provided that they can be absolutely sure that the local state of the wound and the patient's general condition are expertly and frequently monitored throughout the recovery period.

## C. perfringens food poisoning

C. perfringens is normally present in considerable numbers in human faeces. Carrier rates for 'typical food poisoning strains' range from about 2% to more than 30% in different groups that have been surveyed across the world. These bacteria also occur in animals; thus, meat is often contaminated with their heat-resistant spores. When meat is cooked in bulk, heat penetration is slow and subsequent cooling is slow unless special precautions are taken. The heat-resistant spores may survive and, during the cooling period, they will germinate in the anaerobic environment produced by the cooked meat and multiply. Thus, anyone who eats this will consume the equivalent of a cooked meat broth culture of the organism. The organisms are protected from the gastric acid by the protein in the meal and pass in large numbers into the intestine where they sporulate.

Ingestion of large numbers of the viable organisms is necessary for the production of the typical disease syndrome, which is mediated by an enterotoxin that is released when sporulation occurs in the gut. Typical symptoms are abdominal cramps beginning about 8–12 h after ingestion, followed by diarrhoea. Fever and vomiting are not typically encountered and symptoms generally subside within a day or two. No specific treatment is indicated. The carrier state persists for several weeks, but this should not be regarded as an indication for exclusion from any duties, since carriers may be quite numerous in various communities.

The vehicle of infection is usually a precooked meat food that has been allowed to stand at a temperature conducive to the multiplication of C. perfringens. Whilst the heat resistance of spores of typical food poisoning strains ensures their survival in cooked foods and presumably accounts for the association of these strains with most of the reported outbreaks of C. perfringens food poisoning, similar trouble can be caused by classical heat-sensitive type A strains if they gain access to food during the cooling period under conditions suitable for their subsequent multiplication.

## Laboratory diagnosis

This depends upon the isolation of similar strains of C. perfringens from the faeces of patients and from those at risk who have eaten the suspected food, and from the food itself. The isolates can be sent to a reference laboratory for special typing to prove their identity.

## Prevention

The occurrence of this type of food poisoning is an indictment of the catering practices concerned, as food has to be mishandled to allow the chain of events to take place. Nevertheless, C. perfringens food poisoning is quite common.

## C. perfringens enterotoxin-associated colitis

A sporadic diarrhoeal syndrome, usually associated with elderly patients during treatment with an antibiotic, has been described. The circumstances differ substantially from those of *C. perfringens* food poisoning. An enterotoxin with a cytopathic effect can be detected in the patient's faeces.

## Enteritis necroticans (pig-bel)

A subgroup of *C. perfringens* type C produces heat-resistant spores. This organism is the cause of a disease that affects New Guinea natives when they have pork feasts. The method of cooking the pork allows the clostridia to survive. When the contaminated meat is eaten along with a sweet potato vegetable that contains a proteinase inhibitor, a toxin (the β toxin) is able to act on the small intestine to produce a necrotizing enteritis.

## CLOSTRIDIUM SEPTICUM

### Description

This Gram-positive bacillus varies considerably in its appearance. It is generally about $4-6 \times 0.6$ μm, but shorter, longer and filamentous forms also occur. Spores are readily formed and, as they develop, various shapes arise ranging from swollen Gram-positive 'citron bodies' to obviously sporing forms in which the oval spores may be central or subterminal and are clearly bulging. Older Gram-negative cells may be seen.

The organism is actively motile with numerous peritrichous flagella. It is one of the less exacting anaerobes and grows well at 37°C on ordinary media. It is saccharolytic, and glucose promotes growth.

Surface colonies are irregular, transparent and droplet-like, later becoming greyish and opaque, with projecting radiations that are coarser than those of *C. tetani*.

An exotoxin with lethal, necrotizing and haemolytic properties, the α toxin, can be demonstrated in cultures.

### Pathogenesis

*C. septicum* is one of the gas gangrene group of clostridia. The organism also occurs in the human intestine where it is usually harmless. In some circumstances when the integrity of the gut epithelium is impaired, e.g. by leukaemic infiltration, *C. septicum* bacteraemia may occur.

Intramuscular injection of cultures in laboratory animals produces a spreading inflammatory oedema,

with slight gas formation in the tissues. The organisms invade the blood and the animal dies within a day or two. Smears from the liver show long filamentous forms and citron bodies.

### Epidemiology

The primary habitat of *C. septicum* is either the soil or the animal intestine. Areas with large numbers of spores appear to be associated with a higher incidence of *C. septicum* infections in humans and animals than less heavily infected areas.

## CLOSTRIDIUM NOVYI (C. OEDEMATIENS)

This Gram-positive bacillus resembles *C. perfringens* in morphology, but it is larger, more pleomorphic and a much more strict anaerobe; it is readily inactivated when its vegetative cell is exposed to air. It possesses peritrichous flagella, but its motility is inhibited in the presence of oxygen. The spores are oval, central or subterminal. The organism occurs widely in soil and is associated with disease in humans and animals. The *C. novyi* species includes four types – A, B, C and D – distinguished on the basis of the permutations of the toxins and other soluble antigens they produce. Only type A strains are of medical interest as they cause some cases of gas gangrene in humans.

*C. novyi* gas gangrene is associated with profound toxaemia. Culture filtrates are highly toxic and possess at least four active substances (α, β, δ and ε toxins) that account for the various haemolytic, necrotizing, lethal, phospholipase and lipase activities of this organism.

## CLOSTRIDIUM SPOROGENES

This Gram-positive motile bacillus is very widely distributed in nature, e.g. in soil and in the intestines of animals, and is generally regarded as a harmless saprophyte. It is about $6-8 \times 0.8$ μm. Gram-negative forms are frequent in older cultures. Its oval, central or subterminal spores may be highly resistant and the organism is frequently encountered in mixed cultures in the laboratory, even after preliminary heating of these cultures to select heat-resistant pathogens. Its spores may survive boiling for periods ranging from 15 min up to 6 h.

*C. sporogenes* is frequently isolated from wound exudates in association with accepted pathogens. While its presence may accelerate an established anaerobic infection by enhancing local conditions, it does not by itself cause gas gangrene and cannot be regarded as a pathogen in its own right.

## CLOSTRIDIUM TETANI

### Description

The organism generally appears by microscopy as a straight, slender rod with rounded ends. Although it is Gram-positive, Gram-negative forms are usually encountered in stained smears. The fully developed spore gives the organism the appearance of a drumstick with a large round end. The tetanus bacillus is an obligate anaerobe. It is motile and has numerous peritrichous flagella. It grows well in cooked meat broth and produces a thin spreading film when grown on enriched blood agar. The spores may be highly resistant to adverse conditions, but the degree of resistance varies with the strain. Spores of some strains resist boiling in water for up to 3 h. They may resist dry heat at 160°C for 1 h, and 5% phenol for 2 weeks or more. Iodine (1%) in water is said to kill the spores within a few hours, but this should not significantly influence clinical practice. Glutaraldehyde is one of the few chemical disinfectants that are assuredly sporicidal.

### Toxin

*C. tetani* produces an oxygen-labile haemolysin (tetanolysin), but the organism's neurotoxin (tetanospasmin) is the essential pathogenic product. Strains vary in their toxigenicity; some are fiercely toxigenic. Most strains produce demonstrable toxin after culture in broth for a few days.

Tetanospasmin has been separated as a pure crystalline protein with an estimated lethal dose for the mouse of 0.0001 μg. It is composed of a heavy chain and a light chain linked by a disulphide bond. It is toxic to humans and various animals when injected parenterally, but it is not toxic by the oral route. When tetanus occurs naturally the tetanus bacilli stay at the site of the initial infection and are not generally invasive, but the toxin diffuses to affect the relevant level of the spinal cord (local tetanus) and then to affect the entire system (generalized tetanus). These stages, including the intermediate one of 'ascending tetanus', are demonstrable in experimental animals, but the stages tend to merge in their clinical presentation in humans (see below). The toxin is absorbed from the site of its production in an infective focus and is transmitted to the central nervous system via motor nerves and apparently specifically by motor fibres. However, some toxin may be delivered from an infective focus via the blood to all nerves in the body and the subsequent transmission to the central nervous system depends upon uptake through neuromuscular nerve endings and intra-axonal transport. Thus, the tendency for the first signs of human tetanus to be in the head and neck is attributed to the shorter length of the cranial nerves. In fact, descending involvement of the nervous system is seen in humans as the tetanus toxin takes longer to traverse the longer motor nerves and the toxin also diffuses in the spinal cord.

The toxin appears to act by interfering with the normal inhibition of motor impulses exercised by the upper motor neurone over the lower, producing an increase in tonus and tonic spasms. There is a presynaptic block of inhibitory transmission in the cord, with spastic paralysis of the affected muscles as a result of activation of both agonist and antagonist groups. Interference with the synthesis of acetylcholine at presynaptic levels with the resultant loss of a critical feedback control system in the motor pathway is our present, rather inadequate, explanation of the mechanism of action of tetanus toxin.

### Occurrence of tetanus bacilli

*C. tetani* occurs in the intestine of humans and animals, but reported isolation rates are very variable. Tetanus bacilli seem to be derived primarily from animal faeces and indirectly via soil. The organism is especially prevalent in manured soil and, for this reason, a wound through skin contaminated with soil or manure deserves special attention. However, tetanus spores occur very widely and are commonly present in gardens, sports fields and roads, and in the dust and plaster and the air of hospitals and houses, on clothing and on articles of common use.

Spores of *C. tetani* and other anaerobes may be embedded in surgical catgut and other dressings, and this has been the source of infection in some cases in the past, but the sterility of surgical catgut (prepared from the gut of cattle and sheep) is now rigorously controlled.

### Pathogenesis

If washed spores are injected into an animal they fail to germinate and are removed by phagocytosis.

Germination and outgrowth of tetanus spores depend upon reduced oxygen tension in devitalized tissue and non-viable material in a wound so that the $E_h$ is significantly lowered. When infection occurs, often assisted by the simultaneous growth of facultative organisms in a mixed inoculum, the tetanus element remains strictly localized, but tetanus toxin is elaborated and diffuses as described earlier.

Conditions that favour the germination of the spores and their outgrowth are similar to those that have been discussed earlier in relation to gas gangrene (see p. 232–5).

Cases of tetanus have been reported in which the infection was apparently associated with a superficial abrasion, a contaminated splinter or a minor thorn prick. Indeed, gardening enthusiasts form one of the recognized risk groups in the UK at present.

In some cases the site of infection is assumed to be in the external auditory meatus; thus, *otogenic tetanus* may be attributable to over-zealous cleansing of the meatus with a small stick. In other patients, the site of infection remains undiscovered, and this is referred to as *cryptogenic tetanus*. Tetanus infection may also occur in or near the uterus in cases of septic abortion.

*Tetanus neonatorum* follows infection of the umbilical wound of newborn infants (see below). Cases of *postoperative tetanus* have been attributed to imperfectly sterilized catgut, dressings or glove powder, and sometimes to dust-borne infection of the wound at operation.

## Clinical features of tetanus

The onset of signs and symptoms is gradual, usually starting with some stiffness and perhaps pain in or near a recent wound. In some cases the initial complaint may be of stiffness of the jaw (*lockjaw*). Pain and stiffness in the neck and back may follow. The stiffness spreads to involve all muscle groups; facial spasms produce the 'sardonic grin', and in severe cases spasm of the back muscles produces the opisthotonos (extreme arching of the back) beloved of textbook writers. The period between injury and the first signs is usually about 10–14 days, but there is a considerable range. A severe case with a relatively poor prognosis shows rapid progression from the first signs to the development of generalized spasms. Sweating, tachycardia and arrhythmia, and swings in blood pressure reflect sympathetic stimulation, which is not well understood but creates problems of management.

## Treatment

The patient remains conscious and requires skilled sedation and constant nursing. If generalized spasms are worrying, the patient is curarized and ventilated mechanically until the toxin that has been taken up has decayed; this may take some weeks.

The patient is given 10 000 units of human tetanus immunoglobulin (HTIG) in saline by slow intravenous infusion. Full wound exploration and debridement is arranged, and the wound is cleansed and left open with a loose pack. Penicillin and metronidazole are given for as long as considered necessary to ensure that bacterial growth and toxin production are stopped. The antitoxin and the antibiotics are given immediately, and preferably before surgical excision, but delay must be avoided.

## Laboratory diagnosis

Gram smears of the wound exudate and any necrotic material may show the typical 'drumstick' bacilli, but this is not invariably so, and it is only presumptive evidence as other organisms that resemble *C. tetani* have terminal spores. Simple light microscopy is often unsuccessful; immunofluorescence microscopy with a specific stain is possible but is not generally available.

Direct culture of unheated material on blood agar incubated anaerobically is often the best method of detecting *C. tetani*. There are various other tricks that exploit the organism's motility and fine spreading growth; sometimes these are vitiated by overgrowth with *Proteus* species. Material from the wound or from a mixed sporing subculture may be heated at various temperatures and for various times to exclude non-sporing bacteria; the heated specimens are then seeded onto solid media and incubated anaerobically. Tetanus may be produced in mice by subcutaneous injection of an anaerobic culture prepared from wound material; control mice are protected with tetanus antitoxin.

## Epidemiology

Tetanus ranks among the major lethal infections. The incidence varies enormously from country to country, and it is inversely related to socio-economic development and standards of living, preventive medicine, and wound management. There is a direct relationship with fertile soil and a warm climate; thus, people living in the agricultural areas of developing tropical and subtropical countries are exposed to severe challenges associated with poor

**Table 23.2** The reported mortality from tetanus in various countries

| High incidence | | Low incidence | |
|---|---|---|---|
| Country | Mortality per 100 000 of the population | Country | Mortality per 100 000 of the population |
| Haiti | 46.2 | Italy | 0.90 |
| Malaysia | 31.4 | France | 0.78 |
| Panama | 17.7 | Japan | 0.63 |
| Nigeria | 14.6 | New Zealand | 0.45 |
| Philippines | 9.0 | Switzerland | 0.35 |
| Mexico | 6.7 | Australia | 0.33 |
| Venezuela | 6.7 | FRG | 0.30 |
| Fiji | 4.6 | USA | 0.13 |
| Kenya | 4.6 | Finland | 0.09 |
| Thailand | 4.3 | England | 0.05 |
| Sri Lanka | 4.0 | Canada | 0.03 |

From Rubbo S D 1966 New approaches to tetanus prophylaxis. *Lancet* ii: 449–453

hygiene, lack of shoes, neglect of wounds, and inadequate immunization.

In addition, some local customs promote the occurrence of tetanus; for example, treatment of the umbilical cord stump with primitive applications that include animal dung, tying of the umbilical cord itself with primitive ligatures, and ear-piercing and other operations done with unsterile instruments.

In general, and with the exception of neonatal tetanus, which carries a very high mortality, fatality rates range up to 50 or 60%. Case fatality rates can be greatly reduced to less than 10% by modern methods of treatment in specialist centres. Unfortunately, such expensive skilled help is available for only a small proportion of patients; under-privileged people in countries with poorly developed medical services or expensive medical service arrangements are at greatest risk and are least likely to get sophisticated assistance (Table 23.2).

## Prevention and control

Prompt and adequate wound toilet and proper surgical debridement of wounds are of paramount importance in the prevention of tetanus. There is an increased risk that tetanus spores may germinate in a wound if cleansing is delayed and if sepsis develops. Clean superficial wounds that receive prompt attention may not require specific protection against tetanus and it is unreasonable to insist that every small prick or abrasion requires protection with antitoxin or antibiotic.

Routine practice should take account of the local incidence of tetanus and the individual circumstances of the case. It is wise to recommend specific pro-phylaxis for a non-immunized patient with a deep wound, puncture or stab wound, ragged laceration, a wound with much bruising and any devitalized tissue, a wound that is already septic, or a bite wound or other type of wound that is likely to be heavily contaminated. Figure 23.2 shows an approach that reflects current thinking in the UK.

The need for passive immunization is avoided if the patient is known to be properly immunized against tetanus (see Ch. 68).

A patient may be regarded as immune for 6 months after the first two injections, or for 5–10 years after a planned course of three injections (or a subsequent booster injection) of adsorbed tetanus toxoid (see Ch. 68). Tetanus antitoxin should not be given to immune patients, but their active immunity may be enhanced when necessary by giving a dose of tetanus toxoid at the time of injury if the circumstances justify it.

A patient is considered non-immune if there is no history of having had an injection of tetanus toxoid or if only one injection has been given. Take care: a patient may recall having had 'a tetanus shot', but this may have been a previous dose of antitoxin for passive protection (which is transient and cannot be boosted by toxoid). If more than 6 months have elapsed after a course of two injections, or more than 10 years after a full primary course of three injections of adsorbed toxoid (or a booster injection), the patient should be regarded as non-immune. A patient is non-immune if more than 2–3 weeks have elapsed since a previous injection of equine antitoxin, or more than 6–8 weeks in the case of homologous (human) antitoxin. Non-immunity should be assumed if there is any doubt about the immunization history.

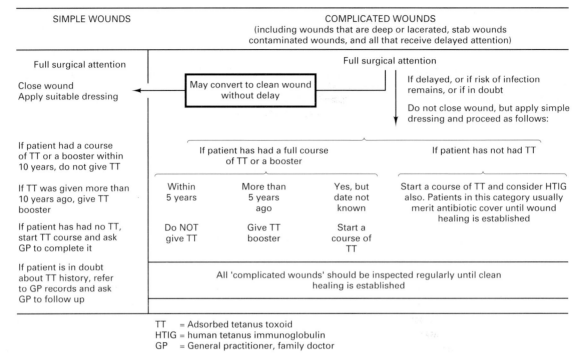

| SIMPLE WOUNDS | COMPLICATED WOUNDS<br>(including wounds that are deep or lacerated, stab wounds<br>contaminated wounds, and all that receive delayed attention) | | |
|---|---|---|---|

Full surgical attention

Close wound
Apply suitable dressing

May convert to clean wound without delay

Full surgical attention

If delayed, or if risk of infection remains, or if in doubt

Do not close wound, but apply simple dressing and proceed as follows:

If patient had a course of TT or a booster within 10 years, do not give TT

If TT was given more than 10 years ago, give TT booster

If patient has had no TT, start TT course and ask GP to complete it

If patient is in doubt about TT history, refer to GP records and ask GP to follow up

If patient has had a full course of TT or a booster

If patient has not had TT

| Within 5 years | More than 5 years ago | Yes, but date not known | Start a course of TT and consider HTIG also. Patients in this category usually merit antibiotic cover until wound healing is established |
|---|---|---|---|
| Do NOT give TT | Give TT booster | Start a course of TT | |

All 'complicated wounds' should be inspected regularly until clean healing is established

TT    = Adsorbed tetanus toxoid
HTIG = human tetanus immunoglobulin
GP    = General practitioner, family doctor

**Fig. 23.2**   Wound management guidelines, with special reference to the prevention of tetanus.

## Passive immunization with antitoxin

Human tetanus immunoglobulin (HTIG) (homologous antitoxin) is available for passive protection and now supersedes equine antitoxin (heterologous antitoxin), which has been associated with occasional adverse reactions in the past. However, equine antiserum should not be prematurely discarded in countries that do not yet have HTIG. The prophylactic dose of HTIG is 250–500 units by intramuscular injection.

## Combined active–passive immunization

A non-immune patient receiving passive protection with HTIG after injury may be given the first dose of a course of active immunization with adsorbed toxoid at the same time, provided that the injections are given from different syringes and into contralateral sites. The active immunization course must be subsequently completed.

## Antibiotic protection

The prophylactic administration of antibiotics to all cases of open wounds is not recommended, but the use of penicillin or erythromycin or an oral cephal-osporin is justified in some cases when there may be a significant risk of infection. This precaution must not replace prompt and adequate sugical wound toilet.

# CLOSTRIDIUM BOTULINUM

## Description

*C. botulinum* is a strictly anaerobic Gram-positive bacillus (about $5 \times 1$ μm). It is motile with peritrichous flagella. Its spores are oval and subterminal. It is a widely distributed saprophyte occurring in soil, vegetables, fruits, leaves, silage, manure, the mud of lakes, and sea mud. Its optimum growth temperature is about 35°C, but some strains have been shown to grow and to produce toxin at temperatures as low as 1–5°C.

The widespread occurrence of *C. botulinum* in nature, its ability to produce a potent neurotoxin in food, and the resistance of its spores to inactivation combine to make it a formidable pathogen of humans and a range of animals and birds. Spores of some strains withstand boiling in water (100°C) for several hours. They are usually destroyed by moist heat at 120°C within 5 min. Spores of type E strains (see below) are usually much less heat-resistant. Insufficient heating in the process of preserving foods is an important factor in the causation of botulism, and great care must be taken in canning factories to ensure that adequate heating is achieved in all parts of the can contents. The resistance of the spores to radiation is of special relevance to food processing.

## Toxins of *C. botulinum*

Botulinal toxins are among the most poisonous natural substances known. Seven main types of *C. botulinum* designated A–G produce antigenically distinct toxins with pharmacologically identical actions. Types A, B and E are those most frequently associated with human disease, but all types can cause disease in humans. The importance of this point is that, if antitoxin is given to a patient in an emergency, only the type-specific antitoxin will be effective.

## Human botulism

Botulism is a severe, often fatal, form of food poisoning characterized by pronounced neurotoxic effects. The disease has been caused by a wide range of foods, usually preserved hams, large sausages of the German variety, home-preserved meats and vegetables, canned products such as fish, liver paste, and even hazelnut purée and honey. Traditional dishes such as fish or seal's flipper fermented in a barrel buried in the ground cannot be recommended by a bacteriologist! Type E strains are particularly but not invariably associated with a marine source, whereas type A and type B strains are usually associated with soil.

Foods responsible for botulism may not exhibit signs of spoilage. The preformed toxin in the food is absorbed from the intestinal tract. Although it is protein, it is not inactivated by the intestinal proteolytic enzymes. The toxin primarily affects the cholinergic system and seems to block release of acetylcholine, chiefly at points in the peripheral nervous system.

## Clinical features

The period between ingestion of the toxin and the appearance of signs and symptoms is usually 1–2 days, but it may be much longer. There may be initial nausea and vomiting. The oculomotor muscles are affected and the patient may have diplopia and drooping eyelids with a squint. There may be vertigo and blurred vision.

There is progressive descending motor loss with flaccid paralysis but with no loss of consciousness or sensation, though weakness and sleepiness are often described. The patient is thirsty, with a dry mouth and tongue. There are difficulties in speech and swallowing, with later problems of breathing and despair. There may be abdominal pain and restlessness. Death is due to respiratory or cardiac failure.

### Wound botulism

Rare cases of wound infection with *C. botulinum* resulting in the characteristic signs and symptoms of botulism have been recorded.

### Infant botulism

The 'floppy child syndrome' describes a young child, usually less than 6 months old, with flaccid paralysis that is ascribed to the growth of *C. botulinum* in the intestine at a stage in development when the colonization resistance of the gut is poor. There are various grades of the syndrome. Some of the cases recorded in the literature have been attributed to the presence of *C. botulinum* spores in honey; when the honey was given as an encouragement to feed, the spores were ingested and were able to germinate and produce toxin in the infant gut.

## Laboratory diagnosis

The organism or its toxin may be detected in the suspected food, and toxin may be demonstrated in the patient's blood by toxin–antitoxin neutralization tests in mice. Samples of faeces or vomit may also yield such evidence. Take care: bear in mind that botulinal toxin is very dangerous – specialist help should be summoned and the laboratory alerted.

## Treatment

The priorities are: (1) to remove unabsorbed toxin from the stomach and intestinal tract; (2) to neutralize unfixed toxin by giving polyvalent antitoxin (with due precautions to avoid hypersensitivity reactions to the heterologous antiserum); and (3) to give relevant intensive care and support.

## Control

Home canning of foodstuffs should be avoided, and commercial canning must be strictly controlled. The amateur preservation of meat and vegetables, especially beans, peas and root vegetables, is dangerous in inexperienced hands. Acid fruits may be bottled safely in the home with heating at 100°C, since a low pH is inhibitory to the growth of *C. botulinum*.

A prophylactic dose of polyvalent antitoxin should be given intramuscularly to all persons who have eaten food suspected of causing botulism. Active immunity in humans can be produced by injecting three doses of mixed toxoid at intervals of 2 months, but the very low incidence of the disease under normal conditions does not justify this as a routine. Active immunization should be considered for laboratory staff who might have to handle the organism or who might have to handle specimens containing the organism or its toxin.

## CLOSTRIDIUM DIFFICILE

### Description

*C. difficile* is a motile Gram-positive rod with oval spores. It occurs quite commonly in the faeces of neonates, but it is not generally regarded as a normal commensal of adults. The organism produces an enterotoxin (toxin A) and a cytotoxin (toxin B).

### Pathogenesis

This organism has a direct relationship with pseudomembranous colitis. There is almost always, but not invariably, a history of prior antibiotic therapy. The lincosamide antibiotics have a special association, but ampicillin and cephalosporins are also high in the league table of incriminated drugs

and there is virtually no antibiotic that has escaped blame. Evidence often suggests that the organism may be acquired from an exogenous source by a patient whose intestinal colonization resistance has been compromised in some way. The condition may be lethal if it is not quickly recognized and treated.

### Laboratory diagnosis

*C. difficile* can be isolated from the faeces by enrichment and selective culture procedures. Toxin can be detected in the patient's faeces by testing extracts against cell monolayers of human embryo fibroblasts or other susceptible cells or by immunological methods, e.g. enzyme-linked immunosorbent assay (ELISA).

### Treatment

It is essential to discontinue the antibiotic that is presumed to have precipitated the disease and to suppress the growth and toxin production of *C. difficile* by giving oral vancomycin or metronidazole.

### Prevention

Clinical awareness is the keynote. If a patient develops unexplained diarrhoea, especially if this is antibiotic-associated, the possibility of *C. difficile* and pseudomembranous colitis should be borne in mind. If several cases occur in a hospital unit, the possibility of cross-infection should be considered and the existing antibiotic policy of the unit should be reviewed.

RECOMMENDED READING

Brazier J S 1995 The laboratory diagnosis of *Clostridium difficile*–associated disease. *Reviews in Medical Microbiology* 6: 236–245
Collee J G, van Heyningen S 1991 Systemic toxigenic diseases (tetanus, botulism). In: Duerden B I, Drasar B S (eds) *Anaerobes in Human Disease*. Arnold, London, pp 372–394
Hatheway C L 1990 Toxigenic clostridia. *Clinical Microbiology Reviews* 3: 66–98
Hobbs B C, Roberts D 1993 *Food Poisoning and Food Hygiene*, 6th edn. Arnold, London

Sakurai J 1995 Toxins of *Clostidium perfringens*. *Reviews in Medical Microbiology* 6: 175–185
Smith J W G, Collee J G 1990 Tetanus. In: Parker M T, Collier L H (eds) *Topley and Wilson's Principles of Bacteriology, Virology and Immunity. Bacterial Diseases* (Smith G R, Easmon C S F, vol eds), 8th edn. Edward Arnold, London, vol 3, pp 331–351
Willis A T, Phillips K D 1983 *Anaerobic Infections. Public Health Laboratory Service Monograph Series 3*, 2nd edn. Her Majesty's Stationery Office, London

# 24

# Neisseria and moraxella (branhamella)

**Meningitis; gonorrhoea; respiratory infections**

*R. J. Fallon and R. C. B. Slack*

Neisseriae are Gram-negative diplococci, of which the pathogenic members, the meningococcus and the gonococcus, are characteristically found inside the polymorphonuclear pus cells of the inflammatory exudate. Although difficult to differentiate on morphological and cultural characters, these two pathogens are associated with entirely different diseases. *Neisseria meningitidis* is the cause of a range of diseases (Table 24.1); acute purulent meningitis (variously called *epidemic cerebrospinal meningitis, cerebrospinal fever* or, because of a purpuric rash which is sometimes present, *spotted fever*) and an acute septicaemic illness with a petechial rash, but without meningitis, are the commonest. About one-third of cases of meningococcal disease present as septicaemia, most others being of meningitis. The term *meningococcal infection* embraces these and other syndromes associated with the organism.

*N. gonorrhoeae* is the cause of the sexually transmitted disease *gonorrhoea*. This commonly presents as a purulent infection of the mucous membrane of the urethra and also the cervix uteri in the female; there may be rectal or pharyngeal infection, and secondary local and metastatic complications, e.g.

epididymitis, salpingitis and arthritis, may occur if the primary infection is not promptly treated. In the newborn the gonococcus may give rise to a purulent conjunctivitis, *ophthalmia neonatorum*, and in young girls a vulvovaginitis. Disseminated gonococcal infection, which is recognized by a rash and evidence of blood spread, may also occur, more commonly in women.

The non-pathogenic or potentially pathogenic members of the genus are common commensals of the upper respiratory tract, which is also the reservoir of the meningococcus. The gonococcus may occasionally be isolated from this site. *N. lactamica* and *N. polysacchareae*, two species of uncertain taxonomic status, have been isolated frequently from the nasopharynx during meningococcal surveys. These organisms have a cultural resemblance to the meningococcus and will grow on selective media, unlike the classical nasopharyngeal commensals. Although similar to the meningococcus in culture, these two neisseriae are of low pathogenicity; *N. lactamica* is occasionally isolated from blood or cerebrospinal fluid (CSF). Additional commensal species include *N. subflava* (of which there are several

**Table 24.1** Clinical manifestations of meningococcal infection

| Site of infection[a] | Common manifestation | Outcome |
|---|---|---|
| Blood | Fulminant septicaemia (Waterhouse–Friderichsen syndrome) | Fatal |
| Blood | Septicaemia, purpuric rash | Mortality 14–50% |
| Blood and CSF | Septicaemia, rash and meningitis | |
| Blood and CSF | Meningitis with no rash | Mortality 2–6% |
| Blood | Chronic meningococcal septicaemia (rash, arthralgia, metastatic sepsis) | Recovery with treatment |
| Blood and site of sepsis | Arthritis, pericarditis, metastatic sepsis | Recovery with treatment |
| Eye | Conjunctivitis | Recovery with treatment |
| Genital tract | Asymptomatic carriage; rarely vulvovaginitis (children), urethritis, proctitis | Recovery with treatment |
| Chest | Pneumonia | Recovery with treatment |

CSF, cerebrospinal fluid.
[a]In most cases of clinical disease the organism is also carried in the nasopharynx.

biovars), *N. sicca*, *N. mucosa* and *N. flavescens*. Two others, *N. elongata* and *N. weaveri* are unusual in being rod-shaped.

Moraxellae are non-fermentative organisms that may be rod-shaped or coccoid. There is still uncertainty as to their taxonomic position. Some strains resemble *Acinetobacter* spp. and other glucose non-fermenters (see Ch. 29). The most important member of the group, *Moraxella catarrhalis* (*Branhamella catarrhalis*), is a common commensal of the upper respiratory tract which may give rise to disease, usually as an opportunist pathogen.

## NEISSERIA

## Description

The two pathogenic neisseriae, *N. meningitidis* and *N. gonorrhoeae*, are very similar in their morphological and cultural characters. They are Gram-negative, oval cocci occurring in pairs with the apposed surfaces flat or even slightly concave (bean shaped) and with the axis of the pair parallel and not in line as in the pneumococcus. In pus from inflammatory exudates, such as CSF or urethral discharge, many diplococci are found in a small proportion of the polymorphonuclear cells. This is more marked with the gonococcus than with the meningococcus. Extracellular cocci also occur and there may be considerable variation in their size and intensity of staining. In cultures the diplococcal arrangement is less obvious and more coccoid forms may be seen in stained films. Faintly staining involution forms are frequent in older cultures.

## Growth requirements

Pathogenic neisseriae are exacting in their growth requirements due, in part, to susceptibility to inhibitory substances in the culture medium. The addition of heated blood or ascitic fluid, or both, to nutrient agar ensures a good growth of colonies from infected material, provided incubation is carried out, preferably at 35–36°C, in a moist atmosphere containing 5–10% carbon dioxide. Growth is rather slow (more so with the gonococcus) but, on a good medium, grey, glistening, slightly convex colonies of 0.5–1.0 mm in diameter appear in 8–24 h. Incubation should, however, be continued for another 24 h, when the colonies will be much larger (2–3 mm), with the gonococcus in particular having a slightly roughened surface and a tendency to crenation of the margins. Gonococci have been divided into four types by Kellogg according to colonial appearance, auto-agglutinability and virulence, as demonstrated by the induction of urethritis in human volunteers. The more virulent strains (Kellogg types T1 and T2) bear numerous fimbriae, whereas the avirulent forms (Kellogg types T3 and T4) are non-fimbriate. Both meningococci and gonococci may bear fimbriae. The relationship between these and disease due to the meningococcus is uncertain but gonococcal fimbriae appear to be associated with attachment of the organism to mucosal surfaces and resistance to killing by phagocytic cells.

Colonies of meningococci and gonococci react quickly in the test for cytochrome oxidase; colonies of non-pathogenic neisseriae react more slowly. Species identification depends on carbohydrate utilization reactions: the meningococcus produces acid from glucose and maltose, although strains may be encountered which ferment only one of these sugars; the reactions may be slow and sometimes occur only after several subcultures. The gonococcus produces acid from glucose only. Neither species ferments lactose or sucrose.

Most strains of *N. lactamica* grow on ordinary serum-free culture medium and produce acid from glucose, maltose and, under optimum conditions, lactose, but not sucrose or fructose. It can be differentiated from the pathogenic neisseriae by its positive reaction in the *o*-nitrophenyl-β-galactoside (ONPG) test for β-galactosidase.

### Serological classification

Meningococci are divisible into three main serogroups: A, B and C. Group A is, in most countries, the serogroup associated with epidemic cerebrospinal meningitis. The ability to cause epidemics seems to be associated with certain genetically defined clones of the organism. Group C strains have been associated with epidemics but more commonly give rise to local outbreaks, while group B meningococci are seen in both epidemic and outbreak situations. Of other serogroups associated with disease (X, Y, Z, 29E (Z') and W-135), W-135 is isolated most frequently in the UK. A few cases due to serogroups X and Y also occur, but disease due to meningococci of serogroups Z and 29E, which are killed by normal human serum, is rare, and then only in patients with underlying disease. Capsulate meningococci of serogroups H, I, J, K and L have been described but do not appear to cause disease.

The serogroup of a meningococcus is determined by its polysaccharide capsular antigen, and the serogroup of a culture can be recognized by a slide agglutination test with absorbed group-specific antisera. Meningococci can be typed with antisera directed against outer-membrane proteins. This is useful in epidemiological studies, but some serotypes are also found to be associated with more severe disease and, in the case of group B meningococci, with outbreaks. These are so-called *epidemic strains* of group B meningococci, which appear to be of a single genotype.

Gonococci are antigenically more heterogeneous than meningococci. Strains can be characterized by *auxotyping*, which recognizes requirements for specific nutrients, such as arginine, proline, hypoxanthine and uracil. Panels of monoclonal antibodies that recognize specific proteins are also used to divide strains into various serovars. Epidemiological typing makes use of both methods.

## MENINGOCOCCAL INFECTION

### Pathogenesis

The natural habitat of the meningococcus is the human nasopharynx. Surveys of normal populations show that around 5–10% are carriers of meningococci, over half of which are non-capsulate strains. In communities in which outbreaks of cerebrospinal meningitis are occurring, the carrier rate of the epidemic strain (capsulate, as are all pathogenic meningococci) may range from 20% to as high as 90%, and some studies have shown that a sharp increase in the carrier rate of group A or other pathogenic groups of meningococci precedes the occurrence of clinical cases. However, the carrier:case ratio varies in different outbreaks and with the strain and population surveyed. Smokers appear to carry meningococci more often than non-smokers.

The route of spread from the nasopharynx to the meninges is controversial: the organism may either spread directly through the cribriform plate to the subarachnoid space by the perineural sheaths of the olfactory nerve; or, much more probably, it passes through the nasopharyngeal mucosa to enter the bloodstream. In favour of the latter route are the frequent positive blood cultures in the early stages of infection, the purpuric rash in many cases with the isolation of meningococci from the skin lesions, and the occurrence, particularly during epidemics, of meningococcal septicaemia with rash but no clinical meningitis.

Cerebrospinal meningitis occurs among only a limited proportion of the population at risk. The absence of bactericidal antibody in the blood is the factor most closely related to susceptibility to clinical infection. Evidence in support of this relationship is:

1. The age distribution of meningococcal disease, which has its highest incidence in infants and young children from 3 months to 3 years of age (see Fig. 24.1), among whom humoral meningococcicidal antibodies are rarely found: the analogy with haemophilus meningitis is obvious.

2. The reciprocal relationship in the appearance of these bactericidal antibodies in older children and adults with the decreasing incidence of cerebrospinal meningitis, except when it occurs in outbreaks among young adults brought together for special reasons, e.g. military training and, in earlier days, in ships and gaols.

3. Prospective studies among military recruits which showed that, whereas only 1% of the total

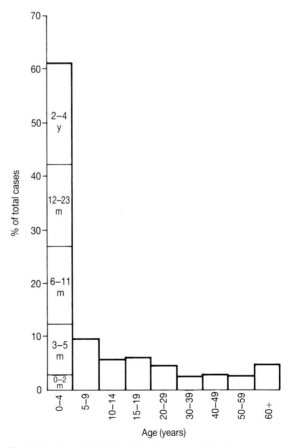

**Fig. 24.1** Age distribution of meningococcal infection (Scotland, 1972–82).

population at risk became clinically affected, 38.5% of those lacking specific bactericidal antibody to the meningococcus, and who became infected with the epidemic group C strain, developed meningococcal meningitis.

4. Patients convalescent from meningococcal infection develop typical immunoglobulin and bactericidal antibody to the infecting strains.

It is clear, nevertheless, from the relatively low incidence of meningococcal infections in young children and their absence in the large proportion of adults lacking specific antibody, that in most persons the first infection of the nasopharynx with a meningococcus leads to antibody production without development of clinical disease. It is possible that colonization with *N. lactamica*, which is common in children, may contribute to such antibody production.

Group-specific antibody is protective and this is the basis of the success of vaccination against meningococcal disease. Antibodies to outer-membrane proteins may also protect, but the range of antigens involved in this particular effect and the role of non-specific defence mechanisms in preventing clinical disease is ill-understood. However, the complement system is important as shown by the recurrent attacks of meningococcal infections in complement-deficient subjects.

Apart from serious clinical disease, meningococci are found in purulent conjunctivitis which, on rare occasions proceeds to systemic disease and occasionally in monarticular purulent arthritis without any preceding evidence of septicaemic infection; rarely, a chronic septicaemic form of disease may occur with both joint and skin involvement. Pneumonia, pericarditis and endocarditis are also unusual clinical manifestations.

## Laboratory diagnosis

In any suspected meningococcal infection, blood culture must be undertaken. If meningitis is suspected, a lumbar puncture must be performed as soon as possible unless signs of raised intracranial pressure render this a dangerous procedure. Lumbar puncture yields more positive cultures than blood culture from patients with meningococcal meningitis.

In meningococcal meningitis, CSF is under pressure and is turbid due to the large number of polymorphonuclear leucocytes present in a typical case. In the very first stages of infection, lumbar puncture may yield unremarkable results due to the fact that the meningeal reaction has not had time to take place, but typically the CSF will contain large numbers of Gram-negative diplococci which can be recognized by microscopical examination of the stained deposit. At a later stage they may be scanty and even apparently absent in films stained by Gram's method. Very scanty organisms may be seen more easily in a film stained with methylene blue. In the early untreated case, Gram-negative diplococci are seen in a proportion of the pus cells; later on many are present.

The CSF is cultured on heated blood (chocolate) agar and on blood agar. In the absence of visible meningococci, glucose broth may be added to the remaining sediment of the centrifuged deposit to facilitate the isolation of very scanty organisms. Cultures are incubated overnight at 37°C in an atmosphere of 5–10% carbon dioxide. If Gram-stained films from the resulting growth either on solid or in liquid medium show Gram-negative diplococci and if colonies on solid medium are oxidase-positive, sugar utilization tests are performed. Direct slide agglutination with specific antisera may be carried out on suspensions of colonies picked from solid medium. As an early aid to diagnosis, the isolate may be subcultured onto medium containing a test carbohydrate plus indicator; alternatively, preformed enzymes may be recognized by the rapid carbohydrate utilization technique. The serogroup may be recognized more readily in some instances if the organism has first been subcultured on blood agar.

For quick differential diagnosis, which is necessary for early chemotherapy, microscopical examination of the CSF is often sufficient. When organisms are scanty, owing to the stage of the disease, or to the institution of chemotherapy, meningococcal capsular polysaccharide may be demonstrated in CSF by counter-current electrophoresis or, less satisfactorily, by latex agglutination. Reference laboratories use the polymerase chain reaction to demonstrate meningococcal DNA in either CSF or blood.

Meningococci may be found in genital sites, and therefore it is particularly important to identify the organisms accurately and differentiate them from gonococci. Cultures should be sent, on slopes of chocolate agar, to a reference laboratory for sero-grouping and serotyping, procedures that provide important epidemiological information.

## Treatment

Almost all clinical isolates of meningococci in the UK are presently sensitive to benzylpenicillin. However, meningococci of reduced susceptibility to penicillin have been reported in some countries and are likely to become more common; therefore, it is important that accurate sensitivity testing is carried out on all meningococcal isolates from clinical disease. Meningococci of group A and 'epidemic' strains of group B are commonly resistant to sulphonamides. Overall, about 15–35% of meningococcal isolates are resistant to sulphonamides, and these drugs are no longer in use.

Penicillin should be given intravenously in the initial treatment of meningococcal infections. Although penicillin does not cross uninflamed meninges, it readily passes into CSF when inflammation is present. Chloramphenicol has long been used as an alternative to penicillin in meningococcal meningitis, but cefotaxime (or ceftriaxone) is at least as effective and avoids the possibility of blood dyscrasia. All three drugs have the advantage of being effective against *Haemophilus influenzae* and *Streptococcus pneumoniae*, the other two principal causes of meningitis in childhood after the neonatal period. In the absence of organisms in the Gram-stained CSF deposit, it is wise to give therapy which would cover all three pathogens. Ampicillin used to be the drug of choice, but the prevalence of resistance in *H. influenzae* is now sufficiently high to preclude its use alone.

At the end of a course of therapy with penicillin it is important to give eradicative treatment with rifampicin, or possibly ciprofloxacin, because penicillin does not eradicate meningococci from the nasopharynx and a patient returning home as a carrier may infect others.

The mortality rate in septicaemic illness may range from 14% up to 50% in some outbreaks. The mortality in meningitis is about 2–6%. Bad prognostic signs are the presence of coma on admission to hospital and a rapidly coalescing purpuric rash, together with signs of shock. Occasionally in the most fulminating forms of septicaemia there may not be time for the rash to develop before death. In such cases meningococci are isolated from the blood in life or post mortem and haemorrhagic adrenals are seen at autopsy, these being characteristic of the *Waterhouse–Friderichsen syndrome*.

## Epidemiology

Meningococcal infections occur world-wide and are notifiable in most countries. In the northern hemisphere, they tend to occur during the winter months. About two-thirds of cases occur in the first 5 years of life, but the peak prevalence of disease is in the 1st year of life (Fig. 24.1). The incidence is higher in males than females. In interepidemic periods the prevalence of meningococcal infection fluctuates (Fig. 24.2).

In recent times there has been an increase in meningococcal infection. There have been dramatic

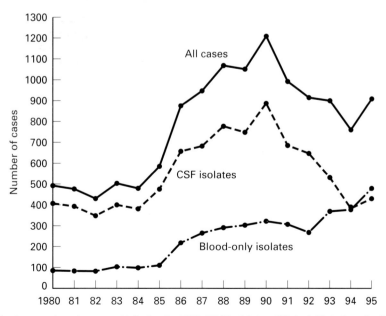

**Fig. 24.2**  Yearly totals of cases of meningococcal infection for 1980–95 (England and Wales). (Data from the Communicable Disease Surveillance Centre.)

epidemics due to group A meningococci in many parts of the world; to group C in Brazil and Africa; and to group B in Norway. In 1994 in England and Wales, 70% of cases of meningococcal meningitis were due to group B strains and 26% to group C. There were over 1800 cases of meningococcal infection in England and Wales in 1995 with 185 deaths.

Outbreaks have occurred frequently among young adult populations recruited for military service, and what might have been limited outbreaks of infection were fanned into great conflagrations of cerebrospinal meningitis in troops in training in both World Wars. Before the introduction of vaccination, localized outbreaks were common in some US army training camps. Small outbreaks have been seen even in recent times in the UK. Outbreak strains have commonly been group C, although there have been some outbreaks of group B.

Intensive studies in these training centres have shown that a high proportion of recruits became nasopharyngeal carriers of meningococci; cases tended to occur as the carriage rate rose, indicating that the critical point at which a patient either becomes ill or immune is at the time of acquiring the organism. Epidemic strains of group A or group B may give rise to a high incidence of disease in susceptible individuals who acquire such a strain. The increase in immunity observed with increasing age is likely to be due to asymptomatic infection with avirulent strains, which are carried by 7–20% of a healthy population, often for many months. Household contacts of a case are 500–800 times more likely to develop meningococcal infection than the general population.

Outbreaks of meningococcal meningitis require at least three factors:

1. The presence of a population of susceptible individuals who lack bactericidal antibodies to the current strains
2. A high transmission rate from person to person
3. A virulent, capsulate strain of meningococcus.

The factors that determine the virulence and communicability of a meningococcus are still not fully understood but only capsulate strains are isolated from systemic infections.

## Control

### Chemoprophylaxis

Outbreaks of disease may be controlled either by chemoprophylaxis alone, thus eradicating the organism from carriers, or combined with vaccination. Until the emergence of resistant strains, sulphonamides were effective, but rifampicin is now the preferred drug although it is effective in eradicating meningococcal carriage in only 80–90% of the population treated. After prophylaxis, rifampicin-resistant strains may be found in a small number of patients and may, on rare occasions, give rise to disease in contacts. Ciprofloxacin is also effective as a prophylactic. All household and other intimate (e.g. mouth kissing) contacts of a case should be given chemoprophylaxis as a routine.

### Vaccination

Resistance to meningococcal infection is closely associated with the possession of bactericidal antibodies that may be maternal in origin or actively produced in response to carriage. Vaccines containing the pure group-specific capsular polysaccharide of meningococci of groups A, C, Y and W-135 are available and are good immunogens. For civilian purposes, a vaccine containing group A and C polysaccharides alone is adequate and is licensed in most countries in the world. Vaccines containing all four polysaccharides are used in some countries for immunization of military recruits. The protection provided by the vaccine is group-specific and lasts for at least 3 years but does not prevent meningococcal carriage. Group C vaccine is unsuitable for children aged under 2 years.

Immunization is recommended for travel to parts of the world in which epidemics due to group A or C meningococci are in progress or are to be expected. One approach to the management of epidemics of meningococcal infection due to group A meningococci has been to vaccinate all the population and to give penicillin to any clinical cases. Any cases that arise before an immune response to the vaccine has commenced are also treated. There is presently no vaccine available against group B meningococci, but this problem is undergoing urgent investigation.

## GONOCOCCAL INFECTION

The name 'gonorrhoea' derives from the Greek words *gonos* (seed) and *rhoia* (flow) and described a condition in which semen flowed from the male organ without erection. It became apparent that gonorrhoea was associated with sexual promiscuity, one of the diseases celebrated by being named after the Roman goddess of love, Venus. Indeed, gonorrhoea is a classical venereal disease, being almost exclusively spread by sexual contact, having a short incubation period and being relatively easy to diagnose and treat.

## Pathogenesis

*N. gonorrhoeae* is exclusively a human pathogen although chimpanzees have been infected artificially. It is never found as a normal commensal although a proportion of those infected, particularly women, may remain asymptomatic. These individuals may develop systemic or ascending infection at a later stage.

The commonest clinical presentation of the disease is acute urethritis in the male a few days after unprotected vaginal or anal sexual intercourse. Dysuria and a purulent penile discharge make most sufferers seek treatment rapidly. A few men have relatively minor symptoms which may disappear rapidly. Truly asymptomatic infection is rare in the active male. However, up to 5% may carry the organism without apparent distress, and this is more common with certain types of gonococci. Rectal and pharyngeal infection is less often symptomatic and may be discovered only after tracing contacts.

In women with vaginal infection, only half may have symptoms of discharge and dysuria. Most seek attention because of their partner's symptoms, as part of contact tracing or screening of high-risk individuals. Asymptomatic carriage in women is common, especially in the endocervical canal. At menstruation or after instrumentation, particularly termination of pregnancy, gonococci ascend to the fallopian tubes to give rise to *acute salpingitis*, which may be followed by *pelvic inflammatory disease* and a high probability of sterility if inadequately treated. Peritoneal spread occasionally occurs and may produce a perihepatic inflammation (*Fitz–Hugh–Curtis syndrome*). Some auxotypes of *N. gonorrhoeae* spread more widely and give rise to disseminated gonococcal infection.

Disseminated infection is seen more commonly in women who may present with painful joints, fever and a few septic skin lesions on their extremities (Fig. 24.3). The diagnosis of a venereal disease may not be obvious and isolation of gonococci from joint fluid, blood culture and skin aspirates requires particular care. The organisms are invariably present in the cervix, but in many cases antibiotics have been given before the diagnosis is considered. Most strains are highly susceptible to penicillin. Rarely, disseminated gonococcal infection may present as endocarditis or meningitis.

Babies born to infected women may suffer *ophthalmia neonatorum*, in which the eyes are coated

**Fig. 24.3** Skin lesions in disseminated gonococcal infection.

with gonococci as the baby passes down the birth canal. A severe purulent eye discharge with periorbital oedema occurs within a few days of birth. If untreated, ophthalmia leads rapidly to blindness. It may be prevented in areas of high prevalence by the instillation of 1% aqueous silver nitrate in the eyes of newborn babies.

In prepubertal girls, vulvovaginitis may be caused by gonococci. This occurs either in conditions of poor hygiene or by sexual abuse; it should always be investigated carefully and the child put in touch with social services and other professionals capable of dealing with this difficult condition.

## Laboratory diagnosis

Cultivation of *N. gonorrhoeae* from sites with scanty commensals, such as the male urethra, rarely presents any problems, and Gram staining of a smear is usually 95% sensitive. *N. gonorrhoeae* is usually intolerant of drying and temperature changes; it readily undergoes autolysis. It is a fastidious microbe, requiring humidity, 5–7% carbon dioxide and complex media for growth. Ideally, exudate is taken directly from the patient onto appropriate preheated, freshly prepared solid media and immediately placed in a carbon dioxide incubator. This is usually possible only in specialized clinics with sufficient patient numbers to justify the expense. Where there is likely to be any delay, transport media must be used to carry the material on swabs.

## Treatment

The susceptibility of isolates of *N. gonorrhoeae* to commonly used antibiotics varies so much that regular testing is essential. The use of sulphonamides in the Second World War led to the rapid development of resistance, but the arrival of penicillin at that time solved the problem. Penicillin, especially in slow-release intramuscular forms, such as procaine penicillin, has remained the preferred therapy. Small decreases in susceptibility occurred in the 1950s and 1960s and were overcome by increasing the size of the single dose. The correlation between increasing minimum inhibitory concentration of penicillin for *N. gonorrhoeae* and failure of a single dose of 300 000 units of penicillin to treat acute gonorrhoea in men (Fig. 24.4) is the clearest example of the relationship between antibiotic susceptibility tests in vitro and the success of a drug in field conditions.

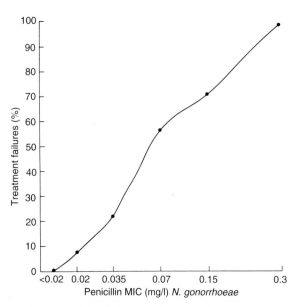

**Fig. 24.4** Correlation between minimum inhibitory concentration (MIC) of penicillin for *N. gonorrhoeae* and failure of treatment with a single dose of 300 000 units of penicillin in the treatment of acute gonorrhoea in men. (Data from Curtis F R, Wilkinson A E 1958 *British Journal of Venereal Diseases* 34: 70–82.)

By the 1970s the dose of penicillin required to cure simple acute gonorrhoea in men in some parts of the world had reached an impossibly large injection. In 1976, penicillinase-producing *N. gonorrhoeae* were first found. These strains may carry different plasmids and have arisen in different parts of the world, but all possess the gene coding for the TEM-type β-lactamase commonly found in *Escherichia coli*.

Single-dose therapy appears adequate for the majority of cases of acute genital gonorrhoea in men and women. There are obvious advantages to this approach in obtaining complete compliance and stopping the chain of infection. In disseminated gonococcal disease and any complicated infection treatment for 7–10 days is necessary.

If penicillin is contra-indicated because of allergy or bacterial resistance there are many alternatives; fluoroquinolones have many advocates. Tetracyclines are effective in most places and also treat concomitant chlamydial infection if given in a sufficiently long course of treatment. Tetracycline resistance in gonococci is increasing in some countries. Newer cephalosporins, in particular ceftriaxone, are extremely active, but have to be given by injection and are expensive. Infection with β-lactamase-producing gonococci in a patient not hypersensitive to penicillins responds to co-amoxiclav; this can be given with a large dose of procaine penicillin to overcome intrinsic penicillin resistance which is not reversed by the β-lactamase inhibitor clavulanic acid.

## Epidemiology and control

Since there should be little difficulty in the diagnosis and treatment of a typical case of acute gonorrhoea, one would expect the disease to be limited in distribution and well controlled. This was the case in much of the world until the 1960s. Venereal diseases were seen in small selected populations such as sailors and prostitutes. The number of new cases in countries which had reliable statistics fell rapidly and many felt that venereal disease would be eradicated. The remarkable changes since the 1960s of travel, migration, sexual licence and wide availability of oral contraceptives rapidly reversed this process so that there was an increase in gonorrhoea and non-specific genital infection (mainly caused by chlamydiae) for every year until scares about the acquired immune deficiency syndrome in the 1980s. Barrier methods, the condom in particular, greatly reduce the rate of transmission.

## MORAXELLA

The genus *Moraxella* is a member of the family Neisseriaceae. The organisms are characterized as asaccharolytic, oxidase-positive, catalase-positive short rods, coccobacilli or, in the case of *M. catarrhalis*, diplococci. They are commensals of mucosal surfaces and occasionally give rise to opportunistic infections. *M. lacunata* is occasionally encountered as a cause of 'angular' blepharoconjunctivitis.

The related genus *Kingella* contains organisms that differ from the moraxellae in being catalase-negative, glucose-fermenting coccobacilli. In common with some other Gram-negative rods, such as *Cardiobacterium hominis*, *Eikenella corrodens* and *Actinobacillus actinomycetemcomitans*, *Kingella* species (usually *K. kingae*) are sometimes found in endocarditis. They have also been implicated in joint infections.

## MORAXELLA (BRANHAMELLA) CATARRHALIS

### Pathogenesis

*M. catarrhalis* is a respiratory tract commensal and, as with other members of the upper respiratory tract flora, such as the pneumococcus and *H. influenzae*, it can gain access to the lower respiratory tract in patients with chronic chest disease or compromised host defences. *M. catarrhalis* is commonly isolated from sputum, and a pathogenic role is suspected only if the sputum contains large numbers of pus cells and Gram-negative diplococci, and if culture yields a heavy growth of *M. catarrhalis* in the absence of other recognized respiratory pathogens.

As well as causing chest infection itself, *M. catarrhalis* may also protect other respiratory pathogens from the action of penicillin or ampicillin by producing β-lactamase.

*M. catarrhalis* has also been incriminated in otitis media and sinusitis, and may be isolated on occasion from blood culture in patients who are immuno-compromised.

### Laboratory diagnosis

Sputum is examined by Gram film. In true infections large numbers of Gram-negative diplococci may be seen dispersed between the pus cells. Sputum is cultured on media suitable for the isolation of other potential respiratory pathogens (e.g. blood agar and chocolate agar) and incubated in 5% carbon dioxide overnight. In situations in which it is held to be pathogenic, *M. catarrhalis* is predominant in culture.

*M. catarrhalis* produces rough, circular, convex colonies which can be lifted off intact with a wire loop from agar culture medium. Colonies are oxidase-positive. In common with other moraxellae, they do not ferment sugars. Growth on nutrient agar at 22°C has been suggested as a differential characteristic, but clinically significant isolates of *M. catarrhalis* may not grow in these conditions. Tests for deoxyribonuclease (DNAase) and for butyrate esterase are positive. Up to 50% of strains produce β-lactamase.

### Treatment

*M. catarrhalis* is sensitive to amoxycilli, combined with clavulanic acid (co-amoxiclav) in the case of β-lactamase-producing strains, and also to cephalosporins, tetracycline and erythromycin.

RECOMMENDED READING

Cartwright K (ed) 1995 *Meningococcal Disease.* Wiley, Chichester

Cartwright K A V, Jones D M 1989 ACP Broadsheet 121. Investigation of meningococcal disease. *Journal of Clinical Pathology* 42: 634–639

Easmon C S F, Ison C A 1987 *Neisseria gonorrhoeae*: a versatile pathogen. *Journal of Clinical Pathology* 40: 1088–1097

Murphy T R 1996 *Branhamella catarrhalis*: epidemiology, surface antigenic structure, and immune response. *Microbiological Reviews* 60: 267–279

Nassif X, So M 1995 Interaction of pathogenic neisseria with nonphagocytic cells. *Clinical Microbiology Reviews* 8: 376–388

Oates J K, Csonka G W 1990 Gonorrhoea. In: Csonka GW, Oates J K (eds) *Sexually Transmitted Diseases.* Baillière Tindall, London, pp 209–226

PHLS Meningococcal Infections Working Group and Public Health Medicine Environmental Group 1995 Control of meningococcal disease: guidance for consultants in communicable disease control. *Communicable Disease Report* 5: R189–R195

Tunkel A R, Scheld M W 1995 Acute bacterial meningitis. *Lancet* 346: 1675–1680

# 25

# Salmonella

**Food poisoning; enteric fever**

*M. J. Lewis*

Salmonellae are a major cause of food-borne infection world-wide. In the statistics for England and Wales kept by the Public Health Laboratory Service, annual salmonella isolations from humans almost trebled from 10 251 to 27 000 between 1981 and 1988. However, this apparently inexorable increase in incidence has not been sustained. Between 1989 and 1995 the number of salmonella infections reported in England and Wales has been steady at about 30 000 infections a year (Fig. 25.1). In the USA the figures are double these, and in both countries many, perhaps most, infections go unrecognized. In the developing countries, where large-scale farming and processing of food animals is not yet the norm, salmonellae are not as important a cause of community-acquired diarrhoea. Nevertheless, the incidence of salmonellosis world-wide must be astronomical.

## DESCRIPTION

Salmonellae are typical members of the Enterobacteriaceae, facultatively anaerobic Gram-negative bacilli able to grow on a wide range of relatively simple media and distinguished from other members of the family by their biochemical characteristics and antigenic structure. Their normal habitat is the animal intestine.

### Antigens

Antigenic structure is important, but in day-to-day practice the demonstration of a small number of biochemical characters (Table 25.1) together with the demonstration of some salmonella antigens is sufficient to decide that the organism is a *Salmonella* species. To give the salmonella a name demands a more complete antigenic analysis.

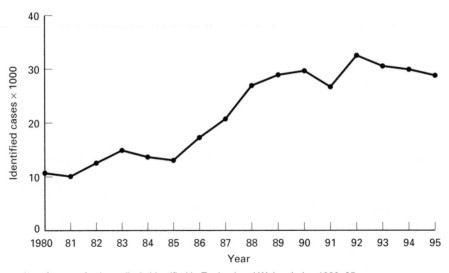

**Fig. 25.1** The number of cases of salmonellosis identified in England and Wales during 1980–95.

**Table 25.1** Biochemical tests that help to differentiate between members of the Enterobacteriaceae

| Test | Salmonella Typhi | Other Salmonella serotypes | Shigella | Escherichia coli | Citrobacter | Klebsiella | Enterobacter[a] | Proteus | Providence |
|---|---|---|---|---|---|---|---|---|---|
| Motility | + | + | − | + | + | − | + | + | + |
| Gas from glucose | − | + | − | + | + | + | + | v | v |
| Acid from lactose | − | − | − | + | + | + | + | − | − |
| Urease | − | − | − | − | − | v | − | + | − |
| Citrate utilization | − | + | − | − | + | + | + | v | + |
| H$_2$S production | + | + | − | − | v | − | − | v | − |
| Indole | − | − | v | + | v | v | v | v | + |
| PPA test | − | − | − | − | − | − | − | + | + |
| Gluconate oxidation | − | − | − | − | − | + | + | − | − |

+, most strains positive; −, most strains negative; v, variable; PPA, phenylpyruvic acid.
[a]Includes *Serratia*.

The typical salmonella possesses two sets of antigens which are readily demonstrable by serological reactions in the laboratory. Heat-stable polysaccharides which form part of the cell wall lipopolysaccharide are known as *somatic* or *O antigens*. *Flagellar* or *H antigens* are formed from the structural proteins which make up the flagella that endow the organism with motility. In most salmonellae the flagella exhibit the property of diphasic variation. That is, the flagellar antigens exist in two alternative forms defined by two different sets of genes in the bacterial genome. When one of these sets is expressed, the flagella consist of one or more *phase 1* antigens, while when the other set is operative two or more *phase 2* antigens are synthesized. Some salmonellae also produce a surface polysaccharide, of which the Vi antigen of *Salmonella* Typhi is the most important example, which can occasionally make detection of the O antigens difficult. The O antigens have been numbered with Arabic numerals. The flagellar antigens of phase 1 have been labelled with lower-case letters, and of phase 2 with a mixture of lower-case letters and Arabic numerals. The antigenic structure of any salmonella is expressed as an antigenic formula which has three parts, describing the O antigens, the phase 1 H antigens and the phase 2 H antigens, in that order. The three parts are separated by colons, and the component antigens in each part by commas. More than 2000 serotypes have so far been described in this way, and almost all have been given names.

When this scheme was being developed by White in 1929 and later modified by Kauffmann, each named serotype was regarded as a separate *Salmonella* species, and the convention was adopted that each new serotype should be given the name of the place where it was first isolated. It is now generally accepted that all salmonellae belong to one species, *Salmonella enterica*, which has seven subspecies. Most of the serotypes which infect mammals are found in subspecies 1 and are named as, for example, *S. enterica* subspecies 1 serotype Enteritidis. For convenience it is usual to abbreviate this to *S.* Enteritidis, or even just Enteritidis. Some of the commoner serotypes are shown in Table 25.2. The Kauffmann–White scheme, which elegantly catalogues

**Table 25.2** The antigenic structure of some representative salmonellae

| Typhi | 9, 12, [Vi] | : | d | : | − |
|---|---|---|---|---|---|
| Paratyphi B | 1, 4, 5, 12 | : | b | : | 1, 2 |
| Typhimurium | 1, 4, 5, 12 | : | i | : | 1, 2 |
| Enteritidis | 1, 9, 12 | : | g, m | : | 1, 7 |
| Virchow | 6, 7 | : | r | : | 1, 2 |
| Kedougou | 1, 13, 23 | : | i | : | 1, w |
| Hadar | 6, 8 | : | Z10 | : | e, n, x |
| Heidelberg | 1, 4, 5, 12 | : | r | : | 1, 2 |
| Infantis | 6, 7, 14 | : | r | : | 1, 5 |
| Newport | 6, 8, 20 | : | e, h | : | 1, 2 |
| Panama | 1, 9, 12 | : | l, v | : | 1, 5 |
| Dublin | 1, 9, 12 | : | g, p | : | − |

this system of description, places the salmonellae into some 30 groups on the basis of shared O antigens, and further subdivides the groups into clusters with H antigens in common. Some salmonellae, such as *S.* Typhi (9, 12, [Vi]: d: –), express only one flagellar phase. Only a small number of salmonellae regularly cause illness in humans.

## HOST RANGE AND PATHOGENICITY

Salmonellae are widely distributed in nature. All vertebrates appear capable of harbouring salmonellae in their gut, and salmonellae have also been isolated from a wide range of arthropods such as flies and cockroaches. Most animal infections seem to be symptomless, or to cause a self-limiting gastroenteritis of variable severity. Many serotypes such as Typhimurium show a wide host range, and can be isolated from many different animal species. A small number of strains, the *host-adapted* serotypes, are much more restricted in the species they inhabit, and show a different spectrum of illness.

### Host-adapted serotypes

Among the host-adapted serotypes, Typhi and Paratyphi A, B and C are primarily human pathogens which are rarely, if ever, isolated from animals other than humans. Paratyphi B, while essentially a human pathogen, is occasionally isolated from cattle, pigs, poultry and other animals, although cycles of transmission in these hosts have not been demonstrated.

Human infection with these organisms is characterized by a long incubation period of 10–14 days, followed by a septicaemic illness, *enteric fever*, quite unlike the diarrhoea and vomiting that are characteristic of food poisoning.

Other salmonellae adapted to particular animal hosts include Cholerae-suis (pigs), Dublin (cattle), Gallinarum-pullorum (poultry), Abortus-equi (horses) and Abortus-ovis (sheep). These are all responsible for considerable morbidity, mortality and economic loss among domestic animals. All can cause illness in humans, but only Cholerae-suis and Dublin do so regularly. The rest of the 2000 or so serotypes of salmonellae show no apparent host preference. The extent to which they cause human infection is determined by the accident of their prevalence in domestic food animals at any particular time and on the opportunity for the contamination of food in which further multiplication can take place. In developed countries most human infections are caused by a relatively small number of locally prevalent serotypes.

## PATHOGENESIS

Salmonella infection is initiated by ingestion of a sufficient number of organisms to overcome the body's defences, in particular gastric acidity, and to colonize the small intestine. The organisms need to be swallowed. Experiments in which volunteers gargled with suspensions of different serotypes without swallowing regularly failed to cause infection.

### Infective dose

The number of salmonellae which must be swallowed in order to cause infection is uncertain, and the widely accepted dictum that large inocula of salmonellae are required for induction of illness in humans is based largely on volunteer studies. In most of these the median infective dose for most serotypes, including Typhi, has varied from $10^6$ to $10^9$ organisms. However, investigation of outbreaks suggests that in natural infection the infective dose is regularly below $10^3$ organisms and sometimes less than 100 bacteria.

Many factors influence the infective dose. There appears to be considerable strain-to-strain variation in virulence even within a single serotype. Systematic variation in pathogenicity between serotypes is less easy to demonstrate outside the host-adapted strains. The vehicle of ingestion also matters. Organisms in water and other drinks may be carried through the stomach relatively rapidly, and thus escape the effect of the gastric acid. Similarly, the administration of antacids, or the effects of gastric resection, reduce the infective dose. Salmonellosis caused by contaminated endoscopes introduced through the stomach into the small intestine is another example of this effect.

### Host factors

Host factors are also likely to be important, although these may be difficult to separate from confounding variables. For example, age-specific isolation rates for salmonellae, as for some other gut pathogens, is higher for children less than a year of age than for any other age group, but this reflects the fact that a higher proportion of infections are investigated in this age group. This is often misinterpreted as revealing a greater susceptibility.

## Initiation of infection

Once the bacteria enter the lumen of the intestine they are able to multiply. Some of the bacteria attach to the microvilli of the ileal mucosa by means of adhesins on the bacterial surface, which adhere specifically to mannose-containing receptors on the epithelium. Attachment is followed by degeneration of the microvilli to form breaches in the cell membrane through which the salmonellae enter the cell. Further multiplication in these cells and in macrophages of the Peyer's patches follows. Some bacteria penetrate into the submucosa and pass to the local mesenteric lymph nodes. All the clinical manifestations of salmonella infection, including diarrhoea, begin after ileal penetration.

## CLINICAL SYNDROMES

Although salmonellae can cause a wide spectrum of clinical illness there are four major syndromes, each with its own diagnostic and therapeutic problems, which are best considered separately. These are enteric fever, gastro-enteritis, bacteraemia with or without metastatic infection, and the asymptomatic carrier state.

## Enteric fever

Enteric fever is most usually caused by Typhi or Paratyphi A, B or C, but can be caused by any salmonella serotype. The clinical features tend to be more severe with Typhi (typhoid fever). After penetration of the ileal mucosa the organisms pass via the lymphatics to the mesenteric lymph nodes, whence after a period of multiplication they invade the bloodstream via the thoracic duct. The liver, gallbladder, spleen, kidney and bone marrow become infected during this primary bacteraemic phase in the first 7–10 days of the incubation period. After multiplication in these organs, bacilli pass into the blood, causing a second and heavier bacteraemia, the onset of which approximately co-incides with that of the fever and other signs of clinical illness. From the gallbladder a further invasion of the intestine results. Peyer's patches and other gut lymphoid tissues become involved in an inflammatory reaction and infiltration with mononuclear cells, followed by necrosis, sloughing and the formation of characteristic typhoid ulcers occurs.

### Onset

The interval between ingestion of the organisms and the onset of illness varies with the size of the infecting dose. It can be as short as 3 days or as long as 50 days, but is usually about 2 weeks. The onset is usually insidious. Early symptoms are often vague: a dry cough and epistaxis associated with anorexia, a dull continuous headache, abdominal tenderness and discomfort are among the most common symptoms. Diarrhoea is not commonly a feature of enteric fever and early in the illness many patients will complain of constipation.

### Progression

In the untreated case the temperature shows a step-ladder rise over the 1st week of the illness, remains high for 7–10 days and then falls by lysis during the 3rd or 4th week.

Physical signs include a relative bradycardia for the height of the fever, hepatomegaly, splenomegaly and often a rash of *rose spots*. These are 2–4 mm in diameter, slightly raised discrete irregular blanching pink macules most often found on the front of the chest. They appear in crops of up to a dozen at a time and fade after 3 or 4 days, leaving no scar. They are characteristic of, but not specific for, enteric fever.

### Relapse

Apparent recovery can be followed by relapse in 5–10% of untreated cases. Relapse is usually shorter and of milder character than the initial illness, but can be severe and may end fatally. Severe intestinal haemorrhage and intestinal perforation are serious complications which can occur at any stage of the illness.

### Morbidity and mortality

Classic typhoid fever is a serious infection which, when untreated, has a mortality approaching 20%. However, it is notoriously unpredictable in its presentation and course. Mild and asymptomatic infections are not uncommon. In areas where typhoid is endemic, and particularly where it co-exists with schistosomiasis, chronic infection can present with fever of many months' duration, accompanied by chronic bacteraemia. Occasionally, diarrhoea may dominate the picture from the outset, particularly in paratyphoid infections, which sometimes present as typical gastro-enteritis no different from that caused by the large majority of salmonella serotypes.

## Gastro-enteritis and food poisoning

Acute gastro-enteritis is characterized by vomiting, abdominal pain, diarrhoea and fever. It can be caused by ingestion of a wide variety of bacteria or their products, several viruses and a number of vegetable toxins and inorganic chemicals. The term *bacterial food poisoning* is conveniently restricted to cases and epidemics of acute gastro-enteritis that are caused by the ingestion of food contaminated by bacteria or their toxins. It is an important feature of bacterial food poisoning that the bacteria need the opportunity to multiply in the food to reach an infective concentration before being eaten. Infections such as hepatitis A or bacillary dysentery, in which food may be an incidental vector, are not usually considered to be examples of food poisoning. Salmonellae are common causes of food poisoning world-wide.

### Clinical features

The most common clinical manifestation of salmonella infection is diarrhoea, often accompanied by headache, malaise, nausea and vomiting. The incubation period is usually 8–48 h, the onset abrupt and the clinical course short and self-limiting. Symptoms vary from the passage of two or three loose stools which may be disregarded by the sufferer, to a severe and prostrating illness with the frequent passage of watery, green, offensive stools, fever, shivering, abdominal pain and, in the most severe cases, dehydration leading to hypotension, cramps and renal failure. Vomiting is rarely a prominent feature of the illness.

Severe infections occur most often in the very young and the elderly, although mild and subclinical infections also occur in these age groups. Salmonella infections in those already ill or debilitated for other causes are also likely to be more severe and life-threatening. In most cases the acute stage is over within 2 or 3 days, although it may be more prolonged. Persistent or high fever suggests bacteraemia, possibly with metastatic infection.

### Bacteraemia and metastatic disease

Bacteraemia is a constant feature of enteric fever, and can occur as a rare complication of any salmonella infection. Transient bacteraemia occurs in up to 4% of cases of acute gastro-enteritis but in most cases the organisms are cleared from the bloodstream without ill effect. Occasionally, dissemination of the bacilli throughout the body results in the establishment of one or more localized foci of persisting infection, especially where pre-existing abnormality makes a tissue or organ vulnerable. Atherosclerotic plaques within large arteries, damaged heart valves, joint prostheses and other implants are all susceptible to metastatic infection. Osteomyelitis is most often found in long bones, costochondral junctions and the spine. Multiple bony sites may be affected, and sickle cell anaemia is an important predisposing factor. Suppurative arthritis can occur either as an extension of contiguous osteomyelitis or as a primary infection. Salmonella meningitis is a particularly serious complication of infection in neonates and very young children. Abscess formation can occur in almost any organ or tissue. Even in the absence of obvious tissue damage the ability of salmonellae to enter and survive within macrophages and other cells, particularly in the liver and biliary tree, but also in bone marrow and the kidney, occasionally leads to persistent infection and the chronic carrier state.

### The prolonged carrier state

Most sufferers from a salmonella infection continue to excrete the organism in their stools for days or weeks after complete clinical recovery, but eventual clearance of the bacteria from the body is usual. A minority of patients continue to excrete the salmonellae for prolonged periods. The term *chronic carrier* is reserved for those who excrete salmonellae for a year or more. Chronic carriage can follow symptomatic illness or may be the only manifestation of infection. It can occur with any salmonella serotype, but is a particularly important feature of enteric fever; up to 5% of convalescents from typhoid and a smaller number of those who have recovered from paratyphoid fever become chronic carriers, many for a lifetime. The bacilli are most commonly present in the gallbladder, less often in the urinary tract, and are shed in faeces and sometimes in urine. The long duration of the carrier state enables the enteric fever bacilli to survive in the community in non-epidemic times and to persist in small and relatively isolated communities.

Age and sex are important determinants of the frequency of carriage, at least of Typhi. After enteric fever, less than 1% of patients under 20 years old become carriers, but this proportion rises to more than 10% in patients over 50 years of age. At all ages women become carriers twice as often as men.

Duration of excretion following infection with other salmonellae has been less well documented, but more than 50% of patients stop excreting the organisms within 5 weeks of infection, and 90% of adults are culture-negative at 9 weeks. The duration of excretion is significantly greater in children less than 5 years old. However, even in small children eventual clearance is the rule, and virtually all permanent carriers are adults.

## LABORATORY DIAGNOSIS

Laboratory diagnosis usually depends on the isolation and identification of the causal salmonella from a specimen of the patient's blood or faeces. Testing the patient's serum for salmonella antibodies is useful only in the diagnosis of enteric fever (see below).

### Blood culture

The definitive diagnosis of enteric fever is made by the isolation of the salmonella by blood culture. The organisms may be recovered from the bloodstream at any stage of the illness, but are most commonly found during the first 7–10 days and during relapses. Most blood culture systems will grow salmonellae rapidly. The organisms can also be recovered from the blood clot from a sample taken for serological examination. The clot is digested with streptokinase or minced, and added to broth which is incubated and examined as in the blood culture technique. Clot culture may be positive even when blood culture is not. The same holds for culture of bone marrow aspirates.

### Stool and urine culture

Specimens of faeces and urine should also be submitted for examination, but the isolation of a salmonella from either of these specimens may merely mean that the patient is a carrier. In typhoid fever, stool cultures are usually positive from the 2nd week and urine cultures from the 3rd week of the infection. In paratyphoid B infections the clinical course may be much shorter than in typhoid, diarrhoea may occur early and stool cultures are often positive in the 1st week of the illness.

Faeces or the centrifuged urine deposit are plated on desoxycholate–citrate agar (DCA) and are also inoculated into fluid enrichment media such as tetrathionate or selenite broth which is subcultured to plates of appropriate selective media after incubation. Suspicious colonies from the culture plates are tested directly for the presence of salmonella O antigens by slide agglutination and subcultured to peptone water for determination of H antigen struc-

ture and for further biochemical analysis. A presumptive diagnosis of a salmonella infection can often be made within 24 h of the receipt of a specimen, but confirmation that the isolate is a salmonella may take another day, and its formal identification to serotype several more days. A negative report must await the result of enrichment cultures, which take at least 48 h.

### Widal test

The interpretation of this test for specific O and H antibodies in the patient's serum is only valid if note is taken of certain findings which may otherwise cause false-positive results. The level of 'enteric' antibodies in the healthy population must be known and may be variable. Previous inoculation with TAB (typhoid, paratyphoid A, paratyphoid B) vaccine can give relatively high titres of specific antibodies, as can previous infection, although only the H antibodies tend to persist at detectable levels. Cross-reacting antibodies from previous exposure to other salmonellae sometimes confuse the picture. As with other serological tests for acute infections, the usefulness of the Widal test is greatest when a four-fold or greater rise in antibody levels is detected on testing a second specimen of the patient's serum some days after the first; by this time the diagnosis has usually been made by isolation of the offending organism from blood culture.

The Widal test was formerly used in the search for typhoid carriers, for example in the routine examination of food handlers and waterworks employees but it is of doubtful value and its use in this context has been abandoned. The detection of persisting Vi antibody in significant titre may be of limited value in the search for long-term carriers after an outbreak of infection.

### Food poisoning

The laboratory diagnosis of bacterial food poisoning depends on the isolation of the causal organism from samples of faeces or suspected foodstuffs. The procedures for isolation and identification of food poisoning salmonellae are identical to those for the enteric fever pathogens. The more common food poisoning serotypes, such as Enteritidis or Typhimurium, may also be subjected to phage typing, so that the isolates from patients may be matched with those from the infected food and from a suspected animal source.

The examination of vomit is rarely of value.

## TREATMENT

### Enteric fever

The introduction of chloramphenicol in 1948 transformed the treatment of enteric fever, turning a life-threatening illness of several weeks' duration and a mortality of more than 20% into a short-lasting febrile illness with a mortality below 2%. Many patients can be treated adequately with oral chloramphenicol from the outset. Initial intravenous therapy with the drug may be necessary for the more severally ill patient, who may have anorexia, abdominal distension and, perhaps, vomiting. The intramuscular route gives inadequate blood levels. Treatment should be maintained for 14 days because relapse is more frequent with a shorter course.

The problem of bone marrow toxicity and, in the 1970s, the widespread emergence of plasmid-mediated chloramphenicol resistance in South America and South-East Asia prompted the search for alternative agents. Among these, the ampicillins and co-trimoxazole are as effective as chloramphenicol, and became widely used. Since 1989, however, simultaneous resistance to all three antibiotics has become increasingly common in strains of Typhi in India, Pakistan and China, and has been found in the Middle East and South Africa. Imported multi-resistant typhoid is being encountered world-wide. Ciprofloxacin has emerged as the drug of choice for the treatment of adult typhoid, and is proving equally effective and free from side-effects in children.

### Gastro-enteritis

Management of salmonella gastro-enteritis includes replacement of fluids and electrolytes and control of nausea, vomiting and pain. Drugs to control the hypermotility of the gut are contra-indicated; they may give symptomatic relief for a while but it is easy to transform a trivial gastro-enteritis into a life-threatening bacteraemia by paralysing the bowel. The role of antibiotics is also limited. Several randomized placebo-controlled double-blind studies have assessed the efficacy of different oral and parenteral antibiotics in the treatment of salmonella gastro-enteritis. None showed any benefit from any antibiotic on the duration and severity of the diarrhoea or the duration of fever, while some seemed to prolong the carrier state. Most authorities agree that antibiotics have no part to play in the management of most cases of salmonella enteritis. However, when a patient is clearly at increased risk of bac-teraemia and generalized salmonella invasion, an antibiotic may protect against this serious complication. Such patients include infants under 3 months of age, patients with malignancies, haemoglobino-pathies, chronic gastro-intestinal disease such as ulcerative colitis, especially when these need treatment with steroids, and patients who are immuno-suppressed for other reasons. Treatment, with an appropriate agent (see above), should continue until the gastro-enteritis has completely resolved.

### Salmonella bacteraemia

Established salmonella bacteraemia requires aggressive antimicrobial treatment with chloramphenicol, co-trimoxazole, high-dose ampicillin or ciprofloxacin. Uncomplicated bacteraemia should be treated for 10–14 days. A careful search for focal metastatic disease should be undertaken, especially when relapse follows cessation of treatment. Surgical drainage of metastatic abscesses may be required, with surgical intervention if heart valves or large vessels are affected. In salmonella meningitis in infancy, treatment with chloramphenicol or ampicillin may be un-successful in up to a third of cases caused by sensitive strains. Since cefotaxime and ceftriaxone penetrate into the cerebrospinal fluid reasonably well and are highly active against most salmonellae, they offer an effective alternative to the more conventional agents.

### Chronic asymptomatic carriers

The chronic carrier state presents a particularly difficult therapeutic challenge. The principal site of carriage is the biliary tract, and concomitant biliary disease has significant implications for therapy. When the patient has chronic cholecystitis or gallstones, antibiotics alone are most unlikely to eradicate the infection. Cholecystectomy together with appropriate antibiotic treatment will result in cure in about 90% of cases, but has significant risk, not least from metastatic infection from dissemination of the organisms during surgery. In the absence of biliary disease, prolonged courses of ampicillin, amoxycillin, co-trimoxazole or ciprofloxacin may cure up to 80% of carriers. However, it is difficult to justify even moderately heroic efforts to cure a condition which has little if any ill effect on the individual and not much direct public health importance. The chronic human carrier is the principal reservoir of enteric fever salmonellae, but even in the developing world direct person-to-person spread by asymptomatic carriers is not common. 'Typhoid Mary', who is reputed to have caused many infections by her cooking, was an exception and must have had peculiar personal habits. Normal personal hygiene, adequate sanitation and a reliable supply of potable water are the real safeguards against enteric fever. Prolonged carriage of other salmonella serotypes is of even less public health importance, and rarely if ever justifies exclusion from any employment, or intrusive efforts to eradicate the infection.

## EPIDEMIOLOGY AND CONTROL

The typhoid and paratyphoid bacilli are essentially human parasites. Humans are the reservoir host and most infections can be traced to a human source, or at least to a source of human sewage. All other salmonellae have animal hosts.

## Enteric fever

### Incidence

In developing countries, Typhi is commonly isolated by laboratories, but data are incomplete. It has been estimated that between 10 and 500 cases of typhoid per 100 000 of the population occur annually throughout the developing world. In 1938 there were almost 1000 notifications of typhoid fever in England and Wales. Within a decade the incidence had fallen to less than 200 cases a year, largely because of the almost universal introduction of chlorination of public water supplies, and improved techniques for the detection of cases and carriers which formed the basis for improved standards of hygiene and sanitation generally. The current incidence throughout most of the developed world is about 0.2 cases per 100 000 of the population. Most contract their infection by travel to endemic areas or by close family contact with excreters. Paratyphoid infections show a similar pattern.

### Sanitation

The control of enteric fever is straightforward. Cases occur from the ingestion of food or water contaminated with human sewage carrying typhoid or paratyphoid bacilli. Outbreaks occur when numbers of people are infected from a primary source, which may be a single meal or a briefly contaminated water supply, or may be from a water supply or source of food contaminated and available for ingestion over a longer period. Secondary transmission from patients infected by the primary source is rare. Control depends essentially on the wide public availability of wholesome drinking water and the provision of adequate means for the proper disposal of human excreta. Enteric fever is a public health problem only where these provisions do not exist, and where, therefore, the organisms can be spread widely from carriers and from convalescent and sick persons, possibly helped by cultural factors such as food habits, occupation and personal behaviour. In such communities the selection of control measures may be difficult, and provision of adequate sanitation and pure water may need to be supplemented by prophylactic immunization.

### Vaccination

Heat-killed, phenol-preserved whole-cell vaccines containing a mixture of cultures of Typhi, Paratyphi A and Paratyphi B (TAB) have been used for many years in countries with a high endemic level of typhoid fever, and field trials have shown that such preparations confer considerable, although not absolute, protection against typhoid itself. There has always been doubt about the value of the paratyphoid components, as well as concern about the unpleasant side-effects associated with the large antigenic load of the triple vaccine, so that monovalent typhoid vaccines are now preferred.

Controlled trials have shown that both heat-killed, phenol-preserved Typhi vaccine and an acetone-killed vaccine preserved in the dry state give 70–90% protection for 3–7 years. Travellers to endemic areas where there are high carriage rates and poor standards of hygiene should be offered immunization, especially if they intend to visit rural areas, or to live rough. However, the risk to the air traveller with full board at a reputable hotel is so small that typhoid immunization is unnecessary. The risk of infection in southern Europe does not justify recommending the vaccine to the many millions travelling there on holiday every year, but vaccination is recommended for travel to eastern Europe, especially for backpacking holidays outside the main tourist areas.

Recent trials of oral live attenuated typhoid vaccines have shown encouraging protection rates.

### Salmonella food poisoning

The problem of zoonotic salmonellosis is altogether different from that of enteric fever. No other zoonosis is as complex in its epidemiology and control as salmonellosis; epidemiological patterns differ greatly between geographical areas, depending on climate, population density, land use, farming practices, food-processing technologies and consumer habits. Also, the biology of different salmonella serotypes differs so widely that discussions on salmonellosis, salmonella infections or salmonella contamination are inevitably complex.

## Sources

The carcasses or products (cooked meats, eggs, milk) of naturally infected domestic animals are the commonest sources of food poisoning. Flesh may be infected when an ill, septicaemic animal is slaughtered, but in most cases the salmonellae important in human infection cause only mild or inapparent infection in their animal hosts and abattoir and shop cross-contamination with intestinal contents from a carrier animal is a more important hazard. Poultry (particularly hens), ducks and turkeys are the most significant reservoirs of food poisoning salmonellae in the UK. Pigs share the honours with poultry in much of northern Europe, while beef cattle are important sources in the USA. Duck eggs have always been a problem, since they can be infected in the oviduct before the egg is shelled. Hen eggs acquire their shells higher in the oviduct, and are less commonly infected in this way, although they can be contaminated on the outside if laid on soil contaminated by infected hen faeces.

## Food contamination

Rats and mice are commonly infected with food poisoning salmonellae and may contaminate human food with their faeces. Food poisoning may occasionally be caused by food contaminated by a human case or carrier. Thus, even if the foodstuff is initially free from salmonellae the chance of contamination 'from the hoof to the home' is high and the more sophisticated the manipulation of the food, the greater the chance of contamination. For example, one egg containing salmonellae, if eaten by an individual, probably will not give rise to an infection. On the other hand, if such an egg is pooled with others free from salmonellae, as in preparing a mayonnaise or a Hollandaise sauce for communal consumption, and if conditions of temperature and time allow multiplication of the salmonellae, there will be the potential for an outbreak of infection among those who eat the contaminated food.

A clean carcass can be contaminated at the abattoir by instruments or by hanging in contact with an infected carcass in the chilling hall or during trans-portation to the wholesale and retail butchers' premises. The aggregation of calves or pigs in holding pens greatly increases the occurrence of cross-infection before slaughter. Infection in pigs is most often due to the feeding of swill containing infected animal matter, a practice that is difficult to prevent.

Numerous studies have demonstrated a close correspondence between the types of salmonellae prevalent in animals, especially pigs and poultry, and the types causing infection in humans. Typhimurium, which is a primary pathogen in a wide variety of animals, is common, and Enteritidis has become prevalent as a result of a widespread epidemic of domestic poultry flocks. Some serotypes such as Heidelberg, Brandenburg, Panama and Virchow are rarely found in animals and yet may be responsible for widespread human infections. More needs to be learned about the epidemiology of such infections.

## Food preparation

Infection of food with salmonellae is not in itself sufficient to cause food poisoning. It is necessary for the infected food to be moist and to be held long enough under conditions which will allow the bacteria to grow, e.g. overnight in a warm kitchen or several days in a cool larder. If the food is then eaten without further cooking, infection will follow. Although cooking of liquid foods will render them safe, cooking of solid foods often fails to do so because of the relatively poor rate of penetration of heat into the food. A cold or chilled joint of meat, a poultry carcass or a large meat pie may be heated in an oven until the surface is well cooked, while the central part is still insufficiently heated to destroy vegetative bacteria.

## Outbreaks

Food poisoning incidents occur most dramatically as explosive outbreaks among members of a community sharing communal meals, as in factories, hospitals or schools or at some celebratory feast, although sporadic incidents affecting a single family or a single person are much more common and much more difficult to track to a source. In the UK, salmonellae account for about 75% of the incidents of food poisoning in which a causal agent is identified. However, this may only reflect the fact that salmonellosis is relatively easy to confirm bacteriologically and is therefore more readily recognized than food poisoning due to other agents, which often escapes diagnosis.

## Prevention

The principles of the prevention of salmonella food poisoning can be readily set out: they are the raising of animals free from infection, the elimination of contamination by rodents at all levels of food production, and the prevention of contamination by human handlers at the wholesale, retail and hotel levels; yet the barriers of economic husbandry, out-of-date premises and, perhaps the most important of all, the need for continuing education of food handlers at all levels of production make implementation of these principles difficult.

To reduce the incidence of food poisoning, whether due to salmonellae or to other bacteria, two basic precepts must be observed. Firstly, raw foodstuffs of animal origin, which are always potentially contaminated, must never have contact, either direct or indirect, with cooked foods. Secondly, if a foodstuff is thought to be contaminated with salmonellae it should be treated or held under temperature conditions which prevent the organisms from growing. Cooked foods should be served and eaten immediately after cooking, and while still hot, or cooled rapidly and held at refrigerator temperature until eaten, so that at least the inoculum eaten by any individual is small.

It is often found that the food incriminated in an outbreak had been cooked several hours or even a day or two before and then left at room temperature before being reheated immediately before serving. This procedure ensures that salmonellae which survived the initial cooking or gained access to the food from contaminated kitchen surfaces or implements had excellent opportunities to multiply in the interval before being warmed up for consumption.

As in most other endeavours to control the spread of infection the human element is the weakest link in the chain, so that health education, particularly of food handlers, is a most important and continuing requirement.

### RECOMMENDED READING

Christie A B 1987 *Infectious Diseases: Epidemiology and Clinical Practice*, 4th edn. Churchill Livingstone, Edinburgh, chs 4 and 5

Levine M M, Ferreccio C, Black R E, Tacket C O, Germanier R, Chilean Typhoid Committee 1989 Progress in vaccines against typhoid fever. *Reviews in Infectious Diseases* 11(suppl 3): S552–S567

Mandel B K 1994 *Salmonella typhi* and other salmonellas. *Gut* 35: 726–728

Mirza S H, Beeching N J, Hart C A 1996 Multi-drug resistant *Salmonella typhi*: a global problem. *Journal of Medical Microbiology* 44: 317–319

Turnbull P C B 1979 Food poisoning with special reference to salmonella - its epidemiology, pathogenesis and control. *Clinics in Gastro-enterology* 8: 663–713

WHO 1988 Salmonellosis control: the role of animal and product hygiene. *WHO Technical Report Series*, No. 774. World Health Organization, Geneva

WHO 1994 Control of salmonella infections in animals and prevention of human foodborne salmonella infections. *Bulletin of the World Health Organization* 72: 831–833

# 26

# Shigella

**Bacillary dysentery**

*M. J. Lewis*

Dysentery, the bloody flux of biblical times, is a clinical entity characterized by the frequent passage of blood-stained mucopurulent stools. Aetiologically it is divisible into two main categories, amoebic and bacillary. Both forms are endemic in most warm-climate countries. Bacillary dysentery, caused by members of the genus *Shigella*, is also prevalent in many countries with temperate climates.

## DESCRIPTION

Shigellae are typical members of the Enterobacteriaceae and are closely related to the genus *Escherichia*. Microscopically, in stained preparations, shigellae are Gram-negative bacilli indistinguishable from other enterobacteria. They are non-motile and non-capsulate. Culturally they are similar to most other enterobacteria except that on MacConkey or desoxycholate–citrate agar (DCA) medium they are non-lactose-fermenting after incubation for 18–24 h. Thus, on such differential media colonies are pale and similar to those of the other common pathogenic

genus, *Salmonella*. The main biochemical reactions which differentiate shigellae from the other members of the Enterobacteriaceae are summarized in Table 25.1 (see p. 253).

The genus *Shigella* is subdivided on biochemical and serological grounds into four species: *Shigella dysenteriae*, *Sh. flexneri*, *Sh. boydii* and *Sh. sonnei* (Table 26.1). One of these, *Sh. dysenteriae*, is unique in being unable to ferment mannitol. Another, *Sh. sonnei*, is a late lactose fermenter, and colonies growing on MacConkey or DCA medium for more than 24 h become pink. The antigenic structure of the shigellae is complex. *Sh. dysenteriae* can be subdivided into 10 and *S. boydii* into 15 specific serotypes. A combination of group- and type-specific antigens allows subdivision of *Sh. flexneri* into six serotypes, each of which can be further subdivided. *Sh. sonnei* strains are serologically homogeneous, and a variety of other markers such as the ability to produce specific colicines or the carriage of drug-resistance or other plasmids are used to discriminate between strains for epidemiological purposes.

---

**Table 26.1**  Some biochemical reactions of *Shigella* species and serotypes

| Organism | Gas from glucose | Acid from | | | ONPG | Indole | Catalase |
| --- | --- | --- | --- | --- | --- | --- | --- |
| | | Lactose | Mannitol | Dulcitol | | | |
| *Sh. dysenteriae* 1 | − | − | − | − | + | − | − |
| *Sh. dysenteriae* 2–10 | − | − | − | − | v | v | + |
| *Sh. flexneri* 1–5 | − | − | + | − | − | v | + |
| *Sh. flexneri* 6 | v | − | v | v | − | − | + |
| *Sh. boydii* | − | − | + | v | − | v | + |
| *Sh. sonnei* | − | (+) | + | − | + | − | + |

v, variable; (+), positive only after incubation for ≥48 h.
ONPG, *o*-nitrophenyl-β-galactosidase.

## PATHOGENESIS

Shigellae are pathogens of humans and other primates. There are anecdotal reports of infection in dogs, but other animals are immune. Infection occurs by ingestion. The infecting dose is small, between 10 and 100 organisms.

Shigellae and entero-invasive *Escherichia coli* (EIEC, see Ch. 27) cause bacillary dysentery by identical invasive mechanisms. The bacteria are relatively unaffected by gastric acid or bile, being protected by a lipopolysaccharide coat. However, the invasive process depends on the presence of certain outer-membrane proteins that are cleaved by pancreatic enzymes during passage through the small intestine; the organisms are temporarily non-invasive while in the small gut.

After reaching the large intestine the organisms multiply in the gut lumen, restoring their outer membrane proteins, before penetrating the mucus layer with the aid of glycosidases produced by the gut normal flora. Many bacteria then adhere to the underlying epithelial cells and induce these cells to ingest them. The shigellae multiply within the epithelial cells and spread laterally into adjacent cells and deep into the lamina propria. The infected epithelial cells are killed and the lamina propria and submucosa develop an inflammatory reaction with capillary thrombosis. Patches of necrotic epithelium are sloughed and ulcers form. The cellular response is mainly by polymorphonuclear leucocytes, which can be seen readily on microscopical examination of the stool, together with red cells and sloughed epithelium. Dysentery bacilli rarely invade other tissues. Transient bacteraemia can occur but septicaemia with metastatic infection is rare.

Although the main determinant of pathogenicity in shigella infection is invasion of the wall of the large bowel, with its consequent inflammatory reaction, many strains have been shown to produce an exotoxin able to cause secretion of water and electrolytes by cells of the small bowel by a mechanism similar to that of cholera and *Esch. coli* toxins. This toxin may be responsible for the brief episode of watery diarrhoea which often precedes the onset of the severe bloody flux of classical dysentery.

## CLINICAL FEATURES

The incubation period is usually between 2 and 3 days, but may be as short as 12 h. The onset of symptoms is usually sudden, and frequently the initial symptom is abdominal colic. This is followed by the onset of watery diarrhoea, and in all but the mildest cases this is accompanied by fever and malaise. Many episodes resolve at this point, but others progress to abdominal cramps, tenesmus and the frequent passage of small volumes of stool, predominantly consisting of bloody mucus. In a typical case of dysentery the symptoms last about 4 days but, exceptionally, may continue for 10 days or more.

The severity of the clinical illness is to some extent associated with the particular species involved. Infection with *Sh. dysenteriae* is usually associated with a severe illness in which prostration is marked and, in young children, may be accompanied by febrile convulsions. The special virulence of *Sh. dysenteriae* has been ascribed to its ability to produce a potent exotoxin; this was formerly described as a neurotoxin because of the neurological effects resulting from vascular endothelial damage produced by the toxin when injected intravenously in experimental animals. However, this toxin, which also has a fluid transuding effect on the intestinal mucosa, is elaborated by many other strains of shigellae, and its role in the pathogenesis of dysentery is uncertain.

*Sh. dysenteriae* type I has also been responsible for many cases of the haemolytic uraemic syndrome accompanying outbreaks of dysentery in several countries. The condition, with its triad of haemolytic anaemia, thrombocytopenia and acute renal failure, can be caused by many pathogens (in particular, *Esch. coli* O157, see Ch. 27). It is associated with complement activation and disseminated intravascular coagulation, and in some parts of the world is one of the commonest forms of acute renal failure in children.

The illness caused by members of the *Sh. flexneri* and *Sh. boydii* groups may be as prostrating as that caused by *Sh. dysenteriae*. At the other end of the clinical spectrum of bacillary dysentery, the illness associated with *Sh. sonnei* in an otherwise healthy person may be confined to the passage of a few loose stools with vague abdominal discomfort, and the patient often continues at school or work. Death from bacillary dysentery is uncommon; it occurs mostly at the extremes of life or in individuals who are suffering from some other disease or debilitating condition.

## LABORATORY DIAGNOSIS

A specimen of faeces is always preferable to a rectal swab. Rectal swabs do not allow adequate macroscopic and microscopic examination of the stool, and unless properly taken and bearing obvious faecal material may be no more than a swab of peri-anal skin. Moreover, because of drying of the swab, pathogenic species die off quite rapidly, and may not survive transport to the laboratory.

Fresh unstained suspensions of faeces should be examined microscopically for the presence of protozoa that may be responsible for the diarrhoea (see Ch. 61) and also to note the character of the cellular exudate.

The faeces are inoculated on DCA or MacConkey agar. Mucus, if present in the specimen, may be used as the inoculum. Suitable cultures should also be set up to detect other possible bacterial pathogens such as *Salmonella* (see Ch. 25) or *Campylobacter* (see Ch. 30) species.

After incubation at 37°C for 18–24 h, pale non-lactose-fermenting colonies from DCA or MacConkey agar are tested for urease production (negative for shigellae), motility (negative) and for the ability to utilize certain sugar substrates. Colonies that give the characteristic reactions must have their identity confirmed by serological investigation with species-specific sera and then with type-specific sera unless the strain is *Sh. sonnei*. It is rarely necessary to take strain identification any further except when investigating major outbreaks in endemic areas. With *Sh. sonnei*, plasmid pattern analysis and colicine typing may help elucidate patterns of spread.

Tests for specific antibodies in the patient's serum are of little value since in an endemic area the patient's serum rarely shows any increased level of specific antibody compared with sera from healthy people.

## TREATMENT

Most cases of shigella dysentery, especially those due to *Sh. sonnei*, are mild and do not require antibiotic therapy. Symptomatic treatment with the maintenance of hydration by use of oral rehydration salt solution (see Ch. 31, Table 31.2) is all that is required. As with salmonella infections, drugs which impair gut motility should be avoided. Treatment with a suitable antibiotic is necessary in the very young, the aged or the debilitated, and in severe infections. Ampicillin, co-trimoxazole, tetracycline or ciprofloxacin is an appropriate choice, provided the drug is shown to be active in vitro; each may be administered orally. There is no evidence that antibiotics reduce the period of excretion of the organisms,

and they should not be used in the asymptomatic person either prophylactically or in attempts to hasten clearance after recovery.

## EPIDEMIOLOGY

The 20th century has seen a steady and remarkable change in the relative frequency of the different *Shigella* species in the UK and other European countries. Infections due to *Sh. dysenteriae*, common before the First World War, are now rare. Between 1920 and 1930 both *Sh. flexneri* and *Sh. sonnei* were endemic and approximately equal in incidence, but by 1940 *Sh. sonnei* had become dominant, increasing in incidence annually to a peak of over 49 000 notifications (99% of all shigellae notified) in 1956. The incidence of Sonne dysentery then declined steadily in the UK to an annual average of about 3000 notified cases between 1970 and 1990. However, the number of cases rose sharply in 1991, when there were several widespread community outbreaks, and continued to rise to a peak of 17 000 cases in 1992, the highest level in the UK for more than 20 years. The incidence has since fallen, but there were still more than 4550 cases in 1995. Infections due to the other shigellae, usually imported, have remained fairly constant at about 800–900 a year for the past decade.

Similar changes have taken place in the USA although more slowly. Up to 1968, *Sh. flexneri* and *Sh. sonnei* were equally common, but *Sh. sonnei* now accounts for 65% of cases and *Sh. flexneri* for about 30%. Over the past several decades the other two *Shigella* species have been responsible for less than 5% of notifications, but there has been a recent increase in cases imported from Asia and South America.

In tropical areas of the developing world, shigellosis is endemic; it has been estimated that some 5 million cases require hospital treatment and about 600 000 die every year. Young children are particularly vulnerable.

### Sources and spread

Bacillary dysentery is usually spread faecal–orally by fingers. The case or carrier, after contaminating his or her hands while cleansing at toilet, touches and thus contaminates the lavatory flush handle, door knobs, washbasin taps, hand towels and other objects which, when handled by another individual, allow transfer of dysentery bacilli to the recipient's hands and thence to the mouth. Such spread is facilitated by separating the washbasin from the lavatory compartment so that the handle of the intervening door acts as an efficient vehicle of infection. The carrier may also touch and thus infect food that is eaten, or eating utensils that are used by another person, who is thereby infected. Dysentery bacilli are also liberated into the air in an aerosol when an infected loose stool is flushed from the toilet, and after settling on the surfaces of toilet seats, furniture and surroundings may survive for some days in a moist atmosphere.

An important feature of the epidemiology of bacillary dysentery in the UK and other countries with good environmental sanitation is that the main patient group involved is school age children and particularly primary school children. Here, unwitting neglect of toilet hygiene by children at school undoubtedly plays a part. The disease is often endemic among adults living in residential institutions where for one reason or another high standards of hygiene are difficult to maintain, and has in the past been a scourge in gaols and in armies in the field. The seasonal distribution of bacillary dysentery in the UK is bimodal, with the highest incidence in spring and a second peak in October and November. The incidence is at its lowest in summer, when schoolchildren are on holiday. Since this is the period when flying insects are most abundant, this suggests that in this country insects play little if any part in transmission. However, in communities without satisfactory methods of sewage disposal, insects can gain access to infected human excreta and transfer shigellae mechanically to foodstuffs. Foods may also be contaminated directly by human cases or carriers.

Occasional epidemics of bacillary dysentery have been traced to water supplies when chlorination of the supply has not been instituted or has been defective. Such water-borne epidemics are usually spectacular in the large numbers of people simultaneously infected and in the speed with which they can be terminated when the water supply is adequately treated. Epidemic infection may also follow the contamination of milk or ice-cream.

# CONTROL

The mild and often fleeting nature of the clinical illness associated with *Sh. sonnei* infection means that frequently the case of bacillary dysentery remains ambulant and follows his or her daily labour and leisure pursuits, remaining in circulation as a disperser of the causal organism. The pressure on toilet facilities, particularly in schools, allows hand-to-mouth spread of the bacilli. The provision of washbasins in the same compartment as the toilet pedestal would allow some reduction in spread, especially if flushing mechanisms and washbasin taps could be operated by foot instead of by hand. However, handwashing, although very important, cannot be guaranteed to remove all the dysentery bacilli from the hands. During diarrhoea, faecal soiling of the fingers can be heavy, and handwashing will at best only reduce the numbers of bacteria present. The normal disinfecting effect of the skin fatty acids and competing skin organisms may take up to half an hour to destroy the rest. For this reason it is important that people with symptoms such that they need to go to stool during a normal working shift should stay off work and as far as possible out of circulation until the symptoms have subsided, especially when their work involves preparation of food or direct contact with other people. Asymptomatic carriers are far less important in the spread of this disease, and seldom if ever need to be excluded from any employment.

## Control of an outbreak

Outbreaks of dysentery in schools and other institutions are notoriously difficult to control. In nursery school outbreaks, infection is usually widespread before the first cases are notified, with considerable environmental contamination. Some children will be incubating the infection; others will have recovered from the diarrhoea but still be excreting the organisms. In this situation the acute case is far more important in the spread of infection than the symptomless excreter. There is little to be gained by trying to ascertain bacteriologically who is infected and who is not, once the cause of the outbreak has been established, since there is little reason to exclude an asymptomatic carrier and it is pointless to seek confirmation of a clearly symptomatic case. The practical course is usually to exclude acute cases but to allow children without symptoms to remain at or return to school.

Having determined the exclusion policy it is important to try to stop hand-to-hand spread among those who remain at school. Supervision of children using the lavatory, supervised handwashing before meals, frequent disinfection of water closets, including seats, lavatory chain and door handles, and the general use of paper towels all play a part. No single measure alone will be sufficient. Staff need support as morale can flag, and they themselves are vulnerable to infection. Outbreaks can persist for weeks despite all measures, and then subside abruptly for little apparent reason.

Similar principles can be applied to outbreaks in residential institutions or a hospital ward. The most important single factor in all these situations is the need for adequate communication. Teachers, nurses, parents and all who are involved in trying to control the outbreak need to have explained to them exactly how the infection spreads, and the reasons for the measures taken or not taken. Finally, the temptation to use antibiotics prophylactically in an attempt to limit the spread must be resisted.

## RECOMMENDED READING

Bennish M L, Harris J R, Wojtyniak B J, Struelens M 1990 Death in shigellosis: incidence and risk factors in hospitalized patients. *Journal of Infectious Diseases* 161: 500–506

Christie A B 1987 *Infectious Diseases: Epidemiology and Clinical Practice*, 4th edn. Churchill Livingstone, Edinburgh, ch 6

Hale T L, Formal S B 1987 Pathogenesis of shigella infections. *Pathology and Immunopathology Research* 6: 117–127

Keusch G T 1979 Shigella infections. *Clinics in Gastro-enterology* 8: 645–662

Sasakawa C 1995 Molecular basis of pathogenicity of *Shigella. Reviews in Medical Microbiology* 6: 257–266

# 27

# Escherichia

**Urinary tract infection; travellers' diarrhoea; haemorrhagic colitis; haemolytic uraemic syndrome**

*M. J. Lewis*

*Escherichia coli* and related Gram-negative 'coliform' bacteria predominate among the aerobic commensal flora in the gut of humans and animals. Widespread, and present wherever there is faecal contamination, *Esch. coli* appears not to lead an independent existence outside the animal body, and for this reason is regularly used by public health microbiologists as an indicator of faecal pollution of water sources, drinking water and food. The species encompasses a great variety of strains that include purely commensal organisms as well as those possessing combinations of virulence determinants that enable them to act as specific pathogens of the gut and of extra-intestinal sites, especially the urinary tract.

## DESCRIPTION

*Esch. coli* is the type species of the genus but several other species have been described. Strains of *Esch. coli* are usually motile and some, especially those from extra-intestinal infections, produce a polysaccharide capsule. They grow well on non-selective media, forming smooth, colourless colonies 2–3 mm in diameter in 18 h on nutrient agar, and large, red colonies on MacConkey agar; there may be haemolysis on blood agar. They grow over a wide range of temperature (15–45°C). Some strains are more heat-resistant than other members of the Enterobacteriaceae and will survive 60°C for 15 min or 55°C for 60 min.

Some of the biochemical reactions which help distinguish *Esch. coli* from other enterobacteria are given in Table 25.1 (see p. 253). Although most strains ferment lactose with the production of acid and gas within 24–48 h, some do so only after extended incubation or are non-lactose fermenters. Many characteristic biochemical reactions, such as indole production and the formation of acid and gas

from lactose and other carbohydrates, take place at 44°C as well as at 37°C.

The term *coliform* is commonly used to refer to any member of the Enterobacteriaceae but in origin meant 'like *Bact.* (later *Esch.*) *coli*', and many workers, especially in fields related to public health, prefer to reserve *coliform* to describe genera or species of enterobacteria which normally ferment lactose, using the term *non-lactose fermenter* (NLF) to describe the rest. Neither term has any taxonomic validity.

Studies of DNA–DNA recombination show that *Esch. coli* and *Shigella* organisms form a single genetic species, and it is therefore to be expected that intermediate strains will occur. Certain of these, which are non-motile and anaerogenic, and often ferment lactose late or not at all, have caused difficulties in classification. They were at one time included in the so-called 'Alkalescens-Dispar' group but these strains are now considered to be atypical *Esch. coli*.

### Antigenic structure

The diagnostic serotyping scheme is based on the distribution of O, H and K antigens, as detected by the reactions obtained in agglutination tests. Over 160 different somatic or O antigens have been described. Agglutination tests must be carried out on boiled or autoclaved cultures to overcome inagglutinability caused by K antigens. Numerous cross-reactions occur between individual *Esch. coli* O antigens, and between these and the O antigens of organisms belonging to the genera *Citrobacter*, *Providencia*, *Salmonella*, *Shigella* and *Yersinia*. In some instances the antigens appearing in the different genera are identical serologically and structurally. In contrast to *Salmonella* and *Klebsiella* species, which produce only neutral O-specific polysaccharide, that produced by *Esch. coli* strains may be neutral or acidic. In most cases the acidic components are hexuronic acids.

**Table 27.1**   K antigens of *Esch. coli*

| Properties | Group I | Group II |
|---|---|---|
| Molecular weight | >100 000 | <50 000 |
| Acidic component | Hexuronic acid, pyruvate | Glucuronic acid, phosphate, KDO, NeuNAc |
| Heat stability (100°C, pH 6) | All stable | Mostly labile |
| O groups | O8, O9 | Many |
| Chromosome site | *His* | *SerA* |
| Expressed at 17–20°C | Yes | No |
| Electrophoretic mobility | Low | High |

KDO, ketodeoxyoctonate; NeuNAc, *N*-acetylneuraminic acid.

More than 50 H (flagellar) antigens are known. Most are monophasic but rare diphasic strains have been reported. There are only a few significant cross-reactions between them and with the H antigens of other members of the Enterobacteriaceae. Before use for H antigen determination it is often necessary to grow cultures in semi-solid agar.

The term 'K antigen' was first used collectively for surface or capsular antigens that cause 'O inagglutinability'. In the past these antigens were divided into three classes (L, A and B) according to the effect of heat on the agglutinability, antigenicity and antibody-binding power of bacterial strains that carry them. In modern usage, 'K antigen' refers to the acidic polysaccharide capsular antigens, and those of *Esch. coli* may be divided into two groups (groups I and II; see Table 27.1) that largely correspond to the old A and L antigens.

Antisera for serotyping purposes are not readily available except for enteropathogenic O groups (EPEC; see below).

Many of the Enterobacteriaceae possess fimbriae (see Ch. 2). Strains may carry both sex pili and more than one type of common fimbriae. Within a culture, there are individual cells with many common fimbriae and others with none, and there is reversible variation between the fimbriate and the non-fimbriate phase. Type 1 fimbriae are able to mediate adhesion to a wide range of human and animal cells that contain mannose residues. Such adhesion might favour pathogenicity and there are some examples of this. The possible role of type 1 fimbriae in urinary tract infection remains controversial.

A number of filamentous protein structures resembling fimbriae have been described in *Esch. coli*. These cause a mannose-resistant haemagglutination, and there is good evidence that they play an important part in the pathogenesis of diarrhoeal disease and in urinary tract infection.

They include the K88 antigen found in strains causing enteritis of pigs, the K99 antigen found in strains causing enteritis of calves and lambs, and the colonization factor antigens (CFAs) found in enterotoxigenic *Esch. coli* of human origin. Fimbriae that are of importance in urinary tract infection and cause mannose-resistant haemagglutination are distinguished according to their receptor specificities. These include the P fimbriae that bind specifically to receptors present on the P blood group antigens of human erythrocytes and uroepithelial cells.

## PATHOGENESIS

Strains of *Esch. coli* possess a battery of virulence determinants. The polysaccharides of the O and K antigens protect the organism from the bactericidal effect of complement and phagocytes in the absence of specific antibodies. However, in the presence of antibody to K antigens alone, or to both O and K antigens, phagocytosis is successful. In a capsulate strain the presence of K antigens exerts only a partial protection against the effect of antibody to O antigens alone.

Many strains form a haemolysin, and a much higher proportion of *Esch. coli* isolated from human extra-intestinal infections are haemolytic than are those from human faeces. Furthermore, haemolytic strains have been found to be more virulent than non-haemolytic ones in animal experiments. It is likely that haemolytic strains obtain iron from the lysed erythrocytes of the host. Cytotoxic activity may also be important in some infections.

Some strains possess the ColV plasmid, which carries the genetic determinants for an aerobactin-mediated iron uptake system, and this may be responsible for enhanced virulence.

## Urinary tract and septic infections

*Esch. coli* is by far the most common cause of acute, uncomplicated urinary tract infection outside hospitals as well as causing much hospital associated urinary tract sepsis. It also causes neonatal meningitis and septicaemia, sepsis in operation wounds and abscesses in a variety of organs.

As many as 80% of *Esch. coli* strains causing neonatal meningitis and 40% of those isolated from infants with septicaemia but without meningitis possess the K1 antigen. Strains possessing the K1 or the K5 antigen may have greater virulence than those with other K antigens since they are very poorly immunogenic because of their structural identity with host components.

Expression of the aerobactin-mediated iron uptake system occurs more frequently in strains from septicaemia, pyelonephritis and lower urinary tract infection than among human faecal isolates.

*Esch. coli* that cause urinary tract infection often originate in the gut of the patient, and the infection is thought to occur in an ascending manner. There is evidence that the ability of *Esch. coli* to infect the urinary tract is associated with fimbriae that specifically mediate adherence to the uroepithelial cells.

### Epidemiology

Urinary tract infection is much commoner in females than in males since the shorter, wider female urethra appears to be less effective in preventing access of the bacteria to the bladder. Sexual intercourse is a predisposing factor. The high incidence in pregnant women can be attributed to impairment of urine flow due partly to hormonal changes and partly to pressure on the urinary tract. Other causes of urinary stagnation that may predispose to urinary tract infection include urethral obstruction, urinary stones, congenital malformations and neurological disorders, all of which occur in both sexes. In men, prostatic enlargement is the most common predisposing factor. Catheterization and cystoscopy may introduce bacteria into the bladder and therefore carry a risk of infection.

Since most urinary tract infections are thought to be caused by organisms originating from the patient's own bowel, each infection is generally regarded as sporadic. However, the prevalence of various serotypes of *Esch. coli* in urinary tract infections varies with geographical location, and this fits well with the view that *Esch. coli* which cause such infections are specific pathogens for the urinary tract. Pathogenic strains, possibly transmitted in contaminated foods, are able to colonize the bowel, and in individuals with predisposing factors may cause a urinary tract infection. The prevalence of infections due to a particular strain may therefore increase for a time in a locality.

### Laboratory diagnosis

Clinical specimens may be stained by Gram's method for microscopical examination, and are cultured on MacConkey agar or other suitable media. In the case of suspected urinary tract infection, culture is semiquantitative; in acute *Esch. coli* infections the organism is generally present in pure culture at a count of $10^5$ or more per millilitre of urine (see Ch. 64).

### Treatment and control

*Esch. coli* is naturally resistant to benzylpenicillin but sensitive to ampicillin and the cephalosporins, and usually to tetracycline, chloramphenicol, aminoglycosides, trimethoprim, and sulphonamides. Many strains, however, have acquired plasmids conferring resistance to one or more of these drugs. Strains resistant to ampicillin, streptomycin, sulphonamides and tetracyclines are particularly common, and strains resistant to chloramphenicol, trimethoprim and cephalexin are no longer rare; the resistances are usually transferable.

Extra-intestinal *Esch. coli* infections are treated with specific antimicrobial therapy, preferably guided by the results of laboratory tests for sensitivity. In particular, bacterial meningitis is a medical emergency and vigorous early treatment is required.

Urinary catheterization and cystoscopy require rigorous aseptic technique to minimize the introduction of bacteria into the bladder. Bladder irrigation and systemic treatment with antimicrobial agents has been used in catheter-associated infections but such treatment is seldom more than palliative and encourages infections with resistant organisms.

## Diarrhoea

*Esch. coli* may cause: acute enteritis of young animals, including human infants, piglets, calves and lambs; acute enteritis in human subjects of all ages occurring mainly in the tropics and including travellers' diarrhoea; a dysentery-like disease affecting humans at all ages; and haemorrhagic colitis or 'bloody diarrhoea'.

**Table 27.2** The major groups of diarrhoea-causing *Esch. coli*

| Pathogenic group | Common serogroups |
|---|---|
| 1. Enteropathogenic *Esch. coli* (EPEC) | O26, O55, O86, O111, O114, O119, O125, O126, O127, O128, O142 |
| 2. Enterotoxigenic *Esch. coli* (ETEC) | O6, O8, O15, O25, O27, O63, O78, O115, O148, O153, O159, O167 |
| 3. Entero-invasive *Esch. coli* (EIEC) | O28ac, O112ac, O124, O136, O143, O144, O152, O164 |
| 4. Vero cytotoxin-producing *Esch. coli* (VTEC) | O157[a] |

[a]VTEC have been found in many other serogroups but these are far less common than O157 in human disease.

Strains that cause diarrhoea fall into at least four groups with different pathogenic mechanisms (Table 27.2):

1. *Enteropathogenic Esch. coli (EPEC).* EPEC were first discovered by serotyping in epidemiological studies. They cause infantile enteritis, especially in tropical countries; outbreaks often occur in hospitals and may have a high mortality, but such outbreaks have become uncommon in industrialized countries.

2. *Enterotoxigenic Esch. coli (ETEC).* These strains produce a heat-stable enterotoxin (ST) or a heat-labile enterotoxin (LT) or both. In addition, they possess colonization factors that are specific for the host animal species and which enable the organisms to adhere to the epithelium of the small intestine.

3. *Entero-invasive Esch. coli (EIEC).* EIEC cause an illness identical to shigella dysentery in patients of all ages.

4. *Vero cytotoxin-producing Esch. coli (VTEC).* *Esch. coli* O157 is the commonest serogroup found in human VTEC infections but others are encountered. VTEC produce one or both of two Vero cytotoxins (VT1 and VT2). VT1 is closely related to the so-called Shiga toxin produced by strains of *Shigella dysenteriae* type 1, and is sometimes called Shiga-like toxin. VTEC cause a range of symptoms from mild, watery diarrhoea to a severe diarrhoea with large amounts of fresh blood in the stool (*haemorrhagic colitis*). An important complication, especially in children, is the *haemolytic uraemic syndrome*.

## Enteropathogenic Esch. coli *(EPEC)*

The fact that EPEC strains were originally identified epidemiologically as being able to cause diarrhoea meant that strains with a diversity of pathogenic mechanisms were inevitably included in what later proved to be a heterogeneous collection of serogroups all labelled EPEC. Of these, a few have been shown to be enterotoxigenic and are best regarded as ETEC, while some produce VT and should be termed VTEC. The term 'EPEC' is best reserved for strains that do not produce ST, LT or VT and are not entero-invasive.

*Pathogenesis.* The ability of EPEC strains to cause diarrhoea has been confirmed by oral administration of the organisms to babies and adults, but the mechanism by which they do so is incompletely understood.

Colonization of the upper part of the small intestine occurs in infantile enteritis associated with EPEC. In many patients, EPEC are seen by electron microscopy to be intimately associated with the mucosal surface and to be partially surrounded by cup-like projections ('pedestals') of the enterocyte surface and in areas of EPEC attachment the brush border microvilli are lost. Many strains are strongly adhesive to intestinal epithelial cells, and this represents an important pathogenic mechanism. Such strains of *Esch. coli* have been termed attaching, effacing *Esch. coli* or entero-adherent *Esch. coli* (EAEC).

Nevertheless, some EPEC strains associated with human diarrhoea possess none of these characters, and their pathogenic mechanism is still unclear.

*Epidemiology.* Since 1971 few epidemics of EPEC enteritis have been reported in the UK or the USA, but a satisfactory explanation for this has not been put forward. Strains isolated recently from sporadic cases in the UK possess the same virulence determinants as those that caused outbreaks in the 1960s and early 1970s. In the absence of epidemics, the incidence of sporadic cases of infantile enteritis in the UK shows a peak in the summer months.

Although EPEC enteritis now appears to be of little importance in areas with good standards of hygiene, it is still common in communities with poor hygiene. In these countries sporadic cases and outbreaks occur very frequently in the general community as well as in institutions.

The importance of EPEC as a cause of enteritis in adults is difficult to evaluate since few laboratories look for these organisms in patients over 3 years of age. However, a few outbreaks have been described.

**Laboratory diagnosis of EPEC.** Stool specimens are plated on media such as MacConkey agar, and lactose-fermenting colonies are examined by slide agglutination with polyvalent antisera for the EPEC serogroups. Those giving positive reactions are subcultured and again tested by slide agglutination with monovalent antisera; identification is finally confirmed by tube agglutination tests. Strains provisionally serogrouped in this way should also be identified as *Esch. coli* because there is widespread sharing of antigens among the Enterobacteriaceae.

Tests for adhesion to HEp-2 cells and DNA probes for the detection of the EPEC adherence factor are available in some laboratories, and serve to discriminate EAEC strains from other EPEC.

## Enterotoxigenic Esch. coli *(ETEC)*

### Pathogenesis.

*Heat-labile enterotoxin (LT).* LT is closely related to the toxin produced by strains of *Vibrio cholerae*. Both are protein complexes consisting of one polypeptide A subunit and five poly-peptide B subunits with molecular weights of about 25 000 and 11 500, respectively. The B subunits are responsible for binding of the toxin to the epithelial cells. After translocation across the membrane of intestinal epithelial cells, subunit A catalyses the nicotinamide adenine dinucleotide (NAD)-dependent activation of adenylate cyclase to cause an increase in the concentration of cyclic adenosine 5'-monophosphate (cAMP). In the intestinal villus cells, cAMP inhibits the absorption of sodium and therefore of chloride and water while in the crypt cells cAMP increases sodium secretion and causes loss of chloride and water, leading to profuse watery diarrhoea.

LT is plasmid encoded in many strains of human and animal origin, and the organization of the operon encoding the A and B subunits is known in detail.

Occasional *Esch. coli* strains produce a heat-labile toxin (LT-II) which has similar biological activity to LT but which does not react with antiserum in neutralization or immunodiffusion tests. The struc-tural genes for LT-II appear to be chromosomal although few strains have been studied.

*Heat-stable enterotoxin (ST).* In contrast to LT, the STs of *Esch. coli* have a low molecular weight and are poorly immunogenic. There are two major classes of *Esch. coli* STs, designated $ST_A$ and $ST_B$ (or ST-I and ST-II). $ST_A$ is detected by an infant mouse test in which secretion occurs in the intestine within 4 h following intragastric administration. This toxin activates guanylate cyclase activity resulting in an increase in the level of cyclic guanosine monophosphate (cGMP). The activity of $ST_A$ is rapid, whereas LT acts after a lag period. The mechanism of secretion caused by $ST_A$, via cGMP, is not known but calcium may play a role.

$ST_A$ is plasmid encoded, and these plasmids may also carry genes for LT, adhesive factors or antibiotic resistance.

$ST_B$ is distinguished from $ST_A$ by its biological activity and by its insolubility in methanol. $ST_B$ stimulates fluid accumulation in ligated intestinal loops of piglets but not in the infant mouse test. The mechanism of action of $ST_B$ is not known but it appears not to act via cAMP or cGMP.

**Adhesive factors.** Enterotoxin alone is not sufficient to enable *Esch. coli* to cause diarrhoea. The organism must also be able to adhere to the mucosal surface of the epithelial cells of the small intestine. This adhesion is usually mediated by fimbriae which bind to specific receptors in the cell membrane. Adhesins or *colonization factors* are antigenic and can be recognized by means of agglutination or immunodiffusion tests. Their presence can also be demonstrated by haemagglutination, by experimental colonization of animal intestines or by tissue or organ culture methods. In contrast to the haemagglutination due to type 1 fimbriae of *Esch. coli*, that due to colonization factors associated with diarrhoeal disease is not inhibited by mannose. Plasmids that simultaneously carry genes for both a colonization factor and enterotoxin production have been described.

The first colonization factor in *Esch. coli*, initially recognized as a surface antigen (K88), is controlled by a transferable plasmid and is fimbrial in nature. Its importance in the pathogenesis of piglet enteritis was demonstrated in experiments in which it was shown that the loss of the K88 plasmid from a strain of *Esch. coli* O141 was accompanied by the loss of its capacity to cause diarrhoea when given orally to piglets. This was restored by introducing a K88 plasmid from another strain of *Esch. coli*. There is a gene in pigs which is inherited in a simple Mendelian manner and which determines the

**Table 27.3** Properties of some important human colonization factors

| Colonization factor | Components | MRHA | | | Fimbrial type | Associated toxin | Associated serogroups |
|---|---|---|---|---|---|---|---|
| | | Human | Bovine | Guinea-pig | | | |
| CFA I | | + | + | – | Rod-like | ST or ST/LT | O4, O7, O15, O20, O25, O63, O78, O90, O104, O110, O126, O128, O136, O153, O159 |
| CFA II | CS1 | (+) | + | – | Rod-like | ST/LT | O6, O139 |
| | CS2 | – | + | – | Rod-like | ST/LT | O6 |
| | CS3 | – | + | – | Fibrillar | ST/LT | O8, O78, O80, O85, O115, O128, O139, O168 |
| CFA III | | – | – | – | Rod-like | LT | O25 |
| CFA IV | CS4 | + | + | – | Rod-like | ST/LT | O25 |
| | CS5 | + | + | + | Helical | ST | O6, O29, O92, O114, O115, O167, O25, O27, O79, O89, O92, O148, O153, O159, O169 |
| | CS6 | – | – | – | None | ST or LT | |

MRHA, mannose-resistant haemagglutinin; CS, coli surface antigen; (+), weak reaction.

presence of receptors for K88 in the pig intestinal epithelium; pigs lacking this receptor are resistant to colonization of the small intestine by *Esch. coli* strains with the K88 antigen.

Several colonization factors have subsequently been discovered in human strains of ETEC and, no doubt, others remain to be discovered. The properties of some of the more important colonization factors are shown in Table 27.3.

***Epidemiology.*** ETEC are uncommon in geographical regions where hygiene and nutrition are good, but occasional outbreaks of diarrhoea and sporadic cases have been reported. In the developing countries, diarrhoeal diseases are a major cause of death in children under 5 years of age, and ETEC cause a large proportion of these. In its most severe form ETEC infection resembles cholera.

ETEC are the commonest cause of travellers' diarrhoea. This is a world-wide illness, usually of brief duration, often beginning with the rapid onset of loose stools and accompanied by variable symptoms, including nausea, vomiting and abdominal cramps. It occurs most frequently among those travelling from areas of good hygiene and temperate climate to areas with lower standards, particularly in warmer countries.

There have been several studies of travellers' diarrhoea in Mexico where 'turista' has an attack rate of 29–48%; in African countries ETEC have been found in 31–75% of Peace Corps volunteers with diarrhoea.

The sources and modes of spread of ETEC infection in warm-climate countries are not well understood but it seems likely that water contaminated by human or animal sewage plays an important part in the spread of infection.

***Laboratory diagnosis of ETEC.***
*Detection of LT.* Tests in tissue cultures of Y1 mouse adrenal cells and Chinese hamster ovary (CHO) cells are accepted as standard methods for the detection of LT, but other cell lines, including Vero monkey kidney cells, are also sensitive to the toxin. Exposure of the cells to culture supernates containing LT or cholera toxin leads to a morphological response which can be seen by microscopy. The response can be regarded as stimulatory or 'cytotonic' in contrast to the cytotoxic effect of VTEC supernates on Vero cells.

Several immunological techniques are available for the detection of LT, including an enzyme-linked immunosorbent assay (ELISA) and a solid-phase radio-immunoassay (RIA). These tests are performed in microtitration trays or in tubes, and the results can be read spectrophotometrically. A precipitin test (the *Biken test*) performed directly on bacterial colonies growing on a special agar medium may be suitable for use in field laboratories. Additionally, a staphylococcal co-agglutination test and a commercially available latex particle agglutination test are useful for screening.

*Detection of ST.* Many enterotoxigenic strains of *Esch. coli* produce only ST and it is essential to include tests for ST production in any survey of enterotoxigenicity. Unfortunately the usual tests for this toxin are cumbersome and time-consuming.

Injection of enterotoxin preparations, both LT and ST, into ligated ileal loops of rabbits leads to the accumulation of fluid. The action of ST can be distinguished from that of LT both by its relative stability to heat and by the rapidity of its action. So far it has proved impossible to devise tissue culture tests for ST, and the most widely used method for detecting $ST_A$ is the infant mouse test. The intestines are removed after the injection of culture supernates, and the ratio of gut weight to remaining body weight is used as an objective measure of fluid accumulation.

The non-antigenic nature of ST at first prevented the development of immunological tests. This problem was overcome by preparing antiserum from toxin coupled to a bovine serum albumin carrier and using the antiserum in an RIA. Subsequently, ELISA tests with monoclonal antibody specific for ST became available.

*Genetic probes.* Gene probes have been developed for the detection of ST or LT in stool, food or water containing ETEC.

## Entero-invasive Esch. coli *(EIEC)*

The very close relationship between *Esch. coli* and shigellae is reflected in the fact that EIEC and shigellae both cause bacillary dysentery by the same mechanisms (see also Ch. 26).

**Pathogenesis.** Both EIEC and shigellae cause disease by invading intestinal epithelium. Infection is by ingestion; only a small number of bacteria need to be swallowed as they are relatively resistant to gastric acid and bile, and pass readily into the large intestine where they multiply in the gut lumen. Passing through the overlying mucus layer the bacteria attach to the intestinal epithelial cells. They then induce the cells to take them up by a process of endocytosis, being carried into the cell in an endocytic vacuole which then lyses. The ability to cause the vacuole to lyse is an important virulence attribute, as organisms unable to do this are unable to spread to neighbouring cells. Following lysis of the vacuole the bacteria multiply within the epithelial cell and kill it. Spread to neighbouring cells leads to tissue destruction and consequent inflammation, which is the underlying cause of the symptoms of bacillary dysentery.

Virulence in shigellae and EIEC depends on both chromosomal and plasmid genes. A large plasmid (120 MDa in *Shigella sonnei* and 140 MDa in other shigellae and in EIEC) carries genes for the expression of outer-membrane proteins that are required for invasion as well as genes that may be necessary for the insertion of these proteins into the cell membrane. Plasmid genes are also required for the ability to escape from the endocytic vacuole and to invade contiguous host cells. Chromosomal virulence genes include those required for the expression of a smooth lipopolysaccharide and genes for an aerobactin iron-binding system.

**Epidemiology.** The epidemiology and ecology of EIEC have been poorly studied, but there is no evidence of an animal or environmental reservoir. Surveys suggest that they cause about 5% of all diarrhoeas in areas of poor hygiene. In the UK and USA, outbreaks are occasionally described, especially in schools and hospitals for the mentally handicapped. Infections are usually food-borne but there is also evidence of cross-infection. The most common serogroup is O124.

**Laboratory diagnosis of EIEC.** The original test for entero-invasive potential is the guinea-pig eye or *Sereny test*. The bacterium is instilled into the conjunctival sac of the guinea-pig, and the animal is examined for up to 7 days for signs of conjunctivitis. Tissue culture methods are also available in which monolayers of HEp-2 or HeLa cells are exposed to suspensions of the organism under test. After an appropriate infection period the cells are washed with a solution containing gentamicin and lysozyme to remove extracellular organisms. After a further period to allow intracellular growth the cells are examined microscopically for the presence of intracellular organisms.

## Vero cytotoxigenic Esch. coli *(VTEC)*

The importance of VTEC in human disease has only become clear since the association was established between VTEC and two diseases of previously unknown aetiology: *haemorrhagic colitis* and *haemolytic uraemic syndrome* (HUS). The ability to cause haemorrhagic colitis has led some workers to refer to these strains as enterohaemorrhagic *Esch. coli*, or EHEC.

Haemorrhagic colitis is a grossly bloody diarrhoea, usually in the absence of pyrexia. It is usually preceded by abdominal pain and watery diarrhoea. Outbreaks were recognized in the USA in 1982 and, since then, outbreaks and sporadic cases have been reported in several other countries. Since 1995 well-publicized major episodes in the USA, Canada, Japan and Lanarkshire, Scotland, have heightened general awareness of the importance of this disease.

HUS is characterized by acute renal failure, micro-angiopathic haemolytic anaemia and thrombocytopenia. HUS occurs in all age groups but is more common in infants and young children and is a major cause of renal failure in childhood. HUS may be classified into two principal sub-groups; 'typical' HUS is associated with a pro-dromal bloody diarrhoea while an 'atypical' form occurs without a diarrhoeal phase. *Esch. coli* O157 is associated with the typical form of HUS.

VTEC infection in humans can be associated with a range of clinical symptoms from mild, non-bloody diarrhoea to severe manifestions such as HUS, and a wide spectrum of illness can occur even within a single outbreak. VTEC infection may also be accompanied by thrombotic thrombocytopenic purpura in which the clinical features of HUS are further complicated by neurological involvement and fever.

VTEC have also been implicated as a cause of disease in animals, particularly calves and pigs.

***Pathogenesis – nature and mode of action of VT.*** When VT was first described it was found to be very similar to Shiga toxin, produced by strains of *Sh. dysenteriae* type 1, in terms of biological properties, physical characteristics and antigenicity. The term 'Shiga-like toxin' (SLT) was therefore used to describe the toxin produced by *Esch. coli* strains, and both terms, VT and SLT, are widely used. VT that is neutralized by anti-Shiga toxin is now designated VT1 and a second VT, first shown in strains of serogroup O157 and not neutralized by anti-Shiga toxin, is termed VT2. VT1 and VT2 are also known as SLT-I and SLT-II.

Like Shiga toxin, VT1 and VT2 are made up of A and B subunits. For both toxins the A subunit possesses the biological activities of the toxin while the B subunits are thought to mediate specific binding and receptor-mediated uptake of the toxin. VT1 and VT2 have the same biological activities as Shiga toxin: cytotoxicity for Vero and HeLa cells, enterotoxicity in ligated rabbit gut loops and mouse paralytic lethality.

The genes controlling production of VT are phage encoded in several *Esch. coli* strains. VT genes have been cloned in *Esch. coli* K12 from phages originating in strains of serogroups O26 and O157, and probes for the VT genes have been developed.

Human umbilical cord endothelial cells have been used in studies of the action of VT1. There is a direct, dose-dependent cytotoxic effect on these cells in culture and actively dividing cells are the most sensitive. Since a micro-angiopathy of the capillaries is a characteristic renal lesion in HUS the results with this model support the hypothesis that vascular endothelial cells are a primary target for VT.

A plasmid in VTEC of serogroup O157 is necessary for the expression of fimbriae that determine the attachment of small numbers of bacteria in tissue culture. However, surface structures other than fimbriae may also mediate attachment. A DNA probe derived from this plasmid has been evaluated for the detection of VTEC.

***Epidemiology.*** VTEC outbreaks have occurred in the community, in nursing homes for the elderly and in day care centres for young children. The most severe clinical manifestations are usually seen in the paediatric and geriatric populations.

Food is an important source of VTEC infection. In several outbreaks of haemorrhagic colitis due to *Esch. coli* O157 in the USA and Canada the causative organism has been isolated from products as diverse as hamburger meat, unpasteurized apple juice, and unpasteurized milk. In the outbreak of infection in Lanarkshire, Scotland, in which a number of elderly people died, cooked meat from an award-winning butcher was implicated, indicating that bacteria have no respect for reputations. *Esch. coli* O157.H7 was also isolated from healthy heifers on the farms associated with the milk-borne incidents, and it seems likely that cattle are a major reservoir of *Esch. coli* O157.H7.

***Laboratory diagnosis.*** The proportion of VTEC in the faecal flora may be low, often less than 1%, so that picking and testing of individual colonies from culture plates may not always detect the presence of VTEC. DNA probes for the VT1 and VT2 genes have been developed, and by using these probes in colony hybridization tests several hundred colonies from each faecal specimen can be examined, giving a considerable increase in sensitivity.

While 95% of *Esch. coli* are sorbitol fermenters, O157 VTEC do not ferment sorbitol in 24 h, and this characteristic has been used as the basis of tests to detect them, e.g. using sorbitol–MacConkey agar for primary culture followed by agglutination with an O157 antiserum. VT production is confirmed by testing strains for a cytotoxic effect on Vero cells.

Evidence for VTEC infection has also been obtained by observing rising levels of VT-neutralizing antibodies or of antibody directed against the O157 lipopolysaccharide in patients' sera.

## Prevention and treatment of Esch. coli enteritis

***General measures.*** As with most diarrhoeal disease, the early correction of fluid and electrolyte imbalance is the most important single factor in preventing the death of the patient in severe infections.

The most effective means of preventing infection is to avoid exposure to the infecting agent. Contaminated food and water are probably the most important vehicles of ETEC infection in developing countries. The provision of safe supplies of water together with education in hygienic practice in the handling and production of food, particularly that given to young children, are essential. Travellers to countries with poor hygiene, especially in the tropics, should select eating places with care and, if possible, should consume only hot food and drinks, or bottled water. Self-peeled fruits are probably safe, but salads should be avoided. Unheated milk should always be considered unsafe.

The spread of infantile enteritis in hospitals and nurseries is mainly from patient to patient, generally on the hands of attendants, or from contaminated infant feeds. It can be prevented only by very strict hygiene. Infected patients, and recently admitted patients suspected of being infected, must be isolated by barrier nursing techniques to prevent faecal spread. In some cases outbreaks can be terminated only by closing the ward or nursery and cleaning thoroughly before re-opening.

It is likely that VTEC infections are acquired most frequently from meat and unpasteurized milk. Such infections should be avoided by normal food hygiene with particular attention to the thorough cooking of raw meats, especially if minced.

*Vaccination.*   The most extensive studies of the use of vaccines have so far been in the veterinary field. A potential vaccine for human use has been prepared by cross-linking a synthetically produced ST with the non-toxic B subunit of LT. Tests in the rat showed that the vaccine protects against subsequent challenge with ST or LT or with organisms that produce them. In human volunteers, oral administration causes an increase in antitoxin levels in serum samples and jejunal aspirates.

*Inhibition of enterotoxin activity.*   A number of substances such as activated charcoal, bismuth subsalicylate and non-steroidal anti-inflammatory drugs (NSAIDs) inhibit or reverse the secretory effects of enterotoxins in experimental animals and may be of value in the prevention or treatment of diarrhoea. Clinical trials have shown some benefit from such substances but more work needs to be done to establish the optimum conditions for their use.

*Antimicrobial prophylaxis.*   A number of antimicrobial drugs reduce the incidence of diarrhoea in travellers to tropical areas. These include doxycycline, trimethoprim, norfloxacin and other fluoroquinolones. However, the widespread use of antibiotic prophylaxis has been criticized both on the grounds of drug toxicity and because of the possibility that the development and spread of drug resistance might be encouraged among a variety of enteropathogenic organisms.

## OTHER *ESCHERICHIA* SPECIES

*Esch. blattae* was first described among bacteria isolated from the gut of the cockroach. It differs from *Esch. coli* both in oxidizing gluconate and fermenting malonate, as well as in failing to form indole, acidify mannitol or sorbitol, or produce β-galactosidase. It would probably be better placed in another genus. The species has not been reported from human clinical specimens. *Esch. fergusonii*, *Esch. hermanii* and *Esch. vulneris* have been recovered from various clinical specimens, especially faeces and wounds, but their clinical significance is usually unclear.

RECOMMENDED READING

Echeveria P, Savarino S J, Yamamoto T 1993 *Escherichia coli* diarrhoea. *Baillière's Clinical Gastroenterology* 7: 243–261
Gross R J 1991 The pathogenesis of *Escherichia coli* diarrhoea. *Reviews in Medical Microbiology* 2: 37–44
Johnson JR 1991 Virulence factors in *Escherichia coli* urinary tract infection. *Clinical Microbiology Reviews* 3: 80–128
Schoolnik G K 1989 How *Escherichia coli* infects the urinary tract. *New England Journal of Medicine* 12: 804–805

Scotland S M 1988 Toxins. *Journal of Applied Bacteriology Symposium Supplement*: 109S–129S
Tarr P I 1995 *Escherichia coli* O157:H7 Clinical, diagnostic and epidemiological aspects of human infection. *Clinical Infectious Diseases* 20: 1–10

# 28

# Klebsiella, enterobacter, proteus and other enterobacteria

Pneumonia; urinary tract infection; opportunist infection

*M. J. Lewis*

The genera described in this chapter conform to the general definition of the Enterobacteriaceae in that they are aerobic or facultatively anaerobic, ferment glucose, and give a positive catalase and a negative oxidase reaction. Together with organisms of the genera *Salmonella* (see Ch. 25), *Shigella* (see Ch. 26), *Escherichia* (see Ch. 27) and *Yersinia* (see Ch. 36),

they are commonly referred to as *enterobacteria*. Species of clinical interest are listed alphabetically in Table 28.1, along with a few of their common synonyms. Numerous tests are used to differentiate the various enterobacteria; a simple scheme that allows presumptive identification to the genus level is shown in Table 25.1 (see p. 253).

**Table 28.1** The principal genera and species of Enterobacteriaceae of clinical interest

| Genus | Species | Synonyms |
|---|---|---|
| Citrobacter | C. amalonaticus | Levinea amalonatica |
| | C. freundii | |
| | C. koseri | C. diversus, L. amalonatica |
| Edwardsiella | E. tarda | E. anguillimortifera |
| Enterobacter | Ent. aerogenes | K. mobilis |
| | Ent. cloacae | |
| Erwinia | Erw. herbicola | Ent. agglomerans |
| Escherichia[a] | | |
| Hafnia | H. alvei | Ent. alvei, Ent. hafniae |
| Klebsiella | K. oxytoca | |
| | K. pneumoniae | |
| | ssp. aerogenes | K. aerogenes |
| | ssp. ozaenae | K. ozaenae |
| | ssp. pneumoniae | K. pneumoniae |
| | ssp. rhino-scleromatis | K. rhino-scleromatis |
| Morganella | M. morganii | Pr. morganii |
| Proteus | Pr. mirabilis | |
| | Pr. vulgaris | |
| Providencia | Prov. alcalifaciens | |
| | Prov. rettgeri | Pr. rettgeri |
| | Prov. stuartii | |
| Salmonella[a] | | |
| Serratia | S. liquefaciens | Ent. liquefaciens |
| | S. marcescens | |
| | S. odorifera | |
| Shigella[a] | | |
| Yersinia[a] | | |

[a]See appropriate chapter.

## KLEBSIELLA

## CLASSIFICATION

The classification of the genus *Klebsiella* has a complex history that must be considered briefly to avoid confusion. In the past the name *Klebsiella aerogenes* was used for the non-motile, capsulate, gas-producing strains commonly found in human faeces and in water. These probably corresponded to strains described in the 19th century as *Bakterium lactis aerogenes,* referred to later as *Bacterium aerogenes*, and subsequently transferred to the genus *Klebsiella*. Unfortunately, the term 'Bact. aerogenes' (later *Aerobacter aerogenes*) was also used by water bacteriologists to refer to organisms that were subsequently shown to be motile and are now classified as *Enterobacter* species. In an attempt to resolve the resultant confusion, some taxonomists adopted '*pneumoniae*' as the species name for the non-motile *aerogenes*-like organisms, although it had earlier been used to designate certain biochemically atypical *Klebsiella* strains isolated from the respiratory tract of humans and animals. This view has now been accepted formally, and the name *K. pneumoniae* appears in the Approved Lists of Bacterial Names while *K. aerogenes* is omitted. In this chapter the name *K. pneumoniae* is therefore used for the species as a whole, but the most frequently encountered, biochemically typical form of it is referred to as *K. pneumonia*e ssp. *aerogenes*. The atypical respiratory strains are included in the subspecies *ozaenae*, *pneumoniae* and *rhinoscleromatis*. A further species, *K. oxytoca*, is occasionally encountered in clinical specimens.

## DESCRIPTION

Members of the genus *Klebsiella* tend to be slightly shorter and thicker than the other enterobacteria, and are straight rods about 1–2 μm long and 0.5–0.8 μm wide. The capsule is often pronounced and can be demonstrated even by Gram's stain. Capsular material is produced in greater amounts in media rich in carbohydrate. In these conditions the growth on agar is luxuriant, greyish white and extremely mucoid (Fig. 28.1). The polysaccharides of the different capsular types are all complex acid polysaccharides, which usually contain glucuronic acid and pyruvic acid. They resemble the K antigens of *Escherichia coli* (see Ch. 27).

Klebsiellae are non-motile but most strains are fimbriate. The organisms grow between 12–43°C (optimum, 37°C) and are killed by moist heat at 55°C in 30 min. They may survive drying for months and, when kept at room temperature, cultures remain viable for many weeks. They are facultatively anaerobic, but growth under strictly anaerobic conditions is poor. There is no haemolysis of horse or sheep red cells.

Members of the genus can be differentiated by simple biochemical tests (Table 28.2). A useful character of practically all strains of *K. pneumoniae*, spp. *aerogenes* and *pneumoniae*, and practically no other members of the Enterobacteriaceae, is the ability to form gas within 4 days from starch.

### Antigenic structure

About 80 capsular (K) antigens are presently re-

**Fig. 28.1** Mucoid (left) and non-mucoid (right) variants of *Klebsiella* species on carbohydrate-rich medium. (By courtesy of George Sharp and Richard Edwards.)

cognized. Among current UK isolates, types K2, K3 and K21 predominate, and the prevalence of these types limits the usefulness of capsular serotyping as an epidemiological tool.

In addition to the capsular antigens, five different somatic or O antigens occur in various combinations with the capsular antigens. Four of the five *Klebsiella* O antigens are identical with or related to *Esch. coli* O antigens. It is therefore possible to divide *Klebsiella* strains into a small number of groups which may be further subdivided into capsular types, but this is of little practical value in the classification of the capsulate members of the genus.

There is some association between antigenic structure, biochemical activities and habitat. Members of

**Table 28.2** Some differential biochemical reactions of medically important *Klebsiella* species

| Property | K. oxytoca | aerogenes | ozaenae | pneumoniae | rhinoscleromatis |
|---|---|---|---|---|---|
| | | | *K. pneumoniae* ssp. | | |
| Gas from glucose | + | + | v | + | − |
| Indole formation | + | − | − | − | − |
| Growth in KCN medium | + | + | + | − | + |
| Malonate fermentation | + | + | − | + | + |
| Methyl red test | v | − | + | + | + |
| Urease formation | + | + | − | + | − |

+, most strains positive; −, most strains negative; v, variable.

capsular types 1–6 occur most frequently in the human respiratory tract.

Considerable overlap occurs between *Klebsiella* antigens and those of unrelated organisms. Capsular type 2, for example, is immunologically similar to the type 2 pneumococcus. Capsular antigens are usually detected by means of the capsular 'swelling' reaction, but agglutination, complement fixation, indirect immunofluorescence and countercurrent immuno-electrophoresis may also be used.

## Other typing methods

Many *Klebsiella* strains produce bacteriocines, which appear to be distinct from colicines because they have no action on *Esch. coli*. They have a narrow range of activity on other klebsiellae and epidemiological analysis may be improved by the use of bacteriocines as an adjunct to capsular serotyping. Phage typing has also been used, and biotyping has been recommended instead of serotyping for use in less well-equipped laboratories.

## PATHOGENESIS

Klebsiellae are a fairly common cause of urinary tract infection and occasionally give rise to cases of severe bronchopneumonia, sometimes with chronic destructive lesions and multiple abscess formation in the lungs (*Friedländer's pneumonia*). Cases are sporadic and usually occur in members of the general population rather than in hospital patients. In many cases there is also bacteraemia, and the mortality is high. This condition is usually but not always associated with members of capsular types 1–5, which are often biochemically atypical.

However, the main importance of klebsiellae as human pathogens is in causing infections in hospital patients; the strains responsible are nearly always biochemically typical members of *K. pneumoniae* ssp. *aerogenes*, most of which belong to higher-numbered capsular types. Clinical sepsis develops in surgical wounds and in the urinary tract; a number of patients have bacteraemic infections and some of them die. Colonization of the respiratory tract is very common in hospitalized patients receiving antibiotics, but its clinical significance is often difficult to assess. Some debilitated patients develop bronchopneumonia in which a klebsiella appears to be the primary infecting agent. In the early days of antibiotic usage, klebsiellae were naturally resistant to the available antibiotics and with the passage of time they acquired resistance

to the newly developed ones. The emergence of klebsiella as an important cause of infection in hospitals is undoubtedly related to the use of antibiotics.

The *ozaenae* and *rhinoscleromatis* subspecies of *K. pneumoniae* take their names from the diseases with which they are associated. Rhinoscleroma is a chronic upper respiratory tract disease that occurs in a number of countries in eastern Europe and other parts of the world, where it is associated with prolonged exposure to crowded and unhygienic conditions. The lesions occur in the nose, larynx, throat and, to a lesser extent, in the trachea, and consist of granulomatous infiltrations of the submucosa. Ozaena is an uncommon, chronic disease in which there is atrophy of the nasal mucosa in which *K. pneumoniae* ssp. *ozaenae* is of doubtful significance.

## Virulence determinants

Bacterial pathogens must multiply in order to establish an infection and in order to multiply they need to acquire iron. *Klebsiella* strains possess two high-affinity iron uptake systems, one employing *aerobactin*, the other *enterochelin*. Production of aerobactin can be correlated with virulence and the genes encoding aerobactin are located on a plasmid.

*Klebsiella* strains show resistance to complement-mediated serum killing and phagocytosis if both K and O antigens are present; resistance to the former seems related to the O antigens and the latter to the K antigens. The virulence of *K. pneumoniae* in animal models varies considerably and does not appear to depend on capsule formation.

## TREATMENT

Clinical isolates of *Klebsiella* are nearly always naturally resistant to ampicillin, amoxycillin and most other penicillins, but usually sensitive to cephalosporins, especially β-lactamase-stable derivatives such as cefuroxime and cefotaxime. Resistance to chloramphenicol and tetracycline varies from strain to strain; they are often sensitive to gentamicin and other aminoglycosides, but transferable enzymic resistance to aminoglycosides and various cephalosporins has become common in strains found in some hospitals.

Klebsiella infection of the urine often responds to trimethoprim, nitrofurantoin, co-amoxiclav or oral cephalosporins. Pneumonia and other serious infections require vigorous treatment with an aminoglycoside or a cephalosporin such as cefotaxime.

## ENTEROBACTER

## DESCRIPTION

*Enterobacter* (formerly *Aerobacter*) species have many features in common with those of the genus *Klebsiella*, but are readily distinguished by their motility. Several species are now recognized; *Enterobacter aerogenes* and *Ent. cloacae* are much the most important clinically.

Although motility is the main distinguishing character between *Enterobacter* and *Klebsiella* species, a few strains that in all other respects resemble *Ent. cloacae* are non-motile. The colonies of *Enterobacter* strains may be slightly mucoid. In general, the fermentative activity of *Enterobacter* strains is more limited than that of typical *Klebsiella* strains. *Ent. aerogenes* and *Ent. cloacae* can be distinguished according to decarboxylase activity: *Ent. aerogenes* is usually able to decarboxylate lysine, but not arginine, whereas *Ent. cloacae* decarboxylates arginine, but not lysine.

## PATHOGENESIS

The normal habitat of *Enterobacter* species is probably soil and water, but the organisms are occasionally found in the faeces and the respiratory tract of humans. In recent years, infection of hospital patients with *Ent. cloacae* and *Ent. aerogenes* has been reported more frequently, but *Enterobacter* species are a much less important cause of hospital infection than *Klebsiella* species. Most infections are of the urinary tract, although members of the genus are an important cause of bacteraemia in some hospitals.

## TREATMENT

*Enterobacter* strains are nearly always highly resistant to penicillins and to the earlier cephalosporins because they produce a chromosomal β-lactamase with cephalosporinase activity. Many are also resistant to tetracycline, chloramphenicol and to streptomycin, although most are sensitive to other aminoglycosides including gentamicin and to fluoroquinolones. Most strains of *Ent. cloacae* appear susceptible to cefotaxime on primary testing, but they often possess an inducible chromosomal cephalosporinase which allows the rapid development of resistance during therapy.

*Enterobacter* strains differ from *Serratia* strains in being sensitive to the polymyxins.

## HAFNIA

## DESCRIPTION

*Hafnia alvei* was formerly placed in the genus *Enterobacter*, but DNA–DNA hybridization studies show that this organism deserves separate generic status. Three DNA-related groups have been recognized among *H. alvei* strains but at present the genus contains only the one species.

Strains grow well on ordinary media, producing greyish convex colonies 1–2 mm in diameter on nutrient agar at 37°C after incubation for 24 h. *H. alvei* ferments a much narrower range of sugars than members of the genus *Enterobacter*. It is not capsulate and does not liquefy gelatin. All *H. alvei* strains are lysed by a single phage, which is without action on any other members of the Enterobacteriaceae. There is an antigenic scheme that includes many serotypes.

## PATHOGENESIS

Strains are isolated from the faeces of humans and other animals and are also found in sewage, soil, water and dairy products. They are occasionally encountered as opportunist pathogens.

## SERRATIA

## DESCRIPTION

Although numerous species of the genus *Serratia* have been described, *S. marcescens* is the one most commonly encountered in clinical specimens. Several others, including *S. liquefaciens* (formerly known as *Ent. liquefaciens*) and *S. odorifera* are sometimes isolated. The size is subject to considerable variation. Even on the same type of medium a single strain may at one time give rise to coccobacilli and at another to rods indistinguishable from other enterobacteria. Capsules are not normally formed, but capsular material has been shown to be formed on a well-aerated medium poor in nitrogen and phosphate. Most *Serratia* strains are motile.

Colonies of *S. marcescens* on agar are usually homogeneous for the first day or two, and then may become differentiated into a convex, pigmented and relatively opaque centre and an effuse, colourless, almost transparent periphery with an irregular crenated edge. Pigment is formed only in the presence of oxygen and at a suitable temperature, which is not necessarily the same as that for optimal growth. Thus, many strains grow best at 30–37°C but form little or no pigment whereas at lower temperatures growth is poorer and pigment formation is abundant.

The red pigment *prodigiosin* is soluble in absolute alcohol and other organic solvents but is insoluble in water. It has been separated into three red fractions and one blue fraction with different absorption spectra. Prodigiosin is also formed by certain organisms unrelated to *S. marcescens*, including an actinomycete, and certain Gram-negative rods from sea water.

## PATHOGENESIS

*S. marcescens* is widely distributed in nature, but faecal carriage is uncommon in the general population. Pigmented strains may cause concern by giving rise to red colours in various foods or by simulating the appearance of blood in the sputum or faeces. Pigmented and non-pigmented strains are found occasionally in the human respiratory tract and in faeces. Most infections occur in hospital patients; they include infections of the urinary and respiratory tracts, meningitis, wound infections, septicaemia and endocarditis. Some strains become endemically established in hospitals and outbreaks of infection are also frequently reported. *Serratia* strains are able to multiply at ambient temperatures in fluids containing minimal nutrients and outbreaks have followed the introduction of the organisms directly into the bloodstream in contaminated transfusion fluids. Only a small proportion of the strains responsible for infection are pigmented.

The other *Serratia* species also occur commonly in the natural environment, especially in water; *S. liquefaciens* and *S. odorifera* are occasionally found in clinical specimens.

## TREATMENT

*Serratia* strains, like *Enterobacter* strains, are commonly resistant to cephalosporins. Resistance to ampicillin and gentamicin is variable, but many strains destroy these antibiotics enzymically.

An aminoglycoside, such as gentamicin, is usually the most reliable first-line choice. Fluoroquinolones or carbapenems may be useful in recalcitrant cases.

## *PROTEUS* AND RELATED GENERA

## CLASSIFICATION

The history of the genera *Proteus*, *Providencia* and *Morganella* is inextricably linked, and they are best considered together. The organism first isolated by Morgan early this century was formerly included in the genus *Proteus*, but genetic evidence and enzyme studies show that a separate genus is justified with a single species, *Morganella morganii*.

There has been similar debate over the taxonomy of the remaining species in this group, with successive proposals to combine and separate the genera *Proteus* and *Providencia*. The organisms once known as biotypes A and B of *Proteus inconstans* are now regarded as separate species of the genus *Providencia*: *Providencia alcalifaciens* and *Prov. stuartii*. As a result of genetic studies, *Proteus rettgeri* has also been transferred to the genus *Providencia* as *Prov. rettgeri*, even though it resembles *Proteus* species rather than other organisms of the genus *Providencia* in producing urease. This leaves only *Pr. vulgaris* and *Pr. mirabilis* in the genus *Proteus*.

## DESCRIPTION

### Morphological and cultural characters

There is considerable morphological variation, but in agar cultures after 24 h the microscopical appearance is much like that of other coliform bacteria with rods 1–3 × 0.6 µm in size.

All grow well on ordinary nutrient media. A notable property of *Pr. vulgaris* and *Pr. mirabilis* strains is the ability to swarm on solid media: the bacterial growth spreads progressively from the edge of the colony and eventually covers the whole surface of the medium. This swarming characteristically takes place in a discontinuous manner, with each period of outward progress followed by a stationary period (Fig. 28.2). A number of methods have been devised to inhibit swarming, mainly to avoid interference with the isolation of clinically more important organisms.

**Fig. 28.2** Swarming growth of *Pr. mirabilis* inoculated centrally onto a blood agar plate and incubated overnight at 37°C. (By courtesy of George Sharp and Richard Edwards.)

## Biochemical activities

*M. morganii* and *Proteus* and *Providencia* species have the almost unique ability to oxidatively de-aminate amino acids, which is shown by growing the organism in a medium containing phenylalanine, from which phenylpyruvic acid is formed (the PPA test). Some other differential characteristics are shown in Table 28.3.

## Typing methods

Phage-, bacteriocine- and serotyping schemes have been developed for *Proteus* and *Providencia* species. Swarming *Proteus* strains exhibit the *Dienes phenomenon* (the mutual inhibition of swarming), and this forms

the basis for a precise method of differentiation among such strains. Test organisms are inoculated onto the surface of an agar plate, and those that show no line of demarcation in areas where the swarming growths meet are regarded as identical.

## PATHOGENESIS

Strains of *Pr. mirabilis* are a prominent cause of urinary tract infection in children and in domiciliary practice. Indole-positive *Proteus* and *Providencia* strains are usually seen in hospital patients, especially in elderly males following surgery or instrumentation. Septicaemia generally occurs only in patients with serious underlying conditions or as a complication of urinary tract surgery, but outbreaks of septicaemia, often with meningitis, may occur among the newborn in hospitals. A variety of other infections, usually of surgical wounds or bedsores, occur in hospitals and are usually considered to originate from the gut flora. Urease-producing organisms such as those of the genus *Proteus* may provoke the formation of *calculi* (stones) in the urinary tract.

*M. morganii* is uncommon in human disease but occasionally causes infections in hospital patients.

## TREATMENT

Most strains of *Pr. mirabilis* do not produce β-lactamase; they are consequently moderately sensitive to benzylpenicillin and fully sensitive to ampicillin, and most other β-lactam antibiotics. *Pr. vulgaris* strains are usually resistant to penicillins and early cephalosporins, although they may be sensitive to β-lactamase-stable derivatives such as cefotaxime. All strains are resistant to polymyxins while susceptibility to chloramphenicol and tetra-

**Table 28.3** Some differential biochemical reactions of *Proteus*, *Providencia* and *Morganella* species

| Test | Pr. mirabilis | Pr. vulgaris | Prov. alcalifaciens | Prov. rettgeri | Prov. stuartii | M. morganii |
|---|---|---|---|---|---|---|
| Ornithine decarboxylase | + | − | − | − | − | + |
| Gas from glucose | + | + | v | − | − | + |
| H₂S production | + | v | − | − | − | − |
| Indole formation | − | + | + | + | + | + |
| Urease formation | + | + | − | + | − | + |

+, most strains positive; −, most strains negative; v, variable.

cycline varies. *Proteus* and *Providencia* strains are inherently sensitive to aminoglycosides but resistance, which may be due to enzymic or non-enzymic mechanisms, is now common.

*Pr. mirabilis* urinary tract infections usually respond to ampicillin or trimethoprim but nitrofurantoin is not effective. Treatment of infection associated with renal stones is often unsuccessful. Serious infection with other *Proteus*, *Providencia* or *Morganella* strains can often be treated with an aminoglycoside or a cephalosporin such as cefotaxime. However, susceptibility is unpredictable and treatment should be guided by laboratory findings.

## CITROBACTER

### DESCRIPTION

The genus *Citrobacter* was first proposed for a group of lactose-negative or late lactose-fermenting coliform bacteria that share certain somatic antigens with salmonellae and were also known as the *Ballerup–Bethesda* group. These organisms are now known as *Citrobacter freundii*. Other species included in the genus are *C. koseri* (known as *C. diversus* in the USA) and *C. amalonaticus* (formerly *Levinea amalonatica*). They grow well on ordinary media, producing smooth, convex colonies 2–4 mm in diameter on nutrient agar. They are not pigmented. Rough or mucoid forms sometimes occur.

### PATHOGENESIS

Members of the genus *Citrobacter* are often found in the faeces of humans and may be isolated from a variety of clinical specimens. They do not often give rise to serious infections. *C. koseri* occasionally causes neonatal meningitis; in this condition there is a high mortality and the formation of cerebral abscesses is common.

### TREATMENT

*C. freundii* is usually sensitive to aminoglycosides and chloramphenicol while sensitivity to ampicillin, tetracycline and cephalosporins varies. *C. freundii* strains are commonly resistant to cephaloridine whereas most *C. koseri* strains are sensitive. Resistance to aminoglycosides occurs frequently among *C. koseri* strains. Choice of treatment should be based on laboratory tests of susceptibility.

## OTHER GENERA

### ERWINIA

*Erwinia herbicola*, an anaerogenic, yellow-pigmented organism, known as *Ent. agglomerans* in the USA, is not uncommon in the human upper respiratory tract and in swabs from superficial lesions. It resembles closely organisms that are frequently isolated from plants and soil, some of which are plant pathogens. It is an occasional pathogen in predisposed human patients, and may be isolated from upper respiratory tract and urinary tract infections. It has also caused bacteraemia when administered in contaminated intravenous fluids.

### EDWARDSIELLA

*Edwardsiella tarda* was first described under the name *Asakusa* to include a group of enterobacteria that appeared to be quite distinct from all others. It grows well on ordinary media but produces only small colonies of 0.5–1 mm diameter after 24 h.

*Edwardsiella* strains are frequently isolated from healthy cold-blooded animals and their environment. They are pathogenic for eels, catfish and other animals, sometimes causing economic losses. *E. tarda* is an occasional pathogen of humans, mainly causing wound infection, but meningitis and septicaemia have also been reported. *E. tarda* is rarely found in the faeces of healthy people, but a higher isolation rate has been found in patients with diarrhoea, and the role of the species in the aetiology of diarrhoea requires further study. Human infections with *E. tarda* probably originate from contact with cold-blooded animals.

## RECOMMENDED READING

Ewing W H 1986 *Edwards and Ewing's Identification of Enterobacteriaceae*, 4th edn. Elsevier, New York

Farmer J J, Wells J G, Griffin P M, Wachsmuth K I 1987 Enterobacteriaceae infections. In: Wentworth B B (ed), *Diagnostic Procedures for Bacterial Infections*, 7th edn. American Public Health Association, Washington, pp 233–296

Lund B M, Sussman M, Jones D, Stringer M R (eds) 1988 Enterobacteriaceae in the environment and as pathogens. *Society of Applied Bacteriology Symposium Series*, No. 17. Blackwell Scientific, Oxford (published as a supplement to *Journal of Applied Bacteriology* 65)

Williams P, Tomas J M 1990 The pathogenicity of *Klebsiella pneumoniae*. *Reviews in Medical Microbiology* 1: 196–204

# 29

# Pseudomonads and non-fermenters

**Opportunistic infection; cystic fibrosis; melioidosis**

*J. R. W. Govan*

The term *pseudomonads* describes a large group of aerobic, non-fermentative, Gram-negative bacilli belonging to over 200 species that were originally contained within the genus *Pseudomonas*. Most are saprophytes found widely in soil, water and other moist environments. Historically, the genus *Pseudomonas* has been used as a microbial repository for a vast range of species, often with diverse phenotypic characteristics. Molecular analyses of the group have led to revised taxonomic classifications, and many species have been allocated to new genera which include *Burkholderia, Comamonas, Stenotrophomonas* and *Brevundimonas* (Fig. 29.1). A few species are pathogenic for plants, insects and animals. *Pseudomonas aeruginosa* is the species most commonly associated with human disease but *Burkholderia* (previously *Pseudomonas*) *pseudomallei* is an important pathogen in some parts of the world. *Burkholderia* (previously

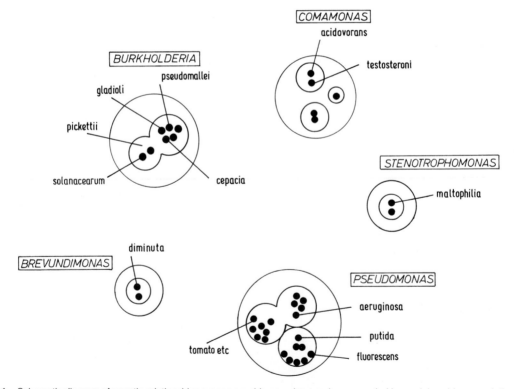

**Fig. 29.1** Schematic diagram of genetic relationships among aerobic pseudomonads as revealed by nucleic acid reassociation. Each large outer circle represents an rRNA homology group, determined by DNA–rRNA hybridizations. The distances between the groups are abitrary. The smaller circles define DNA homology groups. The black dots within each small circle represent species of which the most important are named. (After Palleroni et al 1973 *International Journal of Systematic Bacteriology* 23: 333–339.)

*Pseudomonas*) *cepacia* has emerged as an important pathogen in immunocompromised patients, particularly in individuals with cystic fibrosis or chronic granulomatous disease.

Several other species are occasionally isolated from human clinical specimens as opportunistic pathogens including *Ps. putida*, *Ps. fluorescens*, *Ps. stutzeri* and a number of other glucose non-fermenters. In addition, there is growing evidence that *Stenotrophomonas* (previously *Pseudomonas* or *Xanthomonas*) *maltophilia* has pathogenic potential in immunocompromised patients, with a mortality reaching 60% in patients with haematological malignancies.

The reasons for the pre-eminent status of *Ps. aeruginosa* as an opportunistic pathogen lie in its adaptibility, its innate resistance to many antibiotics and disinfectants, its armoury of putative virulence factors, and in an increasing supply of patients compromised by age, underlying disease or immuno-suppressive therapy.

## *PSEUDOMONAS AERUGINOSA*

### Description

*Ps. aeruginosa* is a Gram-negative bacillus, non-sporing, non-capsulate, and usually motile by virtue of one or two polar flagella (see Fig. 2.9, p. 15). It is a strict aerobe but can grow anaerobically if nitrate is available. The organism grows readily on a wide variety of culture media over a wide temperature range and emits a sweet grape-like odour that is easily recognized. Most strains produce diffusible pigments; typically, the colony and surrounding medium is greenish-blue due to production of a soluble blue phenazine pigment, *pyocyanin*, and the yellow-green fluorescent pigment *pyoverdin*, which acts as the major siderophore; additional pigments include *pyorubrin* (red) and *melanin* (brown). Some 10–15% of *Ps. aeruginosa* strains readily produce pigment only when grown on pigment-enhancing media. Individual colonies can occur as five distinct types ranging from dwarf colonies to large mucoid colonies; the most common colonial form is relatively large, low-convex with an irregular surface, an edge that is translucent and an oblong shape with the long axis parallel to the line of inoculum.

*Ps. aeruginosa* differs from members of the Entero-bacteriaceae by deriving energy from carbohydrates by an oxidative rather than a fermentative metabolism. It appears inactive in carbohydrate fermentation tests, and only glucose is utilized. However, all strains give a positive oxidase reaction and this is a useful preliminary test for non-pigmented strains. Although a few Gram-negative bacilli are also oxidase-positive, none reacts as swiftly as *Ps. aeruginosa*, which gives a positive reaction within 30 s.

Typing for epidemiological purposes, or to investigate clonal relationships between isolates, has traditionally relied on phenotypic markers such as serospecificity of the lipopolysaccharide (LPS), susceptibility to phages and the profile of bacteriocin production. Bacteriocin typing is simple to perform and allows characterization of most isolates, including the mucoid and LPS rough phenotypes. For non-mucoid isolates with smooth LPS, simple LPS-based serotyping methods are commercially available. The problem of instability in the phenotypic markers used in serotyping or bacteriocin typing has been circumvented by the development of restriction endonuclease typing with pulsed-field gel electrophoresis (see p. 34). This is the most reliable and discriminatory of the DNA-based typing methods for investigation of *Ps. aeruginosa* epidemiology.

### Pathogenesis

*Ps. aeruginosa* can infect almost any external site or organ. In the community, infections are mostly mild and superficial, e.g. otitis externa and varicose ulcers; such conditions are often chronic, but not disabling. Recreational and occupational conditions associated with susceptibility to pseudomonas infections include jacuzzi or whirlpool rash (an acute self-limiting folliculitis) and industrial eye injuries which may lead to panophthalmitis.

In hospital patients, pseudomonas infections are more common, more severe and more varied. Infection is usually localized, as in catheter-related urinary tract infection, infected ulcers, bed sores, burns and eye infections. In patients compromised by age, or immunosuppressing diseases such as leukaemia, and in those treated with immuno-suppressive drugs or corticosteroids, pseudomonas infections frequently become generalized, and the organism may be cultured from the blood or from many organs of the body post-mortem. *Ps. aeruginosa* is not a major cause of Gram-negative septicaemia or necrotizing pneumonia but is associated with high mortality in these conditions, and in the case of septicaemia the characteristic black skin lesions of ecythema gangrenosum. The lungs of children with cystic fibrosis are particularly susceptible to infection. In these patients, asymptomatic pulmonary colonization with typical non-mucoid forms eventually leads to the emergence of mucoid variants (Fig. 29.2);

**Fig. 29.2**   Gram-stained sputum from patient harbouring mucoid *Ps. aeruginosa*. Note spawn-like microcolony and adjacent phagocytes.

debilitating episodes of pulmonary exacerbation due to mucoid *Ps. aeruginosa* are the major cause of morbidity and mortality in cystic fibrosis.

Most strains produce two exotoxins, exotoxin A and exo-enzyme S, and a variety of cytotoxic substances including proteases, phospholipases, rhamnolipids and the blue-green pigment pyocyanin; an alginate-like exopolysaccharide is responsible for the mucoid phenotype (Fig. 29.3). The importance of these putative virulence factors depends upon the site and nature of infection: proteases play a key role in corneal ulceration; exotoxin and proteases are important in burn infection; and phospholipases, proteases and alginate are associated with chronic pulmonary colonization. Fluorescein or pyoverdin pigments act as bacterial siderophores. Production of fluorescein in vivo allows *Ps. aeruginosa* to compete with mammalian iron-binding proteins such as transferrin and, in association with pyocyanin, gives rise to the characteristic blue-green pus of pseudomonas-infected wounds, and the old species name *pyocyanea* (Latin = blue pus) as well as the present *aeruginosa* (Latin = verdigris, blue-green). The mechanism of action of exotoxin A is similar to that of diphtheria toxin (see Ch. 18) although the molecular receptors are different.

**Fig. 29.3**   Alcohol extraction of alginate from mucoid *Ps. aeruginosa*.

## Laboratory diagnosis

*Ps. aeruginosa* grows on most common culture media, but for specific investigation material can be cultured on a medium that is selective and enhances the production of the characteristic blue-green pigment, pyocyanin. For culture from water or soil, a selective medium containing acetamide as the sole carbon and nitrogen source may be used. Resultant colonies are usually easily identified. About 10% of isolates do not produce detectable pigment even on suitable media; in such cases a positive oxidase test provides presumptive evidence of the identity. Formal identification can be made with an appropriate multitest system such as API 20NE. Tests for serum antibodies against pseudomonas antigens have no place in diagnosis except in patients with chronic obstructive pulmonary disease, in which increasing antibody levels correlate directly with immune-mediated lung damage.

## Treatment

*Ps. aeruginosa* is normally resistant to most commonly employed antimicrobial agents. Until the 1960s, pseudomonas infections were usually treated with polymyxins, agents that exhibit considerable toxicity. With the development of antipseudomonal β-lactam compounds, like azlocillin, ticarcillin and ceftazidime, and aminoglycosides such as gentamicin and tobramycin, treatment with a combination of an aminoglycoside and a β-lactam was commonly adopted. There is little clinical evidence of the superiority of combined therapy although it has the potential for antibacterial synergy and reduced antibiotic resistance. Monotherapy with broad-spectrum β-lactam agents such as ceftazidime and imipenem is used, but resistance to these agents is observed.

Each of these agents has to be given parenterally; in contrast, fluoroquinolones such as ciprofloxacin can be administered orally. Ciprofloxacin exhibits good activity against *Ps. aeruginosa* and penetrates well into most tissues, but resistance may develop.

Passive vaccination may be useful for the treatment of septicaemia and burn infections due to *Ps. aeruginosa*, which are associated with high mortality; active vaccination to prevent pulmonary colonization would be desirable for patients with cystic fibrosis and a conjugate vaccine is in clinical trial.

## Epidemiology

*Ps. aeruginosa* is a competent and hardy saprophyte and can be isolated from a wide variety of environmental sources. The ability of the species to persist and multiply, particularly in moist environments, and on moist equipment (e.g. humidifiers) in hospital wards, bathrooms and kitchens, is of particular importance in cross-infection control. Consumption of salad vegetables contaminated with pseudomonas is a potential risk for immunocompromised patients in intensive care units.

The organism is resistant to, and may multiply in, many of the disinfectants and antiseptics commonly used in hospitals. It can be a troublesome contaminant in pharmaceutical preparations and may cause ophthalmitis following the faulty chemical 'sterilization' of contact lenses.

Most hospital-acquired infections with *Ps. aeruginosa* originate from exogenous sources but some patients suffer endogenous infection, particularly of the urinary tract. Healthy carriers usually harbour strains in the gastro-intestinal tract, but in the open community the carriage rate seldom exceeds 10%. In contrast, acquisition of *Ps. aeruginosa* in a hospital is rapid, and up to 30% of patients may excrete the organisms within 2 days of admission.

Burned patients are especially at risk; the presence of the organism in ward air, dust and in eschar shed from the burns suggests that infection can be air-borne. However, contact spread has been demonstrated and is probably more important than the air-borne route. Transmission may occur directly via the hands of medical staff, or indirectly via contaminated apparatus. Severely burned patients and those with chest injuries who require artificial ventilation are very susceptible to *Ps. aeruginosa*; pulmonary infection not infrequently precedes septicaemia, which is associated with high mortality. Modern intensive care equipment can be difficult to clean, and there is little doubt that infection can be spread by this source.

Eye infections due to *Ps. aeruginosa* can be particularly severe, and may result from contaminated contact lenses, industrial eye injuries or from introduction of contaminated medicament during ophthalmic procedures. Similarly, in the early days of North Sea oil exploration, diving operations had occasionally to be aborted because of outbreaks of troublesome ear infection. The warm, moist and aerated conditions under which *Ps. aeruginosa* thrives are ideally met in poorly maintained whirlpools or jacuzzis. Ear infections and an irritating folliculitis known as *jacuzzi rash* are typical examples of opportunistic pseudomonas infections that may be acquired from such sources. Epidemics of gastro-intestinal infection can occur in newborn and young infants in maternity units and paediatric wards, and may result from contaminated milk feeds.

## Control

Prevention is easier than cure; once *Ps. aeruginosa* has gained access to the hospital environment, or has established infection, it is notoriously difficult to eradicate. Three guidelines to control infection are offered in the knowledge that it is not always easy to put them into practice:

1. Patients at a high risk of acquiring infection with *Ps. aeruginosa* (e.g. a patient being evaluated for organ transplantation) should not be admitted to a ward where cases of pseudomonas infection are present.

2. Antimicrobial and other therapeutic substances and solutions must be free from *Ps. aeruginosa*, and particular danger exists when multidose ointments, creams or eye drops are used to treat several individuals over a period. Initially, the preparation may be sterile but contamination can easily occur between uses, and *Ps. aeruginosa* can multiply readily at a range of temperatures in many medicaments.

3. In hospital units, episodes of cross-infection due to a single strain may occur as sporadic infections in individual patients over a period of months or years. For this reason, if facilities are available, it is advantageous to monitor all clinically relevant isolates by a suitable typing system to identify epidemic strains.

## BURKHOLDERIA PSEUDOMALLEI

*Burkholderia pseudomallei* is a free-living saprophyte that causes *melioidosis*, a devastating tropical infection of animals and humans that is endemic in eastern Asia and northern Australia. Laboratory-acquired infection is a serious risk: the species is included in hazard group 3 together with the plague bacillus, *Yersinia pestis*, and must be handled with great care under strictly designated conditions. *B. pseudomallei* is easily cultured and produces characteristic wrinkled colonies after several days of growth on nutrient agar; fresh cultures emit a characteristic pungent odour of putrefaction. The organism is oxidase-positive and motile but, unlike some other pseudomonads, does not produce diffusible pigments.

A related organism, *B. mallei*, causes *glanders*, a disease of horses in Asia, Africa and the Middle East. Human cases are rare.

## Melioidosis

*B. pseudomallei* is found in soil and surface water in rice paddies and monsoon drains; isolation rates are highest during the rainy season and in still rather than flowing water. Human infection is mainly acquired cutaneously through skin abrasions or by inhalation of contaminated particles. The clinical manifestations range from a subclinical infection, diagnosed by the presence of specific antibodies, to a benign pulmonary infection that may resemble tuberculosis or fulminating septicaemia with a mortality rate of 80–90%. In north-eastern Thailand, *B. pseudomallei* is responsible for 20% of all community-acquired septicaemia. Virtually every organ can be affected, and hence melioidosis has been called the 'great imitator' of other infectious diseases. Melioidosis commonly presents as pyrexia and, in endemic areas, serological testing for *B. pseudomallei* is important in the evaluation of pyrexia of unknown origin. *B. pseudomallei* can survive intracellularly within the reticulo-endothelial system, and this may account for latency and the emergence of symptoms many years after exposure. Suppurative parotitis is a characteristic presentation of melioidosis in children.

Early diagnosis and appropriate antibiotic therapy are key factors in the successful management of melioidosis. The organism may be observed, usually in very small numbers, as small, bipolar-stained Gram-negative bacilli in exudates, and may be isolated from sputum, urine, pus or blood. Enzyme-linked immunosorbent assay (ELISA) for the detection of specific IgG and IgM antibody to *B. pseudomallei*, as well as an indirect haemagglutination test, are useful serological screening tests in subclinical melioidosis. A polymerase chain reaction (PCR) method has also been described.

## Treatment

Combinations of antimicrobial agents such as tetracycline and chloramphenicol have been widely used, but prolonged treatment is necessary to avoid relapse. The ability of *B. pseudomallei* to survive and multiply in phagocytes may explain the difficulty of treating melioidosis with antibiotics that are effective against the organism in vitro, and the frequent recurrences seen when the duration of treatment is insufficient. Of the newer agents, ceftazidime is especially effective in vitro and in vivo.

## BURKHOLDERIA CEPACIA

*Burkholderia cepacia* was previously best known as the causative agent of soft rot of onions (*cepia*, Latin = onion). It has now emerged as a major opportunistic cause of respiratory infection in patients with chronic granulomatous disease or cystic fibrosis. Among the cystic fibrosis population and their carers, anxiety over *B. cepacia* is based on the innate multiresistance of the organism to antibiotics, its transmissibility by social contact and clinically by the risk of cepacia syndrome, an acute, fatal necrotizing pneumonia, sometimes accompanied by bacteraemia, which occurs in approximately 20% of colonized patients.

*B. cepacia* isolates produce few classic virulence determinants; however, pro-inflammatory cytokines such as tumour necrosis factor are stimulated more by LPS from clinical and environmental isolates of *B. cepacia* than by *Ps. aeruginosa* LPS. Laboratory identification is aided by the use of selective media and by multitest identification systems such as API 20NE.

*B. cepacia* is probably the most nutritionally adaptable of all pseudomonads. It demonstrates an unusual form of antibiotic resistance by an ability to use penicillin as a sole carbon and energy source. In vitro, some strains are susceptible to ceftazidime, or the carbapenem meropenem. However, infections may be particularly intractable.

Isolates from human and environmental sources display considerable phenotypic and genomic heterogeneity. Molecular taxonomic studies of isolates presently identified as *B. cepacia* suggest that most, in particular those colonizing patients with cystic fibrosis, may belong to new bacterial species.

# GLUCOSE NON-FERMENTERS

The heterogeneous group of aerobic Gram-negative bacilli commonly referred to as *glucose non-fermenters* are taxonomically distinct from the carbohydrate-fermenting Enterobacteriaceae and the oxidative pseudomonads. Their clinical relevance is based on their role as opportunistic pathogens in hospital-acquired infections and their intrinsic resistance to many antimicrobial agents. They grow easily on common culture media, but unequivocal identification may be difficult as most species are relatively inert in the biochemical tests used in identification of Gram-negative bacteria.

*Eikenella corrodens* is a commensal of mucosal surfaces which may cause a range of infections, in particular endocarditis, meningitis, pneumonia and infections of wounds and various soft tissues.

*Flavobacterium meningosepticum* is a saprophyte whose natural habitat is soil and moist environments, including nebulizers; it may cause opportunistic nosocomial infections, particularly in infants. As the name suggests, this species is associated with meningitis, and has been responsible for high mortality in epidemic outbreaks.

*Acinetobacter* species are saprophytes found in soil, water and sewage, and occasionally as commensals of moist areas of human skin. The organisms survive well in the hospital environment, and are increasing in importance as opportunist pathogens. Hospital-acquired infections, including pneumonia and other respiratory infections, are most commonly associated with *Acinetobacter baumannii*. Patients in intensive care units are at particular risk. *A. baumannii* isolates are often resistant to many antimicrobial agents, including β-lactam agents (other than carbapenems), aminoglycosides and quinolones.

Two other genera of Gram-negative bacteria, *Alcaligenes* and *Achromobacter*, may be confused with *Pseudomonas* species. Like other non-fermenters, they are saprophytes found in moist environments including those in hospital wards, and are associated with a range of hospital-acquired opportunistic infections, including septicaemia and ear discharges.

Susceptibility to antibiotics of glucose non-fermenters is very variable, and treatment should be based on the results of laboratory tests.

## RECOMMENDED READING

Bergogne-Bérézin E, Towner K J 1996 *Acinetobacter* spp. as nosocomial pathogens: microbiological, clinical and epidemiological features. *Clinical Microbiology Reviews* 9: 148–165

Dance D A B 1991 Melioidosis: the tip of the iceberg? *Clinical Microbiology Reviews* 4: 52–60

Gilligan P H 1995. *Pseudomonas* and *Burkholderia*. In: Murray P R, Baron E J, Pfaller M A, Tenover F C, Yolken R H (eds) *Manual of Clinical Microbiology*. American Society for Microbiology, Washington, DC, pp 509–519

Govan J R W, Brown P H, Maddison J, Doherty C J, Nelson J W, Dodd M, Greening A P, Webb A K 1993 Evidence for transmission of *Pseudomonas cepacia* by social contact in cystic fibrosis. *Lancet* 342: 15–19

Govan J R W, Nelson J W 1993 Microbiology of cystic fibrosis lung infections; themes and issues. *Journal of the Royal Society of Medicine* 86(suppl 20): 11–18

The International *Pseudomonas aeruginosa* Typing Study Group 1994 A multicenter comparision of methods for typing strains of *Pseudomonas aeruginosa* predominantly from patients with cystic fibrosis. *Journal of Infectious Diseases* 169: 134–142

Vasil M L 1986 *Pseudomonas aeruginosa*: biology, mechanisms of virulence, epidemiology. *Journal of Pediatrics* 105: 800–805

# 30

## Campylobacter and helicobacter

Enteritis; gastritis; peptic ulcer

*M. B. Skirrow*

*Campylobacter* and *Helicobacter* are members of a group of spirally shaped flagellate bacteria known as rRNA superfamily VI. Both genera contain bacteria of great medical importance. They are specially adapted to colonizing mucous membranes and are able to penetrate mucus with particular facility. In most industrialized countries, *Campylobacter jejuni* is the commonest cause of infective diarrhoea, and as a result it causes much morbidity and economic loss. The discovery of *Helicobacter pylori* in 1983 has been hailed as the most significant advance in gastroduodenal pathology this century. Infection of the stomach with this bacterium is essentially the cause of 'idiopathic' peptic ulceration and a significant risk factor for the development of gastric cancer.

## CAMPYLOBACTER

Campylobacters were first isolated in 1906 from aborting sheep in the UK. They were thought to be vibrios, and the first species was named '*Vibrio fetus*'. This is now *C. fetus* and the type species of the genus. It is a major cause of abortion in sheep and cattle world-wide, and an occasional cause of bacteraemic infection in people with immune deficiency. It does not cause disease in healthy people, except for rare cases of septic abortion.

The discovery that *C. jejuni* and *C. coli* commonly cause diarrhoea in man was not made until the 1970s, when Butzler, in Belgium, applied veterinary microbiological methods to look for campylobacters in patients with diarrhoea. Several other species, such as *C. upsaliensis* and *C. lari*, are enteropathogenic, but they are less common and found mainly in children in developing countries. *Arcobacter* (formerly *C.*) *butzleri* can cause abdominal pain, with or without diarrhoea, in children. Several species of campylobacter, notably *C. concisus* and *C. rectus*, are associated with periodontal disease.

## CAMPYLOBACTER JEJUNI AND C. COLI

### Description

*C. jejuni* and *C. coli* are small, spiral, Gram-negative rods with a single flagellum at one or both poles (Fig. 30.1), which endows the bacteria with exceptionally rapid motility. They are unusually sensitive to oxygen and superoxides, yet oxygen is essential for growth, so micro-aerophilic conditions must be provided for their cultivation. They grow best at 42–43°C. They do not form spores, but undergo coccal transformation under adverse conditions. They are inactive in many conventional biochemical tests, including metabolism of sugars (asaccharolytic), but they are strongly oxidase-positive.

*C. jejuni* and *C. coli* are closely related, but *C. jejuni* hydrolyses hippurate – the only species of campylobacter to do so. *C. jejuni* accounts for 90–95% of infections in most parts of the world.

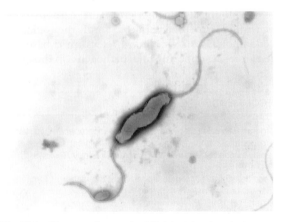

**Fig. 30.1** Electron micrograph of *C. jejuni* showing single unsheathed bipolar flagella. ×11 500. (Photomicrograph by Dr A. L. Curry and D. M. Jones, Manchester Public Health Laboratory.)

## Antigens and strain typing

These campylobacters possess two classes of antigen: heat-stable lipopolysaccharide O antigens, which form the basis of the Penner serogrouping scheme (65 serogroups); and heat-labile surface and flagellar protein antigens, which form the basis of the Lior serogrouping scheme (160 serogroups). Serotyping can be used in concert with biotyping or phage typing to give finer discrimination. Molecular 'fingerprinting' methods are gaining favour for epidemiological studies.

## Pathogenesis

Infection is acquired by ingestion. In volunteer studies, infection has been established with as few as 500–800 organisms. The jejunum and ileum are the first sites to become colonized, but the infection extends distally to affect the terminal ileum and usually the colon and rectum. The organisms are invasive. In well-developed infections, mesenteric lymph nodes are enlarged, fleshy and inflamed, and there may be transient bacteraemia. Histological examination of the mucosa shows an acute neutrophil polymorphonuclear leucocyte response, oedema, and sometimes superficial ulceration. These changes are indistinguishable from those seen in salmonella, shigella, or yersinia infections.

### Immune response

Specific humoral antibody is formed in response to infection. The immunoglobulins IgA and IgM appear within 10 days of onset, and decline within about 2 weeks; IgG appears almost as quickly but persists for several weeks or months.

## Clinical manifestations

The typical features of campylobacter enteritis are shown in Figure 30.2. The average incubation period is 3 days, with a range of 1–7 days. The illness may start with abdominal pain and diarrhoea, or there may be an influenza-like prodrome of fever and generalized aching, sometimes with rigors and sweating. Abdominal pain and diarrhoea are the main symptoms. Nausea is common, but vomiting is seldom pronounced. Severe watery diarrhoea may lead to prostration. Leucocytes are almost always present in the faeces, and frank blood may be apparent. Symptoms usually resolve within a few days, but excretion of bacteria may continue for several weeks. Prolonged carriage occurs only in patients with immunodeficiency. Campylobacter enteritis cannot be distinguished clinically from salmonella or shigella infection, but abdominal pain tends to be more severe in campylobacter infection. Indeed, the most common reason for patients with campylobacter enteritis to be admitted to hospital is suspected acute appendicitis. Occasionally, illness starts with symptoms of colitis without preceding ileitis, which can make it difficult to distinguish from acute ulcerative colitis.

### Complications

Intestinal haemorrhage, toxic megacolon, and haemolytic uraemic syndrome have been reported rarely. Reactive arthritis, or peripheral polyneuropathy (*Guillain–Barré syndrome*), may appear 1–2 weeks after the onset of acute illness. Campylobacter enteritis accounts for about 26% of episodes of the Guillain–Barré syndrome.

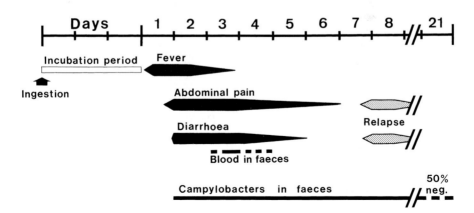

**Fig. 30.2** Typical course of untreated campylobacter enteritis of average severity. There is considerable variation among individual patients.

## Laboratory diagnosis

### Microscopy

The motility and morphology of campylobacters are sufficiently characteristic for a rapid presumptive diagnosis to be made by direct microscopy of faeces, either in wet preparations or stained smears, but in practice this is seldom necessary.

### Culture

Isolation of campylobacters from faeces requires some form of selective culture in order to inhibit competing faecal flora. Early selective media were blood-based and contained agents such as vancomycin, polymyxin and trimethoprim, but charcoal-based blood-free media containing cefoperazone are currently favoured. Culture on non-selective media can be achieved by inoculating cellulose acetate membranes (pore size, 0.45–0.65 µm) laid on the surface of the plate; the slender campylobacters are able to pass through the membrane, which is removed before incubation. This method has the advantage of detecting fastidious campylobacter species that are sensitive to the antimicrobial agents used in selective media.

Plates are incubated in closed jars with the oxygen tension lowered to 5–15% and carbon dioxide raised to 1–10%. Incubation at 42–43°C gives added selectivity against other faecal flora and more rapid growth of *C. jejuni* and *C. coli*, but it may exclude other species of campylobacter. Colonies are typically flat and effuse, with a tendency to spread on moist agar.

### Serology

Serology may be useful in patients presenting with aseptic arthritis or the Guillain–Barré syndrome after a bout of diarrhoea that was not investigated. A complement fixation test and enzyme-linked immunosorbent assay (ELISA) are group-specific tests that can detect recent infection with *C. jejuni* or *C. coli*.

## Treatment

Campylobacter enteritis is usually self-limiting and patients seldom require more than fluid and electrolyte replacement. *C. jejuni* and *C. coli* are moderately resistant to penicillins and most cephalosporins, although several other species are sensitive. All species are usually sensitive to erythromycin, which is effective if given early in the disease. Ciprofloxacin and other fluoroquinolones are also effective, but resistance rates are rising.

Campylobacters are highly resistant to trimethoprim, but many strains are sensitive to metronidazole and other nitroimidazoles, an unusual property among bacteria that are not strict anaerobes.

## Epidemiology

### Incidence

Campylobacter enteritis is the commonest form of acute infective diarrhoea in most developed countries. In the UK, laboratory reports indicate an incidence of about 87 per 100 000 of the population, but the true figure is probably 10-fold higher. The disease occurs in people of all ages. There is high morbidity in young adults, and an unexplained excess of male patients in this group (the male:female ratio is 1.7:1).

In developing countries, infection is hyperendemic, and children are repeatedly exposed to infection from an early age. By the time they are 2–3 years old they have developed substantial immunity that lasts into adulthood. The maintenance of immunity probably depends on continuous exposure to infection.

### Sources and transmission

Animals are the main sources of infection. *C. jejuni* and *C. coli* are found in a wide variety of animal hosts, particularly birds, an adaptation that is reflected in their high optimum growth temperature. There is a constant shedding of the bacteria from wild birds and other animals into the surface water of lakes, rivers and streams, in which they can survive for many weeks at low temperatures. Farm animals are commonly infected from such sources. *C. jejuni* and *C. coli*, like *C. fetus*, can cause septic abortion in sheep and mild diarrhoea in young animals of several species. Cattle are commonly infected, and raw milk often becomes contaminated. The distribution of raw milk and untreated water has caused major outbreaks of campylobacter enteritis affecting several thousand people.

***Poultry and raw meats.*** *C. jejuni* and *C. coli* colonize domestic poultry with particular ease. At least 60% of chickens sold in shops are contaminated with campylobacters, and broiler chickens are thought to account for about 50% of human infections in industrialized countries. Red meats are less often contaminated.

Properly cooked poultry and meats do not pose a risk; it is what happens to them before they are

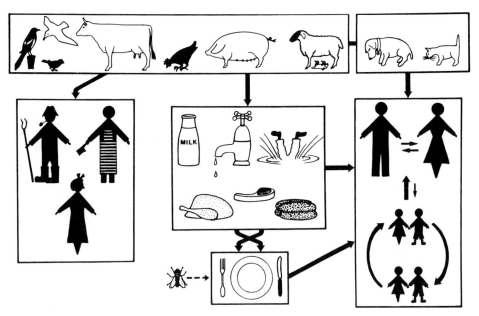

**Fig. 30.3** Sources and transmission of *C. jejuni* and *C. coli*. Top boxes: animal reservoirs and sources of infection (the sheep has just given birth to a dead campylobacter-infected lamb). Left-hand box: transmission by direct occupational contact (farmer, butcher, poultry processor). Right-hand box: transmission by direct domestic contact (puppy or kitten with campylobacter diarrhoea; intrafamilial spread mainly from children). Central box: indirect transmission through consumption of untreated water, raw milk, raw or undercooked meat and poultry, food cross-contaminated from raw meats and poultry; possible transmission from flies. (From document VPH/CDD/FOS/84.1 by permission of the World Health Organization, which retains the copyright.)

cooked that can create problems in the kitchen. Most infections are probably acquired via other foods, such as bread and salads, that become contaminated from raw meats in the kitchen. Unlike salmonellae, campylobacters do not multiply in foods, so explosive food poisoning outbreaks are rare. Most infections are sporadic or confined to one household.

*Other routes of infection.* Direct contact with infected animals or their products can also give rise to infection, as shown in Figure 30.3, which summarizes the principal sources and routes of transmission of campylobacters to man. Spread of infection between humans is of relatively minor importance.

## Control

The wide distribution of campylobacters in nature precludes any possibility of reducing the reservoir of infection. Efforts must be directed to interrupting transmission. The purification of water and the heat treatment of milk are obvious and basic measures. The control of infection in broiler chickens merits high priority, but sufficient resources for research and implementation are lacking. Terminal irradiation of carcasses eliminates campylobacters. Public education on basic hygiene in the handling

of raw meats, especially poultry, needs to be widely promulgated.

## HELICOBACTER

It is remarkable that a bacterium that colonizes roughly one-half of the world's population remained undiscovered until 1983. There are various reasons for this, but the turning point came with the introduction of fibre-optic endoscopy and with it the ability to biopsy the gastric mucosa. The discovery of *H. pylori*, as the organism was later named, was made by Warren and Marshall in Western Australia, and it soon became clear that it was a major factor in the pathogenesis of peptic ulceration.

This led to a search for similar bacteria in animals, and now some 17 species and taxons are recognized within the genus *Helicobacter*. Some colonize the stomachs of animals – the monkey, cat, dog, ferret, cheetah – each with its own species of helicobacter. Others colonize the intestines of a wide range of animals; *H. cinaedi* and *H. fennelliae* are associated with proctitis in homosexual men.

293

'*H. heilmannii*' ('*Gastrospirillum hominis*') is a larger more tightly spiralled bacterium, with up to 12 polar sheathed flagella, which is also found in the human stomach. It is much less common than *H. pylori*, but it is also associated with gastritis. It has not yet been cultured in vitro, so its name remains provisional. A morphologically indistinguishable organism has been observed in the stomachs of dogs and cats.

# HELICOBACTER PYLORI

## Description

*H. pylori* is a Gram-negative spirally shaped bacterium, 0.5–0.9 µm wide by 2–4 µm long. Like campylobacters, it is strictly micro-aerophilic and it requires carbon dioxide for growth, but it has a tuft of sheathed unipolar flagella, unlike the unsheathed flagella of campylobacters (Fig. 30.4; cf. Fig. 30.1). It is biochemically inactive in most conventional tests, but it produces an exceptionally powerful urease, almost 100 times more active than that of *Proteus vulgaris*. It undergoes coccal transformation even more rapidly than *C. jejuni* when exposed to adverse conditions.

## Antigens and strain typing

Although *H. pylori* shows some antigenic diversity, serotyping is of limited practical value. However, its genetic diversity can be exploited by molecular typing based on DNA analysis (see Ch. 3). Such

**Fig. 30.4** *H. pylori* showing multiple sheathed unipolar flagella. ×11 500. (Photomicrograph by Dr A. L. Curry and D. M. Jones, Manchester Public Health Laboratory.)

methods give fine discrimination between strains and are widely used.

## Pathogenesis

### Site of infection

*H. pylori* is a highly adapted organism that lives only on gastric mucosa. Colonization ceases abruptly where gastric mucosa ends, e.g. in areas of intestinal metaplasia in the stomach. Conversely, areas of gastric metaplasia elsewhere in the gut, notably the duodenum, may become colonized with *H. pylori*.

The gastric antrum is the most favoured site, but any part of the stomach may be colonized. The bacteria are present in the mucus overlying the mucosa where the pH is about 7.0 (they are not acid-tolerant). Colonization often extends into gastric glands, but they do not invade the mucosa (Fig. 30.5). Where the bacteria are numerous, the underlying mucosa usually shows a superficial gastritis of the type known as chronic active or type B gastritis, not to be confused with type A atrophic auto-immune gastritis of pernicious anaemia. This is characterized by infiltration with chronic inflammatory cells, but polymorphonuclear leucocytes are also present, hence the designation chronic active gastritis. Mucus-secreting foveolar cells often show damage where the bacteria are numerous.

### The course of infection

After an incubation period of a few days, patients suffer a mild attack of acute achlorhydric gastritis with symptoms of abdominal pain, nausea, flatulence and bad breath. Symptoms last for about 2 weeks, but hypochlorhydria may persist for up to a year. Despite a substantial humoral antibody response, infection and chronic gastritis persist indefinitely, but after several decades there may be a progression to atrophic gastritis. Conditions are then inhospitable for *H. pylori*, which disappears or is much reduced in number.

### Associated disease

Despite the presence of chronic gastritis, most infections are symptomless, and endoscopic appearances of the stomach are normal. However, a minority of infected persons develop peptic ulceration. It is likely that non-ulcer dyspepsia is sometimes caused by *H. pylori*, but there is currently no way of identifying such patients. More importantly, long-standing infection is associated with an increased

**Fig. 30.5** Section of gastric mucosa showing colonization with *H. pylori*. ×1400. Warthin–Starry silver stain. (Photomicrograph by Mr G. H. Green, Worcester Royal Infirmary.)

risk of developing gastric cancer. Moreover, gastric lymphoma although rare, is strongly associated with *H. pylori* infection, and complete regression has been observed after elimination of the organism.

## Peptic ulceration

There is now no doubt that *H. pylori* is actively involved in the pathogenesis of what was once regarded as idiopathic peptic ulceration (ulceration not related to non-steroidal anti-inflammatory agents or the *Zollinger–Ellison syndrome*). Clearly other factors are involved, but the role of *H. pylori* is crucial: infection is virtually a prerequisite for ulceration, and elimination of infection allows healing of ulcers without recurrence, in contrast to short-term treatment with agents that suppress gastric acidity. Any recurrence of ulceration is almost always associated with recrudescence of infection.

The pathogenic mechanism is unknown, but several factors may operate:

1. The production of ammonia by urease, which causes ionic changes in the mucus layer with a consequent back-diffusion of hydrogen ions in the mucosa.
2. The production of toxins or other substances, such as lipopolysaccharides, that activate inflammatory cells.
3. The stimulation of an auto-immune response by the production of antigens that cross-react with antral gastric antigens.

4. The degradation of mucus by a protease.

Infected patients also have hypergastrinaemia which upsets gastrin–hydrochloric acid homeostasis.

## Laboratory diagnosis

### Invasive tests

*H. pylori* can be detected in samples of gastric mucosa obtained by gastroscopy. Sensitivity is enhanced if two or more samples are taken for examination.

***Microscopy.*** *H. pylori* was seen in histological sections of gastric mucosa long before it was cultured, and microscopy remains a sensitive method in experienced hands. Warthin–Starry silver staining, as used for legionella bacteria, shows the organisms most clearly (Fig. 30.5), but many less complex staining methods are satisfactory. The bacteria can be seen in smears of biopsy material stained by Gram's stain.

***Culture.*** As culture is hardly more sensitive than histology, it is only necessary if the organism is required for sensitivity tests, or if strain typing is needed for epidemiological studies. Specimens must be kept moist and ideally should not be more than 2 h old. Selective agars similar to those used for campylobacters are used for primary isolation. Sensitivity is increased if a non-selective medium is used in parallel. Plates are incubated at 37°C in the same atmosphere as is used for campylobacters. High humidity is essential. Plates should be left undisturbed for 3 days and incubated for a week before being discarded as negative. *H. pylori* forms discrete domed colonies unlike the effuse colonies of *C. jejuni* and *C. coli*.

**Biopsy urease test.**   This test can be used at the bedside or in the clinic. *H. pylori* produces such abundant urease that it is detectable in biopsy tissue. A portion of tissue is put into a small quantity of urea solution with an indicator that detects pH changes resulting from the formation of ammonia by the action of urease. A positive result is obtained within a few minutes to 2 h, but the test may not detect light infections. Several versions of the test are marketed commercially.

**Molecular tests.**   DNA hybridization tests with DNA probes, usually with polymerase chain reaction (PCR) amplification, have great potential, but they are not yet sufficiently well developed for routine use.

### Non-invasive tests

**Serology.**   Several serological tests, mostly based on the ELISA principle, can be used to detect antibodies to *H. pylori* or its products. They are sensitive, but false-positive results may be given for a variable period after colonization has ceased, whether from treatment or progression to atrophic gastritis. Thus they are unreliable in the elderly.

**Urea breath test.**   Urea containing an isotope of carbon (carbon-14 or -13) is fed to the patient, and the emission of the isotope as carbon dioxide is measured in the breath. Patients infected with *H. pylori* give high readings of the isotope because of the release of carbon dioxide from urea by the action of the urease. The test has excellent sensitivity and specificity, but analysis is only practicable in centres possessing the complex equipment needed to assay the isotopes.

## Treatment

*H. pylori* is sensitive to most β-lactam antibiotics, macrolides, tetracyclines and nitroimidazoles, but resistant to trimethoprim. It is also sensitive to bismuth compounds.

The eradication of *H. pylori* infection requires the use of at least two antimicrobial agents in combination. The most effective regimen – bismuth subcitrate (or subsalicylate), tetracycline (or amoxycillin) and metronidazole given for 2 weeks – eliminates infection in over 90% of patients and is the standard

against which other regimens are judged. Unfortunately, owing to side-effects and the complexity of the regimen, patient compliance tends to be poor. Moreover, metronidazole-resistant strains are beginning to emerge with disturbing frequency in some regions.

An alternative strategy uses a proton (acid) pump inhibitor, such as omeprazole or lansoprazole, with an antibiotic such as clarithromycin or amoxycillin. Compliance is good, because the proton pump inhibitor makes the patient feel better from the outset. Omeprazole and lansoprazole exert an independent antibacterial effect on *H. pylori* and also enhance the action of antibiotics by raising gastric pH. Clearance rates of about 80% are attainable with this treatment.

## Epidemiology

Man appears to be the sole reservoir and source of *H. pylori*. How infection is transmitted is unknown, but it is presumably by the oral–oral or, possibly, faecal–oral route. *H. pylori* has been detected, with difficulty, in dental plaque, saliva and faeces.

Infection rates are strongly related to poor living conditions and overcrowding during childhood. Cross-sectional surveys show that there is a steady rise in seropositivity with increasing age (about 50% infected by the age of 60 years in industrialized countries), but this may simply mean that older people spent their childhood under poorer conditions than younger people. In developing countries most children become infected by the time they reach puberty. These high rates of infection broadly correlate with high rates of gastric cancer.

Inmates of psychiatric units and orphanages, and professional staff carrying out endoscopy examinations, show higher than average rates. Nosocomial infection from inadequately disinfected endoscopes has also been reported.

## Control

Social deprivation is the dominant factor governing the prevalence of *H. pylori* infection. In Western society, social advancement has brought about a reduction of infection, and peptic ulcer disease is on the decline. However, this is far from the case in developing countries, where a cheap and effective vaccine would be valuable, particularly for the prevention of gastric cancer.

## RECOMMENDED READING

Calam J (ed) 1995 *Helicobacter pylori. Baillière's Clinical Gastroenterology* 9: 415–663

Healing T D, Greenwood M H, Pearson A D 1992 Campylobacters and enteritis. *Reviews in Medical Microbiology* 3: 159–167

Jerris R C 1995 *Helicobacter*. In: Murray P R, Baron J O, Pfaller M A, Tenover F C, Yolken R H (eds) *Manual of Clinical Microbiology*, 6th edn. ASM Press, Washington, DC, pp 492–498

Marshall B J 1994 *Helicobacter pylori. American Journal of Gastroenterology* 89: S116–S127

Mishu Allos B, Blaser M J 1995 *Campylobacter jejuni* and the expanding spectrum of related infections. *Clinical Infectious Diseases* 20: 1092–1101

Nachamkin I 1995 *Campylobacter* and *Arcobacter*. In: Murray P R, Baron J O, Pfaller M A, Tenover F C, Yolken R H (eds) *Manual of Clinical Microbiology*, 6th edn. ASM Press, Washington, DC, pp 483–491

Skirrow M B, Blaser M J 1995 *Campylobacter jejuni*. In: Blaser M J, Smith P D, Ravdin J I, Greenberg H B, Guerrant R L (eds) *Infections of the Gastrointestinal Tract*. Raven Press, New York, pp 825–848

# 31

# Vibrio, mobiluncus, gardnerella and spirillum

Cholera; vaginosis; rat bite fever

## M. J. Lewis

---

### VIBRIO

The genus *Vibrio* is the most extensively characterized and medically important group within the family Vibrionaceae. The genus includes species that are commonly found in aquatic environments, some of which can also cause disease in man as well as in marine vertebrates and invertebrates. In the past the importance of vibrios has been associated almost exclusively with the epidemic and pandemic cholera caused by a particular antigenic form of *Vibrio cholerae*.

Until recently it was thought that man was the only natural hosts of *V. cholerae* and that all infections resulted from direct or indirect contact with human faeces. It is now recognized that *V. cholerae*, like other vibrios, is commonly found as a natural resident of aquatic environments in areas free of cholera, and that its presence is not necessarily associated with faecal contamination. The concept that this organism has only limited potential for survival outside the human intestine has been radically revised.

Other significant changes have occurred in our understanding of vibrios during the last 20 years, and the genus *Vibrio* now includes more than 30 species. The most important pathogens of man are *V. cholerae*, *V. parahaemolyticus* and *V. vulnificus*, but various other species are occasionally implicated as opportunistic pathogens.

## DESCRIPTION

Vibrios are short, Gram-negative rods which are often curved and actively motile by a single polar flagellum. They are fermentative but anaerogenic, and reduce nitrate to nitrite. Nearly all are oxidase-positive and produce indole. The genus can be divided into non-halophilic vibrios, including *V. cholerae* and other species that are able to grow in media without added

salt, and halophilic species which do not grow in these media. They grow readily on ordinary media provided that their requirements for electrolytes are met, and grow best when abundant oxygen is present. Most vibrios grow at 30°C but some of the halophilic species grow poorly at 37°C, whereas *V. cholerae*, *V. parahaemolyticus* and *V. alginolyticus* grow at 42°C.

Vibrios are tolerant to alkali but have a low tolerance to acid. Growth is rapid in the pH range 7.4–9.6 while the limits for growth are approximately pH 6.8 and 10.2.

## VIBRIO CHOLERAE

### Description

The biochemical reactions which differentiate *V. cholerae* from the other main pathogenic *Vibrio* species are shown in Table 31.1. The somatic (O) antigen structure is of fundamental importance in the identification of this organism. More than 130 different O serogroups have been described; the causative organism of epidemic cholera (the so-called *cholera vibrio*) is defined by its possession of the O1 antigen, and is known as *V. cholerae* O1. Strains of other serogroups are collectively known as *non-O1 V. cholerae* and correspond to strains known in the past as *non-agglutinable vibrios* or *non-cholera vibrios*. These have come under closer scrutiny as it has become clear that some of them can cause diarrhoea in man. All *V. cholerae* strains share the same flagellar (H) antigen.

Strains of *V. cholerae* O1 may be further subdivided on the basis of their O antigens into the subtypes *Inaba* and *Ogawa*. Some strains possess determinants of both of these subtypes and are known as subtype *Hikojima*.

There are two biotypes of *V. cholerae* O1: the classical and eltor biotypes. The eltor variant is distinguished

**Table 31.1**    Characteristics distinguishing important pathogenic *Vibrio* species

| Characteristic | *V. cholerae* | *V. parahaemolyticus* | *V. vulnificus* | *V. alginolyticus* |
|---|---|---|---|---|
| Voges–Proskauer | + (–) | – | – | + |
| Fermentation of: | | | | |
|   Sucrose | + | – | – | + |
|   Lactose | (+) | – | + | – |
|   L-Arabinose | – | + | – | – |
|   Cellobiose | – | – | + | – |
|   Salicin | – | – | + | – |
| Growth in: | | | | |
|   0% NaCl | + | – | – | – |
|   3% NaCl | + | + | + | + |
|   6% NaCl | – | + | + (–) | + |
|   10% NaCl | – | – | – | + |

+ (–), usually positive; – (+), usually negative; (+), positive after 3 or more days.

from the classical biotype by its haemolytic activity and its resistance to polymyxin B. The two biotypes can also be recognized by their differential susceptibility to specific phages.

## Pathogenesis

Cholera is typically characterized by the sudden onset of effortless vomiting and profuse watery diarrhoea. Although vomiting is a common feature, the rapid dehydration and hypovolaemic shock, which may cause death in 12–24 h, are related mainly to the profuse, watery, colourless stools with flecks of mucus and a distinctive fishy odour – *rice water stools* – which contain little protein and are very different from the mucopurulent blood-stained stools of bacillary dysentery. Anuria develops, muscle cramps occur and the patient quickly becomes weak and lethargic with loss of skin turgor, low blood pressure and absent or thready pulse. There are, however, all grades of severity, and milder cases cannot be distinguished clinically from other secretory diarrhoeas. Symptomless infections are common.

The sequence of events leading to cholera are confined to the gut. The cholera vibrios are ingested in drink or food and, in natural infections, the dose must often be small. After passing the acid barrier of the stomach the organisms begin to multiply in the alkaline environment of the small intestine, where they produce a potent enterotoxin known as *cholera toxin*. The toxin consists of five B subunits and a single A subunit. The A subunit is made up of two peptides linked by a single disulphide bridge. The B subunit binds to sugar residues of a specific ganglioside receptor on the cells lining the villi and crypts of the small intestine. It is thought that

insertion of the B subunit into the host cell membrane forms a hydrophilic transmembrane channel through which the toxic A subunit can pass into the cytoplasm. The cholera enterotoxin causes the transfer of adenosine diphosphoribose (ADP ribose) from nicotinamide adenine dinucleotide (NAD) to a regulatory protein which is part of the adenylate cyclase enzyme responsible for the generation of intracellular cyclic adenosine monophosphate (cAMP). The result is irreversible activation of adenylate cyclase and overproduction of cAMP. This in turn causes inhibition of uptake of $Na^+$ and $Cl^-$ ions by cells lining the villi, together with hypersecretion of $Cl^-$ and $HCO_3^-$ ions. This blocks the uptake of water which normally accompanies $Na^+$ and $Cl^-$ absorption, and there is a passive net outflow of water across mucosal cells, leading to serious loss of water and electrolytes. Cholera toxin is closely related to the *Escherichia coli* heat-labile toxin (see Ch. 27).

Although cholera toxin is the most important virulence factor in *V. cholerae* O1, the motility of the organism and the production of mucinase and other proteolytic enzymes enable it to overcome the protective mucosal barrier and reach the enterocytes. Once the organism penetrates the mucus layer it must be able to adhere closely to the enterocyte surface, and several adhesive haemagglutinins have been reported.

Some strains of *V. cholerae* O1 which cause diarrhoea do not produce cholera toxin. The toxin responsible differs in antigenic nature, receptor site, mode of action and genetic homology from cholera toxin.

## Laboratory diagnosis

Stool specimens are inoculated into alkaline peptone water, in which vibrios grow rapidly and accumulate on the surface. After incubation for 3–6 h a loopful from the surface is inoculated on a suitable solid medium, such as thiosulphate–citrate–bile salts–sucrose (TCBS). On this medium *V. cholerae* strains appear as yellow sucrose-fermenting colonies which may be tested for oxidase production and for agglutination in O1 antiserum prior to biochemical confirmation.

| Table 31.2 Formulation of oral rehydration solution recommended by the WHO[a] | |
| --- | --- |
| Sodium chloride | 3.5 g |
| Potassium chloride | 1.5 g |
| Sodium citrate | 2.9 g |
| Glucose (anhydrous) | 20.0 g |

[a]To be dissolved in 1 litre of clean drinking water.

## Treatment

Absolute priority must be given to the life-saving replacement of fluid and electrolytes. Oral rehydration therapy is often sufficient, but severe cases may require intravenous rehydration. The World Health Organization (WHO) is promoting the use of oral rehydration therapy in all cases of severe diarrhoea, including that due to *V. cholerae*. The recommended formula is shown in Table 31.2.

Tetracycline, chloramphenicol and co-trimoxazole reduce the period of excretion of *V. cholerae* in the stools of cholera patients, and tetracycline is often given to reduce environmental contamination and to reduce the risk of cross-infection. Strains of *V. cholerae* O1 eltor presently circulating are mainly drug-sensitive, but tetracycline-resistant strains began to appear in the 1970s and were soon followed by the appearance of strains resistant to a wide range of antimicrobial agents, including penicillins, streptomycin, chloramphenicol and trimethoprim.

## Epidemiology

A series of six pandemics of cholera, originating in the Bengal basin, ravaged the world in the 19th and early 20th centuries. Subsequently, cholera was increasingly contained within the endemic foci and surrounding areas of India and Bangladesh until 1961, when a seventh pandemic due to the eltor biotype

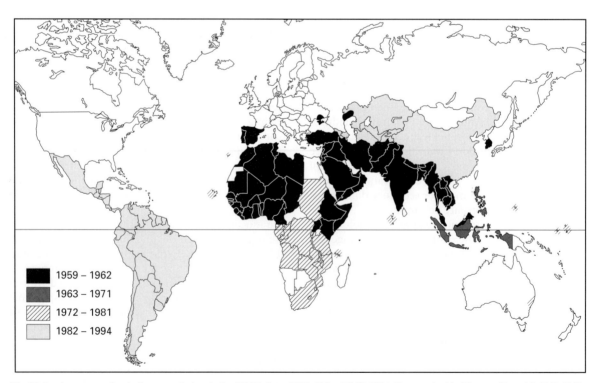

| | |
| --- | --- |
| ■ | 1959 – 1962 |
| ▨ | 1963 – 1971 |
| ▨ | 1972 – 1981 |
| ▧ | 1982 – 1994 |

**Fig. 31.1** Areas reporting indigenous cholera to the WHO since 1959. (After WHO 1991 *Communicable Disease Report* 1: R48–R49 and WHO 1995 *Weekly Epidemiological Record* 70: 202.)

of *V. cholerae* O1 spread from Indonesia to the Far East and then swept back through much of southern Asia. Early in the 1970s the pandemic invaded Africa, and in 1991 it reached South America, where the first epidemic in that subcontinent this century occurred in Peru. By December 1993 more than 820 000 cases of cholera, with almost 7000 deaths, had occurred, and the epidemic had involved all Latin American countries except Uruguay. In the following year the epidemic abated somewhat; a total of 113 684 cholera cases were reported, from 17 countries in the Americas, a reduction of 46% on the numbers reported in 1993, and at the time of writing (January 1996) the number of cases in the Western hemisphere continues to fall. However, during 1994 the WHO received an additional 270 000 notifications of cholera from a further 77 countries, mostly in Africa and Asia, where the downward trend seen since 1992 has not been maintained. The extent of the seventh pandemic of cholera in 1994 is shown in Figure 31.1.

The eltor biotype, originally isolated from pilgrims at the quarantine station known as El Tor, and at first thought to be of doubtful pathogenicity, supplanted the classical biotype in India during the 1960s and spread into Indian states previously free from infection. By 1973 the classical biotype in Bangladesh was also entirely displaced by the eltor biotype, and it remained in obscurity until October 1979 when five cases were reported. During the 1980s the classical biotype once again replaced the eltor biotype as the epidemic strain in Bangladesh, but it does not seem to have spread to other countries.

Infection is generally spread by contaminated water or foods such as uncooked seafood or vegetables. The source of the contamination is usually the faeces of carriers or patients with cholera, but contamination can probably sometimes occur from natural aquatic reservoirs. Cholera is characteristically an infection of crowded communities with poor standards of hygiene, often in low-lying areas. Infection tends to persist in communities with shared communal water supplies such as tanks, ponds, canals or rivers used for bathing, washing and for household use. Outbreaks occur either as explosive epidemics, usually in non-endemic areas, or as protracted epidemic waves in endemic areas. The seasonal incidence is fairly consistent in different endemic regions but the climatic conditions during epidemic waves may be distinctive for each region. For example, in Bangladesh the cholera season (November to February) follows the monsoon rains and ends with the onset of the hot dry months. In Calcutta the main epidemic wave (May to July) rises to its peak in the hot dry season

and ends with the onset of the monsoon but extends inland to neighbouring states during the rainy season.

Spread of infection is facilitated by the high ratio of symptomless carriers to clinical cases, which varies from 10:1 to 100:1 depending on living conditions and biotype. Symptomless carriers occur much more frequently in eltor than in classical infections.

## Control

In general, public health measures used in the control of any disease spread by faecal contamination are of value in the control of cholera. Most important are the provision of safe drinking water supplies and the proper disposal of human faeces.

Knowledge about cholera prevention and control has improved substantially, but the disease still causes fear, especially among travellers to affected areas. They should be reassured; although cholera can be life-threatening it is easily prevented and treated. In 1994, 29 countries that were not affected by endemic cholera reported a total of 283 imported cases, with no deaths. In the context of the millions of people on the move around the world each year this number of cases is insignificant.

### Vaccines

The immune response to cholera is directed against the bacterium rather than the toxin. It is specific for a given serotype. Infection with the classical biotype is followed by almost complete immunity for several years, but infection with the eltor biotype confers little or no immunity. It is not surprising, therefore, that the development of effective vaccines has proved difficult.

The traditional parenteral cholera vaccine conveys incomplete, unreliable protection of short duration, and is not recommended. Inactivated oral vaccines against O1 strains and live attenuated oral vaccines against O1 and O139 strains (see below) give better protection and are available in some countries for use by travellers. No country requires cholera vaccination as a condition of entry.

## *VIBRIO CHOLERAE* NON-O1

These strains are biochemically and genetically identical to *V. cholerae* O1 and may be isolated and characterized by similar techniques. There are over 130 different O serogroups, which occur widely in aquatic environments, and many infections are associated with exposure to saline environments or consumption of seafood. They appear to survive and multiply better than *V. cholerae* O1 in a wide range of foods, and it is likely that food-borne outbreaks occur as with other more common enteric pathogens.

Non-O1 *V. cholerae* causes mild, sometimes bloody diarrhoea, often accompanied by abdominal cramps. Symptoms may occasionally be severe, in which case the disease resembles cholera. Wound infections may occur in patients exposed to aquatic environments, and bacteraemia and meningitis have been reported.

Non-O1 *V. cholerae* strains may elaborate a wide range of virulence factors including enterotoxins, cytotoxins, haemolysins and colonizing factors. A few strains produce cholera toxin.

## Cholera and non-O1 *Vibrio cholerae*

Until 1992 it was accepted that strains of *V. cholerae* of serotypes other than serotype O1 do not cause epidemic cholera. However, in October 1992 unequivocal cases of cholera caused by a new non-O1 strain of *V. cholerae* were reported in Madras, India. By mid-January 1993 similar isolates were found in neighbouring Bangladesh, and these rapidly spread north, following the course of the major rivers and raising fears of a new pandemic. At the time of writing this strain has not spread beyond South Asia, and the number of cases appears to be declining.

The new *V. cholerae* strain does not agglutinate with O1 antiserum or with antisera to any of the other O serogroups. It has been assigned to a new serogroup, O139 Bengal. However, it closely resembles *V. cholerae* O1 eltor biochemically and physiologically, and it is possible that it will eventually attain the status of a subtype (*Bengal*) of that organism alongside the subtypes *Inaba* and *Ogawa* already recognized.

Cholera caused by *V. cholerae* O139 is indistinguishable from that caused by *V. cholerae* O1, and the recommended strategies for the control of epidemics caused by that organism apply.

## *VIBRIO PARAHAEMOLYTICUS*

### Description

*V. parahaemolyticus* was first isolated in 1950 from postmortem specimens of patients who died during an outbreak of food poisoning due to semi-dried sardines in Japan. It is a halophilic vibrio and will not grow in the absence of sodium chloride (see Table 31.1). This property is conveniently demon-

strated by inoculating the organism onto cystine–lactose–electrolyte-deficient (CLED) agar, which supports the growth of non-halophilic vibrios but not halophilic species. Strains of *V. parahaemolyticus* from clinical specimens generally form green, non-sucrose-fermenting colonies on TCBS agar, but sucrose-fermenting strains are found in estuarine and coastal waters.

Strains associated with gastro-enteritis usually cause haemolysis of human red cells in Wagatsuma's agar, a special medium containing mannitol. This haemolysis is known as the *Kanagawa phenomenon*.

### Pathogenesis

*V. parahaemolyticus* can cause explosive diarrhoea, but symptoms usually abate after 3 days. Other symptoms include abdominal pain, nausea and vomiting, and there may be blood in the stools. A few extraintestinal infections have been reported, particularly from wounds.

Kanagawa-positive strains produce a heat-stable cytotoxin and cause diarrhoea in volunteers. In contrast, volunteers have ingested $10^{10}$ cells of Kanagawa-negative strains without ill effects. Kanagawa-positive strains also adhere to human intestinal cells while Kanagawa-negative strains do not. A heat-labile enterotoxin can be separated from the heat-stable haemolysin and causes morphological changes in tissue culture cells resembling those caused by cholera toxin and the heat-labile enterotoxin of *Esch. coli*.

Most strains from seafood and the environment are Kanagawa-negative although positive colonies can usually be found if a sufficient number are tested. It is likely that a few Kanagawa-positive strains multiply selectively in the human intestine as infection develops and predominate in the stools of patients with diarrhoea.

### Laboratory diagnosis

*V. parahaemolyticus* grows well on TCBS, and the faeces of patients with a history of recent consumption of seafood may be examined for *V. parahaemolyticus* by the methods used for *V. cholerae*. In the examination of seafood and sea or estuarine waters for halophilic species, including *V. parahaemolyticus*, enrichment culture in alkaline peptone water containing 1% sodium chloride should be used.

### Epidemiology

*V. parahaemolyticus* is a common cause of diarrhoea in Japan and in Singapore. It has also been reported as a cause of illness associated with seafood in many other countries, including the USA and the UK. The organisms are ubiquitously distributed in fish and shellfish and in the waters from which they are harvested. Infections occur more frequently in the warmer months when the organisms are most prevalent in the aquatic environment. There is a particular risk associated with the consumption of raw seafood prepared and eaten in Japanese-style restaurants.

Extra-intestinal infections are always associated with exposure to the aquatic environment or handling of contaminated seafood.

## Treatment and control

Patients with diarrhoea generally require only fluid replacement therapy. Infection can be avoided by normal food hygiene procedures and by refrigeration of seafood to reduce the possibility of multiplication of *V. parahaemolyticus*.

# VIBRIO VULNIFICUS

## Description

This halophilic species was first recognized formally in a study in 1976 of a number of halophilic organisms differing from known species. The biochemical properties are shown in Table 31.1. Of particular importance are the fermentation of salicin and the production of β-galactosidase as detected by the *o*-nitrophenyl β-galactoside (ONPG) test.

## Epidemiology

Infections occur most frequently in areas where the water temperature remains high throughout the year, such as the mid-Atlantic and Gulf coast states of the USA. They are much more common during the warmer months of the year when *V. vulnificus* is most abundant. Wound infections are associated with injuries sustained in the aquatic environment while septicaemic infections are associated with the consumption of raw shellfish.

## Pathogenesis

There are three distinct clinical syndromes associated with *V. vulnificus* infections:

1. Rapid onset of fulminating septicaemia followed by the appearance of cutaneous lesions. More than 50% of those with primary septicaemia die. The condition is invariably associated with the consumption of raw shellfish. It is thought that the organisms enter the bloodstream by way of the portal vein or the intestinal lymph system. Elderly males with liver function defects due to alcohol abuse are particularly susceptible, but any deficiency in the immune system may also be a contributing factor.

2. A rapidly progressing cellulitis following contamination of a wound sustained during exposure to salt water. Infections of this kind occur in otherwise healthy persons as well as in the debilitated, and are characterized by wound oedema, erythema and necrosis which only occasionally progresses to septicaemia. The infection can be rapidly fatal.

3. Acute diarrhoea following the consumption of shellfish. This is less common; victims generally have mildly debilitating underlying conditions. Mortality is rare.

Virulence is associated with the presence of a polysaccharide capsule that probably contributes to the ability to resist phagocytosis and the killing effects of human serum. Virulent strains are able to use transferrin-bound iron, but not at the level of transferrin saturation normally found in man. This may explain the association of infection with pre-existing liver or other disorders that may result in elevated serum iron levels.

Strains of *V. vulnificus* produce several toxins that may contribute to tissue damage. They include a collagenase and cytolytic and proteolytic substances. A vascular permeability factor has also been described.

# VIBRIO ALGINOLYTICUS

## Description

*V. alginolyticus* is a halophilic organism formerly regarded as biotype 2 of *V. parahaemolyticus*. It fails to grow on CLED agar but grows in the presence of 10% sodium chloride. It forms large, yellow (sucrose-fermenting) colonies on TCBS. There is pronounced swarming on non-selective solid media.

## Pathogenesis

It occasionally causes opportunistic self-limiting infections of wounds. Clinical features include mild cellulitis and a seropurulent exudate. The pathogenic mechanism is unknown.

## Epidemiology

This organism is widely distributed in sea water and seafood and is probably the most common vibrio found in these sources in the UK. It occurs in large numbers throughout the year. Infections are invariably associated with exposure to sea water.

## OTHER VIBRIOS

*V. damsela* is a halophilic, aerogenic marine vibrio found in tropical and semi-tropical aquatic environments. It is associated with severe infections of wounds acquired in warm coastal areas.

*V. fluvialis* (previously known as group F vibrios, one biotype of which is now regarded as a separate species, *V. furnissii*) is easily confused with *Aeromonas hydrophila* because of a superficial phenotypic similarity. It was first recognized as a cause of diarrhoea in the late 1970s and a significant outbreak was reported in Bangladesh in 1980. Patients experienced diarrhoea, abdominal pain, fever and dehydration. *V. fluvialis* can be isolated in low numbers from fish and shellfish, and from sea water in areas where this is warm. It seems likely that infection is from contaminated seafood.

*V. hollisae* has been associated with bacteraemia and diarrhoea, especially in areas of the USA where the sea water is warm, such as the Gulf of Mexico. Infections are strongly associated with the consumption of raw seafood. *V. hollisae* exhibits gene sequences homologous with those encoding the thermostable haemolysin of *V. parahaemolyticus*.

*V. mimicus* occurs in similar environments to *V. cholerae*. Most isolates are from the stools of patients who develop gastro-enteritis after consumption of raw oysters, although a few ear infections have also been reported.

Other aquatic organisms that are probably related to vibrios include *Aeromonas* spp. and *Plesiomonas shigelloides*. *Aeromonas* spp., notably *A. hydrophila*, have been debatably implicated in diarrhoea and occasionally cause more serious infection in compromised individuals. *A. salmonicida* is an economically important pathogen of fish. *P. shigelloides* is an organism of uncertain taxonomic status that sometimes causes water-borne outbreaks of diarrhoea in warm countries.

## MOBILUNCUS AND GARDNERELLA

The name *Mobiluncus* was first proposed for a group of curved, motile, Gram-variable, anaerobic bacteria isolated from the vagina of women with bacterial vaginosis. Although the genus was first placed tentatively in the family Bacteroidaceae its taxonomic position is uncertain. Recent studies of 16S RNA suggest that the genus *Mobiluncus* belongs to the order Actinomycetales, in which it is most closely related to the genus *Actinomyces*.

*Gardnerella vaginalis* (formerly *Corynebacterium vaginale* or *Haemophilus vaginalis*) is often found in association with *Mobiluncus* spp. in bacterial vaginosis and, for convenience, is included here.

## DESCRIPTION

There are two species of *Mobiluncus*, *M. curtisii* and *M. mulieris*. The former is short (mean length 1.5 μm) and Gram-variable while the latter is long (mean length 3.0 μm) and Gram-negative. Both species have multiple flagella originating from the concave aspect of the cells. Cell wall studies show that there is no outer membrane and, although the cell wall is thinner than that of most Gram-positive organisms, it is generally considered that both species are Gram-positive. Two subspecies have been proposed for *M. curtisii*, spp. *curtisii* and *holmesii*.

*G. vaginalis* is a micro-aerophilic, pleomorphic, Gram-variable rod of uncertain taxonomic status.

## BACTERIAL VAGINOSIS

The clinical condition described as non-specific vaginitis or bacterial vaginosis is characterized by the presence of a thin, homogeneous vaginal discharge with a characteristic 'rotten fish' smell. This becomes more pronounced on alkalization, and can be evoked by placing a drop of potassium hydroxide solution on the fresh exudate on a slide or the speculum used for the vaginal examination. In addition, *clue cells* (epithelial cells covered with bacteria) can be seen in fresh unstained smears, and there is a raised vaginal pH (>4.5). The characteristic smell is ascribed to amines which are assumed to be produced by one or more of the bacterial species that form the complex microbial flora of the vagina.

The microbiology of bacterial vaginosis is complex. It appears to be a polymicrobial infection, with certain organisms playing a key role, especially when they overgrow the lactobacilli of the normal flora. *Mobiluncus* species are isolated from less than 50%

of women with bacterial vaginosis, but this almost certainly underestimates the prevalence of these fastidious and slow-growing organisms. By use of DNA probes, *Mobiluncus* species have been found in the vaginal secretions of over 80% of women with vaginosis but rarely in women without vaginosis. *Mobiluncus* are frequently found in association with *G. vaginalis* and with other organisms that may also be of aetiological importance. It appears that both the combination of species and their relative numbers are of importance in the development of the syndrome.

*Mobiluncus* species are occasionally isolated from extragenital sites, especially from breast abscesses.

## TREATMENT

*Mobiluncus* species and *G. vaginalis* are susceptible to most antimicrobial agents, including benzylpenicillin, clindamycin, erythromycin and nitroimidazoles. *M. mulieris* is more susceptible than *M. curtisii* to metronidazole, but treatment with this drug appears to eliminate all *Mobiluncus* species in patients with vaginosis. Oral or topical (intravaginal) metronidazole or clindamycin have been successfully used for the treatment of bacterial vaginosis.

## SPIRILLUM MINUS

The organism commonly known as *Spirillum minus*, one of the causes of rat-bite fever in man, is of uncertain taxonomic position. It was once regarded as a spirochaete but was later placed in the genus *Spirillum*. According to the 8th edition of *Bergey's Manual of Systematic Bacteriology* it does not belong to the genus *Spirillum*, *Oceanospirillum* or *Aquaspirillum*, and it is therefore regarded as a species *incertae sedis*.

## DESCRIPTION

*S. minus* is a short, spiral, Gram-negative organism about 2–5 μm in length and 0.2 μm in diameter. Longer forms up to 10 μm may be observed. The regular short coils have a wavelength of 0.8–1.0 μm. The organisms are very actively motile, showing darting movements like those of a vibrio. The move-

ment is due to polar flagella which vary in number from one to seven at each pole. The organisms can be demonstrated in fresh specimens by dark-ground illumination or by staining with Leishman's or other stains. Although there have been many unconfirmed claims the organism has not been cultivated on artificial media and many of its properties are therefore unknown.

## LABORATORY DIAGNOSIS

In rat-bite fever, *S. minus* may be demonstrated in the local lesion, in the regional lymph glands or in the blood, either by direct microscopical methods or by animal inoculation. Guinea-pigs, white rats and mice are susceptible to infection, and the organism may be detected by microscopy in the peripheral blood following intraperitoneal challenge.

## EPIDEMIOLOGY, PATHOGENESIS AND TREATMENT

*S. minus* occurs naturally in wild rats and other rodents, causing bacteraemia. The clinical syndrome of rat-bite fever begins with an acute onset of fever and chills 1–4 weeks after the animal bite. The bite usually heals before the onset of symptoms but it often re-ulcerates. Local lymphadenopathy and lymphangitis develop with the onset of fever and systemic disease. A generalized rash with large brown to purple macules is usually observed, but some patients present with urticarial lesions. A roseolar rash may spread from the area of the original bite. Fever usually declines within 1 week before returning again after a few days; the fever may then recur in an episodic fashion for months or even years. Endocarditis, meningitis, hepatitis, nephritis and myocarditis are rare complications. In most untreated cases, symptoms resolve within 2 months, after six to eight episodes of fever, although up to 6.5% of untreated cases may be fatal. This form of rat-bite fever occurs mainly in Japan and the Far East and is known as *sodoku*. Cases have been diagnosed, however, in other parts of Asia and in Europe and the USA.

*S. minus* infections respond to treatment with antibiotics, including penicillin and tetracyclines. In the rare case of endocarditis the addition of an aminoglycoside may be of value.

## RECOMMENDED READING

Catlin B W 1992 *Gardnerella vaginalis*: characteristics, clinical considerations and controversies. *Clinical Microbiology Reviews* 5: 213–237

Honda T, Iida T 1993 The pathogenicity of *Vibrio parahaemolyticus* and the role of the thermostable direct haemolysin and related haemolysins. *Reviews in Medical Microbiology* 4: 106–113

Jenkins S G 1988 Rat-bite fever. *Clinical Microbiology Newsletter* 10: 57–59

Kaper J B, Morris J G, Levine M M 1995 Cholera. *Clinical Microbiology Reviews* 8: 48–86

Levett P N 1992 Bacterial vaginosis. *Reviews in Medical Microbiology* 3: 15–20

Nair G B, Albert M J, Shimada T, Takeda Y 1996 *Vibrio cholerae* O139 Bengal: the new serogroup causing cholera. *Reviews in Medical Microbiology* 7: 43–51

Rippey S R 1994 Infectious diseases associated with molluscan shellfish consumption. *Clinical Microbiology Reviews* 7: 419–425

WHO 1995 Cholera in 1994. *Weekly Epidemiological Record* 70: 201–211

# 32

# Haemophilus

**Respiratory infections; meningitis; chancroid**

*M. P. E. Slack*

The major pathogen in this group of organisms is *Haemophilus influenzae*, which is associated with a variety of invasive infections such as meningitis, epiglottitis, pneumonia and septic arthritis and localized disease of the respiratory tract such as bronchitis and otitis media. *H. influenzae* biogroup aegyptius (formerly *H. aegyptius*) is a cause of epidemic conjunctivitis and Brazilian purpuric fever. Other haemophili of medical importance include *H. ducreyi*, the causative organism of chancroid, and *H. parainfluenzae*, *H. aphrophilus* and *H. paraphrophilus*, three organisms which are occasionally encountered in patients with infective endocarditis and a variety of other miscellaneous conditions, including dental infections, lung abscess and brain abscess. The generic name (= 'blood-loving' (Greek)) relates to the inability of this group of organisms to grow on culture media without the presence of whole blood or certain of its constituents.

The first documented observation of haemophili is thought to have been made in 1883 by Robert Koch, who described the microscopical appearance of a profusion of minute rods in pus from patients with conjunctivitis while engaged on cholera research in Egypt. A few years later, during the influenza pandemic of 1889–92, Pfeiffer noted the constant presence of large numbers of small bacilli in the sputum of patients affected with the disease. He had established these organisms in stable subculture by 1892, and in 1893 published a complete account of his work on influenza arguing that the bacillus was the causative agent of the disease.

In the succeeding years, considerable controversy surrounded this issue. It was observed that the influenza bacillus was sometimes absent in the localized outbreaks of infection which followed the pandemic and that the organism could be isolated from the respiratory tract of healthy individuals and from others with diseases in which clinical influenza was absent. The matter was resolved in 1933 when Smith, Andrewes and Laidlaw confirmed that the true aetiological agent was a virus. It still remains a possibility that secondary infection with *H. influenzae* contributed to the high mortality seen in the 1889–92 and 1918–19 pandemics.

## DESCRIPTION

### Morphology

Haemophili are pleomorphic Gram-negative rods. In clinical specimens, *H. influenzae* is most commonly seen as a small, uniform coccobacillus. In some cultures, and occasionally in clinical material, longer, filamentous forms may be seen, often in association with large, spherical or fusiform bodies.

### Encapsulation

Some strains of *H. influenzae* produce a capsule which is demonstrable by capsule stains and a *Quellung* reaction (swelling of the capsule) with type-specific antisera. The capsules are polysaccharide in composition and represent six distinct antigenic types, designated a–f. The most important of these is type b, which is a polymer of ribosyl ribitol phosphate. Strains possessing the type b capsule (Hib) are associated with most invasive infections seen with this species. The six capsular types can be identified with a polymerase chain reaction (PCR) method.

### Growth factors

The dependence on blood for growth on laboratory culture media is based on a requirement for two factors, termed $X$ and $V$. X factor – haemin – is required for the synthesis of the iron-containing respiratory enzymes cytochrome $c$, cytochrome oxidase, catalase and peroxidase. Unlike most bacteria, haemin-dependent haemophili cannot synthesize protoporphyrin from δ-aminolaevulinic acid. V factor is nicotinamide adenine dinucleotide (NAD) or NAD phosphate (NADP) or certain unidentified precursors of these compounds. It is essential for oxidation–reduction processes in cell metabolism. The differential requirements for X and V factors are important criteria for defining *Haemophilus* species: *H. influenzae* requires both; *H. parainfluenzae*, V factor only; and *H. aphrophilus* and *H. ducreyi*, X factor only.

## Growth on laboratory media

Ordinary blood agar contains X and V factors, but growth of *H. influenzae* on this medium is poor. The major growth restriction is due to the lack of availability of V factor, and enhancement of growth is obtained if the medium is supplemented with NAD. Streaking an organism which excretes an excess of this substance (e.g. *Staphylococcus aureus*) across the surface of the agar will produce growth stimulation in its vicinity (*satellitism*). Utilization of V factor in blood agar is also limited by the presence of serum nicotinamide adenine dinucleotidase (NADase). This can be inactivated by heating blood agar for a few minutes at 70–80°C until it turns brown (*chocolate agar*). This process also liberates extra X and V factors from the lysed red cells into the medium. X factor is heat-stable, but heating of media at 120°C for several minutes destroys V factor. Good growth is also obtained on certain transparent media containing blood extracts (e.g. Levinthal agar or Fildes' peptic digest agar). The latter are useful for demonstrating capsulate strains, colonies of which are iridescent when viewed obliquely with transmitted light. Type b capsulate strains can also be detected by the presence of precipitin haloes on transparent media containing hyperimmune *H. influenzae* type b antiserum.

## Metabolism

*Haemophilus* species are aerobic but facultatively anaerobic. Anaerobic growth considerably reduces the haemin requirement of X-dependent species. *H. aphrophilus* is the only species involved in human disease that has a requirement for carbon dioxide and this character may be lost on subculture. *H. influenzae* does not require a carbon dioxide-enriched atmosphere for growth but will often grow better in such conditions.

## Biochemical reactions

Haemophili are generally catalase-positive, oxidase-positive, reduce nitrate to nitrite and ferment glucose.

**Table 32.1** Differentiation of biotypes of *H. influenzae*

| Reaction | Biotype | | | | | | | |
|---|---|---|---|---|---|---|---|---|
| | I | II | III[a] | IV | V | VI | VII | VIII |
| Indole | + | + | – | – | + | – | + | – |
| Urease | + | + | + | + | – | – | – | – |
| Ornithine decarboxylase | + | – | – | + | + | + | – | – |

[a]Indistinguishable from *H. influenzae* biogroup aegyptius.

Patterns of acid production from other carbohydrates are used to identify the species. *H. influenzae* can be divided into eight biotypes on the basis of indole production, urease activity and ornithine decarboxylase reactions (Table 32.1). Biotypes I–III are the most common, and most invasive (type b) organisms are biotype I.

# PATHOGENESIS

## Normal carriage

*H. influenzae* is exclusively a human parasite which resides principally in the upper respiratory tract. Noncapsulate organisms are present in the nasopharynx or throat of between 25 and 80% of healthy people; capsulate strains (about half of which are capsular type b) in 5–10%. Immunization of infants with *H. influenzae* type b conjugate vaccine significantly reduces pharyngeal carriage of Hib, but has no effect on the carriage of other capsular types.

## Invasive infections

Invasive infections, usually caused by capsular type b, are quite distinct from the local (mostly respiratory) infections seen with non-typable *H. influenzae*. Meningitis is the most common invasive disease, followed by epiglottitis, bacteraemia without a clearly defined focus of infection (though often associated with pharyngitis), septic arthritis, pneumonia and cellulitis (Table 32.2).

These infections are unusual in the first 2 months of life, but are otherwise mainly seen in early childhood. Most cases occur in children under 2 years of age, but acute epiglottitis tends to present in slightly older children, having a peak incidence between 2 and 4 years of age.

The polysaccharide capsule is the major virulence factor for type b *H. influenzae*. The rarity of infec-

**Table 32.2**    The clinical presentation of 749 cases of invasive *H. influenzae* type b infections[a]

| Clinical diagnosis | No. of cases | % |
|---|---|---|
| Meningitis | 437 | 56 |
| Epiglottitis | 111 | 14 |
| Bacteraemia | 63 | 8 |
| Cellulitis | 54 | 7 |
| Pneumonia | 41 | 6 |
| Septic arthritis | 37 | 5 |

[a]Data from Public Health Laboratory Service regional *H. influenzae* survey 1990–92.

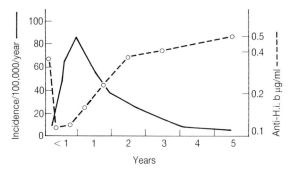

**Fig. 32.1**    The incidence of *H. influenzae* meningitis (continuous line) during the first 5 years of life and the corresponding mean level of anti-*H. influenzae* type b capsular polysaccharide antibodies (broken line). (From Peltola H, Käyhty H, Sivonen A, Mäkelä H 1977 *Haemophilus influenzae* type b capsular polysaccharide vaccine in children: a double blind field study of 100 000 vaccinees 3 months to 5 years of age in Finland. *Pediatrics* 60: 730–737.)

tions in the first 2 months of life correlates with the presence of maternal antibodies to this substance, and the occurrence of infection in early infancy with the absence of antibodies having such specificity. As the prevalence and mean level of capsular antibodies in the population rise, *H. influenzae* type b infections become less common (Fig. 32.1).

What determines whether acquisition of type b organisms in a susceptible host will lead to asymptomatic carriage and the stimulation of protective antibodies, or to the induction of invasive disease, is unclear. However, animal experiments suggest that when invasion occurs, the organism penetrates the submucosa of the nasopharynx and establishes systemic infection through the bloodstream.

The type b capsular polysaccharide has been shown to facilitate all phases of the invasion process. Other virulence factors which may be involved include fimbriae, which assist attachment to epithelial cells;

IgA proteases, which are also involved in colonization; and outer-membrane components, including outer-membrane proteins and lipopolysaccharide which may contribute to invasion at several stages. Initiation of invasive infection may be potentiated by intercurrent viral infection. Host genetic factors and immunosuppression may also play a role. It is unclear whether it is exposure to *H. influenzae* type b, or some other organism (e.g. *Escherichia coli* K100) possessing cross-reacting antigens which usually stimulates natural protective antibody production.

Non-capsulate *H. influenzae* may also be responsible for invasive disease. Meningitis and septicaemia due to non-capsulate *H. influenzae* is sometimes seen in the neonate.

## Non-invasive disease

*H. influenzae* also produces a variety of local infections which are often associated with some underlying physiological or anatomical abnormality. The commonest infections affect the respiratory tract and consist of otitis media, sinusitis and purulent episodes in patients with exacerbations of chronic obstructive airway disease.

Acute sinusitis and otitis media are usually initiated by viral infections. These predispose to secondary infection with potentially pathogenic components of the local resident microbial flora through mechanisms which may involve obstruction to the outflow of respiratory secretions, decreased clearance of micro-organisms via the normal mucociliary mechanism and depression of local immunity. Non-capsulate strains are usually responsible when *H. influenzae* is involved.

Acute exacerbations of chronic obstructive airway disease are similarly initiated by acute viral infections and, again, it is non-capsulate strains of *H. influenzae* that are chiefly responsible. Respiratory viruses compromise an already impaired mucociliary clearance mechanism in patients with chronic lung disease and allow bacterial colonization of the lower respiratory tract. In this situation *H. influenzae* can establish purulent infection and further damages pulmonary function by a direct toxic effect on cilia.

## LABORATORY DIAGNOSIS

### Direct examination

Gram-stained smears of cerebrospinal fluid, pus, sputum or aspirates from joints, middle ears or sinuses can provide a rapid, presumptive identification. Haemophili tend to stain poorly and dilute carbol fuchsin is a better counterstain than neutral red or safranin.

## General considerations

The viability of *H. influenzae* in clinical specimens declines with time, particularly at 4°C. For optimal yield, specimens should be transported to the laboratory and seeded onto appropriate culture media without delay. Chocolate agar represents a good, general purpose medium and can be used without further supplementation for specimens obtained from sites that would normally be expected to be sterile. Plates should be incubated in an aerobic atmosphere enriched with 5–10% carbon dioxide.

## Sputum

Specimens of expectorated sputum inevitably become contaminated by upper respiratory flora. This will commonly include *H. influenzae*, and the finding of the organism in such specimens cannot be automatically taken to imply involvement in a pathological process. Support for the significance of *H. influenzae* is provided if, in a purulent sample, the organism is present as the predominant isolate, or in a viable count of over $10^6$ colony-forming units per millilitre. Addition of bacitracin (10 IU/ml) facilitates the selective isolation of *H. influenzae* from mixed cultures of respiratory organisms. Obtaining bronchial secretions by broncho-alveolar lavage will reduce the problem of contamination with commensal organisms.

## Throat swabs

The temptation to obtain throat swabs in patients with suspected acute epiglottitis should be resisted, since attempts to obtain the sample may precipitate complete airway obstruction. Blood cultures are usually positive in this condition.

## Blood culture

Blood should be drawn for culture from patients with suspected invasive disease. Any good blood culture medium is satisfactory. Visual examination of the bottles cannot be relied upon to indicate positive growth. Bottles must be routinely subcultured onto solid medium, or some other detection system (e.g. fluorescent detection of released carbon dioxide) used.

## Antigen detection

The detection of type b polysaccharide antigen in body fluids or pus can be a useful and rapid diagnostic aid, particularly in patients who have received antibiotics before specimens are obtained. Techniques available include countercurrent immuno-electro-phoresis and agglutination of latex particles coated with rabbit antibody to type b antigen.

In the absence of confirmatory cultures, the results should be regarded with caution as some serotypes of *Streptoccoccus pneumoniae* and *Esch. coli* may share similar antigens.

## Molecular techniques

Techniques, such as PCR, are now being applied to the identification of *Haemophilus* species in clinical specimens and as confirmatory tests on isolates.

## Antibiotic sensitivity tests

Because of the fastidious nature of the organism, accurate determination of the antibiotic susceptibility of *H. influenzae* requires careful standardization of the methodology. Disc tests are less reliable for detecting enzyme-mediated ampicillin and chloramphenicol resistance than microbiological or biochemical techniques that demonstrate antibiotic inactivation.

## TREATMENT

*H. influenzae* is sensitive to a wide range of antibiotics and is usually inhibited by low concentrations of ampicillin (or amoxycillin), chloramphenicol and tetracycline. Early cephalosporins were relatively ineffective against this species, but compounds such as cefuroxime, cefotaxime and ceftazidime are highly active. Other antibiotics active against *H. influenzae* include co-amoxiclav, ciprofloxacin, azithromycin and clarithromycin.

Cefotaxime and related cephalosporins such as ceftriaxone are the antibiotics of first choice for the treatment of meningitis. They are bactericidal for *H. influenzae*, achieve good concentrations in the meninges and cerebral tissues and have proved highly effective in clinical practice.

Chloramphenicol was formerly the treatment of choice. Resistance may be encountered, but in most parts of the world this remains uncommon. Ampicillin is also effective and for a time enjoyed popularity for the primary treatment of bacterial meningitis as it appeared to cover all the pathogens likely to be responsible and avoided the potential toxicity of chloramphenicol. However, resistance to the drug, due to the production of a β-lactamase is now encountered in up to 25% of type b strains in the UK. In view of this level of resistance, ampicillin should no longer be used as a single agent in meningitis if *H. influenzae* is a possibility and the results of sensitivity tests are not available.

Antibiotic therapy is only one component of the clinical management of patients with haemophilus meningitis and full supportive care is required to achieve the most favourable outcome. Skilled medical and nursing care is also vital in the management of acute epiglottitis where maintenance of a patent airway is crucial. Cefotaxime is the antibiotic of choice.

For the treatment of less serious respiratory infections, such as otitis media, sinusitis and acute exacerbations of chronic bronchitis, oral antibiotics such as amoxycillin, co-amoxiclav and clarithromycin are all effective. β-Lactamase-mediated amoxycillin resistance is seen in about 20% of invasive non-capsulate isolates in the UK.

## EPIDEMIOLOGY OF INVASIVE DISEASE

*H. influenzae* is an important cause of serious systemic bacterial disease in children throughout the world. Meningitis is more common in winter months, in families of low socio-economic status and in household contacts of a case. The disease is usually seen in the youngest member of a family and uncommonly in children who have no siblings. Household contacts of patients with invasive disease have an increased risk of acquiring infection if they are under 5 years of age. The risk for children under 2 years of age is 600–800-fold higher than the age-adjusted risk for the general population.

Outbreaks of infection have been described in close communities, such as nursery schools. Contact with a case in a day care centre or nursery has also been associated with increased attack rates in children under 2 years of age although the calculated risk is lower than that seen in household contacts.

Very high rates have been reported in several distinct populations, e.g. Navajo and Apache Indians and Alaskan Eskimos. It is possible that socio-economic considerations are important in determining such racial differences, but host genetic factors may also play a role. Immunosuppression, whether iatrogenic or associated with malignancies (especially

Hodgkin's disease), asplenia or agammaglobulinaemia also predispose to invasive disease.

The mortality associated with *H. influenzae* meningitis is around 5%. Neurological sequelae, especially hearing loss, may be present in 10–30% of survivors.

*H. influenzae* type b conjugate vaccines (see below) have had a dramatic impact on the incidence of *H. influenzae* type b invasive disease. Before the introduction of immunization, *H. influenzae* was the leading cause of bacterial meningitis in the USA, accounting for some 12 000 cases annually. In the 1980s the incidence in the UK was similar; on several occasions the annual incidence of haemophilus meningitis exceeded that due to the meningococcus. Routine immunization with conjugate vaccine has dramatically reduced the incidence of haemophilus meningitis in countries where it has been adopted. Since 1992, when routine immunization was introduced in the UK, *H. influenzae* type b disease in children less than 5 years old has declined by 95% (Fig. 32.2).

## CONTROL

### Active immunization

The early haemophilus vaccines consisted of purified type b capsular polysaccharide. Unfortunately these proved to be poorly immunogenic in children less than 2 years old; the group most at risk of haemophilus meningitis, and in patients with immunodeficiency. Conjugate vaccines have now been developed in which the polysaccharide is covalently coupled to various proteins such as tetanus toxoid, a non-toxic variant of diphtheria toxin, *Neisseria meningitidis* outer-membrane protein, and diphtheria toxoid. These produce a lasting anamnestic response which is not age related, and may also be effective in high-risk patients who give a poor response to polysaccharide vaccine alone. In the UK, *H. influenzae* type b vaccine is routinely offered to infants at 2, 3 and 4 months of age, concurrently with diphtheria, tetanus and pertussis (DTP) immunization (see Ch. 68). There is no booster dose in the 2nd year of life.

### Prophylaxis

Rifampicin in a dosage of 20 mg/kg (up to a maximum of 600 mg) given orally once daily for 4 days is effective in eradicating carriage of *H. influenzae*, and has been used in attempts to prevent secondary

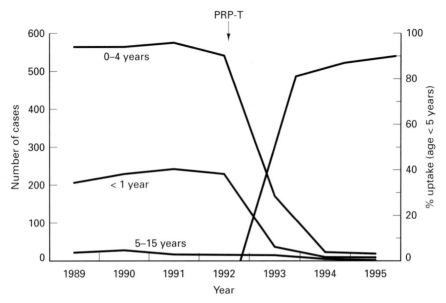

**Fig. 32.2**   Yearly totals of cases of *H. influenzae* type b meningitis and bacteraemia for 1989–95 (England and Wales) and the percentage vaccine uptake of *H. influenzae* type b vaccine (PRP-T) after its introduction as routine immunization in the UK in October 1992. (Data on yearly totals from the Communicable Disease Surveillance Centre; data on percentage vaccine uptake derived from O'Brien H 1994 *Communicable Disease Report* 4(2): R17–R18 and information published quarterly in *Communicable Disease Reports*.)

infection in both household and nursery contacts. Conclusive data regarding its efficacy are not available. Unvaccinated siblings who are more than 4 years old should be immunized with conjugate vaccine. Unvaccinated siblings younger than 4 years old should be given both chemoprophylaxis and vaccine. Children less than 4 years of age with invasive *H. influenzae* type b disease should also be offered both vaccine and chemoprophylaxis to eliminate nasopharyngeal carriage as the disease sometimes fails to induce immunity in the very young. The widespread use of conjugate vaccine may soon render chemoprophylaxis unnecessary.

## HAEMOPHILI OTHER THAN *H. INFLUENZAE*

### *H. influenzae* biogroup aegyptius

This organism, formerly known as the *Koch–Weeks bacillus* and *H. aegyptius*, is now thought to be a subgroup of *H. influenzae*. It is indistinguishable from *H. influenzae* biotype III in routine tests, but can be identified by a PCR method. It causes a purulent conjunctivitis and *Brazilian purpuric fever*, a clinical syndrome that was first recognized in Brazil in 1984, in which conjunctivitis proceeds to an overwhelming septicaemia resembling fulminating meningococcal infection. Ampicillin in combination with chloramphenicol has been successful when treatment has been started sufficiently early.

### *H. ducreyi*

This organism is responsible for a sexually transmitted disease, *chancroid*, which is most prevalent in tropical regions, particularly Africa and South-East Asia. Patients present with painful penile ulcers (*soft sore* or *soft chancre*) and inguinal lymphadenitis. Typical small Gram-negative bacilli can be seen in material from the ulcers or in pus from lymph node aspirates. It is likely that the lesions of chancroid have facilitated the transmission of human immunodeficiency virus in some tropical countries.

Chancroid has traditionally been treated with sulphonamides (alone or in combination with streptomycin), tetracyclines or erythromycin, but resistant strains occur. Newer drugs, including co-trimoxazole, co-amoxiclav, cefotaxime and ciprofloxacin, are effective.

An unrelated Gram-negative rod, *Calymmatobacterium granulomatis*, causes a somewhat similar sexually transmitted disease, *granuloma inguinale*, in parts of the tropics. Intracellular organisms, known as *Donovan bodies* (not to be confused with the Leishman–Donovan bodies of leishmaniasis), can be demonstrated in the stained smears from the lesions. Tetracyclines are usually used in treatment.

## Other haemophili

Various other species of *Haemophilus*, notably *H. parainfluenzae*, *H. aphrophilus*, *H. paraphrophilus* and *H. haemolyticus*, are occasionally implicated in human disease, especially bacterial endocarditis. A combination of ampicillin and gentamicin has been successfully used to treat such cases.

### RECOMMENDED READING

Alphen van L, van Ham S M 1994 Adherence and invasion of *Haemophilus influenzae*. *Reviews in Medical Microbiology* 5: 245–255

Jordens J Z, Slack M P E 1995 *Haemophilus influenzae*: then and now. *European Journal of Clinical Microbiology* 14: 935–948

Powell M 1988 Antimicrobial resistance in *Haemophilus influenzae*. *Journal of Medical Microbiology* 27: 81–87

Swaminathan B, Mayer L W, Bibb W F et al, The Brazilian Purpuric Fever Study Group 1989 Microbiology of Brazilian purpuric fever and diagnostic tests. *Journal of Clinical Microbiology* 17: 605–608

Tree D L, Morse S A 1995 Chancroid and *Haemophilus ducreyi*: an update. *Clinical Microbiology Reviews* 8: 357–375

Wenger J D 1994 Impact of *Haemophilus influenzae* type b vaccines on the epidemiology of bacterial meningitis. *Infectious Agents and Disease* 2: 324–333

# 33

# Bordetella

## Whooping cough

*N. W. Preston and R. C. Matthews*

The genus *Bordetella* constitutes one of the groups of very thin ovoid or rod-shaped Gram-negative bacilli, often described as parvobacteria. The genus contains two human pathogens, *Bordetella pertussis* and *B. parapertussis*, which cause one of the most frequent and serious bacterial respiratory infections of childhood in communities not protected effectively by vaccination.

## The pertussis syndrome

Per-tussis (severe cough) has been recognized as a clinical entity for several centuries. Typically, the child suffers many bouts of paroxysmal coughing each day; during these, with no pause for air intake, the tongue is protruded fully, fluids stream from the eyes, nose and mouth, and the face becomes cyanotic; when death seems imminent, a final cough clears the secretions and, with a massive inspiratory effort, air is sucked through the narrowed glottis, producing a long high-pitched whoop – hence the term *whooping cough*. Such attacks often terminate with vomiting. Between them the patient does not usually appear ill.

If a characteristic attack is witnessed, a clinical diagnosis of pertussis is readily made. However, the illness is often mild and atypical, especially in older children and adults, or in younger children who have been incompletely immunized, or in very young infants partially protected by maternal antibody.

In these cases, the laboratory has a vital role in diagnosis, because similar coughing may be caused by a variety of viruses and such illness is generally mild and of short duration. Here, the term *pseudo-whooping cough* has been applied aptly. False diagnosis may create a popular impression of pertussis as a trivial disease; and it has been recommended that, in the absence of positive bacterial culture, whooping cough should not be diagnosed for paroxysmal coughing lasting less than 3 weeks. With genuine pertussis, the illness is likely to persist for months rather than weeks. Furthermore, because pertussis vaccine cannot be expected to protect against viral infection, estimates of vaccine efficacy require an accurate diagnosis. Thus, a study in the UK by the Public Health Laboratory Service found an efficacy of 93% against pertussis confirmed by bacterial culture, compared with only 82% for cases diagnosed solely on clinical criteria.

## DESCRIPTION

Bordetellae used to be classified in the genus *Haemophilus*. However, growth is not dependent on either of the nutritional factors X and V, and *B. parapertussis* and *B. bronchiseptica* do not require blood for their growth. The three species resemble each other in being small Gram-negative bacilli, in causing infection of the respiratory tract, and in sharing some surface antigens.

### Bordetella pertussis

This is the most fastidious of the bordetellae. It produces toxic products which must be absorbed by a culture medium containing charcoal, or starch, or a high concentration of blood as in the original Bordet–Gengou medium. Because agglutination forms an important part of identification, a smooth growth is essential, and this is best provided by charcoal–blood agar. *B. pertussis* is a strict aerobe, with an optimal growth temperature of 35–36°C. Even under these conditions it usually takes 3 days before colonies are visible to the naked eye.

Typical colonies are shiny, greyish white, convex, and with a butyrous consistency. By slide agglutination, they react strongly with homologous (pertussis) antiserum, and weakly or not at all with parapertussis antiserum, depending on the specificity of the reagent. Subculture reveals no growth on nutrient agar.

**Table 33.1** Differential properties of *B. pertussis* and *B. parapertussis*

| Property | B. pertussis | B. parapertussis |
|---|---|---|
| Duration of incubation to yield visible colonies | 3 days | 2 days |
| Growth on nutrient agar | None | Good |
| Pigment diffusing in medium | None | Brown |
| Slide agglutination with: | | |
| Pertussis antiserum | Strong | Weak |
| Parapertussis antiserum | Weak | Strong |

The organism produces three major agglutinogens (1, 2 and 3) which can be detected by the use of absorbed, single-agglutinin sera. Factor 1 is common to all strains; the three serotypes pathogenic to humans (type 1,2, type 1,3, type 1,2,3) also possess factor 2 or factor 3 or both factors, and these type-specific agglutinogens have a role in immunity to infection.

## Bordetella parapertussis

This organism is readily distinguished from *B. pertussis* by its ability to grow on nutrient agar, with the production of a brown diffusible pigment after 2 days (Table 33.1). It also grows more rapidly than *B. pertussis* on charcoal–blood agar, and is agglutinated more strongly by parapertussis than by pertussis antiserum.

It causes less severe illness than *B. pertussis*, and is uncommon in most countries, though occasionally it has been responsible for outbreaks of whooping cough.

## Bordetella bronchiseptica

Colonies of this species are visible on nutrient agar after overnight incubation; it differs from the other species by also being motile and by producing an obvious alkaline reaction in the Hugh and Leifson medium that is used to differentiate oxidative from fermentative action on sugars. It is therefore placed by some taxonomists in the genus *Alcaligenes*; however, it is readily distinguished from the intestinal commensal *Alcaligenes faecalis* by its rapid hydrolysis of urea.

Although rarely encountered in human infection, *B. bronchiseptica* is a common respiratory pathogen of animals, especially laboratory stocks of rodents. Because it shares antigens with other bordetellae,

animals must be checked for freedom from bordetella antibody before they are used in the preparation of specific antisera. For this reason, sheep or donkeys have sometimes been used in preference to rodents.

## PATHOGENESIS

Whooping cough is a non-invasive infection of the respiratory mucosa, with humans as the only natural hosts. In a typical case, an incubation period of 1–2 weeks is followed by a 'catarrhal' phase with a simple cough but no distinctive features. Within about a week, this leads into the 'paroxysmal' phase, with increasing severity and frequency of paroxysmal cough, which may last for many weeks and be followed by an equally prolonged 'convalescent' phase.

In the initial preventable stage of the infection there is colonization of the ciliated epithelium of the bronchi and trachea with vast numbers of bacteria whose agglutinogens play a vital and type-specific role in attachment. *B. pertussis* produces a tracheal cytotoxin which paralyses the cilia, and leads to paroxysms of coughing as an alternative means of removing the increased mucus. Another bacterial product, called pertussis toxin (PT), is responsible for the characteristic lymphocytosis in uncomplicated whooping cough. A subsequent increase in the number of neutrophils, together with fever, suggests bronchopneumonia or other secondary infection, maybe with pyogenic cocci. Blockage of airways may cause areas of lung collapse, and anoxia may lead to convulsions, though with modern intensive care the disease is rarely fatal.

In developing countries, whooping cough is still a major cause of death; but in developed countries, concern is focused on a very prolonged and frightening illness with possible respiratory and neurological sequelae, on the anxiety and exhaustion of parents, and on the heavy use of hospital and community medical resources.

### Experimental infection in animals

Some, though not all, of the features of human disease have been produced in animals. Thus, marmosets and rabbits develop catarrh during prolonged colonization of the respiratory tract; they produce a similar range of agglutinin response to vaccination, and this immunity shows evidence of serotype specificity.

However, the mouse, which has long been used in the evaluation of pertussis vaccine potency, does not show these features. It can be infected and even killed by degraded organisms of serotype 1, which have lost the type-specific agglutinogens (2 and 3) that are necessary for human infection. It also reveals additional properties of PT that are not seen in humans: histamine sensitization, and islets activation (inducing hyperinsulinaemia and hypoglycaemia). Furthermore, PT and another component of the organism (filamentous haemagglutinin, FHA) are virulence factors in the mouse; but their role in human infection is uncertain. It is therefore necessary to interpret with caution experimental evidence from mice or other small rodents.

## LABORATORY DIAGNOSIS

### Bacterial culture

Because atypical clinical cases occur frequently, laboratory confirmation of the diagnosis is often essential. Bacterial culture has the highest specificity of the tests available. In the absence of really effective therapy, accuracy in the diagnosis is more important than speed. Bacterial culture has the additional advantage that the isolate can be serotyped and genotyped, and thus provide valuable epidemiological information.

So rarely has a positive culture been obtained from a healthy person, other than one incubating the disease, that a false-positive result can be discounted. Moreover, with good technique of swabbing and culture, the organism can be recovered up to 3 months from the onset of illness when coughing persists. This casts doubt on the widespread belief that the bacterium is eliminated in a few weeks, and has implications for the transmission of infection.

Though the disease is mainly in the lower respiratory tract, the organism can be recovered readily from the nasopharynx. 'Cough plates' and postnasal swabs are unsatisfactory because of overgrowth by commensal bacteria. A pernasal swab acquires fewer commensals, and these can be suppressed by penicillin (0.25 unit/ml = 0.15 mg/l) or cephalexin (30 mg/l) in the charcoal–blood agar plate; higher concentrations may suppress bordetellae. Pernasal swabs on flexible wire are available commercially; the tip is directed downwards and towards the midline, passing gently along the floor of the nose for about 5 cm (depending on the patient's age) until stopped by the posterior wall of the nasopharynx.

Practice in swabbing is necessary, initially with a co-operative adult! If old enough, patients should be warned to expect a tickling sensation but no pain; and a child's head should be held steady. Ideally, a segment of the culture plate should be inoculated immediately after withdrawal of the swab. The use of transport medium reduces the isolation rate. A single swab may yield a negative culture, but isolation rates of up to 80% may be achieved by taking specimens on several successive days.

In the laboratory, the inoculum is spread to give separate colonies, and the plate is incubated for at least 7 days before being discarded as negative. Because of the prolonged incubation, the medium should have a depth of 6–7 mm (40 ml in a 9 cm dish); and a bowl of water may be placed in the incubator, to reduce drying of the culture. Cephalexin tends to give 'rough' growth which may have to be subcultured on cephalexin-free medium for reliable serological identification.

### Detection of bacterial antigens

Bordetella antigens may be detected in serum and urine in tests with specific antiserum. Alternatively, bacteria in nasopharyngeal secretions are labelled with fluorescein-conjugated antiserum and examined by ultraviolet microscopy. This method has the theoretical advantage, compared with culture, of detecting dead bordetellae. However, false-negative results are likely unless the patient's own antibody is removed from the bacteria by enzyme, before application of the fluorescent reagent. Moreover, false-positive results may occur because of serological cross-reactions with organisms such as staphylococci, yeasts, haemophili and moraxellae, some of which resemble bordetellae microscopically. Bordetella antiserum should be absorbed with these organisms, but appropriate reagents are not readily available. Reports on the high specificity of this test lack conviction, in the absence of reliable evidence on the true diagnosis.

### Detection of bordetella antibody

Sera and nasopharyngeal secretions can usefully be examined for antibody. However, a negative result does not exclude pertussis because the serological response is often slow and weak, especially in very young children. More importantly, a positive result needs careful interpretation because antigens are shared with other organisms (see above). Even with insensitive tests, such as agglutination, pertussis antibodies are readily detected in the sera of healthy persons. More sensitive techniques, such as enzyme-linked immunosorbent assay (ELISA), are liable to increase the number of false-positive results, and thereby give spurious respectability to a diagnosis that should rightly be 'pseudo-whooping cough'. The need at present in serological diagnosis is not for greater sensitivity but for greater specificity.

## Differential blood count

Although lymphocytosis is a characteristic response to pertussis infection, many cases of true pertussis do not develop a significant increase in circulating lymphocytes; conversely, there are so many other causes of lymphocytosis that a positive result lacks diagnostic specificity.

## TREATMENT

### Antimicrobial drugs

Most antibiotics have little or no clinical effect when the infection is well established, even though the organism may be sensitive in vitro.

The drug of choice is erythromycin, which may reduce the severity of the illness if given before the paroxysmal stage. If given for at least 14 days it sometimes eliminates the organism and so reduces the exposure of contacts. However, positive cultures are frequently obtained after short periods of erythromycin therapy.

Erythromycin may also be given to protect non-vaccinated infants, though it seems unrealistic to expect this treatment to be maintained throughout the several months that the older sibling (or adult) may remain infectious.

Appropriate antibiotics should, of course, be administered to patients who show signs of secondary bacterial infection.

### Other measures

Cough suppressants and corticosteroids may control the paroxysms, but may be harmful by encouraging retention of secretions. Cyanosis and anoxia can be reduced by avoiding sudden noises, excitement or excessive medical examination, which tend to precipitate paroxysms; but mucus and vomit should be removed to prevent their inhalation.

Treatment with pertussis immunoglobulin has been tried, but with limited success – probably because such materials have never been checked for the presence of all three agglutinins.

Because of the dearth of effective therapy for whooping cough, the widespread use of pertussis vaccine is of supreme importance (see below).

## EPIDEMIOLOGY

### Source and transmission of infection

Most new cases arise from patients (usually children, sometimes adults) with typical symptoms, presumably because the paroxysmal cough provides an efficient means of droplet dissemination. Atypical cases have only a minor role in transmission; long-term asymptomatic carriage is unknown. The degree of contact is important: 80–90% of non-immune siblings exposed in the household become infected, compared with less than 50% of non-immune child contacts at school. Antibiotic therapy may reduce transmission, but is not completely effective.

### Incidence and mortality

Pertussis infection occurs world-wide, affects all ages, and is a major cause of death in malnourished populations. In the developed countries, mortality has gradually declined with a combination of improved socio-economic conditions, availability of intensive care in hospitals, and antibiotic therapy to combat secondary infection. However, the latter constitute an unnecessary use of medical resources on a disease that is eminently preventable by vaccination.

The disease is most severe, and the morbidity rate highest, in the first 2 years of life; most fatal cases are in infants under 1 year old. Even very young babies are not immune: maternal antibody does pass to the fetus, but it rarely contains all three agglutinins, and protection is incomplete.

Although one attack usually confers long-lasting immunity, infection with a different serotype of the organism can occur subsequently.

The disease occurs in epidemic waves at about 4 year intervals – the time needed to build up a new susceptible population after the 'herd' immunity produced by an epidemic. Figure 33.1 illustrates the pattern, for England and Wales, where whooping cough has been a notifiable disease since 1940. The maintenance of a 4 year cycle presumably results from the interaction of various factors, such as the degree of artificial immunity produced by high vaccination rates, and the levels of natural immunity that follow either large epidemics or a high back-

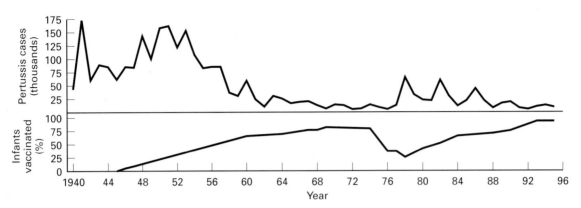

**Fig. 33.1** Whooping cough in England and Wales since 1940.

ground incidence of endemic pertussis in inter-epidemic intervals.

Figure 33.1 also illustrates how variations in the rates of uptake of pertussis vaccine have affected the incidence of whooping cough more than the steady improvement in the general health of the population that continued throughout the period. After the gradual introduction of pertussis vaccination during the 1950s, there was a steady reduction in the size of epidemics until the 1970s. Unfounded fear of brain damage caused a loss of faith in the vaccine, and three large epidemics occurred before the slow restoration of confidence in the vaccine began to take effect.

## Prevalence of serotypes

The three serotypes of *B. pertussis* pathogenic for humans are liable to spontaneous reversible variation,

as shown by the arrows in Table 33.2. Fimbriae are readily demonstrable on strains possessing agglutinogen 2, aiding colonization of the respiratory mucosa; serotypes 1,2 and 1,2,3 predominate amongst the strains isolated from patients in non-vaccinated communities.

In the 1960s, many countries used type 1,2 vaccine, and these two serotypes were suppressed. However, type 1,3 organisms, which have a weak factor 1 component, became predominant in these countries, and caused infection even in vaccinated children before the vaccine was modified in the late 1960s by addition of agglutinogen 3. Similarly, countries which used a vaccine deficient in agglutinogen 2, or in both agglutinogens 2 and 3, saw a predominance of type 1,2 infection, even in vaccinated children.

To be effective, it seems, a vaccine must contain all three agglutinogens, as recommended by the World Health Organization. However, because the

**Table 33.2** Occurrence of serotypes of *B. pertussis* in different communities

|  | Serotypes of *B. pertussis* that cause whooping cough | | |
|---|---|---|---|
|  | 1,2 ⇄[a] | 1,2,3 ⇄[a] | (1)[b],3 |
| Prevalence in non-vaccinated communities | High | | Low |
| Prevalence in communities vaccinated with type 1,2 | Low | | High[c] |
| Prevalence in communities vaccinated with type 1,3 or type 1 | High[c] | | Low |
| Relative incidence in communities vaccinated with type 1,2,3 (prior to complete elimination) | Lower | | Higher |

[a]The arrows indicate spontaneous reversible variation of serotype.
[b]The parentheses (1) indicate a weak factor 1 component, so that type 1,3 does not protect against type 1,2 infection, and vice versa.
[c]Infection occurs even in vaccinated children.

agglutinin 3 response is usually the weakest (when type 1,2,3 vaccine is used), type 1,3 organisms are the last to be eliminated from a community with an effective vaccination programme.

## Genotypes

It is not possible to trace the spread of infection by serotyping isolates, because there are only three serotypes and they undergo spontaneous variation. In contrast, more than 40 genotypes have been demonstrated in macro-restriction profiles by pulsed-field gel electrophoresis of DNA digests. Isolates within a household have been shown to belong to the same genotype, but the technique is probably too expensive and time-consuming for routine use.

## CONTROL

### Treatment and quarantine

Neither the antibiotics nor the immunoglobulins currently available are very effective for the treatment of patients or the prophylaxis of contacts.

Because patients typically disseminate the organism for many weeks or months, and because children are infectious even before the most characteristic symptoms develop, control of the disease by quarantine is unrealistic.

### Vaccination

Vaccination is safe and more than 90% effective and is strongly recommended. The vaccines in general use are suspensions of whole bacterial cells, killed by heat or chemicals, which are administered by deep intramuscular injection. Adsorption of the bacteria onto an adjuvant, such as aluminium hydroxide, enhances the immune response (particularly important with factor 3) and also causes fewer adverse reactions (Table 33.3).

Three conditions are essential for good protection with these vaccines:

1. Presence of all three agglutinogens in the vaccine
2. Use of adsorbed vaccine (i.e. with adjuvant)
3. Minimum of three doses, at monthly intervals.

Since there is little passive protection from the mother, and since effective active immunity cannot be achieved until after the third injection of vaccine, the first dose is given as soon as a good response can be obtained. In many countries, therefore, the first injection is recommended at 3 months of age. But, in the UK and some other countries, concern for the vulnerability of the young infant has prompted an earlier start, at 2 months, although the immune response is somewhat weaker. For these and other aspects of vaccination, see also Chapter 68.

### Safety of pertussis vaccine

Minor adverse reactions occur in up to one-third of vaccinated children, and can be considered as part of the normal immune response. Parents should therefore be warned to expect possible erythema and local swelling, slight feverishness, and crying. Of much more concern are possible neurological sequelae; but the National Childhood Encephalopathy Study in the UK, together with several other studies, showed that pertussis vaccination seems merely to trigger the manifestation of neurological disorders that would occur in any case, and there is no firm evidence that the vaccine causes serious long-term adverse side-effects.

### Contra-indications to pertussis vaccination

Severe adverse reaction to a previous dose is probably the only firm contra-indication. A current feverish illness (not merely snuffles) is cause for postponement until the child is well. Parental concern over a possible neurological contra-indication is due reason for consultation with a paediatrician. Allergy is not a contra-indication; neither is age – children who missed vaccination in infancy may receive the normal three-dose course. Vaccination is also sometimes advised for adults, e.g. nurses and doctors in appropriate hospitals.

### Acellular pertussis vaccine

Although doubts about the efficacy and safety of whole-cell pertussis vaccine have largely passed, the urge to identify the essential protective components persists. Trials in different countries (including one

| Table 33.3 Plain and adsorbed pertussis vaccine | | |
|---|---|---|
| Vaccine | Immune response | Adverse reactions |
| Plain | Weaker | More |
| Adsorbed (onto adjuvant) | Stronger | Less |

with type 1,2 prevalence, and another with type 1,3 prevalence), and with vaccines containing various components, may reveal a correlation between protection of children and the antigenic response to PT, FHA or other antigen in addition to the type-specific agglutinogens. However, a satisfactory acellular vaccine may be too expensive for routine use, especially for developing countries where the need is greatest.

## Eradication

Vaccination aims at a herd immunity, which breaks the cycle of transmission because the organism dies before finding a new susceptible host (see Ch. 68).

In several countries, good vaccine is readily available. Eradication is possible; but, even if high levels of vaccination of infants are maintained, it will be some years before adequate herd immunity is achieved within the child population.

## RECOMMENDED READING

Cherry J D, Brunell P A, Golden G S, Karzon D T 1988 Report of the Task Force on Pertussis and Pertussis Immunization – 1988. *Pediatrics* 81: 939–984

Editorial 1992 Pertussis: adults, infants, and herds. *Lancet* 339: 526–527

Jenkinson D 1995 Natural course of 500 consecutive cases of whooping cough: a general practice population study. *British Medical Journal* 310: 299–302

Khattak M N, Matthews R C 1993 Genetic relatedness of *Bordetella* species as determined by macrorestriction digests resolved by pulsed-field gel electrophoresis. *International*

*Journal of Systematic Bacteriology* 43: 659–664

Preston N W 1993 Eradication by vaccination: the memorial to smallpox could be surrounded by others. *Progress in Drug Research* 41: 151–189

Preston N W, Matthews R C 1995 Immunological and bacteriological distinction between parapertussis and pertussis. *Lancet* 345: 463–464

Thomas M G, Lambert H P 1987 From whom do children catch pertussis? *British Medical Journal* 295: 751–752

Wardlaw A C, Parton R (eds) 1988 *Pathogenesis and Immunity in Pertussis*. Wiley, Chichester

# 34

# Legionella

## Legionnaires' disease; Pontiac fever

*R. J. Fallon*

The Legionellaceae are Gram-negative rods whose natural habitat is water. Man is infected accidentally and the disease is not transmissible from person to person. There are 39 genetically defined species of *Legionella*, much the most important of which is *Legionella pneumophila*. This species can be subdivided on the basis of DNA relationships into three subspecies: *L. pneumophila* ssp. *pneumophila* and *L. pneumophila* ssp. *fraseri*, which have been described in human disease; and *L. pneumophila* ssp. *pascullei*, which has so far been isolated only from the environment. Eighteen *Legionella* species have been associated with human disease (Table 34.1) but most infections are caused by just one of the many serogroups of *L. pneumophila*, serogroup 1 (SG1). Other serogroups, and species such as *L. micdadei* and *L. bozemanii*, account for a few cases; other legionellae are rare causes of infection.

Legionellae give rise to two main clinical syndromes:

1. *Legionnaires' disease*. This is a pneumonia which may progress rapidly unless treated with appropriate antibiotic therapy, and extend to involve two or more lobes of the lung. The incubation period is 2–10 days, and the illness is characterized by high fever and symptoms such as respiratory distress, cough, confusion and focal neurological signs. In previously healthy subjects the mortality is about 10%, but in nosocomial infection the rate may be much higher.

2. *Pontiac fever*. In contrast to Legionnaires' disease, which develops in only a small proportion of the total population exposed to an identified source of infection, Pontiac fever has a high attack rate with no mortality. It is a brief febrile influenza-like illness which may be slow to resolve fully.

Legionellae have rarely been associated with other infections such as prosthetic valve endocarditis or wound infection, but these are usually nosocomial infections. Legionellae are not normally carried by man.

**Table 34.1** *Legionella* species associated with human disease

| Species | Number of serogroups | Autofluorescence under ultraviolet light |
|---|---|---|
| L. anisa | 1 | + |
| L. birminghamensis | 1 | − |
| L. bozemanii | 2 | − |
| L. cincinnatiensis | 1 | − |
| L. dumoffii | 1 | + |
| L. feeleii | 2 | − |
| L. gormanii | 1 | + |
| L. hackeliae | 2 | − |
| L. jordanis | 1 | − |
| L. lansingensis | 1 | − |
| L. longbeachae | 2 | − |
| L. maceachernii | 1 | − |
| L. micdadei | 1 | − |
| L. parisiensis | 1 | + |
| L. pneumophila | >14 | − |
| L. sainthelensi | 2 | − |
| L. tucsonensis | 1 | + |
| L. wadsworthii | 1 | − |

+, blue-white fluorescence; −, no autofluorescence.

## DESCRIPTION

In biological material (e.g. sputum, lung or in water deposits) legionellae are short rods or coccobacilli, but in culture they become longer and sometimes filamentous. Although they are weakly Gram-negative, they are difficult to visualize in biological material by Gram's stain, but may be stained non-specifically using a silver impregnation method. Specific fluorescent antibody stains are used diagnostically. The organisms may be numerous, particularly in patients who are infected in hospital or who are immunosuppressed, but are often present only in very small numbers in the scanty sputum which is characteristic of Legionnaires' disease. They have not been demonstrated in patients with Pontiac fever. Legionellae are exacting in their growth requirements and grow best on buffered charcoal yeast-extract agar (BCYE) which contains iron plus cysteine as an essential growth factor. Some legionellae grow better in the presence of 2.5–5% carbon dioxide at 35–36°C. Colonies do not appear until after incubation for 48 h. Usually they will appear by 5 days, but species other than *L. pneumophila* may take up to 10 days. Colonies have a 'cut-glass' appearance on examination under the plate microscope. Colonies of some *Legionella* species show blue-white (or red – not yet seen in species isolated from man) autofluorescence on illumination with long-wave ultraviolet light (Table 34.1). Species and serogroups within species have specific heat-stable lipopolysaccharide antigens, and further identification depends on serological examination, usually by the fluorescent antibody test or by slide agglutination with specific antisera. Species may be differentiated further, on the basis of serology, into serotypes within serogroups, but this applies, at the present time, almost entirely to *L. pneumophila* SG1. Subtyping is usually by the use of monoclonal antibodies in an immunofluorescence test. Similarities or differences between strains of the same serogroup may be revealed by genetic studies.

## PATHOGENESIS

### Legionnaires' disease

Infection is almost always due to *L. pneumophila* SG1. The disease is most common in those over the age of 40 years with a peak in the 60–70 year age group. Predisposing factors are immunosuppression, smoking and hospitalization. Infection arises as the result of inhalation of an aerosol of fine water droplets containing the organism. There is presently no evidence that ingestion plays a part in pathogenesis, although the demonstration of *L. pneumophila* in bowel contents raises this as a possibility.

Animal models provide some insight into the train of events in the lungs. Guinea-pigs infected by inhalation of an aerosol containing legionellae develop a lobular pneumonia which rapidly becomes confluent. Instillation of a protease produced by *L. pneumophila* into the lungs of guinea-pigs pro-duces a pneumonia which appears to be the same as that caused by inhalation of intact bacteria.

Once infection is established in man the patient develops pneumonic consolidation with an out-pouring of proteinaceous fibrinous exudate, containing macrophages and polymorphs, into the alveoli. Despite the outpouring of cells, patients usually produce little sputum. Apart from the pneumonic consolidation there are distant toxic effects of the infection on the nervous system with confusion, hallucinations and, occasionally, focal neurological signs; renal impairment leading to renal failure may occur. The mechanism of these toxic changes is unknown. The patient develops high fever and the disease may range from a rapidly progressing fatal pneumonia to a relatively mild pneumonic illness.

At the cellular level, legionellae are engulfed by monocytes and can survive therein as intracellular parasites. The duration of intracellular parasitization is unknown but the persistent excretion of group-specific legionella antigen in the urine of some patients, as opposed to its more transient appearance in most cases of legionella pneumonia, suggests that in some patients, intracellular parasitism may be prolonged. There is, however, no evidence of a chronic carrier state or chronic infection. Patients who are debilitated, e.g. by immunosuppression or surgery, are more prone to infections which are usually more severe than those encountered as sporadic cases infected in the community. The deterioration in body defences associated with ageing is also important, the disease being more common in the elderly.

### Pontiac fever

The pathogenesis of this non-pneumonic, non-lethal form of legionella infection is not understood. Living legionellae have been isolated from sources of infection associated with outbreaks of Pontiac fever, and legionella antigen has been demonstrated in the urine of some cases, indicating that appreciable quantities of legionellae have been involved in the infection.

## LABORATORY DIAGNOSIS

The tests used are listed in Table 34.2. As in any case of pneumonia, respiratory secretions (sputum, bronchial aspirate or washings), as well as pleural fluid, lung biopsy or autopsy material, should be examined by microscopy and culture. Gram-stained films are of little value except to demonstrate the

**Table 34.2** Diagnostic tests for legionella infection

| Nature of test | Test | Appropriate specimen |
| --- | --- | --- |
| Detection of whole organism | Culture FAT Gene probes | Sputum or other pathological material |
| Detection of soluble antigen | ELISA | Urine |
| Detection of antibody | FAT RMAT ELISA | Serum |

FAT, fluorescent antibody test; ELISA, enzyme-linked immunosorbent assay; RMAT, rapid micro-agglutination test.

presence of other pathogens and organisms which may interfere with the isolation of legionellae. Legionellae have occasionally been isolated from blood culture, but this is not a rewarding routine procedure.

The preferred diagnostic method is immuno-fluorescent staining with specific monoclonal or polyclonal antisera. Legionellae are usually hard to find in the scanty sputum produced by patients. Specific cultures are made on BCYE medium with and without antibiotics added to suppress other respiratory tract flora. Potentially contaminated material such as sputum or post-mortem material may also be heated at 50°C for 30 min in order to diminish growth by other less heat-stable respiratory tract organisms which have an inhibitory effect on growth of legionellae in culture. In heavy infections, legionellae may appear on BCYE media, but not on standard media, after incubation for 48 h at 36°C in air, preferably enriched with 2.5% carbon dioxide. Some of the less common legionellae may take longer to grow and cultures should not be discarded until after 10–14 days of incubation. Colonies having a 'cut-glass' appearance by plate microscopy or fluorescing blue-white under ultraviolet light are Gram-stained, and single colonies are subcultured onto blood agar or cysteine-deficient medium to show that they will *not* grow on these media. Cultures are identified by use of specific antisera in an immunofluorescence test.

## Antigen tests

The examination of urine for legionella antigen by enzyme-linked immunosorbent assay (ELISA) is a rapid and specific method of identifying *L. pneumophila* SG1 as the likely cause of a pneumonia.

## Serology

Although antibodies take at least 8 days to develop after the onset of infection, some cases may not reach hospital until this period has elapsed so that it is worthwhile to examine serum for antibodies to *L. pneumophila* on admission to hospital. Further sera should be taken at intervals to show the development of antibodies or a rise in antibody titre. Although antibodies usually develop after 8–10 days of illness and then increase in titre, some patients may not produce antibody for some weeks or, rarely, for several months. A four-fold or greater rise in antibody titre or a titre of 256 or more in a typical clinical case indicates infection with legionella. However, in some cases proven by culture, lower titres may be found, especially when death occurs early in the illness. Antibody may persist for months or years and can be a source of confusion, as may cross-reacting antibody produced by some patients with *Campylobacter* infection. At present the only fully validated antibody test is that for infection by *L. pneumophila* SG1, although patients proven by bacterial culture to be infected by other legionellae produce antibodies to the infecting strain.

## TREATMENT

Animal experiments indicate that erythromycin is effective in high dosage and that rifampicin is even more effective. Ciprofloxacin is also very active in vitro, but does not appear to be as good as erythromycin or rifampicin in animal models.

High-dose intravenous erythromycin is the standard therapy in legionella pneumonia. In severe cases this may be supported by rifampicin and, possibly, by the addition of ciprofloxacin, although evidence for the value of this agent is not well documented.

## EPIDEMIOLOGY

In 1976 an outbreak of 182 cases of pneumonia, mainly affecting members of the American Legion, occurred at a convention in Philadelphia. This form of pneumonia became known as *Legionnaires' disease*, and the bacterium associated with it as *L. pneumophila*. Since that time, legionella pneumonia has been recognized as the only acute *bacterial* pneumonia which may occur in outbreak form. This is due to the dissemination of the bacteria in aerosols which may travel for 1–2 km from the source.

Infected aerosols are usually generated from warm water sources, typically:

1. The ponds in cooling towers of refrigeration plants in air-conditioning systems
2. Domestic hot water systems in hotels and hospitals
3. Warm water in nebulizers and oxygen line humidifiers
4. Whirlpool spa baths and showers.

Legionellae are engulfed by, and survive within, free-living amoebae, and the bacteria may be protected from drying and disinfectants when present in the cysts formed by such amoebae. Outbreaks may occur on a fairly large scale in the community, and the source of infection is invariably a cooling tower in which the bacteria are harboured in the water of the pond associated with this apparatus. Smaller outbreaks have been associated with domestic water supplies in hospitals, spas and hotels and also with whirlpool spas. So-called sporadic cases may, on careful epidemiological examination, prove to be associated with cooling towers. About a third of cases in the UK acquire their infection abroad, usually from domestic water supplies in hotels. Legionnaires' disease accounts for a small but significant number of pneumonias admitted to hospital.

In any outbreak, or even one case occurring in hospital, possible sources of an infectious aerosol must be examined by indirect immunofluorescence and cultured to try to identify the source so that it can be eradicated. The disease is more prevalent in the late summer and autumn. This may be due to an increase in bacterial numbers in warm water both in natural sources and cooling towers.

Pontiac fever may affect all age groups, including children, the route and source of infection being the same as in Legionnaires' disease. In Pontiac fever the attack rate is high with almost all of those exposed to the infection source being affected whereas, in Legionnaires' disease, the attack rate is low.

## CONTROL

There is no vaccine. Nevertheless, unlike most forms of bacterial pneumonia, the disease may be prevented by the eradication of *Legionella* species in the various kinds of water source that may give rise to aerosol production. It is therefore important that the disease is identified as the cause of a pneumonia. Information about cases must be notified to epidemiological centres so that any association between cases may be established; once the source is identified, legionellae can be eradicated from water either by heat, or by disinfection with chlorine or other biocides.

Water systems in hotels and hospitals should be managed so that hot water is heated to above 60°C before distribution and does not lie stagnant and cooling in the pipes. As legionellae do not multiply in cold water, cold water supplies should be kept cold (below 20°C) and again not allowed to stagnate, in which situation the water may warm up and allow the multiplication of legionellae. It may be necessary in some infected water systems to chlorinate the water constantly to maintain suppression of growth. Cooling towers should be disinfected by chlorine or other biocides in a way that ensures that the growth of legionellae and possible supporting organisms, such as algae or amoebae, is suppressed.

RECOMMENDED READING

Bartlett C L R, Macrae A D, Macfarlane J T 1986 *Legionella Infections*. Edward Arnold, London
Fallon R J 1996 Legionellaceae. In: Collee J G, Fraser A G, Marmion B P, Simmons A (eds) *Mackie and McCartney Practical Medical Microbiology*, 14th edn. Churchill Livingstone, Edinburgh, pp 489–499
Harrison T G, Taylor A G (eds) 1988 *A Laboratory Manual of Legionella*. Wiley, Chichester

Joseph C A, Watson J M, Harrison T G, Bartlett C L R 1994 Nosocomial Legionnaires' disease in England and Wales 1980–92. *Epidemiology and Infection* 112: 329–345
Winn W C Jr 1988 Legionnaires' disease: historical perspective. *Clinical Microbiology Reviews* 1: 60–81

# 35

# Brucella, bartonella and streptobacillus

Brucellosis; Oroya fever; trench fever; cat scratch disease; rat-bite fever

*J. D. Coghlan*

## BRUCELLA

The genus *Brucella* consists of a group of Gram-negative bacilli that are essentially pathogens of goats, cattle, sheep and pigs. Infection in pregnant animals, particularly cows, leads to abortion, and involvement of the mammary glands may cause the organisms to be excreted in milk for months or even years. Human infections arise through contact with infected animals, including handling of infected carcasses, or through consumption of infected milk or milk products. Brucellosis is a typical zoonosis, and infection does not spread from man to man. Infection may remain latent or subclinical or it may give rise to symptoms of varying intensity. Acute brucellosis in its more severe form sometimes causes the characteristic intermittent waves of temperature that gave the name *undulant fever* to the human disease. This term is misleading since many brucella infections do not manifest this symptom.

## DESCRIPTION

### Morphology

Organisms of the genus *Brucella* appear as cocci, coccobacilli and short bacilli, 0.5–0.7 μm wide by 0.6–1.5 μm long. They occur singly, in groups or short chains. They are Gram-negative, non-motile, non-capsulate and non-sporing.

### Cultural characteristics

*Brucella* spp. are aerobic. However, *Brucella abortus*, when first cultured, is unable to grow without the addition of 5–10% carbon dioxide. All strains grow best in a medium enriched with animal serum and glucose. The optimum temperature for growth is 37°C.

On solid medium the colonies may take several days to appear. They are normally smooth, moist, transparent and glistening. However, the organisms tend to mutate, forming rough colonies. There is a corresponding loss in virulence and some antigenic change, so that they are no longer readily agglutinated by homologous antisera prepared against normal smooth strains.

### Sensitivity and survival

Brucellae are killed by a temperature of 60°C in 10 min. Infected milk is rendered safe by pasteurization. They are very sensitive to direct sunlight and moderately sensitive to acid, so that they tend to die out in sour milk and in cheese that has undergone lactic acid fermentation. They are likely to be destroyed by the acid secretions of the stomach. The organisms can survive in soil and manure for many weeks, and remain viable in dead fetal material for even longer. They have been isolated from butter, cheese and ice-cream prepared from infected milk. They may survive in carcass meat, pork and ham, remaining viable for several weeks after refrigeration.

## CLASSIFICATION

The three main *Brucella* species differ from one another in their choice of animal host, in certain cultural and biological characteristics and in the amount of the two main antigens that they have in common: *B. melitensis* infects goats and sheep; *B. abortus* infects cattle and *B. suis* infects pigs. The host–parasite relationship is not absolute, and both man and domestic animals are susceptible to infection by strains of all three species.

**Table 35.1** Some differentiating biological and biochemical characters of the three main *Brucella* species

| | $CO_2$ requirement | $H_2S$ production | Growth in presence of | | | Urease activity | Agglutination by monospecific serum | |
| | | | Basic fuchsin 1:25 000 | Thionin 1:50 000 | Methyl violet 1:50 000 | | abortus | melitensis |
| --- | --- | --- | --- | --- | --- | --- | --- | --- |
| *B. melitensis* | – | (–) | + | + | + | Variable | – | + |
| *B. abortus* | + | + | + | – | + | Slow[b] | + | – |
| *B. suis* | – | ++[a] | – | + | – | Rapid[c] | + | – |

(–), negative or slight.
[a]Biotype 1, others do not produce $H_2S$.
[b]Demonstrable after 2 h.
[c]Demonstrable within 30 min.

Characteristics that allow the three main *Brucella* species to be readily identified are shown in Table 35.1. Other species that differ from the main ones in their metabolic requirements and antigenic structure include: *B. canis*, isolated from dogs, mainly beagles in the USA, where they cause canine abortion; *B. ovis*, which is responsible for testicular infection of rams and abortion in ewes in Australia and New Zealand; and *B. neotomae*, isolated from the desert wood rat in Utah, USA. Neither *B. ovis* nor *B. neotomae* has been shown to cause human brucellosis; *B. canis* may infect man, but the disease is usually mild.

Within each of the three main species, biotypes (biovars) exist that differ in cultural, biochemical or serological respects from the normal prototype. There are at least nine biotypes of *B. abortus*, three of *B. melitensis* and five of *B. suis*. Biotype 4 of *B. suis*, previously known as *B. rangiferi tarandi*, infects reindeer in Russia and caribou in Alaska. It has been responsible for brucellosis among Eskimos and reindeer breeders.

## PATHOGENESIS

Each of the three main species is pathogenic to man. The incubation period is usually about 10–30 days, but symptoms may be delayed for several months. Brucellae enter the body through skin abrasions, through mucous membranes of the alimentary or respiratory tracts, and sometimes through the conjunctivae, to reach the bloodstream by way of regional lymphatics. The infection may persist for some time without causing any clinical manifestations. Classic undulant fever occurs more frequently with *B. melitensis* than with *B. abortus* or *B. suis*.

Infection by any species may give rise to a variety of symptoms and, without the fluctuating temperature to act as a guide, diagnosis may be difficult. The organisms subsequently localize in various parts of the reticulo-endothelial system with the formation of granulomatous lesions resulting in complications that may involve any part of the body. Brucellae surviving within granulomata may cause relapses of acute disease, or a chronic hypersensitivity condition may develop associated with continued illness and vague symptoms of malaise, low-grade fever, lassitude, insomnia, irritability and swelling around the joints. Such chronic brucellosis may follow an acute attack or develop insidiously over several years without previous acute manifestations.

## LABORATORY DIAGNOSIS

Brucellosis is confirmed in man and animals by isolating the organisms from the blood and by serological and other tests.

### Blood culture

When brucellosis is suspected, blood culture should be attempted repeatedly, not only during the febrile phase. Because the organisms may be scanty, at least 10 ml of blood should be withdrawn on each occasion, 5 ml being added to each of two blood culture tubes containing glucose–serum broth; one tube of each pair should be incubated in an atmosphere containing 10% carbon dioxide. Every few days subculture should be made onto serum–dextrose agar. Blood cultures should be retained for 6–8 weeks before being discarded as negative.

*B. melitensis* and *B. suis* are more readily isolated from blood than is *B. abortus*.

## Serological tests

In the absence of positive blood cultures, the diagnosis of brucellosis depends on serological tests, the results of which tend to vary with the stage of the infection.

The tests used include: the standard agglutination test (SAT); the mercaptoethanol test; the complement fixation test and the anti-human globulin (Coombs') test.

### Standard agglutination test

This test usually becomes positive 7–10 days after infection. During the acute stage of the disease, levels of agglutination associated with both IgM and IgG immunoglobulins continue to rise. Since prozones may occur in the later stages with high-titre sera, it is advisable to make a range of serum dilutions sufficiently great (e.g. to over 1 in 1000) to avoid false-negative results.

### Mercaptoethanol test

Low-titre agglutination due to residual IgM may continue for many months or even years after the infection has cleared. The mercaptoethanol test is carried out simultaneously and in the same manner as the SAT except that the saline diluent contains 0.05 M 2-mercaptoethanol. The agglutinating ability of IgM is destroyed by 2-mercaptoethanol, and therefore agglutination in this test is indicative of the continuing presence of IgG and the likelihood of continuing infection.

### Complement fixation test

As the disease progresses from the acute to the chronic form and the organisms become localized intracellularly in various parts of the body, the IgM antibodies decrease; the agglutination titre falls and may become undetectable even while the patient is still ill. The absence of agglutination therefore does not rule out the possibility of infection. IgG antibodies that remain present in the serum and are no longer capable of agglutinating may be detected by complement fixation tests.

In latent or chronic infection, the complement fixation test is likely to be positive whereas in cases of past infection it is negative.

### Coombs' test

Non-agglutinating (IgG) antibodies may be detected with anti-human globulin serum as in the Coombs' test. This results in the agglutination of a brucella suspension that has been sensitized by the non-agglutinating antibodies in the patient's serum.

Table 35.2 summarizes the interpretation of serological tests.

It should be noted that in some rural communities the sera from a proportion of the normal population agglutinate brucellae in low dilutions because of previous inapparent or latent infections.

The sera of persons who have been immunized against cholera and of those who have antibodies to *Francisella tularensis* may give false-positive reactions in the agglutination test against brucella organisms.

## Brucellin skin test

A delayed hypersensitivity reaction similar to the tuberculin test is sometimes used in the diagnosis of brucellosis, but its interpretation is difficult because, in communities frequently exposed to infection, there may be a high incidence of positive skin reactions as a result of latent infection.

## EPIDEMIOLOGY

### Brucella melitensis

This organism was first isolated in 1886 from the

**Table 35.2**   Results of serological tests used in the diagnosis of brucellosis

| Type of brucellosis | Agglutination test | Mercaptoethanol test | Complement fixation test | Anti-human globulin (Coombs') test |
|---|---|---|---|---|
| Acute | + | | + | |
| Chronic | (–) | + | + | + |
| Past infection | (–) | – | – | (–) |

(–), weak or negative.

spleens of fatal cases by David Bruce, an army doctor serving with the British army on the island of Malta. At that time the disease, known as Malta or Mediterranean fever, had a high incidence among army and navy personnel and among the island's civilian population. The name *Brucella* was subsequently given in honour of Bruce, who established it as the cause of the disease by transmitting the infection to monkeys.

Twenty years later, Zammit, a Maltese bacteriologist, showed that the organism was transmitted to man in goats' milk. Goats' milk and goats' milk products were subsequently prohibited for services personnel, and there followed a spectacular fall in the number of cases, whereas, among the civilian population, who continued to drink goats' milk, the incidence of the disease remained high with a correspondingly high fatality rate.

### Brucella abortus

*B. abortus* infects cattle in many parts of the world. In humans the infection occurs mainly in farming communities, and the disease it causes chiefly affects dairy farmers and veterinary surgeons, although persons who consume unpasteurized milk are also at risk.

Five of the nine biotypes of *B. abortus* (biotypes 1, 2, 3, 4 and 9) were formerly present in dairy herds in various parts of the UK. Since the introduction in 1967 of a compulsory scheme of testing and slaughter of infected animals, the disease has been eradicated. Human cases are now rare and are usually contracted abroad. In countries where the infection still exists, a history of close contact with cattle in a patient with a chronic febrile illness should give rise to a suspicion of brucellosis. However, persons who are no longer infected, but who are repeatedly exposed to brucella organisms, as a result of their work, may maintain high levels of IgG in their sera.

### Brucella suis

Human brucellosis due to *B. suis* is almost entirely an occupational disease arising from contact with infected pigs or pig meat. It has been reported mainly from the USA, chiefly among those who handled raw meat shortly after slaughter. In some European countries, hares may act as reservoir hosts of *B. suis*.

## TREATMENT AND CONTROL

### Chemotherapy

Brucella infections respond to a combination of streptomycin and tetracycline or to rifampicin and doxycycline. Intensive treatment in the acute stage of the illness is advisable in order to prevent the infection from progressing to the chronic form which is less likely to respond to treatment. The effectiveness of therapy should be checked by measuring serum antibody titres during and after the course of treatment.

### Vaccination

Vaccination of young cattle between 6 and 8 months of age with a single dose of *B. abortus* strain S19 protects them from abortion during the first and subsequent four or five pregnancies. Although vaccination cannot completely protect the animals against infection, it is beneficial in limiting its spread and thereby aids eradication.

Vaccination of man is not recommended because of undesirable side-effects and the possibility that hypersensitivity to brucella protein may develop.

### Pasteurization

Pasteurization eliminates the risk of brucella infection arising from the consumption of infected milk or milk products. However, there remains the possibility of infection due to contact with infected cattle or their tissues. Veterinary surgeons and cattle farmers are particularly at risk.

### Eradication

This depends on the elimination of the infection from domestic animals by a policy of compulsory testing of the animals and slaughtering positive reactors.

## BARTONELLA

The genus *Bartonella* consists of several species of very small Gram-negative bacilli, mainly arthropod-borne, that are responsible for feverish illness in humans involving the red blood cells. It includes *Bartonella bacilliformis*, the cause of Oroya fever, spread by sandflies; *Bart. quintana*, the cause of louse-borne trench fever; and *Bart. henselae*, one of the causes of cat scratch disease, the other being *Afipia felis*, which is related to the bartonellae.

Animal pathogens of the genus *Grahamella* are closely related to *Bartonella*, and it is proposed that they should be included in that genus. They are found in the blood cells of mice, voles and other mammals.

## *BARTONELLA BACILLIFORMIS*

In the mountainous regions of Peru, Colombia and Ecuador in South America, *Bart. bacilliformis* is responsible for outbreaks of a severe and often fatal disease of man, known as *Oroya fever*. The name was given after an epidemic of the disease in 1870 during the building of a railway between Lima and Oroya, when 7000 workmen died within a few weeks. The infection is spread by the sandfly *Lutzomyia verrucarum*.

After recovery from Oroya fever the patient may suffer from a skin eruption known as *verruga peruana*. Individuals may act as reservoirs of infection long after recovery from the illness and also after asymptomatic infection.

*Bart. bacilliformis* is pathogenic only to humans.

## Description

*Bart. bacilliformis* is a small Gram-negative coccobacillus, 0.3–1.5 × 0.2–0.5 μm. The organisms occur singly, in pairs, chains or clumps. In older cultures they tend to be extremely pleomorphic. They are motile due to about 10 flagella situated at one end of the cell.

The organism is readily cultured in semisolid nutrient agar containing animal protein in the form of rabbit serum and haemoglobin, similar to that used for the culture of leptospires. *Bart. bacilliformis* is strictly aerobic; the optimum temperature for growth is 25–28°C; the optimum pH is 7.8. Growth is slow, taking up to 10 days to be visible.

## Pathogenicity

After an incubation period of about 20 days, Oroya fever presents as a high fever followed by progressively severe anaemia due to blood cell destruction. There may be enlargement of the spleen and liver and haemorrhages into the lymph nodes.

The case fatality rate may be as high as 40%. Verruga peruana may occur without the initial attack of Oroya fever, or it may develop several weeks after recovery. It consists of a miliary-type skin eruption of round, elevated, hard nodules that may become secondarily infected, producing ulcers and haemorrhagic lesions. The rash may appear mainly on the legs, arms and face, although all parts of the body may be affected. The condition may persist for as long as a year, but it is rarely fatal.

## Laboratory diagnosis

In both Oroya fever and verruga peruana, bartonellosis is confirmed by demonstrating the organisms in blood smears stained by Giemsa. They are seen packing the cytoplasm of the cells and adhering to the cell surfaces.

Blood culture should be carried out at all stages of infection, on semisolid medium containing rabbit serum. Growth is usually apparent within 10 days. It may be difficult to isolate the organisms from the blood when the verruga stage has developed and culture from the skin lesions is rarely satisfactory.

## Treatment

Penicillin, streptomycin, tetracycline and chloramphenicol may be effective in the treatment of the infection and in reducing the mortality rate. Blood transfusion may be necessary in severe cases of anaemia.

## Control

Insecticides such as DDT are used to eliminate the sandfly vector in likely breeding sites inside and outside of houses and the surrounding areas. Since the insects bite only at night, individuals may protect themselves by withdrawing from affected areas at nightfall.

## *BARTONELLA QUINTANA*

This species of small bacilli (0.3–0.5 × 1.0–1.7 μm) was formerly classified among the rickettsiae as *Rochalimaea quintana*. However, unlike the rickettsiae these organisms can grow in cell-free media and they tend to be epicellular rather than intracellular parasites of man.

*Bart. quintana* was first identified as the cause of the febrile illness known as *trench fever* among the troops in the First World War. It is transmitted by the body louse, *Pediculus humanus*, under unhygienic living conditions. Unlike *Bart. bacilliformis* the organism does not possess flagella, although it may exhibit a twitching movement caused by fimbriae.

## BARTONELLA HENSELAE

*Bart. henselae* has been isolated from the blood of patients suffering from *cat scratch disease*, a severe condition of regional lymphadenopathy and fever resulting from the scratch or bite of an infected cat. Although no arthropod vector has been formally identified, it is thought that ticks or fleas may be responsible for transmission.

An organism known as *Afipia felis* is also implicated in cat scratch disease. It is similar to *Bart. henselae*, but differs biochemically and in being culturally less fastidious. Further work is needed to clarify the relationship between these two species.

Both *Bart. quintana* and *Bart. henselae* have been identified in the blood and tissues of individuals suffering from two severe clinical syndromes associated with human immunodeficiency virus (HIV) or other immunosuppressant conditions: *bacillary angiomatosis*, which affects the skin, regional lymph glands and various internal organs; and *bacillary peliosis*, which affects the liver and spleen.

## STREPTOBACILLUS MONILIFORMIS

*Streptobacillus moniliformis* is one of the causes of *rat-bite fever* in man, the other being *Spirillum minus* (see Ch. 31). It is a normal inhabitant of the nasopharynx of rats, and sometimes causes an epizootic disease of mice resulting in multiple arthritis and swelling of the feet and legs.

## DESCRIPTION

*S. moniliformis* is Gram-negative, non-motile, non-capsulate and highly pleomorphic. The organisms appear as short bacilli, 1–3 μm in length, forming chains that are interspersed with long filaments that may show oval or spherical lateral swellings. It is catalase-, oxidase- and urease-negative. It produces acid from glucose, but does not produce indole.

*S. moniliformis* is a facultative anaerobe that benefits from added carbon dioxide and a moist atmosphere. The optimum temperature for growth is 37°C, and growth ceases at 22°C. The optimum pH is 7.6. Culture media must contain blood, serum or ascitic fluid. Loeffler's serum medium is satisfactory. After incubation for 2 days, discrete, granular, greyish yellow colonies, 1–5 mm in diameter are visible on the surface, while minute colonies of 0.1–0.2 mm appear in the depth of the medium. The latter are L-phase variants that have little or no virulence for laboratory animals. They develop spontaneously and are thought to have a defective mechanism for cell wall formation.

In liquid medium, e.g. serum broth, *S. moniliformis* produces no turbidity, but an abundant granular sediment develops, appearing like cotton wool balls that do not disintegrate on shaking.

## Sensitivity

*S. moniliformis* is destroyed by a temperature of 55°C in 30 min. In culture it survives for only a few days, although in serum broth at 37°C it may remain viable for as long as 1 week. With the exception of the L-forms, *S. moniliformis* is susceptible to penicillin, and both forms are sensitive to streptomycin.

## PATHOGENICITY

In man the organism enters the body through the wound caused by a rat bite. It multiplies and invades the lymphatics and the bloodstream, causing a feverish illness with severe toxic symptoms and sometimes complications such as arthritis, endocarditis and pneumonia. Infection may also occur in epidemic form as a result of the ingestion of milk or other food contaminated by rats. This causes *Haverhill fever*, a condition first described in the USA, which is characterized by fever, polyarthritis and erythema. The duration of the illness varies from a few days to several weeks. If untreated the mortality rate is about 10%.

## LABORATORY DIAGNOSIS

*S. moniliformis* can be isolated in culture from the patient's blood during the acute phase of the illness and from the joint fluid of patients who develop arthritis. When growth occurs in a liquid medium the characteristic cotton wool balls are seen on the surface.

Mice are highly susceptible to intraperitoneal inoculation of patient's blood or joint fluid, as a result of which they develop a rapidly fatal generalized condition, or a more progressive disease with swelling of the feet and legs.

Specific agglutinins may be detected in the patient's serum as early as 10 days or as late as several weeks after the rat bite.

## TREATMENT

Penicillin or oral tetracycline are usually effective.

## RECOMMENDED READING

Adal K A 1995 Bartonella: new species and new diseases. *Reviews in Medical Microbiology* 6: 155–164

Corbel M J 1990 Brucella. In: Parker M T, Duerden B I (eds) *Principles of Bacteriology, Virology and Immunity*, 8th edn, vol 2. Edward Arnold, London, pp 339–353

Madkour M M 1989 *Brucellosis*. Butterworths, London

Report 1986 Joint FAO/WHO Expert Committee on Brucellosis, 6th report. *WHO Technical Report Series 740*. World Health Organization, Geneva

Washburn R G 1995 *Streptobacillus moniliformis* (rat-bite fever). In: Mandell G L, Bennett J E, Dolin R (eds) *Principles and Practice of Infectious Diseases*, 4th edn. Churchill Livingstone, Edinburgh, pp 2084–2086

Welsh D F, Slater L N 1995 *Bartonella*. In: Murray P R, Baron E J, Pfaller M A, Tenover F C, Yolken R H (eds) *Manual of Clinical Microbiology*, 6th edn. ASM Press, Washington, DC, pp 690–695

Williams E 1988 Brucellosis in humans: its diagnosis and treatment. *Acta Pathologica Microbiologica et Immunologica Scandinavica Supplement* 3: 21–25

Wullenweber M 1995 *Streptobacillus moniliformis* – a zoonotic pathogen. Taxonomic considerations, host species, diagnosis, therapy, geographical distribution. *Laboratory Animals* 29: 1–15

# 36

# Yersinia, pasteurella and francisella

Plague; mesenteric adenitis; tularaemia

*J. D. Coghlan*

The organisms within these three genera are animal parasites that, under certain conditions, are transmissible to man, either directly or through insect vectors. They are Gram-negative coccobacilli which may show extreme variations in size and shape (*involution forms*), particularly in older cultures. At one time these organisms were all contained within one genus, *Pasteurella*, but differences among the various strains are sufficient to warrant a division into separate genera, each with its own disease manifestations in man and animals.

The main distinguishing features of the most important species are shown in Table 36.1.

parts of the world, burrowing animals such as gerbils and voles act as reservoirs of infection that may be transmitted by fleas to susceptible animals such as bandicoots, marmots and squirrels. The animals suffer from outbreaks of plague, and their fleas may transmit the infection to man, giving rise to sporadic disease referred to as *wild* or *sylvatic plague*. Farmers or trappers who come into contact with infected animals are at risk.

More serious for man, however, is *urban plague*, resulting from the spread of infection among rats, especially the black rat, *Rattus rattus*, that at one time flourished around human habitation. Outbreaks of human plague, following epidemics in rats, have, in the past, sometimes developed into pandemics.

## YERSINIA PESTIS

## INTRODUCTION

*Yersinia pestis* (formerly *Pasteurella pestis*), the *plague bacillus*, is essentially a parasite of rodents. In certain

## DESCRIPTION

### Morphology

*Y. pestis* is a short coccobacillus, $1.5 \times 0.7$ μm, occurring singly, in pairs or, when in fluid culture, in chains. Pleomorphism is marked, especially in old

**Table 36.1** Differentiating characteristics of *Yersinia*, *Pasteurella* and other species of Gram-negative coccobacilli

| | Growth on | | Motility[a] | Acid (no gas) from | | Indole production | Urease activity |
|---|---|---|---|---|---|---|---|
| | Nutrient agar | Bile salt agar | | Maltose | Sucrose | | |
| *Yersinia pestis* | + | + | − | + | − | − | − |
| *Y. pseudotuberculosis* | + | + | + | + | − | − | + |
| *Y. enterocolitica* | + | + | + | +[b] | + | − | + |
| *Pasteurella multocida* | + | − | − | − | + | + | − |
| *P. haemolytica* | + | +/− | − | − | + | − | − |
| *P. pneumotropica* | + | − | − | + | + | + | + |
| *Actinobacillus ureae* | + | − | − | −/+ | + | − | + |
| *Francisella tularensis* | − | − | − | + | − | − | − |

[a]At 22°C, all non-motile at 37°C.
[b]Late maltose fermenter.

cultures in which pear-shaped or globular cells, suggestive of yeast cells, may be seen. The organisms are Gram-negative, non-sporing and non-motile. In smears from exudates and in cultures grown at 37°C they are frequently capsulate. In smears from tissues stained by methylene blue they show characteristic bipolar staining.

## Cultural characteristics

*Y. pestis* grows both aerobically and anaerobically at 14–37°C. It is somewhat sensitive to oxygen, and small inocula may not grow aerobically in ordinary culture media. At the optimum temperature of 27°C, small (<1 mm), slightly viscid, translucent, non-haemolytic colonies develop on blood agar within 24 h. The colony size may reach 3–4 mm on prolonged incubation. Growth occurs on MacConkey's medium, but tends to autolyse after 2–3 days.

## Antigens

There are two main antigenic complexes that include many antigens associated with the virulence and immunogenicity of the organism. One is somatic and heat-stable, the other capsular and heat-labile. Two of the somatic antigens, V and W, appear to enable the organism to resist phagocytosis. The capsular antigen that contains the immunogenic fraction (F1) is necessary for efficient vaccine production.

## Sensitivity

*Y. pestis* is killed at 55°C in 5 min and by 0.5% phenol in 15 min. It is sensitive to drying but may remain viable in moist culture for many months. It is sensitive to many antibiotics, including tetracyclines, aminoglycosides and sulphonamides, but not penicillin.

## PATHOGENESIS

There are three severe forms of human plague: *bubonic*, *pneumonic* and *septicaemic* plague.

## Bubonic plague

The transfer of *Y. pestis* from rats to man through the bites of infected fleas may occasionally result in a localized infection, known as *pestis minor*, with mild constitutional symptoms. More often the lymph nodes draining the area of the flea bite become affected, and the adenitis caused results in painful swellings or *buboes* in the inguinal, axillary or cervical regions, depending on the position of the flea bite. From these primary buboes the plague bacilli may spread to all parts of the body. In the absence of adequate antibiotic therapy administered early in the course of the disease, the case fatality rate may be as high as 50%.

## Pneumonic plague

This develops as a result of droplets infected with *Y. pestis* being passed from person to person. A severe bronchopneumonia develops. The sputum becomes thin and blood stained. It contains numerous plague bacilli that are demonstrable by stained films or culture of the sputum. This type of plague is highly contagious and is usually fatal, unless treated early.

## Septicaemic plague

This may occur as a primary infection or as a complication of bubonic or pneumonic plague. The plague bacilli spread throughout the body and the outcome is invariably fatal.

## LABORATORY DIAGNOSIS

Plague is confirmed by demonstrating the bacilli in fluid from buboes in the case of bubonic plague, in the sputum in pneumonic plague and in blood films and by blood culture when septicaemic plague is suspected.

A smear of exudate or sputum is stained with methylene blue. Characteristic bipolar-stained coccobacilli are confirmed as *Y. pestis* by culturing some of the exudate on blood agar and incubating at 27°C. If some of the exudate is inoculated subcutaneously into guinea-pigs or white rats, or onto their nasal mucosa, infection follows and the animals die within 2–5 days. In septicaemic plague the bacilli may be isolated in blood culture, or from smears of spleen tissue post-mortem.

Characteristic colonies growing on blood agar plates are identified as those of *Y. pestis* by various cultural and biological tests (Table 36.1) and by demonstrating the ability of the bacilli to form chains in broth culture and 'stalactite' growth from drops of oil layered on the surface of fluid medium.

## Serology

The patient's serum may be tested by the complement fixation test or by haemagglutination of tanned sheep red cells to which the capsular antigen F1 has been absorbed.

## TREATMENT

When plague is suspected, whatever the form, antibiotic therapy should be started without waiting for confirmation of the diagnosis. Tetracycline is the drug of choice. It should be given in large doses (4–6 g daily), within 48 h of onset, and continued for 10 days.

## EPIDEMIOLOGY

### History

Plague was introduced into Europe from Asia in the 13th century and led to the great pandemic known as the Black Death, when about a quarter of the population of Europe succumbed to the disease. The infection remained enzootic in European rats and continued to give rise to outbreaks of human plague. After the last major epidemic in England in 1665, plague disappeared spectacularly from Europe, perhaps because the black rat was displaced by the spread of the brown (sewer) rat, *Rattus norvegicus*. *R. norvegicus* is susceptible to plague, but does not commonly frequent human dwellings. Improvements in housing may also have played an important part in the elimination of plague from Europe.

A major outbreak of plague in Hong Kong in 1894 led to a new pandemic, with spread to most major seaports. It was during this outbreak that Yersin first described the plague bacillus.

Strict antirodent measures and the widespread use of DDT to destroy the fleas that transmit the infection have greatly reduced the incidence of urban plague. However, endemic foci of wild rodent plague continue to exist in many rural parts of the world, including North and South America, Africa, South-East Asia, China and southern parts of central Asia (Fig. 36.1). Constant surveillance must be maintained to prevent its spread to urban populations, especially in areas where living conditions are below standard.

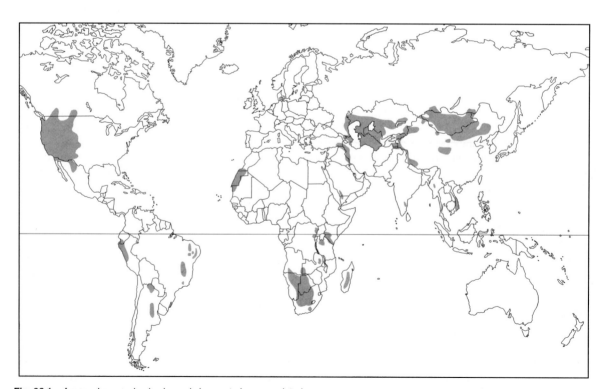

**Fig. 36.1** Areas where endemic plague is known to have persisted.

## Bubonic plague

Bubonic plague is a zoonosis. The bacilli are transmitted from animal to animal and from animal to man by fleas, notably *Xenopsylla cheopis*, an ectoparasite of rats. In cool humid weather, fleas multiply and plague spreads readily among susceptible rats. Hot, dry weather, on the other hand, tends to limit the spread of infection because the fleas die out under those conditions.

When a flea feeds on the blood of a sick animal, plague bacilli are sucked into the insect's midgut, where they multiply to such an extent that they block the proventriculus. On the death of the animal the flea seeks an alternative host, which may be another rodent or man. Because the 'blocked' flea is unable to suck readily, some of the infected blood of the previous host is regurgitated and injected into the bite wound of the new victim.

When the epizootic among rats has reached a stage at which the number of susceptible animals has greatly decreased through death or immunity, it tends to die out, as does any human epidemic associated with it.

## Pneumonic plague

The sputum of persons suffering from pneumonic plague contains large numbers of plague bacilli and under favourable conditions the disease spreads rapidly through the community by droplet infection, independently of rodents or fleas. Epidemics are more likely to occur when overcrowding in unsanitary dwellings allows the infected droplets to spread readily from person to person.

## CONTROL

### Bubonic plague

In areas where the infection is endemic, periodic surveys are advocated to determine the prevalence of rodents and fleas so that control measures can be taken. Rats may be destroyed by rat poison and fleas by the liberal application of insecticide to rat runs.

Other control measures include the construction of rat-proof dwelling houses and buildings such as warehouses in dockland areas. The fumigation of ships and measures to prevent rats gaining access to ships help to prevent the spread of plague from one country to another.

## Pneumonic plague

To control the spread of pneumonic plague, patients should be isolated if possible and overcrowding of dwelling houses avoided. Sulphonamides or tetracyclines administered to immediate contacts may afford some degree of protection.

### Vaccination

Vaccination is sometimes used to protect persons likely to have been exposed to infection. Live vaccine prepared from avirulent strains of *Y. pestis*, and vaccine prepared from inactivated virulent organisms, are available. Neither can be relied upon to confer immunity of more than short duration, and revaccination is necessary at 6-monthly intervals if exposure to infection continues. Reaction to vaccination may be severe.

## YERSINIA PSEUDOTUBERCULOSIS

*Y. pseudotuberculosis* attacks many species of wild and domestic animals and birds, causing a fatal septicaemia. The infection is a zoonosis indirectly transferable to man, resulting in a wide range of illnesses from subclinical to severe, including acute mesenteric lymphadenitis.

## DESCRIPTION

*Y. pseudotuberculosis* is a small, ovoid Gram-negative bacillus which is slightly acid-fast. Like *Y. pestis* it grows on MacConkey's medium, although poorly. The organisms may be differentiated from *Y. pestis* by their motility when grown at 22°C and by their ability to produce urease.

### Sensitivity

*Y. pseudotuberculosis* is sensitive in vitro to tetracyclines, aminoglycosides, sulphonamides and, unlike *Y. pestis*, penicillin.

### Antigens

There are at least six serological types (and a number of subtypes) that possess highly specific thermostable somatic antigens, one of which is common to all types, and thermolabile flagellar antigens present in cultures grown at 18–26°C. A somatic antigen common to all strains is shared with *Y. pestis*, and the two species have many other antigens in common.

About 90% of all human cases appear to be due to strains of serotype 1.

## PATHOGENESIS

*Y. pseudotuberculosis* may give rise to a subclinical infection or a fatal septicaemia. Human infections occasionally result in a severe typhoid-like illness with fever, purpura and enlargement of the liver and spleen which is usually fatal. More frequently it causes mesenteric lymphadenitis, simulating acute or subacute appendicitis, with or without erythema nodosum. This mainly affects young males aged 5–15 years. Recovery is usually uneventful.

## LABORATORY DIAGNOSIS

Infection in man is confirmed by isolation of the organism in culture from blood, local lesions or mesenteric glands, particularly the ileocaecal glands.

Specific serum antibodies are detected and measured by tube agglutination tests carried out during the acute phase of the illness against smooth suspensions of strains of serotypes 1–6 grown at 22°C. The agglutinins decline rapidly and reach low levels within 3–5 months.

An intradermal test, similar to the tuberculin or brucellin tests, becomes positive during the acute infection and remains positive for many years.

## TREATMENT

Mesenteric adenitis is usually self-limiting. Septicaemia demands parenteral treatment with ampicillin or tetracycline.

## EPIDEMIOLOGY

The epidemiology of yersiniosis due to *Y. pseudo-tuberculosis* is still not clear. Many animal species suffer from the infection, but there is little proof of direct transmission to man. Human infections may result from skin contact with water polluted by infected animals, or the ingestion of contaminated vegetables or other food.

## YERSINIA ENTEROCOLITICA

This species resembles *Y. pseudotuberculosis*; it causes gastro-enteritis in man, occasionally with more severe complications.

## DESCRIPTION

Morphologically and culturally, *Y. enterocolitica* resembles *Y. pestis* and *Y. pseudotuberculosis* (see Table 36.1), but it differs from them antigenically and biochemically.

Antigenically the species is very complex; 34 different O antigens and 19 H factors have been identified, so that a large number of serotypes are recognized. Serotypes 3 and 9 account for most human infections in Europe, while serotype 8 is most common in the USA. Other serotypes have been isolated from healthy individuals and are probably non-pathogenic.

Some authorities have divided *Y. enterocolitica* into five different species: *Y. enterocolitica*, *Y. kristenseni*, *Y. intermedia*, *Y. aldovae* and *Y. frederikseni*.

## PATHOGENESIS

*Y. enterocolitica* causes mild and occasionally severe gastro-enteritis, mesenteric lymphadenitis, and septicaemia (often fatal), especially in the elderly. Secondary complications include erythema nodosum, polyarthritis, Reiter's syndrome and meningitis. It affects children and adults of both sexes. In young children the infection may produce fever, diarrhoea, abdominal pain and vomiting. The symptoms may last for several weeks.

It has been isolated from pseudotuberculous lesions and from apparently healthy animals of many species throughout the world. However, it is not a true zoonosis since human disease may result from ingestion of contaminated food or from contact with the environment. Man-to-man transmission also occurs.

## LABORATORY DIAGNOSIS

Infection is diagnosed by isolating the organism from blood, lymph nodes or faeces on blood agar or MacConkey's agar. Identity is confirmed by biochemical tests and motility (Table 36.1). The serotype may be determined by slide agglutination with specific rabbit antisera. Serum antibodies are measured by tube agglutination tests against appropriate O antigens. A significant rise in the titre to 160 or more over a 10 day period indicates acute infection.

## TREATMENT

*Y. enterocolitica* is sensitive to many antibiotics, including tetracyclines, aminoglycosides and chloramphenicol, but it is resistant to penicillins. Treatment is indicated only in severe infection. Tetracycline is probably the drug of choice; β-lactam agents are unreliable.

## PASTEURELLA MULTOCIDA

*Pasteurella multocida* (formerly *P. septica*) is a parasite of many species of domestic and wild animals and birds. Man occasionally become infected, especially following animal bites.

## DESCRIPTION

*P. multocida* organisms are aerobic and facultatively anaerobic coccobacilli, $0.7 \times 0.3–0.6$ μm, i.e. smaller than those of *Yersinia* species. They are arranged singly, in pairs and small bundles, but are pleomorphic in culture. They are Gram-negative, non-motile, non-sporing and capsulate in culture at the optimum temperature of $37°C$. In smears of blood or tissue stained with methylene blue they show bipolar staining. *P. multocida* does not grow on MacConkey's medium.

### Antigens

On the basis of four capsular antigens and 11 somatic antigens, 15 serotypes of *P. multocida* have been identified.

### Sensitivity

*P. multocida* is killed rapidly at $55°C$ and by phenol (0.5%) in 15 min. The organisms may survive and remain virulent in dried blood for about 3 weeks, and in culture or infected tissues for many months if kept frozen.

## PATHOGENESIS

*P. multocida* can be extremely virulent to many species of animals and birds, causing haemorrhagic septicaemia which is usually fatal. It also causes respiratory infections.

The rare human infections take the form of:

1. A local abscess at the site of a cat or dog bite, with cellulitis, adenitis and, sometimes, osteomyelitis.
2. Meningitis following head injury.
3. Infections of the respiratory system such as pleurisy, pneumonia, empyema, bronchitis, bronchiectasis and nasal sinusitis, in which *P. multocida*, although not always the direct cause, may contribute to the severity and duration of the disease.

Cases of appendicitis, in which *P. multocida* has been isolated from pus in pure culture, have also been reported.

## LABORATORY DIAGNOSIS

Swabs from bite wounds, from cerebrospinal fluid in cases of meningitis and from the secretions in suppurative respiratory tract infections are cultured on blood agar. The organisms are identified by various cultural and biochemical tests (see Table 36.1).

## TREATMENT

Infections usually respond to treatment with penicillin. Tetracycline, erythromycin or co-trimoxazole are suitable alternatives. In cases of osteomyelitis following dog or cat bites, antibiotic therapy must be continued for at least 8 weeks.

## EPIDEMIOLOGY

*P. multocida* is carried in the nasopharyngeal region of many species of wild and domestic animals, some of which remain healthy while others suffer septicaemic or respiratory diseases. In human infections following animal bites, the organism passes directly to man in the animal's saliva. Man may also become infected through breathing an atmosphere contaminated by the coughing of animals suffering from respiratory infection.

*P. multocida* may be carried commensally in the human respiratory tract and may cause infection after surgical operation or cranial fracture.

## OTHER *PASTEURELLA* SPECIES

*P. haemolytica*, *P. pneumotropica* and *Actinobacillus ureae* differ from *P. multocida* in certain details of culture, biochemical characteristics and pathogenicity (Table 36.1).

*P. haemolytica* causes pneumonia in sheep and cattle, septicaemia in lambs, and various diseases in domestic animals and poultry. It is apparently non-pathogenic for humans. It differs from *P. multocida* in forming haemolytic colonies on blood agar and by its ability to grow on MacConkey's medium.

*P. pneumotropica* is frequently isolated from the respiratory tract of laboratory animals. In man it has occasionally been isolated from cases of septicaemia, upper respiratory tract infections and from animal bite wounds.

*A. ureae* has been isolated from the sputum of humans suffering from chronic respiratory tract infection and from the cerebrospinal fluid of cases of meningo-encephalitis. It is apparently non-pathogenic for laboratory animals.

## FRANCISELLA TULARENSIS

*Francisella tularensis* produces a disease known as *tularaemia* in man and certain small mammals, notably rabbits and hares.

## DESCRIPTION

When first isolated from infected tissue, *F. tularensis* is a very small, non-motile, non-sporing, capsulate, Gram-negative coccobacillus, $0.7 \times 0.2\,\mu m$. In culture it tends to be pleomorphic, and larger, bacillary, even filamentous forms are present. It stains poorly with methylene blue but carbol–fuchsin (10%) produces characteristic bipolar staining.

## Cultural characteristics

*F. tularensis* is strictly aerobic. It cannot be cultured on ordinary media but requires the addition of either egg yolk or pieces of sterile rabbit spleen. It also grows well on human blood agar containing 2.5% glucose and 0.1% cystine chloride.

## Sensitivity

It is killed by moist heat at 55°C in 10 min, but may remain viable for many years in culture maintained at 10°C, and for many days in moist soil and in water polluted by infected animals.

## PATHOGENESIS

In animals suffering from tularaemia the organisms are present in large numbers within the cells of the liver and spleen, suggesting that they multiply intracellularly.

In man, cases are mostly sporadic, although occasional outbreaks have been reported. After an acute onset with fever, rigors and headache, the disease develops manifestations that vary according to the mode of infection; thus, glandular lesions and ulcers of the skin, sometimes with involvement of the eyes, may result from direct contact with infected animals, whereas indirect contact through tick bites, inhalation of infected dust or ingestion of contaminated meat or water is more likely to lead to typhoid-like or pulmonary illness.

## LABORATORY DIAGNOSIS

Human infections are usually diagnosed by inoculating the discharge from local lesions onto a special enriched medium and identifying any small mucoid colonies characteristic of *F. tularensis*. Alternatively, the exudate may be inoculated into guinea-pigs or mice and the liver and spleen of the infected animals cultured post mortem. The patient's serum is tested for specific antibodies to *F. tularensis* by slide or tube agglutination tests. (Diagnostic antigens and antisera for use in the tests are available from Difco Laboratories.) Serum from cases of brucellosis may cross-react with *F. tularensis*.

## TREATMENT

Streptomycin or gentamicin are the antibiotics of choice in tularaemia. Tetracycline or chloramphenicol are also effective, but relapse may occur with these bacteriostatic agents.

## EPIDEMIOLOGY

Tularaemia has a world-wide distribution. Cases have been reported from North America, from several European countries including Scandinavia, and from Asia. It has not so far been identified in the UK. The infection, which is a typical zoonosis, is mainly tick-borne among the natural hosts, lagomorphs and rodents. It is transmitted to man either directly through the handling of infected animals, e.g. rabbits or hares, or indirectly through tick bites or inhalation of contaminated dust. The organism is highly infectious and laboratory workers are especially at risk through handling infected laboratory animals or cultures of the organism.

Tularaemia is sometimes water-borne as a result of pollution of water with the carcasses or excrement of infected rodents such as water rats or lemmings. Polluted water was probably the cause of the so-called *lemming fever* reported from Norway.

Man-to-man transmission of infection apparently does not occur.

RECOMMENDED READING

Adlam C, Rutter J M 1989 *Pasteurella and Pasteurellosis.* Academic Press, London

American Public Health Association 1990 Plague. In: Benenson A S (ed) *Control of Communicable Diseases in Man*, 15th edn. American Public Health Association, Washington, DC, pp 324–329

Cover T L, Aber R C 1989 *Yersinia enterocolitica. New England Journal of Medicine* 321: 16–24

Evans M E, Gregory D W, Schaffner W, McGee Z A 1965 Tularemia: a 30-year experience with 88 cases. *Medicine* 64: 251–269

Mair N S, Fox E 1986 *Yersiniosis; Laboratory Diagnosis, Clinical Features, Epidemiology.* Public Health Laboratory Service, London

Smith M D, Thanh N D 1996 Plague. In: Cook G C (ed) *Manson's Tropical Diseases*, 20th edn. W B Saunders, London, pp 918–924

# 37

# Non-sporing anaerobes
## Wound infection; periodontal disease

*J. M. Hardie and R. P. Allaker*

The significance of obligate anaerobes in general, and of non-sporing anaerobes in particular, is increasingly recognized. This heightened awareness of the important role that such organisms play, both as part of the normal microbial flora of the body and in a wide variety of infections, has come about largely through the application of greatly improved laboratory techniques for the isolation and cultivation of anaerobic bacteria, and the pioneering efforts of 'anaerobe enthusiasts' in various parts of the world.

A bewildering range of anaerobes is found in the mouth and oropharynx, gastro-intestinal tract and female genital tract of healthy individuals as part of the commensal flora. These include Gram-positive and Gram-negative cocci, rods and filaments, as well as a number of spiral forms (Table 37.1). Most infections with these organisms are of endogenous

origin, except in the case of animal and human bite wounds, where the infecting organisms, usually mixed, are derived from the mouth of the aggressor.

The flora of the lower intestinal tract, in particular, harbours vast numbers of anaerobes; quantitative studies on the bacterial flora of human faeces (Table 37.2) reveal a total content of over $10^{10}$ anaerobes per gram of faeces.

Many of the bacteria isolated from anaerobic infections are opportunistic pathogens. Such organisms are particularly likely to set up infections in damaged and necrotic tissue, when they are translocated to sites other than their normal habitat, or in a host that is compromised or debilitated in some way, leading to impairment of immunological or other defence mechanisms. Anaerobic infections of the head, neck and respiratory tract are often associated with organisms found in the mouth, while infections

**Table 37.1** Anaerobic bacteria found as part of normal flora in man[a]

|  | Skin | Mouth | Gastro-intestinal tract | Genito-urinary tract |
|---|---|---|---|---|
| **Gram-positive bacilli** | | | | |
| *Actinomyces* | − | + | + | + |
| *Bifidobacterium* | − | + | + | + |
| *Clostridium* | − | − | + | + |
| *Eubacterium* | − | + | + | + |
| *Lactobacillus* | − | + | + | + |
| *Propionibacterium* | + | + | + | + |
| **Gram-positive cocci** | | | | |
| *Coprococcus* | − | − | + | − |
| *Gaffkya* | − | − | + | + |
| *Gemmiger* | − | − | + | − |
| *Peptococcus* | + | − | + | + |
| *Peptostreptococcus* | + | + | + | + |
| *Ruminococcus* | − | − | + | − |
| *Sarcina* | − | − | + | − |
| *Streptococcus* | + | + | + | + |

**Table 37.1** (Cont'd)

| | Skin | Mouth | Gastro-intestinal tract | Genito-urinary tract |
|---|---|---|---|---|
| **Gram-negative bacilli** | | | | |
| *Anaerobiospirillum* | – | + | + | (?) |
| *Anaerorhabdus* | – | – | + | (?) |
| *Bacteroides* | – | + | + | + |
| *Bilophila* | – | – | + | + |
| *Butyrivibrio* | – | – | + | – |
| *Centipeda* | – | + | + | (?) |
| *Desulfomonas* | – | – | + | – |
| *Fusobacterium* | – | + | + | + |
| *Leptotrichia* | – | + | + | – |
| *Mitsuokella* | – | + | + | (?) |
| *Porphyromonas* | – | + | + | + |
| *Prevotella* | – | + | + | + |
| *Selenomonas* | – | + | + | – |
| *Succinimonas* | – | – | + | – |
| *Succinivibrio* | – | – | + | – |
| *Wolinella* | – | + | + | – |
| **Gram-negative cocci** | | | | |
| *Acidaminococcus* | – | – | + | + |
| *Megasphaera* | – | – | + | – |
| *Veillonella* | – | + | + | + |
| **Spirochaetes** | | | | |
| *Treponema* | – | + | + | + |
| Other spiral forms | – | + | + | + |

–, not usually found; +, commonly present; (?), presence uncertain (further data required).
[a]Data from various sources.

**Table 37.2** The bacterial flora of faeces of English subjects[a]

| Bacterial group | Mean bacterial count[b] |
|---|---|
| Gram-negative anaerobic rods | 9.8 |
| *Bifidobacterium* spp. | 9.8 |
| *Clostridium* spp. | 5.0 |
| *Veillonella* spp. | 4.2 |
| *Lactobacillus* spp. | 6.5 |
| *Bacillus* spp. | 3.7 |
| Enterobacteria | 7.9 |
| *Streptococcus* spp. | 7.1 |
| *Enterococcus* spp. | 5.8 |
| Total anaerobes | 10.1 |
| Total aerobes | 8.0 |

[a]From Hill M J et al 1971 Bacteria and aetiology of cancer of large bowel. *Lancet* i: 95.
[b]$Log_{10}$ viable organisms per gram of faeces.

in the abdominal and pelvic regions are more commonly associated with gut bacteria.

# FEATURES OF ANAEROBIC INFECTIONS

## Clinical signs

A common, but not invariable, feature is the production of a foul or putrid odour. Foul-smelling pus or discharge should always alert the clinician to the likelihood that anaerobes are present, since no other organisms produce this effect, but the absence of this sign does not necessarily exclude the involvement of anaerobic bacteria. Other clues to the clinical diagnosis are listed in Table 37.3.

## Polymicrobial flora

Infections involving non-clostridial anaerobes are

**Table 37.3** Some clinical signs and indicators of non-clostridial anaerobic infections[a]

- Presence of foul-smelling pus, discharge or lesion
- Production of a large amount of pus (abscess formation)
- Proximity of lesion to mucosal surface or portal of entry
- Failure to isolate organisms from pus ('sterile' pus)
- Infection associated with necrotic tissue
- Deep abscesses
- Gas formation in tissues
- Failure to respond to conventional antimicrobial therapy
- Pus which shows red fluorescence under ultraviolet light
- Detection of 'sulphur granules' in pus (actinomycosis)
- Infection of human or animal bite wound
- Gram-negative bacteraemia
- Septic thrombophlebitis

[a]Adapted from Willis (1983) and Finegold & George (1989).

often polymicrobial. The composition of these mixed infections varies according to the site affected. The complexity may vary from two or three species up to a dozen or more, and may include strict anaerobes, facultatively anaerobic and micro-aerophilic organisms. Such combinations frequently comprise mixtures of Gram-negative rods (such as *Bacteroides*, *Prevotella* and *Fusobacterium* species) and Gram-positive cocci (peptostreptococci or streptococci, or both). In most cases, with the occasional exception of actinomycosis, it is not possible to predict accurately which organisms are present from the clinical presentation, although the detection of red fluorescing pus under ultraviolet light usually indicates the involvement of one of the black-pigmented *Porphyromonas* species.

## LABORATORY DIAGNOSIS

When anaerobic infection is suspected, it is important that adequate clinical specimens are collected and transported as soon as possible to the bacteriology laboratory, preferably under reducing conditions. After direct microscopical examination of the material, appropriate culture media should be inoculated for incubation under good anaerobic conditions, either in an anaerobic cabinet or in anaerobic jars. In some laboratories, gas–liquid chromatography is carried out directly on pus and other clinical specimens in order to detect metabolic products, such as butyric and propionic acids, that are characteristic of certain anaerobes. Since many anaerobes are relatively slow-growing, it is essential that cultures are incubated for several days before being discarded. In mixed infections, fast-growing aerobic or facultatively anaerobic organisms are often detected within 24 h, whereas some anaerobes may require incubation for 7–10 days before their colonies can be recognized.

## NON-SPORING GRAM-NEGATIVE RODS

Gram-negative, anaerobic, non-spore-forming, non-motile rods were previously classified within three genera, *Bacteroides*, *Fusobacterium* and *Leptotrichia*, which constituted the family Bacteroidaceae. The assignment of species was based largely on the profile of metabolic end-products produced after growth in a carbohydrate- and protein hydrolysate-rich medium. Thus, *Leptotrichia buccalis* (*Leptotrichia* is a monospecific genus) produces mainly lactic acid, whereas *Fusobacterium* species produce copious amounts of butyric acid and lower levels of acetic and propionic acids. Organisms that possessed other metabolic end-product patterns were placed in the genus *Bacteroides*, which has now undergone major taxonomic revision. *Leptotrichia* and *Fusobacterium* species may exhibit heterogeneity in biochemical and chemical properties, but taxonomic alterations have hitherto been limited.

Morphologically, *Leptotrichia* and some *Fusobacterium* species tend to form long filamentous rods, often with pointed ends. Such filaments are sometimes described as *fusiform* or spindle-shaped. *Bacteroides* species are usually seen as shorter rods or coccobacilli, but may be pleomorphic.

### *Fusobacterium* spp.

Several new species of *Fusobacterium*, mainly of oral origin, have been proposed. *Fusobacterium nucleatum* now includes the subspecies *nucleatum*, *polymorphum* and *fusiforme*, and *F. necrophorum* includes the subspecies *funduliforme* and *necrophorum*.

Fusobacteria colonize the mucous membranes of humans and animals, and are generally regarded as commensals of the upper respiratory and gastro-intestinal tracts. Species such as *F. nucleatum*, *F. periodonticum*, *F. alocis*, *F. naviforme* and *F. sulci* are generally isolated from the oral cavity and are often associated with infections of this and related sites. *F. nucleatum*, the most studied species, is frequently recovered from mixed infections of the head and neck region, including dental abscesses and the central nervous system, and is also quite commonly isolated from transtracheal aspirates and pleural fluid. *F. necrophorum* is an important animal pathogen. It is associated with infections similar to those caused by *F. nucleatum* in humans but is isolated less often. *F. nucleatum* subspecies *nucleatum* is considered an important periodontal pathogen, particularly during the period when quiescent periodontitis becomes active. *F. mortiferum*, *F. necrogenes*, *F. gonidiaformans* and *F. varium* are generally isolated from the gastro-intestinal and urogenital tracts of humans and animals. These species, together with *F. nucleatum*, are often associated with mixed intra-abdominal infections, perirectal abscesses, osteomyelitis, decubitus and other ulcers and various soft tissue infections. *F. ulcerans* was originally isolated from tropical ulcers but may be found in other sites.

*Fusobacterium* species are susceptible to metronidazole and chloramphenicol. Benzylpenicillin and cefoxitin have comparable efficacy but a few resistant strains occur. Tetracycline is less effective, and erythromycin exhibits poor activity.

## Leptotrichia buccalis

This species was originally classified in the genus *Fusobacterium*, and shares a number of properties with the fusobacteria. Although normally considered to be an oral species, it also occurs outside the oral cavity, but has not been widely studied. The association of *Leptotrichia buccalis* with disease is not clear-cut, although it has been reported in acute necrotizing ulcerative gingivitis (*Vincent's gingivitis*), together with *Treponema*, *Porphyromonas* and *Fusobacterium* species. The antibiotic susceptibility pattern is similar to that of *Fusobacterium* species.

## Bacteroides spp. and related Gram-negative rods

Bacteria that used to be thought of as typical members of the genus *Bacteroides*, especially those isolated from humans, form three broad groups according to whether they are asaccharolytic, moderately saccharolytic or strongly saccharolytic (Table 37.4). The asaccharolytic, pigmented species are now classified in the genus *Porphyromonas*, which includes *Porphyromonas asaccharolytica*, *P. endodontalis* and the important periodontal pathogen *P. gingivalis*. The moderately saccharolytic species that are inhibited by 20% bile and are indigenous to the oral cavity, have been assigned to the genus *Prevotella*. The genus *Bacteroides* is now restricted to *B. fragilis* and related species that are saccharolytic and grow in 20% bile. The taxonomic position of some species, such as *B. ureolyticus* and *B. forsythus*, remains uncertain. *B. gracilis* is now considered to belong to the genus *Campylobacter*.

**Table 37.4** Current taxonomic status of clinically important species previously included in the genus *Bacteroides*

**Saccharolytic group (*B. fragilis* and related species)**

*B. fragilis*, *B. caccae*, *B. distasonis*, *B. eggerthii*, *B. merdae*, *B. ovatus*, *B. stercoris*, *B. thetaiotaomicron*, *B. uniformis*, *B. vulgatus*

**Moderately saccharolytic group (*Prevotella* spp.)**

*Prev. melaninogenica*, *Prev. bivia*, *Prev. buccae*, *Prev. buccalis*, *Prev. corporis*, *Prev. denticola*, *Prev. disiens*, *Prev. heparinolytica*, *Prev. intermedia*, *Prev. loescheii*, *Prev. oralis*, *Prev. oris*, *Prev. oulorum*, *Prev. veroralis*, *Prev. zoogleoformans*

**Asaccharolytic group (*Porphyromonas* spp.)**

*P. asaccharolytica*, *P. gingivalis*, *P. endodontalis*

**Others (uncertain taxonomic status)**

*B. ochraceus*, *B. ureolyticus*, *B. splanchnicus*, *B. forsythus*, *B. capillosus*

To add to the taxonomic complexity of the non-sporing Gram-negative rods, many other former *Bacteroides* species that are usually isolated from non-human sources have been reclassified, and several new genus names have been proposed.

## Infections with Bacteroides *and related species*

*Bacteroides* species and related Gram-negative rods are, together with anaerobic cocci, the commonest cause of non-clostridial anaerobic infections in humans. The *B. fragilis* group are particularly significant, since they are the most commonly isolated and tend to be more resistant to antimicrobial agents than most anaerobes. *B. fragilis* itself is substantially outnumbered by other *Bacteroides* species in the normal bowel microflora, but it is often associated with intra-abdominal and soft tissue infections below the waist. *B. fragilis* is also the most common anaerobe found in bacteraemia, and has even occasionally been reported from head and neck infections, despite its apparent absence from the normal flora of the mouth. Species of the *B. fragilis* group account for about a quarter of all anaerobes isolated from clinical specimens.

Black-pigmented species, including those from the genera *Porphyromonas* and *Prevotella*, occur in abscesses and soft tissue infections in various parts of the body. They are rarely isolated in pure culture. *P. gingivalis* is associated with advanced periodontitis and *P. endodontalis* with dental root canal (endodontic) infections.

*Bacteroides*, *Porphyromonas* and *Prevotella* species are usually sensitive to metronidazole, chloramphenicol, clindamycin and cefoxitin. Resistance to penicillin is common, particularly among the *B. fragilis* group; it is associated with β-lactamase production, and these organisms are usually susceptible to combinations of β-lactam agents with β-lactamase inhibitors (see Ch. 5).

## GRAM-POSITIVE ANAEROBIC COCCI

Classification and nomenclature of strictly anaerobic Gram-positive cocci (as opposed to facultatively anaerobic, micro-aerophilic or carbon dioxide-dependent cocci, which may also be isolated on primary anaerobic culture plates) are still in need of clarification. Consequently, it is not always easy to identify clinical isolates precisely, and they are often described simply as 'anaerobic cocci'.

Most species known to be clinically significant are regarded as belonging to the genus *Peptostreptococcus* (Table 37.5). Distinguishing between *Peptostreptococcus* species depends upon a variety of physiological and biochemical tests, including the analysis of metabolic end-products by gas–liquid chromatography. Many species do not ferment carbohydrate substrates, so that some commonly used identification tests are of little value.

Gram-positive anaerobic cocci comprise part of the normal microbial flora of the mouth, gastro-intestinal tract, genito-urinary tract and skin. They are often isolated from clinical specimens. Other genera, including *Coprococcus*, *Gaffkya*, *Gemmiger*,

**Table 37.5** Currently recognized species of Gram-positive anaerobic cocci

*Peptococcus niger*
*Peptostreptococcus anaerobius*
*Peptostr. asaccharolyticus*
*Peptostr. heliotrinreducens*
*Peptostr. hydrogenalis*
*Peptostr. indolicus*
*Peptostr. lacrimalis*
*Peptostr. lactolyticus*
*Peptostr. magnus*
*Peptostr. micros*
*Peptostr. prevotii*
*Peptostr. productus*
*Peptostr. tetradius*
*Peptostr. vaginalis*

**Table 37.6** Types of infection and clinical specimens from which anaerobic Gram-positive cocci are isolated

- Blood cultures
- Central nervous system (including brain abscesses)
- Head and neck infections (including ear)
- Dental abscesses and infected root canals
- Periodontal diseases
- Human and animal bites
- Pleural infections
- Abdominal infections
- Genito-urinary tract infections
- Decubitus ulcers
- Foot ulcers
- Osteomyelitis

*Ruminococcus* and *Sarcina*, are found as part of the flora of the bowel (see Table 37.1), but are not usually considered to be significant in infections.

## Infections with anaerobic cocci

Anaerobic cocci are isolated from infections in various parts of the body, particularly from abscesses (Table 37.6). They are often found in association with other anaerobes, facultatively anaerobic or aerobic organisms. As with all mixed infections, it is difficult to assess the contribution of each individual organism to the pathogenic process. However, there is sufficient evidence from both clinical and experimental studies to confirm the pathogenic potential of the anaerobic cocci.

## GRAM-NEGATIVE ANAEROBIC COCCI

Among genera recorded as part of the normal flora of the gastro-intestinal tract (see Table 37.1) only *Veillonella* is found regularly at other sites. In the mouth, for example, this genus is a regular component of supragingival dental plaque and of the tongue microflora. Veillonellae are able to use some of the lactic acid produced by bacteria such as streptococci and lactobacilli that potentially induce caries.

The role of *Veillonella* species and other anaerobic Gram-negative cocci in disease, if any, has not been clearly established, although they may be isolated from a variety of clinical conditions. In general, they are regarded as a minor component of mixed anaerobic infections.

## NON-SPORING GRAM-POSITIVE RODS

The spore-forming genus *Clostridium* is well-known

**Table 37.7** Some characteristics of non-sporing Gram-positive rods

| Genus | Sites commonly found | Acid end-products |
|---|---|---|
| Propionibacterium | Skin, mouth, gut, vagina | Propionic acid |
| Bifidobacterium | Gut, mouth, vagina | Acetic and lactic acids |
| Lactobacillus | Mouth, gut, vagina | Lactic acid (major end-product) |
| Actinomyces | Mouth, gut, vagina | Succinic, lactic and acetic acids |
| Eubacterium | Mouth, gut, vagina | Butyric and other acids |

for its involvement in serious infections (see Ch. 23). The role of non-sporing Gram-positive rods, on the other hand, is less well understood, although they are present in significant numbers in the normal flora of the mouth, skin, gastro-intestinal and female genito-urinary tracts, and are isolated from a variety of types of infections. The main genera and some of their characteristics are listed in Table 37.7. As with some other groups of anaerobes, the use of acid end-product analysis by gas–liquid chromatography is an important step in the identification of these bacteria.

## Infections with Gram-positive rods

Any of these bacteria can occur as components of mixed anaerobic infections, and *Actinomyces* species can undoubtedly adopt a pathogenic role. Most cases of actinomycosis are caused by *Actinomyces israelii* and are cervicofacial, although the disease can also occur in the thorax, abdomen and female genital tract (see Ch. 21). *Actinomyces* species are not themselves strict anaerobes, but *A. israelii* requires good anaerobic conditions for primary isolation, and plates should be incubated for 7–10 days.

*Propionibacterium propionicum* is morphologically and biochemically very similar to *A. israelii*. It is particularly associated with infection of the lachrymal canal in the condition called *lachrymal canaliculitis*. The significance of other genera in infections is not clear. Some species are found in acne; they are also occasionally isolated in infective endocarditis, and in infections associated with implanted prostheses. *Eubacterium* species (possibly mistaken for *Actinomyces* species in some reports) may play a role in infections around intra-uterine devices; others may be

involved in human periodontal disease, but further studies are required to confirm these observations. Similarly, there is only limited evidence for the pathogenicity of *Bifidobacterium* species, although *Bif. dentium* has been isolated occasionally from pulmonary infections.

## SPIRAL-SHAPED, MOTILE ORGANISMS

Several *Treponema* species are found in the mouth and elsewhere in the body (see Table 37.1). They are thought to be an important component of the mixed anaerobic infection associated with acute necrotizing ulcerative gingivitis along with fusobacteria and *Prev. intermedia*, and may also contribute to other forms of periodontal disease. The proportion of motile spiral organisms seen by dark-ground microscopy in samples from the gingival pocket increases markedly when there is evidence of periodontal destruction.

Motile, spiral-shaped Gram-negative anaerobes of the genus *Anaerobiospirillum* have been isolated from patients with diarrhoea and from bacteraemia. Although comparatively rarely isolated from humans, they can cause serious infections. The distribution and normal habitat of this and other morphologically similar organisms are not well understood. In some cases the source of infection may be domestic animals and pets.

## TREATMENT

In many infections caused by anaerobes the most important aspect of treatment is surgical. This often involves drainage of pus from abscesses, but may also include debridement, curettage and removal of necrotic tissue. For minor infections surgical drainage alone may be sufficient, but in many cases anti-microbial chemotherapy is also indicated. The main groups of agents used are the penicillins and the nitroimidazoles, particularly metronidazole.

Metronidazole is effective against virtually all obligate anaerobes, but not against facultatively anaerobic or micro-aerophilic bacteria such as actinomyces and streptococci. Many anaerobic species are sensitive to penicillin, but resistance due to β-lactamase production is very common within the *B. fragilis* group.

## RECOMMENDED READING

Duerden B I, Drasar B S (eds) 1991 *Anaerobes in Human Disease*. Edward Arnold, London

Finegold S M, George W L (eds) 1989 *Anaerobic Infections in Humans*. Academic Press, San Diego

Hentges D J 1989 Anaerobes as normal flora. In: Finegold S M, George W L (eds) *Anaerobic Infections in Humans*. Academic Press, San Diego, pp 37–53

Johnson C C, Finegold S M 1987 Uncommonly encountered, motile, anaerobic gram-negative bacilli associated with Infection. *Reviews of Infectious Disease* 9: 1150–1162

Shah H N, Gharbia S E 1993 Ecophysiology and taxonomy of Bacteroides and related taxa. *Clinical Infectious Diseases* 16: 160–167

Skinner F A, Carr J G (eds) 1974 *The Normal Microbial Flora of Man*. Academic Press, London

Willis A T 1983 *Anaerobic Infections*. Update Publications, London

# 38

# Treponema and borrelia

## Syphilis; yaws; relapsing fever; Lyme disease

*A. Cockayne*

---

Members of the genera *Treponema* and *Borrelia* are spirochaetes belonging to the family Spirochaetaceae.

## DESCRIPTION

Spirochaetes are slender unicellular helical or spiral rods (Fig. 38.1) with a number of distinctive ultra-

**Fig. 38.1**  Electron micrograph of *T. pallidum*. The flagella (▼) are inserted at the tip and follow the helical contour of the bacterial cell enclosed within the outer membrane. Bar, 0.1 μm. (Photograph courtesy of Dr C. W. Penn.)

structural features used in the differentiation of the genera (Fig. 38.2). The cytoplasm is surrounded by a cytoplasmic membrane and a peptidoglycan layer contributes to cell rigidity and shape. In *Treponema* species, fine cytoplasmic filaments are visible in the bacterial cytoplasm (Fig. 38.3), but these are absent in *Borrelia* species. Members of both genera are actively motile, and several flagella are attached at each pole of the cell and wrap around the bacterial cell body. In contrast to other motile bacteria, these flagella do not protrude into the surrounding medium but are enclosed within the bacterial outer membrane. Treponemal flagella are complex, comprising a sheath and core (Fig. 38.4), whereas those of *Borrelia* species are simpler and similar to those of other bacteria. The spirochaetal outer membrane is unusually lipid-rich and at least in some treponemes appears to be protein-deficient and to lack lipopolysaccharide. This may account for the susceptibility of these organisms to killing by detergents and desiccation.

Although the treponemes are distantly related to Gram-negative bacteria they do not stain by Gram's method, and modified staining procedures are used. Moreover, the pathogenic treponemes cannot be cultivated in laboratory media and are maintained by subculture in susceptible animals. In contrast, borreliae stain Gram-negative, and many pathogenic species can be cultured in vitro in enriched, serum-containing media.

### Importance as human pathogens

Human diseases caused by *Treponema* and *Borrelia* species (Table 38.1) include those such as syphilis that have been known for thousands of years, and infections such as Lyme disease the prevalence and geographical distribution of which are still being evaluated.

Treponemal infections may be spread from person to person by intimate physical contact, contact with infectious body fluids or, in some instances, by

347

**Fig. 38.2** Schematic representation of the structure of *T. pallidum* in longitudinal and cross-section: C, postulated capsular layer; OM, outer membrane; F, flagellum; CW, cell wall peptidoglycan; CM, cytoplasmic membrane; CF, cytoplasmic filaments (absent in borreliae). Areas of uncertainty, indicated by question marks, concern the existence and form of the capsule, the continuity or otherwise of the outer membrane over the tip of the organism, the nature and form of the tip structure, and the exact juxtaposition of the ends of the cytoplasmic filaments with the bacterial flagellar basal bodies. (After Strugnell et al 1990 *Critical Reviews in Microbiology* 17: 231–250.)

**Fig. 38.3** Electron micrograph of a detergent- and protease-treated *T. pallidum* cell showing cytoplasmic filaments (▼) in the bacterial cytoplasm. Bar, 0.1 μm.

**Fig. 38.4** Electron micrograph of a detergent-treated *T. pallidum* cell showing the complex structure of the treponemal flagellum. Both sheathed (S) flagella and the thinner flagellar cores (C) are visible. Bar, 0.1 μm.

**Table 38.1** Principal human diseases caused by spirochaetes

| Organism | Disease | Distribution | Primary mode of transmission | Animal reservoirs |
|---|---|---|---|---|
| *T. pallidum* | Syphilis | World-wide | Sexual–congenital | None |
| *T. endemicum* | Bejel | Arid, subtropical or temperate areas | Mouth-to-mouth via utensils | None |
| *T. carateum* | Pinta | Arid, tropical Americas | Skin-to-skin contact | None |
| *B. recurrentis* | Epidemic relapsing fever | Central, East Africa; South American Andes | Louse bites | None |
| *Borrelia* spp. | Endemic relapsing fever | World-wide[a] | Tick bites | Yes |
| *B. burgdorferi* sensu lato | Lyme disease | World-wide[a] | Tick bites | Yes |

[a]Distribution governed by presence of tick vectors.

fomites. The treponemes infecting humans are obligate human parasites, and no other natural hosts are known. In contrast, borreliae are transmitted to humans by the bites of infected ticks or lice. The borreliae that cause Lyme disease and endemic relapsing fever also infect many other animal species which act as reservoirs of infection, and humans are an unfortunate incidental host in the natural history of these pathogens.

Characteristically, treponemal and borrelial infections occur in several distinct clinical stages. These may be separated by periods of remission, and each stage may have a particular associated pathology. Commonly the causative organism is detectable in early lesions but is much more difficult to identify in later disease. The pathogen spreads from the initial site of infection to many organs via the bloodstream, and in some untreated cases these infections may be progressive, destructive and, in some instances (e.g. tertiary syphilis), may be fatal. In other cases, however, only the early symptoms are apparent and the later pathology is not seen.

With the exception of the relapsing fevers, in which antigenic variation contributes to bacterial virulence, the pathogenic mechanisms employed by spirochaetes are poorly understood. No extracellular toxins have yet been identified, and the mechanisms that enable these organisms to persist in tissues despite vigorous immune responses remain unclear. It seems likely, however, that the later manifestations of these infections may involve auto-immune phenomena.

In addition to the pathogenic species, many other spirochaetes form part of the normal bacterial flora of the mouth, gut and genital tract. Morphological and antigenic similarities between pathogenic and commensal spirochaetes may cause problems in the clinical and serological diagnosis.

## TREPONEMA

*Treponema* species pathogenic for humans include the causative agents of venereal syphilis, and the non-venereal treponematoses *yaws*, *bejel* and *pinta*. The spirochaetes causing these different infections are micro-aerobic, morphologically identical – tightly coiled helical rods, 5–15 μm long and 0.1–0.5 μm diameter – and show only subtle antigenic differences. Differentiation of these organisms is based primarily on the clinical syndromes they cause and minor differences in the pathology induced in experimental animals.

## *Treponema pallidum* ssp. *pallidum* (*T. pallidum*)

*Treponema pallidum* is the causative agent of syphilis, and was first isolated from syphilitic lesions in 1905. Infection is usually acquired by sexual contact with infected individuals, and is commonest in the most sexually active age group of 15–30 year olds. *Congenital syphilis* usually occurs following vertical transmission of *T. pallidum* from the infected mother to the fetus in utero, but neonates may also be infected during passage through the infected birth canal at delivery. Infection in utero may have serious consequences for the fetus. Rarely, syphilis has been acquired by transfusion of infected fresh human blood.

### Pathogenesis

Untreated syphilis may be a progressive disease with *primary*, *secondary*, *latent* and *tertiary* stages. *T. pallidum* enters tissues by penetration of intact mucosae or through abraded skin. The bacterium rapidly enters the lymphatics, is widely disseminated via the bloodstream and may lodge in any organ. The exact infectious dose for humans is not known, but in experimental animals less than 10 organisms are sufficient to initiate infection. The bacteria multiply at the initial entry site, and a *chancre*, a lesion characteristic of primary syphilis, forms after an average incubation period of 3 weeks. The chancre is painless and most frequently on the external genitalia, but it may occur on the cervix, perianal area, in the mouth or anal canal. Chancres usually occur singly, but in immunocompromised individuals, such as those infected with the human immunodeficiency virus (HIV), multiple or persistent chancres may develop.

The chancre usually heals spontaneously within 3–6 weeks, and 2–12 weeks later the symptoms of secondary syphilis develop. These are highly variable and widespread but most commonly involve the skin where macular or pustular lesions develop, particularly on the trunk and extremities. The lesions of secondary syphilis are highly infectious.

These lesions gradually resolve, and a period of latent infection in which no clinical manifestations are evident but serological evidence of infection persists is entered. Relapse of the lesions of secondary syphilis is common, and latent syphilis is classified as early (high likelihood of relapse) or late (recurrence unlikely). Individuals with late latent syphilis are not generally considered infectious but may still transmit infection to the fetus during pregnancy and their blood may remain infectious.

Late or tertiary syphilis, which may develop decades after the primary infection, is a slowly progressive, destructive inflammatory disease that may affect any organ. The three most common forms of late syphilis are *neurosyphilis*, *cardiovascular syphilis* and *gummatous syphilis* – a rare granulomatous lesion of the skeleton, skin or mucocutaneous tissues. Isolation of *T. pallidum* from patients with late syphilis is usually impossible, and much of the observed pathology may be due to auto-immune phenomena.

## Treponema pallidum ssp. pertenue (*T. pertenue*)

*T. pertenue* is the causative agent of *yaws*, a disease that is endemic among rural populations in tropical and subtropical countries such as Africa, South America, South-East Asia and Oceania. The number of cases of yaws world-wide was estimated at over 50 million in the 1950s, but eradication programmes sponsored by the World Health Organization reduced the number of cases to less than 2 million in the 1970s. Termination of these programmes has led to a resurgence of pockets of disease, particularly in West Africa.

Infection with *T. pertenue* is non-venereal, and occurs following contact of traumatized skin with exudate from early yaws lesions. Infection is usually acquired before puberty. Primary yaws has an incubation period of 3–5 weeks, and the initial lesions usually occur on the legs. The papular lesions enlarge, erode and usually heal spontaneously within 6 months. Eruption of similar lesions occurs weeks to months later, and relapse is common. Secondary lesions may involve bones, particularly the fingers, long bones and the jaw. Late yaws is characterized by cutaneous plaques and ulcers and thickening of the skin on the palms and soles of the feet. Gummatous lesions may also develop. In contrast to syphilis, neurological and cardiovascular damage does not occur in late yaws. As affected individuals acquire infection early in life, they are essentially non-infectious at child-bearing age, and congenital yaws is unknown.

## Treponema pallidum ssp. endemicum (*T. endemicum*)

This organism causes a non-venereal, syphilis-like disease called *endemic syphilis* or *bejel*. Bejel is endemic in Africa, western Asia and Australia, and mainly affects children in rural populations where living conditions and personal hygiene are poor. Transmission is by direct person-to-person contact and by sharing of contaminated eating or drinking utensils.

The initial lesion is usually oral and may not be detected. Secondary lesions include oropharyngeal mucous patches, condyloma lata and periostitis. Late lesions involve gummata in the skin, nasopharynx and bones. As in yaws, the cardiovascular and central nervous systems are not involved, and congenital infection is rare because of the early age of infection.

## Treponema carateum

Unlike the other treponematoses, the manifestations of *pinta*, caused by *T. carateum*, are confined to the skin. Although these lesions are non-destructive, they do cause disfigurement with associated social problems for infected individuals. Pinta is probably the oldest human treponemal infection, whose distribution today is restricted to arid rural inland regions of Mexico, Central America and Colombia.

Spread of infection is by direct contact with infectious lesions. After a 7–21 day incubation period, small, erythematous pruritic primary lesions develop, most commonly on the extremities, face, neck, chest or abdomen. The primary lesions enlarge and coalesce, and once healed may leave areas of hypopigmentation. Disseminated secondary lesions appear 3–12 months later and may become dyschromic. Recurrence of lesions is common up to 10 years after the initial infection. The depigmented lesions are characteristic of the later stages of pinta but do not cause any serious harm.

## Other infections

There are several other human infections in which treponemes are implicated. Commonly, the microbial flora associated with these conditions is complex, and the exact role of the spirochaetes in the aetiology of infection remains to be determined. Moreover, the true taxonomic status of some of these organisms is uncertain.

### Oral infections

*T. denticola*, *T. socranskii* and *T. pectinovorum* form part of the normal flora, and numbers of these organisms increase in acute necrotizing ulcerative gingivitis and chronic adult periodontal disease. *T. vincentii* (or Vincent's spirillum) is similarly associated with ulceromembranous gingivitis or pharyngitis, *Vincent's angina*. Several spirochaetes appear to be involved in the aetiology of a similar condition called *trench mouth*.

## Gastro-intestinal infections

Several as yet unidentified weakly haemolytic spirochaetes have been implicated in the aetiology of persistent diarrhoea and rectal bleeding in certain human populations. A morphologically similar but genetically distinct organism, *Serpulina hyodysenteriae*, is the cause of swine dysentery.

## Skin lesions

*Tropical ulcer* is a chronic skin condition in which spirochaetes of unknown identity have been implicated, usually in association with fusiform bacteria and other organisms.

# LABORATORY DIAGNOSIS

The inability to grow most pathogenic treponemes in vitro, coupled with the transitory nature of many of the lesions, makes diagnosis of treponemal infection impossible by routine bacteriological methods. Although spirochaetes are detectable by microscopy in primary and secondary lesions, diagnosis is based primarily on clinical observations and is confirmed by serological tests. For practical purposes, the serological responses to all these pathogens are identical, and only their use in the serodiagnosis of syphilis will be considered here.

## Direct microscopy

Treponemes can be visualized directly in freshly collected exudate from primary or secondary lesions by dark-ground or phase-contrast microscopy. Although this method allows a rapid definitive diagnosis to be made, it may be rather insensitive because primary lesions may contain relatively few bacteria. In addition, care must be taken to differentiate between pathogenic and commensal spirochaetes that may occasionally contaminate such material. More sensitive and specific results may be obtained using fixed material in an immunofluorescence assay with an anti-treponemal antibody.

## Serological tests

Infection with *T. pallidum* results in the rapid production of two types of antibodies:

1. Specific antibodies directed primarily at polypeptide antigens of the bacterium
2. Non-specific antibodies that react with a non-treponemal antigen called *cardiolipin*.

The mechanism of induction of non-specific antibodies remains unclear. Cardiolipin is a phospholipid extracted from beef heart, and it is possible that a similar substance, present in the treponemal cell or released from host cells damaged by the bacterium, may stimulate antibody production.

Assays for non-specific antibody, because of their low cost and technical simplicity, are routinely used as screening tests for evidence of syphilis infection. Since these tests have relatively low specificity, positive results are confirmed by detection of specific anti-*T. pallidum* antibody.

## Non-specific serological tests for syphilis

The *Venereal Disease Reference Laboratory* (VDRL) test is a non-specific serological test for syphilis which uses a mixture of cardiolipin, cholesterol and lecithin as antigen. IgM or IgG antibody present in positive sera or in cerebrospinal fluid from patients with neurosyphilis causes a suspension of this lipoidal antigen to flocculate, and the result can be rapidly read by eye. This is used as a screening test, and is positive in approximately 70% of primary and 99% of secondary syphilitics, but is negative in individuals with late syphilis. This test can be used quantitatively, and increases in VDRL titre with time may be used to confirm a diagnosis of congenital syphilis.

Since a positive result in the VDRL test usually indicates active infection, it can also be used to monitor the efficacy of antibacterial therapy.

## Tests for specific antibody

*Fluorescent treponemal antibody (FTA-Abs) test.* The FTA-Abs test is an indirect immunofluorescence assay in which *T. pallidum* is used as an antigen. Acetone-fixed treponemes are incubated with heat-treated sera, and bound antibody is detected with a fluorescein-labelled conjugate and ultraviolet microscopy. The serum is first absorbed with a suspension of a non-pathogenic treponeme which removes non-specific cross-reactive antibodies that may be directed against commensal spirochaetes. The FTA-Abs is positive in approximately 80, 100 and 95% of primary, secondary and late syphilitics, respectively, and, unlike the VDRL test, remains positive following successful therapy.

*T. pallidum* **haemagglutination assay (TPHA)**. In this test, *T. pallidum* antigen is coated onto the surface of red blood cells, and specific antibody in test sera causes haemagglutination. As in the FTA-Abs assay, sera are pre-absorbed with a non-pathogenic treponeme to remove antibody against commensal spirochaetes. The TPHA is less sensitive than the FTA-Abs in primary syphilis (positive in 65%), but both give similar results for secondary and late syphilis; the TPHA also remains positive for life following infection. This assay can also be used to detect localized production of anti-treponemal antibodies in cerebrospinal fluid, a marker of neurosyphilis.

*Other antibody tests.* Production of monoclonal anti-*T. pallidum* antibodies has permitted development of assay systems based on the detection of antibody responses to individual treponemal antigens. Such assays use enzyme-linked immunosorbent assay (ELISA) technology, allowing rapid screening of large numbers of samples with potentially enhanced specificity. Assays which detect either IgM or IgG are available.

### Problems in the serological diagnosis of syphilis

Occasionally, both the non-specific and specific tests produce false-positive results. The VDRL assay may give a transient positive result following any strong immunological stimulus such as acute bacterial or viral infection or after immunization. More persistent false-positive results occur in individuals with auto-immune or connective tissue disease, in drug abusers and in individuals with hypergammaglobulinaemia. False-positive results usually become apparent when negative results are found in specific serological tests, but in some cases FTA-Abs results may also be positive or borderline.

Rarely, the FTA-Abs test, may be positive and the non-specific VDRL test negative. Other spirochaetal diseases such as relapsing fever, yaws, pinta and leptospirosis may give positive results in both specific and non-specific tests. Of particular difficulty is the differential diagnosis of syphilis and yaws in immigrants from areas in which yaws is endemic.

Lyme disease (see below) induces antibodies that react in the FTA-Abs but not in the VDRL assay.

Direct detection of spirochaetal DNA in clinical material by molecular methods, such as the polymerase chain reaction, may have a future role in confirming a diagnosis of syphilis in difficult or atypical cases.

## TREATMENT

All the pathogenic treponemes are sensitive to benzylpenicillin, and prolonged high-dose therapy with procaine penicillin has been the traditional method of treatment for primary and secondary syphilis. So far there have been no reports of penicillin resistance. If penicillin allergy is a problem, erythromycin, tetracycline or chloramphenicol may be used. There are reports of treatment failure with erythromycin, and an erythromycin-resistant variant of *T. pallidum* has been isolated. In late syphilis, aqueous benzylpenicillin is used, as this penetrates better into the central nervous system. In neurosyphilis, successful eradication of the organism may not result in a clinical cure. More aggressive and prolonged antibiotic therapy may be required in HIV patients with syphilis due to impairment of immune function.

Antibiotic therapy of syphilitics, particularly with penicillin, characteristically induces a systemic response called the *Jarisch–Herxheimer reaction*. This is characterized by the rapid onset (within 2 h) of fever, chills, myalgia, tachycardia, hyperventilation, vasodilation and hypotension. This response is thought to be due to release of an endogenous pyrogen from the spirochaetes.

## EPIDEMIOLOGY AND CONTROL

### Syphilis

The incidence of all venereal diseases, including syphilis, increased dramatically during the Second World War. The widespread introduction of antibiotic therapy shortly afterwards produced an equally dramatic decrease in the incidence of these diseases, but syphilis remained endemic within the general population. Until the mid-1980s most cases of syphilis in developed countries occurred in male homosexuals. The advent of HIV and the acquired immune deficiency syndrome (AIDS) in the 1980s reduced the incidence among this group due to changes in sexual practices. More recently, there has been a resurgence of syphilis among the heterosexual population in the USA, resulting in an increase in the incidence among women and in the number of cases of congenital syphilis. There were 81 000 cases of syphilis in the USA in 1994, of which over 2000 were congenital. Several possibilities may have accounted for this increase, including:

1. Changes in health care policies and abolition of screening of pregnant women in some states
2. Increased promiscuity associated with drug abuse
3. Changes in antibiotic prescribing for other sexually transmitted diseases which previously resolved many inapparent infections with *T. pallidum*.

Although the incidence of all forms of syphilis in the UK is currently very low (fewer than 500 cases reported per year), this disease still has major implications in relation to public health. In particular, the possibility of congenital infection and the acquisition of syphilis by blood transfusion necessitates large and costly screening programmes of all pregnant women and blood donations.

Control of syphilis is achieved by treating index cases and any known contacts. Treatment of contacts is important as some may be incubating the infection even if they have no overt signs of disease.

## Other treponematoses

The incidence of the other treponematoses is primarily influenced by socio-economic factors. Prevention and control involve treatment of individuals with active or latent disease and contacts, and improvement of living conditions and personal hygiene

## BORRELIA

The two principal human diseases associated with borreliae are *relapsing fever*, caused by *Borrelia recurrentis* and several other *Borrelia* species; and *Lyme disease* or *Lyme borreliosis*, a multisystem infection caused by *B. burgdorferi*.The bacteria causing these infections are morphologically similar helical rods, 8–30 μm long and 0.2–0.5 μm in diameter, with 3–10 loose spirals. Antigenic and genetic differences are used to differentiate the species.

## RELAPSING FEVERS

Relapsing fevers occur virtually world-wide in endemic or epidemic forms. Both are transmitted to humans by arthropod vectors. They are characterized clinically by recurrent periods of fever and spirochaetaemia.

*Endemic* or *tick-borne relapsing fever* is caused by several *Borrelia* species, including *B. duttoni*, *B. hermsii*, *B. parkeri* and *B. turicatae*, and is transmitted to humans by soft-bodied *Ornithodorus* ticks. The natural hosts for these organisms include rodents and other small mammals on which the ticks normally feed. The disease occurs world-wide, reflecting the distribution of the tick vector. In contrast, *B. recurrentis*, the sole cause of *epidemic* or *louse-borne relapsing fever*, is an obligate human pathogen, transmitted from person to person by the body louse, *Pediculus humanus*.

The incidence of epidemic relapsing fever is influenced by socio-economic factors such as lack of personal hygiene, and, historically, increases during periods of social upheaval such as wars and famines. This disease still occurs in central and eastern Africa and in the South American Andes.

The spirochaetes causing the two forms of relapsing fever differ in their mode of growth in the arthropod vector, and this influences the way infection is initiated in humans. *B. recurrentis* grows in the haemolymph of the louse but does not invade tissues. As a result the excrement of the louse is non-infectious and the bacterium is not transferred transovarially to the progeny. Infection occurs in humans when such lice are crushed, releasing the bacteria which then gain entry to tissues through damaged or intact skin or mucous membranes. Spirochaetes causing tick-borne relapsing fever invade all the tissues of the tick, including the salivary glands, genitalia and excretory system. Infection therefore occurs when saliva or excrement is released during feeding. Transovarial transmission to the tick progeny maintains the spirochaete in the tick population.

## Pathogenesis of relapsing fever

In both forms of relapsing fever, acute symptoms, including high fever, rigors, headache, myalgia, arthralgia, photophobia and cough, develop about 1 week after infection. A skin rash may occur, and there is central nervous system involvement in up to 30% of cases. During the acute phase there may be up to $10^5$ spirochaetes per cubic millimetre of blood. The primary illness resolves within 3–6 days, and terminates abruptly with hypotension and shock, which may be fatal. Relapse of fever occurs 7–10 days later, and several relapses may take place. Each episode of spirochaetaemia is terminated as the result of development of specific anti-spirochaete antibody. Subsequent febrile episodes are caused by borreliae that differ antigenically, particularly in outer-membrane protein composition, from those causing earlier attacks. As the cycle of fever and relapse continues, the borreliae tend to revert back to the antigenic types that caused the original spirochaetaemia, and ultimate clearance of the infection appears to be due to antibody-mediated killing.

In general, louse-borne relapsing fever has longer febrile and afebrile periods than tick-borne infection, but fewer relapses. The case fatality rate varies from 4 to 40% for louse-borne infection and from 2 to 5% for tick-borne relapsing fever, with myocarditis, cerebral haemorrhage and liver failure the most common causes of death.

## Laboratory diagnosis

Definitive diagnosis of relapsing fevers is made by detection of borreliae in peripheral blood samples. Thick or thin blood smears may be stained with Giemsa, or other stains such as acridine orange.

Although antibodies to the borreliae are produced during infections, antigenic variation and the tendency to relapse complicates serological tests for these infections, and such tests are not widely available. Serological tests for syphilis are positive in 5–10% of cases.

## Treatment

Tetracycline, chloramphenicol, penicillin and erythromycin have been used successfully. As in the treatment of syphilis, a Jarisch–Herxheimer reaction is produced following administration of antibiotics.

Prevention of these infections involves avoidance or eradication of the insect vector. Insecticides can be used to eradicate ticks from human dwellings, but elimination from the environment is not feasible. Prevention of louse-borne infection involves maintenance of good personal hygiene, and delousing if necessary.

## LYME DISEASE

Lyme disease or Lyme borreliosis, originally called *Lyme arthritis*, was recognized as an infectious condition in 1975, following an epidemiological investigation of a cluster of cases of suspected juvenile rheumatoid arthritis which occurred in Lyme, Connecticut, USA. A common factor in these cases was a previous history of insect bite, and the infectious agent, *B. burgdorferi*, was subsequently isolated from an *Ixodes* tick. Retrospective serological data suggest that Lyme disease was endemic in the USA as early as 1962, and the clinical manifestations of this infection have been known in Europe, including the UK, since the early 1900s. Lyme disease has also been reported in Scandinavia, eastern Europe, China, Japan and Australia.

The natural hosts for *B. burgdorferi* are wild and domesticated animals, including mice and other rodents, deer, sheep, cattle, horses and dogs. The larger animal hosts such as deer are probably more important in maintaining the size of tick populations rather than acting as a major source of *B. burgdorferi*. Infection in these animals may be inapparent, though clinical infection has been observed in cattle, horses and dogs.

*B. burgdorferi* is transmitted to humans by ixodid ticks that become infected while feeding on infected animals. The principal vectors in the USA are *Ixodes dammini* and *I. pacificus*, and in Europe, *I. ricinus*. The life cycle of these ticks involves larval, nymph and adult stages, all of which are capable of transmitting infection, though the nymphal stage is most commonly implicated. In areas endemic for Lyme disease, 2–50% of ticks may carry *B. burgdorferi*. The bacterium grows primarily in the midgut of the tick, and transmission to humans occurs during regurgitation of the gut contents during the blood meal. Transmission efficiency appears to be relatively low, but increases with the duration of feeding.

Lyme disease may be a progressive illness, and is divided into three stages. Although there is general similarity, clinical manifestations may differ in the USA and Europe. This variation has now been shown to be due in part to significant differences in the bacterial strains causing infection in these two continents, and has resulted in the division of *B. burgdorferi* into three distinct genospecies. Although also isolated in Europe, *B. burgdorferi* sensu stricto is the principal organism isolated in the USA where Lyme arthritis is a common complication of infection. In contrast, *B. afzeli* and *B. garinii* are commonly isolated in Europe but not in the USA, and are associated with chronic skin and neurological symptoms of Lyme disease respectively. Several other genetically distinct isolates of *B. burgdorferi* have also been identified in ticks, but their importance in human infection has yet to be established.

*Stage 1* Lyme disease is characterized by a spreading annular rash, *erythema chronicum migrans* (ECM), which occurs at the site of the tick bite 3–22 days after infection. The bacterium also disseminates to a variety of other organs. In the USA, secondary lesions similar to those of ECM are common. Malaise, fatigue, headache, rigors and neck stiffness may also be apparent. ECM and secondary lesions fade within 3–4 weeks and, weeks to months later, some patients develop cardiac or neurological abnormalities, musculoskeletal symptoms or intermittent arthritis, which are characteristic of *stage 2* Lyme disease. Patients with *stage 3* disease, which may occur months to years later, present with chronic skin, nervous system or joint abnormalities.

Congenital infection may occur with serious, potentially fatal consequences for the fetus.

## Laboratory diagnosis

Once a clinical diagnosis has been made, culture of the spirochaete from suitable biopsy material provides a definitive diagnosis, but this is a lengthy, specialized technique that is not widely available. In addition, the difficulty encountered in detecting the organism in histological sections means that serological tests are routinely used for the confirmation of Lyme disease although polymerase chain reaction (PCR) techniques have been been used in some laboratories.

Specific IgM antibodies develop within 3–6 weeks of infection. The earliest response appears to be against the bacterial flagellum and later against outer-surface proteins. Subsequently, IgG antibodies are produced, and the highest titre is detectable months or years after infection.

An indirect immunofluorescence test is available, but ELISA is now widely used. Immunoblotting has been proposed as a method of confirming serological diagnosis. Serological diagnosis of early Lyme disease may still pose problems, as in some individuals antibodies to the bacterium are slow to develop and formation of immune complexes may affect the test results. Antibodies that cross-react with *B. burgdorferi* may be produced after infection with other spirochaetes, and sera from Lyme disease patients may give a positive FTA-Abs test, though the VDRL test is negative.

Serological evidence of infection may also be detectable in the absence of overt disease in apparently normal individuals. The significance of these findings is not yet clear but the possibility that such individuals may develop late complications of Lyme disease merits consideration.

## Treatment

Penicillins, the newer macrolides, cephalosporins and tetracyclines have all been used successfully in Lyme disease. Reports suggest that treatment with tetracyclines produces fewer late complications than penicillin therapy. About 15% of patients experience a Jarisch–Herxheimer reaction after antibiotic therapy. Despite antibiotic treatment, some patients suffer from minor late complications of the disease, which may be immunologically mediated or may indicate low-level persistence of the organisms. An additional complication of antibiotic therapy is the reduction or abolition of the antibody response, which may interfere with the serological confirmation of infection.

## Epidemiology and control

The geographical distribution of Lyme disease is governed by that of the tick vector and its associated animal hosts. Consequently, infection occurs primarily in individuals who frequent these areas. Forestry workers and farmers are particularly at risk, but infection is also associated with recreational activities. In the UK, Lyme disease occurs in areas that support large populations of wild or domesticated animals on which ixodid ticks feed. Infection may also be acquired after travel to countries where Lyme disease is endemic. It is difficult to assess accurately the true incidence of Lyme disease in the UK since infection may be mild or asymptomatic and consequently not detected. In 1993, 44 cases were reported in England compared with over 13 000 in the USA.

Prevention of infection involves avoidance of Lyme disease-endemic areas and education of the public regarding the possible risks of infection in these localities. Eradication of the tick vectors or mammalian hosts from such areas is not feasible.

RECOMMENDED READING

Barbour A G 1990 Antigenic variation of a relapsing fever *Borrelia* species. *Annual Review of Microbiology* 44: 155–171
Barbour A G, Hayes S F 1986 Biology of *Borrelia* species. *Microbiological Reviews* 50: 381–400
Guy E C 1993 The laboratory diagnosis of Lyme borreliosis. *Reviews in Medical Microbiology* 4: 89–96
Holt S C 1978 Anatomy and chemistry of spirochetes. *Microbiological Reviews* 42: 114–160
Hudson M J 1991 The spirochaetes. In: Duerden B I, Drasar B S (eds) *Anaerobes in Human Disease*. Edward Arnold, London, pp 108–132
Larsen S A, Steiner B M, Rudolph A H 1995 Laboratory diagnosis and interpretation of tests for syphilis. *Clinical Microbiology Reviews* 8: 1–21
O'Connell, S 1995 Lyme disease in the United Kingdom. *British Medical Journal* 310: 303–308
Schell R F, Musher D M (eds) 1983 *Pathogenesis and Immunology of Treponemal infections*. Marcel Decker, New York
Steere A G 1989 Lyme disease. *New England Journal of Medicine* 321: 586–596
Szczepanski A, Benach J L 1991 Lyme borreliosis: host responses to *Borrelia burgdorferi*. *Microbiological Reviews* 55: 21–34

# 39

# Leptospira

**Leptospirosis; Weil's disease**

*J. D. Coghlan*

---

Spirochaetes of the genus *Leptospira* are characterized by their slender appearance, numerous coils, hooked ends and active motility. Many different types exist; some are harmless to humans and animals, while others are potential pathogens. The parasitic leptospires are normally carried in the kidneys of rodents and other small mammals and are excreted in the urine. In some parts of the world, wading birds, snakes, frogs and tortoises are infected, although they probably play only a minor role as carrier hosts. The organisms appear to cause no harm to their normal hosts, but if they are transmitted accidentally to other animal species or to humans they may give rise to clinical infections. The disease may be relatively mild or extremely severe. In humans the most virulent types may cause spirochaetal jaundice, known as *Weil's disease* after the German physician who described the syndrome in 1886. In cattle, pigs, sheep, goats and horses, infection may give rise to abortions or stillbirth in pregnant animals and mastitis in lactating cattle. Dogs suffer two forms of leptospirosis, one characterized by an acute and often fatal jaundice, the other a subacute or chronic nephritis, depending on the type of leptospire responsible.

## DESCRIPTION

### Classification

The genus *Leptospira* consists of two species, *Leptospira interrogans* and *L. biflexa*. The former includes the parasitic strains while the latter comprises the free-living saprophytic strains found in fresh water and occasionally in salt or brackish water.

The two species are indistinguishable morphologically but *L. biflexa* strains can grow in simple media without the addition of animal protein, which is normally essential for the growth of parasitic leptospires. Saprophytic strains can also grow at a temperature of 13°C and in the presence of the purine analogue, 8-azaguanine, both of which are inhibitory to strains of *L. interrogans*. The two species may also be differentiated by their DNA composition.

Within the two species serological tests have revealed many antigens, some of which are common to all leptospires, whereas others are restricted to certain strains. On the basis of these more specific antigens, many different serological types, designated *serovars*, have been identified. The serovar is the basic taxon of *Leptospira*. Because of common antigens, certain serovars have, for convenience, been collected into serogroups. Within *L. interrogans*, 23 serogroups are now recognized, comprising over 170 serovars that have been isolated from humans and animals.

## Morphology

Leptospires are spiral bacteria, 6–20 μm long and 0.1 μm broad. They usually appear straight and rigid with one or both ends hooked, although unhooked forms are sometimes seen. The primary coils are so numerous and so closely set together that they are difficult to see in the living state except by dark-ground microscopy (Fig. 39.1). They are so thin that they are capable of passing through a membrane filter with a pore size of 0.22 μm.

Electron microscopy reveals a helicoidal protoplasmic cylinder surrounded by a cell wall consisting of a cytoplasmic–peptidoglycan complex, the whole being enclosed in an outer envelope of at least three layers (Fig. 39.2). Between the cytoplasmic membrane and the outer envelope two flagella-like axial filaments are entwined around the organism, each attached subterminally, one at either end of the cell, to a basal body. The free ends of the axial filaments are directed towards the centre of the leptospire.

**Fig. 39.1** The appearance of living leptospires as seen by dark-ground microscopy. Note the very fine coils and characteristic hooked ends. (From an original painting by Dr Cranston Low, in Low & Dodds 1947 *Atlas of Bacteriology*. Livingstone, Edinburgh.)

## Movement

In a liquid medium, leptospires rotate rapidly along their long axes and also glide across the field with either end foremost, occasionally forming secondary coils and then straightening again into the rigid form that is so characteristic of the group.

## Staining

Leptospires stain poorly with the usual bacterial stains but they can be demonstrated by the silver impregnation techniques of Levaditi and Fontana and by fluorescent antibody techniques.

## Cultural characteristics

Leptospires are obligate aerobes. The optimum growth temperature is 28–32°C, but for primary isolation from infected tissues incubation at 37°C may be advantageous. They grow best in a fluid medium of pH 7.2. Growth is slow, especially in primary culture, and may not be obvious until 2 or 3 weeks after inoculation.

*L. interrogans* strains require the addition of animal protein in the form of serum, or a fraction of bovine serum albumin (fraction V) with polysorbate (Tween 80), to supply the fatty acids that are their main source of energy. This medium, first devised by Ellinghausen and McCullough, is used in a modified form known as EMJH medium for culturing the strains that are used in serological diagnostic tests and for typing newly isolated strains.

A semisolid medium prepared by adding 0.2–0.5% agar to a liquid medium is used for isolating leptospires from animal tissues.

## Sensitivity

Leptospires are killed at a temperature of 50°C in 10 min and at 60°C in 10 s. They are susceptible to desiccation, to hypochlorite disinfectants and to pH

**Fig. 39.2**  Part of an intact leptospire, showing the protoplasmic cylinder, cell wall, outer envelope and axial filaments (transmission electron micrograph).

values outside the range 6.2–8.0. They are especially sensitive to acid urine, non-aerated sewage and polluted water. Unlike saprophytic strains, they do not survive for long in salt or brackish water.

Pathogenic leptospires may survive for several days outside the animal body in moist conditions at a pH of not less than 6.8. They survive for a time in animal tissues kept at low temperature; thus, serovar *canicola* has been isolated from pigs' kidneys on sale in a butcher's shop.

## PATHOGENESIS

The pathogenic leptospires enter the body through cuts or abrasions of the skin or through the mucous membranes of the nose, mouth or eyes. They multiply in the blood and circulate to all parts of the body, affecting any organ, so that the signs and symptoms that characterize the disease vary considerably in their form and intensity. A mild influenza-like illness may develop, sometimes with meningitis and usually with some degree of renal involvement, indicated by albuminuria. *Canicola fever* is an example of this type of 'benign' leptospirosis. At the other extreme the disease may be severe and even fatal, characterized by jaundice and haemorrhages in the eyes, skin and mucous membranes. Any of the pathogenic serovars may cause benign leptospirosis, but the severe form, Weil's disease, is usually due to serovar *icterohaemorrhagiae*. In some parts of the world, other serovars, e.g. *andamana*, *australis*, *bataviae* and *pyrogenes*, may also cause spirochaetal jaundice.

## LABORATORY DIAGNOSIS

Leptospirosis should always be considered as a possible cause of feverish illness, with or without jaundice, in patients whose work, recreation or living conditions are likely to expose them to infection from animal sources.

## Examination of blood

After an incubation period of 5–12 days there is a phase of leptospiraemia that lasts for about a week, during which time live leptospires may be seen by dark-ground microscopy of the patient's blood. Care must be taken not to identify as leptospires the protoplasmic extrusions from red cells that are normally present in blood films and which may undulate, due to Brownian movement, in such a way that they resemble spirochaetes.

To confirm the diagnosis, leptospires are cultured from the blood by inoculation of a liquid medium, or by peritoneal inoculation of the blood into laboratory animals, followed some days later by culture of the animal blood obtained by cardiac puncture.

## Examination of urine

Leptospires may be present in the urine during the 2nd week of illness and continue to be excreted intermittently for 4–6 weeks.

They may be seen by dark-ground microscopy in the deposit of centrifuged urine and may be cultured directly from the sediment in a semisolid medium containing neomycin sulphate to control contaminants, or after animal inoculation. Because leptospires are very sensitive to acid urine, the urine should be examined immediately after being voided.

## Identification of infecting strains

To identify the serovar of strains isolated from blood or urine, use is made of agglutination and agglutinin absorption techniques that have been developed for the purpose. The results are compared with those obtained in parallel tests against reference strains of various serovars and their antisera prepared in rabbits. This is a specialized technique that is best carried out in one of the Leptospira Reference Laboratories recognized by the World Health Organization, to which all new isolates should be sent for identification.

## Serological examinations

Specific antibodies are detectable in the patient's serum towards the end of the 1st week of illness; they continue to rise for several weeks, and then begin to decline. Residual agglutinating antibody may persist for many years. Serum should be examined during the early days of the illness and at 4–5 day intervals thereafter in order to detect the rise in antibody titre that is diagnostic of current infection.

Some serological tests are genus-specific, others are serogroup- (or serovar-) specific.

## Genus-specific tests

These have the advantage of being able, in a single test, to detect, in human serum, antibodies resulting from leptospiral infection, whatever the serovar responsible. A complement fixation test with a genus-specific antigen prepared from a strain known as Patoc 1 of the saprophytic species *L. biflexa* has been widely used. Since complement-fixing antibodies of immunoglobulin class IgM decrease more rapidly than agglutinating IgG antibodies, the test is only suitable for diagnosing current infection, not for survey work.

Other genus-specific tests include haemagglutination and haemolysis of sheep or human red cells treated with erythrocyte-sensitizing substance extracted from the strain Patoc 1, and the slide agglutination test of Mazzonelli and Mailloux. In this simple test, a drop of the patient's serum is mixed with a drop of a dense suspension of a heat-killed culture of strain Patoc 1. Agglutination is clearly visible to the naked eye.

An enzyme-linked immunosorbent assay (ELISA) which is capable of detecting specific IgM and IgG leptospiral antibodies is useful for indicating the stage of the infection.

## Serogroup-specific test

The microscopic agglutination test (MAT) has been widely used for many years to diagnose leptospirosis and to indicate the likely serogroup (and sometimes the serovar) of the infecting strain. A series of dilutions of the patient's serum is tested against a battery of reference strains of different serovars representing all serogroups to which the infecting strain might belong. The reactions are read by low-power dark-ground microscopy. In the early stages of infection the antibodies may cross-react with strains of different serogroups, but subsequent tests usually result in the highest titres being obtained against the specific serogroup and against the serovar that is most likely to be that of the infecting strain.

## TREATMENT

Leptospirosis usually responds to treatment with antibiotics, provided they are administered in large enough doses early in the infection. Benzylpenicillin should be administered intravenously for up to 7 days in a daily dose of 6–8 mega-units (3.6–4.8 g). Penicillin may cause a temporary exacerbation of the symptoms (the *Jarisch–Herxheimer reaction*) but this should not prevent continuation of treatment. Patients allergic to penicillin may be treated with streptomycin, tetracycline or erythromycin.

When there is impairment of kidney function, as sometimes happens in Weil's disease, it may be necessary to resort to renal dialysis to counteract the uraemia which is the main cause of death. Tetracyclines should not be used if there is evidence of renal failure.

## EPIDEMIOLOGY

Leptospirosis is a zoonosis, and humans are unnatural or 'end' hosts and do not transmit the infection further. Each leptospiral serovar appears to have its own particular animal host of election, usually a rodent, although some domestic animals, e.g. dogs, cattle and pigs, may also act as natural reservoirs of infection. Most reservoir hosts remain healthy carriers. Serovar *icterohaemorrhagiae* is normally carried by the brown rat, *Rattus norvegicus*, and serovar *hebdomadis*, first reported as the cause of seven-day fever of field workers in Japan, is carried by the field mouse, *Microtus montebelloi*. However, serovar *canicola*, which causes canicola fever in humans, is carried by dogs, and serovar *hardjo* by cattle; no rodent hosts have been found for these two serovars.

Leptospires are exceptional among pathogenic micro-organisms in being dependent on transmission in the host's urine. They localize in the kidneys, colonizing the convoluted tubules and are periodically washed out in the urine, thereby contaminating the environment. Cattle, pigs and horses become infected through grazing in fields or on fodder contaminated by infected urine. The infection may spread within the herd, again by means of the urine, resulting in herd epizootics. Humans become infected mainly through contact with water, soil or vegetation contaminated by animal urine.

Workers in certain occupations are particularly at risk: farmers, miners working in damp, rat-infested coal mines, sewer workers and fish handlers are all particularly liable to infection by serovar *icterohaemorrhagiae* because the conditions under which they work encourage rat infestation, and the moist conditions allow the leptospires excreted in the rat urine to survive for a considerable time outside the animal body. Agricultural workers are especially at risk in countries where it is customary for them to go bare footed in the fields, as in the rice fields or sugar plantations of tropical countries. The leptospires readily penetrate the skin through cuts and abrasions of the feet and legs.

In the UK, as in other countries where serovar *hardjo* infects cattle, dairy farmers are liable to become infected through inhaling droplets of infected urine during milking.

## CONTROL

Agricultural workers should protect their skin by wearing suitable gloves and boots when digging ditches, harvesting, cleaning out pig pens, cow sheds, kennels, etc. Buildings that house animals or act as work places should be rat-proofed and the floors and work benches kept in a good state of repair and cleanliness. They should be regularly washed down with sodium hypochlorite solution so that any leptospires will be killed.

Persons who seek recreation through water sports, such as bathing, paddling, wind surfing, canoeing or fishing in ponds, canals or rivers that may be fouled by rats or other animals, should be warned of the risk of infection. They should be encouraged to wear protective clothing and to cover any cuts or abrasions of the skin.

In parts of the world where the risk of infection is high among certain groups, e.g. rice field and sugar cane workers, vaccination against local leptospiral strains is being carried out successfully.

In the UK and some other countries, the incidence of human infection by serovars *icterohaemorrhagiae* and *canicola* derived from infected dogs has been reduced by the widespread vaccination of dogs against these two serovars.

RECOMMENDED READING

Alston J M, Broom J C 1958 *Leptospirosis in Man and Animals*. Livingstone, Edinburgh

Faine S (ed) 1982 *Guidelines for the Control of Leptospirosis*. WHO Offset Publication, No 67 World Health Organization, Geneva

Gsell O 1990 The changing epidemiology of leptospirosis in Europe. *International Journal of Medical Microbiology* 273: 412–427

Kmety E, Dikken H 1993 *Classification of the Species* Leptospira interrogans *and History of its Serovars*. University Press, Groningen

# 40

# Chlamydia

**Genital infections; trachoma; psittacosis; pneumonia**

*I. W. Smith*

Chlamydiae are small Gram-negative bacteria which are obligate intracellular parasites like viruses, but differ from them in that they have both RNA and DNA, ribosomes, a cell wall, and divide by binary fission. However, they differ from most true bacteria in that they have no peptidoglycan in their cell wall and lack the ability to produce their own adenosine triphosphate (ATP). They require to use the host ATP – hence the term *energy parasites*. The genus *Chlamydia* is the only one in the family Chlamydiaceae and the order Chlamydiales.

There are four species agreed by an international committee: *Chlamydia trachomatis*, *C. psittaci*, *C. pneumoniae* and *C. pecorum*. *C. trachomatis* can be divided into three biovars:

1. Those causing trachoma and inclusion conjunctivitis (TRIC)
2. Those causing lymphogranuloma venereum (LGV)
3. The one causing mouse pneumonitis (MoPn) (a similar organism has recently been isolated from swine).

Both the trachoma and LGV biovars which infect humans can be subdivided into serovars: the trachoma biovar has 14 (A–K) and the LGV biovar at least three (L1, L2 and L3). Classic trachoma is caused by serovars A, Ba, B and C while inclusion conjunctivitis and genital infections are due to serovars D–K. *C. psittaci* will infect both mammalian and avian species, but some that infect mammals have been reclassified as *C. pecorum*. *C. pneumoniae* can infect humans and animals – the human strains showing variation. On the basis of serology, a link has been suggested between *C. pneumoniae* and coronary heart disease, atherosclerosis and sarcoidosis. Recent demonstration of the organism in atheromatous plaques is circumstantial evidence that *C. pneumoniae* may be influencing the disease although its etiological role is not yet proven.

## DESCRIPTION

### Morphology

Chlamydiae are small non-motile bacteria, 300–350 nm in size, which stain poorly with Gram's stain. They can, however, be demonstrated in preparations stained by Giemsa or other methods. These particles represent the extracellular, infectious, metabolically inert form of chlamydiae known as the *elementary body* (EB). Once the organism infects its host cell it increases in size to 800–1000 nm. This non-infectious but metabolically active particle is known as the *reticulate body* (RB) (Fig. 40.1).

Chlamydiae may also be demonstrated by immunofluorescence when a specific antibody tagged with fluorescein isothiocyanate is applied to smears made from clinical material, e.g. from the cervix or urethra or from infected tissue culture material. The EBs appear as discrete bright apple-green particles, and intracellular inclusions may also be visualized in the ultraviolet microscope. By this technique it is possible to confirm chlamydial infection within 30 min of receiving a specimen.

The four species can be differentiated on the basis of:

1. Growth
2. Nucleic acid profile
3. Presence of plasmids
4. The antigens they express
5. Inclusions in host cells which are morphologically different.

*C. trachomatis* produces a glycogen matrix in its inclusion which stains brown with iodine and has proved useful in diagnostic work.

### Elementary bodies

Chlamydial EBs are 300–350 nm in diameter with very little periplasmic space. Initially, *C. pneumoniae*

**Fig. 40.1** Electron micrograph of a thin section of chlamydial inclusion: ⬉, small elementary body (EB); ⬉, 'reticulate' body (RB). ×15 000. (By courtesy of Dr Douglas R. Anderson, Miami.)

was reported to have a large periplasmic space, giving the EBs a pear-shaped appearance (310–400 nm), but this appears to be strain-dependent.

### Reticulate bodies

The RB of all species is larger and circular in shape (800–1000 nm). As RBs are metabolically active their internal structure will reflect the stage of replication. Early in the cycle many ribosomes are seen. Later the DNA is reorganized into cores for the progeny EB. Glycogen production in the RBs of *C. trachomatis* is detected in the electron microscope about 18 h post-inoculation, and the inclusions are apparent at about 22 h. No glycogen production has been observed with the other three species.

No peptidoglycan is demonstrable between the cytoplasmic membrane and cell wall, as is seen in Gram-negative bacteria.

### Nucleic acid

The molecular weight of the nucleic acid content of

chlamydiae has been estimated to be $660 \times 10^6$. The four species can be separated on the basis of homology as the intraspecies homology does not exceed 19%. Plasmid DNA is also found in most strains of *C. trachomatis*, *C. psittaci* and *C. pecorum*, but the ovine strains of *C. psittaci* and human *C. pneumoniae* do not appear to have plasmids.

### Protein

A small number of proteins are thought to be important to the understanding of antigenicity, pathogenesis and for possible vaccine production.

There are four outer-membrane proteins, of which the major one has species-specific epitopes. These outer-membrane proteins are rich in cysteine, and it is thought that the rigidity of chlamydial EBs is due to disulphide bonding between cysteine residues of these proteins.

Chlamydiae have a heat shock protein, antibody to which cross-reacts with similar-sized proteins from unrelated micro-organisms and host cells, making the interpretation of serological responses to chlamydial infections difficult.

### Lipopolysaccharide

Genus-specific chlamydial antigen may be obtained by the methods used for extraction of lipopolysaccharide (LPS) from Gram-negative bacteria. This material has three epitopic sites, only one of which is specific for chlamydiae. The LPS contains 2-keto-3-deoxyoctonic acid (KDO) and lipid A. These epitopes cross-react with mutants of *Escherichia coli*, *Proteus mirabilis* and *Salmonella typhimurium* and with LPS derived from *Acinetobacter* species. As the LPS is the antigen used in both the complement fixation test and in certain of the enzyme-linked immunosorbent assay (ELISA) detection tests, care must be taken in the interpretation of results.

## LABORATORY PROPAGATION

In the 1930s, Bedson, while studying the replication of the psittacosis strain in mice, was able to elucidate the growth cycle and establish that the organism divided by binary fission. In 1957, *C. trachomatis* was isolated in the yolk sac of embryonated hens' eggs. The presence of the organism in the moribund eggs was confirmed by staining. Although this method is not now widely used for isolation it is used to produce antigen, especially for the micro-immunofluorescence test. Tissue culture isolation was first successful in 1965. For growth of chlamydiae, cell cultures have to be modified to allow productive interaction of the organism and its host cell. This is done by centrifuging the organism onto the cells and inhibiting the host cell by irradiation or by addition of 5-iodo-2'-deoxyuridine or cycloheximide to the medium. Giemsa stain will detect all types of chlamydiae, and iodine can be used to detect the glycogen containing inclusions of *C. trachomatis*. Immunofluorescence with appropriate antisera can detect either genus-specific or species-specific antigens. The different species of chlamydiae have slightly different requirements for growth, but *C. pneumoniae* is the most difficult to cultivate in both eggs and cell culture.

## GROWTH CYCLE

Initially the organism must attach to the host cell. Specific binding proteins have been sought, and a heparin sulphate-like ligand on the surface of the EBs may be a candidate. Not all species of chlamydiae interact easily with their host cells. *C. psittaci* and the LGV biovar attach and saturate the host cell surface but *C. trachomatis* and *C. pneumoniae* are unlikely to do so. This appears to be due in part to the net negative charge of the organism and host cells, causing repulsion at a distance. To overcome this, the addition of a polycation, such as DEAE dextran, increases the adsorption of *C. trachomatis*, while centrifuging *C. trachomatis* or *C. pneumoniae* with their host cells allows hydrophilic bonds to be formed and increases the attachment of both species. These interactions, though successful in vitro, probably do not reflect the situation in vivo.

Once the chlamydiae and host cell have come into contact, the organism enters the cell within a vesicle (Fig. 40.2). Viable chlamydiae entering the host cell cytoplasm inhibit fusion with lysosomal vesicles and so escape degradation.

In the vesicles the EB loses its dense DNA core. The cell wall becomes less rigid due to breaking of the disulphide bonds; the particle increases in size

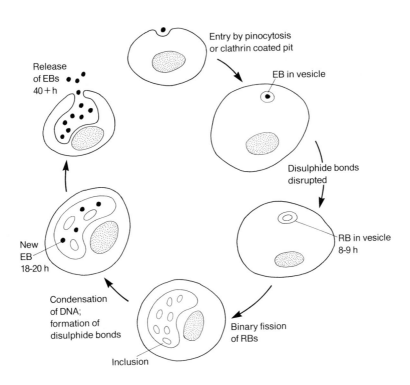

EB = elementary body; RB = reticulate body

**Fig. 40.2** The chlamydia growth cycle.

and becomes an RB. The RBs have no cytochrome and lack the ability to produce ATP, which must be supplied by the host. In the vesicle the RB divides by binary fission to yield pleomorphic organisms. At 18–20 h the DNA condenses, disulphide bonds are formed in the outer-membrane proteins and new EBs are generated within the endosomal vesicle. The release of EBs follows autolysis of the host cell, but whether release is the cause or the effect of autolysis is uncertain.

The need of chlamydiae for specific amino acids may lead to an inhibition of growth which can be reversed on the addition of the essential amino acid. This obviously gives the opportunity for latency since an amino acid-starved infection may lie dormant for a period but reappear on the addition of the essential building block.

## IMMUNOLOGICAL RESPONSE AND PATHOGENESIS

Infections with chlamydiae give rise to both humoral and cell-mediated immune responses, which play varying roles in the recovery from infection, resistance to reinfection and immunopathological sequelae. Human infections cannot be studied easily experimentally, and although animal models have been developed for human infections the reactions may not be typical of those in humans. However, two natural infections, guinea-pig inclusion conjunctivitis (GPIC) and mouse pneumonitis have been exploited. Recovery is delayed if the guinea-pigs are immunosuppressed with either cyclophosphamide or anti-lymphocytic serum, indicating that both humoral and the cell-mediated immune responses are required in recovery from GPIC.

### Initial host response

In human infections, chlamydiae have a predilection for either squamous epithelial cells or for the macrophages of the lung or gastro-intestinal tract. Such infections invoke an inflammatory response with infiltration of neutrophils during the acute stage. The intracellular destruction of chlamydiae by the neutrophils occurs in cells with oxygen-dependent or oxygen-independent enzyme systems. Subsequently, monocytes and lymphocytes appear in the infiltrate. Chlamydiae do not replicate in monocytes but when these cells become macrophages both *C. psittaci* and the LGV biovar can escape the phagolysosomal fusion and produce high

titres of organisms. *C. trachomatis* can also replicate in macrophages but to a lesser extent. It has been suggested that the infected macrophages may be a vehicle for the spread of the chlamydiae within the host.

### Antibody response

Antibody production follows the normal sequence of IgM then IgG, the level of antibody production being dose-dependent. Serum IgA is produced and secretory IgA (S-IgA) is found in the mucosal fluids. The higher the level of S-IgA, the less successful is the isolation of chlamydiae from a genital site. The development of IgM and IgG antibody to *C. pneumoniae* is delayed 6–8 weeks compared with 2–3 weeks following genital infection – a factor which must be considered when using serology for diagnosis.

The importance of mucosal antibody (or rather the lack of it) is seen in neonates who have maternal IgG. Of those infected with *C. trachomatis* in the birth canal, a proportion develop conjunctivitis, despite maternal IgG. If the infection is not appropriately treated, a proportion of these babies develop pneumonitis at 4–12 weeks of age. This is when the maternal antibody is waning and neonates are beginning to produce their own IgM and IgG. The presence of IgM antibody or a rising IgG titre is taken as evidence of chlamydial infection of the respiratory tract of neonates.

Although specific antibody can neutralize chlamydiae in vitro, there is little protection against reinfection of the ocular and genital mucous membranes in patients with circulating IgG antibody. In second or subsequent infections there is a very swift infiltration of neutrophils and lymphocytes. The plasma cells produce antibody, making it difficult to recover the organism. This lack of protection has implications for attempts to produce a successful vaccine.

### Cellular response

Antibody is not the only factor to be considered in reinfection. The cell-mediated response also plays a part which may or may not be of advantage to the host. Whole live chlamydiae, heat-killed organism or even LPS can stimulate the production of lymphokines such as γ-interferon and interleukin-1.

In trachoma, the acute infection results in an inflammatory response with infiltration of neutrophils and lymphocytes. These lymphocytes may clump together and produce a follicle. The centre of the follicle is composed of B cells and macrophages surrounded by T cells, and all are enclosed in a thin layer of epithelial cells. These epithelial cells are sloughed off as the follicle becomes necrotic, and regeneration of fibrotic tissue stimulated by interleukin-1 leads to scarring. With reinfection or restimulation with chlamydial antigen the inflammatory response is quicker, leading to more follicle formation and scarring.

A similar situation pertains in the genital tract where ascending infection can lead to salpingitis. This results in an inflammatory response with infiltration of neutrophils and lymphocytes, deciliation of the epithelium and destruction of the epithelial cells near to the lymphocytes. Repeated infection causes severe tubal damage with follicle formation, more damage to the epithelium and scarring, leading to the obstruction of the fimbriated end of the fallopian tube. Such damage can result in infertility due to interruption of ovum transport and to chronic pelvic inflammatory disease.

## INFECTION OF HUMANS

Table 40.1 summarizes the chlamydial infections of the eye, genital and respiratory tracts.

### Ocular infection

*Trachoma* has been known for thousands of years, and during the 19th century was still found in Europe. The improvement in hygiene led to a decrease in the incidence of the disease in industrially developed countries, but it is still found in countries where standards of sanitation and hygiene are poor and flies abound. *C. trachomatis* A, B, Ba and C are the usual causal agents, and in endemic areas children are often infected before their second birthday. Blindness due to this cause is still a problem in the 'trachoma belt', which stretches from North Africa to South-East Asia. Reinfection and secondary infections play a part in the progression to blindness, which may take 25–30 years. To compare the progress of the disease in different areas a grading scheme was produced for the World Health Organization. Five selected key signs were recorded to illustrate the progression of the disease:

1. Medium trachomatis inflammation in the conjunctiva with follicular inflammation
2. Intense inflammation with diffuse thickening of the conjunctiva
3. Scarring of tarsal conjunctiva
4. Inturned eyelashes
5. Corneal opacity.

The disease is spread by eye-seeking flies, or fingers, from one patient to another (Table 40.2). The children also shed the organism from the respiratory and gastro-intestinal tract, thus constituting another mode of spread.

*Adult inclusion conjunctivitis* (paratrachoma) is caused by serotypes D–K. It is most prevalent in sexually active young people and is spread from genitalia to eye. In the acute stage it presents as follicular conjunctivitis, which, if not treated, persists, together with a mucopurulent discharge. Although

| **Table 40.1** Human chlamydial infections | | |
|---|---|---|
| Site of infection | Disease | Organism (serovars) |
| Eye | Trachoma | *C. trachomatis* (A, B, Ba, C) |
| | Inclusion conjunctivitis | *C. trachomatis* (D–K) |
| | Ophthalmia neonatorum | *C. trachomatis* (D–K) |
| Genital tract | | |
| Male | Urethritis, epididymitis, proctitis | *C. trachomatis* (D–K) |
| Female | Urethritis, cervicitis, proctitis, salpingitis perihepatitis, peri-appendicitis, infertility | *C. trachomatis* (D–K) |
| | Abortion, stillbirth | *C. psittaci* (ovine strains) |
| Male and female | Lymphogranuloma venereum | *C. trachomatis* (L1–L3) |
| Respiratory tract | Pneumonitis of infants | *C. trachomatis* (D–K) |
| | Pharyngitis, pneumonia | *C. pneumoniae* |
| | Psittacosis | *C. psittaci* (avian strains) |
| | Pneumonia | *C. psittaci* (ovine strains) |

**Table 40.2** Modes of spread of chlamydial infections

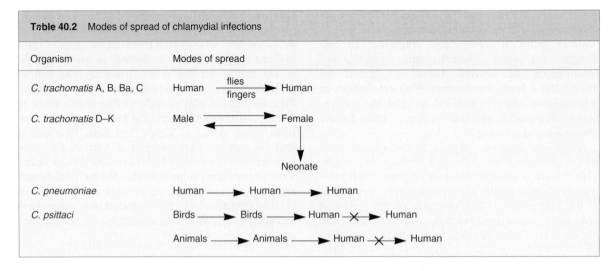

some patients develop scarring, corneal lesions or pannus formation, the disease is usually self-limiting and is not thought to lead to blindness.

*Chlamydial ophthalmia neonatorum* (inclusion blennorrhoea) develops in infants 5–21 days after birth. Follicles are not usually seen but the disease presents as a swelling of the eyelids, hyperaemia and a purulent infiltration of the conjunctiva. If untreated, the disease can linger up to 1 year, and secondary bacterial infection may cause ocular damage and even blindness. A proportion of these untreated neonates develop pneumonia. The source of infection is the infected genital tract of the mother, and the child is infected during passage through the birth canal (Table 40.2).

## Genital infection

### Males

*C. trachomatis* serovars D–K are the commonest cause of non-gonococcal urethritis in males, accounting for at least 30% of cases (Table 40.3).

Varying amounts of mucopurulent discharge are produced in symptomatic patients and, although the condition is usually localized, some may progress to epididymitis, especially in those aged under 35 years. The effect on fertility is not known although acute epididymitis may result in a transient subfertility. *C. trachomatis* may also be isolated from males who do not have clinical signs or symptoms. Unless such patients are identified by laboratory screening they will form an untreated pool of infection.

Members of this group of chlamydia have also been isolated from the rectum of homosexual males and are associated with some cases of proctitis. Rectal pain, rectal bleeding, mucopurulent discharge and diarrhoea have all been described with chlamydial proctitis.

### Lymphogranuloma venereum

*C. trachomatis* serovars L1–L3 can cause LGV in both males and females, with the majority of reported cases in males. It is found in the tropics and subtropics, though isolated cases are imported else-

**Table 40.3** Frequency of isolation of *C. trachomatis* from the genital tract

| Heterosexual males | | Females | |
|---|---|---|---|
| Primary diagnosis | Range (%) | Primary diagnosis | Range (%) |
| Non-specific urethritis | 30–58 | Contacts of chlamydia-positive males | 45–67 |
| Gonorrhoea | 26–35 | Contacts of chlamydia-negative males | 4–18 |
| Asymptomatic | 3–7 | Gonorrhoea | 27–63 |
| | | Attending genito-urinary clinic | 12–30 |
| | | Attending other clinics | 1–19 |
| | | Requesting termination of pregnancy | 10–23 |

where. The disease begins with a genital ulcer followed by lymphadenopathy of the regional lymph nodes. Buboes are seen in men and, should the infection persist, it can spread to the gastro-intestinal and genito-urinary tract, causing strictures and, in some cases, penoscrotal elephantiasis.

## Females

In females, *C. trachomatis* D–K can cause muco-purulent cervicitis and urethritis. It has also been associated with a proportion of cases of vaginitis and vaginal discharge. Many apparently asymptomatic females harbour the organism in their cervix. If untreated, such patients are not only a risk to their sexual partners or offspring (Table 40.2) but also to themselves, as ascending infection can occur. This results in endometritis and salpingitis, which singly or together may be referred to as *pelvic inflammatory disease*. Tubal damage from such infections can result in ectopic pregnancy and infertility. Peri-appendicitis and perihepatitis (*Fitz-Hugh–Curtis syndrome*) may follow salpingitis.

## Infection in pregnancy

There have been a few reported cases in the UK of *C. psittaci* infection in pregnancy leading to mis-carriage or intra-uterine death. The patients developed a febrile prodrome a few days to 2 weeks after contact with sheep. One infant delivered vaginally yielded *C. psittaci* from the liver, lungs and heart. The organism seems to have a predilection for the placenta, causing placentitis. The confirmed infections were all in patients who had been in contact with sheep, so women should be counselled to avoid contact with sheep during pregnancy. Also, as two cases of abortion have occurred at 14 weeks, there is a potential hazard to nursing or medical staff when dealing with unsuspected cases due to the heavy load of organisms in the placenta.

C. trachomatis has also been isolated from abortion products, but its role in abortion, stillbirth, pre-mature birth and premature rupture of membranes is uncertain. A number of patients who yielded *C. trachomatis* from abortion products have sub-sequently developed salpingitis and possible infertility. Similarly, a proportion of patients seeking therapeutic abortion have been shown to harbour the organism pre-evacuation, and these are also at risk of more serious infection. Thus, all such patients should be screened and, if necessary, treated before and during surgical manipulation.

## Respiratory infections

### Chlamydia pneumoniae

*C. pneumoniae* causes pneumonia, pharyngitis, bronchitis, otitis and sinusitis with an incubation period of about 21 days. *C. pneumoniae* was the third or fourth most common cause of pneumonia following *Streptococcus pneumoniae* and *Haemophilus influenzae*. Patients who had been treated initially with penicillin or ampicillin had a recurrence of their pneumonia 3 weeks to 3 months later. Radiological evidence showed that a different part of the lung was affected at the second episode. These patients developed a high IgG response but no IgM response, so the pneumonia was thought to be due to either reactivation or reinfection. Thus, *C. pneumoniae* not only causes acute respiratory infections, it also gives rise to recurrences. Serological surveys have shown that there is a 40–50% prevalence in a number of countries. The antibody to *C. pneumoniae* does not decline with age, in contrast to the find-ings with *C. trachomatis* infections of the genital tract.

### Chlamydia psittaci

*Psittacosis (ornithosis)* in man is caused by infection with avian strains of *C. psittaci*. The incubation period is about 10 days, and the illness ranges from an 'influenza-like' syndrome, with general malaise, fever, anorexia, rigors, sore throat, headache and photophobia, to a severe illness, with typhoidal state, delirium and pneumonia with numerous well-demarcated areas of consolidation; these may resemble bronchopneumonia, but the bronchioles and larger bronchi are involved as a secondary event and sputum is scanty. Although the pneumonic form of the illness may focus clinical attention, the organism is blood-borne through the body, and there may be meningo-encephalitis, arthritis, pericarditis or myocarditis, or a predominantly typhoidal state with enlarged liver and spleen, and even a rash resembling that of enteric fever. Subacute endocarditis resembling that complicating Q fever has also been described. The ovine strain of *C. psittaci* has caused respiratory infection of shepherds.

### Chlamydia trachomatis

A proportion of neonates develop pneumonitis due to *C. trachomatis* acquired during birth from the mother's infected genital tract.

**Table 40.4**  Examples of the range of diseases caused by *C. psittaci* in natural hosts

| Host | Conjunctivitis | Intestinal infections | Respiratory infections | Placental infection and abortion | Seminal infection | Infertility | Polyarthritis | Meningo-encephalitis | Mastitis |
|------|----------------|------------------------|-------------------------|-----------------------------------|-------------------|-------------|----------------|----------------------|----------|
| Birds | +[a] | + | + | – | – | – | – | + | – |
| Sheep | + | + | + | + | + | – | +[a] | – | + |
| Cattle | + | +[a] | +[a] | + | + | + | +[a] | +[a] | + |
| Goats | – | + | + | + | – | – | – | – | + |
| Cats | + | + | + | – | – | – | – | – | – |
| Guinea-pigs | + | – | – | – | – | + | – | – | – |
| Koala bears | +[b] | – | – | – | – | + | – | – | – |

[a]Should be reclassified as *C. pecorum*.
[b]Should be reclassified as *C. pneumoniae*.

## INFECTION OF BIRDS AND MAMMALS

Table 40.4 shows some examples of natural hosts infected and the range of diseases reported to date. Non-human infections are important economically and as a source of infection to humans. Agricultural economy is affected as psittacosis is not confined to psittacine birds: outbreaks have been reported in turkeys, geese and ducks. Abortion in ewes can occur in one-third of a previously uninfected flock, and a continuing 1–2% abortion rate is found in infected flocks. Genital and eye infections of koala bears have been reported in Australia, giving rise to speculation that the species could become endangered due to chlamydia-induced infertility.

Birds with respiratory and intestinal infections shed the organism in nasal secretions and droppings. The nasal secretions contaminate the feathers, where they dry and produce an infected dust in which the organism can survive for months. There are import controls in many countries to restrict the movement of birds which are rendered more infectious by stress.

Similarly, the organism has been found in sheep droppings, in the milk, and on the placenta and fleece of sheep. Aerosols can be produced and are a hazard to shepherds, who may develop a respiratory infection, and to pregnant women, some of whom have miscarried.

## EPIDEMIOLOGY OF HUMAN CHLAMYDIAL INFECTIONS

Unlike *C. psittaci*, for which there is a non-human reservoir of infection, *C. trachomatis* and *C. pneumoniae* only appear to infect humans (see Table 40.2). *C. psittaci* infections of humans are not usually spread from person to person.

In areas hyperendemic for trachoma, such as sub-Saharan Africa and the Middle East, nearly all children become infected with *C. trachomatis*, but the severity of the infection appears to be dependent on the poverty level of the families.

Chlamydial *ophthalmia neonatorum* is caused by the D–K serovars responsible for the sexually transmitted disease which is prevalent in sexually active young people world-wide and can be found in association with gonorrhoea and other sexually transmitted diseases.

*C. pneumoniae* has only recently been recognized, but there have been outbreaks in military establishments and in student populations, indicative of aerosol spread. Serological studies have shown that there is a difference in the age profile of the infection. In the Far East, 10–15% of children under 5 years have evidence of infection, while there is little serological evidence in children in the Western world until they start school. After that the attack rate rises steadily till the late teenage years, and reaches 50% by middle age.

## LABORATORY DIAGNOSIS

### Cultivation

Chlamydiae may be isolated in either embryonated eggs or tissue culture. However, McCoy cells treated with cycloheximide are the most widely used, although *C. pneumoniae* grows better in HeLa or HL cells. The presence of the organism is detected by staining for inclusions or EBs. The disadvantage of culture is that it only detects viable organisms. This requires specimens to be sent quickly to the laboratory in a suitable transport medium (containing no penicillin) at 4°C or after freezing in liquid nitrogen.

## Antigen detection

To overcome the problems of culture, several direct tests have been developed. Staining of smears by fluorescent antibodies will demonstrate EBs, and the ELISA test can detect chlamydial antigens. While these tests have the advantage of not requiring special transport conditions they do suffer from false-positive results due to cross-reactions with antigens of other bacteria. In the ELISA test it is especially important to confirm positive results by the blocking test or by fluorescent staining of a deposit from the specimen.

## Nucleic acid detection

In certain chlamydial infections (or, more correctly, chlamydia-stimulated immunopathological reactions) it is not possible to isolate viable organisms, so either evidence of antigen (as above) or nucleic acid has to be used. This can be in the form of a probe for DNA or mRNA which can identify the infected cells or by amplification of parts of the genome by polymerase chain reaction or ligase chain reaction. These techniques have increased the detection of chlamydia in both complicated and uncomplicated infections.

## Serology

Serology has also been used, especially in respiratory infections. Atypical pneumonia due to *C. psittaci* produces high levels of complement-fixing antibody in serum from patients. This antibody is directed against group antigen and, until recently, adults with high or rising titres were thought to have psittacosis although contact with psittacine birds could not be established in all cases. Now that *C. pneumoniae* has been isolated, it is clear that a number of these cases of 'psittacosis' were in fact due to *C. pneumoniae*. To detect species-specific and serovar-specific antibody, the micro-immunofluorescence test is used with antigens from all chlamydial strains. Serology is also used to confirm the diagnosis of pneumonitis due to *C. trachomatis* in neonates. A high level (>64) of IgM and a rising or high titre (>256) of IgG are taken as diagnostic.

# TREATMENT AND CONTROL

## Immunization

To date, vaccines have not been very successful. The vaccine used against ovine abortion in sheep does not give complete protection, and a suitable replacement is being sought. There are several problems: serum antibody is not completely protective in vivo; mucosal antibody is also required; and the question of cell-mediated immunity must be addressed. Another problem is the choice of antigen: should a genus-specific antigen which stimulates antibody to all four species of chlamydia be used, or should it be a strain-specific antigen with a much narrower spectrum? For a rapid response to challenge, the immune response should be to exposed epitopes.

## Chemotherapy

Antibiotics can be used in the treatment of chlamydial infections. The antibiotic of choice is tetracycline in adults and erythromycin in babies. Penicillin should *not* be used as it is chlamydiastatic (*vide supra*). Similarly, chloramphenicol eye drops, which have been used to treat sticky eyes in babies, are chlamydiastatic, and there is a risk of the baby developing pneumonitis when the drug is discontinued. Because chlamydiae have a prolonged replication cycle and may be suppressed, not eradicated, by short courses of antibiotics, treatment must be given for a minimum of 7 days. Many authorities advocate treatment of 3 weeks' duration, especially for ascending and complicated genital infections in women. Unfortunately, many patients receive inadequate antimicrobial therapy. The advent of azithromycin, which can be given as a single dose, could well overcome this problem.

## Contact tracing

Tracing partners of index cases of chlamydial infection is very important as it is useless to treat the index case only to leave the patient exposed to a risk of reinfection from an untreated partner. Genital infections can be insidious, not causing clinical signs and symptoms. It is therefore essential that the partner should be screened for chlamydiae and treated even if clinically normal. In cases of neonatal infection both parents should be examined and treated. Where these measures have been rigorously applied frequency of genital infection in the developed world has decreased compared to that given in Table 40.3.

## Animal contact

Control of infection may mean avoidance of contact with well-known sources of infection, e.g. sheep at lambing, milking and shearing. Pregnant women are particularly at risk from such infection and so should avoid contact with sheep during pregnancy. The control of importation of psittacine birds has reduced the risk of psittacosis in pet owners and bird fanciers in the UK, although the increasing popularity of exotic pets has lead to an increase in numbers of cases.

## Hygiene

The effect of improved hygiene has been shown by the decrease in trachoma in the Western world so that, in addition to extending medical care, improving standards of hygiene and sanitation should be a prime objective in developing countries.

### RECOMMENDED READING

Barron A L 1988 *Microbiology of Chlamydia.* CRC Press, Boca Raton

Beatty W L, Morrison R P, Byrne G I 1994 Persistent chlamydiae: from cell culture to a paradigm for chlamydia pathogenesis. *Microbiological Review* 58: 686–699

Brunham R C, Peeling R W 1994 *Chlamydia trachomatis* antigens: role in immunity and pathogenesis. *Infectious Agents and Disease* 3: 218–233

Kuo C-C, Grayston J T, Campbell L A, Goo Y A, Wissler R W, Benditt E P 1995 *Chlamydia pneumoniae* (TWAR) in coronary arteries of young adults (15–34 years old). *Proceedings of the National Academy of Sciences of the USA* 92: 6911–6914

Rank R G, Dascher C, Bowlin A K, Bavoil P M 1995. Systemic immunization with Hsp60 alters the development of chlamydial ocular disease. *Investigative Ophthalmology and Visual Science* 36: 1344–1351

Ridgway G L and Taylor-Robinson D 1991 Current problems in microbiology: I. Chlamydial infections: which laboratory test? *Journal of Clinical Pathology* 44: 1–5

Treharne J D, Ballard R C 1990 The expanding spectrum of the *Chlamydia*—a microbiological and clinical appraisal. *Reviews in Medical Microbiology* 1: 10–18

# 41

# Rickettsia, orientia, ehrlichia and coxiella

**Typhus; spotted fevers; scrub typhus; ehrlichioses; Q fever**

## D. H. Walker and K. L. Gage

Few diseases have had a greater impact on the course of human history than epidemic typhus. Hans Zinsser's classic book *Rats, Lice and History* provides a graphic account of how *Rickettsia prowazekii*, the aetiological agent of this louse-borne disease, has caused millions of deaths and much human suffering in conditions of famine, poverty and war. Epidemic typhus has become relatively rare as world conditions have improved, but various other rickettsial diseases are still widely distributed, and deteriorating socio-economic conditions and warfare in parts of eastern Europe such as the former Yugoslavia and USSR raise the spectre of the re-emergence of louse-borne typhus.

As currently classified, the family Rickettsiaceae includes a diverse group of organisms that share such common features as intracellular growth and transmission by arthropod vectors. A family tree based upon sequences of the 16S rDNA reveals that *Rickettsia* species, *Orientia* (formerly *Rickettsia*) *tsutsugamushi* and *Ehrlichia* species evolved from a common ancestor.

Some obligately intracellular Gram-negative bacteria formerly classified with the Rickettsiaceae are no longer considered to be members of the family. *Bartonella* (formerly *Rochalimaea*) *quintana*, the louse-borne aetiological agent of trench fever and bacillary angiomatosis, is a cell-associated bacterium that can be grown in cell-free culture (see Ch. 35). *Coxiella burnetii* is obligately intracellular and can be isolated from arthropods, but does not require an arthropod vector to maintain itself in nature.

## RICKETTSIA AND ORIENTIA

## DESCRIPTION

The genera *Rickettsia* and *Orientia* include organisms responsible for numerous diseases in many parts of the world (Table 41.1). The pioneering research of Ricketts and others in the early 20th century demonstrated the rickettsial aetiology of Rocky Mountain spotted fever. Several other diseases, including epidemic and murine typhus, were later shown to be rickettsial infections. The discovery of a hitherto unrecognized spotted fever in 1984 in Japan and even more recently in Australia led to the subsequent isolation of the aetiological agents, *Rickettsia japonica* and an organism with the proposed name *R. honei*, indicating that much remains to be learned about these organisms. In addition to species known to be associated with human disease, there are a number of presumably non-pathogenic rickettsiae which have been isolated primarily from arthropods and are poorly understood.

*Rickettsia* species are small ($0.3–0.5 \times 0.8–1.0\ \mu m$) Gram-negative bacilli. They are obligate intracellular parasites that reside in the cytosol of host cells (Fig. 41.1). All are associated with an arthropod vector. Species that are pathogenic for humans parasitize endothelial cells almost exclusively. They are highly specialized and can synthesize adenosine triphosphate (ATP) and proteins. ATP, amino acids and metabolic intermediates are also transported from the cytoplasm of the host cell by specific mechanisms.

The genus *Rickettsia* is currently divided into two antigenically distinct groups: the typhus group and the spotted fever group. Typhus and spotted fever group rickettsiae are very closely related, as indicated by DNA–DNA hybridization studies; both have a typical Gram-negative bacterial cell wall, including a bilayered outer membrane that contains the lipopolysaccharide antigens that distinguish the two groups. External to the outer membrane there appears to be a slime layer, probably composed of polysaccharides. Electrophoresis has demonstrated a number of distinct proteins in typhus group rickettsiae. The immunodominant surface protein antigen, designated SPA in both *R. prowazekii* and *R. typhi*, contains both cross-reactive and species-

**Table 41.1**    Human diseases caused by *Rickettsia* and *Orientia* species

| Species and disease | Geographical distribution | Means of transmission | Primary vectors | Important vertebrate hosts |
|---|---|---|---|---|
| **Typhus group** | | | | |
| *R. prowazekii* (epidemic typhus) | Extant foci in Africa, North and South America | Louse faeces | *Pediculus humanus* | Humans, possibly other mammals (flying squirrels) |
| *R. typhi* (murine typhus) | Primarily tropics and subtropics | Flea faeces | *Xenopsylla cheopis* and other fleas | Rodents and other small mammals |
| *R. felis* (cat flea typhus) | North America | Flea, undetermined mechanism | *Ctenocephalides felis* | Opossums |
| **Spotted fever group** | | | | |
| *R. akari* (rickettsialpox) | USA, Ukraine, Croatia, Korea | Bite of mouse mite | *Liponyssoides sanguineus* | House mice (*Mus musculus*), possibly other rodents |
| *R. australis* (Queensland tick typhus) | Australia | Bite of tick | *Ixodes holocyclus* | Unknown |
| *R. conorii* (boutonneuse fever) | Europe, Africa, Middle East, India | Bite of tick | *Rhipicephalus, Amblyomma*, etc. | Rodents and other small mammals |
| *R. japonica* (oriental spotted fever) | Japan | Bite of tick | Unknown tick species | Unknown |
| *R. rickettsii* (Rocky Mountain spotted fever) | North and South America | Bite of tick | *Dermacentor*, etc. | Rodents and other small mammals |
| *R. sibirica* (north Asian tick typhus) | Northern Asia | Bite of tick | *Dermacentor, Haemaphysalis*, etc. | Rodents and other small mammals |
| *R. honei* (Flinders Island spotted fever) | Australia | Bite of tick | Unknown | Unknown |
| **Scrub typhus group** | | | | |
| *Orientia tsutsugamushi* (scrub typhus) | Asia, Australia, islands of SW Pacific and Indian oceans | Bite of larval mite | Chiggers (*Leptotrombidium* species) | Rodents (especially rats) |

**Fig. 41.1**    Electron micrograph of a cell infected with *R. rickettsii*, showing dilation of the endoplasmic reticulum of host cells that occurs as a result of injury associated with infection by spotted fever group rickettsiae.

specific epitopes. The spotted fever group rickettsiae contain the genetically related rickettsial outer-membrane protein B, a 135 kDa protein that is processed from a gene encoding a 168 kDa polypeptide. The other major surface protein of spotted fever group rickettsiae, rickettsial outer-membrane protein A, contains a hydrophilic region of tandem repeat units that determine the diversity of molecular size and antigens largely by the number, order and type of repeat units.

The scrub typhus rickettsiae appear to be fundamentally different and have been classified into a related but distinct genus as *Orientia tsutsugamushi* (Table 41.1). There is no indication of antigenic similarities between *O. tsutsugamushi* and members of the genus *Rickettsia*. The cell wall lacks lipopolysaccharide, peptidoglycan or a slime layer and appears to derive its structural integrity from proteins linked by disulphide bonds. *O. tsutsugamushi* exhibits three or four major antigenic proteins with both strain-specific and cross-reactive epitopes.

## PATHOGENESIS

### Invasion and destruction of target cells

Rickettsiae normally enter the body through the bite or faeces of an infected arthropod vector. They are disseminated through the bloodstream, enter endothelial cells by induced phagocytosis, escape from the phagosome, multiply intracellularly and eventually destroy their host cells. Observations in cell culture systems suggest that the mechanisms of destruction of the host cell differ between the spotted fever and typhus group rickettsiae. After infection with *R. prowazekii* or *R. typhi*, the rickettsiae continue to multiply until the cell is packed with organisms (Fig. 41.2) and then bursts, possibly as a result of phospholipase A activity; before lysis, host cells have a normal ultrastructural appearance.

Spotted fever group rickettsiae behave differently; they seldom accumulate in large numbers and do not burst the host cells, but stimulate polymerization of F-actin tails which propel them through the cytoplasm and into filopodia, from which they escape the cell (Fig. 41.3). Infected cells exhibit signs of membrane damage associated with an influx of water, which is sequestered within cisternae of dilated, damaged rough endoplasmic reticulum (see Fig. 41.1). The means by which rickettsiae damage host cell membranes is uncertain, but there is experimental evidence to suggest a role for free radicals of oxygen, a phospholipase, or a protease.

**Fig. 41.2**  Electron micrograph of a cell infected with *R. prowazekii*. The rickettsiae continue to multiply within the cell until it is completely packed with organisms and bursts. In contrast to cells infected with spotted fever group rickettsiae, the ultrastructural appearance of cells infected with typhus group rickettsiae remains normal until the cell lyses. The region of the cell containing rickettsiae is indicated by the arrow.

**Fig. 41.3**  Electron micrograph of *R. conorii* escaping from a host cell. Note the location of the rickettsiae within host cell filopodia.

Scrub typhus rickettsiae also escape from host cells soon after infecting them, but little is known about the mechanism(s) by which these organisms damage cells.

### Pathological lesions

All members of the genera *Rickettsia* and *Orientia* cause widespread microvascular injury leading to the destruction of infected endothelial cells. The pathological manifestations result more from direct rickettsial injury than by immunopathological mechanisms, mediated via cytokines and cytotoxic T lymphocytes, inflammation, disseminated intravascular coagulation, or endotoxin. Interference with normal circulation and increased vascular permeability following damage of blood vessels can cause life-threatening encephalitis and non-cardiogenic pulmonary oedema.

## Clinical aspects of rickettsial diseases

### Epidemic typhus

Initial symptoms of the disease are headache and fever 6–15 days after being exposed to *R. prowazekii*. A macular rash, often noted 4–7 days after patients become ill, first appears on the trunk and axillary folds and then spreads to the extremities. In mild cases the rash may begin to fade after 1–2 days, but in more severe cases it may last much longer and become haemorrhagic. Severe cases may also develop pronounced hypotension and renal dysfunction. The mental state of the patient may progress from dullness to stupor and, in very severe cases, even coma. Although the prognosis is grave for comatose patients, prompt treatment may be life-saving.

Individuals who survive a primary infection of louse-borne typhus may develop a relatively milder reactivation of latent infection many years later. This is referred to as recrudescent typhus or *Brill–Zinsser disease*. Such individuals are nevertheless immune to a second louse-borne infection.

### Flea-borne fevers

Patients infected with *R. typhi*, the aetiological agent of murine typhus, develop symptoms similar to those of epidemic typhus. Fatal cases are rare but occasionally do occur, particularly in the elderly. Although the disease is much milder than epidemic typhus, it is still severe enough to require several months of convalescence. A novel related species, *R. felis*, an organism that is transovarially maintained in cat fleas, causes a human illness similar to murine typhus.

### Tick-borne spotted fever

There are many clinical similarities among the tick-borne rickettsioses of the spotted fever group. Although all can be life-threatening, the most severe is Rocky Mountain spotted fever. Patients become ill within 2 weeks of being bitten by an infected tick.

Early symptoms include fever and severe headache, often accompanied by myalgia, anorexia, vomiting, abdominal pain, diarrhoea, photophobia and cough. An eschar frequently occurs at the site of the tick bite in all spotted fever group infections except Rocky Mountain spotted fever. A maculopapular rash usually develops within 3–5 days. The rash of spotted fever usually develops first on the extremities rather than on the trunk. Absence of a rash does not exclude rickettsial infection since a disproportionate number of fatal cases of Rocky Mountain spotted fever are of the 'spotless' variety. Spotted fever group rickettsiae are found within the endothelial cells and less often macrophages of vertebrate hosts, but *R. rickettsii* is also capable of invading vascular smooth muscle.

Vascular damage in severe cases may result in haemorrhagic rash, hypovolaemia, hypotensive shock, non-cardiogenic pulmonary oedema and impairment of central nervous system function. A fulminant form of Rocky Mountain spotted fever sometimes kills the patient within 5 days of the onset of symptoms; this form of the disease is more common in black males who are deficient in glucose-6-phosphate dehydrogenase, and may be related to haemolysis in these patients. Infection confers long-lasting immunity.

### Rickettsialpox

Rickettsialpox is a relatively mild infection transmitted by mites. The clinical course is similar to the other spotted fever group infections and includes development of fever, headache and an eschar at the site where the infected mite fed. The rash is initially maculopapular but often becomes vesicular. Fever lasts about a week, and patients usually recover uneventfully.

### Scrub typhus

Human infection with scrub typhus rickettsiae may be mild or fatal, depending on host factors and presumably the virulence of the infecting strain. Symptoms develop 6–18 days after being bitten by infected mite larvae (chiggers). An eschar is often apparent at the site of the bite with enlargement of local lymph nodes. Progression of the disease may be accompanied by interstitial pneumonitis, generalized lymphadenopathy, splenomegaly and rash. Death may result from encephalitis, respiratory failure and circulatory failure. Patients who survive generally become afebrile after 2–3 weeks, or sooner if treated. Scrub typhus confers only transient immunity, and re-infection may occur with heterologous or homologous strains.

## LABORATORY DIAGNOSIS

Timely and accurate diagnosis of rickettsial disease followed by administration of an appropriate antibiotic may mean the difference between death of the patient and uneventful recovery. The lack of widely available, reliable diagnostic tests that can detect the disease in its early stages remains a problem, particularly as symptoms are often non-specific. The rash may appear at a late stage in the infection and may resemble exanthemata of many other diseases. The presence or significance of an eschar, if present, is also commonly overlooked.

### Methods of laboratory diagnosis

#### Serological methods

The oldest and most widely used laboratory method is the *Weil–Felix test*, which relies on agglutination of the somatic antigens of non-motile *Proteus* species. Although widely available, this test is not recommended because of unacceptably low levels of sensitivity and specificity.

More reliable diagnostic tests for detecting antibodies to rickettsiae include immunofluorescence, latex agglutination and enzyme immuno-assay. These tests are commercially available. The detection of specific antibody early in the course of rickettsial infections remains a problem. Serological diagnosis is usually achieved only after the patient is on the way to recovery; death may occur before detectable levels of antibody are present.

#### Isolation of rickettsiae

Isolation of the organism in cell culture or susceptible laboratory animals, such as mice or guinea-pigs, provides conclusive proof of rickettsial infection. However, it is seldom attempted because of lack of facilities or expertise and because of the presumed danger to laboratory personnel of handling rickettsiae-infected tissues. Such dangers have been overemphasized in this era of antibiotics, but use of containment facilities is appropriate.

#### Detection of rickettsiae in tissue

Skin biopsies from the centre of petechial lesions can be examined for rickettsiae by immuno-fluorescence or immuno-enzyme methods. This approach is virtually 100% specific but has a sensitivity of 70%. Rickettsiae can be visualized for up to 48 h after the administration of antirickettsial drugs. Formalin-fixed, paraffin-embedded specimens can also be examined for rickettsiae by immuno-histological methods. This approach is particularly effective for diagnosing rickettsial infection post mortem. A clever method has been developed for capturing detached, circulating endothelial cells by antibody-coated magnetic beads and immuno-cytological detection of intracellular rickettsiae.

Polymerase chain reaction (PCR) techniques that detect rickettsial DNA are more rapid than isolation and allow specific identification, but they exhibit relatively low sensitivity and are not yet generally available.

## TREATMENT

Owing to the difficulties of accurate diagnosis and the risks involved in misdiagnosis, empirical anti-rickettsial therapy is appropriate for patients who have a fever for 3 days or more and a history consistent with the epidemiological and clinical features of rickettsial disease. Tetracyclines are slightly more effective than chloramphenicol. Both are rickettsiostatic and allow the patient's immune system time to respond and control the infection. Sulphonamides should not be administered as they exacerbate rickettsial infections. Intensive nursing care, management of fluids and electrolytes, replacement of platelets to compensate for those consumed as part of the patient's haemostatic response, and administration of red blood cells to patients that develop anaemia may be needed. Surgery may also be necessary to remove digits and extremities that develop ischaemic necrosis.

## EPIDEMIOLOGY

### Typhus group infections

#### Epidemic typhus

*R. prowazekii* is transmitted from human to human by the body louse, *Pediculus humanus*; the organisms are present in the faeces of infected lice and enter through the bite wound or skin abrasions. Lice do not transmit the rickettsiae to their offspring transovarially (adult to offspring via the egg). In fact, *R. prowazekii* causes a fatal infection of the louse, which is therefore incapable of long-term maintenance of the rickettsiae, and humans appear to be reservoirs of epidemic typhus. Individuals who suffer a bout of recrudescent typhus (Brill–Zinsser disease) circulate sufficient rickettsiae in their blood to infect approximately 1–5% of lice that feed on them, and this is sufficient to initiate new epidemics of the disease. The importance of non-human reservoirs of the disease is uncertain, but a number of serologically confirmed cases of *R. prowazekii* infection have been documented among persons in the USA, whose homes harboured flying squirrels, which maintain *R. prowazekii* in an enzootic cycle involving their own fleas and lice. Reports based on serological evidence that ticks and domestic animals are reservoirs of the rickettsiae in Africa have not been confirmed.

## Murine typhus

Murine typhus is widely distributed, particularly in tropical and subtropical coastal regions and port facilities where large numbers of rats are found. This disease is maintained in an enzootic cycle involving rats and their fleas which remain infected for life. Even the inefficient rate of transovarial transmission in fleas may play an important role in maintaining the rickettsiae in nature. Humans are infected by the contamination of abraded skin, respiratory tract or conjunctiva with infective flea faeces, in which the rickettsiae can survive for as long as 3 days under optimal conditions of temperature and humidity. The disease is an occupational hazard of working in rat-infested areas such as markets or ports.

## Spotted fever group infections

### Tick-borne infections

Tick-borne rickettsiae of the spotted fever group are maintained in enzootic cycles involving ticks and their wild animal hosts. Ticks are the primary reservoirs of the rickettsiae, and maintain the organisms by both trans-stadial transmission (larvae to nymph to adult tick) and transovarial or vertical transmission. Some horizontal transmission (rodent to tick to rodent) is likely to be essential to the survival of the rickettsiae in nature because they are pathogenic to ticks.

Humans become infected following the bite of infected ticks or through contamination of abraded skin or mucous membranes. People place themselves at risk of infection when they enter areas infested with infected ticks. Individuals may also become infected if they are bitten by ticks of domestic dogs or by manual deticking of dogs, when the partially fed ticks may rupture, releasing rickettsiae.

### Rickettsialpox

*R. akari* is the only member of the spotted fever group that is transmitted by a mite (*Liponyssoides sanguineus*) rather than ticks. The rickettsiae are maintained in an enzootic cycle that involves house mice (*Mus musculus*) and their mites. As with other spotted fever group infections, the arthropod vector is also the primary reservoir and can maintain the organism by trans-stadial and transovarial transmission. Other rodents and their ectoparasites may be able to maintain the rickettsiae in rural areas, but their importance remains unknown. Rickettsialpox is primarily an urban disease associated with mice-infested buildings.

## Scrub typhus

*O. tsutsugamushi* is transmitted to humans by the larval stages of mites of the genus *Leptotrombidium*. The nymphal and adult stages of the mites do not feed on mammals. The parasitic larvae (chiggers) occur in habitats that have been disturbed by the loss or removal of the natural vegetation. The area becomes covered with scrub vegetation, which is the preferred habitat for chiggers, and gives the disease its name. The disease is often localized because of the restricted habitat of the chiggers and their mammalian hosts. The vertebrate hosts of *Leptotrombidium* mites are usually rats or other small mammals that prefer the scrub vegetation, but humans entering infected areas are also at risk.

## CONTROL

It is virtually impossible to eradicate rickettsial infections because of their enzootic nature. Measures aimed at reducing rodent or ecto-parasite populations may help to reduce the risk of infection. In addition to delousing infested persons, their clothing and bedding should be decontaminated.

Persons entering areas endemic for spotted fever group infections should wear protective clothing treated with repellent. Individuals should also carefully examine themselves for ticks as soon as possible after returning from tick-infected areas. The probability of infection is decreased if the tick is removed soon after it attaches. Transmission may require up to 24 h of feeding, perhaps because starved ticks require a partial blood meal if they are to reactivate the virulence of the rickettsiae.

There is no safe, effective vaccine for any of the rickettsial diseases. The attenuated E strain of *R. prowazekii* induces protective immunity but is not suitable for general use because it causes a mild form of typhus in 10–15% of those inoculated and reverts to a virulent state after animal passage. Inactivated vaccines for Rocky Mountain spotted fever may ameliorate the course of the disease, but none prevents illness completely, and all have been removed from the market. Scrub typhus infections also cannot be prevented by administration of vaccines derived from killed rickettsiae. Recombinant vaccines may be more successful, but will have to include those epitopes that are crucial for stimulating cell-mediated immune mechanisms, which are more important than humoral immunity in rickettsial infection.

Prophylactic use of antimicrobial agents is not recommended, since they are only rickettsiostatic and disease develops as soon as the antibiotic regimen is discontinued. Prolonged prophylaxis with weekly doses of doxycycline is effective against scrub typhus, but is probably inappropriate except under exceptional circumstances, e.g. during military operations.

## EHRLICHIA

### DESCRIPTION

Organisms designated as *Ehrlichia* species (Table 41.2) reside in three clusters determined by 16S rDNA similarity which may be assigned to two or three different genera. At least one human pathogen is a member of each of these three clusters along with organisms currently bearing other genus names: *Cowdria*, *Anaplasma* and *Neorickettsia*. Long recognized as the aetiological agents of veterinary diseases such as bovine and ovine tick-borne fever in the UK, the first human ehrlichial disease was recognized in 1954 when *Erlichia sennetsu* was identified as the cause of an illness resembling glandular fever in Japan (*sennetsu* means glandular fever in Japanese). Ehrlichiae have emerged as the cause of two newly recognized tick-borne diseases in the USA, human monocytic ehrlichiosis (*E. chaffeensis*) and human granulocytic ehrlichiosis (an organism very similar and possibly identical to *E. equi* and *E. phagocytophila*).

Ehrlichiae are small Gram-negative bacteria. They multiply within membrane-bound cytoplasmic vacuoles, usually in various phagocytes, and form characteristic microcolonies resembling mulberries, termed morulae (Latin *morum* = mulberry) (Fig. 41.4). Electron microscopy reveals two distinct morphological forms, larger reticulate and smaller dense-core cells, both of which divide by binary fission, strong evidence against a developmental cycle. Ehrlichiae preferentially metabolize glutamine in the synthesis of ATP.

## PATHOGENESIS

Entry of ehrlichiae into the host is best defined for tick-borne ehrlichiosis. In the Orient, *E. sennetsu* is suspected to be ingested with raw fish. Some related animal pathogens (*Neorickettsia* spp.) are transmitted by ingestion of fish containing certain parasitic flukes that carry the organism.

**Table 41.2** Human diseases caused by *Ehrlichia* species

| Species and disease | Geographical distribution | Means of transmission | Primary vectors |
| --- | --- | --- | --- |
| *E. sennetsu* (Sennetsu ehrlichiosis) | Japan, Malaysia | Unknown (infection of fluke-infested fish?) | Unknown |
| *E. chaffeensis* (Human monocytic ehrlichiosis) | USA, Europe, Africa | Tick bite | *Amblyomma* species |
| *E. phagocytophila*[a] (Human granulocytic ehrlichiosis) | USA, Europe | Tick bite | *Ixodes* species |

[a]Or a closely related species.

**Fig. 41.4** Cells infected with *E. sennetsu*. Arrows indicate a number of infected cells containing an ehrlichia-laden vacuole or morula. (Micrograph by courtesy of Dr J. Stephen Dumler.)

Few details of the pathogenesis of human infections are known. *E. sennetsu* is associated with lymphoid hyperplasia and atypical lymphocytosis. Human monocytic ehrlichiosis causes leucopenia, thrombocytopenia, perivascular lymphohistiocytic infiltrates in many organs and non-necrotizing granulomata in bone marrow and liver. Human granulocytic ehrlichiosis is also often associated with leucopenia and thrombocytopenia. The two latter diseases can be fatal, often owing to opportunistic fungal and viral infections. Ehrlichiae can establish prolonged, even persistent infections in vivo, and some species, including *E. chaffeensis*, can kill heavily infected cells in vitro.

Most data are available for *E. risticii*, an equine pathogen closely related to *E. sennetsu*. It attaches to a macrophage membrane receptor by an unidentified adhesin, enters by phagocytosis and receptor-mediated endocytosis, and inhibits phagosome–lysosome fusion. Antibody to ehrlichiae confers passive protection, and infected macrophages express ehrlichial antigens on the cell surface, a potential target for the immune system. Suppression of cellular immunity by *E. risticii* and *E. phagocytophila*, and neutrophil function by *E. phagocytophila*, may predispose to opportunistic infection.

## LABORATORY DIAGNOSIS

The human ehrlichioses are diagnosed by demonstrating the development of specific antibodies during convalescence. Indirect immunofluorescent methods use cell culture-propagated organisms. *E. chaffeensis* and the human granulocytic ehrlichia are detected diagnostically by PCR with specific primers to amplify the ehrlichial DNA. Human granulocytic ehrlichiosis can often be diagnosed by identification of characteristic morulae in Giemsa-stained peripheral blood neutrophils; *E. chaffeensis* is rarely detected in monocytes in blood smears.

## TREATMENT

Doxycycline is very effective in shortening the course of infection and reduces the mortality of human monocytic and granulocytic ehrlichioses.

## EPIDEMIOLOGY

Deer and ticks are probably involved in the ecology of both human monocytic and granulocytic ehrlichioses. *Amblyomma americanum* ticks appear to be the major vector of *E. chaffeensis*, and *Ixodes ricinus*-like ticks seem to be the vectors of the human granulocytic ehrlichia. Whether deer or rodents are the most important reservoirs of these two species remains to be determined. Immature ticks obtain ehrlichiae from the blood of infected animals; the organisms are maintained transstadially, but not transovarially, and are transmitted during a subsequent blood meal. Human infections have been associated strongly with the season of tick activity and a history of actual tick bite.

## COXIELLA

## DESCRIPTION

Query or Q fever was first identified as a distinct clinical entity in 1935 after an outbreak of typhoid-like illness among abattoir workers in Australia. Subsequent studies have shown that this disease is the most widespread of all rickettsial infections with an almost global distribution. The aetiological agent, *C. burnetii*, is an obligately intracellular prokaryote, but genetic analysis suggests it is more closely allied to *Legionella* species.

**Fig. 41.5**  Immunoperoxidase staining of *C. burnetii* in alveolar macrophages in a patient with Q fever. A cell containing many *Coxiella* organisms is indicated by the arrow. (Micrograph by courtesy of Dr J. Stephen Dumler.)

*C. burnetii* is a pleomorphic, coccobacillary bacterium. It is approximately 0.3 μm wide and 1.0 μm long, and ultrastructural studies reveal a Gram-negative cell wall. The organisms typically grow within the phagolysosome of macrophages of the vertebrate host (Fig. 41.5). Structurally distinct large and small cell variants of *C. burnetii* have been described, suggesting that it has a developmental cycle. In acidic conditions, similar to those found within a phagolysosome, it actively metabolizes a variety of substrates and can accomplish significant levels of macromolecular synthesis. Prolonged in-vitro cultivation results in a change in antigenic composition, known as phase variation. Phase I organisms are representative of strains isolated from nature, whereas phase II organisms appear in laboratory cultures and are avirulent for laboratory animals. The basis for the phase variation is structural differences in the lipopolysaccharides analogous to the smooth to rough transitions observed in other bacteria. *C. burnetii*, unlike *Rickettsia* species, has been found to contain plasmids.

## PATHOGENESIS

Human infection usually follows inhalation of aerosols containing *C. burnetii*. Entry into the lungs results in infection of the alveolar macrophages and a brief rickettsaemia. Many infections are subclinical. The incubation period for the acute form of the disease is usually about 2 weeks but can be longer. In addition to a non-specific febrile illness, the patient may suffer pneumonitis, hepatic and bone marrow granulomata, meningo-encephalitis and endocarditis. Chronic infections can develop, with the organism persisting in cardiac valves and possibly other foci. Endocarditis is rare, but potentially fatal, and may be accompanied by glomerulonephritis, osteomyelitis, or central nervous system involvement. Reactivation of latent *C. burnetii* infections of pregnant women may occur, and the organism is shed with the placenta or abortus.

## LABORATORY DIAGNOSIS

Diagnosis relies on the demonstration of specific antibodies in a complement fixation test (CFT) or indirect immunofluorescence assay. Immunofluorescence assay titres peak earlier (4–8 weeks) than those of the CFT (12 weeks) and thus are more sensitive early in the course of the disease. Use of the CFT is also hindered by the anti-complementary activity of some sera.

Isolation of *C. burnetii* from patient specimens is a specialized procedure and is not generally recommended because of the extremely infectious nature of the organism.

## TREATMENT

Most *C. burnetii* infections resolve without antibiotic treatment, but administration of doxycycline reduces the duration of fever in the acute infection and is definitely recommended in cases of chronic infection. In Q fever endocarditis, long-term administration of a tetracycline (in combination with co-trimoxazole, lincomycin or rifampicin) has been suggested. All antibiotics tested to date are rickettsiostatic within the acidic phagolysosome, and *C. burnetii* may be recovered from some patients after months or even years of continuous treatment. In addition to antibiotic therapy, the haemodynamic status should be monitored. Valve replacement may be necessary in some cases of Q fever endocarditis.

## EPIDEMIOLOGY

Q fever has been found on all continents except Antarctica, but most cases are reported from the UK and France. Elsewhere, the disease often goes unreported, is misdiagnosed, or causes such mild infections that persons fail to seek treatment. The primary reservoirs of the disease are wild and domestic ungulates, including cattle, sheep and goats. Ticks can maintain *C. burnetii* by trans-stadial and transovarial transmission. Faeces of infected ticks contain very large numbers of *C. burnetii*, but these arthropods are not necessary to maintain the infection in nature.

*C. burnetii* may be the most infectious of all bacteria. Humans generally become infected after inhalation of aerosols or following direct contact with the organisms in the milk, urine, faeces or birth products of infected animals. *C. burnetii* can survive on wool for 7–10 months, in skim milk for up to 40 months and in tick faeces for at least 1 year. Most individuals acquire the disease as an occupational hazard. Cases are common among abattoir workers and those associated with livestock rearing or dairy farming. Although Q fever normally occurs as isolated, sporadic cases, a number of well-documented outbreaks have been reported.

## CONTROL

Elimination of infected reservoir hosts is probably impossible because of chronic infections among the animals and the ability of the organism to survive for long periods in the external environment. Exposure can be reduced by construction of separate facilities for animal parturition, destruction of suspect placental membranes, heat treatment of milk (74°C for 15 s), and efforts to reduce the tick population. Abattoir workers should take care while handling carcasses, especially in the removal and dissection of mammary glands and inner organs. Animal hides should be kept wet until the salting procedure begins. Appropriate containment procedures should be observed in laboratories working with this highly infectious organism.

Vaccines have been developed from formalin-killed whole cells, attenuated *C. burnetii*, and trichloroacetic acid-extracted antigens. Vaccines derived from phase I organisms generate a much greater protective response than similar ones prepared from phase II organisms.

## RECOMMENDED READING

Aitken I D, Bogel K, Cracea E et al 1987 Q fever in Europe: current aspects of aetiology, epidemiology, human infection, diagnosis and therapy. *Infection* 15: 323–327

Audy J R 1968 *Red Mites and Typhus*. Athlone Press, London

Baca O G, Paretsky D 1983 Q fever and *Coxiella burnetii*: a model for host–parasite interactions. *Microbiological Reviews* 47: 127–149

Kass E M, Szaniawski W K, Levy H et al 1994 Rickettsialpox in a New York City hospital, 1980 to 1989. *New England Journal of Medicine* 331: 1612–1617

McDade J E, Newhouse V F 1986 Natural history of *Rickettsia rickettsii*. *Annual Review of Microbiology* 40: 287–309

Marrie T J 1990 *Q Fever*. CRC Press, Boca Raton

Raoult D 1991 Rickettsioses in the Mediterranean – a problem for travellers. *Reviews in Medical Microbiology* 2: 115–120

Rikihisa Y 1991 The tribe *Ehrlichieae* and ehrlichial diseases. *Clinical Microbiology Reviews* 4: 286–308

Walker D H 1988 *Biology of Rickettsial Diseases*. CRC Press, Boca Raton

Walker D H 1989 The rickettsia–host interaction. In: Moulder J W (ed) *Intracellular Parasitism*. CRC Press, Boca Raton

Walker D H, Dumler J S 1996 Emergence of the ehrlichioses as human health problems. *Emerging Infectious Diseases* 2: 18–29

Winkler H H 1990 *Rickettsia* species (as organisms). *Annual Review of Microbiology* 44: 131–153

# 42

# Mycoplasmas

**Atypical pneumonia; genital tract infection**

## D. Taylor-Robinson

Mycoplasmas are the smallest prokaryotic organisms that can grow in cell-free culture media. They are found in humans, animals, plants, insects, soil and sewage. The first to be recognized, *Mycoplasma mycoides* ssp. *mycoides*, was isolated 100 years ago from cattle with pleuropneumonia. As other pathogenic and saprophytic isolates accumulated from veterinary and human sources they became known as *pleuropneumonia-like organisms* (PPLO), a term now superseded by *mycoplasmas*. 'Mycoplasma' (Greek: *mykes* = fungus; *plasma* = something moulded) refers to the filamentous (fungal-like) nature of the organisms of some species and to the plasticity of the outer membrane resulting in pleomorphism.

The class Mollicutes ('soft-skins') comprises four orders and five families: Mycoplasmataceae, Entomoplasmataceae, Spiroplasmataceae, Acholeplasmataceae and Anaeroplasmataceae. The family Mycoplasmataceae is subdivided into the genus *Mycoplasma*, which contains about 100 named species, and the genus *Ureaplasma*, which provides a separate status for urea-hydrolysing organisms, trivially termed *ureaplasmas*. These were known originally as *T strains* or *T mycoplasmas*; 'T' for 'tiny' to describe the size of the colonies. Many animals are infected by ureaplasmas but the genus presently contains only six species. Ureaplasmas of avian, bovine, canine and feline origin are antigenically distinct from the human strains and have been placed in separate species. Ureaplasmas of human origin belong to the species *Ureaplasma urealyticum*, which comprises at least 14 serotypes. Members of the family Acholeplasmataceae (trivially termed *acholeplasmas*) do not depend on sterol for growth, and belong to a single genus, *Acholeplasma*, comprising at least 13 species, of which *Acholeplasma laidlawii* was the first to be named. The genus *Spiroplasma* of the family Spiroplasmataceae contains helical, motile organisms (trivially termed *spiroplasmas*) that cause disease in plants and insects. *Anaeroplasma* species are strict anaerobes found in the rumen of cattle and sheep. The term 'mycoplasma'

is used often, as here, in a trivial fashion to refer to any member of the class Mollicutes, irrespective of whether they belong to the genus *Mycoplasma*, although the term 'mollicute' is also used.

Mycoplasmas are distributed widely in nature, and various species cause economically important infections in cattle, goats, sheep, swine, other mammals and birds as well as humans. In addition, mycoplasmas are of concern to those who use cell cultures because of the problems of contamination.

## DESCRIPTION

### Reproduction

Mycoplasmas multiply by binary fission. However, cytoplasmic division may not always be synchronous with genome replication, resulting in the formation of multinucleate filaments and other shapes. Subsequent division of the cytoplasm by constriction of the membrane at sites between the genomes leads to chains of beads which later fragment to give single cells. Budding occurs when the cytoplasm is not divided equally between the daughter cells. The minimal reproductive unit of mycoplasmas is a roughly spherical cell about 200–250 nm in diameter. It is from organisms of this order of size, whatever the shape, that growth is initiated in cell-free medium; such organisms also make up, with larger forms (0.5–1.0 μm diameter), the substance of the characteristic agar-embedded colonies.

### Morphology

Cell morphology varies with mycoplasmal species, environmental conditions and the stage of the growth cycle. Light microscopy reveals pleomorphic organisms, which may range from spherical through coccoid, coccobacillary, ring and dumb-bell forms,

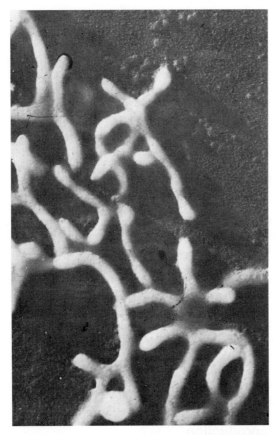

**Fig. 42.1** Electron micrograph of *M. mycoides* spp. *mycoides* (bovine origin), gold shadowed, to show branching filaments. ×28 800. (From Rodwell and Abbot 1961 *Journal of General Microbiology* 25: 201.)

to short and long branching (Fig. 42.1), beaded or segmented filaments. The helical shape of spiroplasmas is characteristic but not always seen.

Several mycoplasmas, including *M. genitalium* (Fig. 42.2), *M. pneumoniae* and *M. penetrans* of human origin, have specialized structures at one or both ends by which they attach to respiratory or genital tract mucosal surfaces. Sections of the terminal structures of the two former mycoplasmas may exhibit a dense rod-like core when viewed by electron microscopy.

The mycoplasma cell is limited by a membrane, 7.5–10 nm wide, in which two electron-dense layers are separated by a translucent one (Fig. 42.3). Some species have an extramembranous layer which, in the case of *M. mycoides* ssp. *mycoides*, for example, comprises galactan and has a dense capsular appearance. Some others, e.g. *M. gallisepticum*, *M. genitalium*, *M. pneumoniae*, *M. pulmonis* and *Spiroplasma citri*, have surface spikes (sometimes described as a 'nap'), somewhat coarser than those seen on myxoviruses, which may contribute, through adhesin proteins, to attachment to eukaryotic cells. *M. gallisepticum*, *M. genitalium* and *M. pneumoniae* attach to neuraminic acid receptors. Close adherence enables the mycoplasma to insert nucleases and other enzymes into the cell and to take from it the products of enzyme action, such as nucleotides. Adherence to erythrocytes (*haemadsorption*), tissue culture cells, spermatozoa and other eukaryotic cells may be demonstrated with certain mycoplasmas (Fig. 42.4).

The electron-lucent part of the membrane comprises lipids with the long chains of the fatty acids arranged inwards and polar groups to the external

**Fig. 42.2** Electron micrograph of *M. genitalium* (human origin), negatively stained, to show flask-shaped appearance and terminal specialized structure covered by extracellular 'nap'. ×120 000. (From Tully et al 1983 *International Journal of Systematic Bacteriology* 33: 387.)

**Fig. 42.3** Electron micrograph of *M. pulmonis* (murine origin); thin section illustrating trilaminar membrane (arrow). ×75 000

transport mechanisms. Cholesterol, or carotenoid/ carotenol, is interspersed between the phospholipid molecules and plays an important part in maintaining membrane integrity in the face of varying external osmotic pressures and in the absence of the rigid cell wall that is found in bacteria. However, the presence of cholesterol renders the cell membrane susceptible to damage with agents like saponin, digitonin and some polyene antibiotics (filipin, amphotericin B) that complex with sterols. As expected, mycoplasmas are completely resistant to antibiotics that act on bacterial cell wall synthesis and also to lysozyme.

The cytoplasm of mycoplasmas does not contain endoplasmic reticulum but it is packed with ribosomes; nuclear material (unbounded without nucleoli) in fibrillar form (3 nm thick) is centrally placed or dispersed. The ribosomes have a sedimentation coefficient of about 70S and protein synthesis is inhibited by antibiotics such as tetracyclines, aminoglycosides, erythromycin and chloramphenicol.

The genome of *M. genitalium* has been fully sequenced and is not much larger than that of a large poxvirus, an indication of the small amount of genetic information needed for a free-living existence and the reason why mycoplasmas have a paucity of biochemical activity and are nutritionally fastidious.

and internal parts of the organisms; the electron-dense layers consist of protein and carbohydrate. The mycoplasma membrane is the site of many metabolic reactions involving membrane-bound enzymes and

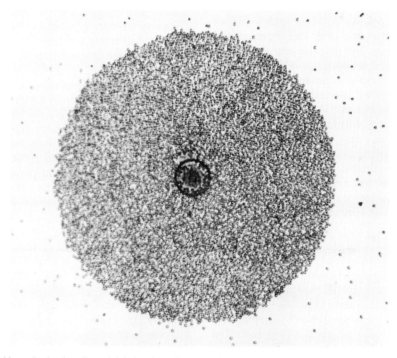

**Fig. 42.4** Colony of *M. agalactiae* (caprine origin) showing adherent guinea-pig erythrocytes (phenomenon of haemadsorption).

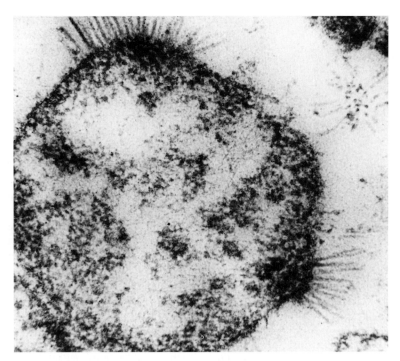

**Fig. 42.5**  Rod-shaped virus particles (75 × 7.5 nm) radiating from the surface of an *A. laidlawii cell.* ×100 000.

## *Viruses and plasmids*

Fourteen viruses have been identified: six in *Acholeplasma*, four in *Mycoplasma* and four in *Spiroplasma* species. They are rod-shaped (Fig. 42.5) or enveloped spheres that bud from the mycoplasma membrane surface, or are polyhedral with a tail. Those that have been examined in detail contain single- or double-stranded DNA in either a circular or linear form. There is evidence for integration of the viral genome into the mycoplasmal chromosome, especially in spiroplasmas, and this may provide a mechanism for the promotion of genetic diversity. The release of the viruses is continuous and not accompanied by cell lysis. Plasmids, so far regarded as cryptic, have been detected in *Acholeplasma*, *Mycoplasma* and, most frequently, *Spiroplasma* species.

## Cultivation

Mycoplasmas have limited biosynthetic abilities, so that they need a rich growth medium containing natural animal protein (usually blood serum) and, in most cases, a sterol component. Serum supplies not only cholesterol but also saturated and unsaturated fatty acids for membrane synthesis, components that the organisms cannot synthesize. A widely used isolation medium contains bovine heart infusion (PPLO broth) with fresh yeast extract and horse serum. However, these components vary in their ability to support growth and success may depend on use of different batches of the components, sera from other animal species, or the addition of various supplements.

Cultivation of spiroplasmas is more difficult. The development of a medium designated SP-4 has been helpful in the isolation of spiroplasmas as well as *M. genitalium* and other fastidious mycoplasmas. Although various specific formulations have been described for isolation of ureaplasmas, most mycoplasma media are suitable. The sterol-independent organisms also grow readily on these media but serum, which often promotes growth, is not usually essential.

Mycoplasmas are grown in fluid media and on the same media solidified with agar. Incorporation of an appropriate substrate (glucose, arginine or urea) and a pH indicator (e.g. phenol red) and observance of a colour change in fluid media aids the detection of mycoplasmal growth. Most mycoplasmas are facultatively anaerobic but, since organisms from primary tissue specimens frequently grow only under anaerobic conditions, an atmosphere of 95% nitrogen and 5% carbon dioxide is preferred for primary isolation. Continued propagation sometimes requires quite stringent anaerobic conditions and, of course, these are needed for *Anaeroplasma* species. The optimum temperature for most mycoplasmas and ureaplasmas from humans or animals is 36–38°C, but is lower for acholeplasmas and spiroplasmas.

## Colonial morphology

On agar, mycoplasmas produce colonies that have a 'fried egg' appearance, with an opaque central zone of growth within the agar and a translucent peripheral zone on the surface (Fig. 42.6). The size of the colonies varies widely: colonies of some bovine mycoplasmas and most acholeplasmas may exceed 2 mm in diameter, and are easily visible to the naked eye, whereas those of the ureaplasmas are characteristically small (15–60 μm in diameter) because they usually lack the peripheral zone of growth. Size and appearance also depend on the constituents and degree of hydration of the medium, the agar concentration, atmospheric condition and age of the culture.

## Biochemical reactions

Mycoplasmas use either glucose (and some other carbohydrates) or arginine as a major source of energy;

a few use both, and others do not metabolize either substrate. In most mycoplasmas the respiratory pathways are flavin terminated so that the haem compounds, cytochromes and catalase, are absent. The distinctive feature of ureaplasmas is the conversion of urea to ammonia by urease. The various biochemical reactions are used to detect mycoplasmas and as a first step in identification and classification (see below).

*Mycoplasma*, *Ureaplasma*, *Entomoplasma* and *Anaeroplasma* species depend on sterol. They fail to grow in serum-free media and are inhibited by digitonin, distinguishing them from the species that do not require sterol. In addition, most *Mycoplasma* species and ureaplasmas produce hydrogen peroxide, which causes some lysis of guinea-pig or other erythrocytes when these are suspended in agar over developing colonies. *M. pneumoniae* produces clear zones of β-haemolysis. About one-third of all *Mycoplasma* species exhibit haemadsorption (see Fig. 42.4).

## Antigenic properties

DNA analysis has made a fundamental contribution to the taxonomy of mycoplasmas. Nevertheless,

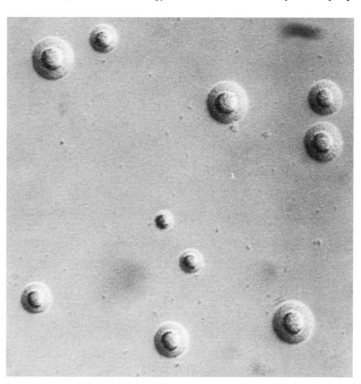

**Fig. 42.6** Colonies of *M. hominis* (human origin) (up to 110 μm in diameter) with typical 'fried egg' appearance. Oblique illumination. ×150.

identification and species classification still rest largely on antibody responses to mycoplasmas, which in turn reflect their antigenic composition. The Western blot technique is useful in assessing the importance of particular antigens, but examination of specific antisera by gel diffusion and immuno-electrophoresis techniques is important for studying the antigenic structure of mycoplasmas and the relationships between them. For sero-epidemiological studies and for serological diagnosis, more sensitive tests, such as indirect haemagglutination, an enzyme-linked immunosorbent assay (ELISA) and micro-immunofluorescence, are used.

The way in which different antigens function is exemplified by considering *M. pneumoniae*. The glucose- and galactose-containing membrane glycolipids of the organism are haptens, which are antigenic only when bound to membrane protein. They induce antibodies that react in complement fixation, metabolism inhibition and growth inhibition tests. Glycolipids with fortuitously similar structure have been found in the human brain. Their cross-reactivity with antibodies to *M. pneumoniae* could account for the neurological manifestations of *M. pneumoniae* infection (see below). Furthermore, the ability of the organisms to alter the I antigen on erythrocytes sufficiently to stimulate anti-I antibodies (*cold agglutinins*) leads to an auto-immune response and damage to erythrocytes. *M. pneumoniae* has two major surface proteins, including the P1 protein involved in attachment, which are recognized by the host; antibody to them is detected in convalescent sera and in respiratory secretions. Variation in the P1 protein has led to the recognition of two subtypes of strains which may vary epidemiologically and in pathogenicity.

Variable membrane lipoproteins of several mycoplasmas form an antigenic variation system providing a means of escaping from the host immune response; the variations are restricted to a small number of protein antigens and do not appear to alter the total cell protein profiles of the organisms.

## PATHOGENESIS

Thirteen species in the genus *Mycoplasma*, two in the genus *Acholeplasma* and one in the genus *Ureaplasma* have been isolated from humans (Table 42.1), mostly from the oropharynx. Five unequivocally cause disease, or are strongly associated with disease: *M. fermentans*,

**Table 42.1**  Some properties of mycoplasmas of human origin

| Mycoplasma | Frequency of detection in | | Metabolism of | Preferred pH of medium | Haemadsorption (chick red blood cells) |
|---|---|---|---|---|---|
| | Respiratory tract | Urogenital tract | | | |
| *M. buccale* | Rare | Not reported | Arginine | 7.0 | − |
| *M. faucium* | Rare | Not reported | Arginine | 7.0 | + |
| *M. fermentans* | Common | Rare | Glucose and arginine | 7.5 | − |
| *M. genitalium* | Rare | Rare[a] | Glucose | 7.5 | + |
| *M. hominis* | Rare | Common | Arginine | 7.0 | − |
| *A. laidlawii* | Rare | Not reported | Glucose | 7.5 | − |
| *M. lipophilum* | Rare | Not reported | Arginine | 7.0 | − |
| *A. oculi* | ? | Not reported | Glucose | 7.5 | − |
| *M. orale* | Common | Not reported | Arginine | 7.0 | + |
| *M. penetrans* | Not reported | Rare | Glucose and arginine | 7.5 | + |
| *M. pirum* | Not reported | ? | Glucose and arginine | 7.5 | ? |
| *M. pneumoniae* | Rare[a] | Very rare | Glucose | 7.5 | + |
| *M. primatum* | Not reported | Rare | Arginine | 7.0 | − |
| *M. salivarium* | Common | Rare | Arginine | 7.0 | − |
| *M. spermatophilum* | Not reported | Rare | Arginine | 7.0 | − |
| *U. urealyticum* | Rare | Common | Urea | ≤ 6.0 | +[b] |

[a]Rare, except in disease.
[b]Serotype 3 only.

*M. genitalium*, *M. hominis*, *M. pneumoniae* and *U. urealyticum*.

## Respiratory infections

### Mycoplasma pneumonia

Pneumonias not attributable to any of the common bacterial causes were labelled historically as *primary atypical pneumonias*. In one variety associated with the development of cold agglutinins, a filterable micro-organism, first called the *Eaton agent*, was isolated in embryonated eggs. Serious doubts about the possibility of the agent being a virus arose when its growth was found to be inhibited by chlortetracycline and gold salts, and cultivation on cell-free medium in the early 1960s finally clinched its mycoplasmal nature. The organism was subsequently named *M. pneumoniae*, and its importance as a cause of respiratory disease was confirmed by numerous studies based on isolation, serology, volunteer inoculation, and vaccine protection.

***Epidemiology.*** Infection occurs world-wide. Although endemic in most areas, there is a preponderance of infection in late summer and early autumn in temperate climates; in some countries, such as the UK, epidemic peaks have been observed about every 4 years. Spread is fostered by close contact, e.g. in a family. Overall, *M. pneumoniae* may cause only about one-sixth of all cases of pneumonia, but in certain populations, such as military recruits, it has been responsible for almost half the cases of pneumonia. Children are infected more often than adults, and the consequence of infection is also influenced by age. Thus, in school-aged children and teenagers, about a quarter of infections culminate in pneumonia, whereas, in young adults, fewer than 10% do so. Thereafter, pneumonia is even less frequent, but severity tends to increase with the age of the patient.

***Clinical features.*** Infections often have an insidious onset with malaise, myalgia, sore throat or headache overshadowing and preceding chest symptoms by 1–5 days. Cough, which starts around the 3rd day, is characteristically dry, troublesome and sometimes paroxysmal, and becomes a prominent feature. However, patients usually do not appear seriously ill and few warrant admission to hospital. Physical signs, such as rales, become apparent, frequently after radiographic evidence of pneumonia. Most often this amounts to patchy opacities, usually of one of the lower or middle lobes. About 20% of patients suffer bilateral pneumonia, but pleurisy and pleural effusions are unusual. The course of the

disease is variable, but cough, abnormal chest signs, and radiographic changes may extend over several weeks and relapse is a feature. A prolonged paroxysmal cough simulating the features of whooping cough may occur in children. Very severe infections have been reported in adults, usually in those with immunodeficiency or sickle cell anaemia, although death is rare.

Disease is limited usually to the respiratory tract. Extrapulmonary manifestations include: the Stevens–Johnson syndrome and other rashes; arthralgia; meningitis or encephalitis (and other neurological sequelae); haemolytic anaemia; myocarditis; and pericarditis. Haemolytic anaemia with crisis is an auto-immune phenomenon brought about by cold agglutinins (anti-I antibodies). Some of the other complications, such as the neurological ones, may arise in a similar indirect way, although *M. pneumoniae* has been isolated from cerebrospinal fluid.

***Laboratory diagnosis.*** Because the clinical manifestations are not sufficiently distinct for definitive diagnosis, laboratory help is required. A non-specific (cold agglutinin) or, more often, a specific (usually complement fixation) serological test is relied upon in routine practice. A four-fold or greater rise in antibody titre in either test, with a peak at about 3–4 weeks, is indicative of a recent infection. The cold agglutinin test is less sensitive than the complement fixation test, which enables a rise to be detected in about 80% of cases. Neither test is completely specific; cross-reactivity with *M. genitalium* may be a problem with the complement fixation test. Western blotting may be used to check specificity in dubious cases. Because paired sera are not always available, a single antibody titre of 64 or more with either test, in a suggestive clinical setting, should be sufficient to institute therapy.

Attempted isolation of *M. pneumoniae* (and *M. fermentans*) requires the use of mycoplasmal broth supplemented with penicillin and glucose, and with phenol red as a pH indicator. After inoculation with sputum, throat washing, pharyngeal swab, or other specimen, the fluid medium is incubated at 37°C, and a colour change (red to yellow), which may take up to 3 weeks or longer, indicates fermentation of glucose due to multiplication of the organisms. The broth is then subcultured on agar medium for specific identification by growth inhibition or immunofluorescence techniques.

Isolation is not often attempted because of the time required. However, the polymerase chain reaction (PCR) assay is rapid, sensitive and specific. If an isolate is required, a sensible approach is to test specimens by both the PCR assay and culture and to continue the latter only for those specimens that prove to be PCR-positive.

Diagnostic procedures for the other mycoplasmas that might be found in the respiratory tract are considered under urogenital infections.

***Treatment***. *M. pneumoniae*, like other mycoplasmas, is most sensitive to the tetracyclines in vitro, but is more sensitive to erythromycin than some of the other mycoplasmas of human origin. In practice these antibiotics have proved less effective for treating pneumonia than they have in planned trials, probably because disease is often well established before treatment begins. Nevertheless, it is worthwhile administering a tetracycline to adults and erythromycin to children and pregnant women. The newer macrolides, such as clarithromycin and azithromycin and the newer quinolones are at least as active in vitro, and quinolones may have some cidal effect. Failure to kill the organisms probably explains persistence in the respiratory tract long after clinical recovery as well as relapse in some patients. Furthermore, a functioning immune system is important in eradication so that in some hypogammaglobulinaemic patients the organisms may persist for months or years.

Antibiotic treatment of *M. pneumoniae* or other mycoplasma-induced infection should start as soon as possible, based on clinical suspicion rather than waiting for laboratory confirmation, and a 3 week course is justified, particularly if supported by serological or other evidence of infection.

## Respiratory infection in the newborn

*M. hominis* and ureaplasmas occasionally cause respiratory disease in the newborn, particularly in those of very low birth weight, the infections often being acquired in utero. The likelihood of death or chronic lung disease in infants of less than 1000 g with a ureaplasmal respiratory tract infection within 24 h of birth is double that of uninfected infants of similar birth weight, or heavier infants.

## Other respiratory infections

*M. hominis* produces sore throats when given orally to adult volunteers; however, it does not seem to cause naturally occurring sore throats in children or adults. Recent observations suggest that *M. fermentans* is associated more with the respiratory tract than, as previously thought, with the urogenital tract. By use of the PCR it has been found in the throat and has been associated with adult respiratory distress syndrome with or without systemic disease, and with

pneumonia in a few children with community-acquired disease. *M. genitalium* has been isolated, together with *M. pneumoniae*, from the respiratory secretions of a few adults but its role, if any, in respiratory disease seems small.

# Urogenital infections

*M. fermentans*, *M. genitalium*, *M. hominis*, *M. penetrans*, *M. pneumoniae*, *M. primatum*, *M. salivarium*, *M. spermatophilum* and *U. urealyticum* have been isolated from the urogenital tract; *M. hominis* and ureaplasmas occur most frequently.

## Urogenital infections in men

Although *M. hominis* may be isolated from about 20% of patients with non-gonococcal urethritis (NGU), it has not been incriminated as a cause. On the other hand, there is some evidence to implicate ureaplasmas as one cause of non-chlamydial acute NGU. The proportion of cases for which ureaplasmas may be responsible is unclear, but their occurrence in the urethra of asymptomatic men suggests that only certain serotypes are pathogenic or that predisposing factors, such as impaired mucosal immunity, exist in those who develop disease. *M. genitalium* has also been implicated in acute and chronic NGU, but there is no evidence that this or other mycoplasmas are a cause of acute or chronic prostatitis. *M. genitalium* has not been sought in epididymitis, but there is evidence that ureaplasmas may occasionally cause the disease. It is not thought that ureaplasmas are a cause of male infertility.

## Urinary infection and calculi

*M. hominis* has been isolated from the upper urinary tract of patients with acute pyelonephritis and probably causes about 5% of such cases. Ureaplasmas do not seem to be involved in pyelonephritis. However, the fact that they produce urease, induce crystallization of struvite and calcium phosphates in urine in vitro and produce calculi experimentally in animal models raises the question of whether they cause calculi in the human urinary tract. Ureaplasmas are found more often in the urine and calculi of patients with infective stones than in those with metabolic stones, suggesting that they may have a causal role.

## Reproductive tract disease in women

*M. hominis* organisms and, to a lesser extent, ureaplasmas are found in much larger numbers in the vagina of women who have bacterial vaginosis than in healthy women and, with various bacteria, may contribute to the condition. However, evidence that ureaplasmas alone contribute to the development of the urethral syndrome is weak.

Bacterial vaginosis, and hence the bacteria associated with it, may lead to pelvic inflammatory disease (PID). M. hominis has been isolated from the endometrium and fallopian tubes of about 10% of women with PID, together with a specific antibody response. However, its significance is difficult to judge when several micro-organisms are present. Ureaplasmas have also been isolated directly from affected fallopian tubes, but the absence of antibody responses and failure to produce salpingitis in subhuman primates make them an even less likely cause of disease at this site.

The pathogenic potential of M. genitalium is greater; antibody responses in some patients with PID and the production of salpingitis in subhuman primates suggest that it may have an important role.

The minor part that M. hominis plays in PID makes its role, if any, in infertility as a result of tubal damage inevitably small. The suggestion that ureaplasmas might cause involuntary infertility, or affect sperm, remains speculative.

## Diseases associated with pregnancy and the newborn

M. hominis and ureaplasmas have been isolated from the amniotic fluid of women with severe chorio-amnionitis who had preterm labour. Similarly, ureaplasmas have been isolated from spontaneously aborted fetuses and stillborn or premature infants more frequently than from induced abortions or normal full-term infants. Isolation of ureaplasmas from the internal organs of aborted fetuses, together with some serological responses and an apparent diminished occurrence following antibiotic therapy, support a role for these organisms in abortion. However, bacterial vaginosis is strongly associated with preterm labour and late miscarriage and as M. hominis and ureaplasmas are part of the extensive microbial flora of bacterial vaginosis, it is possible that they do not act independently but as part of this flora. The same may be said about the role of genital mycoplasmas, particularly ureaplasmas, in causing low birth weight in otherwise normal infants. Bacterial vaginosis has been largely ignored in defining the association and a study in which women given erythromycin in the third trimester delivered larger babies than those given a placebo has not been confirmed in later trials. Although there is obvious

uncertainty surrounding this issue, premature infants are prone to meningitis caused by M. hominis or ureaplasmas within the first few days of life.

After an abortion, M. hominis has been isolated, apparently in pure culture, from the blood of about 10% of febrile women; half of them exhibit an antibody response. The organism was not found in the blood of aborting afebrile women, or normal pregnant women, although it has been recovered from the blood of about 5–10% of women with postpartum fever. Similar observations have been made for ureaplasmas and it seems that both micro-organisms induce fever by causing endometritis.

## Laboratory diagnosis of urogenital infections

Material from urethral, cervical or vaginal swabs or centrifuged deposit from urine is added to separate vials of liquid mycoplasmal medium containing phenol red and 0.1% glucose, arginine or urea. M. genitalium metabolizes glucose and changes the colour of the medium from red to yellow. M. fermentans additionally, converts arginine to ammonia, as do M. hominis and M. primatum. The ureaplasmal urease also breaks down urea to ammonia. In each case, the pH of the medium increases, and there is a colour change from yellow to red. The colour change produced by ureaplasmas occurs usually within 1–2 days, that caused by M. hominis well within a week, while that for M. genitalium may take a month or longer or not occur at all. Subculture to agar medium results usually in the formation of characteristic colonies. On ordinary blood agar, M. hominis, but not ureaplasmas, produces non-haemolytic pinpoint colonies. M. hominis also multiplies in most routine blood culture media; the inhibitory effect of sodium polyanethol sulphonate, included as an anticoagulant, can be overcome by the addition of gelatin (1% w/v). Serological tests are used for definitive identification. Kits designed to isolate and identify ureaplasmas and M. hominis are available commercially and are of particular value if the need to detect these micro-organisms arises infrequently.

DNA primers specific for M. fermentans, M. genitalium and U. urealyticum have been developed and used for amplification by the PCR. This technique is much more sensitive than culture for detecting the two former mycoplasmas.

Genital mycoplasmal infections stimulate antibody responses, but the various techniques to detect them are rarely used diagnostically.

## Treatment of urogenital infections

Treatment must take into account the fact that several different micro-organisms may be involved and that a precise microbiological diagnosis may not be attainable. Patients with NGU should receive one of the tetracyclines which inhibit chlamydiae, ureaplasmas and *M. genitalium*. However, at least 10% of ureaplasmas are resistant to tetracyclines, and patients who fail to respond to such therapy should then be treated with erythromycin, to which most tetracycline-resistant ureaplasmas are sensitive. A tetracycline should also be included for the treatment of PID to cover chlamydiae and *M. hominis*. However, since about 20% of *M. hominis* strains are resistant to tetracyclines, other antibiotics, such as lincomycin or clindamycin, may need to be considered. Azithromycin, which is being used increasingly for chlamydial infections, is also active against a wide range of mycoplasmas. Fever following abortion or childbirth often settles within a few days but if it does not, tetracycline therapy should be started, while keeping tetracycline resistance in mind.

## Joint infections

There is evidence that ureaplasmas are involved in the aetiology of sexually acquired reactive arthritis based on synovial fluid mononuclear cell proliferation in response to specific ureaplasmal antigens. They also have a role in arthritis in hypogammaglobulinaemic patients (see below). There are isolated reports of *M. genitalium*, detected by a PCR assay, in the joints of patients with Reiter's disease and rheumatoid arthritis. *M. fermentans* has been found by a PCR assay in the joints of 21% of patients with rheumatoid arthritis and in those of patients with other inflammatory rheumatic disorders.

## Infections in immunocompromised patients

*M. pneumoniae* may cause severe pneumonia in immunodeficient patients and may persist for many months in the respiratory tract of hypogammaglobulinaemic patients, despite apparently adequate treatment. A few hypogammaglobulinaemic patients develop suppurative arthritis, and mycoplasmas are responsible for at least two-fifths of the cases. The mycoplasmas involved have been *M. pneumoniae*, *M. salivarium* (usually regarded as non-pathogenic), *M. hominis* and, particularly, ureaplasmas. In some cases involving ureaplasmas, the arthritis has been associated with subcutaneous abscesses, persistent urethritis, and chronic cystitis. Although responding sometimes to tetracyclines, the organisms and disease may persist for many months despite concomitant use of anti-inflammatory and γ-globulin replacement

therapy. Administration of specific mycoplasmal anti-serum prepared in an animal (e.g. the sheep or rabbit) may aid clinical and microbiological recovery.

Septicaemia due to *M. hominis* has occurred after trauma and genito-urinary manipulations, and the mycoplasma has been found in brain abscesses and osteomyelitis. Haematogenous spread leading to septic arthritis, surgical wound infections and peritonitis seems to occur more often after organ transplantation and in other patients on immunosuppressive therapy. Particularly common are sternal wound infections caused by *M. hominis* in heart and lung transplant patients.

It has been suggested that infection of human immunodeficiency virus (HIV)-positive subjects with *M. fermentans* might lead to more rapid development of the acquired immune deficiency syndrome, and that *M. penetrans* is associated uniquely with HIV-positivity and possibly with Kaposi's sarcoma. However, convincing evidence has not been forthcoming.

## MYCOPLASMAS AND CELL CULTURES

Only about 1% of primary cell cultures become infected with mycoplasmas, but continuous cell lines do so frequently. The mycoplasmas currently most responsible are *M. arginini*, *M. fermentans*, *M hyorhinis*, *M. orale*, *M. salivarium* and *A. laidlawii*. The effects of contamination include those caused by mycoplasmal enzymes and toxins, and those resulting from the use of media components, or from changes in pH. Despite the presence of up to $10^8$ organisms per millilitre of culture fluid, there may be little effect on viral propagation, although it may decrease the yield. Occasionally, the yield may be increased as, for example, with vaccinia virus in *M. hominis*-infected cells.

Culture and an indicator cell system with staining (e.g. Hoechst DNA dye) are used to detect contamination, but these may be superseded by PCR methods. Numerous procedures have been described to eliminate mycoplasmas from cell cultures, but none is consistently successful. Whenever possible it is easier to discard the cultures, replace them with mycoplasma-free cells and adhere to simple guidelines to prevent contamination. If it is imperative to save cells, treatment with an antibiotic that is likely to have mycoplasmacidal activity, such as a fluoroquinolone, identification of the contaminant and use of a specific antiserum, or a combination of these methods is most likely to be successful.

## RECOMMENDED READING

Barile M F, Razin S (eds) 1979 *The Mycoplasmas. Cell Biology.* Academic Press, New York, vol 1

Cassell G H (ed) 1986 Ureaplasmas of humans: with emphasis upon maternal and neonatal infections. *Pediatric Infectious Disease* 5(suppl): S221–S354

Furr P M, Taylor-Robinson D, Webster A D B 1994 Mycoplasmas and ureaplasmas in patients with hypogammaglobulinaemia and their role in arthritis: microbiological observations over 20 years. *Annals of the Rheumatic Diseases* 53: 183–187

Glatt A E, McCormack W M, Taylor-Robinson D 1990 The genital mycoplasmas. In: Holmes K K, Mårdh P-A, Sparling P F, Wiesner P J (eds) *Sexually Transmitted Diseases*, 2nd edn. McGraw Hill, New York, p 279

Maniloff J, McElhaney R N, Finch L R, Baseman J B (eds) 1992 *Mycoplasmas. Molecular Biology and Pathogenesis.* American Society for Microbiology, Washington, DC

Mårdh P-A, Møller B R, McCormack W M (eds) 1983 *Mycoplasma hominis* – a human pathogen. *Sexually Transmitted Diseases* 10(suppl)

Razin S, Barile M F (eds) 1985 *The Mycoplasmas. Mycoplasma Pathogenicity.* Academic Press, New York, vol 4

Razin S, Tully J G (eds) 1995 *Molecular and Diagnostic Procedures in Mycoplasmology. Molecular Characterization.* Academic Press, London, vol 1

Symposium 1993 The changing role of mycoplasmas in respiratory disease and AIDS. *Clinical Infectious Diseases* 17(suppl 1)

Taylor-Robinson D 1995 The history and role of *Mycoplasma genitalium* in sexually transmitted diseases. *Genitourinary Medicine* 71: 1–8

Taylor-Robinson D 1995 *Mycoplasma* and *Ureaplasma.* In: Murray P R, Baron E, Pfaller M A, Tenover F C, Yolken R H (eds) *Manual of Clinical Microbiology*, 6th edn. American Society for Microbiology, Washington, DC

Taylor-Robinson D 1996 Mycoplasmas and their role in human respiratory tract disease. In: Myint S, Taylor-Robinson D (eds) *Viral and Other Infections of the Human Respiratory Tract.* Chapman and Hall, London, p 319

Taylor-Robinson D, McCormack W M 1980 The genital mycoplasmas. *New England Journal of Medicine* 302: 1003–1010, 1063–1067

Tully J G, Razin S (eds) 1996 *Molecular and Diagnostic Procedures in Mycoplasmology. Diagnostic Procedures.* Academic Press, London, vol 2

Tully J G, Whitcomb R F (eds) 1979 *The Mycoplasmas. Human and Animal Mycoplasmas.* Academic Press, New York, vol 2

# Part 4

# VIRAL PATHOGENS AND ASSOCIATED DISEASES

# 43

# Adenoviruses

**Respiratory disease; conjunctivitis; gut infections**

*C. R. Madeley and J. S. M. Peiris*

Adenoviruses have been described as the weeds in the virological garden; always present, not valued for themselves, sometimes decorative and felt to be of only limited interest to serious clinical virologists. As all gardeners will know, a plant is only a weed if it is in the wrong place, and much of the interest in a wild area is provided by 'weeds'. They can also be valued for themselves and, with increasing doubts that viruses are always pathogens, the epidemiology of adenoviruses is becoming of greater interest.

They were named from their original source, *adenoid tissue* removed at operation and cultured as explants in vitro. Cellular outgrowth occurred readily, but this often deteriorated rapidly a week or 10 days later. The cause of the deterioration was found to be *adenovirus(es)* present in the original tissue and which replicated enthusiastically in the new cells growing from the explant.

This discovery initiated much research which established that there were a considerable number of serotypes, or species, and that they were mostly associated with mild *upper respiratory tract infections*. In addition, there were occasional serious (and even fatal) childhood *pneumonias* and infrequent *eye infections*. Some of these infections, mostly in children and not always symptomatic, could persist for weeks or months. The focus of adenovirus research then shifted away from clinical virology with the discovery that some species could cause malignancies in laboratory rodents. As a result, virologists have thoroughly investigated adenovirus structure, replicative mechanisms and oncogenicity during the last 25 years.

Clinical interest revived in the middle 1970s with the discovery of two new serotypes (subsequently numbered types 40 and 41) linked (with several other previously unknown viruses) to that previously elusive entity '*viral gastroenteritis*'. This revival of clinical interest has now been extended by the discovery in rapid succession of six new serotypes (numbered 42–47), most of them in patients with acquired

immunodeficiency syndrome (AIDS). This was unexpected, the more so because it is only rarely that adenoviruses have been noted as opportunist invaders of immunosuppressed patients. Why they do not exploit more the vulnerability of these patients is unknown at present. Although they may be present in the stools of congenitally immunodeficient children, adenoviruses rarely damage their human hosts seriously, but their activities and epidemiology should have important lessons for medicine, and investigations into their interactions with our immune mechanisms are overdue. This last point is now very relevant because the use of adenoviruses as vectors in gene therapy is being explored. They are able to carry a DNA insert of up to 7 kb, but using a virus capable of replicating (and therefore of inducing an immune response) presents practical difficulties yet to be overcome.

## DESCRIPTION

Adenovirus virions provide a very good example of an *icosahedron*. Figure 43.1a shows a group of typical adenovirus particles while Figure 43.1b and c compare a single virus particle, as seen in the electron microscope, with a model. The particles in Figure 43.1a lack the fibres projecting from the apices (they are rarely seen in situ in the electron microscope) but otherwise the particles in Figure 43.1a and b resemble the model closely. Indeed, the adenovirus is one of the few viruses of which a convincing model can be made.

The virion is 70–75 nm in size, depending on whether it is measured across the 'flats' or the apices, and there are probably minor variations between preparations and, possibly, serotypes. The surface has 252 visible surface knobs, the capsomers: 12 apical capsomers, each surrounded by five others, are known as *pentons*; 60 peripentons surround the

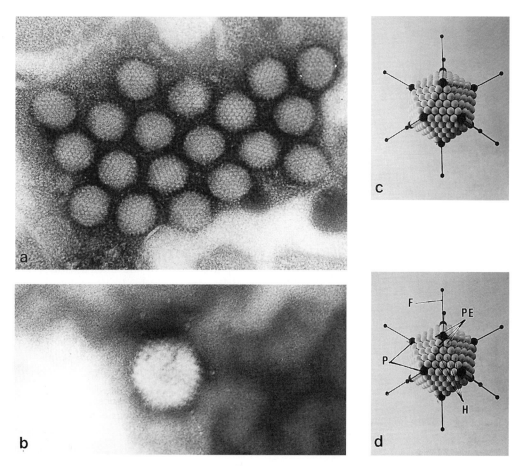

**Fig. 43.1**  **a** Group of adenovirus particles from a stool extract. These show the typical adenovirus morphology, although apical fibres are not visible. Individual capsomers are visible as surface 'knobs'. These particles should be compared with the model seen in **c**. Negative contrast, 3% potassium phosphotungstate, pH 7.0 ×160 000. **b** Single adenovirus particle showing some of the apical fibres. This is an uncommon finding. Negative contrast, 3% potassium phosphotungstate, pH 7.0 ×280 000. **c** Photograph of a model of an adenovirus for comparison with the electron micrograph. **d** The same model with pentons (P), peripentons (PE) and hexons (H) indicated. Note that the fibres (F) are attached to the penton.

pentons and 180 other capsomers make up the major part of the faces (Fig. 43.1d). Except for the pentons, all the other capsomers are surrounded by six others, and are therefore called *hexons*, while the apical capsomers are called pentons by the same logic.

From each penton projects an apical *fibre*. The fibres vary greatly in length between 9 and 31 nm. Collapse of particles on storage or on exposure to some negative stains can release visible fibres in large amounts. Some avian types have double fibres but human strains all have single ones.

Adenoviruses contain a single piece of double-stranded DNA 33–45 kb in size which codes for a considerable number of proteins with molecular weights between 7500 and 400 000. They include both structural and non-structural proteins. The 10

structural ones include three polypeptides which make up each hexon, one which forms the penton base and a glycoprotein for the fibre. These five lie on the surface of the particle while the others are internal.

The pentons and fibres bear antigenic determinants that are 'type' specific, and antibody binding to them results in neutralization of virus infectivity. The hexons also have some type-specific antigenic determinants, but carry group-specific antigens as well. The same group antigens are found on all the mastadenoviruses (see below), the genus to which the medically important human adenoviruses belong. These group-specific antigens provide a basis for tests to detect adenoviruses and antibodies to them (by immunofluorescence, enzyme immuno-assays, complement fixation, etc. – see below).

## Classification

The family Adenoviridae comprises two genera:

1. *Mastadenovirus*, whose members infect mammalian species, including humans
2. *Aviadenovirus*, whose members infect avian species.

The two genera are completely distinct antigenically. Human adenoviruses are further subdivided into six subgenera (A–F) (Table 43.1), based on DNA homology. By definition, those with above 50% homology are members of the same subgenus, while those of different subgenera have below 20% homology.

Within each subgenus, adenovirus serotypes are defined by cross-reactivity in neutralization tests. There are 47 recognized serotypes of human adenoviruses at present, of which types 40–47 have only been recognized within the last 15 years. There may be more types yet to be discovered. Some virologists refer to species rather than serotypes, but most clinical virologists refer to serotypes, and this term will be used here.

## REPLICATION

The virus attaches to susceptible cells by the apical fibres and is then taken into the cell, losing both fibres and pentons in the process. It then passes to the nucleus, losing the peripentons at the nuclear membrane. Inside the nucleus the DNA is released and the process of replication initiated.

The first messenger RNAs (mRNAs) code for non-structural proteins which shut off most host cell activities while switching on the host cell DNA-dependent DNA polymerase, which is required to replicate viral DNA. About 20 of these 'early' proteins are produced, most of which are not incorporated in new particles (i.e. they are non-structural).

Following production of new viral DNA, the remaining genes are transcribed from it to form 'late' proteins. These are produced in quantity in the cytoplasm, are mostly structural and are later transported back to the nucleus where new virus particles are assembled, normally as crystalline arrays. They are assembled on a scaffold protein, initially as empty shells into which the nucleic acid is inserted afterwards. The effects of the shutting down of the host cell metabolism and the accumulation of thousands of new virions results in rupture (lysis) and death of the infected cell with release of the particles.

In cell cultures this process causes the cells to round up, swell and aggregate into clumps resembling bunches of grapes. The cells then disintegrate as they lyse.

**Table 43.1** Properties and classification of adenoviruses of subgenera A–F

| Subgenus[a] | Serotypes | No. of small fragments[b] | Haemagglutination pattern[c] | Oncogenicity in newborn hamsters | Tissues most commonly infected |
|---|---|---|---|---|---|
| A | 12, 18, 31 | 4–5 | IV | High | Gut (no symptoms) |
| B | 3, 7, 11, 14, 16, 21, 34, 35 | 8–10 | I | Low | Respiratory tract Kidney |
| C | 1, 2, 5, 6 | 10–12 | III | None | Respiratory tract Lymphoid tissue (tonsils and adenoids) |
| D | 8, 9, 10, 13, 15, 17, 19, 20, 22–30, 32, 33, 36–39, 42–47 | 14–18 | II | None | Conjunctiva Gut Respiratory tract (?) |
| E | 4 | 16–19 | III | None | Conjunctiva Respiratory tract |
| F | 40, 41 | 9–12 | IV | None | Gut |

[a] >50% DNA homology between members.
[b] Restriction endonuclease digestion. Some small fragments probably not included.
[c] I, complete agglutination of monkey erythrocytes; II, complete agglutination of rat erythrocytes; III, partial agglutination of rat erythrocytes; IV, agglutination of rat erythrocytes only after addition of heterotypic serum

**Table 43.2** Disease associated with adenovirus serotypes

| Disease | Those at risk | Associated serotypes |
|---|---|---|
| Acute febrile pharyngitis | | |
|   Endemic | Infants, young children | 1, 2, 5, 6 |
|   Epidemic | Infants, young children | 3, 4, 7 |
| Pharyngoconjunctival fever | Older school-age children | 3, 7 |
| Acute respiratory disease | Military recruits | 4, 7, 14, 21 |
| Pneumonia | Infants | 1, 2, 3, 7 |
| Follicular conjunctivitis | Any age | 3, 4, 11 |
| Epidemic keratoconjunctivitis | Adults | 8, 19, 37 |
| Haemorrhagic cystitis | Infants, young children | 11, 21 |
| Diarrhoea and vomiting | Infants, young children | 40, 41 |
| Intussusception | Infants | 1, 2, 5 |
| Disseminated infection | Immunocompromised, e.g. AIDS, renal, bone marrow and heart–lung transplant recipients | 5, 34, 35, 43–47 |

# CLINICAL FEATURES

Table 43.2 lists the more common associations of serotypes with disease. However, this does not tell the whole story. On the one hand, the great majority of infections with adenoviruses are probably undiagnosed and the full extent of pathogenesis is not known. On the other hand, virus infection and replication is not invariably associated with disease. For example, a wide variety of serotypes are isolated from faeces without evidence of gut pathology, and prolonged tonsillar carriage in children is common. However, some well-recognized disease syndromes are caused by adenovirus infections.

## Respiratory disease

### In childhood

These are usually mild upper respiratory tract infections with fever, a runny nose and a cough. The majority are due to types 1–7, although higher serotypes may be involved sporadically. Types 1, 2, 5 and 6 are more commonly associated with endemic infections while types 3, 4 and 7 are more epidemic. In Newcastle upon Tyne, in the period March 1989 to March 1990, types 1, 2, 5 and 6 accounted for 71 of 103 adenovirus infections (69%), types 3, 4 and 7 for 12 (12%) and other types for 20 (20%). The associated clinical diagnoses included 'upper respiratory tract infection (URTI)', 'increased secretions', 'wheezy', 'cold and cough' and 'failure to thrive'.

These infections are rarely serious but, occasionally and unpredictably, may progress to a pneumonia which is both extensive and frequently fatal. The majority of these pneumonias occur in young children.

In older children and young adults a proportion of these will be labelled as 'colds' but epidemics of adenoviral infection with respiratory symptoms and fever are common in, for example, US military recruit camps, where violent exercise and close proximity combine to make the victims more vulnerable and facilitate spread. These outbreaks can be severe in both numbers and extent of disease; severe enough, in fact, to warrant preparation of a trial vaccine. Eye involvement is a common feature (see below), leading to such outbreaks being called pharyngoconjunctival fever. Types 3 and 7 are associated with these outbreaks but other serotypes are found from time to time.

Adenovirus infections are said to mimic whooping cough in some patients, and dual infections with *Bordetella pertussis* have been found. However, there is little doubt that genuine whooping cough is due to the bacterium.

## Eye infections

Adenoviruses have been associated with several outbreaks of conjunctivitis in the UK, frequently referred to as 'shipyard eye' because it was originally thought to be caused by steel swarf thrown up from welding and grinding. It was later shown that adenovirus was being transmitted through fluids, eyebaths and other instruments used to treat eye injuries in the shipyard first aid clinic and which had become contaminated by virus from the index case. Use of properly sterilized instruments and single-dose preparations of eye ointment have now made this uncommon. Most such outbreaks were due to adenovirus type 8 (although types 19 and 37 may also be involved). This is not one of the easiest types to isolate, and sporadic cases may not be identified as readily as outbreaks, which inevitably attract a more concentrated effort at diagnosis. Eye infections with type 8 do not usually cause systemic symptoms.

As indicated above, conjunctivitis caused by other serotypes may form part of outbreaks of pharyngo-conjunctival fever. It is a follicular conjunctivitis which resembles that due to chlamydiae, from which it should be differentiated, but the usual marked adenovirus respiratory symptoms provide a clue.

## Gut infections

The common respiratory serotypes (1–7) are frequently isolated from faeces, and, in young children, the same serotype may be recovered from both ends of the child. Despite some anecdotal reports there is little evidence to link such isolates with disease of the gut. However, when faecal extracts from children with diarrhoea were examined by electron microscopy, typical adenoviruses were seen in a proportion of cases, often in very large numbers. Surprisingly, these morphologically typical viruses could not be isolated in cell culture. It is now clear that these belonged to two hitherto unknown serotypes, 40 and 41. These are associated with a significant proportion of endemic cases of childhood diarrhoea and, in numbers of cases, are second only to rotaviruses. Estimates of the proportion vary between different laboratories but they may contribute up to a third of such cases in which a virus is found. As with other viruses found in diarrhoeal faeces, such adenoviruses may also be present less frequently in the faeces of apparently normal babies, but there is no doubt of their pathogenic potential for the gut. How they differ from the other non-pathogenic types in the gut is unknown, nor is it known whether they cause respiratory infections.

The role of adenovirus(es) in mesenteric adenitis and intussusception is uncertain. Even when the former is identified at laparotomy it is not usual to excise a node for diagnosis, and direct evidence is lacking. Finding a coincidental adenovirus in faeces is not proof of involvement, nor is it clear how often adenitis precedes (and possibly initiates) intussusception. Where any such temporal association has been recorded it has involved the common serotypes 1, 2, 5 and 6. Probably the appropriate verdict is the old Scots one of 'not proven'!

Six new serotypes (42–47) have been found, five of them (43–47) in the faeces of patients with AIDS. The sixth was isolated from the faeces of a normal child. Chronic diarrhoea is, in any case, a feature of AIDS and the role of these adenoviruses, if any, in causing it awaits further investigation. Interestingly, these new serotypes were isolated and identified in cell culture, suggesting they are indeed 'new'. If so, their origin and significance are both unknown.

## Other diseases

Infrequently there have been reports of adenovirus (types 11 and 21 mostly) recovered from the urine of children with haemorrhagic cystitis. Finding virus provides a (possible) retrospective cause.

There are reports in the literature of recovery of adenoviruses from both the male and the female genital tracts. They may be sexually transmitted but are not the cause of a major sexually transmitted disease.

There is no good evidence of adenoviruses being involved in central nervous system disease nor in human tumour production. Experimentally, adenoviruses may induce transformation of hamster cells in culture and such transformed cells will produce tumours in laboratory animals. There is no evidence that this can occur in humans although it has been diligently sought. Under laboratory conditions adenoviruses can also form hybrids with simian virus 40 (SV40), a papovavirus which contaminated early stocks of polio vaccine grown in monkey kidney cells. The hybrids, carrying part of the SV40 genome, are neither pathogenic nor oncogenic in humans.

## PATHOGENESIS

Adenoviruses are mostly infectors of mucosal surfaces (respiratory tract, gut and eye) but it is clear that by no means all such infection leads to overt disease. Different serotypes appear to prefer different regions. It is not known what this means at a molecular or cellular level but it may reflect the presence or absence of particular receptors. Infection of an individual cell will cause its death but several studies have documented prolonged respiratory and gut excretion in healthy children lasting weeks or months. Such respiratory 'carriage' is probably in lymphoid tissue (tonsils and adenoids) and gut carriage may be in the equivalent Peyer's patches, although this has not been documented.

Most infections with adenoviruses, whatever the primary site, probably spread to include the gut. 'Respiratory' strains are frequently recovered from faeces and it seems very improbable that this results solely from overflow from the upper respiratory tract. It is much more likely that faecal excretion follows a secondary gut infection, albeit asymptomatic in most cases.

The role of the five newly discovered serotypes (43–47) in patients with AIDS is not known at present. All were recovered from faeces by culture and had not been identified before. They extend the unanswered questions about adenoviruses to include where new types could come from and whether they can arise by mutation and/or recombination.

## LABORATORY DIAGNOSIS

### Direct demonstration of 'virus'

#### Electron microscopy

Virus particles may be seen directly in stool extracts by electron microscopy, although this will not identify serotypes. Nonetheless, where virus is seen this will usually be types 40 or 41, particularly where large numbers are present (the level may reach more than $10^{10}$ particles per gram of faeces). Finding virus in faeces by electron microscopy does not mean that virus must also be present in the nasopharynx or eye.

#### Virus antigen

The presence of viral antigen in the nasopharynx may be identified by immunofluorescence with group- specific antibodies (polyclonal or monoclonal) directly on aspirates (*not* swabs), provided they contain respiratory cells. The presence of such infected cells usually indicates a significant infection, in contrast to asymptomatic carriage. Alternatively, viral antigen may be detected by enzyme immuno-assays. However, these detect virus antigen alone without indicating where it was located. Hence they cannot distinguish between a significant presence in respiratory cells (indicating invasion of the mucosal surface) and mostly silent (and clinically insignificant) carriage, probably in the tonsils and adenoids.

#### Viral DNA

It is also possible to detect viral DNA directly from faeces by polyacrylamide gel electrophoresis. The intact DNA forms a single band found near the top of the gel but its identity as definitely adenovirus in origin can be confirmed only after digestion with restriction endonucleases and repeat electrophoresis. A characteristic 'ladder' of DNA fragments separated by size confirms the diagnosis, distinguishes between types 40 and 41 (and identifies others) and can also indicate subtypes. This approach is particularly useful to identify types 40 and 41, which are difficult or impossible to isolate in cell culture, and for laboratories without access to electron microscopy.

### Culture

Virus can be grown in cell culture from respiratory specimens (nasopharyngeal aspirates, and nose and throat swabs), eye swabs, faeces and, occasionally, urine. The speed of isolation can provide a pointer to the significance of the finding. If it takes longer than 12 days it is less likely to be clinically significant, particularly with types 1, 2, 5 and 6.

Isolation of an adenovirus in cell culture from the faeces of patients with diarrhoea is by itself of little significance. As mentioned earlier, diarrhoea-causing adenoviruses are not readily isolated in culture, and cultivable adenoviruses in the stool are not usually those associated with diarrhoea. Nevertheless, the diarrhoea-associated adenoviruses go through partial replication in G293 cells (an adenovirus-transformed human embryo kidney cell line), and the antigens induced in these cells are type-specific. They may be identified by immunofluorescence using type-specific antibodies.

### Serology

A rise in antibody levels indicates recent infection (though not its site or nature) but absence does not exclude it, especially in babies. Complement fixation is the test most frequently used, and it provides only a group-specific diagnosis. Group- and type-specific enzyme immuno-assays have also been developed but are not used widely. Neutralization tests are both type-specific and more sensitive, but are not available as routine tests; neither is haemagglutination inhibition widely available. However, both tests may be used by reference laboratories or in research.

## TREATMENT

There are no antiviral drugs available for the treatment of adenoviral infections. Since adenovirus infections are usually self-limiting and there is little evidence that they provide frequent or major problems in the immunocompromised, demand is likely to be too small to warrant development of a drug.

## EPIDEMIOLOGY

Adenoviruses are endemic and types 1–7 spread readily between individuals, presumably by droplets. Faecal–oral transmission can also occur and probably does in underdeveloped areas, particularly where there is also overcrowding. However, it is probable that types 40 and 41, which are widespread causes of diarrhoea even in highly developed countries, also spread via droplets.

Subtyping, which has shown, for example, eight subtypes of adenovirus type 7 (the prototype 7p, and seven variants 7a–7g), has also shown geographical variations in their distribution. Such detailed analysis is not done routinely, however, and no information on subtype distribution of types 40 and 41 is available.

It is probable that only a minority of adenovirus infections are diagnosed virologically. What is known about their epidemiology is therefore only the tip of a considerable iceberg. Using the earlier analogy to weeds, like them they will always be with us, providing a more luxuriant overgrowth from time to time as circumstances allow. It is probable that some individuals are more vulnerable than others to their activity, e.g. some young children who develop pneumonia, and, possibly, patients with AIDS. There is a need for more information about these viruses whose range of activities is wide.

## CONTROL

For the same reasons discussed earlier under treatment, there is little demand for a vaccine. How well it would work can be questioned because circulating antibody may not prevent reinfection, although volunteer studies indicate that reinfection rarely results in disease. Nevertheless, the problems with adenoviruses encountered by US armed forces in recruit camps led them to experiment with a live virus vaccine administered orally in enteric capsules. It provided adequate protection from disease and was licensed for use but only in military personnel. The plethora of serotypes, their widespread presence and their generally benign outcome makes extension to the general public unlikely to be worthwhile.

A careful and rigorous attention to aseptic technique and single-dose vials of materials for use in the eye is the best approach to preventing outbreaks of adenovirus eye infections. As a component of pharyngoconjunctival fever, conjunctivitis is not preventable.

## ADENOVIRUS-ASSOCIATED VIRUSES

The adenovirus-associated viruses (AAVs) are members of the parvoviridae. They are about 22 nm in diameter, appear to be more hexagonal than circular in outline and contain insufficient single-stranded DNA to replicate on their own. They form a genus, *dependoviruses*, indicating their dependence on adenoviruses (or herpes simplex virus) to provide the missing functions.

True AAV (also known as adenovirus satellite virus) has not been implicated in clinical disease. However, as with any other virus found in faeces, large numbers of parvovirus-like particles have been seen in extracts of diarrhoeal faeces, sometimes (but not invariably) combined with smaller numbers of adenoviruses. Neither virus grows in cell culture, leaving the significance of these observations obscure (see Ch. 48 on parvoviruses).

RECOMMENDED READING

Dorin J 1996 Somatic gene therapy (editorial). *British Medical Journal* 312: 323–324
Madeley C R 1986 The emerging role of adenoviruses as inducers of gastroenteritis. *Pediatric Infectious Disease Journal* 5(suppl 1): 563–574

Sharp I R, Wadell G 1995 Adenoviruses. In: Zuckerman A J, Banatvala J E, Pattison J R (eds) *Principles and Practice of Clinical Virology*, 3rd edn. Wiley, Chichester

# 44

# Herpesviruses

Herpes simplex; varicella and zoster; infectious mononucleosis; cytomegalovirus disease; roseola infantum; Kaposi's sarcoma; herpes B

*M. M. Ogilvie*

The herpesviruses, a large family infecting many animal species, share a number of features, including their structure and mode of replication and the capacity to establish lifelong latent infections from which virus may be reactivated.

**Latent infection.** This has been defined as 'a type of persistent infection in which the viral genome is present but infectious virus is not produced except during intermittent episodes of reactivation'.

**Reactivation.** Reactivation from the latent state may be restricted to asymptomatic virus shedding.

**Recurrence or recrudescence.** These terms are used when reactivated virus produces clinically obvious disease.

At present eight human herpesviruses are recognized, and infection with each of the first seven has been shown to be common in all populations; studies with the eighth are awaited:

1. Herpes simplex virus 1      HSV-1
2. Herpes simplex virus 2      HSV-2
3. Varicella–zoster virus      VZV
4. Epstein–Barr virus          EBV
5. Cytomegalovirus             CMV
6. Human herpesvirus 6         HHV6
7. Human herpesvirus 7         HHV7
8. Human herpesvirus 8         HHV8

The herpes B virus of monkeys can be transmitted to humans accidentally. These viruses, the infections caused by them, and associated diseases will be described here.

## DESCRIPTION

Herpesviruses have a characteristic morphology visible in electron microscopical studies (Fig. 44.1). Negative staining reveals the icosahedral protein capsid of average diameter 100 nm, consisting of 162 hollow hexagonal and pentagonal capsomeres, with an electron-dense core containing the DNA genome. Outside the capsid in mature particles is an amorphous proteinaceous layer, the *tegument*, surrounded by a lipid *envelope* derived from cell membranes. Projecting from the trilaminar lipid envelope are *spikes* of viral glycoproteins. Cryo-electron micrographs indicate that the capsid is organized into at least three layers, with viral DNA inserted in the innermost layer. The average enveloped particle diameter is approximately 200 nm.

The genome of herpes virions is linear double-stranded DNA, varying in length from 125 to 240 kb, with a base content ranging from 42 to 69 G + C mol% for the human herpesviruses. The presence of long and short unique regions bounded by repeated and inverted short segments allows recombination and isomeric forms in some cases (Fig. 44.2). Genes coding for viral glycoproteins, major capsid proteins, enzymes involved in DNA replication and some transcripts associated with latency have been identified. Conserved sequences appear in certain regions, and some genes show homology with regions of human chromosomes. Restriction endonuclease analysis permits epidemiological comparison of strains ('fingerprinting') within herpes species.

Some herpesviruses are predominantly neurotropic (HSV and VZV) or lymphotropic (EBV, HHV6 and HHV7).

## Biological classification

The family Herpesviridae comprises three broad groups (subfamilies):

1. Alphaherpesviruses, e.g. HSV, VZV and B virus; rapid growth, latency in sensory ganglia
2. Betaherpesviruses – CMVs; slow growth, restricted host range
3. Gammaherpesviruses, e.g. EBV; growth in lymphoblastoid cells.

Of the newer human herpesviruses, HHV6 and HHV7 have been classified with CMV as betaherpes-

**Fig. 44.1** Electron micrograph of HSV. Negative staining (2% PTA). Bar, 100 nm. (Prepared by Dr B. W. McBride.)

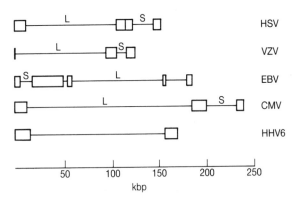

**Fig. 44.2** Diagrammatic comparison of herpesvirus DNAs. Lines indicate long (L) or short (S) unique sequences, and repeated regions are boxed.

viruses, and the most recently identified HHV8 is a gammaherpesvirus like EBV.

The viruses are relatively thermolabile and readily inactivated by lipid solvents such as alcohols and detergents.

## Replication

After attachment to receptors, the envelope of herpes virions fuses with the cell membrane. The nucleocapsids cross the cytoplasm to the nuclear membrane; replication of viral DNA and assembly of capsids take place within the nucleus. With HSV, it is

known that tegument protein transactivates expression of the first set of genes. Between 65 and 80 viral proteins are synthesized, in an orderly sequence or cascade.

These proteins are of three types:

1. Immediate early ($\alpha$) – mainly regulatory functions
2. Early ($\beta$) – includes many enzymes involved in DNA replication
3. Late ($\gamma$) – structural proteins of capsid, glycoproteins.

The viral capsid proteins migrate from the cytoplasm to the nucleus where capsid assembly occurs and new viral DNA is inserted and located in the inner shell. Viral glycoproteins are processed in the Golgi complex and are incorporated into cell membranes from which the viral envelope is acquired, usually from the inner layer of the nuclear membrane as the virus buds out from the nucleus (Fig. 44.3). It then passes by way of membranous vacuoles to reach the cell surface. Productively infected cells generally do not survive.

## HERPES SIMPLEX VIRUS

HSV is ubiquitous, infecting the majority of the world's population early in life and persisting in a

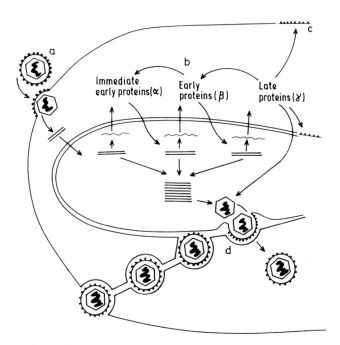

**Fig. 44.3** A summary of events in herpesvirus replication: a, entry; b, viral DNA transcription and replication, showing cascade of proteins synthesized; c, glycoprotein expression on cell membranes; d, assembly and egress of new virions. (By courtesy of J. P. Vestey, Dermatology, Royal Infirmary, Edinburgh.)

latent form from which reactivation with shedding of infectious virus occurs, thus maintaining the transmission chain.

## Description

The virus has the general structure and chemical composition already described. In contrast to other members of the group, HSV can be grown in cells from a wide variety of animals relatively easily, so that far more extensive studies have been undertaken with this virus.

There are two distinct types of HSV, named type 1 (HSV-1) and type 2 (HSV-2). These two types are generally (but not exclusively) associated with different sites of infection in patients (see below); type 1 strains are associated primarily with the mouth, the eye and the central nervous system, while type 2 strains are found most often in the genital tract.

## HSV glycoproteins

The envelope of HSV contains several glycoproteins which have been studied in detail both at the structural and functional level. At least 11 glycoproteins are known. Three of the glycoproteins are essential for production of infectious virions – gB and gD,

which are involved in adsorption to and penetration into cells, and gH, involved in the release of virus. Some of the glycoproteins have common antigenic determinants shared by HSV-1 and HSV-2 (gB and gD) whilst others have specific determinants for one type only (gG).

## Pathogenesis

### Primary infection

The typical lesion produced by HSV is the *vesicle*, a ballooning degeneration of intra-epithelial cells. The underlying layer of basal epithelium is usually intact, vesicles only occasionally penetrate the subepithelial layer. The base of the vesicle contains multinucleate cells (sometimes called *Tzanck cells*, seen in Giemsa-stained preparations) and infected nuclei contain eosinophilic *inclusion bodies*. The roof of the vesicle breaks down, and an ulcer forms: this happens rapidly on mucous membranes and non-keratinizing epithelia; on the skin the ulcer crusts over, forming a scab, and then heals. A mononuclear reaction is normal, with the vesicle fluid becoming cloudy, and cellular infiltration in the subepithelial tissue. After resorption or loss of the vesicle fluid the damaged epithelium is regenerated. Natural killer cells play a significant role in early defence. Synthesis of herpesvirus gly-coproteins during the virus growth cycle is followed by the insertion of the glycoproteins into the cell membranes, and some are secreted into extracellular fluid. The infected host responds to all these foreign antigens, producing cytotoxic T cells (CD8$^+$), and helper T lymphocytes (CD4$^+$), which activate primed B cells to produce specific antibodies and are also involved in the induction of delayed hypersensitivity. The different glycoproteins have significant roles in generating these various cell responses; probably all of them induce neutralizing antibody.

During the replication phase at the site of entry in the epithelium, virus particles enter through the sensory nerve endings which penetrate to the parabasal layer of the epithelium, and are transported, probably as nucleocapsids, along the axon to the nerve body (neurone) in the sensory (dorsal root) ganglion by retrograde axonal flow. Virus replication in a neurone ends in neuronal cell death; however, some of the herpesvirus reaching the ganglion cells is able to establish a *latent infection* in which the neurones survive but continue to harbour the viral genome. Neurones other than those in sensory ganglia can be the site of herpes latency. Whether true latency occurs at epithelial sites is not yet clear; there is some evidence of persistence of virus at peripheral sites, but this may be due to a reactivation with a low level of virus replication.

Antibody does reduce the severity of infections, although it does not prevent recurrences. Neonates receiving maternal antibody transplacentally are protected against the worst effects of neonatal herpes. HSV-2 infection seems to protect against HSV-1, but prior HSV-1 infection only partly modifies HSV-2 disease.

## Latent infection

Latent infection of sensory neurones is a feature of the neurotropic herpesviruses HSV and VZV. Most of the information available about the latent state has been obtained from studies of HSV-1 latency. Of the latently infected neurones, only a small proportion (about 1%) of cells in the affected ganglion carry the viral genome, which is in a different state to that found in virions. In latency, viral DNA exists as free circular *episomes* – perhaps about 20 copies per infected cell. Very few virus genes are expressed in the latent state; in HSV some viral RNA transcripts (latency-associated transcripts) are found in the nuclei but no virus-coded proteins have been demonstrated in the cells, so these infected neurones are not recognized by the immune system. Latent herpes simplex genomes

have been detected in postmortem studies on excised ganglia and other neuronal tissues. HSV-1 is regularly detected in the trigeminal ganglion; it has also been found in other sensory and autonomic ganglia (e.g. vagus), in adrenal tissue and in the brain. HSV-2 latency in the sacral ganglia has been demonstrated. Either type may become latent in other ganglia.

## Reactivation and recrudescence

Reactivation processes are still not understood. It is suggested that in some way herpesvirus DNA passes along the nerve axon back to the nerve ending where infection of epithelial cells may occur. Not all reactivation will result in a visible lesion; there may be asymptomatic shedding of virus only detectable by culture.

Whilst some progress has been made in the molecular biology of the latent state in the neurone, the factors influencing the development of recrudescent lesions are not yet clearly identified. An increase of CD8$^+$ suppressor cell activity is common at the time of recurrences. Spread of the virus may be enhanced by some mediators, e.g. prostaglandins, and a temporary decrease in immune effector cell function, particularly delayed hypersensitivity. Certainly the known triggers for recurrences are accompanied by a local increase in prostaglandin levels; depression of cell-mediated immunity predisposes to herpes recurrence. The mechanism of reactivation is not known, but the event can be accurately predicted in those known to harbour latent virus. Thus, following bone marrow transplant or high-dose chemotherapy, herpes simplex recurs in 80% at a median interval of 18 days in the absence of prophylaxis.

However reactivation is achieved, it is a feature of HSV infection. It occurs naturally, and can be induced by a variety of stimuli such as ultraviolet light (sunlight), fever, trauma and stress. The interval between the stimulus and the appearance of a clinically obvious lesion is 2–5 days, as has been regularly demonstrated in patients undergoing neurological interference with their trigeminal ganglion, a common site of herpes latency.

## Clinical features

***Primary infection.*** Primary herpetic infection, as the name indicates, is the patient's first experience of HSV and occurs therefore in those with no antibody to the virus. It usually involves the mucous membranes of the mouth, but may include the lips, skin of the face, nose or any other site, including the eye and genital tract.

**Table 44.1** Types of herpes simplex virus infection

| Type of infection | Immune status of patient |
|---|---|
| *Primary* – first HSV infection (any type at any site) | Seronegative |
| *Latent* – no symptoms | Seropositive |
| *Recurrent* – recrudescence of the latent HSV type(s) | Seropositive |
| *Initial (non-primary)* – first episode of the heterologous HSV in a seropositive patient | Seronegative for infecting type; seropositive for latent type |
| *Reinfection (exogenous)* – with a strain that differs from the latent HSV type | Seropositive |

***Recurrence or recrudescence.*** Symptomatic recurrence is heralded by a *prodrome* in two-thirds of people, who experience pain or paraesthesia (tingling, warmth, itch) at the site, followed by erythema and a papule, usually within 24 h. Progression to a vesicle and ulcer, with subsequent crusting, takes 8–12 days before natural healing. Because of their association with febrile illness the lesions are popularly known as 'cold sores' or 'fever blisters'. The most common site is at the mucocutaneous junction of the lip, seldom inside the mouth. Other sites frequently involved are on the chin and inside the nose. However, recurrent lesions will manifest at any site innervated by the affected neurone, determined by the site of initial infection.

HSV infections may be differentiated according to the immune status of the patient (Table 44.1).

Severe pain, extensive mucosal ulceration and delayed healing are features of recurrent herpes in severely compromised patients. The ulcers provide entry for other infections. Herpes simplex viraemia after reactivation is uncommon, even in the immuno-compromised, but can lead to disseminated infection in internal organs. Some sufferers experience *erythema multiforme* following their recurrent herpes. This is associated with reaction to certain herpes antigens, and may take the form of the Stevens–Johnson syndrome. Prophylaxis to prevent the herpes recurring has proved useful.

## Oral infection

Classically, the first infection presents as an acute, febrile *gingivostomatitis* in pre-school children. Vesicular lesions which rapidly ulcerate can be seen in the front of the mouth and on the tongue. Gingivitis is usually present. Vesicles may also develop on the lips and skin around the mouth, and cervical lym-phadenopathy occurs. The child is miserable for 7–10 days in an untreated case before the lesions heal. However, the majority of primary infections go unrecognized, the episode being attributed to teething or mistaken for 'thrush' (candida infection). Herpetic stomatitis also occurs in older children and adults acquiring a primary infection. There may be an associated mononucleosis in the older patient; pharyngitis is noted. Viraemia with dissemination of herpes to internal organs is rare except in pregnancy (primary infection) or the neonate (see later) or the immunocompromised patient.

## Skin infection

***Herpetic whitlow.*** Hand infections with HSV are not uncommon. Three presentations may be seen: the classical primary lesion on the fingers or thumb of the toddler with herpetic stomatitis, due to auto-inoculation; another classical and often primary infection is acquired by accidental inoculation in health care workers. These infections may recur; the majority are HSV-1. The commonest hand lesions are, however, recurrent, associated with HSV-2 and genital herpes and seen in young adults. Pain and swelling occur, and the vesicles become pustular, but, if in well-keratinized areas, do not always ulcerate. Associated lymphangitis is common. Primary lesions take up to 21 days to heal, recurrent ones only 10 days.

***Eczema herpeticum.*** A severe form of cutaneous herpes may occur in children with *atopic eczema* – eczema herpeticum or Kaposi's varicelliform eruption. Vesicles resembling those of chickenpox may appear, mainly on already eczematous areas. Extensive ulceration results in protein loss and dehydration, and viraemia can lead to disseminated disease with severe, even fatal, consequences. A similar picture is occasionally seen in adults with pemphigus who develop herpes simplex. Patients with burns are also at risk. In each instance early recognition and antiviral therapy can be life-saving.

## Eye infection

HSV infection of the eye may be initiated during a childhood primary infection or occur from transfer of virus from a cold sore. There may be simply conjunctivitis, or keratoconjunctivitis associated with corneal ulceration. Typically, branching or dendritic corneal ulcers are found, and recur, resulting in corneal scarring and impairment of vision. More extensive ulceration occurs if steroids have been used, but deeper infiltrates are common in long-standing cases and benefit from combined steroid and antiviral therapy. The presence of typical herpes vesicles on eyelid margins is a useful clinical guide but not always seen. The majority of eye infections are HSV-1, and most patients with recurring eye disease are aged over 50 years. More than half of the corneal grafting performed in the UK is for HSV corneal scarring, but the disease may recur in the graft. Recently, acute retinal necrosis associated with HSV-2 has been recognized.

## Central nervous system infection

HSV may reach the brain in a variety of ways. Viraemia has been detected during primary herpetic stomatitis, and infection may be carried by cells into the brain and meninges. Direct infection from nasal mucosa along the olfactory tract is another possibility, but the most likely route is central spread from trigeminal ganglia.

*HSV encephalitis (HSVE).* This is a rare condition, but is the commonest sporadic fatal encephalitis recognized in developed countries (affecting approximately 1 in 500 000 persons each year). The infection has a high mortality rate and significant morbidity in survivors of the acute necrotizing form. HSVE presents at any time of year, and can occur at any age. Occasionally it is seen in the young, but is more frequent in those in the 50–70 year age group; 70% of cases are in people with serological evidence and often a clinical history of previous herpes simplex. However, recurrent lesions are seldom apparent at the same time as HSVE. A prodromal fever and malaise is followed by *headache* and *behavioural change* sometimes associated with a sudden focal episode such as a *seizure*, or *paralysis*; *coma* usually precedes death. The *temporal lobe* is most frequently affected, and virus replication in neurones, followed by the oedema associated with the inflammatory response, accounts for the haemorrhagic necrosis and space-occupying nature of this form of the disease. More *diffuse*, milder disease has been recorded. Brain stem encephalitis is another serious manifestation.

Clinical recognition leading to early specific antiviral therapy will significantly reduce the 70% mortality and serious morbidity of untreated cases but therapy must be started as soon as possible, before the patient progresses from a drowsy state into coma. Diagnostic confirmation used to be most reliably provided by examination of brain biopsy tissue for virus antigens, virus particles and the characteristic histopathology. Brain biopsy is now seldom performed for suspected HSVE in the UK, but should tissue be available in the course of intracranial pressure monitoring it should

be examined. Cerebrospinal fluid (CSF) collected in the acute stages of HSVE should be sent to a laboratory offering DNA amplification by polymerase chain reaction (PCR). This highly sensitive technique is now established in several reference centres, and unlike previous attempts to find HSV in CSF by culture or antigen detection, can demonstrate the presence of HSV DNA in the majority of cases within the first 10 days of onset. Diagnosis can be confirmed in the convalescent period after therapy by the demonstration of intrathecal synthesis of HSV antibody. For this purpose CSF and peripheral blood taken on the same day are required.

The majority by far of HSVE cases where virus has been identified (outside the neonatal period – see below) have been due to HSV-1. HSV-2 encephalitis does occasionally occur in immunocompromised adults and may be seen more frequently in those infected with the human immunodeficiency virus (HIV).

## Genital tract infection

Both types of HSV can infect the genital tract. Although the more common association has been with type 2 strains, type 1 infection is not infrequent, particularly in young women, where it may account for more than half of genital infections. Genital infection may be acquired by auto-inoculation from lesions elsewhere on the body, but most often results from intimate sexual contact, including orogenital contact. The lesions are vesicular at first but rapidly ulcerate. In the male, the glans and shaft of the penis are the most frequent sites of infection, while in the female, the labia and vagina or cervix may be involved. Lesions may spread to surrounding skin sites.

The incubation period following exposure to virus is 2–20 days, with an average of 7 days. A primary infection is usually the most severe, especially in women. Fever and malaise are accompanied by regional lymphadenopathy; urethritis and vaginal discharge may be present. The whole episode lasts 3–4 weeks, and high titres of virus are shed. In some cases a lymphocytic meningitis develops, and urinary retention can also be a problem. Both of these are manifestations of sacral radiculopathy. Where the infection is an initial (non-primary) genital herpes the attack is generally less severe, but lasts around 2 weeks.

*Recurrent genital herpes.* This can be as frequent as six or more episodes a year. Although the attacks are milder and shorter (around 7–10 days) than first episodes, the results are socially and psychologically distressing. Prodromal symptoms in the distribution of the sacral nerves are experienced by some but the patient is already infectious at that stage. Virus shedding from the genital tract is often asymptomatic, and recurrent lesions may not be recognized by the patient or general practitioner as herpetic in origin, so that in many instances the risk of transmission to sexual partners is not apparent. HSV-1 genital infection recurs less often than HSV-2, and thus carries a better prognosis. Either type is capable of transmission from mother to infant. Transplacental passage resulting in intra-uterine damage to the fetus has been recorded but is very rare, and is probably limited to cases with substantial maternal viraemia. Ascending infection from the cervix may be more significant, especially when the membranes are ruptured for some time before delivery.

Genital herpes increased in incidence during the 1970s and 1980s. It appears to have decreased now, as reflected in genito-urinary clinic and laboratory reports in the UK. However, the increased role of general practitioner consultations and treatment may be affecting these numbers. Genital herpes can be a significant problem in immunosuppressed patients, and is seen as persistent severe perianal lesions with or without proctitis in many HIV-infected male homosexuals. Genital herpetic ulcers may predispose patients to infection with HIV.

## Neonatal herpes

A rare but very serious infection, untreated neonatal herpes has a case fatality rate exceeding 60%, with half of the survivors severely damaged. Virus, commonly HSV-2, is acquired by passage through an infected genital tract at birth. The greatest risk, with 50% transmission rate (because there is more virus present and no antibody transfer), occurs with a primary infection in the mother at the time of delivery. With recurrent herpes at term, the transmission rate is only 8% or less. Neonatal infection usually presents about the 6th day post partum. It is important to note that skin lesions are not always present, that they may be very few and that they are commonly located on the presenting part, e.g. scalp. Virus dissemination to internal organs is the most serious complication, in which the infant shows signs of general sepsis, including fever, poor feeding and irritability. Pneumonia and jaundice develop, with or without signs of meningitis or encephalitis. Progressive liver failure with coagulopathy leads to death around the 16th day, in this the most serious disseminated form. Occasionally, infection is restricted to skin or mucosae, including the conjunctiva, or involves the central

nervous system with or without dissemination to internal organs. Early antiviral therapy is the key to survival with minimal morbidity, although local recurrent lesions can be expected especially at skin sites in the first year.

The prevention of neonatal herpes is difficult, the vast majority of infections occurring in babies born to women with no past history of genital herpes and in whom the infection at term has either been asymptomatic or has gone unrecognized clinically. Routine preterm screening for virus shedding, particularly as applied to those with a past history, does not predict the babies at risk. Once type-specific antibody tests become available routinely, susceptible women at risk of acquiring HSV-2 from partners could be identified. If any suspicious lesions are seen during labour, swabs for virus culture and a rapid detection test should be taken. Caesarean section is only likely to reduce the risk of infection if performed in the early stages of labour. If the mother is known to have moderate levels of antibody, the baby is unlikely to develop the disease. Some cases of neonatal herpes are acquired just after birth from contact with sources of HSV other than the mother's genital tract. The clinical presentation is similar, although the virus is likely to be type 1 from oral or skin lesions of attendants or relatives. In the case of suspected neonatal herpes without skin lesions, nasopharyngeal secretions, CSF and blood lymphocytes should be cultured.

## Laboratory diagnosis

Virus detection and serological studies both have their place in the diagnosis of infection with HSV. In all instances of acute infection, be it primary or recurrent, virus detection is the method of choice, for antibody responses are naturally later and much less informative. Indeed, in recurrent episodes the antibody titre may not vary. Sensitive assays for IgG antibody, including type-specific antibody, have an important place in prospective testing.

## Herpes virus detection

Direct diagnosis of HSV infection is available, and should be sought in cases where there is any doubt as to the clinical diagnosis, or where rapid confirmation is required to support the choice of therapy or other management. Virus isolation is suitable for most common herpes infections, direct diagnosis being reserved for the atypical or serious situations.

Isolation of HSV from an infected patient is now most usually attempted in cultures of human diploid fibroblast cells. Growth is rapid, and within 24 h a cytopathic effect (CPE) may be visible, presenting as rounded, ballooned cells in foci which later expand and eventually involve the whole cell sheet. Virus is released from infected cells into the culture fluid, hence the rapid spread of infection from the initial foci.

Herpes virions may be demonstrated by electron microscopy in vesicle fluid or tissue preparations. Detection of viral antigens in cells (by immuno-fluorescence, for example) provides a rapid diagnosis on cells scraped from the base of lesions. Unfortunately, in the most serious infections it is often not possible to have easy access to the site of infection. Detection of amplified viral DNA by PCR in CSF or other samples is proving a most sensitive and specific method of diagnosis. The two HSV types can be differentiated either by using type-specific primers in the PCR, or using common primers followed by analysis with restriction enzymes or hybridization probes for each type.'

### Antibody tests for HSV

Complement fixation tests (CFT) are still useful in the diagnosis of primary infections when a significant change in antibody titre can be expected. The titre of antibody may not be high, especially in genital infection, and the test measures total antibody, not differentiating type-specific antibodies. In the case of herpes encephalitis, a serological diagnosis depends on demonstration of intrathecal synthesis of antibody to HSV. CFT can be used, testing serum and CSF in parallel against HSV antigens and another unrelated antigen. In health there is no antibody detectable by such tests in the CSF. If the serum antibody:CSF antibody ratio is diminished from the normal 200:1 to 40:1 (or less), and the blood–CSF barrier integrity is confirmed by other antibody (or albumin) being excluded from the CSF, intrathecal antibody synthesis is demonstrated. It is also helpful to check for the possible transfer of antibody from blood to CSF by means of an IgG index performed on the same serum and CSF samples by the biochemists or immunologists. Tests on serum alone cannot confirm HSVE.

Enzyme immuno-assays are much more sensitive and specific than CFT. When type-specific antigen preparations based on glycoprotein G are used, type-specific antibody can be detected. Immunoblotting similarly can demonstrate type-specific antibody, and can be used to study changes in the profile of antibodies seen in sequential samples at intervals after infection. Therapy often results in delay in these type-specific antibodies appearing, and late conva-lescent samples, at 6 weeks, should be included. To date, type-specific assays have only been available on a research basis, but enzyme immuno-assays for total antibody to HSV are supplied commercially.

## Treatment

Specific antiviral therapy has revolutionized the management of HSV infections over the last 15 years. Prior to the development of agents suitable for systemic use, topical application of the relatively non-selective idoxuridine was used successfully in the treatment of eye and skin infections. *Vidarabine* and *acyclovir* have better therapeutic ratios and were proven effective, when used early enough, in appropriate dosage, for the whole range of acute HSV infections. Latency is not eradicated by these agents, which inhibit viral DNA synthesis. Prophylactic use of acyclovir is now an established part of the management to prevent reactivation in the immuno-compromised, e.g. transplant recipients. Long-term suppressive therapy with acyclovir has been particularly successful in the management of frequently recurring genital herpes, and HSV-related erythema multiforme. Patient-initiated early treatment can also abort or modify recurrences.

Acyclovir is the most widely used antiherpes treatment, having an excellent safety record and being available in preparations for topical, oral and intravenous use. Use in pregnancy continues to be monitored for any adverse outcome in the infant. Topical cream or ointment is suitable only for mild epithelial lesions, such as recurrent cold sores or genital herpes or corneal ulcers. Oral or intravenous therapy with acyclovir should be given for:

1. Any deeper lesions
2. Disease in immunocompromised hosts
3. Any of the serious manifestations.

Intravenous therapy is required for central nervous system and other systemic infection.

Dosage varies considerably, depending on the site of infection and whether the aim is suppression of recurrence or therapy of established disease. Because the level of acyclovir achieved in the CSF is only half that in plasma, the dosage for the treatment of encephalitis has to be twice that for other systemic disease. It is important to maintain therapy until clinical signs indicate a favourable response. In serious systemic disease, or in the severely immuno-compromised, therapy will need to continue for 2 weeks or longer.

The poor bio-availability of acyclovir given by mouth has stimulated the development of a pro-drug, *valaciclovir*, which is rapidly converted into acyclovir, producing significantly higher plasma levels after oral dosage. Another effective antiherpes agent, penciclovir, which is activated and inhibits HSV DNA synthesis in a similar fashion, is given in the form of an oral pro-drug, *famciclovir*. Both of these new agents are licensed for treatment of genital herpes, and may be administered less frequently than acyclovir.

Resistance to acyclovir does develop in some instances; so far this has not been a significant clinical problem in relation to strains with deficient or altered thymidine kinase (TK), which are unable to phosphorylate acyclovir, but it is on the increase, particularly in severely immunocompromised hosts with the acquired immunodeficiency syndrome (AIDS) or following bone marrow transplant. A few resistant viruses with altered DNA polymerase have also been isolated and were associated with clinical disease. With widespread use of acyclovir, more resistant strains may be expected to arise, and monitoring of the antiviral sensitivity of herpes isolates will be necessary. Strains resistant to acyclovir are generally also resistant to famciclovir, and may need to be controlled with an agent such as foscarnet which does not require activation by viral TK.

## Epidemiology

HSV is probably transferred by *direct contact*. Many children, especially in overcrowded conditions, acquire oral HSV-1 infections in the first years of life. Spread may not occur so readily in better social conditions, with the result that primary infection is delayed to young adulthood. This is the usual time of exposure to genital herpes and, as a result, primary infections may be HSV-2 or HSV-1.

Sensitive immuno-assays have shown that 60–90% of adults have had HSV-1 infections. Type-specific serology has also revealed that many more women have had HSV-2 infection than give a history of genital herpes. However, neonatal herpes is still a rare complication in the UK; the British Paediatric Surveillance Unit reported 37 confirmed neonatal herpes infections over a period of 42 months. Eleven of the infants died within the 1st month, and several of the survivors suffered adverse sequelae. The rate of cases has increased in some populations as genital herpes has become more common. Herpes encephalitis outside of the neonatal period occurs sporadically at a rate of about 1 per 500 000 of the population per annum.

The role of HSV in human carcinomata, particularly carcinoma of the cervix, is not clear; the ability of the virus to transform cells in vitro is well

known, although permissive cells are usually destroyed before any effect can be shown.

## Control

Transmission of herpes simplex can be reduced by alleviating overcrowding, practising simple hygiene, and education regarding the infectious stages. Sexual transmission may be significantly reduced by the use of condoms. Exposure of the infant at birth can be avoided if delivery by caesarean section is performed in the early stage of labour, but this is only to be recommended when lesions are present in the mother or virus has been demonstrated at that time. Reference has already been made to the use of prophylactic antiviral regimens to control predictable recurrence. Progress in understanding latency and reactivation will provide approaches to preventing reactivation. Protection from ultraviolet light and the use of inhibitors of prostaglandin synthesis may be useful in this context.

Experimental vaccines are under investigation, but none is licensed for use in the UK at present. Research into subunit vaccines based on the viral glycoproteins or other significant viral proteins may lead to an appropriate preparation to elicit the immune responses important in control of herpes simplex.

## VARICELLA–ZOSTER VIRUS

Infection with VZV presents in two forms. The primary infection *varicella* (or chickenpox) is a generalized eruption, whereas the reactivated infection *zoster* (or shingles) is localized to one or a few dermatomes.

## Description

The viruses isolated from varicella or zoster are identical, and this has now been confirmed by molecular epidemiological studies on viruses isolated from individual patients. The virus has the morphology of all herpesviruses. Seventy genes code for 67 different proteins, including five families of glycoprotein genes. The glycoproteins gE, gB and gH (previously named gpI, gpII and gpIII, respectively) are particularly abundant in infected cells, and are present in the viral envelope (Fig. 44.4).

Virus replication takes place in the nucleus, and histological examination of infected epidermis reveals typical nuclear inclusions and multinucleate giant cells identical to those of herpes simplex. Human fibroblast

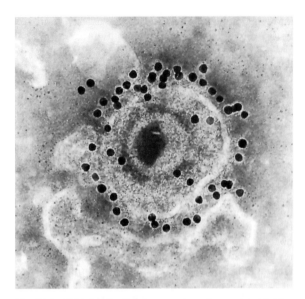

**Fig. 44.4** VZV showing the virus envelope glycoprotein I (gE) labelled with monoclonal antibody and goat anti-mouse IgG conjugated with 15 nm colloidal gold. ×150 000. (Micrograph taken by C. Graham, supplied by Dr E. Dermott, Department of Microbiology and Immunobiology, Queen's University, Belfast.)

cell cultures are most often used for isolation, but VZV can grow in a variety of human and simian cell cultures. The enveloped virions released from the nucleus remain closely attached to microvilli along the cell surface, and this 'cell-associated' characteristic, with infection being passed from cell to cell, has limited studies with this virus compared to the lytic HSV. The typical cytopathic effect appears in cell cultures in 3 days to 2 or 3 weeks.

There is only one antigenic type of VZV known, but 'fingerprinting' of the DNA can be used in some cases to identify isolates from epidemiologically linked sources. Antibodies to the three main glycoproteins all neutralize virus infectivity. One of these glycoproteins, gB, shares 49% amino acid identity with gB of HSV, and this accounts for the cross-reactive anamnestic antibody response that may be detected during infections with either virus.

## Pathogenesis

### Varicella

This is a disease predominantly of children, characterized by a vesicular skin eruption. Virus is thought to enter through the upper respiratory tract, or conjunctivae, and multiply in local lymph tissue for a few days before entering the blood and being distributed throughout the body. Following replication in reticulo-endothelial sites, a second viraemic stage precedes the appearance of the skin and mucosal lesions. Mucosal lesions are less noticeable and ulcerate early, and the skin rash is readily recognized.

These vesicles lie in the middle of the epidermis, and the fluid contains numerous free virus particles. Within 3 days the fluid becomes cloudy with the influx of leucocytes; fibrin and interferon are also present. These pustules then dry up, scabs form, and they desquamate. It is a noticeable feature that lesions in all stages are present at any time while new ones are appearing. The clearance of virus-infected cells is dependent on functional cell-mediated immune mechanisms, cytotoxic T cells and antibody-dependent cell cytotoxicity in particular. Persons deficient in these responses and in interferon production have prolonged clear-vesicle phases and great difficulty in controlling the infection.

### Zoster

The pathogenesis of zoster is not so well established as that of HSV recurrence. Nucleic acid probes have revealed VZV sequences in sensory ganglia, and explant cultures of ganglia produce some VZV proteins, although not fully infectious virus. The latent virus is found in neurones and in satellite cells in sensory ganglia, and more than one region of the genome is transcribed, but the state of the latent VZV is not known. It seems likely that virus reaches the ganglion from the periphery by travelling up nerve axons, as HSV does, but there is also the possibility that during viraemia some virus enters ganglion cells. Another difference from HSV latency lies in the persistent VZV expression that has been detected in some mononuclear cells, which may have a role in VZV disease such as postherpetic neuralgia (see below).

Reactivation of VZV manifested as zoster can occur at any age in a person who has experienced a primary infection which may or may not have been clinically apparent. The rate is much increased in persons aged 60 years or over and, as most primary infection takes place before the age of 20 years, there is usually a latent period of several decades. However, a much shorter latent period is seen in immunocompromised patients, and also in those who acquired primary infection in utero (see below). More than one episode of zoster is uncommon in any individual. The stimulus to reactivation is not known, nor the details, but virus does appear to travel from sensory ganglia to the peripheral site. The zoster is usually limited to one dermatome and, in adults, this is most commonly in the thoracic or upper lumbar regions or in the area supplied by the ophthalmic division of the trigeminal nerve. This distribution is thought to be related to the density of the original varicella rash. There are associations with preceding trauma to the dermatome – injury or injections for instance with an interval of 2–3 weeks before the zoster appears. (An inquiry usually elicits some such association in immunocompetent hosts.) There is an associated suppression of specific cell-mediated responses in acute zoster, but rapid secondary antibody responses are usually found. Reactivation occurs more commonly in T cell immunodeficiency states.

Viraemia may occur in the course of zoster but is not usual, pre-existing immunity normally being rapidly boosted. In the immunocompromised, however, viraemia leads to dissemination of zoster, either to internal organs or in a generalized manner similar to varicella.

## Clinical features

### Varicella

The incubation period averages 14–15 days but may range from 10 to 20 days. The patient is infectious for 2 days before and up to 5 days after onset, while new vesicles are appearing.

The rash of varicella is usually centripetal, being most dense on the trunk and head. Initially macular, the rash rapidly evolves through papules to the characteristic clear vesicles ('dew drops').

Presentations vary widely – from the clinically inapparent to only a few scattered lesions, or to a severe febrile illness with a widespread rash, especially in secondary cases in older members of a household. Whilst commonly a relatively mild infection in the young child, the complications of varicella are serious and account for significant morbidity, requiring hospitalization of normal children and adults, unlike the other herpesvirus infections.

Secondary bacterial infection of skin lesions is the commonest complication, mainly in the young child, and it increases the amount of residual scarring. Thrombocytopenic purpura occurs, especially in immunocompromised hosts. A variety of organs may be affected, producing myocarditis, arthritis, glomerulonephritis and appendicitis. The two most frequent problems are related to the lungs and the central nervous system.

**Pneumonia.** In varicella, viral pneumonitis is a most serious complication, even in normal people. It occurs as a subclinical feature evident only by radio-graphy in a proportion of adults, but is increasingly being recognized for the danger it brings, especially to smokers. Cough, dyspnoea, tachypnoea and chest pains begin a few days after the rash. Nodular infiltrates are seen in the lungs on radiography. Specific antiviral therapy is only successful if used early in sufficient dosage, and should be instituted at the first sign of pneumonia in an adult with chickenpox. Early investigations (radiography and gas exchange) are indicated in all smokers with chickenpox. Immuno-compromised patients are even more at risk of varicella pneumonia.

**Central nervous system.** Neurological compli-cations include the common but benign cerebellar ataxia syndrome. Acute encephalitis is rare but more serious, and occurs more commonly in immuno-compromised patients. This may be confused with postinfectious encephalopathy, which with other post-infectious manifestations, such as transverse myelitis or Guillain–Barré syndrome, is immunologically mediated and not related to viral cytopathogenicity.

**Varicella in pregnancy.** Varicella virus can cross the placenta following viraemia in the pregnant woman, and infect the fetus. The infection may be more serious for the mother herself in pregnancy, with pneumonia the major problem. Two types of intra-uterine infection are noted:

1. *The fetal varicella syndrome* is a consequence of fetal infections with VZV in the first half of pregnancy. The birth of infants so infected has been rarely reported but the features include characteristic scarring of the skin, hypoplasia of limbs, and chorioretinitis. The maternal infection is usually varicella but in one case at least it was disseminated herpes zoster. Fetal infection is not inevitable. Silent intra-uterine infection can also occur: no damage is seen, but the baby is born with latent VZV infection, having recovered from infection.

2. *Neonatal (congenital) varicella* occurs when varicella develops within the first 2 weeks of life, following maternal varicella in late pregnancy, depending on the interval between maternal viraemia and delivery of the baby. If the rash in the mother begins 7 days or more prior to delivery, her antibody response will have developed and been transferred across the placenta so that the baby does not develop disease. However, varicella occurring 6 days or less before delivery (or up to 2 days after) allows viraemic spread across the placenta, without any antibody being transferred, and places the infant at serious risk. Because the usual respiratory entry route has been bypassed, the incubation period is reduced to 10 days on average. If infection occurs, disseminated

disease with pneumonitis and encephalitis may be found. The rate of transmission is 1 in 3, but there is no way of knowing which mother will transmit, and in this situation protection of the neonate with passive immunity (see VZIG 413) and early antiviral therapy is indicated.

## Zoster

This is the manifestation of reactivated VZV infection. It takes the form of a localized eruption, and is unilateral and typically confined to one dermatome. Prodromal paraesthesia and pain in the area supplied by the affected sensory nerve are common before the skin lesions develop; these are identical to those of varicella except in their distribution. The evolution of the rash is similar, with some new vesicles appearing while the earliest ones are crusting; however, the whole episode in the majority of cases is confined to the affected dermatome and heals in 1–3 weeks. Acute pain is not always a feature, but its presence should alert to the possibility of zoster, and a search for early lesions, perhaps internal, is indicated. Occasionally there are no skin lesions – 'zoster sine herpete'.

Dissemination of zoster is indicated by lesions appearing in the skin at distant sites or, more seriously, by involvement of internal organs such as the lung and brain. In the immunocompromised this results in severe disease, with occasional fatalities.

**Postherpetic neuralgia (PHN).** This is the most common complication of zoster, a risk in 50% of patients aged over 60 years, and results in significant morbidity in around 20%. PHN is defined as intractable pain persisting for 1 month or more after the skin rash. Constant pain at the site, or stabbing pains or paraesthesiae may continue over 1 year or much longer in a number of individuals. This is an exhausting and disabling condition for which no satisfactory cure has been found. The indications are that adequate early antiviral therapy may reduce the incidence.

**Ophthalmic zoster.** Involvement of the ophthalmic division of the trigeminal nerve occurs in up to one-quarter of zoster episodes, with ocular complications in more than half the patients. Corneal ulceration, stromal keratitis and anterior uveitis may result in permanent scarring, so this complication may threaten sight when the nasociliary branch is involved. Ocular complications are reduced in patients given oral acyclovir early in ophthalmic zoster. Occasionally acute retinal necrosis associated with VZV is identified.

A contralateral hemiparesis due to granulomatous cerebral angiitis in the weeks following acute ophthalmic zoster is a recognized neurological complication. Other postinfection manifestations are seen, and more acute ones such as the *Ramsay-Hunt syndrome* (facial palsy with aural zoster vesicles) suggest that motor neurones can also be involved. Sympathetic ganglia may also be the site of latency, as indicated by cases where the initial recrudescence has been in gastric mucosa, with subsequent dissemination.

**Recurrent and chronic VZV.** Immunodeficient patients, most particularly those with CD4+ lymphopenia due to HIV infection, may develop recurrent and chronic infection. New lesions continue to appear, or reappear after acyclovir therapy, often presenting an atypical hyperkeratotic appearance. Acyclovir-resistant VZV has been isolated in this situation.

## Laboratory diagnosis

Typical presentations of varicella or zoster seldom need laboratory confirmation; however, atypical presentations merit investigation, especially in the immunocompromised. Vesicular rashes due to enterovirus are sometimes confused with varicella and, in compromised patients, various vesicular lesions may be mistaken for zoster. A common misdiagnosis is the assumption that localized vesicular lesions other than on the face or genitalia are due to zoster. In fact, many are due to herpes simplex recurrences, and this is readily shown by antigen detection and virus isolation.

## Virus detection

Early vesicular lesions provide the best diagnostic material. Vesicle fluid can be collected in a capillary tube or aspirated with a fine needle and syringe. Direct examination by electron microscopy will reveal herpes particles; some of the fluid can be diluted in virus transport medium and inoculated into tissue culture for virus isolation, which takes from 5 days to 3 weeks. More rapid detection is possible with centrifugation-enhanced cultures ('shell vials'). If cells from the base of lesions are available, or biopsy tissue, virus antigens may be sought directly in them, using immunofluorescence tests with monoclonal antibodies. VZV DNA amplification by PCR is also proving valuable for detection of VZV in CSF or aqueous humour.

## Serological diagnosis

Antibody testing with varicella–zoster antigens is useful in confirming a diagnosis of varicella by demonstration of seroconversion or rising titres of antibody between acute and convalescent serum samples; complement fixation is still a useful test for this purpose. However, the test is not sufficiently sensitive to determine past infection and, to assess immune status, assays need to be based on enzyme or radio-labelled methods, or immunofluorescent staining of varicella–zoster-infected cells. For demonstration of IgM antibody, IgM capture systems have been shown to be useful. IgM to VZV is detectable in both varicella and zoster, appearing early in zoster.

## Treatment

*Acyclovir* given intravenously is effective in the treatment of varicella and zoster in immunocompromised patients. Oral acyclovir can be used to accelerate healing and reduce new lesion formation in zoster in healthy patients if given early enough and may lower the rate of postherpetic neuralgia. VZV is not as sensitive to acyclovir as HSV, with 50% inhibitory dose ($ID_{50}$) values ranging from 4 to 17 μM acyclovir compared with 0.1–1.6 μM acyclovir for HSV, so higher dosage is required. For the intravenous preparation this means 10 mg/kg given every 8 h. Oral therapy has to be with the high-dose 800 mg five times a day regimen. Newer preparations such as the oral pro-drugs valaciclovir and famciclovir offer the advantage of less frequent dosing. Trials have shown that high-dose oral acyclovir can shorten the course of varicella in healthy children and adults by 1 day if commenced within 24 h of the onset of the rash. The practical difficulties of achieving this rule out routine treatment for all cases of varicella in healthy children, but consideration should be given to treating all adults, and where possible adolescents and family contact cases, who are known to develop more extensive disease. Treatment of VZV infection is given primarily to all 'high-risk of complication' groups:

1. Neonates (within the first 3 weeks of life)
2. Immunocompromised patients
3. Those with ophthalmic zoster
4. Healthy patients with varicella when there is an additional complicating factor such as smoking or pneumonia.

## Epidemiology

Varicella is partly seasonal, being spread mainly by the respiratory route in winter and early spring. Some cases which result from contact with zoster occur sporadically at any season. The majority of

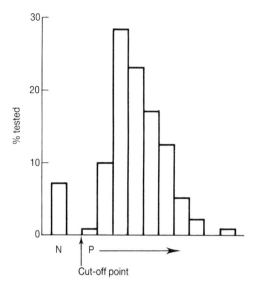

**Fig. 44.5** Distribution of antibody (IgG) to VZV in a young adult population (southern England). Percentage confirmed negative (N) was 7.8%; P →, increasing positive result.

children contract varicella between the ages of 4 and 10 years in Western countries, with around 8% of young adults remaining susceptible (Fig. 44.5). However, a much higher proportion of young adults remain susceptible in subtropical countries. Mortality from varicella is surprisingly high in normal adults, particularly smokers, who develop pneumonia. Zoster is associated with decreased T cell function, and occurs with increasing incidence in old age, the pre-AIDS phase of HIV infection, and after organ transplantation and chemo- or radiotherapy for lymphoma or leukaemia.

## Control

### Passive immunization

Passive immunity is partly protective for varicella, as seen in infants with maternal antibody or patients given *varicella–zoster immunoglobulin* (VZIG) within 72 h of exposure. VZIG (in the UK) or another similar high-titre antibody preparation is available for neonates, non-immune pregnant contacts or immuno-compromised contacts at risk of varicella. As the majority of pregnant contacts will in fact be immune, testing for antibody after exposure may prevent unnecessary use of VZIG. Current preparations will seldom prevent infection, but will modify disease. Recent review of intervention with VZIG in exposed antenatal patients showed that the rate of transmission to the fetus was decreased significantly.

## Varicella vaccine

A live attenuated varicella vaccine has been in use for some years in Japan and some European countries, and was recently licensed in the USA. This vaccine, given by intramuscular injection, has been found to be immunogenic in children with leukaemia in remission and in healthy children and adults; vaccinees have resisted infection on close exposure to varicella. Some symptoms are noted around 10 days post vaccine, and vesicles can occasionally develop. Immunization does not prevent latency developing; however, the incidence of zoster in vaccinees compared to the naturally infected is not increased. Whether vaccination will ever boost immunity to prevent zoster is not yet known. Subunit vaccines would remove the risks of transmission, and latency inherent in the live vaccine.

# EPSTEIN–BARR VIRUS

Epstein, Barr and Achong in 1964 described herpesvirus particles in cells from a common lymphoma in African children studied by Burkitt, who suspected a viral aetiology of the tumour. The link between that new herpesvirus – the *Epstein–Barr virus* – and a variety of lymphoproliferative diseases is now clearer. EBV is, however, most often involved in asymptomatic infections early in childhood or in the classical infectious mononucleosis (*glandular fever*) of adolescents in the developed world. Humans are the only natural host, but EBV infection can be transmitted to some subhuman primates.

## Description

The characteristic morphology seen on electron microscopy placed EBV with the herpesviruses. This virus cannot be grown in human fibroblast or epithelial cell lines and there is no completely productive or permissive system for culture of EBV.

## Replication

The full replication (productive, or lytic) cycle of EBV is now known to take place in differentiated epithelial cells. EBV receptors (the CD21 molecule) are expressed on mature resting B lymphocytes, and similar receptors on cells of stratified squamous epithelium – in the oropharynx, salivary glands and ectocervix for instance. Viral production, however, is restricted to the differentiated cells of the granular layer and above, and virus is shed from the superficial cells. Technical difficulties in growing differentiating epithelia in culture have limited these studies to date, and most work on the lytic cycle of EBV has been done in lymphoblastoid cell lines, in which a proportion of the EBV-infected cells can be induced to produce virions.

The organization of the EBV genome differs from HSV, and some genes are present in one and not the other. Approximately 80 proteins are encoded; some glycoproteins are known, including the major glycoprotein gp350/220, which mediates attachment to CD21, and gp85, which is involved in membrane fusion. The latent (non-productive) state of EBV infection is maintained in B lymphocytes, which have been extensively studied, and perhaps in certain epithelial cells. In the B lymphocytes the EBV genome is maintained as multiple full-length copies in the form of circular episomes. A variable number of EBV genes are expressed in the latent state; these are principally genes coding for nuclear antigens (EBNAs) and a gene encoding a latent membrane protein which hardly extends beyond the plasma membrane but may be involved in recognition by immune T cells. It may also have a role in cell transformation.

The EBV nuclear antigen 1 (EBNA 1) is responsible for maintaining the replication of the EBV episome. EBNA 2 is necessary for transformation of B lymphocytes; there are two alleles of this gene, originally designated EBNA 2A and EBNA 2B. The two EBV strains are now termed EBV-1 and EBV-2. The genes of the latent EBV are replicated by host cell DNA polymerase.

The full lytic cycle of EBV replication is accompanied by production of virus structural antigens and assembly of virions. Although EBV does encode a viral thymidine kinase, acyclovir is phosphorylated by cellular TK in cells producing EBV. The viral DNA polymerase is very sensitive to acyclovir triphosphate, and treatment with acyclovir will reduce EBV production but has no effect on latency or the proliferation induced by the virus.

## Pathogenesis

Infection of oropharyngeal epithelial cells occurs initially, then infection of B lymphocytes, which disseminate through the circulation, with the potential to enter a productive phase and release virus elsewhere in the body. Most shedding of virus, however, takes place in the oral cavity and this can be detected regularly in the saliva of asymptomatic hosts, increasing in immunosuppressed states. How B cells become infected is not proven, but there are opportunities for close contact between lymphocytes and epithelial cells in the nasopharynx.

A proportion of infected B lymphocytes undergo transformation and continue to proliferate in vitro as a lymphoblastoid cell line (*immortalization*). Activated B lymphocytes secrete immunoglobulin, and EBV is a potent polyclonal activator of antibody production by B cells, independent of any accessory cells. IgM-producing lymphocytes predominate, and IgM antibody is found in high levels, but detectable IgG (especially the IgG3 subclass), IgA and IgD have also been found.

Recovery from primary EBV infection is associated with humoral and cellular responses; any delay in cellular control, or over-vigorous responses contribute to the 'disease' associated with the infection. Thus, large initial infective doses result in high numbers of circulating infected B lymphocytes, followed by a marked T cell response. The polyclonal activation of B cells results in transient antibodies (predominantly IgM) appearing, directed against a wide range of self and heterophile antigens. The cellular response is detected as large numbers of 'atypical lymphocytes' in the blood and infiltrating many tissues. These cells have been shown to be mainly cytotoxic/suppressor T cells. The suppression is manifested as a general depression of immune responses. The cytotoxic elements carry the ability to kill EBV-infected cells, and this is not entirely human leucocyte antigen (HLA) restricted (Fig. 44.6).

Antibody responses following EBV infection make a characteristic pattern, with the initial IgM response to virus capsid antigens persisting for some months. The EBNA complex elicits antibodies in late convalescence only, perhaps after release from B cells lysed by the cytotoxic T cells (Fig. 44.7). Failure to produce antibody to EBNA is a feature of immunodeficiency states. This may be associated with increased levels of antibodies to EBV lytic cycle antigens (EA, early antigen, and VCA, viral capsid antigen), reflecting a high virus replication rate. High IgA levels to EBV VCA are found in those at risk of developing nasopharyngeal carcinoma (see later).

## Clinical features

Primary infection with EBV is usually mild and unrecognized in the vast majority who acquire it in the first years of life.

### *Infectious mononucleosis*

The disease known as *infectious mononucleosis*, or *glandular fever*, is a primary EBV infection seen

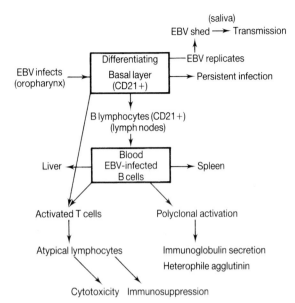

**Fig. 44.6** Simplified outline of EBV infection of cells in the oropharynx and interaction with lymphocytes.

**Fig. 44.7** Appearance and duration of diagnostic antibodies following primary EBV infection.

predominantly in the 15–25 year age group. The incubation period is 30–50 days, and the onset is abrupt with a sore throat, cervical lymphadenopathy and fever, accompanied by malaise, headache, sweating and gastro-intestinal discomfort. Pharyngitis may be severe, accompanied by a greyish white membrane and gross tonsillar enlargement. Lymphadenopathy becomes generalized, often with splenic enlargement and tenderness, mild hepatomegaly in some cases and clinical jaundice in 5–10%. Intermittent fevers with drenching sweats occur daily over 2 weeks. A faint transient morbilliform rash may be seen; a maculopapular rash may follow ampicillin administration due to immune complexes with antibody to ampicillin. The illness can last several weeks, and fatigue and lack of concentration are common in the aftermath.

## Complications of glandular fever

Complications are rare but some are serious. Acute airway obstruction may occur as a result of the lymphoid enlargement and oedema; this merits emergency tracheostomy in some cases, but usually responds well to corticosteroids. Splenic rupture is also rare. Neurological complications include meningitis, encephalitis and the Guillain–Barré syndrome.

## Other EBV-associated disease, tumours and immunodeficiency

EBV is associated with an increasing number of diseases, including malignant tumours, some of which are listed in Table 44.2. The role played by EBV in each of these is not entirely clear in all cases. Cellular immunodeficiency states lead to lack of control over the proliferative phase of EBV infection, and a risk of development of lymphomata. In some situations, as in African Burkitt's lymphoma, EBV infection at an early age accompanied by chronic immunosuppression due to endemic malaria proceeds to a highly aggressive tumour.

## Laboratory diagnosis

Infectious mononucleosis is accompanied by production of heterophile agglutinins which may be readily detected by a rapid slide agglutination test or the *Paul–Bunnell* test. Agglutination of horse or sheep red cells by serum absorbed to exclude a natural antibody is the basis of this test. Atypical lymphocytes, accounting for 20% of the lymphocytosis common in this condition, are seen in blood films. Definitive diagnosis requires the demonstration of IgM antibody to the EBV viral capsid antigen (VCA), or seroconversion if an earlier serum lacks IgG antibody. These tests, using indirect immunofluorescence, are generally available. Other serological tests are applicable in special situations.

EBV isolation is generally confined to research laboratories. Saliva or throat washings are suitable specimens. Tissues can be stained for EBNA, or probed for EBV DNA, but these approaches are not yet routinely available.

## Treatment

Acyclovir therapy does reduce EBV shedding in acute infections, and there may be a place for it in patients suffering from, or at risk of, complications associated with an ongoing viral lytic cycle.

## Epidemiology

Infection with EBV is known to be transmitted by saliva, and requires intimate oral contact. Transmission has rarely been reported following transfusion of fresh blood to seronegative recipients. Infection is

**Table 44.2**  Diseases associated with EBV

| Disease | Cells infected | Link |
|---|---|---|
| Infectious mononucleosis ('glandular fever') | B lymphocytes and nasopharyngeal epithelium | Causal; acute primary infection |
| Oral hairy leucoplakia (seen in AIDS) | Differentiated epithelium along edge of tongue | Causal; productive recurrence in immunocompromised host |
| Nasopharyngeal carcinoma (especially in South-East Asia and China) | Undifferentiated nasopharyngeal epithelium (long latent period; 30+ years) | 100% EBV-positive cells; cofactor(s) + genetic risk |
| Burkitt's lymphoma (endemic African form) | Monoclonal B cell tumour (short latent period; 5+ years) | 100% EBV-positive; immunocompromised by malaria |
| Immunoblastic lymphoma (post-transplant/AIDS; X-linked syndrome) | B lymphocytes | 70–100% EBV-positive cells; immunodeficiency states genetic defect |
| Hodgkin's disease | Hodgkin and Reed–Sternberg cells | 30–90% EBV-positive cells in subsets of disease |
| T cell lymphoma | T lymphocytes | 30–100% EBV-positive cells in subsets of disease |

widespread, with most of the population infected from early in life, even in developed countries. Increased numbers of severely immunocompromised hosts are at risk of developing EBV-associated malignant lymphomas.

## Control

A subunit vaccine, based on the major membrane glycoprotein gp350/220 is undergoing trials. It has been shown to protect marmosets against tumour-inducing doses of EBV. Screening for IgA to EBV VCA is used in populations at risk of nasopharyngeal cancer to detect preclinical cases.

## CYTOMEGALOVIRUS

There are CMVs specific to other animals, and the full name for the virus infecting humans is human cytomegalovirus (HCMV). This will be used only in the description where features of HCMV specifically are given, otherwise the more usual CMV will be used. The name 'cytomegalovirus' was chosen on account of the swollen state of infected cells as seen in culture and in tissues. Nuclei of productively infected cells contain a large inclusion body, giving a typical 'owl's eye' appearance.

## Description

The CMVs have the same general structure as other members of the herpes group.

Human fibroblast cells are required for isolation of HCMV in vitro, but in vivo the virus replicates in epithelial cells – in salivary glands, renal and respiratory epithelium particularly. CMV remains highly cell associated, and is sensitive to freezing and thawing. Virus shed in urine is stable at 4°C for many days.

## Replication

The temporal regulation of viral protein synthesis in the growth cycle is more obvious in laboratory culture of the slower-growing CMV than with HSV. Immediate early (non-structural) protein (p72) appears in nuclei within 16 h of inoculation, whilst late (virion-structural) proteins are produced after DNA synthesis, and the typical cytopathic effect is often not recognizable for 5–21 days. Foci of swollen cells slowly expand as infection passes from cell to cell (Fig. 44.8). Passage and storage of virus are best achieved by trypsinization and passage as infected cells.

**Fig. 44.8** A focus of CMV infection (arrowed) in a tissue culture monolayer of human embryo fibroblasts.

HCMV does not produce a virus-specified thymidine kinase; the protein kinase product of gene UL97 carries out initial phosphorylation of ganciclovir in CMV-infected cells, and cellular kinases produce the triphosphate, which inhibits CMV DNA polymerase.

There are several families of glycoproteins in CMV, and these are important antigenic targets. Most neutralizing antibody is directed against gB.

## Pathogenesis

Primary infection with CMV may be acquired at any time, possibly from conception onwards.

CMV persists in the host for life. Reactivation is common, and virus is shed in body secretions such as urine, saliva, semen, breast milk and cervical fluid. Mononuclear cells are thought to carry the latent virus genome since viral RNA transcripts of early genes have been detected in them, but the nature and site of latency are not yet clear. Whether any virus persists in epithelial cells is not known.

Recurrent infections may follow reactivation of latent (endogenous) virus, or reinfection with another (exogenous) strain. Isolates can be distinguished by restriction endonuclease analysis. Endothelial giant cells (multinucleate cells) have been found in the circulation during disseminated CMV infection. These cells are fully permissive for CMV replication.

## Intra-uterine infection

Maternal viraemia may result in fetal infection in approximately one out of three cases of primary CMV during pregnancy, and this may lead to disease in the fetus. Infection may also be acquired in utero when the mother has a reactivation, but this rarely results in disease. Transplacental infection is probably carried by infected cells, and transmission is associated with high viraemic load.

## Perinatal infection

This is predominantly acquired from infected maternal genital tract secretions or from breast-feeding (3–5% of pregnant women in Europe reactivate CMV). Rarely, perinatal blood transfusion is the source.

## Postnatal infection

This can be acquired in many ways. Saliva containing CMV is profusely distributed amongst young children, and shared by intimate kissing. Semen can have high titres of virus, and may be a source of sexual transmission or artifical insemination-associated infection. Blood transfusion and donated organs are important sources of CMV. As it is not known which donors are most likely to transmit infection, all antibody-positive ('seropositive') donors are considered potential transmitters as the presence of antibody implies the presence of persistent virus.

## Host responses

The host response to primary CMV includes IgM, IgG and T cell responses. Some of the T cell responses may contribute to immunopathology by reacting with HLA molecules induced by CMV. CMV early genes transactivate other viral and cellular genes and this may be an important interaction with HIV, leading to the production of HIV from latently infected cells. Because CMV infects mononuclear cells, there is a degree of immunosuppression associated with the acute infection. Cell-mediated responses are crucial to control of CMV, as shown by the serious consequences of disseminated infections in those deficient in effector cell functions. The incubation period for primary infection is 4–6 weeks; reactivation, post transplantation for instance, appears from 3 weeks onwards.

## Clinical features

### Congenital CMV infection

This is asymptomatic in 95% of infected babies, but around 15% of these will go on to show sensorineural deafness or intellectual impairment later. Progression of the persistent CMV infection may be involved. All congenitally infected infants excrete abundant virus in urine during the first year. The 5% symptomatic infants have 'cytomegalic inclusion body disease'. Growth retardation, hepatosplenomegaly, jaundice and thrombocytopenia are common to various congenital infections. Central nervous system involvement is the significant problem with CMV; microcephaly, encephalitis and retinitis may be noted at birth. Some changes may even be detectable on ultrasound scanning in utero.

### Mononucleosis

Postnatal infection with CMV is seldom recognized clinically, unless virus is isolated. Respiratory tract infection is common in infancy. A *mononucleosis syndrome* is seen occasionally, especially in young adults or when CMV is acquired from blood transfusion. Hepatitis, fever and atypical lymphocytosis are noted, but pharyngitis and lymphadenopathy are unusual and heterophile agglutinins are not found (see EBV – infectious mononucleosis). This syndrome is also seen in some HIV-infected patients before the development of AIDS, and should prompt HIV-related investigations.

### Infection in the compromised patient

Immunocompromised patients may develop symptoms as the result of primary or recurrent CMV infection. Dissemination of the virus in the blood as indicated by a hectic fever is a bad prognostic sign. The complications of CMV infection in cellular immunodeficiency include:

1. Pneumonitis – has a high mortality in bone marrow allograft recipients
2. Encephalitis – like pneumonitis this may be fatal
3. Retinitis – which may occur on its own (10–40% of AIDS patients)
4. Oesophagitis/colitis – 5–10% of AIDS patients
5. Hepatitis
6. Pancreatitis or adrenalitis.

Primary CMV infection in transplant recipients is a significant cause of morbidity and loss of graft. Mortality is high, particularly in allogeneic marrow recipients who develop an immunopathological pneumonitis associated with graft versus host disease.

Retinitis due to CMV recurrence is a feature of late-stage AIDS, when the CD4 cell count is less than 50/µl, and early recognition, antiviral treatment and maintenance therapy are important in slowing the progression towards blindness.

## Laboratory diagnosis

Detection of CMV is the objective, and, if possible, to show its presence at the site of disease. Samples should include urine, saliva, broncho-alveolar lavage fluid or biopsy tissue if available, and peripheral blood collected in anticoagulant. In the neonate, urine samples taken in the first 2 weeks of life are sufficient for diagnosis of congenital infection.

### Virus detection

Rapid diagnostic methods will detect virus DNA in the samples with PCR or a hybridization assay, or CMV early antigen in cell cultures 24 h post inoculation (Fig. 44.9), while conventional culture will be used to isolate virus. High titres of CMV will produce a cytopathic effect very quickly, but most cultures require 2–3 weeks. CMV isolation from urine does not of course prove that the virus is the cause of the disease being investigated. To demonstrate congenital infection, virus must be shown in a sample taken within the first 2 weeks of life; later samples may reflect postnatally acquired virus. Additional confirmation that CMV is related to a disease process comes from showing that the virus is replicating in the affected tissues (perhaps by cytology), and in some cases that a primary infection has occurred. The demonstration of CMV in the circulation is a significant prognostic finding, whether based on detection of DNA or of a late phosphoprotein antigen (pp65), and is predictive of clinical disease.

### Serology for CMV

This is increasingly important, and sensitive screening tests are widely available. Complement fixation tests are adequate for showing seroconversion after primary infection in competent hosts. To screen for 'seropositive' status a more sensitive assay, such as enzyme immuno-assay for CMV IgG antibody or latex agglutination assay, is appropriate. These tests can be done urgently for donor–recipient assessment. CMV IgM is found after primary or secondary infection, but it is not always possible to detect IgM in the neonate or immunocompromised patient.

## Treatment

Some antiviral agents for CMV infections are available but serious side-effects limit their use to life- or sight-threatening complications. Ganciclovir is the agent most often used for serious CMV disease, given

**Fig. 44.9** CMV early antigen demonstrated in nuclei of human embryo fibroblasts by immunofluorescence after incubation for 24 h following centrifuge-assisted inoculation.

intravenously twice a day. Marrow toxicity results in neutropenia, and there is a potential for long-term loss of spermatogenesis. Clinically, treatment has been successful in CMV colitis and encephalitis, and progression of CMV retinitis in AIDS has been controlled with prolonged maintenance therapy, which may now be given orally. Ganciclovir-resistant virus has been found. Foscarnet (phosphonoformate) is an alternative agent that does not require phosphorylation. Acylovir is not effective therapy for CMV, but some benefit from high-dose prophylaxis of CMV in transplant recipients has been noted.

## Epidemiology

Primary CMV infection is acquired by 40–60% of persons with limited exposure by mid-adult life, and by over 90% of those with multiple intimate exposures. Less than 5% of units of blood from seropositive donors result in transmission to seronegative recipients, whilst 80% of kidneys transmit infection from seropositive donors. The full extent of congenital CMV disease is not known, but this infection occurs in approximately 3 out of 1000 live births in the UK.

## Control

Some preventive action is undertaken by way of screening organ donors and recipients to avoid, where possible, a seronegative recipient receiving an organ from a seropositive donor. This has been shown to reduce morbidity and mortality significantly in all forms of allogeneic transplant. Blood donor screening to select CMV seronegative units for support of seronegative patients in transplant programmes is important but not always available. The heavy demands for blood do not allow for such a provision generally, but a special case can be made for any seriously compromised host or any very premature baby to receive screened blood (from CMV seronegative donors) or leucocyte-depleted blood.

No CMV vaccine is licensed for use. Experimental live attenuated vaccines have been tried, but hopes rest on subunit vaccines.

# HUMAN HERPESVIRUSES 6 AND 7

## Description

The existence of further herpesviruses infecting humans was not suspected until one was first isolated in 1986 from the blood of patients with lymphoproliferative disorders, some of whom had AIDS. Electron microscopy revealed a virus with characteristic herpes group features. DNA sequence studies showed this virus, now officially named human herpesvirus 6 (HHV6), to be distinct from the five known human herpesviruses, but closer to HCMV, with which it has some homology. Two variants have been identified on sequence analysis, HHV6A and HHV6B. Although first isolated from B cells, HHV6 was shown to infect CD4$^+$ T cells preferentially, and HHV6A can be propagated in T cell lines in the laboratory. HHV6B is now known to be the cause of a common disease of infancy called *exanthem subitum* or *roseola infantum*, while variant 6A has no clear disease association.

In 1990 another new human herpesvirus was isolated in similar circumstances, and has been shown to be sufficiently distinct to be called HHV7. Primary infection with HHV7 has been identified in some cases of roseola infantum also. There is a proposal that a new genus *Roseolovirus* be established for these two viruses, which are members of the subfamily betaherpesviruses.

## Pathogenesis and clinical features

### Roseola infantum (exanthem subitum)

This disease was long considered to be an infection caused by a virus, and transmission by blood was confirmed experimentally years before HHV6 was isolated. The infection is extremely common in the first years of life, presenting between 6 months and 3 years of age with a sudden onset of fever (40°C). The child is not usually ill, remaining alert and playful, with some throat congestion and cervical lymphadenopathy. Sometimes more pronounced respiratory symptoms occur and febrile convulsions have been reported. Fever persists for 3 days, when the temperature suddenly falls, and a widespread macular rash appears in around a third of cases. HHV6B has been isolated from peripheral blood in the acute febrile phase, in patients who subsequently produced a rash and some who did not. Seroconversion from an antibody-negative to antibody-positive state is noted in convalescence, confirming a primary infection with HHV6. Some cases are associated with HHV7 infection, but as yet no other disease association has been found for HHV7.

Complications of primary infection with HHV6 have been noted, and in the rare adult case hepatitis, lymphadenopathy and neurological features have been found. Reactivation in immunocompromised hosts is commonly diagnosed on the basis of serology, but the extent of disease in the transplant recipient for instance has still to be established.

Both HHV6 and HHV7 infect T lymphocytes, indeed HHV7 uses the same receptor (CD4) as HIV. The potential significance of these interactions has still to be established with regard to effects on the progression of AIDS.

## Laboratory diagnosis

Isolation of HHV6 or HHV7 involves co-cultivation of peripheral blood lymphocytes with mitogen-activated cord blood lymphocytes. The infected lymphocytes do survive for some time but are not immortalized. Very large refractile multinucleate cells are produced in culture, and many intact enveloped virions are released into the culture medium. These viruses may be isolated from saliva, particularly HHV7 which is persistently shed in saliva. DNA amplification by PCR is also used in diagnosis.

Laboratory diagnosis of HHV6 or HHV7 is currently available only from specialist laboratories. Antibody tests are becoming more widely used. Antibody avidity tests can help to establish whether a primary infection has occurred, and this method has proven useful in establishing the correct diagnosis of HHV6-associated roseola infantum in a proportion of suspected cases of infant measles.

## Treatment

HHV6 is sensitive to ganciclovir, but not to acyclovir. Treatment is seldom indicated however.

## Epidemiology

Antibody analysis to date has been based mainly on immunofluorescence studies with cells infected with either HHV6 or HHV7 as antigen. High antibody titres to HHV6 are found in young children in the first 4 years of life, reflecting recent primary infections in this group. Primary infection, with viraemia and seroconversion, has also been detected in seronegative transplant recipients of liver or kidney from seropositive donors. Possible transmission by blood transfusion has not been excluded. Infection with HHV7 is said to occur a few years later on average. Older persons have lower levels of antibody, but more sensitive enzyme immuno-assay tests reveal almost universal seropositivity. The spectrum of disease associated with these viruses and the extent of asymptomatic shedding remain to be established.

## HUMAN HERPESVIRUS 8 (KAPOSI'S SARCOMA-RELATED HERPESVIRUS)

Sequences of DNA representing a completely new human herpesvirus were identified in 1994 in studies of tissue from the epidemic form of Kaposi's sarcoma in patients with AIDS. The DNA fragments unique to the tumour tissue were found to have some homology with the gammaherpesvirus subfamily, including EBV. This is undoubtedly a new virus, officially named HHV8, but also referred to as *Kaposi's sarcoma-associated herpesvirus* (KSHV).

### Kaposi's sarcoma

Whether the new virus is the cause of Kaposi's sarcoma is not established yet, but the evidence is quite strong. This mucocutaneous neoplasm is the commonest tumour in one group of HIV-infected individuals, and was one of the two initial indicators of AIDS , along with *Pneumocystis carinii* pneumonia. The classical form was described as a rare finding in elderly patients; a rather more aggressive endemic form is seen in Africa and in some post-transplant patients, but the aggressive epidemic form has been a feature of the HIV-infected, homosexual male patients in particular. A transmissible agent was long suspected on epidemiological grounds, transmitted sexually but rarely by blood, with faecal-oral contact as a risk factor. Endothelial cells of vascular or lymphatic origin are involved; they have a characteristic spindle shape and are arranged in bundles. Although multilocalized in skin, lymph glands and gastro-intestinal tract, and able to cause functional problems, the tumour itself does not lead to death. Local radiotherapy or systemic chemotherapy have been used in treatment. Lesions on the exposed parts are obvious on account of their blue-pink or red-brown appearance in plaques, sometimes raised, and this is a cause of considerable concern for the affected individual.

### Laboratory diagnosis

At present DNA amplification by PCR is the method of detection of HHV8. Only recently has it been reported that lytic growth of HHV8 can be induced in a latently-infected B cell lymphoma line, and until reagents for antibody testing are available the epidemiology of infection with this new herpesvirus remains unknown.

## CERCOPITHECINE HERPESVIRUS 1 (B VIRUS)

### Description

This virus, antigenically related to HSV, commonly infects Old World (Asiatic) macaque monkeys, causing a mild vesicular eruption on the tongue and buccal mucosa analogous to primary herpetic stomatitis in humans. The infection rate in monkeys increases markedly if they are kept in crowded conditions and, whilst relatively benign in the monkey, this virus is highly pathogenic for humans.

Human infection with B virus is rare. It has usually been acquired from a bite or from handling infected animals without appropriate protective wear. In one instance the wife of an infected monkey handler became infected through contact with her husband's vesicles, and B virus has also been transmitted in the laboratory from infected monkey cell cultures. Within 5–20 days of exposure, local inflammation may appear at the site of entry, usually on the skin, accompanied by some itching, numbness and vesicular lesions. Ascending myelitis or acute encephalomyelitis may follow. Delay in specific therapy leads to a high mortality rate and serious neurological sequelae in survivors.

### Diagnosis and treatment

Diagnosis is by isolation of the virus from blood, vesicle fluid, conjunctival swabs and CSF. Herpes virions may be detectable on electron microscopy of vesicle fluid. Definitive identification of the virus is available in special reference laboratories, using PCR for DNA, or monoclonal antibodies. Demonstration of specific antibodies is complicated by cross-reacting HSV antibody. B virus is not as sensitive to acyclovir as HSV, requiring concentrations equivalent to those used for VZV. Treatment needs to be given promptly to be effective, and intravenous acyclovir for 14 days or longer is recommended. Ganciclovir should be used when there is evidence of central nervous system involvement. Because of the small number of cases the best therapeutic regimen is not well established.

### Prevention of B virus infection

Guidelines have been issued for the protection of those handling monkeys or monkey tissues. These include: recommendations for training to prevent exposure; safe handling and protective wear procedures; care of wounds; and information as to the risks and nature of the infection. Prophylaxis in the event of possible exposure involves wound washing, cleansing with 10% iodine in alcohol, and a course of oral acyclovir (high dose, 800 mg five times a day for 3 weeks) with a prolonged observation period, as the onset of infection may be delayed.

### RECOMMENDED READING

Fields B N, Knipe D M, Howley P M (eds) 1996 *Virology*, 3rd edn. Lippincott-Raven, Philadelphia

Fox J D, Tedder R S, Briggs E M 1994 Human herpesviruses 6 and 7. In: Zuckerman A J, Banatvala J E, Pattison J R (eds) *Principles and Practice of Clinical Virology*, 3rd edn. Wiley, Chichester

Khanna R, Burrows S R, Moss 1995 Immune regulation in Epstein–Barr virus-associated diseases. *Microbiological Reviews* 59: 387–405

Lakeman F D, Whitley R J, The National Institute of Allergy and Infectious Diseases Collaborative Antiviral Study Group 1995 Diagnosis of herpes simplex encephalitis: application of polymerase chain reaction to cerebrospinal fluid from brain-biopsied patients and correlation with disease. *Journal of Infectious Diseases* 171: 857–863

Nahmias A J, Keyserling H, Lee F K 1989 Herpes simplex viruses 1 and 2. In: Evans A S (ed) *Viral Infections of Humans*, 3rd edn. Plenum Press, New York

Revello M G, Furione M, Zavattoni M, Gerna G 1994 Human cytomegalovirus infection; diagnosis by antigen and DNA detection. *Reviews in Medical Microbiology* 5: 265–276

Stevens J G 1989 Human herpesviruses: a consideration of the latent state. *Microbiological Reviews* 53: 318–332

# 45

# Poxviruses

Smallpox; molluscum contagiosum; parapoxvirus infections

*T. H. Pennington*

The world's last naturally occurring case of smallpox was recorded in Merca, Southern Somalia, in October 1977. This momentous event marked the end of a long campaign against smallpox, which in its 'modern' phase started with the introduction of vaccination by Edward Jenner at the end of the 18th century. With the eradication of smallpox – which has joined the dodo and the great auk by becoming extinct in the wild at the hand of humans – the importance of poxviruses in medical practice may appear to be much diminished, as the other naturally occurring viruses in this family that infect humans nearly always restrict themselves to causing self-limiting and trivial skin lesions. Smallpox, on the other hand, caused a generalized infection with high mortality, and fell into that small group of viruses (including viral haemorrhagic fevers and, now, human immunodeficiency virus) which differ from the majority – which usually cause mild or subclinical infections – because their infections are commonly severe and frequently lethal. Notwithstanding their minor role today as human pathogens, poxviruses retain their importance, and their place in this book, for three reasons.

*Firstly*, the successful smallpox eradication campaign is important in its own right as a major achievement. It is also important because it highlights the principles and problems associated with projects that aim to control infections by eradicating the pathogen. Smallpox was the first disease to fall to this approach and remains the only successful example to date.

*Secondly*, work on the molecular biology of poxviruses has led to the identification of distinctive properties and the development of techniques and approaches which have made it possible to move significantly towards constructing single-dose vaccines which protect simultaneously against a wide range of diseases. Genes coding for foreign non-poxvirus antigens have been inserted into the poxvirus genome so that the antigens are expressed during virus infection and induce immunity.

*Thirdly*, no account of virus diseases in general and poxvirus infections in particular is complete without consideration being given to the events which followed the introduction of myxomatosis into Australia, by far the best studied example to date of the evolution of a new virus disease.

## DESCRIPTION

### Classification

A large number of different viruses belonging to the family Poxviridae have been described. They infect a wide range of vertebrate and invertebrate hosts. The subfamily Chordopoxvirinae contains all the viruses that infect vertebrates; it is divided into six genera, each containing related viruses which generally infect related hosts. Thus, members of the genus *Leporipoxvirus* infect rabbits and squirrels, *Avipoxvirus* members infect birds, *Capripoxvirus* members infect goats and sheep, *Suipoxvirus* members infect swine, and *Parapoxvirus* members infect cattle and sheep. Some viruses, including that of molluscum contagiosum, which infects humans, remain unclassified. By far the most intensively studied poxvirus is vaccinia virus, the Jennerian smallpox vaccine virus. This virus has been placed in the genus *Orthopoxvirus* together with smallpox virus and some viruses which infect cattle and mice.

### The virion

Poxviruses are the largest animal viruses. Their virions are big enough to be seen as dots by light microscopy after special staining procedures. They are much more complex than those of any other viruses (Figs 45.1 and 45.2). They are also distinctive in that they do not show any discernible symmetry. The core contains the DNA genome and 15 or more

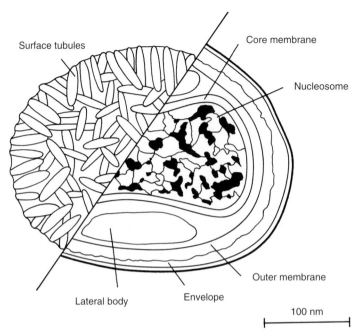

**Fig. 45.1** The structure of the vaccinia virion. Right-hand side, section of enveloped virion; left-hand side, surface structure of non-enveloped particle. (From Fenner F et al 1988 *Smallpox and its Eradication*. World Health Organization, Geneva.)

enzymes which make up a transcriptional system whose role is to synthesize biologically active poly-adenylated, capped and methylated virus messenger RNA (mRNA) molecules early in infection. The core has a 9 nm thick membrane, with a regular sub-unit structure. Within the virion, the core assumes a dumb-bell shape because of the large lateral bodies. The core and lateral bodies are enclosed in a protein shell about 12 nm thick – the outer membrane – the surface of which consists of irregularly arranged tubules, which in turn consist of a small globular subunit. Virions released naturally from the cell are enclosed within an envelope which contains host cell lipids and several virus-specified polypeptides, including the haemagglutinin; they are infectious. Most virions remain cell-associated and are released by cellular disruption. These particles lack an enve-lope so that the outer membrane constitutes their surface; they are also infectious. More than 100 dif-ferent polypeptides have been identified in purified virions.

## The genome

Their DNA genomes range in mass from 85 MDa (parapoxviruses) to 185 MDa (avipoxviruses). The vaccinia virus genome has 186 000 base pairs (123 MDa). The poxvirus genome is distinctive in that covalent links join the two DNA strands at both ends of the molecule, the genome thus being a single uninterrupted molecule that is folded to form a linear duplex structure. The occurrence of invert-ed terminal sequence repetitions is also a charac-teristic feature, identical sequences being present at each end of the genome.

## REPLICATION

Poxviruses are unique among human DNA viruses in that virus RNA and DNA synthesis takes place in the cytoplasm of the infected cell. Because of this they have been intensively studied by workers on gene expression. After entry into the cell the core is uncoated. It starts to synthesize mRNA immediately. About half the genome is transcribed. Genes that are transcribed at this time are called early genes and map throughout the length of the genome. Only a few of their products have been characterized. They include enzymes needed for replication and tran-scription of viral DNA, such as DNA polymerase. Virus DNA replication starts at about 90 min after infection and goes on for several hours. It takes place in well-defined areas in the cytoplasm called factories. As soon as DNA replication starts, a

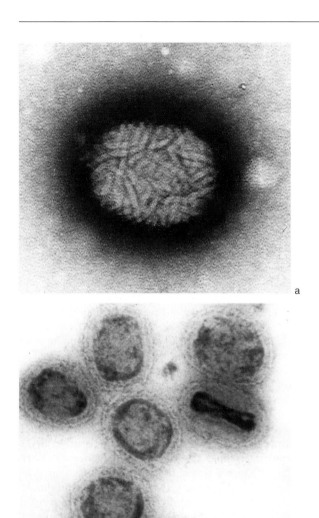

**Fig. 45.2** Electron micrographs of poxviruses. **a** Molluscum contagiosum virus (MCV). ×15 000. **b** MCV showing internal structure. ×75 000. (Prepared by N. Atack.) **c** Parapoxvirus: orf. Bar, 100 nm. (By courtesy of Dr D. W. Gregory.)

dramatic change in viral gene expression occurs. Nearly all the genome now becomes available for transcription, and regulatory mechanisms come into play which lead to the synthesis of a new class of gene product, the late polypeptides. Soon after the onset of synthesis of these polypeptides the expression of most of the early genes is turned off. Most virion structural polypeptides are made late. Virion assembly takes place in the cytoplasm and proceeds in a series of steps which include the formation of spherical immature particles. The onset of virus macromolecular synthesis is accompanied by irreversible inhibition of host protein synthesis due to the functional inactivation and degradation of host cytoplasmic RNA molecules. It is probable that this effect on the host, which leads to the death of infected cells, is a major factor in the causation of tissue damage during infection.

## CLINICAL FEATURES

Smallpox virus had no animal reservoir and spread from person to person by the respiratory route. After infecting mucosal cells in the upper respiratory tract without producing symptoms it spread to the regional lymph nodes and, after a transient viraemia, infected cells throughout the body. Multiplication of virus in these cells led to a second and more intense viraemia which heralded the onset of clinical illness. During the first few days of fever the virus multiplied in skin epithelial cells leading to the development of focal lesions and the characteristic rash. Macules progressed to papules, vesicles and pustules, leaving permanent pockmarks, particularly on the face. Two kinds of smallpox were common in the first half of the 20th century. These were called variola major and variola minor, or alastrim. Variola major virus caused classical smallpox, which had case fatality rates varying from 10 to 50% in the unvaccinated. Variola minor caused a much milder disease and had case fatality rates of less than 1%. The viruses are very similar but can be distinguished in the laboratory by restriction enzyme fragment length polymorphisms of their genomes.

## CONTROL OF SMALLPOX

### Before vaccination

Before the introduction of vaccination, the control of smallpox relied on two approaches, variolation and isolation. Variolators aimed to induce immunity equivalent to that after natural infection. Susceptible individuals were deliberately infected with smallpox pus or scabs by scratching the skin or by nasal insufflation. Although the virus was not attenuated, infections had lower case fatality rates (estimated to be 0.5–2%) and were less likely to cause permanent pockmarks than those acquired naturally. Variolation was first recorded in China nearly 1000 years ago, and was practised in many parts of the world. Variolators were active until very recent times. In Afghanistan, Pakistan and Ethiopia their activities caused problems towards the end of the smallpox eradication programme in the 1970s because they spread virus in a way which evaded the measures erected to control natural virus transmission.

### Vaccination

Edward Jenner vaccinated James Phipps with cowpox virus on 14 May 1796 and challenged him by variolation some months later. He repeated this 'trial', as he called it, in other children, and the description of these events in his 'Inquiry' in 1798 led to the rapid world-wide acceptance of vaccination. Introduction of the vaccine virus into the epidermis led to the development of a local lesion and the induction of a strong immunity to infection

with smallpox virus which lasted for several years. Although the essentials of *Jennerian vaccination* remained unchanged for the rest of its history, early vaccinators developed their own vaccine viruses, which became known as vaccinia. The origin of these viruses is obscure, and modern vaccinia viruses form a distinct species of orthopoxvirus, related to but very clearly distinct from the viruses of both cowpox and smallpox.

### The eradication campaign

Routine vaccination of children – compulsory in some countries – combined with outbreak control by isolation and selective vaccination gradually brought smallpox under control in Europe, the former USSR, North and Central America, and Japan, and the virus had been eradicted from all these areas by the mid-1950s. In 1959 this achievement prompted the World Health Organization (WHO) to adopt the global eradication of smallpox as a major goal. At this time 60% of the world's population lived in areas where smallpox was endemic. A slow reduction in disease was maintained for the next few years, but epidemics continued to be frequent. Consequently the WHO initiated its Intensified Smallpox Eradication Programme. This started on 1 January 1967 when the disease was reported in 31 countries. It had the goal of eradication within 10 years. The goal was achieved in 10 years, 9 months and 26 days. From a starting point of 10 million to 15 million cases annually (Fig. 45.3) and against a background of civil strife, famine and floods, success came because of a major international collaborative effort – aided by some virus-specific factors (Table 45.1). At the beginning of 1976 smallpox occurred only in Ethiopia (Fig. 45.4). Transmission was interrupted there in August of that year, although an importation of virus into Somalia and adjacent countries had occurred by then. This was the last outbreak. The last case occurred on 26 October 1977. In the final years of the programme its emphasis moved from mass vaccination to a strategy of surveillance and containment. This strategy rapidly interrupted transmission. It was possible because cases were easy to detect due to the characteristic rash, because patients usually transmitted disease to only a few people – and only to those in close face-to-face contact – because only persons with a rash transmitted infection, and because outbreaks could be successfully contained in most areas by isolation of cases and vaccination of contacts and people in the immediate vicinity. The WHO Global Commission for the Eradication of Smallpox formally

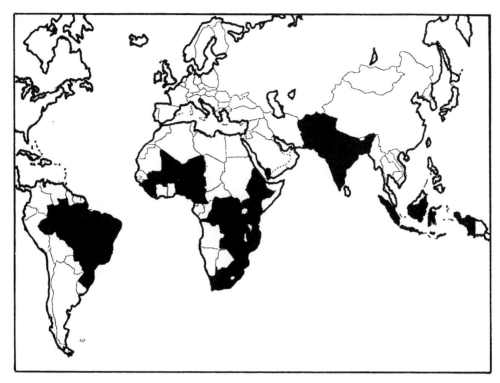

**Fig. 45.3** Smallpox in the world, 1967. The map shows the 31 countries with endemic smallpox. (From Fenner et al (1988) – see Fig. 45.1 for reference.)

**Fig. 45.4** Smallpox in the world, 1976–77. (From Fenner et al (1988) – see Fig. 45.1 for reference.)

**Table 45.1** Features of smallpox that facilitated its eradication

| Feature | Importance |
|---|---|
| Disease severe | Ensured strong public and governmental support for eradication programme |
| Detection of cases easy because of characteristic rash and subsequent development of facial pockmarks | Facilitated containment of outbreaks and audit of success of programme |
| Slow spread and poor transmissibility | Faciitated containment of outbreaks by vaccination/isolation |
| Transmission by subclinical cases not important | Meant that control of spread by isolation of cases was an an effective procedure |
| No carrier state in man | Meant that control of spread by isolation of cases was an effective procedure |
| No animal reservoir | Meant that control of spread by isolation of cases was an effective procedure |
| Vaccine technically simple to produce in large amounts, in high quality and at low cost (in skin of ungulates) | Meant that vaccine availability was not an important constraint in the eradication programme |
| Vaccine delivery simple and optimized by use of reusable, cheap, specially designed needles to deliver a standard amount of vaccine to scratches in skin | Meant that failure at the point of vaccination was not an important constraint in the eradication programme |
| Freeze-dried vaccine stocks were heat-stable with very long shelf life in tropics | Meant that vaccine viability under adverse environmental conditions was not an important constraint in the eradication programme |

certified that smallpox had been eradicated from the world on 9 December 1979.

## OTHER POXVIRUS INFECTIONS OF HUMANS

### Molluscum contagiosum

The lesions of this mild disease are small copper-coloured warty papules which occur on the trunk, buttocks, arms and face. It is spread by direct contact or by fomites. The lesion consists of a mass of hypertrophied epidermis which extends into the dermis and protrudes above the skin. In the epithelial cells very large hyaline acidophilic granular masses can be observed. They crowd the host cell nucleus to one side, eventually filling the whole cell. When material from the lesions is crushed, some of the inclusions burst open, and from them large numbers of virions escape. These have the size, internal structure and morphology of vaccinia virus. The infection has been transmitted experimentally to human subjects, but the virus has not been grown in cultured cells. The development of immunity is slow and uncertain. Lesions can persist for as long as 2 years, and reinfection is common.

### Monkeypox

This has been occasionally implicated in a smallpox-like condition in equatorial Africa. It may be fatal in unvaccinated individuals, but is less transmissible from person to person than smallpox.

### Parapoxvirus infections

The virions of parapoxviruses are characterized by a criss-cross pattern of tubes in the outer membrane (see Fig. 45.2c), and genomes that are considerably smaller – 85 MDa – than those of other poxviruses. They infect ungulates and cause the occupational diseases in humans of orf and milker's nodes. The lesions of orf (which causes a disease in sheep known as contagious pustular dermatitis) are often large and granulomatous. Erythema multiforme is a relatively frequent complication. The lesions of milker's nodes are highly vascular hemispherical papules and nodules. Both diseases are self-limiting, are commonest on the hands and are contracted by contact with infected sheep (orf) or cows (milker's nodes). They are occupational diseases, and are mainly seen in farm workers such as shepherds, slaughterhouse workers or butchers.

# VACCINIA VIRUS AS A VACCINE VECTOR

The vaccinia virus genome can accommodate size-able losses of DNA in certain regions, to the extent that as many as 25 000 base pairs can be lost without lethal effect. By replacing this non-essential DNA with foreign genes it has been possible to construct novel *recombinant virus strains* which express the foreign genes when they infect cells. These genes have been inserted into the vaccinia genome by standard gene manipulation techniques, recombination and transfection.

When a cell is infected with more than one poxvirus strain, recombination can take place between them if they are closely related genetically. Recombination takes place even if one of the poxvirus genomes enters the cell in the form of naked DNA: techniques exist that optimize this process, which is known as *transfection*. Recombination has been used to insert foreign genes into the region of the vaccinia genome that codes for the non-essential enzyme thymidine kinase (TK). A fragment of vaccinia virus DNA containing this gene is taken and by use of gene manipulation techniques the foreign gene is inserted into the TK region, with a vaccinia virus promoter next to it to ensure gene expression. This DNA is then introduced by transfection into cells infected with wild type (TK$^+$) vaccinia virus. Recombination takes place at the TK gene, producing viruses whose genomes now contain the foreign gene. Because this is inserted into the TK gene the latter is non-functional (TK$^-$). Selection procedures for the absence of TK activity are now applied, aiding the identification of recombinant viruses. Recombinant vaccinia strains containing as many as four foreign genes, coding for combinations of bacterial, viral and protozoal antigens, have been constructed.

The advantages of this ingenious way of developing new vaccines are its applicability to many different antigens, the possibility of constructing multivalent vaccines that could give protection against several diseases after a single 'shot', and the ease of administration and cheapness of vaccinia as a vaccine. A strain which expresses the rabies glycoprotein antigen is being used in Europe to protect foxes. Serious disadvantages remain for humans, however. These are primarily those associated with vaccinia virus itself, whose use carried with it a number of serious complications. The most important of these were *progressive vaccinia*, a fatal infection which occurred in immunodeficient individuals, *eczema vaccinatum*, a serious spreading infection which occurred in eczematous individuals, and *postvaccinal encephalitis*, which, although rare, was severe and occurred in normal healthy individuals. These disadvantages preclude the use of vaccinia as a vector for foreign antigens in humans, and work is being done on the modification of its virulence to get round these problems. So far, studies on virulence genes have shown that poxviruses code for an impressive array of factors interfering with host defences. These include proteins which bind complement components, act as receptors for interleukin-1β, interferon, and tumour necrosis factor, and synthesize steroids. These factors are all exported from infected cells. Ones that act inside cells include proteins that block the action of interferon, inhibit the post-translational modification of interleukin-1β, and prevent the synthesis of a neutrophil chemotactic factor. It is possible that abrogation of virulence factors such as these may lead to safer vaccines.

# MYXOMATOSIS: AN EVOLVING DISEASE

As a rule, virus infections are mild and self-limiting. Viruses are obligate parasites and it is easy to understand that it is not in their interests to cause the extinction or massive reductions in size of host populations. It is reasonable to suppose that the type of disease caused by a virus reflects the outcome of a process in which host and virus have co-evolved to levels of resistance and virulence optimal for the maintenance of their respective population numbers. The high mortality of classical smallpox is considered by some to have been a major factor in the restriction of human population size, and this has been used to support the hypothesis that the association between smallpox and humans has been established – in evolutionary terms – only in recent times, co-evolution of the relationship being a long way from equilibrium. It is impossible to test this hypothesis directly, but a dramatic example with many parallels has been provided by the relationship between another poxvirus – myxoma virus – and the rabbit in Australia. This is the only example of co-evolution where changes in an animal host and virus and the evolution of a disease have been studied in real time.

Myxoma virus is South American. It causes a benign local fibroma in its natural host, the rabbit *Sylvilagus brasiliensis*, but causes *myxomatosis* in the European rabbit, *Oryctolagus cuniculus*. This is a generalized infection with a very high mortality rate.

Field trials to test its efficacy as a measure for controlling the European rabbit were done in Australia in 1950. The virus escaped and caused enormous epidemics in the years that followed. The original virus caused infections with a case mortality rate greater than 99%, and rabbits survived less than 13 days. Within 3 years virus isolates from epidemics had become much less virulent, causing infections with mortality rates of 70–95% and survival times of 17–28 days. Changes in the resistance of the rabbit also occurred, with mortality rates of infection falling (from 90 to 25% following challenge with strains of virus with modified virulence, for example) and symptomatology becoming less severe. In myxomatosis, natural selection favoured virus strains with intermediate virulence because such strains are transmitted more effectively than highly virulent strains, which kill their hosts too quickly, and non-virulent strains, which are poorly transmitted.

## RECOMMENDED READING

Baxby D 1981 *Jenner's Smallpox Vaccine*. Heinemann, London
Fenner F, Ratcliffe F N 1965 *Myxomatosis*. Cambridge University Press, Cambridge
Fenner F, Henderson D A, Arita I, Jezek Z, Ladnyi I D 1988 *Smallpox and its Eradication*. World Health Organization, Geneva
Fields B N, Knipe D M (eds) 1995 *Virology*, 3rd edn. Lippincott–Raven, Philadelphia
Jenner E 1798 *An Inquiry into the Causes and Effects of the Variolae Vaccinae*. Sampson Low, London

# 46

# Papovaviruses

**Warts: warts and skin cancers; progressive multifocal leuco-encephalopathy**

*H. Cubie*

The *papillomavirus*, *polyomavirus* and simian virus 40 (SV40), the *vacuolating* virus of rhesus monkeys, are a group of small DNA viruses which are currently classified in two genera (*Papillomavirus* and *Polyomavirus*) of the family Papovaviridae, the name being derived from the first two letters of the names of each of the aforementioned members. Papovaviruses are all small DNA tumour viruses with icosahedral capsid structure, but the molecular biology and pathogenesis of the two genera differ considerably.

*Papillomavirus.* These are species-specific DNA viruses that infect the squamous epithelia and mucous membranes of vertebrates, including man. They are responsible for many varieties of *warts* and fibro-papillomata. Although the lesions are usually benign, their association with tumours of man and other animals is now well documented. The first evidence for oncogenic properties came from the study of the virus types infecting animals. In the 1930s Shope found that the cottontail rabbit papillomavirus caused benign warts with 25% of the lesions undergoing malignant change within a year. Viral DNA remained detectable within the tumours. In domestic rabbits, however, up to 75% of lesions progressed to cancer. Application of tar to the lesions led to more rapid malignant change. Bovine papillomavirus (BPV) causes tumours of the alimentary canal and bladder in cattle fed on a diet containing bracken fern. The tumours are preceded by infection with BPV types 4 and 2, respectively, but the virus is not detected after malignant transformation. These studies show that malignant progression can be influenced by both genetic composition and exposure to chemicals.

*Polyomavirus.* The name is derived from 'poly' (many) and 'oma' (tumour). The viruses are species-specific, and although tumour induction is well described in experimental animals, there is to date no documented association with any naturally occurring tumour of man. Recognized members of this group include the mouse polyomavirus, SV40 of monkeys and two viruses of man – JC virus (JCV) and BK virus (BKV), both named after the initials of the people from whom they were first isolated.

## PAPILLOMAVIRUSES

The papillomaviruses are 52–55 nm in diameter and have an icosahedral capsid composed of 72 capsomeres (Fig. 46.1). The genome is a supercoiled double-stranded circle of DNA, with a single coding strand, a molecular weight of approximately $5 \times 10^6$ and consisting of about 8000 base pairs (bp).

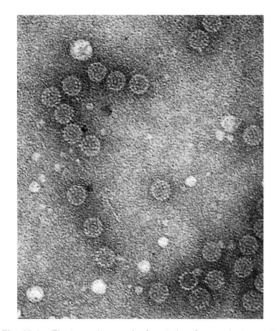

**Fig. 46.1** Electron micrograph of wart virus from a plantar wart. PTA stain. ×100 000. (By courtesy of Dr M. M. Ogilvie.)

**Table 46.1** HPV types associated with specific lesions

| Lesion | HPV type |
| --- | --- |
| **Cutaneous sites** | |
| Deep plantar warts (*verruca plantaris*) | 1, 4 |
| Common warts (*verruca vulgaris*) | 2, 4, 7 |
| Plane or flat warts | 3, 10 |
| Epidermodysplasia verruciformis-like macular lesions | 5, 8 |
| **Mucocutaneous sites** | |
| Genital warts (*condyloma acuminatum*) | 6, 11 |
| Flat condyloma and intra-epithelial neoplasia | 16, 18, 31, 33 |
| Laryngeal papillomata | 6, 11 |
| Oral papillomata | 2, 6, 11, 16, 18, 57 |
| Oral hyperplasia | 13, 32 |

There are over 70 types of the human papillomavirus (HPV), which are distinguished on the basis of the homology between their genomes measured by cross-hybridization between the separated DNA strands. A new type must exhibit less than 50% homology with any other known type. The appearance of the lesions produced or the tissues commonly infected is associated with specific virus types. Types 1, 2, 3 and 4 commonly infect the keratinized epithelium of the hands and feet, producing the common warts frequently seen in young children and adolescents. Type 7 is found in skin warts affecting meat workers (butchers' warts). HPV types 6, 11, 16, 18, 31 and 33 are mucotropic and infect the genito-urinary tract and oral cavity. Types 2 and 57 can infect both skin and genital mucosa. Table 46.1 shows the lesions commonly associated with different virus types.

## Replication

While viral DNA can be found in the basal cells of the epithelium whole virions are found only in the uppermost cell layer in terminally differentiated keratinocytes. It is this close association of viral replication with tissue differentiation which has made the development of tissue culture systems difficult. Understanding of the events in the replication cycle has been deduced therefore from knowledge of comparable viruses. Viral DNA can be found as an episome in productively infected cells and is frequently integrated at random sites into a host chromosome in malignant lesions.

The E (early) region of the viral DNA contains open-reading frames (ORFs), which code for proteins concerned with DNA replication, transcription and transformation while the L (late) region contains two ORFs which code for the viral capsid proteins. The E1 and E2 proteins are both essential for replication. The long control region (LCR) is concerned with the control of transcription. Binding of the E2 protein to an enhancer site on the LCR can up-regulate transcription of E6 and E7, the genes responsible for transformation. Inactivation of E1 leads to integration of viral DNA into the host chromosomes at random sites. E4 causes the collapse of the cellular cytoskeleton, and E5 has transforming activity in some HPV types.

## Clinical features and pathogenesis

### Cutaneous warts

Cutaneous warts are found most frequently in childhood and the viruses commonly associated with such lesions are HPV types 1 and 4 (plantar warts), 3 and 10 (flat warts), and 2, 4 and 7 (common warts) (Table 46.1). Histologically, the lesions are benign with hypertrophy of all the layers of the dermis and hyperkeratosis of the horny layer (Fig. 46.2). The lesions will usually disappear spontaneously within

a

b

**Fig. 46.2** Histology of a wart.

2 years of onset but may be resistant to treatment. Regrowth of the lesions after treatment is thought to be due to persistence of the virus in the skin surrounding the original wart.

Although both humoral immune and cell-mediated immune responses can develop in papilloma infections, regression is usually the result of cellular responses. In patients with primary or secondary cell-mediated immunodeficiency, there is an increased risk of developing warts which can be extensive, persistent or recurrent and likely to progress. For example, in people suffering from the rare genetic skin disorder, *epidermodysplasia verruciformis* (EV), where there is a selective depletion of T cells, large plane warts associated with virus types not usually found in the normal population (HPV types 5 and 8 and others) develop and persist for life. Similarly, up to 40% of renal allograft recipients will develop cutaneous warts within a year of the graft, rising to more than 90% in those with graft survival greater than 15 years.

## Genital warts

These lesions (also known as *condylomata acuminata*) are commonest in sexually active adults. In women they are found on the vulva, within the vagina and on the cervix. Vulvar and vaginal warts are usually plainly visible, but on the cervix they may be indistinguishable from the normal mucosa without the aid of a colposcope to magnify the cervical epithelium. The application of 5% acetic acid causes whitening of epithelium in which there is a high concentration of nuclear material and under these conditions subclinical lesions are revealed as areas of densely white whorled epithelium known as flat or non-condylomatous warts while normal mucosa remains pink.

Subclinical infection of the genital tract may become clinically apparent if the immune response is disturbed. During pregnancy warts may appear on vulvar epithelium and disappear postpartum. It is not known whether this is a hormonal effect or due to the alteration of the immune response that occurs during pregnancy.

Studies of apparently normal people have shown that the papillomaviruses can also be latent since they are detectable in normal epithelia in the absence of lesions. Review of several studies has suggested that about 12% of women with normal cytology carry HPV DNA in the cells from cervical scrapes. The prevalence rate is 3–5 times higher in women aged under 35 years than in older women, and HPV16/18 is more commonly found than HPV6/11.

In men the favoured sites for lesions are the shaft of the penis, peri-anal skin and the anal canal. Subclinical infection of the genital tract may also occur in men and will be visible only if the penis is painted with 5% acetic acid and examined with a magnifying glass or colposcope.

HPV types 6 and 11 are commonly found in benign vulval or penile warts. Cervical and anogenital warts may be due to HPV types 16 or 18, both of which are associated with malignant and premalignant lesions of the cervix and anogenital tract. Some other types, including types 31, 33 and 35, also have an association with genital cancers and their precursor lesions.

## Recurrent respiratory papillomatosis

This rare condition is characterized by the presence of benign squamous papillomata on the mucosa of the respiratory tract, most commonly on the larynx. Recurrent respiratory papillomatosis (RRP) has a bimodal age distribution with peaks of incidence in children under 5 years of age and adults after the age of 15 years. It is caused by infection of the respiratory mucosa with HPV types 6 and 11. Children acquire the disease by passage through an infected birth canal, while adults acquire the disease from orogenital contact with an infected sexual partner. The transmission rate is low. RRP presents with hoarseness of voice or, in children, with an abnormal cry. As the lesions grow they may cause stridor and upper airway obstruction which can be life-threatening and require emergency surgery. Recurrence following treatment is common and extension of the disease to the bronchial tree may occur, particularly after tracheostomy. Involvement of the alveolar membrane, causing the formation of multiple cysts, is uncommon but is usually fatal. Malignant conversion of laryngeal papillomas has been described, usually after radiotherapy to treat the initial lesion.

## Oral papillomatosis

A variety of papillomata and benign lesions associated with HPV occur on the oral mucosa and tongue. Several HPV types including types 2, 7, 13 and 32 have been found, the last two in *focal epithelial hyperplasia* or *Heck's disease* common in Eskimos. Subclinical lesions can be detected on the oral mucosa of normal adults after the application of acetic acid. The virus types here are those more commonly found in the genital tract and infection is acquired during orogenital contact with an infected sexual partner. Multiple lesions may develop on the buccal mucosa, a condition known as *oral florid papillomatosis*. Malignant coversion of oral papillomata has been observed.

## Human wart viruses and cancer

### Premalignant lesions of the genital tract

Malignant disease of the cervix is preceded by neoplastic change in the surface epithelium, a condition known as *cervical intra-epithelial neoplasia* (CIN). A similar pattern of events takes place in other sites in the genital tract of both men and women, known respectively as penile (PIN), vulval (VIN) or vaginal (VaIN) intra-epithelial neoplasia. The initial transforming event takes place in the deepest layer of the epithelium, the germinal layer, and abnormal cells spread through the surface layers. This condition increases in severity from grade 1 to grade 3 (Fig. 46.3), which is characterized by the presence of abnormal cells in all layers of the epithelium with loss of stratification and differentiation. Mitotic figures are present in the uppermost layers of the epithelium. CIN3 has been shown in two prospective studies to progress to *invasive cancer* in 35–50% of affected individuals over a period of 10 years. Lesser degrees of CIN have a lower malignant potential than this, and *regression* may occur spontaneously at all stages. HPV DNA can be detected in all grades of the premalignant lesions of the female and male genital tract. HPV types 6 and 11 are most commonly found in low-grade CIN, VIN, VaIN and PIN whereas HPV types 16 and 18 are more commonly associated with lesions of greater severity and invasive cancer.

### Squamous cell carcinomata

There is a well-documented association of wart viruses with invasive cancers of the skin, larynx and genital tract. Malignant conversion of skin warts occurs in about one-third of EV patients at a relatively young age on skin exposed to sunlight. HPV type 5 or 8 is found in over 90% of the squamous cancers in EV. Malignant conversion of cutaneous warts in renal allograft recipients has also been documented, and some of these tumours contained HPV5/8 or other EV-related types. Squamous cell carcinoma (SCC) of the aerodigestive tract, particularly the tonsils, has recently been shown to harbour HPV, principally HPV16, but including more than 20 other types.

The commonest association with invasive cancer, however, is with tumours of the anogenital tract. Approximately 95% of invasive cervical cancers contain HPV DNA, predominantly HPV16. However, the proportion of cancers containing different HPV types varies around the world and the incidence shows wide demographic, ethnic and socio-economic variation. In Indonesia, for example, HPV18 predominates whereas in Europe HPV16 is by far the most common. HPV18 also predominates in the more aggressive adenocarcinomata. In-situ DNA

**Fig. 46.3** Histological appearances of CIN1 (left) and CIN3 (right).

hybridization of tumour biopsies has shown that the HPV DNA is unevenly distributed throughout the tumour, suggesting that these cancers are polyclonal in origin.

In most animal cancers associated with papillomavirus there is an identifiable cofactor. In humans, the genetic background of the individual, smoking, seminal fluid factors and immune status, have all been implicated as cofactors in HPV-associated genital tract malignancies. Thus, CIN is commoner in relatives of affected women than in the population at large. Women who smoke are at increased risk of CIN and cancer of the cervix as are women who are immunosuppressed, whether due to drug treatment (transplant recipients) or secondary to haematological malignancies (leukaemias) or to infection with human immunodeficiency virus. Further risk factors in the development of genital carcinomata include sexual activity and age at first intercourse, smoking, oral contraceptive use and occurrence of other sexually transmitted infections. It is, however, extremely difficult to assess the relative interdependence of all risk factors.

In the development of HPV-related SCCs at other sites, exposure to ultraviolet or ionizing radiation, smoking, chewing of betel-quid, immunosuppression and genetic make-up are all likely to be important.

## Transmission and epidemiology

Clinical studies of the incidence of skin warts show that infection is common in early childhood and is acquired by direct contact with an infected person. Fomites may also be important, as shown by outbreaks of hand warts from the use of gymnastic apparatus and plantar warts acquired from swimming pool surrounds. Mild shearing trauma is necessary to allow the virus to reach the basal layers of the skin.

Transmission of genital warts occurs during sexual activity. It is becoming increasingly evident that genital wart types can also be acquired non-sexually. There is poor concordance of genital HPV types between heterosexual partners, and genital HPV DNA has been detected in virgins. HPV6-induced juvenile laryngeal papillomatosis occurs as a result of acquisition during passage through the mother's infected birth canal, but high-risk HPV types can also be detected in newborns and infants. A recent study has shown 50% of children born to HPV16-infected mothers to be positive at 24 h and 25% still positive at 6 weeks, while another study showed 19% of infants to have HPV16 in the buccal cavity.

## Laboratory diagnosis

HPV infection may be readily diagnosed when there are typical clinical lesions. Subclinical infection however requires laboratory confirmation using histological, cytological, immunocytochemical and increasingly, DNA hybridization methods. Histological examination of a biopsy taken from an identifiable lesion will show the characteristic features of HPV infection (see Fig. 46.2). These include papillomatosis, hyperkeratinization of the surface layer, hypertrophy of the basal layers and a degree of disorganization of the epidermal structure (acanthosis). Cellular changes seen in the epithelium include the presence of vacuolated cells with atypical enlarged hyperchromatic nuclei described as koilocytes; multinucleate cells are also seen. Viral antigens can be demonstrated in cervical smears and tissues using specific antibodies.

### DNA hybridization

There is currently much debate about the clinical usefulness of HPV testing as part of national cervical screening programmes, with the hope that women who have lesions which are more likely to progress can be identified earlier. Amplification of HPV DNA by polymerase chain reaction (PCR) using consensus primers to detect a wide range of HPV types has been widely used and attempts are underway to automate the procedure. New methods of hybridization in solution involving capture of the hybrid on a solid surface and immunochemical detection of the hybrid also have potential as diagnostic tools, and ligase chain reaction could provide an alternative amplification method. In-situ hybridization on tissue sections or exfoliated cells provides histological information at the same time as HPV detection, and Southern blot hybridization on DNA extracted from cellular material is sometimes performed, but is not always sensitive enough.

### Serology

The lack of native antigen has hampered the development of serological assays for many years, but recent production of virus-like particles in eukaryotic expression systems using baculovirus or vaccinia recombinants has allowed the detection of antibodies to specific HPV types. Such assays are more useful for showing evidence of past exposure rather than current infection. Assays with recombinant proteins or synthetic peptides from the E6 or E7 gene have been used to demonstrate a correlation between antibody presence and poor prognosis.

## Treatment and control

In most immunocompetent people, warts are a cosmetic nuisance and will eventually disappear spontaneously. Simple topical treatment with salicylic acid is as successful as more invasive methods. Chemicals such as trichloracetic acid and formalin are sometimes used. Alternatively, warts may be destroyed by cryotherapy with dry ice or liquid nitrogen or by electrodiathermy or laser evaporation. In pregnant women, vaginal warts may occasionally grow to such a size that the birth canal is obstructed and surgical removal is required.

Agents such as interferon or inosine pranobex may assist the immune system to eradicate the virus and decrease the likelihood of recurrence. In particular, interferons have been used to treat recurrent CIN or laryngeal warts after reduction of tumour load by laser vaporization or surgery, but it is expensive, lesions recur when the interferon is stopped and side-effects are common. Cytotoxic agents such as podophyllin, bleomycin and 5-fluorouracil have been used in specific types of warts, but require close monitoring.

All of these treatments will remove the lesions but do not always eradicate the virus from surrounding normal epithelium. Incomplete treatment is the commonest cause of recurrence of warts and all of a patient's warts must have disappeared with restoration of normal skin texture before a cure is considered.

Prevention of spread of wart viruses can be achieved by avoiding contact with affected individuals. Thus, the use of condoms will diminish the risk of spread of genital warts. Although HPV DNA has been found on vaginal specula, no woman has been shown to have been infected by this route. Autoclaving of vaginal specula will prevent spread of infection.

There are a number of vaccines available for use in cattle and rabbits. Trials of genetically engineered human therapeutic vaccines which might achieve regression of tumours are being considered, but many problems remain to be solved.

## POLYOMAVIRUSES

The virions are 42–45 nm in size with a 72-capsomere icosahedral capsid. The genome has a molecular weight of $3.4 \times 10^6$ and is approximately 5000 bp in length. Like the papillomaviruses, it is a double-stranded supercoiled loop of DNA, but both strands code for virus proteins.

## Replication

The replicative cycles of both BKV and JCV have been extensively studied. JCV is not only species- but also tissue-specific, replicating only in human embryo glial cell cultures. After infection, the first antigens (small t and large T) are detectable in the nucleus and arise from genes in the early region of the DNA. There is an accumulation of these antigens and then a switch to transcription of the late region and production of the structural proteins VP1, VP2 and VP3. The growth cycle in culture is 36–44 h long, and the release of mature virus particles follows lysis of the cell.

## Clinical features and pathogenesis

BKV has been mainly isolated from immuno-compromised individuals and, with one exception, this has been from urine or kidney. BKV has very rarely been isolated from normal children probably experiencing their first infection. DNA hybridization studies, however, would suggest that BKV can also be found in tonsils, lung, lymph nodes and spleen. In contrast, JCV has been isolated principally from the brain, but also from urine and the renal tract of immunocompromised individuals. The genome has been identified in lung, liver, spleen and lymph nodes and, recently, in leucocytes.

Primary polyomavirus infection is a rare diagnosis and has not been associated with any specific clinical syndrome. There are a few reports of children with primary BKV infection showing acute respiratory disease or haemorrhagic cystitis. Polyomavirus infections due to both BKV and JCV are quite common in pregnancy, with viruria being detected in 3–7% of women, especially during the second and third trimesters. The majority of infections are due to reactivation of latent virus and although there are no specific associated symptoms, women with persistent viruria have more illnesses and their babies are more often premature or jaundiced. There is no evidence to confirm that polyomaviruses are transmitted transplacentally in humans.

### Progressive multifocal leuco-encephalopathy

This condition was first described in 1958 in patients with *Hodgkin's lymphoma* and *chronic lymphocytic leukaemia*. It is usually a late complication in people immunocompromised due to therapy or disease. It is more frequent in later life, but recently cases in younger people, such as renal allograft recipients and AIDS patients, have been found. Progressive multifocal leuco-encephalopathy (PML) patients have multiple foci of demyelination, usually in the cerebral hemispheres, but occasionally elsewhere in the central nervous system. There is a unique combination of pathological changes in PML identifiable histologically. Grossly abnormal, swollen oligodendrocytes with hyperchromatic nuclei and occasional basophilic inclusions are found in the peripheral zone surrounding areas of demyelination, but are absent from the centre of the lesion. Polyoma virions can be found in these cells. Astrocytes have an almost neoplastic appearance and may be transformed by virus, although tumour formation is absent and virions have not been seen within such cells. Malignant gliomata and lymphomata have been described in PML patients and are usually found near the areas of demyelination. JCV is consistently associated with PML and is the cause of the demyelination. Replication of the virus occurs in the nucleus of the oligodendrocyte, causing cell destruction and breakdown of the myelin sheath. The presence of low levels of JCV DNA has recently been reported in patients without clinical evidence of PML. Whether this indicates a latent state or a preclinical stage of PML is unknown.

The clinical features depend on the areas affected. Symptoms include visual, mental and speech impairment, hemiplegia, loss of memory and dementia. Death usually occurs within 6 months of the disease first becoming manifest. Similar symptoms can have other causes and differential diagnosis is essential.

### Polyomavirus infection and transplant recipients

In renal transplant recipients, polyomavirus infection appears to be as common as cytomegalovirus infection. Most infections appear to be due to reactivation of BKV, although primary infection with JCV has been recognized with the donor kidney as the likely source of virus. Half of the infections occur between 4 and 8 weeks after transplantation, but subclinical reactivations of virus occurring up to 12 months after transplantation are not uncommon. Polyomavirus infection is associated with a transient decrease in graft function. If this is wrongly interpreted as being a rejection episode and managed by further immunosuppression, complications may occur. Polyomavirus infection of the transplanted ureter results in cell proliferation leading to *ureteric stenosis* and occasionally to obstruction. Both BKV and JCV have been implicated in this condition. Obstruction can occur up to 300 days postoperatively and may

not be recognized until nephrectomy or postmortem is performed. In bone marrow transplant recipients, 38% of a study group in the USA were found to be excreting polyomavirus in their urine, with the highest incidence in patients with acute myeloid leukaemia. Excretion of BKV appears much more common than of JCV. Although not associated with graft versus host disease, some patients had a transient post-transplant hepatitis and late-onset BKV viruria has been linked to haemorrhagic cystitis.

## Laboratory diagnosis

Isolation of BKV and JCV is too difficult for routine diagnostic use. Detection of virus particles by electron microscopic examination of negatively stained urine deposits or brain homogenates is possible. Viral antigen can be detected using indirect immuno-fluorescence on exfoliated cells from urine or in acetone-fixed brain smears. Detection of viral DNA by in-situ hybridization has been used, with positive cells showing characteristic morphological changes of swollen oligodendrocytes in the brain with foamy cytoplasm and enlarged nuclei or inclusion-bearing transitional cells in urine. PCR has been useful in detecting JCV DNA in cerebrospinal fluid and when combined with intrathecal antibody detection provides a sensitive non-invasive diagnostic procedure. The most common serological assay to measure antibody to BKV and JCV is haemagglutination inhibition. Rising titres and the presence of IgM are diagnostic of recent infection. Failure to detect antibody to JCV nearly always excludes a diagnosis of PML.

## Treatment

There is no established treatment for PML, although many antiviral agents have been tried. Cytarabine may allow some improvement especially if given intrathecally for a long time. Reducing the level of immunosuppression is likely to be beneficial, but this may not be possible because of the underlying disease.

## Epidemiology

Serological studies in the UK show that BKV infection is a relatively common event in early childhood. By 3 years of age 30% of children have antibody to the virus, and this rises to 90% by the age of 5 years. The pattern of infection is similar in other countries.

Serological evidence suggests that JCV circulates independently of BKV in the community and acquisition of antibodies is slower and more variable. In the UK, 5% of the preschool population have antibody, this proportion rising to 30% by the age of 17 years, and to 60% in adults. In Japan, infection is more rapid and widespread, with two-thirds of children seropositive by aged 6 years, rising to 90% of adults.

## RECOMMENDED READING

Anderson M C, Brown C L, Buckley C H et al 1991 Current views on cervical intra-epithelial neoplasia. *Journal of Clinical Pathology* 44: 969–978

Bunney M H, Benton E C, Cubie H A 1992 *Viral Warts – Biology and Treatment*, 2nd edn. Oxford University Press, Oxford

Knowles W 1994 Human polyomaviruses In: Zuckerman A J, Banatvala J E, Pattison J R (eds) *Principles and Practice of Clinical Virology*, 3rd edn. Wiley, Chichester

Stern P L, Stanley M A 1994 *Human Papillomaviruses and Cervical Cancer – Biology and Immunology*. Oxford University Press, Oxford

Zur Hausen H, de Villiers E-M 1994 Human papillomaviruses. *Annual Review of Microbiology* 48: 427–447

# 47

# Hepadnaviruses

**Hepatitis B infection; delta virus infection**

*J. F. Peutherer*

The family Hepadnaviridae includes the human hepatitis B virus (HBV) and the woodchuck, ground squirrel and Pekin duck viruses: others have been identified, but these are the best known and studied. The viruses share a number of important features in relation to the structure of their virions and associated particles, the size, nature, organization and replication of the DNA genome, their ability to cause both acute and chronic infections in their natural hosts and their association with hepatocellular carcinoma.

## PROPERTIES

### Structure

Three different particles can be seen in the blood in HBV infection (Figs 47.1 and 47.2). The predomi-

nant form is a small, spherical particle with a diameter of 22 nm. Filaments are also present with a diameter of about 22 nm. Both types of particle are composed of lipid, protein and carbohydrate; they are not infectious and consist solely of surplus virion envelope. The particles carry the hepatitis B surface antigen (HB$_s$Ag). The third type of particle, the virion or *Dane particle*, has a diameter of 42 nm: enclosed within the envelope is the core (27 nm), which contains the viral DNA and polymerase within a shell composed of hepatitis B core antigen (HB$_c$Ag). There may be as many as $10^{13}$ of the small particles and filaments per millilitre. The virions are present in much smaller numbers, usually by a factor of 10 000 or more, and the proportion varies considerably in different stages of the disease. The viral DNA is about 3200 nucleotides long and is circular (Fig. 47.3). The long strand is complete, but there

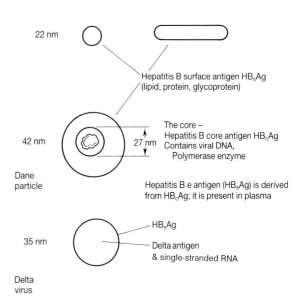

**Fig. 47.1** Electron micrograph of the particles in the blood of a patient infected with HBV. ×130 000. (By courtesy of Dr A. Keen, University of Cape Town.)

22 nm

Hepatitis B surface antigen HB$_s$Ag
(lipid, protein, glycoprotein)

42 nm

Dane particle

27 nm

The core –
Hepatitis B core antigen HB$_c$Ag
Contains viral DNA,
Polymerase enzyme

Hepatitis B e antigen (HB$_e$Ag) is derived from HB$_c$Ag; it is present in plasma

35 nm

HB$_s$Ag

Delta antigen
& single-stranded RNA

Delta virus

**Fig. 47.2** The particles and antigens of HBV and delta virus.

**Fig. 47.3** The gene organization of HBV DNA.

is a gap of variable length of about 1000 nucleotides in the complementary strand: this can be closed via the action of the virion polymerase.

There are four overlapping genes coding for the core, surface and polymerase proteins and an X protein which may act as an activator of transcription. The hepatitis B e antigen (HB$_e$Ag) is derived from the HB$_c$Ag, and is found in the plasma, especially at times when there is active viral replication reflected by the presence of Dane particles in the plasma. The surface antigen gene is transcribed to produce three mRNAs, L, M and S. These are translated to give three proteins: each contains the S protein. The product of the M mRNA consists of the S and pre-S$_2$ proteins. The protein from the L mRNA comprises pre-S$_1$, pre-S$_2$ and S. The L product is present only in the virion, while the M and S proteins are found in each type of particle.

Antigenic and sequence overlap can be shown among the members of the hepadnavirus family, particularly in the core and polymerase proteins. The surface particles are more type-specific although, within HBV, antigenic diversity is recognized in the surface antigens. Thus, HB$_s$Ag particles contain a common 'a' antigen, linked to two sets of mutually exclusive determinants, 'd' or 'y' and 'w' or 'r', giving the four main types – adw, adr, ayw and ayr. These phenotypic variations reflect genomic differences and can be used in epidemiological studies. There are differences in the geographical distribution of the types and also to some extent with the means of transmission in the UK as ayw is associated with parenteral drug misusers. No differences in infectivity or pathogenicity can be associated with each type. However, the 'a' determinant is dominant, and

immunity induced by one phenotype will protect against other types. This means that only one antigenic type is needed in vaccines.

## Stability

It is difficult to assess the stability of HBV due to the lack of a suitable laboratory culture system. Indirect evidence has been obtained from the study of recipients of blood products treated in various ways. Thus, it was established that heating to 60°C for 10 h inactivates virus by a factor of 100–1000-fold. Chimpanzee inoculation experiments show that treatment with hypochlorite (10 000 ppm. available chlorine) and 2% glutaraldehyde for 10 min will inactivate virus 100 000-fold. Studies based on the survival of HB$_s$Ag show that this is much more resistant to destruction.

## Replication

Replication of viral nucleic acid starts within the hepatocyte nucleus where viral DNA can be either free, extrachromosomal or integrated at various sites within the host chromosomes. However, integration is not essential for viral replication. There are some parallels between the hepadnaviruses and the retroviruses, in that:

1. Both synthesize DNA from an RNA template
2. There is base sequence homology between the enzymes involved.

To replicate hepadnavirus DNA, a full-length RNA copy is enclosed in core protein in the hepatocyte nucleus. This is copied to DNA by the polymerase, the RNA is destroyed and the DNA copied, to form double-stranded DNA, as the virion matures.

## CLINICAL FEATURES

The broad range of clinical features associated with HBV infection is summarized in Figure 47.4. The incubation period varies widely from 40 days to 6 months, but is often about 2–3 months. A prodromal illness occurs in some patients, who complain of malaise and anorexia accompanied by weakness and myalgia. Arthralgia also occurs and may be accompanied by an urticarial or maculopapular rash. These features may be related to circulating immune complexes containing HB$_s$Ag, which have been implicated in the rarer complications of polyarteritis nodosa and glomerulonephritis.

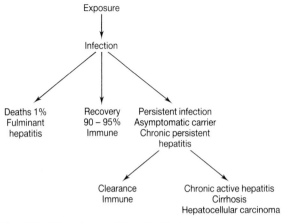

```
                    Exposure
                       │
                       ▼
                   Infection
              ╱        │        ╲
            ╱          │          ╲
          ╱            ▼            ╲
   Deaths 1%       Recovery      Persistent infection
   Fulminant       90 – 95%      Asymptomatic carrier
   hepatitis        Immune       Chronic persistent
                                     hepatitis
                                ╱            ╲
                              ╱                ╲
                            ▼                    ╲
                        Clearance          Chronic active hepatitis
                         Immune                 Cirrhosis
                                         Hepatocellular carcinoma
```

**Fig. 47.4**   The outcome of hepatitis B infection.

Complexes are usually present also in the plasma in cases of fulminant hepatitis B. In an acute case, hepatocellular damage is detectable biochemically before the onset of jaundice and persists after it has resolved. The patient usually begins to feel better when the jaundice appears, accompanied by pale stools and dark urine. Carriers of HBV are initially symptom-free, and many will remain so. Some carriers develop the clinical features of chronic hepatitis and cirrhosis, and eventually hepatocellular carcinoma.

## PATHOLOGY

All types of viral hepatitis produce similar changes at the histological level. In the acute stage there are signs of inflammation in the portal triads: the infiltrate is mainly lymphocytic. In the liver parenchyma, single cells show ballooning and form acidophilic (*Councilman*) bodies as they die. In healthy carriers, the inflammatory response is mild, and the affected hepatocytes are pale-staining and glassy.

In chronic hepatitis, damage extends out from the portal tracts, giving the piecemeal necrosis appearance. Some lobular inflammation is also seen. As the disease progresses fibrosis develops and, eventually, cirrhosis.

### Pathogenesis

#### Acute disease

HBV replicates in the hepatocyte, reflected in the detection of viral DNA and $HB_cAg$ in the nucleus and $HB_sAg$ in the cytoplasm and at the hepatocyte membrane. However, $HB_cAg$ and $HB_eAg$ are also present at the cytoplasmic membrane. Both B and T cell responses are induced by these antigens; damage to the hepatocyte could result from both antibody-dependent, NK and cytotoxic T cell action. Expression of MHC class I antigens is poor in hepatocytes but can be enhanced as interferons are produced in response to the infection. This in turn leads to increased antigen recognition and lysis of the infected hepatocytes. HBV is thought to be non-cytocidal without the assistance of the host's immune system and the disease is usually milder in the immunocompromised. In the asymptomatic carrier there may be no evidence of cell damage, despite the presence of integrated HBV DNA and $HB_sAg$ in the liver and plasma. Cell-mediated responses to $HB_cAg$ are often detectable in patients with chronic active hepatitis. Auto-immune reactions may also contribute to the damage as various liver-specific antigens are induced as the result of HBV infection. Superinfection with the delta virus (see later) may predispose to progression to cirrhosis.

It is not yet clear what determines that an individual will progress to the carrier state. The absence, or relative inefficiency, of the immune system is important, as shown by the increased likelihood of the carrier state in the very young and the immuno-compromised. In the Far East, 90% of children born to infectious mothers will become carriers although acute hepatitis is uncommon in this age group. In the neonate, infection occurs in the presence of maternal IgG anti-$HB_c$ and tolerance to $HB_eAg$ which may cross the placenta. This will have the effect of masking $HB_cAg$ on hepatocyte membranes and thus will prevent its recognition by cytotoxic T cells. The presence of HBV in peripheral blood mononuclear cells and in precursor cells in the marrow may also be important.

### Persistence of hepatitis B

Persistence of hepatitis B:

1. Is indicated by $HB_sAg$ present for more than 6 months
2. Occurs in 5–10% of adult, 30% of childhood and 90% of newborn infections
3. Is more frequent in males
4. Is more likely in the immunocompromised.

### Hepatocellular carcinoma

Hepatocellular carcinoma (HCC) is one of the 10 most frequent tumours in the world, and there is considerable evidence that chronic infection with HBV is an important aetiological factor. Thus, the highest rates of HCC are found in areas where HBV is highly endemic and where infection occurs at a very early age. This is necessary as there may be an interval of 30–40 years between infection and tumour development. Integrated viral DNA can be found in the tumour cells but the site differs in different tumours, although the tumour is clonal in origin in each individual. The integrated DNA is extensively rearranged and regions may be deleted. The mechanism of carcinogenesis is not yet clear, although it is usually associated with cirrhosis. As with other tumours, infection with the HBV may be only one factor and others, such as genetic or chemical, may be necessary.

## LABORATORY DIAGNOSIS

The virology laboratory can test for a wide range of HBV antigens and antibodies, using radio-immuno assays and enzyme-linked immunosorbent assays (ELISAs). The standard test is for HB$_s$Ag, which if present in the serum indicates that the patient is infected with HBV, either as a recent acute infection or as a carrier.

### Acute infection

In an acute case (Fig. 47.5), HB$_s$Ag is present for some weeks before the onset of symptoms and is at maximum titre at the height of liver damage. In most cases HB$_s$Ag cannot be detected beyond 3–4 months. In a few patients, antigenaemia is of short duration and may not be detectable at the onset of clinical symptoms. In such cases the presence of anti-HB$_c$, especially IgM anti-HB$_c$, and anti-HB$_e$ may be the only indications of HBV infection. If successive serum samples are examined, the development of anti-HB$_s$ will confirm the timing of the

infection, although there is considerable variation in the appearance of this antibody.

Typical responses shown by at least three-quarters of cases are outlined in Figure 47.5. HB$_e$Ag is produced when virus is replicating and thus it is usually found soon after HB$_s$Ag. IgM anti-HB$_c$ is the next response to be detected. HB$_e$Ag is correlated strongly with the detection of viral DNA, virions and viral DNA polymerase in the serum. IgM anti-HB$_c$ is a transient response and if present in high titre indicates a recent acute infection. The response declines with time and is usually absent by 6 months. Tests for HB$_e$Ag and anti-HB$_e$ during an acute infection can be helpful in that the disappearance of HB$_e$Ag and replacement with anti-HB$_e$ indicates that the patient is responding to the infection and will clear HB$_s$Ag. Ninety per cent of patients develop anti-HB$_s$; in a few cases it is present at the same time as HB$_s$Ag, but usually there is a gap of up to 6 months before the anti-HB$_s$ appears. Once present, the patient is immune to further infection with HBV.

### Chronic infection

A patient becomes a carrier if HB$_s$Ag is detectable beyond 6 months. As illustrated (Fig. 47.6), a carrier is almost always HB$_e$Ag-positive beyond 6 months. During this time IgM anti-HB$_c$ will disappear, to be replaced by IgG anti-HB$_c$. This is typical of the early replicative phase of chronic infection. It may be succeeded by the loss of HB$_e$Ag and the appear-

**Fig. 47.6** The sequence of events in a patient who becomes a carrier of HBV.

**Fig. 47.5** HBV antigens and antibodies in a patient recovering from acute infection.

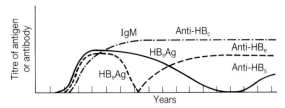

**Fig. 47.7** The sequence of events in a hepatitis B carrier who clears the virus.

ance of anti-HB$_e$ (Fig. 47.7): the change happens at a variable time, but each year from 5 to 20% of HB$_e$Ag-positive carriers will convert, when there is often biochemical evidence of a short-lived increase in liver damage. Eventually, 1–2% of carriers clear HB$_s$Ag each year.

## Surface and core variants

Virus with mutations in the HB$_s$Ag gene have been detected in immunocompromised children born to infected mothers and in a liver transplant patient given antibody to the *a* determinant to prevent reinfection. In both, the variant appears to be an escape mutant. Precore and core variants have been described in patients from the Mediterranean area and the East, who are chronic carriers without HB$_e$Ag reactivity and in a few fulminant cases.

## TREATMENT

Much effort has been focused on the treatment of the chronic carrier with the twin aims of preventing progression of liver disease and of reducing the possibility of transmission to others.

Immunosuppression and anti-inflammatory treatment are not indicated in the long-term management of chronic hepatitis B, but various regimens involving interferon and antiviral compounds are under study. As such treatment can only inhibit viral replication it is usual to select patients with evidence of chronic active hepatitis and continuing viral replication with HB$_e$Ag, viral DNA and DNA polymerase in the serum. The response to therapy varies: in some there is transient loss of serum HBV DNA and DNA polymerase during therapy; in others there is a permanent cessation of HBV replication, but antigenaemia continues and, least often, there is a complete response and DNA replication ceases, HB$_s$Ag disappears and anti-HB$_s$ develops. Interferons have shown promise, particularly α-interferons alone and in combination with other antiviral drugs. If a response occurs this is usually signalled by exacerbation of liver cell damage after 6–10 weeks of therapy. The factors associated with a favourable response to therapy are:

1. Recent infection (less than 2 years)
2. Adult patient
3. Caucasian
4. Chronic viral replication
5. Healthy immune system
6. Therapy maintained for more than 4 months.

If patients are selected according to these criteria, a response to interferon can be expected in 50% of patients.

Another approach is liver transplantation in which the recipient is usually given anti-HB$_s$ in an attempt to prevent infection of the new liver from sources such as peripheral blood cells.

## EPIDEMIOLOGY

HBV is present in the blood and also in body fluids such as semen, vaginal secretions and saliva, although the level is only about 1/1000 of that in blood. Even so, this may still represent a large number of virions. It was recognized from a very early stage that there was a type of hepatitis related to blood transfusion or the use of blood products – hence the name *serum hepatitis*. It was also apparent that very small quantities of blood could transmit infection as occurs in needlestick injuries. Sexual transmission is also recognized, as is that which occurs between family members, siblings, peers and residents in institutions for the mentally handicapped. In these circumstances there will be frequent contact with blood and saliva: the virus will gain entry through cuts and abrasions or across mucous membranes. Biting and scratching are also important. Vertical transmission from mother to child is one of the most important routes. Transmission occurs when maternal blood contaminates the newborn mucous membranes during birth. Transplacental infection is thought to be quite rare.

The prevalence of HBV infection varies widely in different parts of the world:

*Highest rates.* HB$_s$Ag 10–15%: anti-HB$_s$ 70–90% in South-East Asia, China, equatorial Africa, Oceania and South America. Vertical and horizontal transmission are both common.

*Intermediate rates.* HB$_s$Ag 5%: anti-HB$_s$ 30–40% in Eastern Europe, around the Mediterranean, South America and the Middle East.

*Lowest rates.* HB$_s$Ag 0.1–0.5%: anti-HB$_s$ not more than 5% in Western Europe, North America and Australia.

Overall, it is estimated that there are 200 million to 300 million carriers in the world, with a preponderance of males in all populations. In areas of low endemicity the risk of infection varies widely in different groups according to behaviour (Table

**Table 47.1** Factors predisposing to increased risk of hepatitis B infection

1. Parenteral drug injection
2. Many sexual partners – both homosexual and heterosexual
3. Geography: highly endemic in various parts of the world
4. Patients in residential homes for the mentally handicapped
5. Patients in haemodialysis, haemophilia and other units
6. Sexual partner has one of the above risk factors
7. Babies born to mothers who are at risk
8. Health care personnel, especially those in surgery, obstetrics, dental surgery and those caring for patients in categories 4 and 5

The relative importance of each category varies in different parts of the world and also within countries.

**Table 47.2** Acute hepatitis B in health care workers in England[a]

| Staff | 1975–79 | 1980–84 | 1985–88[b] |
|---|---|---|---|
| Surgeons | 12 | 25 | 0 |
| Physicians | 12 | 11 | 2 |
| Laboratory staff (medical) | 27 | 16 | 0 |
| Laboratory staff (scientific) | 18 | 37 | 10 |
| Nurses | 7 | 4 | 2 |
| Mental handicap staff | 31 | 27 | 10 |
| Dentists | 17 | 17 | 16 |

[a] Rate per 100 000 per annum.
[b] Public Health Laboratory Service Communicable Diseases Report (unpublished).

47.1). Most cases occur in parenteral drug injectors who share scarce needles and syringes: sexual transmission by both homosexual and heterosexual routes is also important. Screening of all blood donations has virtually eliminated transmission by transfusion and blood products. Some groups of patients are at increased risk of infection and of becoming carriers. These include patients on maintenance haemodialysis and in homes for the mentally handicapped. Finally, health care personnel and laboratory workers are at risk, although the degree of risk varies with the nature of their work and the care with which it is performed (Table 47.2).

The reduction in the rate of reported acute hepatitis B infections in the period 1985–88 probably reflects an increased awareness of the need to adopt good working practices and the introduction of active immunization (see below).

Surgery, including dental surgery, obstetrics and procedures involving sharp instruments, etc., and

the spilling of patient's blood all increase the risk of transmission. Changes in incidence also occur: in the UK, cases of hepatitis B linked to drug abuse increased to a peak from 1980 to 1984. Patients are also at risk from staff, and several episodes have been identified where a surgeon, gynaecologist, dentist or other staff member has transmitted the virus to their patients during invasive procedures, especially in difficult operations where the operator's hands are hidden and needles and instruments are guided by touch. Apart from small outbreaks linked to a common source, such as surgery or haemodialysis, epidemics of hepatitis B are rare. In the past, before specific tests were available, a few outbreaks were described following the use of blood products prepared in bulk from large numbers of donations. There was a large outbreak in the US armed forces during the Second World War due to the use of yellow fever vaccine stabilized with infectious human plasma.

## CONTROL

Broadly, there are two approaches to the prevention of infection with HBV. Firstly, the possibility of transmission can be reduced or removed by modifying risky behaviour. The measures include the reduction of the number of sexual partners, the use of condoms and avoidance of sharing needles by injecting drug misusers. Implementation of sensible control of infection policies can reduce the risks considerably to health care personnel. It is essential, of course, that blood for transfusion is screened. However, there are limits to these approaches, and immunization, both passive and active, offers many advantages, not least in situations where the prevention of infection is otherwise difficult or impossible. In areas of high endemicity the prevention of transmission of HBV from mother to child and between young children can only be attempted by large-scale immunization programmes, which present considerable problems, not least in the cost and delivery of vaccine.

### Passive immunization

Hyperimmune hepatitis B immunoglobulin (HBIG) is prepared from donors with high titres of anti-$HB_s$. Doses of 300–500 IU in 3 ml are given intramuscularly after accidental exposure, as may occur by needlestick or when broken skin and mucous membranes are splashed with blood from an infected patient.

HBIG must be given as soon as possible after the incident and preferably within 48 h. A second dose is usually given 4 weeks after the first. Such a regimen does not provide absolute protection, but an efficacy of 76% has been reported. Serological studies of patients protected by passive immunization show that a transient antigenaemia can occur but the patient remains well. Protection against the development of the carrier state is also provided. Passive immunization is also effective in reducing the risk of the carrier state in babies born to infectious mothers. HBIG must be given as soon as possible, preferably at birth but no later than 12 h after birth. When this is repeated at monthly intervals for up to 6 months, the proportion of babies who become carriers can be reduced by about 70%. However, even greater protection is provided by combined passive and active immunization in post-exposure prophylaxis. It is advisable, though, to give the injections into different sites. Babies have been shown to respond to the vaccine, and the first dose of the course of active immunization can be given at the same time as the HBIG; the protective efficacy of this combined treatment is 90%. Passive immunization is still necessary for those exposed to HBV if they have not been actively immunized; have not yet completed the course; have failed to respond to the full course of vaccine; or several years have elapsed since the completion of the course of vaccine.

## Active immunization

Much effort has been devoted to the development of vaccines for long-term protection against hepatitis B. Two preparations have been used. The first contained the small 22 nm particles of $HB_sAg$ purified from the plasma of carriers. The particles were separated by ultracentrifugation and treated with proteinase, 8 M urea and formaldehyde.

The product is immunogenic and safe, as the various steps in its preparation inactivate hepatitis B virions and viruses of all other groups. There were fears, however, that HIV might be present in the donors of the plasma. There is no foundation for this fear as, even if present in the pooled plasma, HIV could not survive the manufacturing process. Current hepatitis B vaccines are produced by cloning the surface antigen gene in yeast cells. The product is particulate and resembles the small particles seen in patients, although it is not glycosylated. Both vaccines are administered with alum as adjuvant and are injected intramuscularly; care should be taken to avoid injection into fat as this can produce poorer seroconversion rates. For this reason, injection into the deltoid muscle of the upper arm is recommended. Both vaccines are free from major side-effects; local swelling and reddening may occur in up to 1 in 5 recipients with a slight fever in only a few cases.

Three doses of vaccine are given at 0, 1 and 6 months. The seroconversion rate is dependent on a number of factors, the most important of which are the age and sex of the vaccinee. Rates in excess of 95% are seen in young women, whereas the rate may drop to 80% in older men. Immunosuppressed patients show even lower rates, e.g. only 50–60% in patients on maintenance dialysis. Because virus challenge doses and the infectivity of sources can vary considerably it is impossible to define a minimum protective level of anti-$HB_s$ but levels should be greater than 100 IU/l. If vaccine is used selectively to protect particular groups in the population, it is reasonable to check the response within a few months of the third dose of vaccine. The duration of the response to vaccine is variable and dependent on the level of anti-$HB_s$ after the completion of the course. Vaccinees whose anti-$HB_s$ titres are in excess of 500 IU/l are likely to maintain adequate levels for at least 4–5 years. If the initial response is between 100 and 500 IU/l, then a boost at 3 years is required. If less than 100 IU/l, a booster dose should be given. Low or non-responders need to be identified and told that they are not protected and that they must seek prophylaxis by passive immunization if they suffer accidental exposure. Those who are known to have responded can be given a booster if they are exposed to the virus, although the need for this will depend on the level of anti-$HB_s$ and the interval since completion of the course.

## Who should be immunized?

The aim of immunization is to prevent transmission of HBV by the routes described in the epidemiology section. In the UK, vaccine is offered to: health care personnel, especially those in direct contact with blood and sharp instruments, etc.; patients and staff in homes and hospitals for the mentally handicapped; sexual partners of those known to be infected with HBV; individuals with many sexual partners; parenteral drug misusers; some members of the police, fire and ambulance services; patients at particular risk, e.g. those requiring frequent blood transfusion and blood products and on maintenance dialysis. The introduction of active immunization may already have contributed to the observed reduction in reported cases of hepatitis B in most groups of health care workers (Table 47.2). In the UK and other areas where the prevalence of anti-HB$_s$ is low, it is not cost effective to test for anti-HB$_s$ before immunization. However, it may be useful to test potential vaccinees who are at increased risk for a particular reason such as drug misuse, as many will already be immune. Babies born to infected mothers are an important group to identify as transmission is likely to lead to the carrier state and all its complications. Mothers may be at risk because of their geographical or ethnic origin, by the misuse of drugs or by sexual exposure; they can be defined by selective testing or by routine screening of all antenatal patients. The greatest risk of transmission occurs with carrier mothers who are HB$_e$Ag-positive or develop acute hepatitis B late in pregnancy. Combined passive and active immunization should be started at birth. Active immunization alone has an efficiency of 70–85%. There is less risk of transmission if the mother is negative for HB$_e$Ag, but it may be advisable to immunize all babies born to mothers who are HB$_s$Ag-positive as there may be another source, either father or sibling in the immediate family. In areas of moderate and high endemicity, the main approach must be widespread use of the vaccine. In the East, where neonatal transmission is common, vaccine should preferably be given to all babies at birth. Studies in Africa indicate that many children are infected at a later age and, in this situation, immunization of infants can be expected to reduce the carrier rate in the population. Eradication of hepatitis B is a desirable objective, and the vaccine is now incorporated into the schedules in many countries. Alternative vaccines are also under development. Incorporation of the pre-S$_1$ and pre-S$_2$ proteins and HB$_c$Ag has been proposed, as this might enhance the range and scope of the response. Alternative approaches such as the use of synthetic peptides and hybrid virus vaccines are also under investigation.

## THE DELTA AGENT (HEPATITIS DELTA VIRUS)

When first discovered, the delta (δ) antigen was thought to be another antigen of HBV. It is now known that it is part of another virus which cannot replicate without assistance from HBV (or another hepadnavirus). The virus is a small (35–37 nm) enveloped particle containing a single small circular molecule of RNA of 1.7 kilobase pairs. The internal protein – the δ antigen – has a molecular weight of

68 000. The envelope of the virus is the same as that of HBV (see Fig. 47.2). The origin of the virus is unknown and it is has no homology with HBV DNA. The closest relatives are the satellite viruses of plants.

## Clinical features and pathogenesis

HDV can only infect simultaneously with HBV or as a superinfection of a chronic HBV carrier. The symptoms are similar to those of acute and chronic hepatitis B. The presence of hepatitis delta virus (HDV) may increase the severity of the clinical features compared with those seen with HBV alone. This is reflected in a 10% risk of fulminant hepatitis with simultaneous HBV and HDV infection and a 20% risk in superinfections.

Overall, HDV can be found in up to half of all cases of HB$_s$Ag-associated fulminant hepatitis B. In about 1 in 10 cases, co-infection with HDV and HBV results in a biphasic illness. HDV superinfection of an HBV carrier can cause clinical acute hepatitis and may lead to persistence of both HBV and HDV. The risk of chronic liver disease is increased if this occurs – even to the extent of 50–90% of cases in areas where HDV is common. The rate of progression of the liver disease is also increased so that cirrhosis may be apparent within 5 years.

## Diagnosis

Tests are available for δ antigen and antibody. The sequence of appearance of the various markers in a patient co-infected with HBV and HDV is illustrated (Fig. 47.8). The initial antibody to HDV is of the IgM class. In cases of superinfection, the test results are as illustrated (Fig. 47.9). During the episode of acute hepatitis there may be a drop in the HB$_s$Ag titre and, although it is usually still detectable, it may disappear temporarily in a few cases.

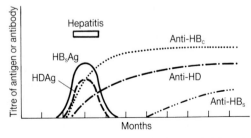

**Fig. 47.8** Test results in a patient simultaneously infected with HBV and HDV.

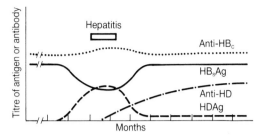

**Fig. 47.9** Test results in a hepatitis B carrier superinfected with HDV.

This can cause some confusion if the episode is the first presentation of the patient.

## Epidemiology

HDV is not a new virus as there is evidence of infection in the 1930s at least. Overall the prevalence of HDV reflects that of HBV, except that it is low in the East. The highest prevalence (1 in 5 carriers of HBV) has been seen in South America in the Amazon basin, but there is considerable variation and HDV is not found uniformly throughout the population. Infection is important also in Italy and the Middle East and some parts of Africa. In areas of low HBV endemicity, HDV is associated with drug misusers in whom the prevalence in HBV carriers may be 50% or more. Sexual transmission is recognized but does not appear to be as frequent as via blood, e.g. in drug misusers and haemophiliacs. In a number of episodes HDV has spread rapidly among a population of HBV carriers, causing hepatitis, death from fulminant hepatitis and chronic illness.

## Treatment and control

There is no established treatment for HDV infection although there is evidence that interferons may induce a temporary improvement in δ antigen levels. The same general control measures for HBV are also relevant to HDV. HBV vaccines will prevent HDV co-infection but there is no means of protecting existing HBV carriers against the potentially serious consequences of superinfection with HDV. Only the avoidance of exposure can help.

---

### RECOMMENDED READING

Bonino F, Smedile A, Verme G 1987 Hepatitis delta virus infection. *Advances in Internal Medicine* 32: 345–358

Carman W F, Thomas H C 1993 Viral genetic variation: hepatitis B virus as a clinical example. *Lancet* 341: 349–353

Chisari F V, Ferrari C 1995 Hepatitis B virus immunopathogenesis. *Annual Review of Immunology* 13: 29–60

Expert Advisory Group on AIDS 1990 *Guidance for Clinical Health Care Workers: Protection Against Infection with HIV and Hepatitis Viruses*. HMSO, London

Fields B N, Knipe D M, Howley P M (eds) 1996 *Virology*, 3rd edn. Lippincott-Raven, Philadelphia

Thomas H C 1995 The emergence and precore/core variants of hepatitis B virus: the potential role of antibody selection. *Journal of Hepatology* 22 (suppl): S1–S8

# 48

# Parvoviruses

**B19 infection; erythema infectiosum**

*J. R. Pattison*

There are three genera in the family parvoviridae. Viruses in the genus *Densovirus* infect insects but do not infect humans or other vertebrates. The members of the genus *Dependovirus* infect a number of species, and serology shows that adeno-associated viruses 1-4 are common human infections although they have not yet been associated with any human disease.

The third genus, *Parvovirus*, contains the *autonomous* parvoviruses, which are widespread in nature and frequently cause disease in their natural hosts (Table 48.1). Some of these viruses (feline parvovirus (FPV) and canine parvovirus (CPV)) are so important in veterinary medicine that immunization

against them is a routine practice in developed countries. At present there is only one parvovirus (B19) that is important in human medicine, although in the future some of the small round viruses seen in human faeces may be shown to be parvoviruses and may prove to be pathogenic.

## DESCRIPTION

Parvovirus virions (Fig. 48.1) are uniform isometric particles 20–25 nm in diameter lacking an envelope. They have a characteristic buoyant density in caesium chloride, ranging from 1.41 to 1.45, and the capsid consists of two proteins. The genome consists of a single strand of DNA which has a characteristic structure. There is a linear coding region bounded at each end by terminal palindromic sequences. Throughout the parvoviruses there is variation in

**Table 48.1** The autonomous parvoviruses, their natural hosts and the diseases they cause

| Virus | Host | Disease |
|---|---|---|
| H1 | Rat | Subclinical |
| Minute virus of mice (MVM) | Mice | Subclinical |
| Feline parvovirus (FPV) | Cat | Enteritis<br>Leucopenia<br>Cerebellar ataxia |
| Simian parvovirus (SPV) | Monkey | Anaemia |
| Mink enteritis virus (MEV) | Mink | Enteritis |
| Canine parvovirus (CPV) | Dog | Enteritis<br>Myocarditis |
| Porcine parvovirus (PPV) | Pigs | Reproductive failure |
| Aleutian disease virus (ADV) | Mink | Pneumonitis<br>Hypergammaglobulinaemia<br>Renal failure |
| B19 | Man | Respiratory tract illness<br>Aplastic crisis<br>Erythema infectiosum<br>Hydrops fetalis |

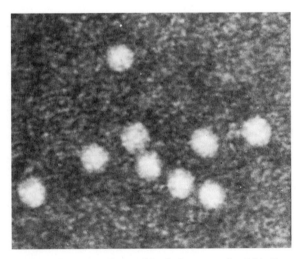

**Fig 48.1** Parvovirus B19 particles in the serum of a child with sickle cell anaemia suffering an aplastic crisis. ×300 000.

the size of the genome and whether plus and minus strands are packaged into mature virions. In the case of B19 the genome is 5.5 kilobase pairs in length, making it one of the largest parvovirus genomes, and both plus and minus strands are packaged with equal efficiency so that the DNA spontaneously anneals into a double-stranded form when extracted from the virions.

Many animal parvoviruses can be grown in cell culture and the appearance of intranuclear inclusions is characteristic. Such inclusions can be seen in B19-infected tissue specimens in human disease (see below).

The individual parvoviruses appear to be very host-specific, although mink enteritis virus (MEV) is very closely related to FPV, and CPV more distantly so. These viruses are probably a set of host range variants of the same virus. Otherwise, each species, including humans, is affected by a genetically and antigenically stable virus. As a consequence, infection with B19 virus is followed by life-long immunity in normal individuals.

## PATHOGENESIS

Autonomous parvoviruses are so called because they do not require the presence of a helper virus for replication. However, they do depend on certain cellular helper functions which are expressed transiently in the cell during the late S or early $G_2$ phase of mitosis. Therefore, virus replication will be relatively extensive in rapidly dividing tissues, and it is not surprising that diseases of the intestine, the haemopoietic system and the fetus feature frequently as consequences of parvovirus infections in animals. There is also evidence that susceptibility to parvovirus infection is related to a particular stage of differentiation of the cell. Thus, very distinct clinical syndromes such as cerebellar ataxia in kittens and aplastic crisis in humans are also a feature of parvovirus infection.

### Animal diseases

In the cat, FPV causes ataxia in kittens if infection occurs in the perinatal period, since the cells of the external granular layer of the cerebellum are dividing rapidly at this stage and become a target for virus-induced damage. As the animals are weaned, the crypt epithelial cells develop a cell cycle time of 8–12 h, and are thus susceptible to FPV. As a consequence, infection is associated with enteritis.

In the dog the distinct clinical syndrome of perinatal infection by CPV is myocarditis, since in the very young pup there is rapid growth of the myocardium and the mitotic index is high. If infection occurs in older puppies, enteritis is a consistent feature. The white blood cells are also a target for infection by FPV and CPV, and so kittens and puppies of 2–4 months of age tend to suffer leucopenia and enteritis.

In mink infected with MEV, severe enteritis is the most consistent feature, and there is not a distinct clinical syndrome associated with perinatal infection. However, mink are the natural host of another parvovirus, Aleutian disease virus (ADV). In newborn kits this causes an acute respiratory disease due to infection of type II alveolar cells, which are only susceptible to productive infection in the early stages of life. In later life ADV establishes a persistent infection in the germinal centres of lymph nodes, a plasmacytosis in many organs, hypergammaglobulinaemia and death due to chronic renal failure as a consequence of immune complex glomerulonephritis. This syndrome occurs earlier and more regularly in Aleutian mink due to the linkage of the Aleutian coat colour gene to a gene associated with a lysosomal abnormality of the Chédiak–Higashi type, leading to a failure to destroy immune complexes following phagocytosis.

In rodents, parvoviruses appear to be asymptomatic in their natural hosts, and the same was thought to be true of porcine parvovirus (PPV), a very common infection of pigs. However, the virus was found in tissue, vaginal and seminal samples from pig herds affected by reproductive failure and it was subsequently shown that infection in early pregnancy leads to transplacental infection, stillbirth, mummification or resorption of the piglets.

A new simian parvovirus (SPV) was discovered in cynomolgus monkeys in 1994. The monkeys presented with severe anaemia associated with persistent SPV infection, and it is probable that this was the consequence of immunosuppression due to co-infection with simian retrovirus.

### Human disease

#### Volunteer studies

Experimental infection of healthy volunteers has revealed the steps in the pathogenesis of B19 infection (Fig. 48.2). The virus is infectious when given in the form of nasal drops. One week later there is an intense viraemia and virus is excreted in the nasal secretions. The viraemia lasts for only a few days before there is a brisk antibody response, initially of the IgM class but followed rapidly by the appearance of IgG antibody.

Haematological changes take place in the 2nd week following inoculation. Erythroid precursors are absent from the bone marrow of normal individuals 10 days after inoculation, and there is consequent disappearance of reticulocytes from the peripheral blood and a small fall in the haemoglobin level (Fig. 48.2). Lymphocyte, neutrophil and platelet levels sometimes fall transiently, but this is not due to lack of precursors in the bone marrow. Studies with cultured bone marrow cells confirm the in-vivo observations. B19 selectively inhibits erythroid colony formation but has no effect on the cells of the myeloid series.

The *rash* and *arthralgia* associated with B19 infection occur in infected volunteers during the 3rd week after inoculation. As yet there are no studies of the pathology of either of these features, but since they follow the disappearance of the viraemia and occur at a time when there is an easily detectable immune response it is assumed that the rash and arthralgia are immune mediated.

The viraemia that is characteristic of B19 infection gives ample opportunity for infection of the placenta and fetus if it occurs during pregnancy. In infected fetuses there appears to be a persistent infection with damage to haematopoietic cells, leading to anaemia, which is one of the factors responsible for *hydrops fetalis*. The other situation in which persistent infection occurs is in the immunosuppressed. The reason is that such individuals produce only small amounts of antibody in response to infection and none of it is capable of neutralizing the virus.

The cell receptor for parvovirus B19 is the P antigen. This is present on red blood cells, vascular endothelium and fetal myocytes. Thus the distribution of the cell receptor is linked to the clinical manifestations of disease.

## Clinical diseases due to B19

There is a spectrum of clinical consequences of B19 infection (Table 48.2). These depend in part on the natural variation in symptomatology that occurs with common childhood infections and in part on recognizable host factors.

*Minor illness.* In children, in whom B19 infection is most common, asymptomatic infection accounts for about half of all infections. Non-specific respiratory tract illness is the next most common illness, at least in boys. This can mimic influenza and coincides with the viraemic phase of the infection.

*Rash illness.* B19 virus causes an erythematous maculopapular rash, which in its most clinically distinct form is called *erythema infectiosum* (EI). EI is common in children aged 4–11 years, and is sometimes called *fifth disease* since it was the fifth of six erythematous rash illnesses of childhood in an old classification. Classically, it starts with an intense

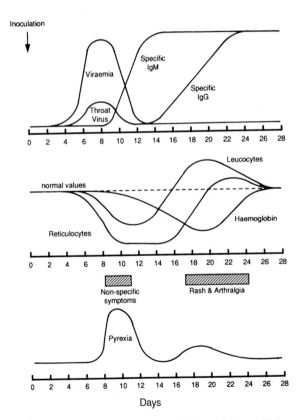

**Fig. 48.2** The virological (upper trace), haematological (middle trace) and clinical events (lower trace) following inoculation of B19 virus. (Reproduced with permission of Wiley, Chichester.)

**Table 48.2** Spectrum of disease due to B19 related to host factors

| Disease | Host |
|---|---|
| Asymptomatic Respiratory tract illness Rash illness Arthralgia | Normal |
| Severe anaemia | Chronic haemolytic anaemia Immunosuppressed Intra-uterine infection |

erythema of the cheeks, hence another of its names – 'slapped-cheek disease'. The rash then proceeds to involve the trunk and limbs. It lasts only a day or two, although transient recrudescences may occur when the individual is hot. The rash on the limbs tends to have a lacy or reticular appearance. There may be associated lymphadenopathy and joint symptoms.

It is now clear that B19 is a cause of rash illness world-wide, but such illnesses are not always diagnosed clinically as EI. The erythematous rash illness is often very similar to rubella. Erythema of the cheeks is not always prominent and the rash often does not have a lacy appearance. It sometimes occurs on the palms and soles. In the absence of laboratory tests the most frequent clinical diagnoses made are rubella, allergy and 'viral illness', unless there is an outbreak in young children associated with red cheeks in which case the diagnosis of EI is often made. In a few cases of B19 infection the rash is purpuric in nature. In most of these the platelet count is normal but a transient thrombocytopenia occasionally occurs.

*Joint disease.* Symptoms and signs of joint involvement occur frequently in B19 infection. Approximately 80% of adult females will report joint symptoms, although the figure is only approximately 10% in childhood cases. Like the rash, the arthropathy of B19 infection is very similar to that seen with rubella, being a symmetrical arthralgia or arthritis involving the small joints of the hands with wrists, knees and ankles affected in some cases. There is a tendency for the arthropathy to be more severe in children. The symptoms and signs usually resolve within 2 weeks, but in a few cases they will persist for months and very occasionally for years. Some of these patients may be classified clinically as early benign rheumatoid arthritis but they will be found to be rheumatoid factor-negative, and B19 virus is not related to rheumatoid arthritis in any way.

*Aplastic crisis.* An aplastic crisis is a transient, acute event which complicates chronic haemolytic anaemia. There is a fall in haemoglobin from steady-state values, a disappearance of reticulocytes from the peripheral blood and a virtual absence of red blood cell precursors in the bone marrow at the beginning of the crisis. The cessation of erythropoiesis lasts 5–7 days, and patients present with symptoms of worsening anaemia. Blood transfusion is required in the acute phase, but after a week or so the bone marrow recovers rapidly, there is a reticulocytosis and the haemoglobin concentration returns to steady-state values.

Throughout the world B19 infection is responsible for 90% of cases of aplastic crisis. It most commonly occurs in children with sickle cell anaemia but also in patients with hereditary spherocytosis, pyruvate kinase deficiency, β-thalassaemia intermedia and a dyserythropoietic anaemia (hereditary erythroblastic multinuclearity with a positive acid serumlysis – HEMPAS).

*B19 infection in the immunosuppressed.* Cases of persistent B19 infection have been described in patients with underlying immunodeficiency states (Nezelof's syndrome, acute lymphatic leukaemia and human immunodeficiency virus (HIV)-positive individuals). The illness is characterized by either persistent anaemia or a remitting and relapsing anaemia. Viraemia occurs and recurs in periods of anaemia, and only a weak humoral immune response can be detected. The bone marrow picture is typical of that seen in aplastic crisis complicating haemolytic anaemia.

*B19 in pregnancy.* No evidence of B19 infection can be found in sera taken during the 1st month of life from infants with birth defects and as yet there is no evidence of late developmental abnormalities in children exposed to B19 in utero. However, early studies of B19 infection in women known to be pregnant suggested that the spontaneous abortion rate was high. Recent studies indicate that there is not an excess number of abortions in the first trimester of pregnancies complicated by B19 infection compared to controls. However, approximately 1 in 10 of pregnancies complicated by B19 infection end in spontaneous abortion during the second trimester, and this is approximately 10 times the incidence in controls. The pregnancy is lost, on average, 4–6 weeks after the onset of symptoms of EI in the mother.

The majority of pregnancies complicated by B19 continue to full-term delivery of normal infants. However, damage sometimes occurs as a consequence of second or third trimester infection, and in these cases *fetal hydrops* appears to be a consistent feature. Maternal B19 infection appears to occur 2–12 weeks prior to the diagnosis of hydrops fetalis. There is a chronic infection in the fetus which leads to anaemia, which is, together with myocarditis, responsible for the hydrops. Overall, B19 infection probably accounts for 10% of cases of non-immunological hydrops fetalis.

## LABORATORY DIAGNOSIS OF B19 INFECTION

In acquired infection the diagnosis of B19-associated disease follows the classical principles for acute systemic virus infections. The viraemia and throat virus excretion coincide with haematological changes, and detection of virus is a useful diagnostic test in cases of aplastic crisis. Rash and arthralgia occur some days after the end of the short period of circulation and excretion of virus, so in these cases diagnosis by the detection of virus-specific IgM antibody is the best method.

## Detection of virus

Serum is the specimen of choice for the detection of virus since the highest concentrations (up to $10^{11}$ particles per millilitre) of virus are found in this fluid and, if virus is not detected in the sample, it can serve as an acute-phase serum for antibody assays. Counterimmuno-electrophoresis (CIE) using a human convalescent serum as the detector antibody is a simple and rapid technique and detects virus in 30% of sera taken within 3 days of the clinical presentation of aplastic crisis. The more sensitive techniques of immuno-assay or nucleic acid hybridization will increase this percentage to 60% in such samples.

## Antibody detection

Most cases have detectable B19-specific IgM within a day or two of the onset of the rash, although in some cases it is necessary to wait for 7 days after the onset in order to be able to demonstrate such antibody in convincing amounts. Once B19-specific IgG has appeared in the serum it rapidly reaches peak concentrations and persists in decreasing amounts for 2–3 months. High concentrations of IgM antibody are usually found a month or two after infection and in most instances detectable IgG antibody persists for life. Diagnosis of recent infection can also be made by demonstrating seroconversion or increasing amounts of IgG antibody.

## Infection in the fetus

The diagnosis of B19 in a fetus depends upon the detection of virus in fetal specimens. Maternal infection is likely to have been some weeks previously and there may be no specific IgM in maternal serum. In most instances the infected fetuses have not been specific IgM-positive, but there is frequently a persistent viraemia. Thus, the diagnosis can be made by detection of virus in fetal blood samples or in fetal tissues taken at autopsy from which DNA has been extracted or detected by in-situ hybridization on formalin-fixed, paraffin-embedded tissue sections.

## TREATMENT

Most cases of B19 infection are mild and self-limiting and specific treatment is not required. However, there are three situations (Table 48.2) in which severe anaemia occurs as a consequence of B19 infection, and in each of these blood transfusion is indicated. In cases of aplastic crisis the transfusion tides patients over the relatively short period of erythroid aplasia before the immune response rapidly clears the virus infection. In the immunosuppressed there is a failure to produce neutralizing antibody so treatment consists of transfusion plus the administration of human normal immunoglobulin for 10 days. This leads to disappearance of the viraemia, sometimes permanently, sometimes only temporarily. The failure of the fetus to eliminate the virus is presumably associated with its inability to mount an immune response. Intra-uterine transfusion has been used to correct the anaemia, and the full-term delivery of normal infants has followed in these cases.

## EPIDEMIOLOGY

B19 infection has been found in all countries (Europe, North America, Scandinavia, Australia and Japan) in which appropriate diagnostic tests have been applied and it is almost certainly world-wide in distribution. Diseases due to B19 infection cluster in childhood, although some complications such as arthralgia occur more commonly in adult cases. Serological studies indicate that infection is most commonly acquired between 4 and 10 years of age and at least 60% of adults are seropositive. B19 virus infections are endemic throughout the year in temperate climates, but there is a seasonal increase in frequency in late winter, spring and early summer months. There are also longer-term cycles of B19 infection with a periodicity of about 4–5 years. The majority of B19 infections are transmitted by the respiratory route, but the occurrence of high-titre viraemia creates the possibility of transmitting this infection by blood or blood products and this has been shown to occur in haemophiliacs.

## CONTROL

Prevention of disease by isolating susceptible individuals is impractical since infections may be subclinical and symptomatic individuals are infectious before any sign of illness. Theoretically, susceptible individuals with chronic haemolytic anaemia or immunocompromised children could be temporarily protected by the administration of human immunoglobulin but this has not been tried. There is as yet no vaccine against B19 disease but, by analogy with the animal viruses, such a strategy would be very effective once sufficient quantities of viral antigen capable of stimulating neutralizing antibody are produced.

## RECOMMENDED READING

Fields B N, Knipe D M, Howley P M (eds) *Virology*, 3rd edn. Lippincott–Raven, Philadelphia, pp 2173–2198

Pattison J R 1994 Human parvoviruses. In: Zuckerman A J,

Banatvala J E, Pattison J R (eds) *Principles and Practice of Clinical Virology*, 3rd edn. Wiley, Chichester, pp 653–666

# 49

# Picornaviruses

**Meningitis; paralysis; rashes; intercostal myositis; myocarditis; infectious hepatitis; common cold**

*S. M. Burns*

The family Picornaviridae contains small (pico) viruses with a diameter of 27–30 nm and containing single-stranded RNA. It is subdivided into four genera, two of which are of considerable importance to humans. Viruses in the genus *Enterovirus* infect via the gut, and include the echo-, coxsackie- and polioviruses and the virus of hepatitis A. The members of the other genus, *Rhinovirus*, are the most important cause of the common cold. The properties of enteroviruses and rhinoviruses are compared in Table 49.1.

## ENTEROVIRUSES

### Description

The polioviruses, coxsackieviruses and echoviruses are described as enteroviruses because they are all found in the intestines and excreted in the faeces. New enteroviruses continue to be isolated, but they are no longer subdivided into the three named groups. Instead they are called enterovirus and numbered, e.g. enterovirus 71. Hepatitis A virus has been classified as enterovirus 72.

**Composition.** The RNA genome constitutes about one-quarter of the virion. The RNA is single stranded and of positive sense, and thus it can be translated directly by host ribosomes. The capsid consists of a protein shell arranged in icosahedral symmetry around the RNA molecule, the complete sequence of which is now known for several strains. Four major peptides are recognized in the shell, VP1, VP2, VP3 and VP4, and are formed from a single precursor protein, VP0, by proteolytic cleavage. Specific neutralizing antibodies are considered to be the major mechanism of protection against infection, and a major antigenic site on the VP1 protein of polio type 3 has been identified.

In addition to the properties listed in Table 49.1, the three groups of viruses and those designated enteroviruses 68–71 have a number of features in common:

1. They all replicate in the intestinal tract
2. They commonly cause asymptomatic immunizing infections which protect against future infections with the same virus
3. They can give rise to viraemia
4. They occasionally cause infection of the central nervous system
5. They are commoner in children than adults
6. In temperate climates they cause infections usually in the summer and autumn.

**Table 49.1** Some properties of picornaviruses

| Property | Enteroviruses | Rhinoviruses |
|---|---|---|
| Size (nm) | 22–30 | 30 |
| Capsid | | |
|     Form | Icosahedral | Icosahedral |
|     Polypeptides | VP1, VP2, VP3, VP4 | VP1, VP2, VP3, VP4 |
|     RNA type | Single-stranded, positive-sense | Single-stranded, positive-sense |
|     RNA molecular weight | $2 \times 10^6$–$2.6 \times 10^6$ | $2.6 \times 10^6$ |
| Acid | Stable (pH 3–9) | Labile (pH 3–5) |
| Optimal temperature for growth (°C) | 37 | 33–34 |
| Density in caesium chloride (g/ml) | 1.34 | 1.39–1.42 |

***Reactions to physical and chemical agents.***
Enteroviruses are among the most stable viruses.
They are insensitive to ether and detergents, which
destroy enveloped viruses. In faeces, virus can
survive for months at 4°C, and years at −20 or
−70°C. In faeces at room temperature the virus
can remain infective for several weeks, depending
on the amount of virus present, the amount of
moisture present and other environmental conditions.
The virus is readily killed by moist heat at 50–55°C
but less effectively in the presence of organic
material.

Virus in foodstuffs may survive exposure to 60°C,
and the flash method of pasteurization is necessary
to render the foodstuffs safe.

The inactivation of poliovirus is inhibited by
magnesium chloride, and this has been incorporated
into live polio vaccine as a stabilizer. Enteroviruses
are rapidly inactivated by ultraviolet light, and usually
by drying.

***Chemical inactivation.*** Poliovirus is rapidly
inactivated by 0.3% formaldehyde, 0.1 M hydrochloric acid and solutions giving a free residual
chlorine concentration of 0.3–0.5 ppm. Higher concentrations are necessary to inactivate virus in the
presence of organic matter, e.g. in swimming bath
water.

## Polioviruses

There are three types of poliovirus, identified by
neutralization tests, their RNA molecules differing
by 50% in hybridization studies. Two outstanding
characteristics of the viruses are their affinity for
nervous tissue and the narrow host range with, only
humans and primates susceptible. Cynomolgus and
rhesus monkeys can be infected by the oral route,
and develop paralysis; in chimpanzees the infection
is often asymptomatic. Under the influence of
cortisone, monkeys become more susceptible to
small parenteral doses of the virus.

The prototype strains are: type 1, the Brunhilde
and Mahoney strains; type 2, which includes the
rodent-adapted strains, the Lansing and MEFI
strains; and type 3, the Leon and Saukett strains.
The three types are antigenically distinct, but
overlap occurs in neutralization tests. Type 1 is the
common epidemic type, type 2 is usually associated
with endemic infections, but type 3 has caused
recent epidemics. The size, chemical and physical
properties, and the resistance of the three types are
all identical, and so their antigenic properties
provide one of the main methods of differentiating
them.

## Echoviruses

Echoviruses were identified by cell culture of faeces
of patients suffering from paralytic and non-paralytic
illness. There are over 30 serotypes of the *enteric
cytopathic human orphan* viruses and, true to their
name, there is still no clear association of all types
with specific disease.

***Pathogenicity for animals.*** None of the main
echovirus types produces clinical illness in laboratory
animals, although some strains of echovirus 9 which
have been adapted to cell culture can produce myositis
in newborn mice (see coxsackievirus infections).

***Haemagglutination.*** Haemagglutination of human group O erythrocytes is caused by certain types,
e.g. 3, 6, 7, 11, 12, 13, 19, 20, 21, 24, 25, 29, 30 and
33. The virus reacts with a receptor present on group
O cells, although not all strains of a particular type
may do so. This property is influenced by temperature, pH and the age of the red blood cell donor.

***Antigenic characters.*** Thirty-three distinct
antigenic types have so far been distinguished by
neutralization tests in cell cultures. Cross-reactions
occur between types 1, 8, 12 and 13 in neutralization
tests. Antigenic variation is known to occur in types
4, 6 and 9, and may be a common occurrence under
natural conditions. The specificity of strains may be
altered by cultivation in the presence of heterologous
antiserum.

## Coxsackieviruses

This group (of 30 serotypes) was named after the
place in New York state where the first member was
isolated. Coxsackieviruses are pathogenic for newborn
mice and hamsters. During the first 48 h of life these
animals are fully susceptible to infection; thereafter,
they acquire a natural resistance and, by the age of
5 days, can no longer be infected. By definition,
coxsackieviruses are unable to infect adult mice.
Two groups of the viruses are recognized according
to the histological nature and the sites of the lesions
they produce in mice (Table 49.2):

**Table 49.2**  Features of coxsackievirus infection in the laboratory

|  | Types | Growth in MK cell culture | Effect in suckling mice |
|---|---|---|---|
| Coxsackie A virus | 1–24[a] | + | Paralysis |
| Coxsackie B virus | 1–6 | + | Spasticity |

MK, monkey kidney.
[a]Coxsackievirus A23 now classified as echovirus 9.

1. *Coxsackie A viruses.* Group A viruses, of which there are 24, cause widespread severe myositis of skeletal muscles in mice. The principal muscles to be involved are of the hind limbs, and in life the mice appear to have flaccid paralysis. Usually the signs of infection appear 4 or 5 days after inoculation and progress until the animal dies 4 or 5 days later.

2. *Coxsackie B viruses.* Group B viruses, of which there are six, cause widespread lesions in many organs of mice. The myositis produced is characterized by focal lesions and gives rise to tremors, incoordination and a paralysis resembling the spastic type. The viruses also cause areas of necrosis in the brown fat lobules, especially those in the interscapular and cervical pads of fat. They also cause meningo-encephalitis and pancreatitis. The incubation period of group B infection in mice is prolonged, and symptoms may not be obvious until 10 days after inoculation. Inoculated mice must be kept under observation for 3 weeks.

*Growth in culture.* All group B coxsackieviruses grow readily in monkey kidney cell cultures. Of group A coxsackieviruses, only A7 and A9 grow in monkey kidney cells, and coxsackievirus A21 can be grown in HeLa, HEp2 or human embryonic kidney cell cultures. The viruses which grow in cell culture produce a cytopathic effect similar to polio- and echoviruses. Identification of the isolate is made by neutralization tests.

The other type A viruses are isolated by the inoculation of suckling mice; thereafter, some can be adapted to cell culture. In monkeys, coxsackieviruses do not usually produce clinical disease, but after inoculation a viraemia develops, and later the virus is excreted for several weeks in the faeces. Types A7 and A14 can cause a mild paralysis in monkeys, with lesions in the central nervous system resembling those of poliomyelitis. Type A7, which has caused paralytic disease in humans, is identical with the Russian AbIV strain, which was at first thought to constitute a fourth type of the poliomyelitis virus.

*Antigenic characters.* Thirty antigenic types have been defined by cross-neutralization tests in mice or cell culture, and cross-complement fixation reactions. Twenty-three have the features of group A and six have those of group B. Each of the six group B types is subject to antigenic variation, and sera from convalescent cases may show heterotypic responses. Coxsackievirus A23 has now been reclassified as echovirus 9.

## New enteroviruses

Detailed examination of the characteristics of the viruses in cell culture and their ability to infect laboratory animals, which had been the basis of classification into polio-, coxsackie- or echoviruses, showed that these were not reliable features. New isolates are simply called enterovirus and given the next available consecutive number. Thus, enteroviruses types 68, 69, 70, 71 and 72 are now recognized.

## Replication

This description of virus multiplication is based on observations of poliovirus growing in cell culture. The virion attaches to specific cellular receptor sites which interact with the protein capsid. Blocking experiments with monoclonal antibodies have shown that all three polioviruses use the same receptor, which is distinct from that for other enteroviruses, e.g. group B coxsackieviruses. The poliovirus receptor sites have been characterized and are glycoproteins on the cell membrane and the presence or absence of these specific receptors determines whether the cell is susceptible to infection by the virus. Once the virus particle is attached to the cellular receptor, VP4 is lost, the virion is taken into the cell and the viral RNA is released from the protein capsid. The viral RNA consists of about 6000 nucleotides, capable of producing genetic information to code for 2000 amino acids or 12 proteins. The viral RNA is polyadenylated and has a protein (VPg) attached at the 5' end; it is a polycistronic messenger RNA and is translated to produce one large polyprotein. This is then cleaved, by proteolytic enzymes, to specific proteins (P1, P2 and P3 – see Fig. 49.1). Viral RNA is synthesized from a negative-strand copy via the action of the viral RNA-dependent RNA polymerase; this occurs in the replicative intermediate complex associated with the smooth endoplasmic reticulum of the cell. Within the complex several new viral positive strands are synthesized on the virus template at any time. The VPg is added at this time, and probably plays a part in packaging of the viral RNA into newly formed capsids which are assembled from VP0, VPI and VP3. Once the RNA is enclosed, the final maturation occurs when VP0 cleaves to VP2 and VP4. Yields of many thousands of virions are normal when the cell bursts to release the progeny virions after an interval of 5–10 h. Only a small fraction, perhaps 1 in a 1000, of the new particles are infectious.

The synthesis of cellular RNA and protein ceases in infected cells, which die and release virus particles.

Vpg

viral RNA

poly A

5' ———————————————————— 3'

↓ Translation

———————————————————— Polyprotein

|
Cleaved

P1      P2      P3

VP0   VP1   VP3        protease; VPg; RNA polymerase

VP2   VP4

**Fig. 49.1**  The synthesis of poliovirus proteins.

| **Table 49.3**  Factors predisposing to paralytic poliomyelitis |
|---|
| Violent muscle exercise |
| Pregnancy (particularly third trimester) |
| Immunization |
| Tonsillectomy |

## Clinical features and pathogenesis

The enteroviruses are associated with a wide variety of clinical presentations, although the majority of infections are asymptomatic. The sites affected are the central nervous system (meningitis, paralysis), the skin (rashes) and muscle (intercostal myositis, myocarditis).

### Polioviruses

There are three types of poliovirus infection:

1. Asymptomatic infection or a mild, transient 'influenza-like' illness; this is the most likely outcome with only 1% of infections resulting in recognizable clinical illness. The virus is excreted in the faeces for a limited time, and an immunological response develops which protects against reinfection with the same strain.
2. Infections with the same symptoms as above and evidence of the involvement of the central nervous system with headache, neck stiffness and back pain (meningitis). Rapid and complete recovery in less than 10 days is usual.
3. Paralytic poliomyelitis in which the patient develops paralysis; this is the most dramatic form of the infection but it is very uncommon, occurring in 1 in 1000 of poliovirus infections in children, although 1 in 75 in adults may be affected. The paralysis is usually flaccid due to destruction of lower motor neurones, although invasion of the brain stem by the virus can lead to inco-ordination of muscle groups and painful spasms. Paralysis occurs early in the illness but the extent is variable. Often the paralysis is greatest initially; some function may return over the next 6 months. Damage to the nerve cells in the brain stem (bulbar paralysis) can lead to the inability to swallow and breathe.

The time between infection with the virus and development of symptoms is usually 14 days but can range from 3 to 21 days. During this period several factors are known to have an adverse effect on the outcome of infection (Table 49.3). Severe muscular activity can lead to paralysis of the limbs used, possibly due to increased vascularity, either in the limb or the appropriate area of the spinal cord, and increased access of virus to nerve endings. Pregnant women in the third trimester of pregnancy can have severe disease, but there is no firm evidence of congenital defects in infants born to mothers with poliomyelitis. Maternal infection acquired late in pregnancy may lead to perinatal infection and disease of the newborn.

Injection of adjuvant-containing vaccines, and irritant substances such as heavy metals, can result in paralysis occurring in the limbs which received the inoculation. Paralysis develops (incidence 1 in 37 000 injections) when poliovirus is contracted within 1 month of receiving the inoculation. Patients who have had their tonsils removed have a higher chance of developing bulbar poliomyelitis. This has been attributed to the reduction of secretory IgA which occurs in the pharynx, and the resultant reduced neutralization of the virus. Paralytic poliomyelitis is recognized as a rare complication of oral polio vaccine or following infection from contact with a vaccinee excreting virus.

Non-polio enteroviruses have also been associated with central nervous disease and paralysis (e.g. echovirus 4 and enterovirus 71); as with polio, paralysis is a rare manifestation of infection.

### Echoviruses

Most echovirus infections cause few or no clinical symptoms, but some have been associated with clinical syndromes (Table 49.4).

Infection can be widespread in a community, although only a few suffer from clinical illness. Symptoms occur following a short incubation period of 3–5 days (simple fever, upper respiratory symptoms or diarrhoea may occur). Non-specific rashes of fleeting duration have been reported. Lymphocytic meningitis can occur in epidemics.

| **Table 49.4** Clinical syndromes associated with echoviruses |
| --- |
| **Main syndromes** |
| Aseptic meningitis |
| Paralysis |
| Rash |
| Respiratory disease |
| **Other features** |
| Pericarditis and myocarditis |
| Neonatal infection |

**Table 49.5** Features of coxsackievirus infection in man

| Coxsackie-virus group | Type | Clinical illness |
| --- | --- | --- |
| A | 1–24 | Aseptic meningitis |
| | | Febrile illness |
| | | Herpangina |
| | | Hand, foot and mouth disease |
| B | 1–6 | Neonatal disease |
| | | Bornholm disease |
| | | Myocarditis, hepatitis |
| | | Meningitis |

The onset of meningitis is abrupt, with severe headache and vomiting. Symptoms are self-limiting, and after a variable convalescent period a full recovery is made, although rare cases of paralysis have been reported.

Most of the echovirus types have been associated with sporadic cases of *aseptic meningitis* or one of the other disease patterns already mentioned. A number of types, notably 4, 6, 9, 16, 20, 28 and 30, have considerable epidemic potential, and the clinical features are very varied. As examples, echovirus 9 epidemics have been common in Europe and North America as large outbreaks of a biphasic fever, with a sore throat, rash on face, neck and chest and, less commonly, on the lower trunk and extremities. A minority of patients show clinical signs of meningitis, but many without distinct clinical signs have a pleocytosis in the cerebrospinal fluid.

Echovirus 16 epidemics have been called *Boston fever* after the city where the illness was first reported. Clinically, the infection starts with a sharp fever, abdominal pains and a mild sore throat. After 24–48 h there appears in children a pink, discrete macular or maculopapular rash, mostly on the face, chest and back. Echovirus 4, 6 and 30 epidemics have been associated with considerable numbers of cases of meningitis in children and adults. Echoviruses 6, 9 and 11 have caused severe and fatal infections in newborn infants. The virus is probably transmitted during birth or postnatally from the mother or nursery attendants who are asymptomatic. Circulatory collapse, hepatitis and meningo-encephalitis occur in the infant, and infection can spread rapidly to other infants in the nursery or special care baby unit. Infection is usually caused by the type of virus circulating in the community at the time.

Echovirus 18 has been recovered from the faeces of many infants in an outbreak of diarrhoea. The children had no rash and no severe involvement of the central nervous system or meningeal reaction.

Several echoviruses, including types 1, 11, 19, 20 and 22, have been isolated from cases of respiratory illnesses in children in whom symptoms include pneumonia, bronchiolitis and upper respiratory tract illness.

## Coxsackieviruses

*Group A viruses.* These viruses give rise to a number of different illnesses (Table 49.5). *Aseptic meningitis*, indistinguishable clinically from that caused by other enteroviruses, is caused by a number of types, e.g. 2, 4, 7, 9 or 23. Type A7 has given rise to epidemics of paralytic disease in Scotland, the former USSR and elsewhere. *Herpangina* is an acute feverish disease, usually in young children, characterized by lesions in the mouth consisting of papules on the anterior pillars of the fauces; these papules become vesicles and finally shallow ulcers with a greyish base and punched-out edge. There are usually 5–10 lesions, and the illness lasts about 4 days. Types 2, 4, 5, 6, 8, 10 and 23 have been isolated at various times from these infections. Outbreaks may be seen in nurseries and schools. *Hand, foot and mouth* disease presents as a painful stomatitis with a vesicular rash on the hands and feet. Typically, it lasts about a week; most of the cases are seen in the summer in children aged 1–10 years, and cases can occur in clusters, and in families. The viruses usually implicated are types 5 and 16.

Coxsackievirus A21 (COE) has caused epidemics of colds in camps of military recruits.

*Group B viruses.* *Epidemic myalgia* or *Bornholm disease*, first described on the Danish island of Bornholm, is characterized by fever and the sudden onset of agonizing stitch-like pains in the muscles of the chest, epigastrium or hypochondrium. Although the disease is most frequently recognized in its epidemic form, many sporadic cases occur. Epidemic myalgia may be complicated by pleurisy and pericarditis.

In newborn infants, severe and often fatal *myocarditis* has been reported, and the virus can be found in high concentrations in the mycocardium at autopsy. Epidemics have occurred in nurseries when there is evidence of group B virus activity in a community. The baby is presumed to be infected by its mother and is highly susceptible to the virus, like the infant mouse. Myocarditis and pericarditis can occur in children and adults, and virus has been isolated from pericardial fluid.

Coxsackie B viruses are a major cause of human *myopericarditis*. Although severe in the neonate, it tends to follow a more benign course in the adult. The initial symptoms are often of an upper respiratory or 'influenza-like' illness followed 7–10 days later by clinical heart disease. Chest pain is a feature and electrocardiogram abnormalities such as tachycardia and arrhythmias have been found. On clinical examination, murmurs, rubs and, occasionally, pericardial effusion are detected. Other features of coxsackie B virus infection can be present at the same time in the individual.

*Aseptic meningitis*, sometimes with cases of paralysis, is a common manifestation of infection due to group B virus. Occasionally a rash is present.

Coxsackie B viruses have been implicated in the condition known as the *postviral fatigue syndrome*. This is a postinfectious complaint in which fatigue, profound muscle weakness and lack of concentration are cardinal features. It was first described following an outbreak involving staff at the Royal Free Hospital, London in 1955. Several viruses have been incriminated, including coxsackie B viruses. The condition and its cause remain to be clearly defined.

B strains have been associated with 'influenza-like' illnesses, upper respiratory infections, bronchitis and pneumonia in young children.

## New enteroviruses (Table 49.6)

***Enterovirus 70.*** In 1969 outbreaks of *acute haemorrhagic conjunctivitis* (AHC) spread throughout Africa and Asia; more recently the disease has occurred in Mexico. AHC is highly infectious and has a short incubation period of 24–48 h. Attack rates are very high where there is overcrowding and poor sanitation. Although subconjunctival haemorrhage is a complication, most cases recover within 7 days.

***Enterovirus 71.*** Like other enteroviruses, enterovirus 71 produces infections that are usually inapparent. It was first recognized in 1969 in California, when it was isolated from the faeces of a 9-month-old infant suffering from encephalitis. Since then it has been isolated from cases showing a spectrum of

**Table 49.6** Illness associated with recently identified enteroviruses

| Enterovirus type | Clinical illness |
| --- | --- |
| 68 | Pneumonia and bronchiolitis |
| 69 | Isolated from an ill person in Mexico |
| 70 | Acute haemorrhagic conjunctivitis |
| 70, 71 | Paralysis, meningo-encephalitis |
| 71 | Hand, foot and mouth disease |
| 72 | Hepatitis A |

illness. During an epidemic of enterovirus 71 disease in Bulgaria in 1975, there was a high incidence of paralytic disease. The majority of the paralytic cases occurred in children under 5 years of age.

## Pathogenesis

All enterovirus infections follow a similar pattern as illustrated in Figure 49.2 for poliovirus, with differences in the target organs, e.g. central nervous system, skin or muscle. Due to the potential severity of infection, and the availability of an animal model, most is known about poliomyelitis, although it is reasonable to assume that similar features are seen with echo- and coxsackieviruses.

Virus is ingested and multiplies initially in the lymphoid tissue of the tonsil or Peyer's patches in the small intestine and then the local lymph nodes, e.g. cervical or mesenteric. In fatal cases, the Peyer's patches and the mesenteric lymph nodes are found to be greatly swollen and inflamed and to contain large amounts of virus. Virus released from the nodes reaches the blood, and then the central nervous system. The paralytic effect of poliovirus results from infection of motor neurone cells in the anterior horns of the spinal cord or bulbar regions. Localization in the motor neurones is probably due to the presence of receptors for the poliovirus. Once within the brain or cord, spread can occur directly to neighbouring cells, or via the cerebrospinal fluid to more remote areas.

The viraemic phase marks the end of the incubation period, and is manifest in the patient by fever and generalized symptoms; it is followed by a period of about 48 h of relative well-being (the disease is biphasic) while the virus is invading nerve tissue and then, in serious cases, the signs of paralysis appear. Viraemia has been proven to occur after experimental infection of monkeys and has been demonstrated on several occasions in humans. It is probable that the process can be arrested at various stages so that virus may multiply in the intestine without ever reaching the bloodstream. If antibody is present in

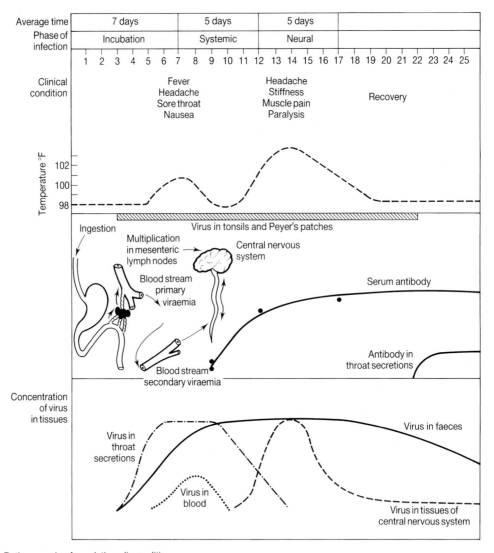

**Fig. 49.2** Pathogenesis of paralytic poliomyelitis.

the blood, virus can be prevented from reaching the central nervous system.

Enteroviruses are lytic, destroying the infected cell within a few hours to days. They are non-enveloped so are unlikely to induce cytotoxic T cell responses. However, cell damage will trigger an inflammatory response; the resultant oedema may affect neurones other than those infected with the virus. As the oedema resolves, function will recover in these cells, thus explaining the apparent improvement in the degree of paralysis in the weeks to months after the acute stage.

Experimentally, it has been shown that the virus can travel along nerves. In most circumstances this

is probably not an important route to the central nervous system, but may explain the increased risk of paralysis associated with muscular activity, tonsillectomy and the use of adjuvant vaccines.

## Laboratory diagnosis

### Culture

Virus isolation is the most useful method for establishing a diagnosis. Examination of cerebrospinal fluid is an essential part of the laboratory diagnosis of meningitis. The sample is directly inoculated into cell culture. Faecal samples should also be submitted, although isolation can be made from rectal and throat swabs. Since virus excretion can be intermittent, two specimens should be collected on successive days, as early as possible in the illness, ideally within 5 days of the onset.

Virus is detected by the development of a cytopathic effect usually within a few days; the isolate is identified by neutralization tests with type-specific antisera. In the UK, poliovirus isolates are likely to be attenuated vaccine strains, which can be differentiated from wild-type virus by several genetic markers.

In paralytic poliomyelitis, the virus can be found in the faeces for a few days preceding the onset of acute symptoms, and is present in over 80% of cases in the faeces during the first 4 days. After 3 weeks some 50% of patients still excrete the virus, and 25% at 5–6 weeks. Only a few cases continue to excrete the virus after the 12th week. No permanent carriers are known but prolonged excretion is recognized in immunocompromised hosts. The virus can be isolated from the oropharynx of many cases for a few days before and after the onset of the illness. Isolation from the cerebrospinal fluid is seldom successful in cases of paralytic poliomyelitis.

Echoviruses, coxsackie B viruses and coxsackie A9 virus are readily isolated from nose and throat swabs, stools or cerebrospinal fluid; they are present in 80% of cases in the faeces for at least 2 weeks after the onset. If the other coxsackie A viruses are to be isolated, the specimens are inoculated by the intracerebral and/or intraperitoneal routes into newborn mice (under 24 h of age). The mice are examined for signs of paralysis. Identification is by neutralization with reference antisera. Animal inoculation is likely to be superseded by detection of RNA by the polymerase chain reaction.

Isolation of virus from the cerebrospinal fluid is a significant finding. However, the relevance of virus isolation from faeces is not always clear, as enteroviruses can be excreted for some time after inapparent infection.

### Serological tests

Although specific IgM and IgG assays for enteroviruses are available their use is limited by the heterotypic and anamestic responses associated with infections. Early and rapid diagnosis of enterovirus disease can now be made by detection of RNA in serum by reverse-transcription polymerase chain reaction.

## Treatment

This is symptomatic. A number of antiviral agents were investigated many years ago for the treatment of paralytic poliomyelitis but they were of no practical value due to the rapid emergence of drug resistance.

## Epidemiology and transmission

The only natural source of poliovirus is humans. The virus is spread from person to person, and no intermediate host is known. Virus is excreted in faeces and, rarely, in oropharyngeal secretions. Since the widespread use of polio vaccines began epidemic poliomyelitis has virtually disappeared, and cases of infection usually occur in areas such as the tropics where the disease is still endemic. The numbers of reported cases considerably underestimate the true prevalence of disease, and countries such as Africa and India still have a significant number of cases. Other countries with low immunization coverage, such as Algeria and Morocco, continue to have cases with a peak incidence every few years.

Prior to the use of vaccines, the disease was endemic in young children with periodic epidemics, usually in the late summer in Europe, America and Australia. Where standards of hygiene were high the spread of the virus was impeded and individuals or whole communities escaped infection for many years. A large proportion of these populations had no immunity and when poliovirus was introduced an epidemic could develop rapidly. In 1978 the Netherlands experienced an outbreak of 110 cases of poliomyelitis, of whom 80 developed paralysis, among a religious group of 70 000 individuals who had refused any sort of immunization. In addition to the cases, poliovirus type 1 was also isolated from the faeces of 70% of their unvaccinated contacts, but not from vaccinated contacts. Later in 1978, six cases of poliomyelitis were reported in Canada, again in a religious group, related to the Netherlands group. The introduction of a strain of higher virulence may also be a factor in epidemic spread, as illustrated by an outbreak of nine cases of paralytic poliomyelitis and one non-paralytic case in Finland between August 1984 and January 1985; these were the first cases seen for 20 years. Intensive immunization reaching 95% of the population halted the outbreak very quickly. A strain of poliovirus type 3 was isolated which was immunologically different from the type 3 vaccine strain, which is known to induce weak responses.

Echovirus and coxsackievirus infections have a similar epidemiology to poliovirus although no vaccines are available.

### Transmission

All enteroviruses are excreted in large numbers from the gut: direct transfer on fingers is common, but eating utensils and food or drink can also be vehicles. Entry through the conjunctiva may also occur occasionally. Outbreaks are often seen in closed communities and schools. In the acute phase of infection, virus is present in the throat and, while droplet spread could occur, the faecal–oral route is the usual means of transmission. After the acute phase, it is the only possible route. Cases are most infectious late in the incubation period but infection can be transmitted at any time during virus excretion in the faeces.

Infection rates can equal 100% in close communities and in households, particularly where children are involved. Social factors, such as standards of hygiene, overcrowding and the age of contacts, are also important. Sewage can contain polioviruses, particularly when there is infection in a community. Enteroviruses can survive for several months in river water, but are unlikely to survive in chlorine-treated water or swimming pools where the recommended level of chlorination (without protein contamination) is achieved. Flies and cockroaches have been found to harbour viruses, but their role in transmission is minimal. Close contact and hygienic standards remain the most important factors.

## Prevention and control

After natural infection, immunity is permanent. Virus-neutralizing antibodies are formed early during the disease (often before the 7th day) and persist for several decades. Secretory IgA is produced in the gut. There is some doubt about the duration of immunity to some of the coxsackieviruses.

## Immunization

There are two types of polio vaccines:

1. *Inactivated polio vaccine (IPV)*. IPV (Salk) was introduced in 1956 for routine immunization. The vaccine contains strains of the three types of virus grown in monkey kidney cell culture and inactivated by exposure to formaldehyde. The batches of vaccine are tested for the presence of residual live poliovirus and must be free of contaminants. Inactivated vaccines are used in Sweden, Finland, Iceland and Holland. With acceptance rates in excess of 90%, these countries have virtually eliminated poliovirus. The circulation of poliovirus in the community has been dramatically reduced despite the fact that inactivated vaccine does not induce much secretory IgA in the alimentary tract. A high rate of immunization is necessary and antibody levels need to be maintained because it has been shown in children that the

outcome of exposure to virus is directly related to the level of antibody at the time of exposure. In the recent outbreak of poliomyelitis in Finland, the strains of poliovirus type 3 were antigenically slightly different from the type 3 poliovirus vaccine strains. Finland has recently introduced a higher-potency vaccine which has been shown to produce a good immunological response to all three poliovirus types and it seems likely that this vaccine will give good, long-lasting protection. It was concluded that the outbreak was not due to failure of inactivated vaccine in general but to the poorly immunogenic preparation previously used. The vaccine should be administered by deep subcutaneous or intramuscular injection, and is not associated with local or general reactions. A course of three injections given with intervals of 6–8 weeks between the first and second doses and 4–6 months between the second and third doses produces long-lasting immunity to all three poliovirus types. Inactivated vaccine is recommended for immuno-compromised individuals and their contacts and others for whom a live vaccine is contra-indicated.

IPV may be used simultaneously with the triple vaccine for diphtheria, pertussis and tetanus. Booster doses of polio vaccine can be given at the same time as diphtheria/tetanus and also with the combined mumps, measles, rubella (MMR) vaccine.

2. *Live attenuated polio vaccines (OPV)*. Attenuated live oral (Sabin) vaccine replaced the Salk vaccine for routine use in the UK in 1962 and is used extensively in many other countries. It contains live but *attenuated* strains of poliovirus types 1, 2 and 3, grown either in cultures of monkey kidney cells or human diploid cells. The strains were obtained by growing less virulent polioviruses which had been isolated in the wild and, after passage, selecting strains which had lost their neurovirulence. The strains most commonly used were developed by Sabin in 1959.

The vaccine is administered orally and parallels natural infection with stimulation of both local secretory IgA in the pharynx and alimentary tract and circulating IgG, thereby producing local resistance to subsequent infection with wild poliomyelitis viruses. Herd immunity is important in preventing the circulation of the wild-type virus and high levels of immunization uptake are necessary. This is aided by the wide circulation of vaccine virus, which helps to maintain immunity in the community. However, vaccine strains are not completely stable and studies of sequential isolates of virus from vaccine recipients show that changes can be detected very rapidly. There is therefore the theoretical possibility that vaccine virus, attenuated by serial passage in culture, could revert to neurovirulence with multiple rounds of replication in the vaccinee and after transmission to contacts. Cases of vaccine-associated poliomyelitis have been reported in recipients of OPV at a rate of 1 in 2 million doses: it has also been seen in contacts of recipients. It is not possible to predict who will become affected, although the extended replication which occurs in the immunocompromised should be avoided as the rate of vaccine-associated polio-myelitis in such patients is 10 000 times greater than in normal people. Non-immunized parents and household contacts of children receiving primary immunization should be immunized against polio-myelitis at the same time as the children.

OPV is recommended for infants from 2 months of age. The primary course consists of three separate doses given at the same time as diphtheria/tetanus/pertussis vaccine (see Ch. 68). Each dose contains all three strains. In infants three drops are dropped from a spoon directly into the mouth, which may be open in response to the simultaneous administration intramuscularly or subcutaneously of diphtheria/tetanus/pertussis vaccine. Breast-feeding does not interfere with the antibody response to OPV and should continue. A reinforcing dose is given to the children at school entry, but it is not necessary for adults unless they are at special risk, e.g. through travel or occupational exposure. The effectiveness of live vaccine is shown by the experience in the USA where the number of paralytic cases has dropped from 21 000 to 5–10 per annum. In the UK, an average of three cases per annum have been notified in recent years.

When a case of paralytic poliomyelitis is diagnosed a dose of OPV should be given to all persons in the immediate neighbourhood of the case who are immunocompetent, whether or not they have a history of previous vaccination against poliomyelitis. This should be followed by completion of the primary course in those not immunized. If the source of the outbreak is uncertain it should be assumed to be a 'wild-type' virus until proven otherwise.

***Poliovirus immunization in the tropics.*** Serological studies in Africa have shown that children will have been infected with two or three types of poliovirus by the age of 5 years. The rate of paralytic disease is low in young children, but significant numbers occur as the infection is widespread. The disease is known as *infantile paralysis*. Through the expanded programme on immunization the World Health Organization has increased the rate of polio immunization chiefly with the use of OPV. Although this is cheaper than IPV, it must be stored at 0–4°C

and thus requires the existence of an effective cold chain to ensure successful immunization. Apart from inactivation of the vaccine, other explanations for low rates of seroconversion include interference from other enteroviruses, malnutrition and the presence of inhibiting factors in the gastro-intestinal contents. Failure to control poliomyelitis in under-privileged countries is also due to not reaching a sufficiently high proportion of the population, and thus is due to a failure of organization rather than vaccine. Recent experience in Brazil, where a national pro-gramme of OPV vaccine distribution has resulted in a dramatic decrease in disease, supports this possibility.

***Prospects for the future.*** When the incidence of poliomyelitis falls dramatically, as in the USA for example, the proportion of cases attributable to vaccine becomes increasingly significant. Recent work has identified the amino acid sequence of antigenic sites which are important for neutralization of the virus. Information concerning the viral factors necessary for virulence is also available. Therefore, it may be possible to develop modified vaccine viruses which cannot revert to neurovirulence. WHO has targetted polio as a disease that could be eradicated by widespread use of vaccine. To achieve this immunization campaigns are being mounted.

## Enterovirus 72 (hepatitis A virus)

Epidemic jaundice has been recognized for centuries; many large epidemics have occurred related to wars, including the Second World War. The virus was first detected by electron microscopical examination of faeces from cases. In the laboratory, infection can be transmitted to the marmoset.

Hepatitis A virus (HAV), the causative agent of *infectious hepatitis*, is now classified as enterovirus 72. It is an unenveloped virus, containing linear, single-stranded RNA. It has similar polypetides to the four major polypeptides of the enterovirus family and shares the same properties of resistance to physical and chemical agents. Recently, it has been adapted to cell culture; it will grow only in cells of primate origin.

### Clinical features

The illness caused by HAV is usually mild, and occurs after an incubation period of 14–45 days (median, 28 days). There is a prodrome of malaise, muscle pain and headache and there may be a low-grade fever. The symptoms usually improve and disappear as jaundice develops. Serological tests show that many patients have a subclinical illness, but fulminating hepatitis and liver failure can also occur (overall, less than 0.5%). There are no carriers of the virus. Infection is mildest in young children, often accompanied only by nausea and malaise. Of children under 3 years of age, only 5% develop jaundice, but this rises progressively to more than 50% in adults. The fatality rate also rises with age to 2% in adults. Some patients develop diarrhoea and some appear to have a relapse a few weeks after the onset. Arthritis and aplastic anaemia are rare complications.

## Pathogenesis

Like other enteroviruses, HAV probably infects cells in the gut and then spreads to the liver via the blood. The histopathology is similar to that of hepatitis B, with periportal necrosis and infiltration of mononuclear cells; viral antigens are seen in the cytoplasm of the hepatocytes. Virus is excreted via the bile into the gut 1–2 weeks before the onset of jaundice, excretion then declines rapidly over the next 5–7 days. Virus is also present in the urine of clinical and subclinical cases during the same period.

## Laboratory diagnosis

Although the virus has been grown in cell culture, it is not possible to do this routinely from the faeces of cases. Diagnosis relies on the demonstration of specific IgM antibody to HAV, which develops very early in the course of infection and is generally present by the time the patient is investigated. It is detectable in the serum for 2–6 months after the onset of symptoms (Fig. 49.3). IgG antibody usually persists for many years and is a useful indicator of immunity.

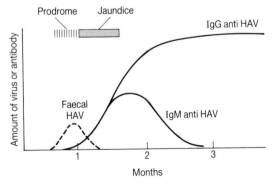

**Fig. 49.3** Events in hepatitis A infection.

## Epidemiology

Only one major type of HAV has been recognized. Serological tests have made it possible to study the rate of infection in different populations throughout the world. Such studies confirm that, since the virus is spread by the faecal–oral route, it is prevalent in countries where sanitation is poor, and children are infected early in childhood. Serological studies also show that, even in developed countries, more than half the population have been infected with HAV. However, lower rates may also be seen, and are reflected in the appearance of increased numbers of acute cases. In young adults and older patients there may be a history of recent travel to an endemic area.

Outbreaks of HAV infection have been associated with food. Shellfish have often been incriminated, particularly when they are harvested from coastlines adjacent to sewage outlets. The mussel, for example, is a filter feeder and can concentrate the virus. Shellfish are eaten raw or partially cooked, thus protecting the virus. Contaminated raspberries were incriminated in another notorious outbreak in which uncooked frozen raspberries were eaten many months after picking. Infection is assumed to have come from an infected raspberry picker. Because there is only a transient viraemic phase, only a few infections have been recognized after blood transfusion.

## Prevention and control

Hepatitis A vaccine was licensed for use in the UK in 1991. It is a formaldehyde-inactivated vaccine prepared from Hepatitis A grown in human diploid cells. A primary course of two doses (or, more recently, a single dose) of vaccine given intramuscularly produces good levels of neutralizing antibody which are likely to persist for at least 10 years. The vaccine is an alternative to human normal immunoglobulin for frequent travellers and those whose occupation takes them to endemic areas abroad.

# RHINOVIRUSES

The viruses of this genus are responsible for the most frequent of all human infections, the 'common cold'. Most people suffer from two to four colds every year and, although the primary infection is not a severe one, secondary bacterial infection often follows with symptoms that may be more severe than the original cold. Sinusitis and otitis media are

**Fig. 49.4** Human rhinovirus. This virus is indistinguishable in appearance from other picornaviruses. Approximate size 25–30 nm. (From Madeley C R, Field A M 1988 *Virus Morphology*, 2nd edn. Churchill Livingstone, Edinburgh.)

quite common. These viruses cause the loss of many million human-hours of work.

## Properties

As the name rhinovirus implies, the genus is associated with the nose. They can be distinguished from the enteroviruses by their acid lability and thus their inability to reach and infect the intestinal tract. There are over 100 serotypes of rhinoviruses; all are fastidious in cell culture. Electron microscopy cannot differentiate them from other family members (Fig. 49.4). Some primates may be susceptible to human viruses, and there are related viruses in cattle, cats and horses. The genomes of some rhinoviruses have 45–60% homology with polioviruses in hybridization tests.

The capsid of rhinoviruses appears to be less rigid than that of the enteroviruses. This loose packing is consistent with its greater buoyant density and sensitivity to acid.

### Cultivation

Rhinoviruses show a distinct preference for cells of human origin, especially fetal lung or kidney. Previously, they were divided into three groups according to the source of the cells in which the virus had been grown. Thus 'M' strains grew in both *m*onkey and human cells, the 'H' strains grew only in *h*uman cells and lastly the 'O' strains could only be grown

in *o*rgan cultures of nasal or tracheal ciliated epithelium. Since many of the 'H' strains could be adapted to grow in monkey cells and many of the 'O' strains could be adapted to grow in human cells this classification was abandoned.

### Stability

Inactivation of rhinoviruses occurs below pH 6.0 and is more rapid the lower the pH. Complete inactivation occurs at pH 3.0.

Some rhinoviruses may survive heating at 50°C for 1 h. They are relatively stable in the range from 20–37°C and can survive on environmental surfaces such as door knobs for several days. They can be preserved at −70°C.

Rhinoviruses are resistant to 20% ether and 5% chloroform, but are sensitive to aldehydes and hypochlorites.

## Replication

Rhinoviruses attach to cell receptors that are members of the Ig superfamily. Most types appear to use the same receptor. The viruses replicate in the cytoplasm of infected cells to give a cytopathic effect (CPE) which coincides with release of the virus in the same way as other picornaviruses. If the infected cultures are incubated at 37°C the yield is reduced to 30–50% of that at 33°C.

## Clinical features and pathogenesis

The typical illness is generally referred to as a common cold. The onset, after contact with infection, is usually within 2–3 days, sometimes as long as 7 days. There is a clear watery nasal discharge which often becomes mucoid or purulent due to secondary bacterial infection, and sneezing and coughing are common. Sore throat, headache and malaise may occur. The symptoms are most severe for 2–3 days when nasal virus titres are maximal and, although recovery is usually complete within a week, symptoms can persist for 2 weeks or longer. The ratio of symptomatic to asymptomatic infection is about 3:1, and the illness is generally worse in cigarette smokers. Rhinoviruses have frequently been isolated from patients during acute exacerbations of chronic obstructive airway disease, and they are the most common viruses to be associated with wheeze in pre-school children.

It should be remembered that all respiratory viruses may cause the symptoms of the common cold and that laboratory diagnosis is necessary to establish the aetiological agent.

Experimental rhinovirus infection in healthy human volunteers and studies on rhinovirus-infected organ cultures have helped to show their pathogenic potential. Humans have proved to be the more sensitive assay as illness can occur when virus cannot be detected by culture in the inoculum. In organ cultures, it has been shown that the virus settles on the ciliated nasal epithelial cells, enters, infects and spreads from cell to cell in the epithelium. The cilia become immobilized, and both cilia and cell degenerate as the virus replicates. Bacterial invasion of the damaged epithelium can then occur. Interferon is usually detectable shortly after the peak of virus shedding and probably plays a part in recovery. When specific antibody is first detected in nasal secretions, virus shedding ceases, suggesting that this may be the main factor leading to recovery. Little is known of the importance of cell-mediated immunity. The symptoms probably relate to the local inflammatory response and interferon release. Rhinoviruses have been recovered in pure culture from sinus fluids collected from patients with acute sinusitis, but secondary bacterial infection is thought to be the usual cause.

Lower respiratory tract infection may occur on some occasions since (1) patients with colds may also have lower respiratory tract symptoms with abnormal lung function, (2) children who develop colds may develop wheeze and (3) adults with colds may suffer exacerbations of chronic obstructive airway disease.

### Immunity

After the acute illness, neutralizing antibody can be detected both in serum and nasal secretions, may continue to rise in titre for 4–5 weeks after infection and persist for up to 4 years, although some infections may provoke only a poor response, leaving the patient susceptible to the same serotype after a few weeks or months.

## Laboratory diagnosis

### Culture

Nose and throat swabs in virus transport medium are the specimens of choice for the recovery of virus from all age groups. Nasopharyngeal aspirates are excellent specimens from children. Specimens should be taken as early in the illness as possible, preferably within the first 3 days.

Cell cultures of human origin such as MRC5 or WI38 are preferred for the isolation of rhinoviruses.

Organ cultures are not used routinely. Cultures are incubated at 33°C and observed microscopically for a cytopathic effect (CPE).

The majority of isolates are apparent within 2 weeks of inoculation although some may take longer. Identification of an isolate as a rhinovirus may be made by considering the cells in which the CPE develops, the appearance of the CPE and the demonstration of acid lability.

### Serology

Serological methods cannot be used in the routine diagnosis of rhinovirus infections because of the multiplicity of serotypes and the lack of a common antigen.

## Epidemiology and transmission

Rhinoviruses can be isolated from patients with respiratory illnesses throughout the year but in temperate climates the incidence of colds due to rhinoviruses increases in the autumn and spring and is at its lowest in the summer months. In the tropics the peak incidence occurs in the rainy season. Deliberate exposure of volunteers to wet and chilling does not increase their susceptibility to colds. Rhinoviruses may be transmitted by inhalation of droplets expelled from the nose of a patient. During the acute phase of the illness high concentrations of virus are present in nasal secretions and may contaminate the fingers, and thereafter the contaminated finger may touch the eye or nasal mucosa. Colds in the home are often introduced by pre-school children in whom the incidence of rhinovirus infections is highest. People who are in contact with young children appear to suffer from more colds than others.

Colds are mostly trivial and are an inconvenience; however, they do cause considerable morbidity and absence from work.

## Treatment and control

Although inactivated vaccines can be produced, there remains the considerable problem of deciding on the antigenic composition. Much effort has been devoted to the development of suitable antiviral therapy and, although compounds such as those related to the benzimidazoles have antiviral activity, no useful drugs are available. Isolation of the infected person, although perhaps desirable, is not a practical method of preventing the spread of infection. Attention to personal hygiene in those with colds and their contacts might help.

## RECOMMENDED READING

Andre F E 1990 Inactivated candidate vaccines for hepatitis A. *Progress in Medical Virology* 37: 72–95

Grist N R, Bell E J 1984 Paralytic poliomyelitis and non-polio enteroviruses. Studies in Scotland. *Reviews of Infectious Diseases* 6(suppl 2): S385–S386

Her Majesty's Stationery Office 1996 *Immunization Against Infectious Disease.* HMSO, London

Roebuck M O 1976 Rhinoviruses in Britain. *Journal of Hygiene* 76: 137–146

Thoren A 1994 PCR for the diagnosis of enteroviral meningitis. *Scandinavian Journal of Infectious Diseases* 26: 249–254

# 50

# Orthomyxoviruses

**Influenza**

*S. Sutherland*

World-wide, people are familiar with *influenza*, the disease caused by the orthomyxoviruses. The family Orthomyxoviridae comprises influenza A, B and C viruses. Formerly the orthomyxoviruses and the paramyxoviruses were grouped together in the myxovirus (Greek, *myxa* = mucus) family. While there are some general similarities in structure and the diseases they cause, the viruses differ in a number of fundamental features. For this reason they were separated into the two families – the Orthomyxoviridae and Paramyxoviridae.

Influenza A viruses can infect a variety of different host species, an ability that is of great importance in determining their ability to cause pandemic infection in humans. Influenza B only infects humans. Influenza C is little studied, and, although assumed to be primarily a human infection, it has recently been isolated from pigs in China.

Influenza virus type A was the first to be isolated, this being achieved in 1933 by the unlikely process of intranasal instillation in the ferret. Thereafter, type B was isolated along with type A in cell culture in 1940. One of the most prominent features of the influenza viruses is their ability to change antigenically either gradually over years (*antigenic drift*) or suddenly (*antigenic shift*). Only influenza A virus has the potential to shift, whereas all three types may drift antigenically, although only very minor changes have been demonstrated in influenza C.

**Fig. 50.1** Influenza A/Dunedin/27/83 $H_1N_1$ virus. Spikes which make up the fringe are also seen in the end-on view, covering the surface of the virus particles and giving them a 'spotty' appearance. Approximate size 80–120 nm. (From Madeley C R and Field A M 1988 *Virus Morphology*, 2nd edn. Churchill Livingstone, Edinburgh.)

## THE VIRUSES

The virions are spherical, 80–120 nm in diameter, but may be filamentous, sometimes up to several micrometres in length (Fig. 50.1). They have a helical nucleocapsid comprising eight segments of single-stranded RNA with a total molecular weight of $5 \times 10^6$. Also present within the virion is the viral RNA-dependent RNA polymerase: this is essential for infectivity as the virion RNA is of negative sense and therefore has to be transcribed to produce viral messenger RNA (mRNA). The nucleocapsid is surrounded by an M1 protein shell, immediately exterior to which is a lipid envelope derived from the host cell. The M2 protein projects through the envelope to form ion channels which allow pH

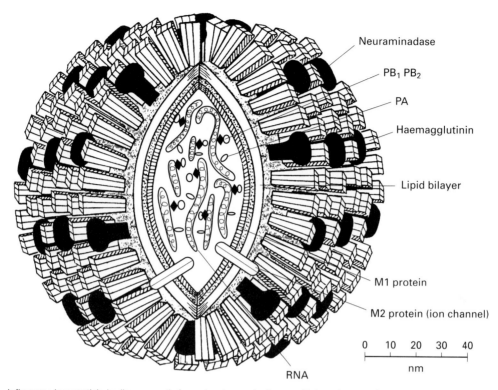

**Fig. 50.2**  Influenza virus particle in diagrammatic form showing projections and internal compositon.

changes in the endosome. Projecting from the envelope are two types of spikes (Fig. 50.2) the *haemagglutinin* (H) and the *neuraminidase* (N). The haemagglutinin, so called because the virus agglutinates certain species of erythrocyte, is about 10 nm in length, with a molecular weight of 225 000, and consists of trimers of identical glycoprotein subunits, each consisting of two polypeptide chains, HA1 and HA2. HA1 contains 328 amino acids, and HA2, 221. The two polypeptides are linked in each subunit by a single disulphide bond between residues 14 of HA1 and 137 of HA2. In the virus particle the haemagglutinin molecule is associated with the lipid membrane by a hydrophobic region near the carboxyl terminus of HA2. Influenza viruses bind to cells by the haemagglutinin interacting with membrane receptors containing *N*-acetylneuraminic acid (sialic acid). The epitopes involved in receptor-binding show great variability due to mutations in the RNA causing amino acid substitutions at several sites on the HA1 molecule. These changes can be located in the three-dimensional structure of the molecule and are found only at a few well-defined sites close to the

attachment site. The HA contains a fusion peptide which at neutral pH is buried within the spike but at low pH a conformational change occurs which exposes the peptide. Together with several other trimers the fusion peptides form a fusion pore which inserts into the cell lipid layer causing the viral and cell membranes to fuse.

Between the haemagglutinin spikes are the mushroom-shaped protrusions of neuraminidase. The head is box-shaped and is assembled from four roughly spherical subunits attached to the stalk containing the hydrophobic region by which it is embedded in the viral envelope. The enzyme catalyses the cleavage of sialic acid and an adjacent sugar residue in glycoproteins found in mucus. This action allows the virus to permeate mucin and escape from these so-called 'non-specific' inhibitors. The neuraminidase also destroys the haemagglutinin receptors on the host cell. Neuraminidase activity is also thought to be important in the final stages of release of new virus particles from infected cells. Sialic acid is always present in newly synthesized virions, and its removal by neuraminidase prevents the new virus particles agglutinating, thus increasing

**Table 50.1** Influenza virus proteins

| Gene segment | Proteins | Molecular weight ($\times 10^3$) | Location in virion | Function | Comments |
|---|---|---|---|---|---|
| 1 | PB2 | 0.87 | Internal | RNA transcription | Polymerase proteins; highly conserved |
| 2 | PB1 | 0.96 | | | |
| 3 | PA | 0.85 | | | |
| 4 | HA1 | 47.5 | Spikes | Binding to cell receptors envelope fusion to endosome | Glycoprotein; haemagglutinin varies antigenically |
| | HA2 | 28.8 | | | |
| 5 | NA | 48–63 | Spikes | Neuraminidase | Glycoprotein enzyme activity |
| 6 | NP | 50–60 | Internal | Subunit of nucleocapsid | Nucleoprotein helical arrangement; type-specific |
| 7 | M1 | 0.28 | Beneath lipid bilayer of envelope | Major structural component | Involved in assembly and budding |
| | M2 | 11–15 | Transmembrane | Ion channel | Changes pH in endosome; blocked by amantadine |
| 8 | NS1 | 0.25 | Internal | mRNA transport inhibition; splicing | Non-structural proteins |
| | NS2 | 0.13 | | Unknown | |

the number of free virus particles and hence spread of the virus from the original site of infection. The viral genes and their functions are shown in Table 50.1.

## Nomenclature

The World Health Organization (WHO) system of nomenclature includes the host of origin, geographical origin, strain number and year of isolation; then follows in parentheses the antigenic description of the haemagglutinin and the neuraminidase, e.g. A/swine/ Iowa/3/70 ($H_1N_1$). If isolated from a human host the origin is not given, e.g. A/Scotland/42/89 ($H_3N_2$). There are 13 different H antigens and nine N antigens. Only $H_{1-3}$ and $N_{1-2}$ have been found so far in viruses from humans, the others being recovered from animals and birds.

## Physical characteristics

The influenza virus withstands slow drying at room temperature on articles such as blankets and glass: it has been demonstrated in dust after an interval as long as 2 weeks. When contained in allantoic fluid or in infected tissues immersed in glycerol saline it will survive for several weeks at 4°C. Virus can survive in cold sea water for a similar period. It can be preserved for long periods at −70°C, and remains viable indefinitely when freeze dried.

Exposure to heat for 30 min at 56°C is sufficient to inactivate most strains; the few which survive this treatment are killed by exposure to the same temperature for 90 min. The viruses are inactivated by a variety of substances such as 20% ether in the cold, phenol, formaldehyde, salts of heavy metals, detergents, soaps, halogens and many others.

## REPLICATION

Following specific attachment of the viral haemagglutinin to *N*-acetylneuraminic acid-containing receptors, viruses enter cells by endocytosis. Fusion of the viral envelope with the membrane of the endosome depends on a specific fusion sequence exposed by the partial unfolding of the haemagglutinin at the low pH found in the endosome. This leads to release of the viral ribonucleoprotein (RNP) and associated RNA polymerase into the cell cytoplasm. Transcription of the viral RNA molecules produces 10 mRNA species (Table 50.1) as RNA segments 7 and 8 both have two reading frames. mRNA molecules are processed in the cell nucleus, where poly(A) sequences are removed from host mRNA molecules and added to the viral transcripts.

Unlike most other RNA viruses, assembly of the new viral RNP takes place in the nucleus of the host cell.

The viral matrix (M) proteins migrate to the cell membrane and are joined by the haemagglutinin and neuraminidase glycoproteins. RNP and polymerase locate at the areas of the cell membrane with matrix protein. Release occurs by budding, aided perhaps by the viral neuraminidase. To be infectious the haemagglutinin protein is cleaved into the components HA1 and HA2, which together form the haemagglutinin molecule.

## CLINICAL FEATURES

### Influenza A

In classical influenza the incubation period is short, 2 days, but it may vary from 1 to 4 days. The illness is characterized by a sudden onset of systemic symptoms such as chills, fever, headache, myalgia and anorexia. Respiratory symptoms are also common but take second place to the systemic effects, especially early in the illness. Many patients have both upper and lower respiratory tract infection, often with a troublesome, dry cough. The main physical finding is pyrexia, which rises rapidly to a peak of 38–41°C within 12 h of onset. Fever usually lasts 3 days, but it can be present for 1–5 days. During the 2nd and 3rd days of the illness the systemic effects diminish, and by the 4th day the respiratory symptoms and signs are predominant, with pharyngitis, laryngitis and tracheobronchitis. In adults, systemic illness without respiratory symptoms is common, as are febrile convulsions in children. About one-third of patients will suffer only a common cold-like illness, and it has been shown that as many as 20% of cases are subclinical. A long convalescence is common, and cough, lassitude and malaise may last for 1–2 weeks after the disappearance of other manifestations. It should be remembered that many other respiratory viruses can cause typical influenza-like illnesses, although the severity of the systemic symptoms is usually greatest with influenza virus. The similarity of the prodromal stages of several infections to influenza has led to the use of the term 'flu-like' to describe these features.

### Influenza B

Symptoms closely resemble those associated with influenza A infections, consisting of a 3 day febrile illness with predominantly systemic symptoms. It is generally thought, however, that overall the infection is somewhat milder, and some studies have shown more involvement of the gastro-intestinal tract, with the coining of the term 'gastric flu'.

### Influenza C

Clinically, influenza C causes an afebrile upper respiratory tract infection usually confined to young children: outbreaks are not recognized.

### Complications of influenza

Primary *influenza pneumonia* may occur especially in young adults during an outbreak, and can be fatal after a very short illness of sometimes less than 1 day. A similar rapid illness can occur in the elderly. More commonly a bacterial pneumonia caused by *Staphylococcus aureus* or *Streptococcus pneumoniae* may occur late in the course of the illness, often after a period of improvement resulting in a classical biphasic fever pattern. The incidence of chest complications is related to the age of the patient, increasing progressively after the age of 60 years. Severe infections and sudden death can occur, especially if there is some underlying disease, such as cerebrovascular, cardiovascular or chronic respiratory disease. In recent years a controversial epidemiological association between influenza in pregnancy and the subsequent development of schizophrenia in the individual exposed as a third-trimester fetus has been postulated. There may have been a weak correlation with the 1957 influenza epidemic, but this has not been shown satisfactorily for any other outbreak investigated.

## PATHOGENESIS

Inhaled virus is deposited on the mucous membrane lining the respiratory tract or directly into the alveoli, the level depending on the size of the droplets inhaled. In the former site, it is exposed to mucoproteins containing sialic acid which can bind to the virus, thus blocking its attachment to respiratory tract epithelial cells.

However, the action of neuraminidase allows the virus to break this bond. Specific local secretory IgA antibodies, if present from a previous infection, may neutralize the virus before attachment occurs, provided the antibody corresponds to the infecting virus type. If not prevented by one of these mechanisms, virus attaches to the surface of a respiratory epithelial cell and the intracellular replication cycle is initiated.

The major site of infection is the ciliated columnar epithelial cell. The first alteration is the disappearance of the elongated form of these cells, which become round and swollen, the nucleus shrinks, becomes pyknotic and fragments. Vacuolization of the cytoplasm may occur. As the nucleus disintegrates, the cytoplasm shows inclusion bodies, and the cilia are lost.

Release of the virus from the cells allows it to spread via the mucus blanket to other areas of the respiratory tract. The cell damage initiates an acute inflammatory response with oedema and the attraction of phagocytic cells. The earliest response is the synthesis and release of interferons from the infected cells: these can diffuse to and protect both adjacent and more distant cells before the virus arrives. It appears that interferons released in this way cause many of the systemic features of the 'flu-like' syndrome. While viral components are absorbed and trigger the immune system, the virus itself is confined to the epithelium of the respiratory tract. Specific antibody will help to limit the extracellular spread of the virus, while T cell responses are directed against the viral glycoproteins on the surface of infected cells, leading to their destruction by cytotoxic T cells and also by antibody-dependent cell cytotoxicity.

## Immunity

After an attack of influenza the ensuing immunity to the particular subtype of infecting virus is of long duration. It is related to the amount of local antibody (IgA) in the mucous secretions of the respiratory tract together with the specific IgG serum antibody concentration. Immunity to infection, especially with type A, is subtype-specific, giving little or no protection from subtypes possessing immunologically distinct H or N proteins.

## LABORATORY DIAGNOSIS

### Virus isolation and detection

For primary isolation the most suitable cells are primary monkey kidney or human embryo kidney cells, but since these tissues are scarce most laboratories now use secondary baboon kidney cells or Madin–Darby canine kidney cells. The presence of virus may be detected in baboon kidney cell cultures incubated at 33°C as early as 18 h after inoculation, by haemadsorption with human group O, fowl or guinea-pig red blood cells. Usually, if viable viruses are present in the clinical specimen, isolation is made within 7 days. The virus may then be identified by the fluorescent antibody technique.

## Rapid diagnosis

Since the advent of antivirals with activity against influenza viruses, rapid diagnosis has increased in importance, particularly in the hospital or institutional context, such as homes for the elderly, so that attempts can be made to limit the spread of the virus by a combination of patient isolation, vaccination and prophylaxis.

Immunofluorescent detection of influenza antigens in respiratory specimens either directly or following amplification in cell culture for 24 h has speeded up diagnosis considerably. The best specimens are nasal aspirates or nasal washes, but nasal or throat swabs taken vigorously to obtain cells and put in viral transport medium can be satisfactory if taken in the first few days of illness.

It is still important in the early stages of an outbreak or in sporadic cases that viruses should be isolated and analysed antigenically for epidemiology and vaccine production, but for patient management and control of infection, rapid antigen detection is more useful. Detection of influenza RNA by reverse-transcriptase polymerase chain reaction may be more sensitive than antigen detection but is not widely available in diagnostic laboratories.

Serological confirmation of the clinical diagnosis is obtained when a four-fold or greater rise in antibody titre can be shown to any one type of virus. Complement fixation tests (CFTs) are still widely used. This test uses nucleocapsid antigens which are type-specific and can distinguish A from B and C infections. Strain differences can be demonstrated by means of haemagglutination inhibition and neutralization assays or strain-specific CFTs. Single, high CFT titres are difficult to interpret in some patients, especially those with chronic respiratory disease since many may exhibit high titres for many years. In patients who are normally healthy a high titre found during an outbreak could, with more assurance, be related to a recent illness.

## TREATMENT

Oral amantadine hydrochloride was introduced in the early 1980s, followed later by a derivative, rimantadine. These drugs work by blocking the ion channels in the envelope thus preventing the pH changes that precede the membrane fusion step essential for nucleocapsid release. Unfortunately, these compounds only have activity against influenza virus type A but not B or C. Therefore, it is essential to know the type of virus responsible for the illness or outbreak. A clinical diagnosis can be fairly confidently made in a typical case seen during an epidemic due to a known type, but is impossible in sporadic or milder cases. Amantadine is effective when given prophylactically but also therapeutically in patients treated within 24 h of onset of illness. Viruses resistant to amantadine and rimantadine may appear within a few days of drug administration; however, resistant strains show no increased pathogenicity or transmissibility.

Tribavirin given by nebulized aerosol, which has proved useful in the treatment of respiratory syncytial virus infections in babies, has shown limited success in the treatment of influenza A and B infections. Computer-aided design techniques using the crystalline structure of the influenza neuraminidase have produced drugs which inhibit both influenza A and B in cell culture and in animal models. One of these sialidase inhibitors, 4-guanidino-Neu5Ac2en, demonstrated 1000 times greater efficacy than amantadine against influenza A.

| Year | Subtype |
|------|---------|
| 1890 | $H_2N_2$ |
| 1900 | $H_3N_8$ |
| 1918 | $H_1N_1$ Swine like |
| | Spanish influenza |
| 1957 | $H_2N_2$ |
| | Asian influenza |
| 1968 | $H_3N_2$ |
| | Hong Kong influenza |
| 1977 | $H_3N_2 + H_1N_1$ |
| 1990 | $H_3N_2 + H_1N_1$ |

**Fig. 50.3** Sequential changes in influenza A antigens associated with antigenic shift. Antigenic drift occurs after the appearance of a new subtype.

## EPIDEMIOLOGY

Epidemics which must have been caused by influenza viruses have been described for over 2000 years. Typically, there is a sudden appearance of cases of respiratory disease; these occur for several weeks and then suddenly cease. The epidemics occur frequently at irregular intervals and were thought at one time to be under the influence of the stars, hence the term *influenza* (Italian for influence). It is well recognized that epidemics vary in severity. The great pandemic of 1918–19 was particularly severe, killing between 20 million and 40 million people as it spread around the world. It was because of this that a great effort was directed into trying to identify the cause of the illness. Success came in 1933 when Sir Christopher Andrewes and others isolated influenza A virus. Continued isolation studies and analysis of isolates have given an understanding of how the epidemic behaviour relates to changes in the virus. Also, it is possible to deduce which viral antigens circulated before virus isolation was possible by virtue of the phenomenon of *original antigenic sin*. This means

that infection with a current virus type stimulates antibody to earlier strains. Thus we can deduce what antigenic components were prevalent back to the end of the last century by antibody studies of older people (Fig. 50.3).

The major pandemics are associated with *antigenic shifts* – when the viral H or N, or both, are changed. This is too extensive to be the result of mutation, and analysis of the viral RNA indicates that shift results from the acquisition of a complete new RNA segment 4 and/or 5. In the laboratory it is easy to show that if a cell is infected with two different strains, the progeny will include virus whose RNA molecules are derived from each parent. Thus, a 'new' virus can result from the process of *re-assortment*. All the H and N antigenic subtypes are found in aquatic birds (both seabirds and ducks), but in these the viruses vary little. The genetic reassortment may take place in pigs from which certain subtypes may transmit to humans. Receptor specificity of haemagglutinin depends on the host species from which they are isolated. The amino acid at site 226 in human and some swine $H_3$ viruses is different from that in avian or equine viruses. Passage of human

H1and H3 viruses in eggs alters the receptor-binding specificity and the antigenicity of the new viruses to have avian virus characteristics.

Until 1977 it was the rule that when a 'new' virus appeared the 'old' one disappeared, but since that time two subtypes have been circulating concurrently, namely $H_3N_2$ and $H_1N_1$. The latter antigens had not been found since the 1950s. The reappearance of $H_1N_1$ in 1977 and the absence of new reassortants in humans since 1968 may indicate that there may be a limited range of antigenic types that can infect humans.

Influenza B viruses do not undergo antigenic shift as there is no animal reservoir and, although epidemics do occur at 3–6 year intervals, they never reach pandemic proportions, and their extent is usually limited to small communities such as boarding schools or residences for the elderly. The antigenic changes result from mutation, as do those seen in influenza A after the appearance of 'new' virus strains; the changes are the cause of antigenic drift.

Influenza may occur as pandemics, epidemics or sporadically. A pandemic develops and spreads world-wide, as in 1918, 1957 and 1968 (Fig. 50.3), when a new reassorted virus appears against which there is no immunity in the population. Pandemics have often started in the East, possibly because of the close association of a high-density population with ducks and pigs, and within 2–3 years spread world-wide involving all age groups. Epidemics result from *antigenic drift* which has drifted so far that the H and N antibodies in the community can no longer prevent large numbers of the population from becoming infected. WHO-designated laboratories monitor influenza A and B throughout the world to check for the appearance of variants. In the UK, influenza activity is monitored in several ways. Spotter general practitioners regularly report the levels of influenza-like illness in their patients. The excess deaths due to respiratory causes rise dramatically over a short period during an influenza epidemic and so are regularly calculated to provide a sensitive measure of increased influenza activity. Laboratories regularly report virus isolations and send isolates to reference laboratories for antigenic analysis.

High rates of infection are found in pre-school children, thereafter the rates are lower even in the elderly. However, elderly patients in residential homes, if not protected, are at particular risk from acute illness and sudden death. Thus, even if the attack rate is low, the case fatality rate is high. Infection may be introduced by staff, visitors or other patients.

Influenza virus type C is not associated with epidemics but gives rise only to mild upper respiratory tract infections, especially in young children. Most infections are asymptomatic.

## CONTROL

The aim of immunization is to produce haemagglutination inhibition or neutralizing antibody in all vaccinees. This protects them against infection, but only with strains closely related to those in the vaccine. Vaccine efficacy in the elderly is about 70%, but uptake is poor, about 5%.

All types of vaccine rely on adequate quantities of virus with the appropriate H and N antigens being produced in the allantoic cavity of embryonated hens' eggs inoculated with seed virus. Reassortment of two strains, one a high-yielding laboratory-adapted strain and the other containing the required H and N antigens, is employed to produce an appropriate inoculum for growth in eggs so that vaccine is prepared as quickly as possible. Separated whole virus particles are inactivated either by formalin or β-propiolactone. Whole virus vaccine should not be given to those who are allergic to egg protein. The H and N antigens may be separated from the whole virus by treatment with detergent, and these subunit or split-virus vaccines are found to be better tolerated, especially in young children. In the UK, influenza vaccines contain three virus strains, two type A and one type B, representing the strains currently circulating in the world. The current vaccines (1996/97) contain an $H_1N_1$ strain (A/Singapore/6/86), an $H_3N_2$ strain (A/Wuhan/359/95) and a B variant (B/Beijing/184/93).

Other types of vaccines have been tried in the past, e.g. live attenuated vaccines given intranasally. These vaccines have been generally effective in provoking a good local (IgA) antibody response but have not gained in popularity. Vaccines containing adjuvants, usually oil-based, have been investigated, but this approach has been abandoned due to the development of very unpleasant local reactions at the site of injection.

## RECOMMENDED READING

Andrewes C 1989 *Viruses of Vertebrates*, 5th edn. Ballière Tindall, London

Fields B N, Knipe D M, Howley P M (eds) 1996 *Virology*, 3rd edn. Lippincott-Raven, Philadelphia

Francis T 1953 Influenza: the new acquaintance. *Annals of Internal Medicine* 39: 203–221

Nichol K L, Margolis K L, Wuorenma J, Von Sternberg T 1994 The efficacy and cost effectiveness of vaccination against influenza among elderly persons living in the community. *New England Journal of Medicine* 331: 778–784

Webster R G, Bean W J, Gorman O T, Chambers T M, Kawaoka Y 1992 Evolution and ecology of influenza A viruses *Microbiological Reviews* 56: 152–179

Wiselka M 1994 Influenza: diagnosis, management and prophylaxis. *British Medical Journal* 308: 1341–1345

# 51

# Paramyxoviruses

**Respiratory infections; mumps; measles**

*C. R. Madeley and J. S. M. Peiris*

The paramyxoviruses are a family of enveloped viruses containing single-stranded RNA as a single piece. They resemble the orthomyxoviruses in both morphology and an affinity for sialic acid receptors on mammalian cells, but they are larger and more fragile (Fig. 51.1a).

Within the family Paramyxoviridae there are three genera, each with several members: *Paramyxovirus* (parainfluenza viruses, mumps virus, Newcastle disease virus (NDV) and simian virus 5 (SV5)); *Morbillivirus* (measles virus, canine distemper virus, rinderpest virus, an equine morbillivirus and several strains recently isolated from seals, dolphins and porpoises); and *Pneumovirus* (respiratory syncytial (RS) virus). Originally, they were all classified together because they were thought to be similar in structure and function. Neither property is constant throughout the family but there are similarities. For example, parainfluenza, mumps and measles viruses, are identical as seen in the electron microscope (and as described below), while pneumovirus, although very similar, has slightly longer surface spikes and is more difficult to visualize.

Functionally there are other differences. Parainfluenza viruses, NDV and mumps virus have a surface haemagglutinin and neuraminidase, while measles virus has a haemagglutinin but no neuraminidase, and pneumovirus has neither. In addition, measles virus has a haemolysin not possessed by the others, while RS virus has a large surface glycoprotein, G, which has a similar cell-attaching function to a haemagglutinin.

## PARAINFLUENZA VIRUSES

### Description

Parainfluenza viruses, mumps virus, NDV and SV5 are indistinguishable in the electron microscope.

a

b

**Fig. 51.1** **a** Electron micrograph of a typical paramyxovirus. **b** Separate internal helical nucleocapsid. Negative contrast microscopy, ×200 000.

Negatively stained virions vary in size from 80 to 350 nm; occasionally there are filamentous forms and giant forms up to 800 nm in diameter. The outer surface of the virion is a pleomorphic envelope consisting of a lipoprotein membrane derived from host cell membrane and covered by projections 12–14 nm long and 2–4 nm wide. Although generally similar, orthomyxoviruses and paramyxoviruses are morphologically distinct. Paramyxovirus particles are easily deformed by external forces, may assume a variety of shapes and break up more easily than orthomyxoviruses.

The envelope surface projections are of two kinds, the HN and F glycoproteins. The former carries both haemagglutinin (H) and neuraminidase (N) functions, in contrast to orthomyxoviruses, in which these functions are on separate spikes. F or fusion proteins cause cell membranes to fuse, leading to the formation of syncytia, and are found on all paramyxoviruses. There are also matrix proteins, M, which line the inner surface of the envelope. All the paramyxoviruses carry an RNA-dependent RNA polymerase within the virion.

Within the enveloped virion is a genome of single-stranded negative-sense RNA complexed with protein to form a helical nucleocapsid. This has a basic length of about 1 µm, and the RNA has a size of 16.5 kilobase pairs (kb), but some particles contain more than one copy. The envelope ruptures readily when the virus is prepared for electron microscopy, releasing the helical nucleoprotein, which has a herring-bone or 'zipper'-like appearance (Fig. 51.1b). This is more easily recognized in the electron microscope than the complete particle; it is 15–19 nm wide with a pitch of about 6 nm.

## Classification

There are four types of parainfluenza viruses (1–4) which have antigenically distinct epitopes. Nevertheless, there are conserved antigenic sites on the paramyxovirus envelope proteins, which are the reason for the serological cross-reactions that occur between the parainfluenza viruses, mumps virus and SV5. These are particularly close between parainfluenza type 1 and a mouse variant (Sendai) which was used for some time as the antigen in complement fixation tests for antibody to the former. However, it became apparent that there were other cross-reactions which made the results of serological tests virtually uninterpretable. Responses to previously experienced paramyxoviruses as well as the currently infecting virus are found. This phenomenon of response to 'original antigenic sin'

has been seen with other viruses such as influenza and coxsackie B viruses. In addition, type 4 has two subtypes, 4a and 4b, which can be distinguished by neutralization or haemadsorption inhibition.

NDV infects chickens and other domestic birds. Its severity varies considerably from inapparent to fatal. Because some strains can cause major outbreaks with high mortality, an effective live vaccine based on avirulent strains has been developed. NDV is a typical paramyxovirus, and has been shown to be a rare cause of conjunctivitis in humans but only as a result of a laboratory accident. SV5 is often present in normal uninfected monkey kidney cell cultures but does not appear to reduce their sensitivity to other viruses. Other parainfluenza viruses are natural pathogens for cattle and other domestic species; they are not known to infect humans.

## Replication

Parainfluenza viruses attach via the haemagglutinin to sialic acid-containing receptors on the cell surface. The F protein then fuses the viral envelope with the cell membrane, releasing the nucleocapsid into the cell. The negative-strand genome cannot act as messenger RNA (mRNA) and the RNA-dependent RNA polymerase carried within the virion is required to produce subgenomic-sized mRNA transcripts, which are translated to produce some of the early virus-specific polypeptides. These include a second RNA polymerase which copies the genome into full-length positive complementary strands which are in turn copied back into negative strands for transcription of later mRNA (coding for structural proteins) and for incorporation into new virions.

The viral components are assembled beneath the cell membrane and the surface HN and F proteins are incorporated into a stretch of membrane, converting it to viral envelope. This evaginates and buds off, enclosing as it does so a nucleocapsid to form a new virion. This is probably released from the host cell by the action of the neuraminidase component of the HN spikes. The incorporation of the HN protein into the cell membrane of infected cells allows red blood cells to adhere to their surface – the phenomenon of *haemadsorption*.

## Clinical features and pathogenesis

The parainfluenza viruses are mostly associated with *croup*, a harsh brassy cough in children familiar to many mothers as a middle-of-the-night irritant. It is due to a combination of tracheitis and laryngitis, but parainfluenza viruses may also cause minor upper respiratory tract illness, as well as some cases of *bronchiolitis* and 'failure to thrive'. They are responsible for 6–9% of respiratory infections for which a virus cause can be identified. The incubation period is from 3 to 6 days, during which the virus spreads locally within the respiratory tract.

Many infections occur in infants in the presence of circulating maternal antibody which does not appear to be protective nor to make the illness worse.

## Laboratory diagnosis

Rapid diagnosis may be made by immunofluorescent staining of exfoliated respiratory cells separated from well-taken nasopharyngeal secretions. Preparation of adequately specific polyclonal sera is time-consuming but practicable, although it may not be possible to separate type 4 positives into subtypes. Preparing satisfactory monoclonal reagents to each type has not proved easy, and available commercial and other kits often offer only a polyvalent one. This reflects the problems of generating and identifying good type-specific monoclonal antibodies against a background of significant antigenic overlap between parainfluenza viruses.

Similar antiviral antibodies may also be used in enzyme immuno-assays to identify viral antigen in specimens from the patient. They have the advantage of requiring only antigen to be present in the specimen while other assays require intact infected cells (for immunofluorescence) or infective virus (for culture). However, enzyme immuno-assays give no information on the quality of the specimen nor the extent of infection.

Virus may be isolated in monkey kidney cells. Visible cytopathic effects in the cell sheets are minimal and it will usually be necessary to show infection of the cells by the haemadsorption of 1% guinea-pig or human group O red blood cells. The infecting virus can be typed (or subtyped) by reacting the cell cultures with type-specific antisera before adding the red cells. The appropriate antibody inhibits the haemadsorption. The typing can be confirmed by a neutralization test or by immunofluorescence, but this is not usually necessary.

Serology is not used routinely in diagnosis. Type-specific antibodies may be detected by neutralization or haemadsorption inhibition but these tests are too complex for routine use. Others such as complement fixation are difficult to interpret because of cross-reactions between parainfluenza viruses with mumps virus and, possibly, SV5 (see above).

## Epidemiology and transmission

Epidemiologically, parainfluenza type 1 infections are more frequent in the winter while type 3 is a summer infection, with small epidemics appearing reliably each year. Type 2 and 4a and 4b infections are more infrequent, in Newcastle upon Tyne at least, although elsewhere in Britain type 2 can be another summer visitor. Type 4 infections are under-diagnosed from a lack of suitable reagents but reported figures are too low for epidemiological patterns to be clear. The reasons underlying these individual epidemiological patterns are unknown.

Numerically, parainfluenza infections are far fewer than those due to RS virus (q.v.) and most diagnosed infections are in pre-school and primary school children. Fatalities are very rare, and reinfections occur.

The viruses are present in respiratory secretions and are expelled during coughing and sneezing. Infection is acquired by inhalation and by person-to-person contact.

## MUMPS

## Description

Mumps virus is a typical paramyxovirus, indistinguishable in appearance from parainfluenza viruses, measles virus and NDV. A similar herring-bone or zipper-like ribonucleoprotein is frequently seen to leak from the virions in preparations examined by electron microscopy, and may be the only unequivocally virus-like material seen. However, if it is found in cerebrospinal fluid it is diagnostic of mumps meningitis because the only other similar virus found in the central nervous system, measles, does not reach levels detectable by electron microscopy in cerebrospinal fluid.

The spikes on the envelope carry either a combined haemagglutinin and neuraminidase (HN) or a fusion (F) protein. The envelope also contains a matrix (M) protein. There is only one serotype, although monoclonal antibodies have shown minor variations in the various surface antigenic epitopes.

## Replication

This is indistinguishable from that already described for parainfluenza viruses. Infected cells show haemadsorption but little obvious damage. New virus is released by budding.

## Clinical features and pathogenesis

Mumps is an 'iceberg' disease which, although common as a childhood infection, is often subclinical. Although the salivary glands are often involved, inapparent or minor infections are more common. Difficulty in recovering the virus and ambiguity in serology mean that infections are rarely confirmed by the laboratory. The USA was the first country to propose a vaccine to control mumps, but elsewhere surprise was expressed that anyone should bother. More complete monitoring of its activity suggests otherwise, and it is a full partner in the MMR vaccine (see below), not an afterthought.

Infection is probably by droplet into the respiratory tract. The incubation period is 14–18 days and is followed by a generalized illness with localization in the salivary glands, usually the parotids. The generalized phase is the usual 'flu-like' illness with fever and malaise, followed by developing pain in the parotid glands which then swell rapidly. Much of the swelling is due to blockage of the efferent duct and the sucking of a lemon in front of a sufferer is a refined form of torture!

Neurological involvement is common in mumps (over 50% of infections), though the majority of cases are not clinically apparent. However, clinical meningitis remains the most common serious complication of mumps, occurring in 1–10% of patients with mumps parotitis. Meningitis (like any other complication of mumps) can occur before, during, after or in the absence of salivary gland involvement. Mumps virus and the enteroviruses (q.v.) account for virtually all the cases of aseptic meningitis in the UK. Of these, the mumps virus is more commonly involved than any other individual virus. Both meningitis and meningo-encephalitis have been described, with the former being very rarely fatal with otherwise complete recovery. The latter is much rarer, carries a poorer prognosis and may result in long-term neurological sequelae or in death. Deafness and tinnitus have also been described, but are very rare.

In prepubertal children the acute illness usually subsides in 4–5 days with complete recovery. The best known complication, in postpubertal males, is *orchitis*. This, though painful and causing softening and atrophy of the affected testicle, is usually unilateral and rarely causes sterility. *Oophoritis* also occurs in girls, and should be distinguished from a ruptured cyst or acute appendicitis. Both orchitis and oophoritis usually develop as the parotitis resolves, and a history of previous parotid pain and swelling will usually provide the clue.

The role of mumps in pancreatitis is difficult to establish. There may be abdominal pain in acute mumps but the levels of serum amylase do not correlate with the clinical picture. High levels may provide supportive evidence but are not diagnostic. Though uncomfortable it is not fatal.

## Laboratory diagnosis

Typical mumps does not usually require laboratory confirmation but mild cases with little parotid swelling may not be noticed until complications develop. By this time virus may not be plentiful in the oropharynx. Direct demonstration by immuno-fluorescence on secretions is very rarely successful, and the diagnosis will depend on growing the virus from throat swabs, from saliva from affected glands or from the cerebrospinal fluid. Collection of infected saliva is difficult but throat swabs provide a satisfactory specimen, although the virus may take up to a week to grow. Virus may be present in urine but not reliably so. The detection of ribonucleoprotein helix in cerebrospinal fluid by electron microscopy is diagnostic, but the small quantities of fluid usually taken make this impractical.

Growth of virus in cell cultures (usually monkey kidney or HEp2 cells) produces little cytopathic effect, but the virus can be detected by haemadsorption, which can be inhibited by specific anti-serum to confirm the presence of mumps virus.

The diagnosis can be made serologically by showing a rise in antibody between acute and convalescent specimens. Complement fixation is the usual test, using soluble (S) and viral (V) antigens. Antibodies to the S antigen are said to develop early, within a week of onset, followed by anti-V antibodies, which persist longer. However, these patterns are not invariable, and only a rise in titre to both antigens can be relied on. A rise to only one antigen in the absence of typical illness will be difficult to interpret and may reflect infection with other paramyxoviruses. Low rises or low static titres in cases of meningitis should also be interpreted with caution – cross-reactions with other paramyxoviruses provide traps for the unwary, and only isolation of the virus provides unequivocal evidence.

Other serological tests have been used, based on enzyme immuno-assays and single radial haemolysis. They have not been used as widely as complement fixation, being more often used in serological surveys or to complement other assays. Neutralization and haemagglutination inhibition tests are more complex to carry out and do not offer any advantages in routine diagnosis.

## Epidemiology

Mumps is a world-wide disease, with humans the only known reservoir. Most infections are in school-age children, with those in adults being more severe and more likely to develop complications. Although epidemics occur, mumps is less infectious than measles or chickenpox. Infection appears to confer life-long immunity, and second infections do not occur.

## Control

Some, but not very reliable, protection can be given by passive immunization; it may prevent severe orchitis even when given at the stage of parotitis.

Generally, mumps has not been thought to warrant a vaccine on its own, although one has been available in the USA for several years. This vaccine, based on the *Jeryl Lynn* or *Urabe* strains, has now been incorporated into a triple vaccine against measles, mumps and rubella (MMR). All three components are live attenuated viruses, and the mumps component induces good antibody levels, lasting long enough to suggest that the recipients will not become susceptible as adults. A few cases of mild post-vaccine meningitis have been described but have not caused serious concern.

## MEASLES

### Description

Measles virus, a *morbillivirus*, is morphologically in-distinguishable from parainfluenza viruses, mumps virus and NDV, although there are important functional differences. The ribonucleoprotein helix is readily released from the virion and may, as with the others, be the only identifiable virus structure seen in the electron microscope.

The spikes on the measles virus envelope carry a haemagglutinin but not a neuraminidase. There is an F protein which is also a haemolysin. A matrix protein, M, is also present below the envelope lipid bilayer.

There is only one serotype of measles virus and no subtypes have yet been recognized, although monoclonal antibodies show that there may be differences between wild and cultivated strains.

Human morbilliviruses are related to a number of animal strains. *Canine distemper* and *rinderpest* in cattle are well-known relatives, but in the past few years other similar viruses have been isolated from seals (of several species), dolphins and porpoises, and an equine morbillivirus has reappeared which has apparently been transmitted to humans in contact, fatally in one. All are distinct but can cause serious illness in their natural species though survivors develop solid immunity. There is partial cross-protection in ferrets between measles and canine distemper viruses.

## Pathogenesis

Measles is an acute febrile illness, mostly in childhood, after an incubation period of 10–12 days. The onset is 'flu-like', with high fever, cough and conjunctivitis. *Koplik's spots* (red spots with a bluish white centre on the buccal mucosa) may be present at this stage. After 1–2 days the acute symptoms decline with the appearance of a widespread maculopapular rash. Viral antigen but not complete virus may be found in the spots. The rash can be inhibited by local injections of immune serum, but will not appear in those who are severely immuno-compromised, and this has been thought to point to an immunopathological (T cell-mediated) mechanism.

Over the next 10–14 days, recovery is usually complete as the rash fades with considerable desquamation. Complications include a giant cell pneumonia, more common in adults, otitis media and a postmeasles encephalitis. The pneumonia is due to direct invasion with virus, but the role of virus in the other two is uncertain. Measles encephalitis can cause severe and permanent mental impairment in those it does not kill. It is rare but disastrous.

The mortality of uncomplicated measles in immunocompetent well-nourished children is low but rises rapidly with malnourishment (marked in Africa), in the immunocompromised and, to a much lesser extent, with age. It has also been devastating in isolated populations into whom it was introduced as a 'new' disease.

One further complication of measles is *subacute sclerosing panencephalitis* (SSPE), which occurs in children or early adolescents who have had measles early in life, usually under 2 years of age. It is a progressive and inevitably fatal degenerative disease. Within infected cells is a defective form of measles virus which, because it is unable to induce the production of a functional M protein, is not released as complete virus from the cells. Patients deteriorate over several years, losing intellectual capacity before motor activities. Oligoclonal antibodies to measles virus proteins appear in the cerebrospinal fluid, but the virus cannot be cultivated unless it is 'rescued' by co-cultivating neuronal cells with a susceptible cell type.

The virus has been linked with multiple sclerosis, Paget's disease of bone and Crohn's disease. In each case, tubular structures resembling measles nucleocapsids have been seen, and immuno-fluorescence has been used to demonstrate measles 'antigens' in biopsy material. Serum from about 50% of adults aged over 50 years, however, will fix complement with measles antigen although the individuals give no history suggestive of recent measles, and it is possible that auto-antibodies to a measles-like protein can be induced with age. If so, its significance is unknown but would be a factor in assessing measles involvement in older patients with chronic diseases. At present, the evidence linking measles virus in the aetiology of these diseases is less than compelling.

## Laboratory diagnosis

Most cases of measles are diagnosed clinically, usually in the patient's home. Direct virological confirmation is often not attempted and is difficult to do in general practice. In hospital and particularly in immuno-compromised patients, in whom the disease will often be rashless, the diagnosis may be made rapidly by immunofluorescence on exfoliated respiratory cells in well-taken nasopharyngeal secretions. The presence of a large number of giant cells, particularly in patients on cytotoxic drugs, is a bad prognostic sign.

Other immuno-assays have been developed but give no feedback on the extent of the infection. Otherwise the virus may be grown in human fibro-blasts, primary monkey cells and vero cells although it does not grow readily.

Measles induces a good antibody response and a rise in complement-fixing antibody is diagnostic. However, complement-fixing antibody in older patients is often detected and its significance is unknown. Other tests for antibody have been dev-eloped but are not used widely because diagnosis is usually made clinically. As measles vaccine (see below) is used more widely, clinical measles is becoming rarer and the need for laboratory con-firmation of probable cases is rising. Antibody tests for measles-specific IgM and IgG on specimens of saliva are now available in some countries and avoid the need for venesection.

## Epidemiology

Transmission is person to person, probably by respiratory droplets, but the associated conjunctivitis may also be a source. Despite some anecdotal evidence, there is no good evidence that distemper in dogs can be a source of measles in humans.

Measles epidemics occur every 2 years in dev-eloped countries in the absence of widespread use of the vaccine. This periodicity will be absent in isolated populations too small to maintain trans-mission (<400 000), in poverty and overcrowding and following widespread use of vaccine. The disease is ubiquitous throughout the world and, although a candidate for eradication, this may be difficult to achieve.

In tropical areas, particularly Africa, children become infected under the age of 1 year, and the mortality rises in consequence, reaching as high a figure as 42% in children under 4 years of age. Mal-nutrition is one of the main underlying causes of this excess mortality. The attack rate is also very high in isolated populations which have not ex-perienced the disease for some years. In the Faroes in the 1840s, three-quarters of the population were infected although the mortality was low. Most of those who were not infected were aged over 65 years, the interval since the last time the disease had been present in the islands, and confirms that infection gives prolonged immunity.

In the USA, where a serious attempt to eradicate measles has been made, the number of cases was reduced from over 500 000 per year to about 2000 (a reduction of over 99%), but outbreaks in immi-grants and high-school students have recently em-phasized the problems of preventing imported cases and of keeping up a high level of immunization.

## Control

The first measles vaccine was a formalin-inactivated one. Although inducing circulating antibody, it was found that vaccinees exposed to natural measles were likely to develop atypical disease. The rash was more peripheral, involving the palms and soles, and pneumonia was common. It was later recognized that the vaccine had failed to induce adequate levels of antibody to the haemolytic F protein, and the immunity induced did not inhibit cell-to-cell spread of the virus. Consequently it was withdrawn and replaced with a live attenuated one. Early versions of the latter were only partially attenuated and were thought only to offer a choice of when to have measles, but with the added uncertainty over whether the resulting immunity was as long-lasting as that following natural measles. Later versions, containing the *Edmonston B* or *Schwarz* strains, have been better attenuated while giving a seroconversion rate of over 90%. So far (over about 20 years) the immunity induced by the vaccine has persisted and may be life-long.

In the UK, vaccine uptake has been relatively low until recently, when its use was promoted more strongly. A nationwide campaign was promoted in 1994–95 to avert a predicted epidemic. High levels were achieved, and no epidemic occurred. In contrast, eradication has been attempted in the USA, where evidence of vaccination or clinical disease is a legal requirement for school entry. This has reduced the disease incidence substantially but importation has frustrated any hopes of interrupting transmission completely.

Measles vaccine has now been combined with those against mumps and rubella to form the MMR vaccine. This combination of three attenuated viruses has been shown to induce good immunity to all three. Introduced initially in the USA, it is now the preferred vaccine in the UK for administration between 12 and 18 months.

Immunization in the high-endemic regions of Africa still presents problems, however. Because many infants are infected before their first birthday, the vaccine has to be given under 6 months to have any effect. Passively transferred maternal antibody often interferes with the immune response to a live vaccine, and such early immunization does not always produce adequate immunity. A second dose at 12–13 months is then probably necessary but adds to the cost and the logistic difficulties. Solutions to both will have to be found before progress is made towards measles eradication in the developing world.

## RESPIRATORY SYNCYTIAL VIRUS

### Description

Superficially RS virus resembles other paramyxoviruses, with a similar pleomorphic envelope studded with surface spikes which may be seen more clearly in the electron microscope than those on the parainfluenza viruses, mumps and measles. The spikes may also be slightly longer, but neither the complete virus particles nor the nucleoprotein helix (with a similar diameter to parainfluenza viruses of 17 nm) are easy to visualize in the electron microscope. However, individual particles are generally larger than other paramyxoviruses (Fig. 51.2).

RS virus is placed in a separate genus – *Pneumovirus* – because of these minor physical differences

**Fig. 51.2** Electron micrograph of respiratory syncytial virus. Phosphotungstic acid stain, ×200 000.

and the lack of a haemagglutinin, a haemolysin or a neuraminidase. The nucleic acid is negative-sense single-stranded RNA of 15 kb, coding for both structural and non-structural proteins. RS virus has no haemagglutinin but has a G glycoprotein instead. It is a receptor for cell attachment but not to red blood cells, and differs in chemical composition from the HN protein of other paramyxoviruses. There are fusion (F), matrix (M), polymerase and nucleocapsid proteins. The F protein induces the syncytia in cell cultures from which the virus gets its name, and is probably responsible for both virus penetration and spread in the host. The virus is relatively fragile and may not survive even snap-freezing to −70°C. Specimens for isolation should not be frozen.

For most purposes there is only one serotype, although the advent of monoclonal antibodies has confirmed that there are two subtypes, A and B. In Newcastle upon Tyne, strains of subgroup A have been prevalent every year since 1974, but subgroup B strains have been more erratic and have not been active in every winter. The reason for this phenomenon is unknown. Analysis of the genome has revealed further minor differences which appear unimportant in diagnosis (i.e. do not represent major antigenic variations) but which have allowed various strain lineages to be recognized. These may reflect selection pressure by immunity but new ones are found widely distributed in the world at the same time and their significance is not yet clear.

RS virus is also a significant pathogen in cattle and infects chimpanzees readily – early isolates were termed *chimpanzee coryza agent*. Both goats and sheep may be infected naturally, and there is evidence that several other domestic and rodent species are susceptible, either naturally, or after some adaptation.

## Clinical features and pathogenesis

The most serious illness caused by RS virus is *bronchiolitis* in young babies, but it is also associated with minor upper tract infections and non-specific 'failure to thrive'. The peak incidence is in those under 1 year of age, and there are (possibly as a consequence) annual winter epidemics. This infection is potentially life-threatening, particularly in those with bronchopulmonary dysplasia or congenital heart defects. In normal babies it is rarely fatal where medical staff have the experience and facilities for appropriate management. RS virus has been recovered from some victims of the *sudden infant death syndrome* (SIDS). Although it may have contributed to the death it is clear that other factor(s) also contribute.

In older children and adults, the virus causes only minor infections, possibly because their air passages are larger. Reinfections are common and in adults may cause no more than a cold. However, the failure of acute infections to immunize, even in the immunocompetent, highlights the difficulty of producing a vaccine.

The main clinical feature is bronchiolitis, but the upper respiratory tract remains infected, and this makes it possible to confirm the diagnosis. If RS virus is present in the nasopharynx and there is clinical evidence of lower respiratory tract involvement, RS virus is likely to be responsible.

Recovery is apparently complete, although it has been suggested that the infection predisposes to chronic respiratory tract disease (asthma, bronchiectasis, etc.). This has yet to be confirmed although studies are in progress.

The sequelae to the use of an inactivated vaccine (see below) have led to the suggestion that some of the severity of bronchiolitis is due to hypersensitivity induced by an earlier infection. Studies in various centres have neither confirmed this theory nor fully excluded it. There is much still to learn about the pathogenesis of RS virus.

There have been reports of severe illness, with some fatalities, in old people's homes. Compared with those associated with influenza, outbreaks of RS virus are reported infrequently, although this may be due to difficulties in diagnosis. A neurological syndrome has also been described, but whether RS virus is the cause is unproven.

## Laboratory diagnosis

During the acute phase of illness virus may be readily demonstrated in nasopharyngeal secretions (which are usually copious) by immunofluorescence, enzyme immuno-assays or culture.

Rapid diagnosis in less than 1 h with commercially available conjugated monoclonal antibodies can be made reliably by immunofluorescence, provided an adequate number of desquamated respiratory cells are collected in the secretions. Generally similar results can be obtained with enzyme immuno-assays. Such assays may be less sensitive when compared to culture, but the virus is slow-growing and positive results will come too late to influence management. This is still true even when the cultured cells are examined by immunofluorescence for the development of virus antigen after a few days' incubation.

Serology is not helpful. Many of the patients are too young to respond reliably and even adults do not always produce a detectable rise in serum antibody levels. Hence, few laboratories offer a serological test. Secretory antibodies may develop more reliably but no routine test is yet available.

## Treatment

Appropriate management includes use of oxygen, if indicated, and tube feeding to maintain energy intake if the baby has difficulty in suckling. Most babies can be managed symptomatically by these measures. The only specific antiviral drug available for chemotherapy is tribavirin. In vivo there is some evidence of efficacy when given as a small-particle aerosol, although it is apparently not effective when given by intravenous infusion. The evidence of efficacy by any route is not overwhelming. This may be because the most affected parts of the lungs are also the least well aerated and therefore least accessible to the aerosolized drug. The drug is expensive and its recommended use is confined to those babies who are at high risk from RS virus because they have congenital heart or lung abnormalities. Even in these babies the damage may be done by the virus before the drug can be given.

## Epidemiology

In temperate climates in both the northern and southern hemispheres, RS virus causes a substantial winter epidemic every year. In the Newcastle upon Tyne/Tyne and Wear conurbation (total population about 1 million) the annual number of virologically confirmed diagnoses regularly exceeds 500. Similar figures are obtained elsewhere where adequate facilities for diagnosis exist. Most infected babies reach hospital, and the failure to recover it from babies with 'colds' attending well-baby clinics in Newcastle upon Tyne has suggested that comparatively few cases go unrecognized.

Why it induces an epidemic every October/November is unknown. In other regions of the world the pattern can be markedly different. In Hong Kong, a semitemperate area, there is an equally clear epidemic, but in the hot and humid months of the summer. Therefore, RS virus epidemics do not always correspond to the same short-term climatic factors (temperature, humidity, etc.), and sporadic cases occur anyway throughout the year. The virus is distributed over all the world, but its activities in tropical, overcrowded and poor areas are under-recorded so far.

The significance, if any, of subtypes in explaining these RS virus phenomena is still under investigation.

## Control

A formalin-inactivated crude whole-virus vaccine was tried in the 1960s. It induced good levels of circulating antibody but failed to protect the recipients, who actually became more ill than placebo controls when subsequently exposed to RS virus. As with measles, this may have been due to the vaccine failing to induce the right protective antibodies. Subsequently, several live vaccines based on cold adaptation, temperature-sensitive mutants or administration by a different route (intramuscularly) were tried but none has proved satisfactory (through insufficient attenuation or inadequate immunogenicity).

A major obstacle in developing a good vaccine is the fact that the peak of disease occurs within the 1st year of life, and thus a safe vaccine immunogenic to such young and largely immunologically immature recipients is difficult to prepare. In the future, genetic engineering offers new ways to prepare vaccines which contain only the relevant antigens in an appropriate viral or bacterial vector, but at present there is no satisfactory vaccine.

RECOMMENDED READING

Evans A S (ed) 1989 *Viral Infections of Humans; Epidemiology and Control*, 3rd edn. Plenum Press, New York
Zuckerman A J, Banatvala J E, Pattison J R (eds) 1994

*Principles and Practice of Clinical Virology*, 3rd edn. Wiley, Chichester

# 52

# Arboviruses: alphaviruses, flaviviruses and bunyaviruses

**Encephalitis; yellow fever; dengue; haemorrhagic fever; miscellaneous tropical fevers; undifferentiated fever; rubella; hepatitis C**

## D. M. McLean, P. Morgan-Capner and J. F. Peutherer

The name 'arbo' (arthropod-borne) virus has been used for many years to define viruses transmitted by arthropod (mainly insect) vectors. However, it is now recognized that there are many different viruses transmitted by arthropods. Indeed, there are more than 500 individual arbovirus serotypes which are now officially classified in five different virus families. As there are many similarities in their behaviour, they will be considered together in this chapter. Arboviruses were defined by a World Health Organization Scientific Group as:

> viruses that are maintained in nature principally, or to an important extent, through biological transmission between susceptible vertebrate hosts by haemotophagous arthropods or through transovarian and possible venereal transmission in arthropods; the viruses multiply and produce viraemia in the vertebrates, multiply in the tissues of arthropods, and are passed on to new vertebrates by the bites of arthropods after a period of extrinsic incubation.

Additional serotypes within the five families are not transmitted by arthropods, but are maintained in nature within rodent reservoirs which may transmit infection directly to humans. They include hantaviruses (family Bunyaviridae), discussed in this chapter, and viruses in the families Arenaviridae and Filoviridae, discussed in Chapter 53.

## DESCRIPTION

### Classification

Arboviruses are classified within five families (Table 52.1). Most serotypes are assigned to the families Togaviridae, Flaviviridae and Bunyaviridae; some

**Table 52.1** Characteristic properties of arboviruses

| Property | Arbovirus family (principal genus) | | | | |
| | Togaviridae (*Alphavirus*) | Flaviviridae (*Flavivirus*) | Bunyaviridae (*Bunyavirus*)[a] | Rhabdoviridae (*Rhabdovirus*)[b] | Reoviridae (*Reovirus*)[c] |
|---|---|---|---|---|---|
| Symmetry[d] | Cubic | Cubic | Helical | Bullet shaped | Cubic |
| Total diameter (nm) | 60–65 | 40–50 | 90–100 | 170 × 70 | 60–80 |
| Nucleic acid | (+)ssRNA | (+)ssRNA | (−)ssRNA | (−)ssRNA | dsRNA |
|    Molecular weight ($\times 10^6$) | 4.2–4.4 | 4.2–4.4 | 0.4–5.0 | 3.5–4.6 | 0.2–3.0 |
|    No. of molecules | 1 | 1 | 3 | 1 | 10–12 |
| No. of serotypes | 28 | 69 | 253 | 63 | 77 |
| Inactivation by diethyl ether or sodium deoxycholate | + | + | + | + | − |

ssRNA, single-stranded RNA; dsRNA, double-stranded RNA.
[a]Other important genera: *Nairovirus*, *Phlebovirus* (arthropod-borne); *Hantavirus* (not arthropod-borne).
[b]See Chapter 58.
[c]See Chapter 54.
[d]All have enveloped virions (except Reoviridae).

are assigned to the families Reoviridae (the genus *Orbivirus* and Colorado tick fever virus) and the Rhabdoviridae (members of the genus *Vesiculovirus*, e.g. vesicular stomatitis virus). Within the Togaviridae, only one genus, *Alphavirus*, contains arthropod-borne serotypes; another genus, *Rubivirus*, which contains rubella virus, is not arthropod-borne. Rubella virus is described in a separate section later in this chapter. The hepatitis C virus, one of the main causes of non-A, non-B hepatitis, is now classified within the Flaviviridae, and is also described in a separate section.

Individual serotypes of arboviruses are distinguished from each other by neutralization tests. Clusters of serotypes which show antigenic overlap in haemagglutination inhibition (HI), enzyme immuno-sorbent assay (ELISA) or complement fixation (CF) tests are termed serogroups. Table 52.2 lists some of the important members.

## Properties

Arboviruses share common biological attributes (see Table 52.1):

1. All induce fatal encephalitis 1–10 days after intracerebral inoculation of suckling mice aged less than 48 h; some also induce fatal encephalitis after intracerebral inoculation of weaned mice aged 3–4 weeks. Encephalitis does not occur after inoculation of virus plus serotype-specific antiserum (neutralization).

**Table 52.2**    Some important arboviruses

| Family and genus | Number of members | Some important members | Comments |
|---|---|---|---|
| Togaviridae<br>  *Alphavirus* | 28 | Western equine encephalitis<br>Eastern equine encephalitis<br>Venezuelan equine encephalitis<br>Chikungunya<br>Ross River | Mosquito-borne<br>Serogroup A |
| Flaviviridae<br>  *Flavivirus* | 68 | St Louis encephalitis<br>Japanese B encephalitis<br>Murray Valley encephalitis<br>Yellow fever<br>Dengue<br>Ilheus<br>West Nile | Mosquito-borne<br>Serogroup B |
| | | Louping ill<br>Powassan<br>Tick-borne encephalitis<br>Kyasanur Forrest<br>Omsk haemorrhagic fever | Tick-borne<br>Serogroup B |
| Bunyaviridae<br>  *Bunyavirus* | 212 | La Crosse<br>Snowshoe hare<br>Oropouche | California (CAL) serogroup |
| *Phlebovirus* | | Rift Valley fever<br>Punta Toro<br>Sandfly fever<br>Toscana | |
| *Nairovirus* | | Crimean–Congo haemorrhagic fever | |
| *Hantavirus* | | Sin Nombre (not arthropod-borne) | |

2. Haemagglutinin for erythrocytes of geese or newly hatched chicks. Haemagglutination is inhibited by antiserum against virus serotypes within the same serogroup, but not dissimilar serogroups. Antigen can also be detected by ELISA and CF tests.

3. Many arboviruses multiply in continuous polyploid tissue cultures of mammalian cells incubated at 37°C, such as grivet monkey kidney (Vero) and baby hamster kidney (BHK).

4. Many arboviruses such as dengue and Ross River viruses multiply in continuous tissue cultures of *Aedes albopictus* mosquito cells when incubated at 28°C or lower temperatures; multiplication is detected by immunofluorescence tests.

5. Mosquito-borne arboviruses multiply after oral feeding or intrathoracic injection of several *Aedes* and *Culex* mosquito species after incubation at 4–28°C (depending on the mosquito species), and mosquitoes transmit virus by biting susceptible vertebrates; virus multiplication in mosquito tissues is revealed by specific immunofluorescence, particularly in salivary glands and in central nervous tissue. Susceptibility of mosquitoes to dengue and California serogroup agents is 10–100 times higher than mammalian tissue cultures or suckling mice.

Some arboviruses, notably bunyaviridae of the California and *Phlebovirus* serogroups and some rhabdoviridae (*Vesiculovirus*) are also transmitted transovarially.

Mosquito-borne arboviruses are not transmitted by ticks; tick-borne arboviruses are not transmitted by mosquitoes. Sandfly-borne viruses are transmitted only by sandflies (*Phlebotomus* sp. and *Lutzomyia* sp.).

6. Tick-borne arboviruses multiply after oral feeding to larval or nymphal ixodid ticks (hard-shelled ticks of the genera *Dermacentor* and *Ixodes*). The virus is transferred trans-stadially to the next development stage of tick (nymph or adult respectively), which then transmits virus by biting susceptible vertebrates.

## REPLICATION

The replication of the various arboviruses differs significantly and is one of the features used in their classification.

## Alphaviruses

The virus attaches to cellular receptors by means of the envelope glycoproteins E1 and E2, and virus enters the cell by endocytosis. The viral RNA is a linear single-stranded molecule. It is polyadenylated and acts as a messenger molecule. Approximately two-thirds of the genome codes for non-structural proteins: the remaining third codes for the capsid and envelope proteins. Viral RNA is replicated from a negative-strand copy catalysed by the viral-specified RNA polymerase. The virus is released by budding from membranes: an essential step in this process is the conversion of a precursor protein to E2.

## Flaviviruses

Flaviviruses are similar to alphaviruses in several respects, but they differ in the composition of the envelope glycoprotein and virion RNA. The virions mature in internal vesicles.

## Bunyaviruses

The virions of bunyaviruses are larger than the alpha- and flaviviruses. They differ fundamentally in their nucleic acid, which is present as three molecules (L, M and S strands) of circular single-stranded RNA. The RNA is of negative sense; the virion contains an RNA polymerase to initiate transcription. The envelope glycoproteins G1 and G2 are derived from the M molecules of RNA: the nucleocapsid protein (N) from the S molecule, which also codes for non-structural protein; the L molecule is presumed to code for the polymerase. Although classified in the same family, there are a number of differences between the phleboviruses and the bunyaviruses.

## PATHOGENESIS

Arboviruses induce high titres of *viraemia* in susceptible vertebrates 1–2 days after parenteral inoculation or following bites by infected arthropods; viraemia persists for several days and serves as a source of infective blood meals for other biting arthropods. The primary site of virus replication is not known but is likely to be in the reticulo-endothelial cells in lymph nodes, liver and spleen or endothelial cells of blood vessels. Release of virus from these sites may be associated with non-specific 'flu-like' symptoms. During this period of viraemia, usually at about 5–7 days after exposure, virus enters the target sites of the central nervous system, skin, etc. There may be a brief period of relief after the initial symptoms – before the onset of the specific

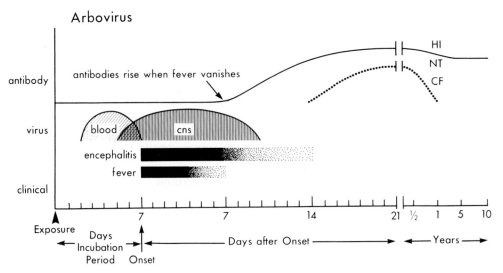

**Fig. 52.1** Pathogenesis of arbovirus infection: time course of clinical features, virus detection and antibodies. NT, neutralization. Antibodies measured by ELISA parallel the time course for HI and NT antibodies. (From McLean D M 1980 *Virology in Health Care*. Williams and Wilkins, Baltimore, p 167.)

features. Thus, the presentation is a biphasic illness. Symptoms of encephalitis begin 7–10 days after exposure to infection and persist for 1 week or more, followed either by remission or by death. Wild birds and mammals regularly exhibit viraemia without symptoms.

Antibodies are first detected when the fever subsides, usually within 2 days after the onset of encephalitis, and persist for many years (Fig. 52.1). Antibodies are of the IgM class for 1–7 weeks after infection, subsequently they are of the IgG class.

Within the central nervous system, arboviruses multiply in and induce necrosis of neurones, which in turn become surrounded by microglia, forming glial knots (Fig. 52.2). Perivascular cuffing with mononuclear cells affects many cerebral blood vessels. Usually there is concomitant meningitis with accumulation of mononuclear cells in the subarachnoid space and hyperaemia of adjacent capillaries. It is important to note that although many subjects become infected with encephalitis viruses, relatively few develop illness manifested as meningitis or encephalitis. There is little information about the role of the immune system, although it may have a role in the pathogenesis of the dengue haemorrhagic shock syndrome, which is seen in young children who are experiencing a second dengue virus infection. Antigen–antibody complex formation has been thought to underlie the syndrome, which is associated with increased capillary permeability and shock,

often with haemorrhage. However, it is known that the uptake of virus into macrophages is enhanced in the presence of antibody, as the virus–antibody complexes bind to Fc receptors. In this way there is likely to be a great increase in the uptake of virus and hence the release of virus from macrophages.

## CLINICAL FEATURES

Arbovirus infections of humans become clinically manifest according to the target organ principally infected (Table 52.3). These include the following syndromes.

### Encephalitis

Encephalitis typically comprises the sudden onset of fever and headache, followed by neck stiffness, nausea or vomiting, drowsiness, and disorientation, frequently advancing into stupor or coma after an incubation period of 4–14 days. Convulsions may be an important feature of the acute illness. Rigidity or weakness of the limbs may occur, together with absent or irregular deep tendon reflexes and upgoing plantar reflexes. Symptoms are most severe 2–5 days after onset, after which the patient may die or the fever and other symptoms may retrogress slowly during the next 2–3 weeks. Characteristically, the

**Fig. 52.2** Powassan virus infection in the brain of a fatal case from whom the prototype LB strain was isolated. Haematoxylin and eosin stain, ×100. **A** Perivascular cuffing of cerebral blood vessel; **B** focus of inflammatory cells around effete neurone (glial knot). (From McLean D M 1980 *Virology in Health Care*. Williams and Wilkins, Baltimore, p 168.)

cerebrospinal fluid shows pleocytosis with a predominance of leucocytes, but sugar and protein levels remain normal. The peripheral blood leucocyte count usually does not exceed $8 \times 10^9$/l and shows a predominance of leucocytes. During most outbreaks of arboviral encephalitis, a proportion of cases develop aseptic meningitis only, without significant neuronal involvement.

## Yellow fever

Yellow fever is characterized by the sudden onset of headache and fever with temperatures exceeding 39°C, accompanied by generalized myalgia, nausea and vomiting, after an incubation period of 3–6 days. Jaundice may appear by the 3rd day of illness, but frequently this is mild or absent. Haematemesis and

**Table 52.3** Clinical syndromes associated with selected arboviruses and their geographical distribution

| Syndrome | Genus | Serogroup (vector) | Causative arbovirus serotype | | Geographical distribution |
|---|---|---|---|---|---|
| Encephalitis or aseptic meningitis | *Alphavirus* | A (mosquito) | EEE | eastern equine encephalitis | Eastern Canada, USA, Caribbean |
| | | | VEE | Venezuelan equine encephalitis | Central and South America |
| | | | WEE | western equine encephalitis | Western Canada and USA, Caribbean |
| | *Flavivirus* | B (mosquito) | JBE | Japanese B encephalitis | Orient (Japan to Malaysia) |
| | | | MVE | Murray Valley encephalitis | Australia |
| | | | SLE | St Louis encephalitis | Canada, USA, Central America |
| | | B (tick) | LI | louping ill | Scotland, Northern Ireland |
| | | | POW | Powassan | Canada, Northern USA |
| | | | TBE | tick-borne encephalitis complex | Central and northern Europe, Siberia |
| | *Bunyavirus* | CAL (mosquito) | LAC | La Crosse | USA |
| | | | SSH | snowshoe hare | Canada |
| Yellow fever | *Flavivirus* | B (mosquito) | YF | yellow fever | Tropical Africa, Caribbean, tropical South America |
| Dengue | *Flavivirus* | B (mosquito) | DEN | dengue (4 types) | Entire tropical zone |
| Haemorrhagic fever | *Alphavirus* | A (mosquito) | CHIK | chikungunya | East Africa, India, South-East Asia |
| | *Flavivirus* | B (mosquito) | DEN | dengue (4 types) | India, Philippines, South-East Asia, Oceania |
| | | B (tick) | KFD | Kyasanur Forest disease | India |
| | | | OMSK | Omsk haemorrhagic fever | Siberia |
| | *Nairovirus* | CHF-CON (tick) | CON | Congo haemorrhagic fever | Central and Southern Africa |
| Miscellaneous tropical fevers | *Alphavirus* | A (mosquito) | CHIK | chikungunya | East Africa, India, South-East Asia |
| | | | RR | Ross River | Australia, Oceania |
| | *Flavivirus* | B (mosquito) | ILH | Ilheus | Caribbean, South America |
| | | | WN | West Nile | Central and Northern Africa |
| | *Bunyavirus* | SIM (mosquito) | ORO | Oropouche | Caribbean, South America |
| | *Phlebovirus* | PHL (mosquito) | RVF | Rift Valley fever | Northern, Eastern and Southern Africa |
| | | PHL (sandfly) | PT | Punta Toro | Central America |
| | | PHL (sandfly) | SFN | sandfly fever – Naples | Mediterranean |
| | *Vesiculovirus* | VS (sandfly) | VSI | vesicular stomatitis – Indiana | USA, Central America[b] |
| Undifferentiated fever | *Coltivirus* | CTF (tick) | CTF | Colorado tick fever | Western USA[c] |

[a]Ross River virus infections frequently exhibit polyarthralgia.
[b]See Chapter 58.
[c]See Chapter 54.

melaena may occur from bleeding into the gastro-intestinal tract and epistaxis and bleeding gums may also be noted. Albuminuria and oliguria may also begin suddenly during the 1st week of illness. In severe cases, death may occur 3 days or more after the onset of illness, and midzonal necrosis is observed in the liver. The case fatality rate is estimated at 20%. Mild cases may develop fever, headache and myalgia only, without gastro-intestinal upsets, jaundice or albuminuria. In such cases, the diagnosis is frequently achieved only by the isolation of virus from the blood or demonstration of rising levels of antibody.

# Dengue

This presents as an acute febrile illness with chills, headache, retro-ocular pain, body aches and arthralgia in more than 90% of cases, accompanied by nausea or vomiting and a maculopapular rash resembling measles lasting 2–7 days in about 60% of cases. Illness usually persists for 7 days or longer, with fever remitting after 3–5 days followed by relapse ('*saddleback fever*'), and pains in the bones, muscles and joints sufficiently severe to earn the epithet '*breakbone fever*'. Rash occurs more commonly in patients aged less than 14 years. Complete recovery is the rule. The incubation period is 5–11 days.

# Dengue haemorrhagic fever

This is a less common manifestation of dengue, affecting mainly children. It is occasionally accompanied by a shock syndrome with a case fatality rate of 50%. After an acute onset, fever of 40°C, accompanied by vomiting and anorexia, enlarged liver and petechiae persists for 5–10 days. This is followed by a complete recovery unless shock supervenes; this occurs in 7–10% of cases from 2 to 7 days after onset, usually accompanied by haematemesis and melaena. Although dengue haemorrhagic fever with shock syndrome was initially recognized in South-East Asia in 1951, it has since occurred in the south-west Pacific, Puerto Rico and Cuba.

# Miscellaneous tropical fevers

These comprise elevation of temperature beyond 39°C, together with any combination of headache, myalgia, malaise, nausea or vomiting, and sometimes accompanied by maculopapular rash or polyarthralgia, i.e. a dengue-like syndrome, but without haemorrhagic manifestations or the shock syndrome. Tropical fevers arise from infection with a wide variety of arboviruses (Table 52.3).

# Undifferentiated fever

A US example is Colorado tick fever (genus *Coltivirus*) in which symptoms of chilliness, headaches, retro-orbital pain and generalized aches, especially in the back and limbs, appear 3–6 days after bites by infected *Dermacentor andersoni* ticks in wooded areas of the Rocky Mountain region. Fever with a temperature of 39–40°C often shows a biphasic course, with eventual defervescence within 1 week, followed by complete recovery.

# Hantavirus pulmonary syndrome

This syndrome, due to the newly described hantavirus Sin Nombre, was first recognized in south-western USA during 1993. Sudden onset of fever, myalgia, headache, cough and nausea or vomiting is accompanied by rapid respirations exceeding 20 per minute, temperature above 38°C and hypotension. Extensive interstitial and alveolar infiltrates are observed on radiographic examination of the lungs, accompanied by reduced oxygen saturation below 90 mm Hg. Fatal cases develop progressive pulmonary oedema with hypoxia and severe hypotension (systolic blood pressure below 86 mm Hg) and die 2–16 (mean 8) days after onset of symptoms; the case fatality rate may exceed 50%. Non-fatal cases usually recover within 1–3 weeks.

# General principles

Certain epidemiological principles apply to human illnesses induced by arboviruses:

1. For each syndrome, several different serogroups may be involved, as in encephalitis due to western equine encephalitis (WEE), Powassan (POW) or La Crosse (LAC) virus infections.

2. There is a high proportion of subclinical infections to clinical illnesses, e.g. 64:1 to 209:1 for St Louis encephalitis (SLE) virus, but this proportion is considerably lower for dengue and miscellaneous tropical fevers.

3. There may be localization of a particular serotype within a particular geographic zone such as: (a) POW virus in forested areas of eastern North America; (b) WEE virus in irrigated farmlands of western North America, where SLE virus is also prevalent; and (c) Murray Valley encephalitis (MVE) virus in Australia. However, dengue is distributed widely throughout tropical regions of each continent and in Oceania.

4. Virus transmission by the bite of culicine mosquitoes or ixodid ticks occurs after ingestion of relatively small titres (0.1–10 plaque-forming units) of virus in blood meals from naturally infected viraemic vertebrates after extrinsic incubation periods of 1–3 weeks at usual summertime temperatures.

5. Viraemia develops asymptomatically in birds (alphaviruses and mosquito-borne flaviviruses) and in mammals (bunyaviruses and tick-borne flaviviruses and orbiviruses) at titres sufficient to infect mosquitoes or ticks which imbibe blood meals from them.

## LABORATORY DIAGNOSIS

Diagnosis of arbovirus infections depends on the isolation of virus from, or on detection of arbovirus-specific RNA in, blood, cerebrospinal fluid or tissues, or on serology. Whenever possible, attempts should be channelled towards virus isolation, especially in febrile illnesses.

### Virus isolation

The causative virus can be isolated from blood collected during the initial 3 day febrile illness induced by serotypes such as dengue, Ross River and yellow fever, when viraemia titres are at a maximum. Collect cerebrospinal fluid or brain biopsy during life, or brain at autopsy of fatal cases of encephalitis. Obtain liver from fatal cases of yellow fever. The isolation procedures are as follows:

1. Inoculate mammalian tissue cultures, e.g. Vero or BHK, and incubate at 37°C under agarose overlay until plaques appear after 7–14 days. Determine the serotype in an extract of an excised plaque by neutralization, immunofluorescence or ELISA tests using appropriate monoclonal antibodies.

2. Inoculate continuous cultures of *A. albopictus* mosquito cells and incubate at 28°C for up to 10 days; examine cells for arbovirus antigen by immunofluorescence.

3. Inoculate acute-phase blood from dengue patients intrathoracically into male mosquitoes and incubate at 30°C for 14 days. Detect viral antigen in head squashes by direct immunofluorescence.

4. Inoculate acute-phase blood, or brain or liver suspensions, intracerebrally into suckling mice aged less than 48 h and examine daily up to 14 days for development of encephalitis (hunching, ruffled fur, convulsions, spasticity and, eventually, death). Remove brains from moribund mice and perform preliminary serogrouping by haemagglutination inhibition tests on sucrose–acetone extracts of brain suspension, followed by final serotypic identification by neutralization tests in suckling mice or by plaque reduction in Vero or BHK tissue cultures.

### Arbovirus-specific RNA detection

Extract viral RNA from serum, suspensions of tissues from patients or tissue culture cells, or mosquito homogenates using a guanidinium isothiocyanate-phenol mixture. Prepare complementary DNA using reverse transcriptase (RT). Amplify the base sequences by the polymerase chain reaction (PCR) using appropriate primers. Analyse the reaction products or their restriction products by gel electrophoresis and compare with nucleotide sequences within fragments of nucleocapsid specific for known arbovirus serotypes.

### Serology

Serological tests frequently offer the only available means of laboratory diagnosis of encephalitis. The detection of a four-fold or greater rise of antibody titre by HI or ELISA tests on paired sera collected during the initial week and several days later after defervescence provides good evidence of concurrent infection. Antibodies detected by CF first appear 2 or more weeks after onset and become undetectable by 3 years. Serotype-specific IgM antibody may be detected within 1 day after onset using an IgM capture ELISA test. IgM antibody wanes 6 weeks after onset and is replaced by IgG antibodies.

## TREATMENT

Currently, no specific anti-arboviral therapeutic agent is available. Patients with encephalitis are managed supportively, using anticonvulsants as required, and ice-packs are applied when indicated to reduce hyperthermia. Similarly, in dengue and haemorrhagic fevers supportive nursing measures are employed, including intravenous infusions when indicated to replace fluids and electrolytes.

## EPIDEMIOLOGY

### Natural cycles

Arboviruses are maintained in nature by one of five natural cycles of infection involving mosquitoes, ticks or sandflies as arthropod vectors and birds or mammals as vertebrate reservoirs, with humans infected tangentially to these cycles (Fig. 52.3). In the arthropod, during the extrinsic incubation period, the virus multiplies initially in gut tissues after an infected blood meal, it then enters the haemocoelic fluid, in which it is carried to the salivary glands where further multiplication occurs, following which it is injected along with saliva into capillaries of new vertebrate hosts through bites. Vertebrates develop viraemia 1–2 days after arthropod bites, and this

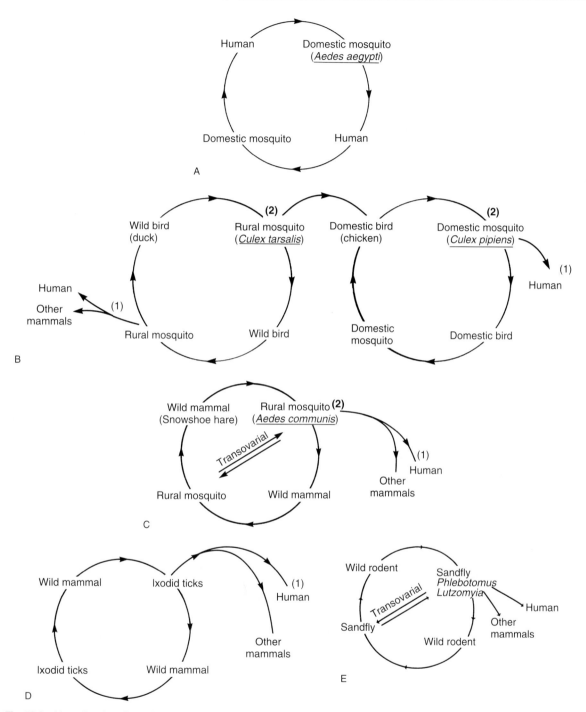

**Fig. 52.3** Natural cycles of arbovirus infection. **a** Human–mosquito cycle of infection, e.g. dengue virus. **b** Bird–mosquito cycle of infection, e.g. western equine encephalitis; transmission of infection to humans may be prevented by (1) repellants and protective clothing and (2) mosquito abatement (larviciding, adulticiding). **c** Mammal–mosquito cycle, e.g. California serogroup viruses. **d** Mammal–tick cycle of infection, e.g. Powassan virus. **e** Mammal–sandfly cycle of infection, e.g. phlebovirus. (From McLean D M 1980 *Virology in Health Care*. Williams and Wilkins, Baltimore, pp 170–174; McLean D M 1988 *Virological Infections*. Thomas, Springfield, Illinois, pp 229–230.)

provides infective blood meals for fresh arthropods. The minimum infective dose of dengue and California serogroup viruses for mosquitoes is 10–100 times smaller than the dose required to infect mice or tissue cultures.

Examples of natural cycles (illustrated in Fig. 52.3) are:

1. Human–mosquito cycle as in dengue and urban yellow fever (Fig. 52.3a). Vectors are typically the highly domesticated *Aedes* mosquito species *A. aegypti*, but peridomestic *A. albopictus* has also been implicated; humans are the sole vertebrate reservoir.

2. Mosquito–bird cycle as in WEE (Fig. 52.3b). Vectors are typically *Culex tarsalis*, which breeds in grass-lined sloughs and irrigation run-offs; reservoirs are typically wild ducks which inhabit these locations; humans are infected tangentially to this rural cycle. Some infected *C. tarsalis* may infect domestic chickens, which in turn may be a source of viraemic blood for domestic *C. pipiens* mosquitoes; these may also transmit infection to humans.

3. Mosquito–mammal cycle, as in California serogroup viruses such as snowshoe hare (SSH) virus in the Canadian Arctic (Fig. 52.3c). Vectors are typically *A. communis*; reservoirs are snowshoe hares or ground squirrels; humans are infected tangentially to this rural cycle. With cool summer-time arctic temperatures, mosquitoes transmit SSH virus after extrinsic incubation at 13°C. Virus is maintained from summer to summer by transovarial transmission; mosquitoes are not prevalent during the winter freeze-up. Birds are insusceptible to SSH virus.

Sylvan yellow fever is maintained in the forest canopies of tropical jungles year-round by a cycle involving *Haemagogus* spp. mosquitoes and arboreal primates; humans become infected during tree felling, when these forest canopy mosquitoes are brought to ground level.

4. Tick–mammal cycle as in POW virus (Fig. 52.3d). Vectors are *Ixodes* spp. ticks, reservoirs are groundhogs or tree squirrels; humans are infected tangentially to this cycle. Comparable natural cycles maintain louping ill virus in Scotland and tick-borne encephalitis viruses throughout northern Europe.

5. Sandfly–human cycle as in sandfly fever of southern Europe and northern Mediterranean areas (Fig. 52.3e). *Phlebotomus* spp. are the vectors and humans are reservoirs; transovarial transmission maintains virus from one summer to the next. Rodents are reservoirs of some phleboviruses.

Epidemiological aspects of arbovirus infections with major impact on human health are described according to syndrome and infecting serotype (see also Table 52.2).

## Alphaviruses

### Western equine encephalitis (WEE) virus

This was first isolated from the brain of a horse with fatal encephalitis. WEE is found from the Mississippi Valley to California and northwards to western Canada. The mean incidence of WEE cases throughout the USA between 1966 and 1985 was 17 per year, constituting 7% of the total reported cases of arbovirus encephalitis. Cases occur only during June to September, when mosquitoes are abundant. Outbreaks of infection occur at intervals of a few years and are preceded by epizootic peaks of encephalitis among horses. The principal mosquito vector species in Canada and the western USA is *C. tarsalis*. Ducks and other water birds constitute the principal natural reservoirs.

Although all age groups may be involved, encephalitis due to WEE virus and California serogroup agents commonly affects children in whom the disease is often severe; SLE virus is most often seen in persons aged 55 years or more.

### Eastern equine encephalitis (EEE) virus

This was also first isolated from the brain of a horse with fatal encephalitis. Human and horse cases of encephalitis have occurred repeatedly during the summer in Atlantic coastal areas extending from Massachusetts and New Jersey southwards to Florida and Texas. Occasionally, disease extends northwards into the Province of Quebec, Canada. During the 20 year period 1966–85 in the USA, EEE caused a mean of four cases of encephalitis per year, constituting 2% of the total cases of arbovirus encephalitis. Illness affected mainly humans aged under 14 years and over 55 years, with overall case fatality rates as high as 69%. Surviving cases will have severe neurological sequelae. Most human cases occur during late August and September, about 3 weeks after the peak of horse cases. Principal mosquito vectors are *Culiseta melanura*, which breeds in freshwater swamps; *Coquillettidia perturbans* and *A. sollicitans* are additional vectors during epidemic periods. Birds such as grackles and pheasants are important vertebrate reservoirs of infection. Human and horse cases have been identified in Central and South America, but antigenic differences have been demonstrated between North American and South American EEE isolates.

## Venezuelan equine encephalitis (VEE) virus

This occurs from Mexico through Central and South America to northern Argentina, including the Caribbean islands. In 1971 it was seen in Texas during a major outbreak in Central America accompanied by neurological disturbances of varying severity, with case fatality rates of 0–33%. In 1995, following a prolonged rainy season, a major outbreak due to subtype IC afflicted over 13 000 humans and numerous equines in the Guajira peninsula of northern Venezuela and neighbouring Columbia, after VEE activity had been absent since 1973. Large numbers of horses develop fatal encephalitis before and during the occurrence of human cases. Principal mosquito vectors during recent Central American epidemics were *Psorophora confinnis* and *C. taeniopus*. Vertebrate reservoirs include cotton rats, pigs and horses, and also a variety of birds. There are nine antigenic subtypes of VEE virus which vary in their virulence for humans and horses.

## Ross River (RR) virus

This is found in Australia throughout coastal regions of Queensland and New South Wales, and the arid Pilbara region of Western Australia, where it has caused epidemics of fever, maculopapular rash and arthralgia. It is maintained in nature by a cycle involving *C. annulirostris* and *A. vigilax* as the principal mosquito vectors, with flying foxes and marsupial mice as reservoirs; humans are infected tangentially. Overwintering between epidemics is by transovarial transfer.

Epidemics of polyarthritis with mild fever, sometimes accompanied by rash, have been attributed to RR virus in Fiji and American Samoa, New Caledonia, Wallis Island and also on Rarotonga where *A. polynesiensis* was confirmed virologically as the vector species.

## Flaviviruses: mosquito-borne

### St Louis encephalitis (SLE) virus

This was first isolated from the brain of a person dying with acute encephalitis in St Louis, Missouri. SLE activity is widely distributed throughout the USA from the Ohio and Mississippi Valleys and extending westwards through Colorado to California and Washington, northwards into the contiguous Canadian Provinces of Ontario, Manitoba and Saskatchewan, eastwards to Ohio and southwards to Florida and Texas. In common with WEE, SLE soon becomes prevalent in arid areas of the northwestern and south-western USA which have been opened up for irrigation farming, due to the breeding of massive populations of the principal mosquito vector *C. tarsalis* in semipermanent collections of water in grassy locations. During the largest outbreak of the past quarter-century, in 1975, when 1815 of 2113 (86%) of confirmed cases of arbovirus encephalitis were due to SLE virus, the Chicago metropolitan area was heavily affected for the first time. Substantial SLE outbreaks affected the Houston, Texas, metropolitan area in 1964 and 1986, where attack rates and case fatality rates were highest among persons over 55 years of age. Metropolitan Los Angeles in coastal southern California was first affected by SLE virus with 26 human cases of encephalitis in 1984. Mosquito vectors in California, the Rocky Mountains and plains states comprise mainly *C. tarsalis*, but *C. pipiens* and *C. quinquefasciatus* are important along the Mississippi Valley and eastwards. The salt marsh mosquitoes *C. restuans* and *A. sollicitans* may be important vectors in some localities.

### Japanese B encephalitis (JBE) virus

The virus was first isolated from the brain of a fatal case of encephalitis in Tokyo, Japan. JBE virus continues to cause epidemics of encephalitis, affecting children, particularly in Japan, Korea, China, South-East Asia and Indonesia, with case fatality rates often exceeding 20%. *C. tritaeniorhynchus* mosquitoes are the principal vectors in Japan when maximum virus isolation rates from mosquitoes during late July occur simultaneously with human and equine epidemics. Important vertebrate reservoirs are black-crowned night herons and other water birds, but pigs may also serve as vertebrate reservoirs. In Malaysia, *C. gelidus* is an important vector as well as *C. tritaeniorhynchus*. In northern Thailand about 1500 cases of encephalitis due to JBE virus have been diagnosed each year since the late 1960s with most cases occurring during the rainy season in June, July and August. The case fatality rate of virologically confirmed cases is 33%, and about 1:300 humans infected with JBE virus develops encephalitis.

### Murray Valley encephalitis (MVE) virus

This was first isolated from the brain of a fatal case of encephalitis at Mooroopna, Victoria, Australia. MVE caused epidemics of encephalitis in irrigated farming regions of the Murray-Darling River basin of south-eastern Australia during the summer months (January to March) of 1951 and 1974, with case fatality rates approaching 40%. MVE virus was isolated from *C. annulirostris* mosquitoes only during 1974 but not during intervening years, which suggests epidemic introduction of virus into this dry temperate region. In the irrigated Ord River region of Western Australia, encephalitis due to MVE virus has been recognized in 1974, 1978, 1981 and 1986, although the virus is endemic in this tropical region. Another endemic focus exists in the Gulf of Carpentaria region of Queensland. Natural cycles of transmission of MVE virus involve *C. annulirostris* as the principal mosquito vector and water birds as reservoirs.

## Yellow fever (YF) virus

This was first isolated in Ghana, West Africa, from the blood of a male patient with fever, headache, backache and prostration. YF virus is prevalent throughout tropical Africa and tropical Central and South America, including the Caribbean islands. There are two epidemiological patterns of YF. In the sylvan cycle, virus is transmitted between monkeys by *Haemagogus* mosquitoes. Man is infected tangentially when entering the area, e.g. to work as foresters. In the urban cycle, human-to-human transmission is via *A. aegypti*, which breeds close to human habitation in water, in pits and scrap containers such as oil drums.

In the Americas, a mean of 135 cases of YF were reported each year from Bolivia, Brazil, Columbia, Ecuador and Peru, and from Trinidad-Tobago and Venezuela only between 1978 and 1980. During 1988, 196 cases of YF were reported in Peru with 167 deaths, but no human cases of YF were reported in Trinidad despite deaths of howler monkeys. In South America, most cases occurred in males aged 15–45 years, particularly colonists and temporary workers on agricultural and forestry projects in enzootic areas, as well as residents of those areas. The incidence usually peaks during March and April when populations of *Haemagogus* mosquitoes are highest during the rainy season.

In Africa, YF is endemic throughout West, Central and East Africa, principally between latitudes 15°N and 15°S, extending northwards into Ethiopia and Sudan. Continuing activity has been encountered in Senegal and the Gambia along the west coast and in Burkina Faso. Attack rates of 3–4% have been recorded with a case fatality rate of 19%, and the ratio of inapparent to apparent infections is about

12:1. In Ethiopia between 1960 and 1962, a major YF epidemic involved about 100 000 cases with a case fatality rate of about 30%. Spread of infection occurred both in irrigated cultivated areas, and in forests and arid areas. The forest mosquito vector was *A. africanus*, but in villages the mosquito vector was probably *A. simpsoni*, which breeds in peridomestic situations; *Colobus* monkeys served as natural reservoirs.

## Dengue (DEN) virus

The infection is endemic in all tropical regions between latitudes 23.5°N and 23.5°S. Typical dengue is induced by any of four serotypes of DEN virus. However, arboviruses from other genera such as the alphavirus serotypes chikungunya (CHIK) and Ross River (RR), bunyavirus serotypes including Oropouche (ORO) and phlebovirus serotypes such as Rift Valley fever (RVF) and Toscana (TOS) have also induced dengue-like disease. These latter agents are differentiated from the dengue virus by serological procedures.

Dengue is maintained in nature by a cycle involving humans as both reservoirs and definitive hosts, and domestic mosquitoes, principally *A. aegypti*, as vectors. However, the peridomestic mosquito species *A. albopictus* is recognized increasingly as a significant dengue vector in many urban localities.

Dengue has caused numerous outbreaks throughout the south-west Pacific region since it was first encountered among servicemen during the Second World War, when the average monthly attack rate of 54 per 1000 peaked to 197 per 1000 during the wet season. Subsequently, in the south-west Pacific, several serotypes of dengue have affected Tahiti with haemorrhagic dengue first encountered in 1971. In addition to *A. aegypti* other species have been implicated as vectors, including *A. scutellaris hebrideus* in New Guinea, *A. polynesiensis* in Tahiti and *A. cooki* in Niue. Cases of imported dengue occurred in Hawaii during 1943 and 1944, probably through the inadvertent transport of dengue-infected mosquitoes on ships returning from dengue-endemic Pacific islands. Currently, with the absence of *A. aegypti*, Hawaii is dengue-free. Also during the Second World War, dengue was imported into the Japanese port cities of Kobe, Nagasaki and Osaka.

Dengue activity continues in tropical countries of the Pacific rim, including Australia. Most South-East Asian countries, including Indonesia, Malaysia, Thailand, Vietnam, China, the Philippines and India, experience repeated epidemics of dengue due to all four serotypes, with most cases occurring between June and November. Mostly children are affected, 25% or more of whom may develop haemorrhagic fever. Most epidemics occur in urban areas and villages where *A. aegypti* is abundant, but not in rural environments.

Dengue is endemic throughout tropical Africa, including Nigeria in the west and Mozambique in the east, and also in Middle Eastern countries such as South Yemen.

Caribbean countries have been involved by 10 epidemic waves of dengue between 1827 and 1969, with little evidence of clinical dengue during interepidemic periods. All four dengue serotypes have been implicated in outbreaks affecting residents of Caribbean islands and adjacent portions of Central and South America. There were 43 435 cases reported in the Caribbean region in 1984. Cases of dengue have been frequently imported into the continental USA following visits to dengue-endemic Caribbean countries, including 67 cases during 1984. During 1986, dengue was reported in 233 cases in the USA. Although most infections occurred among travellers returning from the Caribbean, nine cases of indigenous dengue occurred among residents of Texas where *A. aegypti* is prevalent during the 9 warmer months each year. Since 1985, *A. albopictus* has been introduced into metropolitan communities of Texas and mid-west, north-east and north-west states along with used motor tyre casings which have been imported for retreading from Japan, South Korea and several South-East Asian countries. The peridomestic mosquito *A. albopictus* was first identified as a dengue vector in Malaysia during the 1960s, and it transmits dengue both in the human–mosquito cycle and by transovarial transfer. These factors raise serious concerns that both *A. aegypti* and *A. albopictus* may transmit dengue indigenously in the USA, which hitherto has been considered to be dengue-free.

## Flaviviruses: tick-borne

### Powassan (POW) virus

This, the sole North American tick-borne flavivirus, was first isolated from the brain of a fatal human case of encephalitis in Powassan, Ontario, Canada. To date, POW virus has been recognized as the cause of 25 cases of encephalitis and four deaths among residents of forested areas of Ontario, Quebec and Nova Scotia in Canada, plus Massachusetts, New York State and Pennsylvania in the USA. All cases occurred between May and October. Principal tick vector species in Ontario are *Ixodes cookei*,

which feeds on groundhogs, and *I. marxi*, which feeds on tree squirrels; both these mammals serve as reservoirs.

### Tick-borne encephalitis (TBE) viruses

These agents, related to but distinct from POW virus, have regularly been incriminated as causes of encephalitis or aseptic meningitis from Scotland, Scandinavia, central and northern Europe and Siberia to the Kamchatka Peninsula. Human infections may range in severity from mild biphasic meningoencephalitis, which is characteristic of the central European TBE viruses and the Scottish louping ill virus (so named because it induces a leaping gait in infected sheep), to a severe form of polioencephalomyelitis with a case fatality rate of 2–30%, which is characteristic of far-eastern Russian spring–summer encephalitis virus. In Scotland and other European countries, natural cycles involve *I. ricinus* ticks as vectors, and mice, shrews and other small rodents as reservoirs, with infection transferred tangentially to sheep or other farm animals, and also to humans. In Siberia, *I. persulcatus* ticks serve as vectors.

## Bunyaviruses: *Bunyavirus* genus

### California (CAL) serogroup

There are more than 10 serotypes, and the viruses are related antigenically to the prototype California encephalitis virus. In the USA, encephalitis and aseptic meningitis arise commonly from infections with La Crosse virus (LAC), which was first isolated from the brain of a fatal case of encephalitis at La Crosse, Wisconsin. Other serotypes occasionally associated with aseptic meningitis are snowshoe hare (SSH) virus, which was first isolated from the blood of a snowshoe hare in Montana, and Jamestown Canyon (JC) virus, which was first isolated from *Culiseta inornata* mosquitoes collected at Jamestown Canyon, Colorado. In central Europe, febrile illness sometimes associated with aseptic meningitis arises from infection with Tahyna (TAH) virus, which was first isolated from *A. caspius* mosquitoes collected near Tahyna, in the former Czechslovakia.

Currently, CAL serogroup viruses are the commonest arboviruses associated with encephalitis in the USA, including 76 of 99 virologically confirmed cases in 1994. The highest attack rates occur in states adjoining the Great Lakes from Minnesota and Wisconsin through Illinois and Indiana to Ohio, affecting mainly children aged less than 15 years. Abundant tree holes in wooded areas provide optimum breeding sites for the principal mosquito vector *A. triseriatus*, but rainwater collected in disused motor tyres has proved a suitable breeding ground for *A. triseriatus* in suburban locations. Since adult mosquitoes die in winter, CAL serogroup viruses survive through transovarial transmission. Principal vertebrate reservoirs are tree squirrels and chipmunks.

### Snowshoe hare (SSH) virus

This CAL serogroup agent is endemic throughout the boreal forest and arctic regions of Canada. Rarely, SSH virus has caused human cases of aseptic meningitis. Principal mosquito vectors are *A. communis* throughout the short arctic summer of June and July, with *Cs. inornata*, an additional springtime vector, and *A. hexodontus*, a late summer-time vector. Overwintering of virus is by the transovarial route. Natural vertebrate reservoirs comprise snowshoe hares and arctic ground squirrels.

### Oropouche (ORO)

This virus was first isolated in Trinidad but is also endemic in tropical forest surrounding the mouth of the Amazon River. Large outbreaks of febrile illness were attributed to ORO virus in Belem, Brazil, during 1961, 1968 1987–88 and in the upper Amazon region of Peru during 1995.

## Bunyaviruses: *Phlebovirus* genus

### Rift Valley fever (RVF) virus

This virus was first isolated from sheep during an epizootic causing abortion and death in the Rift Valley near Lake Niavasha, Kenya, but is present from South Africa to Egypt. Severe epidemics affected sheep, cattle and humans in South Africa during 1951 when *A. caballus*, *A. circumluteolus* and *C. theileri* were found to be vectors, with sheep, cattle, buffaloes and rodents as reservoirs. Outbreaks of RVF occurred in Egypt during 1977, and in tropical West Africa from 1987 onwards.

### Sandfly fever (phlebovirus) group

These viruses are distributed throughout the European and North African countries surrounding the Mediterranean Sea, extending eastward through Israel and Iran to West Pakistan and central India. Sandfly fever – Naples (SFN) and Sicilian (SFS) viruses were first isolated from the sera of US servicemen in those localities during an outbreak during the Second World War.

Epidemics of dengue-like fever occur during the sandfly season (June to September) and affect mainly newcomers rather than long-term residents. Natural vectors are *Phlebotomus papatasi* and other phlebotomine sandflies. Isolation of virus from male sandflies collected during July suggests transovarial transfer of virus. The natural cycle of sandfly fever appears to involve solely man as definitive host and reservoir, with sandflies as vectors.

### Toscana (TOS) virus

This virus was first isolated from sandflies collected in Tuscany, Italy. TOS virus is antigenically distinct from SFN and SFS viruses within the phlebovirus antigenic group. It is transmitted by *Phlebotomus perniciosus* sandflies, and is transferred transovarially. Natural reservoirs of TOS virus appear to be small rodents (*Apodemus sylvaticus*). Imported infections have been identified in persons returning to Sweden and the USA following visits to TOS-endemic regions.

## Bunyaviruses: *Nairovirus* genus

### Crimean–Congo haemorrhagic fever (CCHF) virus

There are two antigenically identical arboviruses within the genus *Nairovirus*. Prototype Crimean haemorrhagic fever (CHF) virus was isolated from the serum of a man with fatal haemorrhagic fever near Samarkand, Uzbekistan; Congo (CON) virus was first isolated from the serum of a child with fever and arthralgia in Zaire. CCHF is distributed widely throughout tropical Africa, from Mauritania and Senegal eastwards through Upper Volta, Nigeria, Congo, Zaire, Uganda, Kenya, the Middle East and West Pakistan, and southwards to South Africa. Haemorrhagic fever due to CCHF virus is also prevalent around the Black Sea and Caspian Sea. The geographic distribution of CCHF virus corresponds to that of *Hyalomma* sp. ticks, which have yielded numerous virus isolations from field-collected specimens. Hares are the natural vertebrate reservoirs in Africa and former USSR.

## Bunyaviruses: *Hantavirus* genus

Hantaviruses are typical examples of rodent-associated viruses. They are not arthropod-borne.

Rodents (mainly mice or voles) are the principal natural reservoirs, and excrete virus in urine for prolonged periods. Virus is transmitted to humans by contact with fomites contaminated by rodent urine.

### Hantaan (HTN) and Puumala (PUU) viruses

These antigenically related serotypes induce either: (i) severe illness termed *haemorrhagic fever with renal syndrome* (HFRS) due to HTN virus in Japan, Korea, China and Siberia and PUU virus in Scandinavia; or (ii) mild illness termed *nephropathia epidemica* due to PUU virus in Scotland, France, Belgium and Germany, the Balkans and Greece. Principal vertebrate reservoirs comprise *Apodemus agrarius* rodents in Asia and *Clethrionomys glareolus* (bank vole) in Europe.

### Sin Nombre (SN) virus

This newly described serotype induces hantavirus pulmonary syndrome (HPS), a severe acute respiratory illness with a case fatality rate exceeding 50%. Initially encountered in May 1993 in the Four Corners region of the USA (Arizona, Colorado, New Mexico and Utah), additional cases have since occurred elsewhere in the USA and Canada. The principal rodent reservoir is *Peromyscus maniculatus* (deer mouse).

This was the first occasion on which molecular methods were employed successfully to identify an unknown virus before the virus was isolated. Hantavirus group antibodies were detected in sera from human cases and rodents. Total RNA was extracted from lung or liver of fatal human cases and seropositive rodents. Positive bands were detected by RT–PCR using primers designed to detect Prospect Hill (North American) and PUU-like hantaviruses, but not Hantaan and Seoul-like (Asian) hantaviruses, within 3 weeks after death of the initial human cases. Several months later, Sin Nombre (SN) virus, genomically distinct from Prospect Hill and other hantaviruses, was isolated from tissue suspensions, initially from *P. maniculatus* and subsequently from humans, by intraperitoneal plus intranasal inoculation of laboratory-reared *P. maniculatus*. Virus was detected in mouse lungs by RT–PCR, and subsequently passaged in continuous Vero E6 (monkey kidney) tissue cultures, when virus replication was detected by immunofluorescence.

# CONTROL

Strategies for prevention of arbovirus infections depend on either vector control or active immunization with vaccine.

## Vector control

This is possible for mosquito-borne viruses in urban and suburban localities; suppression of populations of vector mosquito species can halt virus transmission during epidemics. This can be achieved by:

1. The use of insecticides to kill adult mosquitoes ('adulticiding'), e.g. aerial sprays of Malathion, although this may kill many other species.

2. The elimination of breeding sites of domestic *A. aegypti* by removal of objects such as tin cans and motor tyres that could contain rainwater, both near human habitations and in public parks and drainage systems, has prevented occurrence of dengue in Singapore and urban yellow fever in metropolitan areas in Caribbean countries.

3. The chemical control of larvae, termed 'larviciding', by use of Temephos granules or Malathion in oil for even coverage of small breeding sites, has reduced mosquito vector populations substantially in irrigated localities in California and elsewhere.

4. The biological control of larvae is attempted by microbiological agents such as *Bacillus thuringiensis israeliensis*, larvivorous fish, flatworms or mermethid nematodes, or insect growth regulators such as the juvenile hormone mimic Methoprene.

5. Personal protection against bites by mosquitoes involves a combination of wearing protective clothing, preferably impregnated with permethrin, screening of dwellings to prevent entry of mosquitoes and frequent application of mosquito repellants such as diethyl toluamide to exposed skin areas. For tick-borne viruses, protective clothing should be worn outdoors, followed by rigorous inspection to remove attached ticks from skin.

## Vaccines

Prevention of illness following exposure to arbovirus infections is restricted to relatively few serotypes.

### Encephalitis viruses

Human and animal infections due to VEE and JBE viruses have been prevented by immunization with live and killed vaccines, respectively. Although effective killed vaccines have been developed for prevention of WEE in horses, these are unsatisfactory for administration to humans.

### VEE vaccine

This is a live attenuated strain. Widespread vaccination of horses at the advancing edge of epizootics is highly effective in protecting against encephalitis in both horses and humans.

### Yellow fever

Prevention of clinical attacks of yellow fever has been outstandingly successful during the past half century through the use of attenuated YF vaccine. The 17D strain, used exclusively in the Americas, and extensively in Africa, was derived from a virulent prototype strain. Each dose of lyophilized vaccine contains 1000 mouse $LD_{50}$ of the 17D virus, which is administered subcutaneously. Vaccine recipients have demonstrated immunity to natural challenge by YF virus commencing 10 days after vaccination and persisting for at least 10 years. The FN strain derived from mouse brain-passaged YF virus has been used successfully for many years for YF immunization by scarification in certain equatorial regions of Africa. However, adverse reactions, such as fever and occasional encephalopathy, occur more commonly after vaccination with the FN strain than the 17D strain.

## RUBELLA

Rubella (German measles) was first described in the 18th century and was considered a mild illness with only occasional complications until 1941, when the association between maternal rubella in pregnancy and congenital abnormalities in the infant was described by an Australian ophthalmologist, Sir Norman Gregg. He noted an increased incidence of congenital cataracts in children. When questioned the mothers gave a history of having had rubella in early pregnancy when there had been an epidemic in Australia. Since then the importance of maternal rubella for the fetus has been confirmed by many studies.

### Description

Rubella virus was first isolated in cell culture in 1962. It is a single-stranded RNA virus with an envelope, and is classified as a togavirus, being the only member of the genus *Rubivirus*. Virions are pleomorphic in appearance and 50–70 nm in diameter with a nucleocapsid of icosahedral symmetry. Rubella

is inactivated by many chemical agents. The single-stranded RNA is infective, and replication occurs in the cytoplasm of infected cells. Virions acquire the envelope by budding from cell membranes either into intracellular vesicles or to the exterior. There are three major virion polypeptides, C and the envelope glycoproteins E1 and E2. No major antigenic difference between virus strains has been demonstrated. The virus envelope carries a haemagglutinin (E1), present as 5–6 nm projections, which will agglutinate the erythrocytes of 1-day-old chicks, pigeons, sheep and humans, a characteristic which is utilized in the haemagglutination inhibition test for specific antibodies. Experimentally, infection can be transmitted to rhesus monkeys, rabbits and some other animals, but humans are the only naturally infected species. Virus can be isolated in a range of primary and continuous cell lines, e.g. Vero, RK13 and BHK-21 cells, but in only some cell lines, such as RK13, does a cytopathic effect occur. In other cell lines the presence of virus must be demonstrated by immunofluorescence with specific antibody or by resistance to superinfection with another unrelated virus such as echovirus 11. Only one antigenic type of rubella virus is recognized, although minor differences can be found between strains.

## Clinical features and pathogenesis

### Postnatal rubella

The incubation period for postnatal primary rubella is 12–21 days, with an average of 16–17 days. Virus may be excreted in the throat for up to a week before and after the rash and this covers the period of infectivity. The characteristic clinical feature is a macular rash which usually appears first on the face and then spreads to the trunk and limbs. Particularly in childhood the rash may be fleeting and perhaps 50% of infections in children are asymptomatic. In adults, asymptomatic rubella is less common. General features such as minor pyrexia, malaise and lymphadenopathy also occur, with the suboccipital nodes being those most commonly enlarged and tender.

Arthralgia is uncommon in children but may occur in up to 60% of adult females. The joints commonly involved are the fingers, wrists, ankles and knees and, although arthralgia usually only lasts a few days, it may occasionally persist for some months. Encephalitis and thrombocytopenia are rare complications of rubella and usually recovery is complete. Unlike a number of other virus infections, rubella appears to present little danger to the immunocompromised patient, in whom the clinical features are similar to those seen in normal individuals.

Rubella reinfection is diagnosed when an antibody response is demonstrated in someone who has either had natural rubella or has been successfully immunized. Such reinfections are seldom clinically apparent and are usually found when someone is investigated after contact with rubella. It is very uncommon for fetal infection and damage to occur in subclinical reinfection. It can be difficult, however, to distinguish serologically between subclinical primary rubella, which is of major risk to the fetus, and reinfection. The rare reinfection which is clinically apparent must be assumed to present a risk to the fetus similar to that of primary rubella.

Rubella is notoriously difficult to diagnose clinically, as other virus infections, such as some enteroviruses and human parvovirus B19, can present with identical clinical features. For correct diagnosis laboratory investigation is essential and a history of rubella is an unreliable indicator of immunity unless it has been serologically confirmed.

## Congenital rubella

If the fetus is infected during a primary maternal infection a wide spectrum of abnormalities may occur. The classical congenital rubella syndrome (CRS) triad consists of abnormalities of the eyes, ears and heart. Abnormalities of the eyes, which may be bilateral or unilateral, include cataracts, micro-ophthalmia, glaucoma and pigmentary retinopathy, which may result in blindness. Bilateral or unilateral sensorineural deafness may be present at birth, although it may not be detected until later in life; it may increase in severity as the child gets older. There are many possible heart defects, with patent ductus arteriosus, pulmonary artery and valvular stenosis, and ventricular septal defect being most common.

The baby will often have a low birth weight due to intra-uterine growth retardation. A purpuric rash due to thrombocytopenia may be present at birth but this usually resolves, as does hepatosplenomegaly. Microcephaly, psychomotor retardation and behavioural disorders are manifestations of central nervous system involvement. Rarely, a persistent infection of the central nervous system occurs called *progressive rubella subacute panencephalitis*, which is similar clinically to the *subacute sclerosing panencephalitis* due to measles virus. Other problems which may not be present at birth but which may present later in life include pneumonitis, diabetes mellitus, growth hormone deficiency and abnormalities of thyroid function.

The fetus may be so severely affected that intra-uterine death with abortion or stillbirth occurs. Many infected babies, however, are born with no abnormalities, and the risk to the fetus depends on the gestational period in which primary rubella occurs. If maternal rubella occurs in the first trimester the risk is considerable, as more than 70% of babies will be affected and have some or many of the abnormalities described above. If rubella occurs in the 4th month of pregnancy the risk reduces to approximately 20%, and the only abnormality likely to be seen is sensorineural deafness. Maternal rubella before conception is unlikely to harm the fetus. After the 16th week of pregnancy, although fetal infection still occurs, congenital abnormalities are very infrequent and no more likely to occur than in an apparently uncomplicated pregnancy.

## Pathogenesis

Rubella virus is transmitted by the air-borne route. Infection is established in the upper respiratory tract, and, towards the end of the incubation period, a viraemia occurs and seeds the target organs such as the skin and joints. Most of the clinical features are probably a consequence of the host's immune response to the virus, e.g. virus can be demonstrated not only in individual lesions of the macular rash but also in unaffected skin. During the viraemia the virus is able to infect the placenta and cross this barrier to infect the differentiating cells of the fetus. If such fetal infection occurs in early pregnancy a persistent infection is likely. The congenital abnormalities arise from a number of effects of the virus infection. Cell division is slowed, cell differentiation is disordered and damage to small blood vessels may occur. Such effects may lead to the abnormalities seen at birth, but the persistence of infection may result in the clinical problems presenting later in life, either due to direct damage, such as late-onset deafness, or due to immunopathological mechanisms, such as pneumonitis. Virus can persist for many years in babies infected during early gestation, but persistent infection is rare in later pregnancy when the babies are not damaged.

## Diagnosis

### Postnatal rubella

Clinical diagnosis is notoriously unreliable, and laboratory investigation is required if a diagnosis of

**Fig. 52.4**  Serological response in primary rubella.

rubella has important implications, such as in the pregnant patient. As subclinical rubella may occur, pregnant women should also be investigated if they are exposed to someone with possible rubella. Investigation by virus isolation is not indicated as it is unreliable and time-consuming. Serological diagnosis is the method of choice, using techniques to detect total rubella antibody or rubella-specific IgG, and rubella-specific IgM. In primary rubella, specific antibody becomes detectable about the time of the rash, although there may be a delay of 7–10 days, and rapidly increases in concentration (Fig. 52.4). Specific IgM usually, but not always, precedes specific IgG by 1–2 days, but unlike specific IgG, which persists for life, specific IgM is usually only detectable for 1–3 months. Thus, seroconversion may be demonstrated if a serum is obtained soon after contact, prior to the illness, and is examined in parallel with a sample collected at or soon after the rash; primary infection is confirmed by the development of specific IgM. If serum is collected after the rash or more than 12–14 days after contact, any total rubella antibody or specific IgG may have resulted from recent infection or infection many years previously. Tests for specific IgM must be used to determine if the infection was recent.

Tests for total rubella antibody or rubella-specific IgG are also used for serological screening to ascertain susceptibility and whether rubella immunization is indicated. Many assays of appropriate sensitivity and specificity are available. False-positive results must be avoided as a susceptible woman would not be immunized and may not be investigated if contact or illness occurs.

### Congenital rubella

The majority of babies with congenital rubella syndrome excrete large amounts of virus for the first few months of life and, indeed, are highly infectious for their attendants. Thus, virus isolation in cell culture from throat swab or urine is indicated although many laboratories may not have appropriate cell lines readily available. A more sensitive and widely available technique in the first 3–6 months of life is serological testing for specific IgM. Maternal IgM does not cross the placenta so the detection of specific IgM is diagnostic of intra-uterine infection. Specific IgG crosses the placenta from the mother so its detection in the early months of life is no help in diagnosis. Maternal IgG has a half-life in the infant of 3–4 weeks, however, so persistence to the age of 9–12 months is diagnostic of congenital rubella. It is uncommon for the specific IgM to persist to 1 year of age. Occasionally, if an older child presents with deafness, a diagnosis of possible congenital rubella may be suspected. It is impossible, however, to discriminate specific IgG resulting from intra-uterine infection from that persisting after postnatal infection, so the reliable diagnosis of congenital infection in older children is impossible.

## Epidemiology

Rubella has a world-wide distribution with infection being endemic in all countries which have not had a highly successful infant immunization policy. Outbreaks usually occur in spring and early summer, with major epidemics occurring every 4–8 years. Infection is common in childhood. Before immunization in the UK, 80–85% of young adults would have had rubella. With rubella vaccine being offered to all adolescent girls in the UK only approximately 2–5% of young adult females are now susceptible, compared with 15% of young adult males.

## Control

### Passive prophylaxis

There is little evidence that administering normal human immunoglobulin after contact reduces the risk of maternal rubella and fetal infection, although it may attenuate the illness.

### Active prophylaxis

Attenuated live rubella virus vaccines have been widely available since the early 1970s. They are safe, although occasional fleeting rashes and arthralgia occur. Seroconversion occurs in over 95% of susceptible vaccinees and protection persists for more than 15 years. Although vaccine virus may be isolated from the throat of vaccinees, there is no evidence of transmission to susceptible contacts. As it is a live virus vaccine, administration in pregnancy is contra-indicated, and pregnancy should be avoided for the month following immunization. Although the vaccine virus has been shown to infect the fetus, there is no evidence of teratogenicity, so if a susceptible pregnant woman is inadvertently immunized she should be reassured that the risk to her baby is very remote. It is advisable, however, that all women of child-bearing age are screened for rubella antibody before immunization so that only susceptible women are offered vaccine.

The objective of rubella immunization is to eradicate congenital rubella. Two possible approaches are possible. In the UK it was decided in the early 1970s to target the vaccine at girls aged 11–14 years and susceptible adult women, identified by screening all pregnant women and women attending such facilities as family planning clinics, occupational health services and on the initiative of general practitioners. Such a policy was adopted because of uncertainties about the duration of protection and the belief that women would have better protection from having had natural rubella; 50% of adolescent girls would have had natural rubella. It was also thought that vaccine-induced protection would be boosted by occasional exposure to natural rubella. It became apparent in the late 1980s that such a policy would never achieve eradication as 10–20 cases of congenital rubella and 100–200 terminations of pregnancy still occurred each year in the UK. In the second approach, which was adopted in 1988, all children are immunized in an attempt to eradicate rubella from the community and so avoid exposure of any pregnant woman who is susceptible. Thus, the immunization schedule was augmented by offering rubella vaccine together with mumps and measles vaccine (MMR vaccine) to all children at 15 months of age. For a few years, mumps, measles and rubella vaccine were also offered to children at school entry. Support for such a strategy comes from the success achieved in almost eliminating congenital rubella in the USA by offering rubella vaccine to all children in the 2nd year of life. To achieve such success, however, means that there must be at least a 90% uptake of vaccine in infancy.

## HEPATITIS C AND RELATED VIRUSES

Once reliable diagnostic tests for hepatitis A and B infections had been developed it was evident that there were other, presumed viral, causes of infectious hepatitis. The cumbersome name *non-A, non-B hepatitis* (NANB) was coined for these conditions. Epidemiological studies established that there were two routes of transmission of NANB hepatitis; thus enteric (see hepatitis E virus, p. 528) and parenteral or post-transfusion forms were recognized. Hepatitis C virus is now established as the major cause of the parenteral type. More recently, other related agents, including hepatitis G virus, have been identified. The ability of hepatitis C virus to infect chimpanzees was used to define the basic features of the virus: a diameter of less than 80 nm and susceptibility to organic solvents. High-titre plasma from infected chimps was the starting point for the identification of the virus. RNA was extracted from the plasma, and reverse transcribed to give a DNA copy; this was then cloned and expressed in *Escherichia coli*. Numerous clones had to be tested before one was found whose protein product reacted with antibody present in the sera of well-documented cases of NANB hepatitis. It is this antigen and others discovered in the same way that are used in antibody assays for the diagnosis of infection. The complete genetic sequence has now been determined.

## Description

### Classification

Based on genetic analysis, hepatitis C and G viruses are related to the *flaviviruses*, and it is now proposed that these viruses should be placed in a third genus of the Flaviviridae to be called *Hepacivirus*. Further classification into subgenera awaits further information. The grounds for the classification are: similar genome size (9379 bases); viral-encoded glycoproteins in the envelope; viral RNA of positive sense and containing one large open-reading frame; the polyprotein produced is cleaved by cell and viral proteases to produce structural (core and envelope) and six non-structural proteins; similar structure of those parts of the genome involved in replication (located in untranslated regions at both ends of the genome). In general, hepatitis C virus resembles the pestiviruses more closely than the flaviviruses (*Pestivirus* being the other genus in the family).

Electron microscope images are not clear, but it appears that the virus has a diameter of 55–65 nm and consists of a core containing the viral RNA enclosed within an envelope containing glycoproteins as short spikes.

Comparison of the genomes of different viruses shows that there are variable regions that can be used to divide them into six genotypes with about 70% sequence identity, with related subtypes.

The viruses are readily inactivated by organic solvents, detergents and heat. It has proved to be very difficult to grow the virus in cell cultures.

## Clinical features

The disease has an incubation period of 6–10 weeks and is usually mild; it may often only be diagnosed by biochemical studies of liver function. Only 5% of patients become jaundiced, and fulminant hepatitis is rare. Chronic infection occurs in 80% of cases and typically runs a variable course with fluctuation in the extent of liver damage. Chronic liver damage can progress to cirrhosis and hepatocellular carcinoma. Progression is slow, taking 10 years for cirrhosis and 15 years for carcinoma to develop. Some patients may have persistent mild hepatitis for 30 years. Progression can be more rapid in the immunocompromised.

## Pathogenesis

Histologically, hepatitis C virus causes a range of changes in the liver, although a specific diagnosis is not always possible. In chronic cases, 40% show persistent features, 40% chronic active hepatitis and 20% cirrhosis. Viral proteins and RNA can be detected in the cytoplasm of hepatocytes, but only 1% of cells are productively infected.

Antibody and T cell responses can be detected, but are usually unable to clear the virus and do not protect against reinfection even with the same strain of virus. Variation of the envelope glycoproteins may aid persistence as may the binding of virus to lipids. Immunosuppressed patients show enhanced liver disease indicating a direct cytotoxic effect of the virus.

Viral replication can be detected in lymphoid cells. Infection has been linked to several other states, such as immune complex deposition (vasculitis and glomerulonephritis) and Sjögren's disease.

## Laboratory diagnosis

The presence of antibody to various viral antigens indicates that the patient has been infected with the virus and in most cases this means that there is a chronic infection. Commercial ELISAs are available using recombinant proteins or peptides as antigens. Reactive results should be confirmed by different assays. Currently available assays will detect chronic infections but are less sensitive in the early stages of

infection when there may be a 'window' of up to 3 months before tests become positive.

An alternative approach is to detect viral RNA by amplification of DNA after reverse–transcription polymerase chain reaction (RT–PCR).

## Epidemiology

### Transmission

The disease was first recognized in recipients of blood and blood products such as factor VIII and immunoglobulin. The prevalence of infection varies considerably in different parts of the world. In areas with a low prevalence, intravenous drug use is a risk factor, with most infected. Older haemophiliacs are usually infected, but the introduction of donor screening and heat treatment of blood products has eliminated this risk. Transplanted organs and needlestick injuries have been implicated in transmission. There is a small risk through sexual contact and mother-to-baby transfer is also low. However both risks may be increased in the immunocompromised.

### Geographical variation

Infection appears to have been introduced into Europe and North America in the 1960s and is found in about 1% of blood donors. In other parts of the world the virus is more widespread, although it is not known how the virus is transmitted. Infection with genotypes 1, 2 and 3 is common in Europe and North America although they are present world-wide, with the types found in different age groups. Type 4 is frequent in Central Africa, with a prevalence of 20–30% in Egypt. Type 5 is found in South Africa; in the East, type 6a has a restricted location in Hong Kong and Vietnam.

## Control

Neither active nor passive immunization is available. Screening of blood donations, exclusion of those identified as at risk and heat treatment of blood products should eliminate the risk of transmission from this source. Transmission risk exists among injecting drug users and from the re-use of unsterile needles.

### Antiviral treatment

α-Interferon is widely used to treat chronic cases, but high doses (3–6 mega-units, thrice weekly) and long-term treatment (6–12 months) are needed.

The response to interferon is shown by improved liver enzyme levels and reduced viral load in the blood. However, only 50% will respond initially with about 50% of this group relapsing when therapy stops. Overall about 20% will show a sustained response. Combination therapy of interferon with drugs such as tribavirin may give a better result. As interferon is expensive and has significant side-effects, it would be a major advance to be able to select for treatment only those patients who have the greatest chance of responding. Factors such as age, length of carriage, virus genotype, cirrhosis and virus load can influence the outcome. In particular, infection with type 1b, cirrhosis and high virus load are associated with a poor response.

## Liver transplantation

A transplant may be necessary in those with advanced disease, both cirrhosis alone or accompanying hepatocellular carcinoma. Infection of the graft usually occurs.

## Other viruses

Viruses known as GBV-A and GBV-B were isolated from tamarin monkeys inoculated with the blood of a surgeon ('G.B.') who had a chronic hepatitis of unknown cause. These viruses are related to hepatitis C virus on sequence analysis but are believed to have come from the monkey. Another virus, GBV-C, and hepatitis G virus have been found in humans with chronic hepatitis; these viruses are probably identical. Little is known about the association of the human viruses with disease. Infection is more frequent in injecting drug users and haemophiliacs. A link with fulminant hepatitis has been claimed. Hepatitis G virus does not appear to elicit a strong immune response.

There are reports of the detection of further viruses, but these are not yet substantiated; their role in disease is also not established.

## RECOMMENDED READING

Best J M, Banatvala J E 1994 Rubella. In: Zuckerman A J, Banatvala J E, Pattison J R (eds) *Principles and Practice of Clinical Virology*, 3rd edn. Wiley, Chichester

Brown J L 1995 Hepatitis C; the structure and biology of the virus and diagnostic tests. *Journal of Infection* 30: 95–101

Davis G L, Lau J Y 1995 Choice of appropriate end points of response to interferon therapy in chronic hepatitis C virus infection. *Journal of Hepatology* 22 (1 Suppl): 110–4

Ksiazek T G, Peters C J, Rollin P E et al 1995 Identification of a new North American hantavirus that causes acute pulmonary insufficiency. *American Journal of Tropical Medicine and Hygiene* 52: 117–123

McLean D M 1988 *Virological Infections*. Thomas, Springfield, IL

Miller E, Cradock-Watson J E, Pollock T M 1982 Consequences of confirmed maternal rubella at successive stages of pregnancy. *Lancet* ii: 781–784

Miller C L, Miller E, Waight P A 1987 Rubella susceptibility and the continuing risk of infection in pregnancy. *British Medical Journal* 294: 1277–1278

Public Health Laboratory Service Working Party 1988 Laboratory diagnosis of rubella. *PHLS Microbiology Digest* 5: 49–52

Report 1985 *Arthropod-Borne and Rodent-Borne Viral Diseases. WHO Technical Report Series*, No. 719. World Health Organization, Geneva

Simmonds P 1995 Variability of hepatitis C virus. *Hepatology* 21: 570–583

Vodkin M H, McLaughlin G L, Day J F, Shope R E, Novak R J 1993 A rapid diagnostic assay for eastern equine encephalomyelitis viral RNA. *American Journal of Tropical Medicine and Hygiene* 49: 772–776

# 53

# Arenaviruses and filoviruses

**Lassa fever; Marburg and Ebola fevers**

*J. F. Peutherer*

Members of the two unrelated RNA virus families Arenaviridae and Filoviridae cause severe infections in humans. The clinical features can include fever and haemorrhage, and so they are causes of *viral haemorrhagic fever*. Other viruses associated with a similar presentation are described in Chapter 52 on insect-borne viruses.

## ARENAVIRUSES

## PROPERTIES

In the virions of this family the RNA is single stranded and of negative sense and exists as two molecules, the L and S segments. The total molecular weight is between $3.2 \times 10^6$ and $4.8 \times 10^6$ and there is an associated RNA transcriptase. Morphologically the virions consist of an envelope enclosing the helical RNA nucleocapsid; they vary considerably in size, ranging from about 100 to 150 nm in diameter (Fig. 53.1). The virions usually enclose some cell ribosomes during assembly and thus gain their characteristic grainy appearance in the electron microscope (*arena* is the Latin for sand). There are at least four virion polypeptides, some of which are glycosylated and found in the envelope as short surface projections. The arenaviruses of importance to man are the South American *Junin* and *Machupo* viruses; several others are grouped as the *African Tacaribe complex*. However, *Lassa fever virus* is the important virus in Africa. Antigenic cross-reactions can be shown between the viruses. *Lymphocytic choriomeningitis (LCM) virus* has been much studied in the laboratory because of the effect of the age of the animal and its immune status on the

a          b

**Fig. 53.1** **a** Lassa fever virus. **b** Lassa fever virus cross section showing granular appearance of cell ribosomes.

disease presentation after experimental inoculation. It is not a major human pathogen although cases of meningitis have been described. It is world-wide in distribution.

## REPLICATION

Viruses can be grown in several mammalian cell cultures, but vero (grivet monkey kidney) and BHK (hamster kidney) are widely used. A minimal cytopathic effect is produced, and cytoplasmic inclusion bodies are formed. A role for the cell nucleus in viral replication has been proposed and nucleocapsids can be detected within the nucleus. The coding on the genome is antisense; this means that genes can be expressed and regulated independently. Thus the expression of the nucleocapsid (N) protein can be separated from that of the envelope glycoprotein (GPC) although both genes are on the S strand of RNA. Hairpin sequences are present in the viral RNA and the complementary strand, and these may interrupt the progression of the viral RNA polymerase and thus affect gene expression. It has been shown that during infection RNA molecules consisting of sequences from both the viral RNA and host cell ribosomal RNA (rRNA) are produced. Both the L and S molecules contain sequences which bind the 18S subunit of rRNA.

The N protein is the major component of the virion and of infected cells where it is detectable within a few hours after infection and remains so even after virus synthesis has declined. Viral glycoproteins are detectable on cell membranes also within a few hours of infection. Persistently infected cultures arise readily.

## CLINICAL FEATURES AND PATHOGENESIS

### South American haemorrhagic fevers

Argentinian and Bolivian haemorrhagic fevers are caused by Junin and Machupo viruses, respectively. The incubation period is 1–2 weeks with a 'flu-like' prodromal illness. In serious cases, petechiae develop and the patient bleeds from the gastro-intestinal tract. Fluid is lost from the circulation, and hypotension and oliguria may ensue. Encephalopathy occurs in many patients. The mortality rate varies in different outbreaks, but is within the range 5–30%, usually with death due to hypovolaemic shock.

The viruses are widespread in the body, and at post mortem there is evidence of lymphadenopathy, lymphocyte loss from the spleen and bone marrow and endothelial damage in small blood vessels. Haemorrhage is related to the capillary damage and platelet dysfunction. During the earlier stages, there is a drop in the number of circulating leucocytes and platelets, resulting from infection of bone marrow precursor cells. About half of those infected have evidence of neurological damage, with tremor as a feature in most cases. There is some evidence that there are differences in tissue tropism, in that neurological involvement may be a feature with some virus strains.

### Lassa fever

The incubation period is 1–3 weeks, with an insidious onset of fever, headache, muscle and joint pain: pharyngitis is usually present, with an unproductive cough. Electrocardiogram abnormalities are common. Within a few days the fever increases, and the patient complains of abdominal and retrosternal pain, diarrhoea and vomiting. The patient is lethargic, with oedema of the face and neck and lymphadenopathy. The blood pressure is often low. Recovery is within 1–3 weeks. In fatal cases the fever is maintained, and deterioration occurs rapidly within the first 2 weeks. This is associated with hypovolaemia, pleural effusion, ascites and anuria. At post-mortem examination there is often liver damage. A poor prognosis is associated with bleeding from the nose, gums, gut and vagina, linked to platelet dysfunction which is associated with an inhibitory factor in plasma. Neurological complications are also a poor prognostic sign, particularly an encephalopathy rather than the tinnitus and deafness seen in about one-third of patients. The disease is especially severe in the later stages of pregnancy with a mortality rate of 20%, which is reduced if the pregnancy terminates.

There is an early drop in the lymphocyte and platelet counts. Endothelial cells are damaged, leading to a loss of fluid from the circulation. Specific antibodies are produced to the virus but, unlike the South American fevers, this is not associated with clearance of the virus: neutralizing antibodies are usually absent. Viraemia can persist for some weeks in those who make a slow recovery and rises to high levels in fatal cases. The level of viraemia is greater in Lassa fever than in South American haemorrhagic fevers.

## Lymphocytic choriomeningitis virus

LCM virus occurs throughout the world in rodents, and most recognized human infections have been acquired from contact with laboratory animals such as mice and hamsters. Clinically apparent infections are rare but may present as a non-specific febrile illness, meningitis or encephalitis. The incubation period is 1–2 weeks, and the illness is usually of short duration. Long-term effects have been described, and include headache, paralysis and psychological changes. There is little evidence for the involvement of the host immune system in the pathogenesis of the disease, and the effects are probably due to virus replication. LCM virus can be isolated directly from the brain at post-mortem.

In contrast, LCM virus infection of mice has been studied extensively due to the importance of the immune response in pathogenesis. Thus, if mice are infected within 24 h of birth they do not develop acute disease but become carriers for the rest of their lives. This reflects the lack of an effective immune response at this stage of development of the mouse. In contrast, inoculation of the adult mouse leads to a fatal choriomeningitis due to the activity of cell-mediated immune responses directed to a region of CP2, one of the envelope glycoproteins expressed on the surface of infected cells. Mice infected early in life do not become tolerant to the virus as specific antibody is produced. However, this may be difficult to detect as it is bound in antigen–antibody complexes in the circulation; some of these are deposited in tissues such as the kidney to cause a chronic nephritis.

## DIAGNOSIS

It is important to remember that the viruses of the Tacaribe complex and Lassa fever virus are classified as hazard group 4 pathogens because of the severity of the diseases they cause. This means that they can only be cultured in specially secure laboratories. Suspicion of the diagnosis must depend on the history and clinical features, although these may be difficult to distinguish from those of other infections such as malaria, typhoid fever, *Streptococcus pyogenes* infection, trypanosomiasis, listeriosis and typhus. Laboratory tests to exclude these infections must also be carried out in designated laboratories.

Both virus isolation and serology are useful in establishing the specific diagnosis. Lassa fever virus can be grown in Vero cells inoculated with blood and urine, both in the acute stages and for some months thereafter. Viral antigen detection in blood is also possible. The titre of the viraemia is of prognostic significance, as is the level of the aminotransferase enzymes released from the damaged liver. Serological tests show that IgM appears early in the response, to be replaced by IgG; paired sera should be collected for examination. Reverse-transcriptase polymerase chain reaction can be used for early diagnosis.

In human cases of LCM virus infection, the cerebrospinal fluid shows the changes associated with viral meningitis. Virus can be grown from the cerebrospinal fluid, blood and brain.

## TREATMENT

Passive immunization with plasma has been shown to be effective if given within the first few days of infection with Junin virus and in some cases of Lassa fever. Specific therapy with tribavirin can be beneficial. In severe cases it is given intravenously and, if started within 6 days of the fever, the prognosis is improved five-fold. Exchange transfusion has been associated with marked clinical and laboratory improvement.

## EPIDEMIOLOGY AND TRANSMISSION

All the arenaviruses infect rodent species. With LCM virus, mice and hamsters are the reservoirs. The route of transmission to man is probably from urine through breaks in the skin or mucous membranes; the oral route is also a possibility.

Field voles are the reservoir of Junin virus, and another species of vole is the host for Machupo virus. Seasonal variations in the incidence of human cases can be related to peaks in the host population numbers. As with LCM virus, the routes of transmission are not established.

Lassa fever was first recognized in 1969 in Nigeria; the initial case, a nurse, may have become infected from a patient, and probably herself infected two of the staff who cared for her. The virus also infected one of the laboratory investigators who made the first isolation. Further outbreaks based on case-to-case transmission in hospitals occurred. Several outbreaks have been recorded with mortality rates in excess of 40% associated with transmission within hospitals, all in West Africa. The natural host is the multimammate rat, *Mastomys natalensis*, which is widely distributed in the region. A persistent infection is established in rats soon after birth, and they excrete virus thereafter, especially in the urine. It is now established that infection of man is widespread in endemic areas, with only a 1–2% mortality; however, this will produce many deaths. As described, infection may be acquired directly from patients, but the virus is not readily transmitted by the respiratory route. Person-to-person transmission is associated with blood and body fluid contact and inoculation injuries.

## CONTROL

Candidate vaccine strains to protect against Junin virus have been produced, but require further development. It is not possible at present to control the natural reservoirs, although the increases in human cases noted when the rodent population increases suggest that it might be a useful approach. The only protection available is against contamination with rodent excreta. This ought to be possible in colonies of laboratory animals to protect handlers against LCM virus infection but is a very difficult task in the endemic areas of Africa and South America for the haemorrhagic fever viruses.

Suspected and confirmed cases must be cared for in strict isolation in designated hospitals to prevent exposure of the attendant staff to the high levels of virus present in acutely ill patients, especially those with Lassa fever.

## FILOVIRUSES

## PROPERTIES

The two members of the family Filoviridae, *Marburg* and *Ebola* viruses, are enveloped, single-stranded negative-sense RNA virions. The RNA is a single molecule with a molecular weight of between $3.5 \times 10^6$ and $4.5 \times 10^6$, and the helical nucleocapsid is enclosed within an envelope. Overall the virion is tubular in appearance, with a diameter of 80 nm but varying in length from 800 to several thousand nanometres, and may sometimes have a branched or ring structure (Fig. 53.2). The surface spikes are 7 nm high. The nucleocapsid has a dense central core and regular cross-striations. There are seven peptides associated with the virion, including nucleoproteins, transcriptase and membrane proteins. There is minor antigenic overlap between Marburg and Ebola viruses.

**Fig. 53.2**  Ebola virus.

## REPLICATION

Virus can be cultured in the Vero cell line, and in many other cell types. The strategy of replication is similar to that of the paramyxo- and rhabdoviruses. Nucleocapsids accumulate in the cell cytoplasm to form inclusion bodies; virus matures and is released by budding of the nucleocapsid from the plasma membrane. Large numbers of virions are released from cells which are destroyed in the process.

## CLINICAL FEATURES AND PATHOGENESIS

The first features of infection are of a non-specific 'flu-like' illness with fever, malaise, muscle aches and headache: conjunctivitis and bradycardia also occur. The onset is rapid, as is the progression with increased myalgia and diarrhoea with abdominal pain: some patients develop a rash. Death can ensue rapidly in 50–80% of cases. The incubation period is 3–7 days; bleeding starts at about 5–7 days and death at 7–16 days.

The liver is a major site of infection, although the virus can infect most tissues in the body, resulting in high levels of virus in the blood. The cause of death is shock associated with fluid or blood loss into the tissues. Petechiae and bleeding are linked to abnormal platelet function and damage to the vascular endothelium. One of the early features is a severe loss of lymphocytes from the circulation while, at the same time, the polymorph count may rise to $20 \times 10^9/1$.

The fatality rate does vary and appears to be greatest in primary cases acquired from animal sources; cases arising from person-to-person transfer may not have such a high mortality.

Circulating antibodies are produced within 10–14 days, but it is difficult to demonstrate neutralizing antibodies in convalescent cases. This implies that cell-mediated immune responses must be important in recovery, although the virus is directly cytotoxic.

In the infected tissues, filamentous structures can be seen in the cytoplasm of cells: the lungs, kidneys and liver show the greatest involvement and virions are present in large numbers in the damaged hepatocytes and in the bile canaliculi.

## DIAGNOSIS

Virus isolation from blood samples can be made by inoculation of cell cultures; cytoplasmic inclusion bodies develop in which viral antigen accumulates. Although guinea-pigs are susceptible, Vero cells are suitable for virus cultures. The virions can be seen by electron microscopical examination of the blood in the early acute stage of Ebola fever. Antibodies are usually detectable 7–10 days after the onset. As these viruses are hazard group 4 pathogens, virus culture must only be attempted in designated national laboratories.

## TREATMENT

Supportive treatment is all that can be offered to patients as there is no specific therapy. No vaccines are available to give long-term protection. Passive immunization immediately after exposure and interferon therapy have been used, but their value is not established.

## EPIDEMIOLOGY AND TRANSMISSION

The routes of transmission of the viruses are unknown, as are their natural hosts. Both occur in Africa. The Marburg virus was isolated from a patient with a severe haemorrhagic illness in 1967. This was one of 31 cases which occurred in Marburg, Germany, and the former Yugoslavia in persons who had been in contact with the blood and tissues from a batch of African green monkeys from Uganda. In total, seven patients died. Spread to hospital staff occurred and transmission via sexual intercourse was identified in one case 83 days after the initial illness in the index patient. Ebola fever was first described in 1977, when an outbreak occurred in Zaire and Sudan. More recently, extensive outbreaks have been seen in Zaire. There was a high fatality rate – both in the cases and their hospital contacts who were probably infected by the use of contaminated injection equipment and close contact with blood and other body fluids. Several small outbreaks and sporadic cases were recognized in Africa. The natural host is not known as most primates suffer a severe infection like humans. There is no serological evidence of infection in wild monkeys. Human infection with recovery is implied by the finding of antibodies in some human populations. Studies in the Central African Republic showed a 24% prevalence of antibodies to Ebola and 3% to Marburg virus. An outbreak has been recognized in wild chimpanzees in the Ivory Coast.

## CONTROL

The only approach to the control of these dangerous infections is by application of strict precautions in patient management, and in the laboratory. The handling of primates and their tissues can be made safe by quarantine of the animals before use. The most difficult decision in the control of hospital-acquired infection is when to institute rigorous isolation of a patient who may present with non- specific clinical features and a history of travel to equatorial Africa.

---

## RECOMMENDED READING

Evans A S 1989 *Viral Infections of Humans; Epidemiology and Control*, 3rd edn. Plenum Press, New York

Fields B N, Knipe D M Howley P M (eds) 1996 *Virology*, 3rd edn. Lippincott-Raven, Philadelphia

# 54

# Reoviruses

**Gastro-enteritis**

*U. Desselberger*

Reoviridae is a diverse family of viruses that infect humans, other vertebrates (including birds), plants and insects. The genus *Rotavirus* is recognized as the most important cause of infantile gastro-enteritis throughout the world. Viruses in the genera *Orbivirus* and *Coltivirus* infect various species of insects and can thus be described as arboviruses; they are discussed in Chapter 52.

transcribes the negative strand and as isolated RNA is not infectious. All reoviruses replicate in the cytoplasm of infected cells and form intra-cytoplasmic inclusion bodies. Whereas orthoreo-viruses and rotaviruses are relatively stable over a wide pH range, orbiviruses and coltiviruses lose infectivity at low pH.

## CLASSIFICATION

Four out of the nine genera of the family Reoviridae infect humans:

- *Orthoreovirus* – reovirus types 1, 2, and 3
- *Orbivirus* and *Coltivirus* – various serogroups
- *Rotavirus* – several groups, multiple serotypes.

All reoviruses have a double-shelled capsid, no envelope and measure 75–80 nm in diameter. The main features are listed in Table 54.1. The RNA genome consists of 10–12 segments of double-stranded RNA. Functionally, reoviruses can be regarded as negative-stranded viruses, as the virion-associated RNA polymerase early in replication only

## REPLICATION

Attachment is via a specific protein component of the outer capsid, e.g. σ1 of orthoreoviruses or VP4 of rotaviruses, to a cellular receptor (the β-adrenergic receptor and sialoglycoproteins for orthoreoviruses, and sialoglycoproteins for rotaviruses). The viral protein–receptor interaction leads to a conformational change in the viral capsid, which enters the cell by receptor-mediated endocytosis or direct penetration. In the cytoplasm the outer capsid is removed (uncoating), but the viral RNA remains in the inner capsid (subviral particle, SVP). RNA is transcribed by the virion-associated, RNA-dependent RNA polymerase complex to produce messenger RNA (mRNA)

**Table 54.1** Classification and features of genera of the Reoviridae infecting man

| | Reovirus genus | | | |
| --- | --- | --- | --- | --- |
| | *Orthoreovirus* | *Rotavirus* | *Orbivirus* | *Coltivirus* |
| Size (nm) | 80 | 75 | 80 | 80 |
| No. of RNA segments | 10 | 11 | 10 | 12 |
| Molecular weight of genomes (Da) | $15.5 \times 10^6$ | $12.2 \times 10^6$ | $12.7 \times 10^6$ | $\sim18 \times 10^6$ |
| Host range | Humans, other vertebrates | Humans, other vertebrates | Humans, other vertebrates, arthropods | Humans, other vertebrates, arthropods |

molecules from each RNA segment. The mRNA molecules leave the SVP and are translated to generate the various viral proteins, but also act as templates for RNA replication, which is completed within new core structures by the associated RNA polymerase complex. Particle assembly takes place in the cytoplasm, and aggregates of core particles and SVP may be detected histologically as inclusion bodies. Mature virions (double-shelled particles) are formed in the endoplasmic reticulum and are released after cellular lysis.

## CLINICAL FEATURES AND EPIDEMIOLOGY

The first human isolates of this virus family were made from both respiratory secretions and faeces but could not be associated with disease – hence the name *reoviruses* (*r*espiratory *e*nteric *o*rphan) was proposed. However, orthoreoviruses cause systemic disease (meningitis and encephalitis) in mice, and this virus–host system has been used extensively to dissect different steps and mechanisms of viral pathogenesis at a molecular level.

Viral pathogenicity turns out to be a multifactorial phenotype. Although most of the population is exposed to and develops antibodies against orthoreoviruses from an early age, there is still no clear link between these viruses and illness in humans.

The orbiviruses include several serogroups which infect humans and which are transmitted by a variety of insects (ticks, midges and mosquitoes). In the blood the virus is associated with erythrocytes, and in this way hidden from immune responses. Clinically, patients experience a febrile illness, with rashes in 10% and leucopenia in two-thirds of the cases. Infections of the central nervous system leading to meningitis or encephalitis are seen in 3–7% of laboratory-certified cases.

## ROTAVIRUSES

Rotaviruses are the main viral cause of acute gastro-enteritis in infants and young children, and although the infection is usually mild it has a high mortality in developing countries. Rotaviruses also cause diarrhoea in the young of a wide variety of mammals and birds. Since the early 1980s outbreaks of diarrhoea in children and adults have been observed in different parts of China and have been found to be caused by a rotavirus (*a*dult *d*iarrhoea *rota*virus, ADRV).

## Description and classification

Morphologically, rotaviruses are polyhedrons of 75 nm diameter displaying characteristic sharp-edged double-shelled capsids which in electron micrographs (Fig. 54.1) look like spokes grouped around the hub of a wheel (Latin, *rota*), and the name 'rotavirus' was derived from this appearance, which is pathognomonic. More detailed structural studies have shown (Figs 54.2 and 54.3) that the double-shelled capsid is penetrated by a large number of channels and that it carries on the surface 60 protrusions which consist of dimers of VP4 (viral protein 4) molecules (see below).

The genome of rotaviruses is located inside the inner core and consists of 11 segments of double-stranded RNA (Table 54.1) which can be easily extracted from viruses and separated by polyacrylamide gel electrophoresis (Fig. 54.4). All segments except one code for only one virus-specific protein (VP), and gene–protein assignments have been completed for several rotavirus strains.

RNA segments 1, 2 and 3 code for the inner core proteins VP1, VP2 and VP3, respectively; VP2 is the main scaffolding protein (inner layer). RNA segment 6 codes for the inner capsid protein, VP6, which forms a middle layer interacting with the core protein VP2 and the outer capsid proteins (see below) and carries epitopes specifying groups and subgroups. So far, seven different groups (A–G) have been identified, for groups A–E complete lack of serological cross-reactivity has been proven. Within a group, all viruses share common VP6 antigens but may be further differentiated into subgroups. Thus, within group A there are at least four subgroups (I; II; I+II; non-I, non-II) which are identified by specific antisera and monoclonal antibodies. Most of the human rotaviruses are of group A; the Chinese ADRV is of group B; group C rotaviruses cause occasional outbreaks in humans. The outer capsid (third layer) is formed by two proteins, VP7, a glycoprotein (coded for by RNA 7, 8 or 9, depending on strain), and VP4 (coded for by RNA 4). Both surface proteins carry neutralization-specific epitopes which define serotypes. VP4 is post-translationally cleaved into the VP5* and VP8* subunits; proteolytic cleavage is essential for infectivity. Five non-structural proteins (NSP1–NSP5) are coded for by RNAs 5, 7, 8 or 9 (depending on strain), 10 and 11, and have various functions during replication.

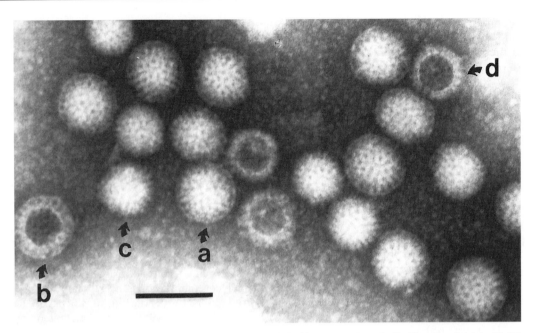

**Fig. 54.1**   Rotavirus particles in the faeces of a child admitted to hospital with acute gastro-enteritis. Negative staining with 2% potassium phosphotungstate, pH 7.0. The scale bar represents 100 nm. Examples of four different morphological forms are arrowed: **a**, double-shelled (ds) particle containing RNA; **b**, ds particle without RNA ('empty'; core penetrated with stain); **c**, single-shelled (ss) particle containing RNA; **d**, ss empty particle. (By courtesy of M. Jenkins, Regional Virus Laboratory, East Birmingham Hospital.)

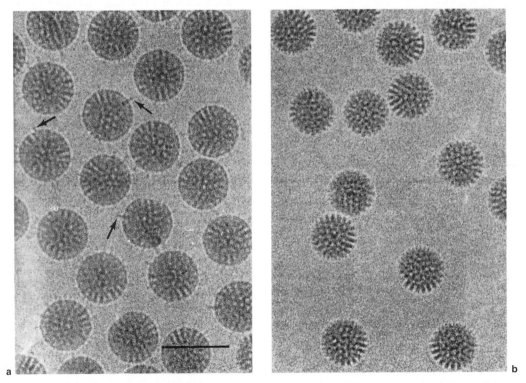

**Fig. 54.2**   **a** Double-shelled and **b** single-shelled rotavirus particles visualized by cryo-electron microscopy. The arrows indicate spikes (VP4) protruding from the surface of double-shelled particles. The scale bar represents 100 nm. (From Prasad et al 1988 *Journal of Molecular Biology* 199: 269–275, with permission from the authors and publishers.)

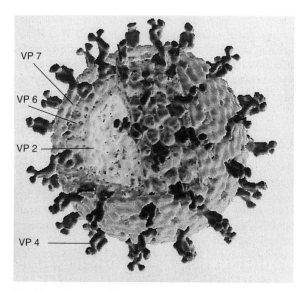

**Fig. 54.3** Diagram of the three-dimensional structure of rotavirus particles derived from cryo-electron microscopy images. Core layer (VP2); inner capsid (VP6); outer capsid (VP7; with inserted dimeric VP4 spikes) shown as a whole particle with partial removal of capsid layers to illustrate the interaction of VP2 with VP6, VP6 with VP7, VP4 with VP7 and VP6. The outer and inner capsids are perforated by 132 holes of three types of symmetry. (From Yeager M et al 1994 *EMBO Journal* 13: 1011–1018 by permission of Oxford University Press.)

**Fig. 54.4** Profiles of genomic RNA of rotaviruses. RNA extracted from purified rotavirus particles was separated by electrophoresis on a polyacrylamide gel. RNA segments (1–11) are labelled at both sides. A 'short' electropherotype RNA is shown in track 1; two 'long' electropherotype RNAs differing in the migration rate of corresponding segments are shown in tracks 2 and 3. (By courtesy of F. Hundley, Institute of Virology, Glasgow.)

So far, 14 different VP7-specific serotypes (G types, derived from *g*lycoprotein) and over 20 different VP4-specific types (P types, derived from *p*rotease-sensitive protein) have been distinguished. Not all P types have been confirmed as serotypes yet, and the P serotype designation is different from the P genotype designation. As VP7 and VP4 are coded for by different RNA segments, they can segregate independently, and a large variety of different G–P-type combinations of rotaviruses have been observed after reassortment in vitro and in nature in vivo. For example, G3 types carry P determinants of at least five different P types (P2, P3, P8, P12 and P16), and P8 types at least four different G types (G1, G3, G4 and G9). Certain G and P types are only found in humans (e.g. G9, G12; P4, P6, P8) or only in animals (e.g. G11, G13; P7, P15, P16); other G and P types are found in *both* humans and animals (e.g. G3, G6, G10; P3, P11), and certain combinations (e.g. G3P3, G4P6 or G10P11) have been observed in *both* humans and animals, raising the possibility of zoonotic transmission (see below). Animals from which rotavirus has been isolated are cattle, sheep, horses, pigs, dogs, cats and mice.

Electrophoresis of genomic RNA segments has been used to establish so-called 'electropherotypes' of rotavirus isolates (Fig. 54.4). Besides 'long' and 'short' electropherotypes (differing in the rates of relative migration of RNA segments 10 and 11), various minor differences in the migration of corresponding segments have been recognized. These differences have been utilized extensively in epidemiological studies, but for many surveillance purposes and for vaccine development, serological classification remains essential.

## Pathogenesis

Rotaviruses replicate exclusively in the differentiated epithelial cells at the tips of the villi of the small intestine. New virus is produced after 10–12 h. Progeny virus is released in large numbers into the intestinal lumen ready to infect other cells. Biopsies show atrophy of the villi with reactive crypt hyperplasia and lymphocytic infiltrates in the lamina propria. The cellular damage leads to malabsorption of nutrients, electrolytes and water, and the crypt hyperplasia to hypersecretion. An osmotic and secretory diarrhoea with vomiting and dehydration results. It has been established that the product of RNA 4, VP4, holds a central position for replication, spread and pathogenicity of rotaviruses, but that products of other RNA segments also contribute to the development of disease. The infection is followed by a local, humoral and cell-mediated immune response and is normally overcome within a week. IgA in the gut is the best known correlate of protection. Infection with one serotype seems to provide homotypic and partial heterotypic protection. In the immunodeficient host, however, a persistent infection can occur with severe chronic diarrhoea.

## Clinical features

The onset of symptoms is abrupt after a short incubation period of 1–2 days. Diarrhoea and vomiting are seen in the majority of infected children and last for 2–6 days. Although symptoms of respiratory tract infection are frequently observed at the time of rotavirus infections, there is no evidence that rotaviruses replicate in the respiratory tract. The clinical symptoms can range from mild to very severe, in part depending on the rotavirus strain. Asymptomatic infections of neonates with 'nursery strains' are not uncommon. It has been estimated that about half of all gastro-enteritis cases requiring admission to hospital are caused by rotaviruses. Infection has been detected in older children and adults, but these are usually asymptomatic. Only in the elderly have rotavirus diarrhoea outbreaks been observed. The disease is especially grave and protracted in immunodeficient children. If children are already malnourished, rotavirus infection can be life-threatening. Five million children under the age of 2 years die each year from diarrhoeal disease in developing countries: rotavirus infections contribute to these deaths to the extent of about 20%.

## Laboratory diagnosis

At the peak of the disease as many as $10^{11}$ virus particles per millilitre of faeces are present. Therefore, the diagnosis is not difficult. Agglutination tests using latex particles coated with rotavirus-specific antibody and different forms of enzyme-linked immunosorbent assay (ELISA) are most commonly used. Electron microscopy, when routinely applied to the diagnosis of viral diarrhoea in infants and young children, will easily detect the characteristic virus particles (see Fig. 54.1). Group, subgroup and G and P serotypes of rotaviruses are determined by ELISA with monoclonal antibodies and, more recently, by reverse-transcription polymerase chain reaction with gene- and type-specific primers. Most human group A rotaviruses are of subgroup II, serotypes G1P8, G3P8 or G4P8, or of subgroup I serotype G2P4. In the majority of cases there are sufficient numbers of virions in faeces to allow identification of RNA profiles by PAGE (Fig. 54.4). Although fastidious, it is possible to isolate rotaviruses in cultures of secondary or continuous monkey kidney cells. To ensure success it is necessary to incorporate trypsin in the culture medium.

## Epidemiology

Rotavirus infections occur world-wide. Most symptomatic infections are seen in children under 2 years of age; by the age of 3 years, more than 90% of children have been infected by most of the major serotypes. In family outbreaks there may be evidence of subclinical infection in older children and adults who may be the source for infection of young children in family or nursery outbreaks. The release of enormous numbers of virions during the acute stage contributes to the easy transmission of the virus. Only a few virus particles are sufficient to cause disease in the susceptible host. Longer-lasting outbreaks may be maintained by the ability of the virus to survive outside the body for some time. In temperate climates there is a pronounced seasonal incidence, with peaks in the winter months occurring with 'clockwise precision'. In tropical areas, on the other hand, infections occur evenly throughout the year. Various surveys in different parts of the world have shown that at any time there is co-circulation of genomically and serologically different rotaviruses.

At the molecular level, several factors have been identified which can explain the genomic and antigenic variability of co-circulating rotavirus strains:

1. Like the genomes of other viruses that depend on virion-associated RNA-dependent RNA polymerases for their replication, rotavirus genomes undergo frequent point mutations which accumulate in time.

2. Rotaviruses, like other segmented RNA viruses, undergo extensive reassortment events in doubly infected cells. This has been shown to occur both in vitro and in vivo. If RNA segments coding for subgroup- and serotype-specific proteins are involved, antigenic shift can occur in reassortants (mechanisms 1 and 2 are also seen in influenza A viruses; see Ch. 50).

3. Rotaviruses may be introduced into humans from animal species, and this may contribute to the genomic variability. Human group A rotavirus isolates have been described, the genome of which is very closely related to that of cat and cattle rotaviruses. The group B ADRVs may have been derived recently from animals. Human group C rotaviruses are significantly different from animal group C rotaviruses.

4. Rotaviruses establishing chronic infections in immunodeficient hosts undergo various forms of genome rearrangements, resulting in highly atypical RNA profiles. Evidence is now emerging that such rearrangements may occur more frequently than originally thought.

5. Various combinations of these factors may occur, e.g. reassortment of viruses with rearranged genomes, or point mutations combined with reassortment.

## Treatment and control

Therapy consists mainly of oral, sometimes intravenous, rehydration with fluid of the appropriate electrolyte and glucose composition (see Table 31.2, p. 300).

As with any infectious agent transmitted by the faecal–oral route, attention to hygienic measures such as handwashing and disinfection of contaminated surfaces and faeces is very important. For a variety of reasons, rotavirus infections have so far resisted prevention by widespread vaccination. Co-circulation of several serotypes at a time occurs in populations at risk (see above), which is also reflected in polytypic serum antibody responses. Furthermore, it is not fully clear to what extent vaccination with one rotavirus serotype cross-protects against other serotypes. However, polyvalent 'cocktail' vaccines containing two or more different serotypes have been shown to have a significant effect on preventing severe disease. A number of candidate vaccines of live attenuated rotavirus of bovine or simian origin and of bovine and simian rotavirus reassortants carrying human VP7 genes of different serotypes are currently being evaluated, and it is hoped that efficient rotavirus vaccines will be available in the near future.

### RECOMMENDED READING

Burke B, Desselberger U 1996 Rotavirus pathogenicity. *Virology* 218: 299–305

Desselberger U 1989 Molecular epidemiology of rotaviruses. In: Farthing M J G (ed) *Viruses and the Gut*. Swan Press, London, pp 55–65

Desselberger U 1996 Genome rearrangements of rotaviruses. *Advances in Virus Research* 46: 69–95

Fields B N, Knipe D M, Howley P M (eds) 1996 *Virology*, 3rd edn. Lippincott-Raven, Philadelphia

Kapikian A Z (ed) 1994 *Viral Infections of the Gastrointestinal Tract*, 2nd edn. Marcel Dekker, New York, pp 131–470

Ramig R F (ed) 1994 *Rotaviruses*. Springer-Verlag, Berlin

Rennels M B, Glass R I, Dennehy P H et al 1996 Safety and efficacy of high-dose rhesus–human reassortant rotavirus vaccines – report of the National Multicentre Trial. *Pediatrics* 97: 7–13

# 55

# Retroviruses

**Leukaemia; lymphoma; acquired immune deficiency syndrome**

*J. F. Peutherer*

The family Retroviridae contains many viruses from widely different host species. They have been studied in the laboratory for many years, mainly because some are associated with tumour production in their natural hosts. Indeed, a wide variety of tumours are caused by the oncovirus genus, including leukaemias and lymphomas, sarcomas, breast and brain tumours, auto-immune disease and blood disorders. The host species include birds, mice, cats, cattle, pigs and several primates. Despite intense effort, it was not until 1980 that the first human retrovirus was isolated from the T cells of patients with T cell leukaemia – the *human T lymphotropic virus type I* or HTLV-I. Since then, the cause of the acquired immune deficiency syndrome or AIDS has been shown to be a retrovirus, also with a predilection for T cells but differing significantly from HTLV-I. It is known as the *human immunodeficiency virus* or HIV.

**Fig. 55.1**  Electron micrograph of HIV. Thin section of T lymphocyte. There are numerous virions lying outside the cell membrane.

## DESCRIPTION

All retroviruses have an outer envelope consisting of lipid and viral proteins; the envelope encloses the core, made of other viral proteins, within which lie two molecules of viral RNA and the enzyme reverse transcriptase, an RNA-dependent DNA polymerase. The virions have a diameter of about 100 nm and, in thin section, differences can be seen in the appearance of the core – those with a central condensed structure are known as type C particles while those with an eccentric bar structure are type D particles (Fig. 55.1).

### Virus stability

HIV is inactivated by:

1. Heat – it is destroyed in the autoclave and hot air oven.

2. Glutaraldehyde 2%.

3. Hypochlorite (10 000 ppm. available chlorine): this is equivalent to a 1 in 10 dilution of domestic bleach.

4. Several other disinfectants, including alcohols. The chemicals will kill at least $10^5$ units of virus within a few minutes, but it is important to remember that disinfectants may not be effective in the presence of organic material.

The survival of HIV has been investigated in some detail. It has been shown that:

1. At room temperature virus may survive for up to 15 days

2. At 37°C virus can survive for 10–15 days

3. Over 60°C virus is inactivated by a factor of 100-fold each hour.

It must be emphasized that these are the limits of survival, as the starting titres of virus were much greater, by a factor of 1000 times or more, than the levels found in the blood of patients. However, they do indicate the need for cleanliness in dealing with HIV.

**Table 55.1** Classification of Retroviridae

| | Subfamily | | |
| --- | --- | --- | --- |
| | Oncovirinae | Lentivirinae | Spumavirinae |
| Growth | Some may transform cells. May cause tumours if they carry oncogenes or by activation of cell oncogene by provirus | Can be lytic. If lytic, destroy host cells. | Foamy degeneration of cells in culture |
| Disease association Examples | Leukaemias and sarcomata Many species, including: Simian T lymphotropic virus Human T lymphotropic virus types I and II | Cause 'slow' infections. Visna/maedi of sheep Equine infectious anaemia Caprine infectious anaemia Feline immunodeficiency virus Simian immunodeficiency virus Human immunodeficiency virus (types 1 and 2) | Not associated with disease Found in many species, including primates and man |

## Classification

The family Retroviridae is divided into the sub-families *Oncovirinae*, *Spumavirinae* and *Lentivirinae* (Table 55.1).

The oncoviruses include the viruses that cause tumours and a number of endogenous non-tumour producing strains. The human viruses are HTLV-I and HTLV-II. A simian virus (STLV-I) is widely distributed in old world monkeys: it can cause lymphomata in some primates and is 90% homologous with HTLV-I.

The spumaviruses have been detected in various species, including cats and primates, but are not associated with disease. The name is derived from the foamy or vacuolated appearance of infected cells in culture.

The lentiviruses are so named due to their association with slowly progressive diseases. *Visna* and *maedi* of sheep were the first to be recognized: they are different clinical presentations of the same virus. The genus includes a virus causing arthritis and encephalitis in goats, equine infectious anaemia virus, and feline, bovine and simian viruses. HIV-1 and HIV-2 are included. By hybridization they show 40% homology of their nucleic acids. HIV-2 is more closely related to *simian immunodeficiency virus* (SIV), with which it has 75% homology. The genome organization is similar for all retroviruses in that their genomes contain in the same order the genes *gag*, *pol* and *env*, which code for the three groups of structural proteins (Fig. 55.2). There are important differences between the types in the nature and arrangement of the genes involved in the regulation of the replication cycle. There are at least six *regulatory genes* in HIV and at least two in

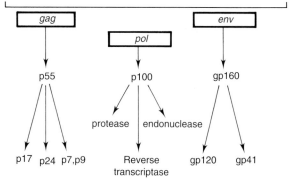

**Fig. 55.2** The genomic organization of HIV structural genes and their protein products.

HTLV-I. In HIV the genes interact – thus *tat* codes for a protein that has a general stimulating effect on the synthesis of all viral proteins, the *nef* gene product has the opposite effect, and the *rev* gene has a regulatory effect, switching on viral protein synthesis by favouring the production of full-length RNA molecules rather than the spliced RNA from the regulatory genes. The long terminal repeat sequences (LTR) at both ends of the genome contain promotor and enhancer sequences. The regulatory products for the *tat* and *rev* genes produce their effect by interacting with regions in LTR. There is evidence that the product of other transactivating genes, such as that of cytomegalovirus (CMV), can also act on the same sequence within the LTR of HIV. HIV-1 and HIV-2 differ in their control genes. The LTR sequences are involved in the integration of the DNA provirus into the host chromosome.

gp120
gp41
p17
p24
Reverse transcriptase complex
RNA + protein (p7, p9)

**Fig. 55.3** Diagram of HIV to show location of structural proteins.

The *gag* gene of HIV codes for four proteins, all found within the virion (Fig. 55.3). The *pol* gene products are a protease, endonuclease, integrase and reverse transcriptase. The *env* gene codes for a large protein which is glycosylated; this is cleaved to gp41, the transmembrane component, and gp120, the external envelope glycoprotein. gp120 is present as a trimer, with many glycosylation sites. On the basis of sequence variation it is possible to divide HIV-1 isolates into subtypes A to F.

## REPLICATION

Retroviruses differ from other RNA viruses in that they replicate and produce viral RNA from a DNA copy of the virion RNA. The best studied method of attachment of HIV to cells is by the interaction of the external envelope glycoprotein gp120 with part of the CD4 molecule of T helper lymphocytes and other cells. Attachment is followed by entry of the virus by fusion of the two membranes, a function dependent on gp41. Once the RNA is released, the reverse transcriptase acts to form the double-stranded DNA copy, which is circularized, enters the nucleus and is spliced into the host cell DNA (see Ch. 12). Once inserted into the host DNA, infection with HIV is permanent. The virus may stay latent or enter a productive cycle. Transcription of messenger RNA (mRNA) from the provirus is by the host RNA polymerase to produce viral mRNA and RNA. Virions are assembled at the cell membrane where envelope and core proteins have located. The internal structure of the virion matures as the virion buds from the cell. In the productive growth cycle the host cell is destroyed.

## CLINICAL FEATURES AND PATHOGENESIS

### HTLV-I infection

Adult T cell leukaemia/lymphoma was first recognized in Japan, and the isolation of the virus HTLV-I reported in 1980. The disease is an acute T cell proliferative malignancy; clinically, the features are leukaemia, generalized lymphadenopathy, hepato-splenomegaly associated with bone marrow and skin involvement. It is now clear that other less dramatic forms exist, including a variant which runs a slow course, associated with adenopathy and splenomegaly. Another disease, a non-Hodgkin T cell lymphoma, is also recognized. The T cells involved carry the CD4 antigen. HTLV-I is also the cause of a neurological disease, *tropical spastic paraparesis*, a slowly progressive myelopathy presenting with spastic or ataxic features. Pathologically, areas of demyelination with lymphocytic infiltration and perivascular cuffing are seen.

The period of latency between infection with the virus and leukaemia or myelopathy lasts for many years. No acute disease is recognized at the time of seroconversion.

There is a clear association of the virus with the tumour cells which contain monoclonally integrated HTLV-I provirus at random sites. There are no virion-transforming genes; the T cell proliferation may be the result of the protein coded by the viral transactivating or *tax* gene. It is not known what triggers the T cell proliferation after the long latency in the small proportion (1–4%) of those infected who develop disease. During the latent period viral proteins are expressed as there are steady high titres of antibody to various viral proteins, particularly to the *gag* proteins. HTLV-II is not linked to a particular disease, although the initial isolation was from a man with the rare T hairy-cell leukaemia.

### HIV and AIDS

In contrast to HTLV-I, a great deal is known about the association of HIV with disease; Figure 55.4 summarizes some of the clinical stages. The *acute seroconversion* illness associated with HIV-1 resembles glandular fever with adenopathy; it is recognized in 5–10% of patients. A few cases of encephalitis have also been reported. The average incubation period to AIDS onset is about 10 years. Overall, almost half of those who have been diagnosed as AIDS cases are dead. Untreated, the median survival is

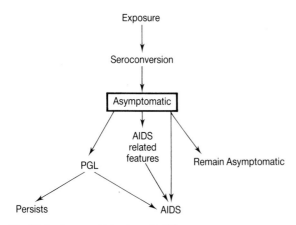

**Fig. 55.4** Stages of infection with HIV.

**Table 55.3** Group IV disease (Communicable Disease Surveillance Centre, London)

**Not AIDS indicator disease**

1. Zoster
2. Oral candidiasis
3. Oral hairy leucoplakia
4. Seborrhoeic dermatitis
5. Other infections – stronglyloidiasis, nocardiasis, pulmonary tuberculosis
6. Constitutional symptoms (e.g. wasting disease)
7. Peripheral neuropathy and myelopathy
8. Thrombocytopenia

**AIDS indicator disease**

1. Bacterial infection, multiple or recurrent in child aged less than 12 years
2. Candidiasis of oesophagus, trachea, bronchi, lungs
3. Coccidioidomycosis
4. Cryptococcosis
5. Cryptosporidiosis
6. Histoplasmosis
7. Isosporiasis
8. Mycobacteriosis – disseminated or extrapulmonary
9. *Pneumocystis carinii* pneumonia
10. Toxoplasmosis of brain
11. Salmonellosis – recurrent septicaemia
12. CMV, e.g. retinitis
13. HSV more than 1 month; or bronchi, lung or oesophagus involved
14. Progressive multifocal leuco-encephalopathy
15. HIV dementia
16. Kaposi's sarcoma
17. Lymphoma – Burkitt's or immunoblastic or primary in brain
18. Lymphoid interstitial pneumonia/pulmonary lymphoid hyperplasia in child aged less than 12 years
19. Wasting syndrome

about 1 year from the time of diagnosis, and 95% are dead within 5 years. There is evidence that the latent period of HIV-2 is even longer than with HIV-1.

## Persistent generalized lymphadenopathy

Persistent generalized lymphadenopathy (PGL) is present in 25–30% of patients who are otherwise asymptomatic (Table 55.2). The enlarged lymph nodes are painless and symmetrical in distribution. The rate of progression of patients with PGL to AIDS seems to be no greater than those without adenopathy. PGL must be distinguished from other causes of adenopathy such as the lymphomata.

## Clinical features of late stages of infection

The enormous variety of infections – including protozoan, fungal, bacterial and viral infections – and tumours indicate clearly the extent of the immuno-suppression that develops and the magnitude of the diagnostic and therapeutic problems presented by these patients (Table 55.3). The features classified as group IV include what was known as the *AIDS-related complex* or ARC. This label was applied to

patients with constitutional symptoms of fever, weight loss and diarrhoea and minor opportunistic infections. Such patients may progress rapidly to AIDS.

*Oral hairy leucoplakia.* This appears to be unique to HIV-infected patients. The margins of the tongue show white ridges of fronds on the epithelium. An association with Epstein–Barr and papilloma-viruses has been proposed.

*Kaposi's sarcoma.* This was one of the earliest features used to define AIDS. It is often aggressive and arises in many sites, including the skin, mouth, gut and eye. The tumours arise from endothelial cells of blood vessels causing bluish purple, raised irregular lesions. The aetiology is now attributed to human herpesvirus 8. It was seen almost entirely in homosexual men; the incidence has declined since it was first recognized. There is also an increased incidence of B cell lymphomata and other tumours.

**Table 55.2** Classification of HIV infection and AIDS (Communicable Disease Center, USA)

| | |
|---|---|
| Group I | Seroconversion illness |
| Group II | Asymptomatic |
| Group III | Persistent generalized lymphadenopathy |
| Group IV | A – Constitutional disease |
| | B – Neurological disease |
| | C – Secondary infectious disease |
| | D – Secondary cancers |
| | E – Other conditions |

***HIV dementia.*** Dementia develops in 25% of patients with AIDS and is marked by a gradual loss of cognitive functions, progressing to overt dementia. In some patients it is the main feature of the disease. Brain scan shows a loss of tissue, with widening of the sulci and ventricles.

***Features in developing countries.*** The features described above are associated with HIV infection in developed countries. In developing countries the clinical presentations may differ in that the types of opportunistic infections reflect those endemic in the region. Many patients show profound weight loss, perhaps accompanied by chronic diarrhoea; the term *slim disease* is applied to this presentation.

### Paediatric AIDS

The features of paediatric AIDS include many of the infections seen in older patients. However, children are also at risk of recurring bacterial infections, lymphoid interstitial pneumonia and pulmonary lymphoid hyperplasia.

## PATHOGENESIS OF AIDS

Patients with AIDS are profoundly immunosuppressed. It was recognized early that the ratio of T helper to T suppressor (T4:T8 or CD4:CD8) lymphocytes in the blood was upset. In fact, the number of T helper cells declines during the asymptomatic period until it reaches a level where resistance to infection is seriously impaired. This can be demonstrated also by the loss of skin hypersensitivity to various standard test antigens. Monitoring the number of T4 cells is a useful guide to the onset of AIDS; in addition, the number of T8 cells increases as disease develops. In the circulation the virus is found in T4 cells and also in monocyte–macrophage cells, which may act as a reservoir for virus. Macrophages are also important in carrying the virus into the central nervous system across the blood–brain barrier. The proportion of infected T4 cells rises as the infection progresses. Virus is also present in the plasma, and this increases with time too. Titres rise as the patient becomes symptomatic. Activation of latently infected lymphocytes can be achieved by contact with foreign antigen and lectins such as phytohaemagglutinin (PHA). There is laboratory evidence too that co-infection or superinfection of cells carrying HIV with other viruses such as CMV and human herpesvirus 6 can lead to HIV replication. Activation of uninfected T4 cells is also important in increasing their sensitivity to infection.

Destruction of T4 cells is achieved by:

1. Viral replication
2. Syncytium formation via membrane gp120 binding to cell CD4 antigen
3. Cytotoxic T cell lysis of infected cells
4. Cytotoxic T cell lysis of T4 cells carrying gp120 released from infected cells
5. Natural killer cells
6. Antibody-dependent cell cytotoxicity.

A few cases have been described in whom T cell responses to viral components appear to be present in the absence of detectable anti-HIV or virus.

Analysis of the viral genomes from a patient shows that there are several different variants present at any time and that these change with time. However, isolation of HIV in T4 cell cultures yields virus that may be different from the predominant genomic variants in the blood. Viruses isolated in the later stages of infection have been shown to grow more rapidly and to higher titres and to form syncytia more readily than strains isolated in the early stages. Regions of the envelope glycoproteins show most variation and this could affect the ability of neutralizing antibody to react with the variant viruses. While this could be relevant to the progression of the disease, it obviously has implications for the development of vaccines. Different HIV-subtypes are linked to different populations and transmission routes.

Observed immunological changes in HIV infection include:

1. Decreased production of interleukin-2, γ-interferon and other lymphokines
2. Impaired function of lymphocytes and macrophages
3. Reduced natural killer cell activity
4. B cell activation.

HIV infection also has effects on the nervous system. HIV is present in the brain predominantly in macrophages but also in microglial, oligodendroglial and capillary endothelial cells. There is expression of viral antigens in these cells and virus can be isolated from them. Virus from such sources may be more able to infect macrophages in culture than virus recovered from peripheral T cells.

There may also be host genetic differences in the risk of disease progression, e.g. HLA haplotype A1B8DR3 has been linked to the rapid development of severe disease. There also appears to be an age effect with evidence of faster progression in some

**Table 55.4** Laboratory markers associated with progression of HIV infection

1. Number of T4 lymphocytes:
   <200, 80% develop AIDS within 4 years
   200–400, 40–50% develop AIDS within 4 years
2. Increasing proportion of infected T4 cells
3. Increasing titre of virus in plasma
4. p24 antigen in plasma
5. Isolation in culture of virus — rapid growth, high antigen levels
6. Loss of antibody to p24
7. Elevated $\beta_2$-microglobulin level
8. Elevated serum neopterin level
9. Elevated serum soluble interleukin-2 level
10. Loss of cutaneous hypersensitivity

infants, the median age at onset being 8 months of age. Table 55.4 lists a number of laboratory markers that are associated with an increased probability of disease progression. The absolute number of CD4-positive cells is the most useful, although it can vary considerably between samples. However, a downward trend in successive samples indicates that the infection is progressing. An absolute level of below 200 is an indication of AIDS. The presence of p24 antigen in the plasma, the ease of virus culture and the loss of antibody to p24 are all correlated with progression (see also Fig. 55.5) but it must be emphasized that these features are not seen in all patients. The final proportion of those infected who will develop AIDS is not known, although the estimates continue to be revised upwards. In the cohorts studied for the longest times, the proportions with AIDS were 5% within 3 years, 20–25% at 6–7 years, and more than 50% at 10 years. It has been estimated that from 2 years after seroconversion

from 5 to 10% of patients will develop AIDS each year.

## LABORATORY DIAGNOSIS

### HIV infection

A specific virological diagnosis of HIV infection can be achieved by:

1. Isolation of the virus in culture
2. The detection of viral components, e.g. p24 antigen, by direct assay in the plasma or detection of proviral DNA or RNA (after reverse transcription) and amplification by the polymerase chain reaction (PCR)
3. The presence of antibody to HIV antigens in the serum.

The various tests are used in different circumstances. Thus, to date the main approach to the diagnosis of infection in patients and for screening populations, e.g. blood donors, has been by assaying for anti-HIV.

### Tests for anti-HIV

This was the first practical approach and many different assays are now available, most using enzyme tracing of the reaction (enzyme-linked immunosorbent assay or ELISA). Originally, the antigen for these tests was prepared from infected T lymphocyte cultures; however, it was impossible to exclude all lymphocyte-derived material from these preparations, and therefore false-positive reactions occurred. Later tests have used antigens prepared by recombinant DNA technology in *Escherichia coli*, or synthetic peptides and monoclonal antibodies. *Western* or *immunoblotting* has been used extensively as a confirmatory assay. Most assays can detect antibody to both HIV-1 and HIV-2 antigens. It is important that a positive test is confirmed by at least two other different assays. A second serum sample should be checked to ensure that the original sample was labelled correctly.

As all who are infected with HIV remain so, a positive test for antibody indicates that the patient is infected. Most patients will seroconvert within 2–3 months (Fig. 55.5) but some may take longer. Thus, there is a gap before antibody tests can detect infection. There have been reports that some patients may remain seronegative for much longer periods (6–9 months); transmission from such individuals has been seen.

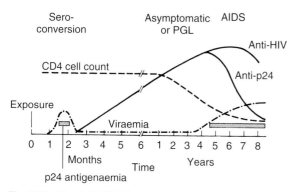

**Fig. 55.5** Events in HIV infection. ▢ p24 antigenaemia

## Tests for p24 antigen

p24 antigenaemia is usually of short duration at the time of initial infection, and is not always detected (Fig. 55.5). As the antibody response builds up antigen tests become negative. However, late in the infection, p24 antigen may reappear until most patients with AIDS give a positive test.

## Virus isolation and detection

Isolation of the virus is a slow process, taking from 3–6 weeks. The usual sample is blood, from which the lymphocytes are separated and co-cultured with PHA-stimulated donor lymphocytes. Virus presence is detected by assays for reverse transcriptase and p24 antigen in the culture fluids.

Amplification by PCR can be a useful diagnostic tool in the investigation of patients with indeterminate serological results, and to detect infection in the early stages as in the partners of infected cases. The diagnosis of infection in babies born to infected mothers may require the use of several approaches. All babies will be positive for anti-HIV for up to 18 months until maternal IgG disappears; if antibody persists beyond this time, this indicates infection. However, some babies do not produce anti-HIV. Detection of p24 antigen or a positive culture establishes that the baby is infected, but the PCR may be invaluable in confirming infection.

## HTLV-I infection

Assays for the detection of antibody to HTLV-I are available; as with HIV, confirmation by other assays or immunoblot must be attempted, although the interpretation can be difficult with some sera. Current tests do not distinguish between HTLV-I and HTLV-II. Culture and PCR can also be used.

# TREATMENT

## HTLV-I infection

There is no specific therapy. If T cell leukaemia develops then this is managed by various drug therapies; interferon has a role in the management.

## HIV infection and AIDS

Various approaches have been tried in the hope of halting or at least slowing the progression of HIV infection to AIDS. The most widely used drug is a nucleoside analogue, azidothymidine or *zidovudine*. The drug is inactive until phosphorylated, when it can block the viral reverse transcriptase, although it also has some effect on host DNA polymerase. The initial studies showed that treatment with zidovudine could improve the symptoms and survival of patients with AIDS, although about a quarter of patients developed serious side-effects, in some cases requiring frequent blood transfusions and cessation of therapy. Treated patients usually show reduced viral load, and the CD4 cell count rises and the plasma p24 antigen level declines. The patient feels better and may put on weight, but the improvement is seldom maintained beyond 6 months. However, the use of zidovudine and the prompt, appropriate treatment of infections as they arise can prolong survival of AIDS patients for up to 3 years or more. There is no evidence that the early introduction of zidovudine can delay the development of AIDS. Therapy is usually started on the basis of the clinical state, CD4 cell count, and other prognostic markers listed in Table 55.4. Resistance to zidovudine has been shown to develop quickly, and is associated with mutations at certain sites in the *pol* gene. The dideoxynucleoside analogues, e.g. dideoxycitidine (zalcitabine, ddC) and dideoxyinosine (didanosine, ddI), didehydrodeoxythymidine (stavudine) and deoxythiacytidine (lamivudine) are available, although toxic effects do occur. Soluble CD4 has not proved effective. More encouraging results have been shown with protease inhibitors such as saquinavir and ritonavir. A synergistic effect has been shown between nucleoside analogues, and combination therapy is now accepted. Combined treatment using a nucleoside and a protease inhibitor also shows promise. The role of treatment to improve immune function is not yet clear.

Apart from specific therapy directed against HIV the most important advances in management have come from the prophylaxis of *Pneumocystis carinii* and *Toxoplasma gondii* and other infections.

# EPIDEMIOLOGY AND TRANSMISSION

## HTLV-I and HTLV-II

HTLV-I is endemic in the Southern islands of Japan and around the Caribbean – in the West Indies, the northern countries of South America, Central America and the southern states of the USA. There are varying reports of infection in some tropical countries in

Africa. Immigrants from these areas will show a similar prevalence, which can be up to 10–15% in Japan and 5% in Jamaica. The prevalence in some populations of the southern USA is 2–3%. In most studies, the seroprevalence rises with age. Other groups found to carry the virus are parenteral drug misusers and prostitutes in the USA and other areas. In some groups, the prevalence can reach 30-50%, the highest figures being found in drug misusers.

In prostitutes, rates up to 25% have been reported. Drug misuse cannot account for all the infections in these studies and transmission by sexual intercourse is the likeliest explanation. As with any venereal infection, the risk rises with the number of sexual partners. This is reflected in the association of infection with other sexually transmitted diseases. HTLV-I can be isolated from semen and the amount of virus may rise with age and, especially, in patients who develop leukaemia and lymphomata. The relative rate of male-to-female transmission is 10 times greater than female-to-male infection. In most population studies therefore, infection is more frequent in females. The pattern of infection with HTLV-I suggests that transmission is difficult and the evidence indicates that the transfer of infected lymphocytes is the means of infection. Transfusion of infected blood can also lead to infection. Mother-to-child transfer is the other major route, although the exact mechanism is not known. Virus has also been demonstrated in lymphocytes in breast milk and this is a possible source of infection for the child. No evidence of occupational exposure of health workers has been obtained.

## HIV-1 and HIV-2

The World Health Organization estimates that there have been 8 million cases of AIDS in all parts of the world, and that more than 40 million will be infected with HIV by the year 2000. To date, most of those infected are in Africa, but the numbers are now increasing rapidly in Asia.

### Routes of transmission of HIV

1. By unprotected, penetrative sexual intercourse
2. From mother to child
3. By blood or blood products.

AIDS was first recognized in homosexual men in the USA and, to date, almost two-thirds to three-quarters of notified AIDS cases were infected by homosexual contact. Most early studies established that anal intercourse and numerous sexual partners were major risk factors, particularly to the recipient partner in anal intercourse. Among homosexual men, the seroprevalence of HIV reached 60–70% in some groups in San Francisco and New York, while the rate in Europe is lower at 20–40% in Denmark and London.

Intravenous drug misuse is a risk factor in about a quarter of AIDS cases in the USA. Heterosexual transmission, paediatric cases and the use of contaminated blood and blood products account for most of the remainder. In Europe the pattern is similar, although about 10% of cases are patients of African origin. In the UK all the major groups are represented, although homosexually acquired cases account for more than 80% of AIDS cases so far. In drug misusers the virus was introduced earlier in the USA, mainly in the east coast cities of New York and New Jersey where up to 60–70% of some groups tested have antibody to HIV. In Europe, drug misusers represent an important group. The virus spread among Swiss, Italian and Spanish drug misusers between 1981 and 1982 while, in the UK, London and other major English cities have shown only a slow increase in prevalence, starting from about 1984–85. As in the USA, there are geographical variations: in Edinburgh the virus was introduced some time in 1983 and spread rapidly thereafter until, by 1984, 40–50% of drug injectors had been infected. This rapid build-up reflects the practice of sharing syringes and needles for injection, at a time when there was an 'epidemic' of intravenous drug misuse. Similar high seroprevalences have been identified in Dublin and Stockholm and may be due to transfer from the foci in southern Europe. In contrast, haemophiliacs in all areas have shown an almost identical pattern of infection from the early 1980s. Heterosexual transmission to partners occurs from infected male and female drug misusers, from bisexual men and from haemophiliacs and others infected through contaminated blood and blood products. A further source in Europe is sexual contact with partners infected in Africa. Although infection has been acquired after a single exposure, there are many instances where frequent unprotected contact has not led to transmission.

The other route of infection is from mother to child. Most infections are acquired at birth, with a few in utero. Breast-feeding accounts for others. The transmission rate has varied in different studies, ranging from almost 50% to less than 10%. The greatest risk of transmission is seen if the mother has already given birth to an infected child or is in the later stages of infection.

In Africa equal numbers of males and females are infected. Seroprevalence studies show that 1–20% of some populations are infected, with female prostitutes showing very high rates of infection of up to 80%. Analysed according to age, the peaks of antibody prevalence are in those aged under 1 year and between 16 and 30 years. This is consistent with a sexually transmitted infection. The presence of the virus in the child-bearing age group also indicates that mother-to-child transfer occurs frequently. Alternative routes include contaminated blood transfusions, inadequately sterilized syringes and needles used to give vaccines and drug injections. The evidence from serological studies is that infection built up during the 1970s. HIV-2 has a more restricted distribution than HIV-1. It is found in West Africa and in some European countries such as Portugal with old colonial links to the area. The routes of transmission appear to be the same as for HIV-1. More recently HIV-1 has been introduced into India and South-East Asia, with a rapid rise in infection acquired through drug use and heterosexual contact. HIV-1 subtypes are associated with certain areas and routes of transmission. Thus of the 10 main subtypes, B is predominant in Europe and North America, whereas subtypes A and C to J are found in developing countries in Africa and the East. In Thailand, subtype B is linked to transmission by drug use, and subtype E to sexual contact.

Virus can be isolated from blood, semen and cervical and vaginal secretions, and these three sources are important in transmission, although breast milk and donated organs have caused infection. Virus may also be present in cerebrospinal fluid, saliva, tears and urine, but usually to a lower titre than in blood. There is no epidemiological evidence that infection can be acquired from these sources. Free virus is known to increase in the plasma in the later stages of infection and this correlates with the epidemiological evidence of the increased risk of transmission at this time.

Transmission during sexual contact is increased in the presence of ulcerative genital disease or other sexually transmitted diseases. Any trauma during intercourse will also facilitate spread, although neither factor is essential for infection. The risk of transmission by blood is related to the volume transferred. The transmission risk is between 1 in 200–300 after needlestick injuries, but must be considerably higher in drug injectors who share contaminated injection equipment, although the frequency of exposure will also have an effect. Factor VIII prepared from large volumes of plasma from many unscreened donors is obviously an effective vehicle, as shown by the high rate of infection in haemophiliacs.

To date, most infected patients can be shown to have been exposed to infection by one of the recognized routes of transmission. There is clear evidence that HIV is *not* spread by casual contact, contamination of intact skin or by inhalation.

## CONTROL

The emphasis in control must be on risk reduction. For both homosexual men and heterosexuals, reduction in the number of sexual partners and the use of condoms, perhaps supplemented with spermicides such as nonoxynol-9 are important measures. Unfortunately, this advice is difficult to accept when the risk of infection appears to be very low. It has to be emphasized that the only way to slow or stop wide dissemination of the virus is by these means, starting now. Drug injectors of course can remove the risk by not injecting or can reduce the risk by not sharing injecting equipment. Screening of all blood donors for risky behaviour and testing all donations should almost eliminate the possibility of infection. Factor VIII is now heated to inactivate any virus present. All organ donors must be screened before transplantation of tissues.

Cases of occupational infection have been documented. The most frequent means of exposure is by accidental injury with a contaminated needle or sharp object. Blood is the usual inoculum. Occupational risk can be controlled by the implementation of straightforward measures to prevent accidental injury and contamination with blood. These will include the use of gloves, masks and eye protection if bleeding and spattering are likely and will be difficult to control, as in major surgical procedures, for example. In other situations the risk must be assessed and the appropriate simple precautions taken. Safe disposal of needles, blades and other sharp objects is obviously a fundamental requirement. The sensitivity of HIV to heat and various disinfectants has been described on page 518. There is now some evidence that zidovudine prophylaxis starting within 1–2 h of an accidental exposure is worthwhile.

### Vaccines

Much effort has been devoted to the development of a vaccine to provide protection. By analogy with hepatitis B, most efforts have been directed to the development of vaccines containing the viral *env* protein gp160, gp120 or gp41 prepared by recombinant DNA cloning and expression, or synthetic peptides identified as being important epitopes for neutralizing antibodies. The presentation of the vaccine components will also be important. Despite the difficulties several vaccines are under trial; proper evaluation will require large-scale trials.

## RECOMMENDED READING

Connolly K J, Hammer S M 1992 Antiretroviral therapy: strategies beyond single agent reverse transcriptase inhibitors. *Antimicrobial Agents and Chemotherapy* 36: 509–520

Fields B N, Knipe D M, Howley P M (eds) 1996 *Virology*, 3rd edn. Lippincott–Raven, Philadelphia

UK Health Departments 1990 *Guidance for Clinical Health Care Workers: Protection Against Infection with HIV and Hepatitis Viruses.* HMSO, London

Weiss R A, Tailor C S 1995 Retrovirus receptors. *Cell* 82: 531–533

# 56

# Caliciviruses and astroviruses

**Diarrhoeal disease**

*W. D. Cubitt*

The introduction of electron microscopy for the examination of faecal samples led, in the 1970s, to the discovery of a number of viruses which cause *diarrhoeal disease* in humans and animals. The viruses discussed are *Norwalk agent*, and morphologically similar agents, collectively referred to as '*small round structured*' viruses (SRSVs) and human *caliciviruses* (HuCV), which are now both placed in the family Caliciviridae; and viruses belonging to the family Astroviridae. Evidence that they cause diarrhoeal disease has been provided by epidemiological surveys, human volunteer experiments and laboratory investigations.

Diagnosis of these agents is still dependent on the use of electron microscopy, except in a few research laboratories which have developed in-house enzyme immuno-assays (EIA) or reverse-transcription polymerase chain reactions (RT–PCRs). The application of these techniques is providing increasing evidence that caliciviruses and astroviruses have a world-wide distribution and that outbreaks of infection involving infants and the elderly are common. Caliciviruses are emerging as important causes of food- and water-associated outbreaks of diarrhoea and vomiting, affecting individuals of all age groups. Hepatitis E, another member of the Caliciviridae, is a cause of epidemic water-borne hepatitis.

Recently, astroviruses have been implicated as a cause of extensive outbreaks of food-borne infection in Japan.

## DESCRIPTION

The properties of the viruses are summarized in Table 56.1.

## Morphology

HuCVs have a characteristic surface morphology (Fig. 56.1), formed by the 32 cups or 'calices' formed by 90 dimers arranged in a *T*=3 symmetry. Three distinct appearances can be observed depending upon the orientation of the particles (Fig. 56.2). Factors such as freezing and thawing, the presence of proteolytic enzymes, or incorrect staining can affect the appearance of the particles, which may then be

**Table 56.1** Properties of HuCV, SRSVs and astrovirus

|  | HuCV | SRSV | Astrovirus |
|---|---|---|---|
| Nucleic acid | ssRNA | ssRNA | ssRNA |
| Protein | VP1 | VP1 | VP1, VP2, VP3? |
| Molecular weight | 65 000 | 60 000–70 000 | 29 000–39 000 |
| Lipid | None | None | None |
| Buoyant density (g/cm$^3$) | 1.38–1.4 | 1.38–1.41 | 1.36–1.38 |
| Morphology | See Figs 56.1 and 56.2 | See Fig. 56.3 | See Fig. 56.4 |
| Diameter (nm) | 28–35 | 30–38 | 28–30 |
| Antigenic strains | 5 | >12 | 8 |
| Replication | Cytoplasm | ? | Cytoplasm |
| Host range | Man | Man | Man |
| Transmission | Faecal–oral, air-borne, contaminated food, and water | | |

ssRNA, single-stranded RNA.

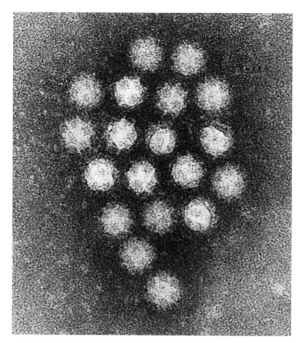

**Fig. 56.1**   HuCVs, displaying characteristic cupped surface morphology. ×300 000. (From Cubitt W D et al 1987 *Journal of Infectious Diseases* 156: 806–813.)

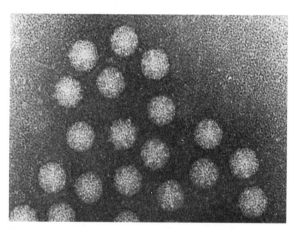

**Fig. 56.3**   SRSVs resembling Norwalk agent. ×300 000. (From Cubitt W D et al 1987 *Journal of Infectious Diseases* 156: 806–813.)

**Fig. 56.4**   Astroviruses, showing surface star. ×280 000.

indistinguishable from SRSVs. The morphology may be masked also by the presence of antibodies. Norwalk virus has a similar structure when studied by cryo-electron microscopy but the tips of the capsomeres are bent and partially obscure the hollows, resulting in an amorphous surface structure with a ragged outline (Fig. 56.3). Complete virions measure 35–40 nm in diameter with a solid inner shell at a radius of 11.5–15.5 nm surrounding the RNA.

Astroviruses can be recognized by a five- or six-pointed star on their surface (Fig. 56.4), but this is

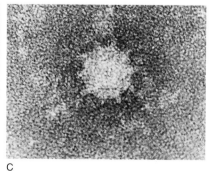

A                              B                              C

**Fig. 56.2**   Electron micrograph showing calicivirus morphology when viewed (A–C) along the two-, five- and three-fold axes of symmetry. ×450 000. (From Cubitt W D et al 1979 *Journal of Clinical Pathology* 32: 786–793.)

generally evident on only a minority of particles in a preparation. The detailed structure of the virion is still unknown.

## Physicochemical and physical properties

The properties of particles which have the appearance of typical HuCVs are identical to those of SRSVs (Table 56.1). Astroviruses have similar properties but appear to be more resistant to inactivation, withstanding acid (pH 3.0), 50°C for 1 h and 60°C for 5 min.

## Genome organization

It is now known that morphologically typical HuCVs and many SRSVs are members of the family Caliciviridae. The genomic organization of two groups of caliciviruses affecting man are shown in Figure 56.5a. Each is distinct, although, in each, non-structural proteins are encoded by ORF1 and structural proteins by ORF2. The exact function of ORF3 is not known. All three groups possess highly conserved regions within ORF1 encoding a helicase (2C), a protease (3C) and the RNA-dependent RNA polymerase 3D. These serve as suitable sites to direct primers for RT-PCR.

The results of sequencing suggest that many of the morphologically typical caliciviruses have a genomic organization similar to HuCV/Manchester whereas most of the caliciviruses previously classified as SRSVs have an organization similar to Norwalk virus.

**Fig. 56.5 a** Genomic organization of two distinct groups of human caliciviruses. **b** Genomic arrangement of astrovirus. (From Murphy et al 1995 by kind permission of Springer-Verlag publishers.)

Astroviruses have a unique genomic arrangement (Fig. 56.5b) and constitute a new family, the Astroviridae.

## Antigenic properties

Several strains of morphologically typical HuCV have been recognized including the prototype HuCV/Sapporo. The use of hyperimmune guinea-pig antisera raised against HuCV/Sapporo indicates that at least four of the strains are antigenically related, whereas immune electron microscopy (IEM) showed them to be antigenically distinct.

The use of IEM and EIA has shown that there are numerous strains of human calicivirus which were previously classified as SRSVs. Three distinct strains have been recognized in the USA, Norwalk virus which falls within genogroup I and Snow Mountain and Hawaii viruses which fall with genogroup II. Representatives of both genogroups have been found in the UK and Japan.

There are eight strains of astrovirus which have been identified with specific antisera. The use of a monoclonal antibody has shown that all serotypes share a group antigen. Types 6–8 were first reported in 1994–95.

## Host range

In-vivo studies with strains of HuCV and Norwalk virus suggest that they are not readily transmitted to other species, although other caliciviruses have been identified in primates, domestic and farm animals, birds, fish, reptiles, amphibians and insects, and some are known to cross species barriers. There are two reports suggesting that primates can undergo sub-clinical infection when fed with HuCV or Norwalk agent. In both these cases, animals showed a significant antibody response and were found to be excreting small numbers of virus particles in faeces. Similar experiments have not been conducted with human astroviruses.

Human volunteer studies with caliciviruses (Norwalk, Hawaii and Snow Mountain agents) and astroviruses have shown that some adults became infected after they had been challenged with faecal filtrates containing virus. Pre-existing antibody to Norwalk virus did not confer immunity to subsequent challenge with the virus.

## Replication

Attempts to propagate enteric caliciviruses in vitro have generally been unsuccessful.

Astroviruses can be readily propagated in a human intestinal cell line CaCo2, and in HT-29 cells provided trypsin is incorporated in the medium. Immunofluorescence shows that replication occurs within the cytoplasm and that a protein is present in the nucleolus at an early stage in the replication cycle. Electron microscopical examination of thin sections of infected cells shows the presence of crystalline arrays of particles adjacent to cytoplasmic vacuoles.

## PATHOGENESIS AND CLINICAL FEATURES

Human volunteer studies with Hawaii and Norwalk viruses have shown that replication occurs in the jejunum. Light microscopy showed that the villi in the proximal part of the small intestine were broadened and blunted and the enterocytes covering the damaged villi were cuboidal and vacuolated. At the same time the numbers of intra-epithelial lymphocytes and neutrophils were increased. Electron microscopical studies showed that epithelial cells remained intact but the microvilli were disarranged and reduced in length. A similar histopathological picture has been found in calves experimentally infected with a bovine calicivirus 'Newbury agent 2'.

The only data on astrovirus infection in humans come from the examination of duodenal biopsies obtained from infants with symptoms of gastroenteritis. Electron microscopical examination of thin sections showed the presence of arrays of virus particles in epithelial cells of the lower third of the villi.

### Clinical features

The clinical features of infection with calicivirus and astrovirus are shown in Table 56.2. The symptoms are similar but vomiting, sometimes projectile, is more frequently reported in calicivirus infections. In some outbreaks of calicivirus infection involving adults the illness resembles 'gastric flu' i.e. diarrhoea, headache, fever, aching limbs and malaise.

The incubation period for HuCVs is between 12 and 72 h, and slightly longer, 3–4 days, for astrovirus. Illness lasts typically for between 1 and 4 days with excretion of detectable numbers of particles for the same period. Occasionally, symptoms may persist for periods of up to 2 weeks.

In patients with severe combined immune deficiency disease, persistent excretion of calici-, astro- and rotaviruses can occur, either individually or simultaneously; in one report a patient was found to be excreting five different enteric viruses over a period of several weeks, before he eventually died.

Symptoms of illness are generally mild and seldom require hospitalization. However, when outbreaks occur among debilitated elderly patients or infants with other underlying problems, intravenous rehydration may be necessary; fatalities are extremely rare.

## LABORATORY DIAGNOSIS

### Specimens required

Faecal samples should be collected as soon as possible after the onset of symptoms and stored at 4°C. Paired serum samples should be obtained, the first taken as soon as possible after onset of symptoms and a further sample 10–14 days later. Blood samples from infants can be obtained by finger or heel pricks and dried on filter papers.

**Table 56.2** Clinical features recorded in outbreaks

| Virus | No. of cases | Cases presenting with symptom (%) | | | | | | |
|---|---|---|---|---|---|---|---|---|
| | | V | D | F | AbP | N | AcL | H |
| HuCV/Norwalk[a] | 30 | 66 | 83 | 47 | 70 | 100 | 73 | 83 |
| HuCV/Snow Mountain[a] | 59 | 71 | 70 | 32 | 67 | 72 | NS | 68 |
| HuCV/UK4 | 181 | 52 | 66 | 65 | 60 | NS | 56 | NS |
| HuCV/UK1 | 9 | 100 | 22 | NS | 33 | NS | NS | NS |
| HuCV/Japan | 250 | 42 | 96 | 18 | 77 | NS | NS | NS |
| Astrovirus | 14 | 74 | 30 | 30 | 49 | NS | NS | NS |

V, vomiting; D, diarrhoea; F, fever; AbP, abdominal pain; N, nausea; AcL, aching limbs; H, headache. NS, not stated.
[a]Morphological appearance = SRSV.

## Laboratory tests

The only widely available test for the diagnosis of calici- and astroviruses is electron microscopy, which requires skilled operators and expensive capital equipment. All the viruses are small and are often difficult to recognize. The use of solid phase immune electron microscopy (SPIEM), which relies on particles being captured by antibodies which have been bound to the grid, can increase the sensitivity of electron microscopy and enables virus particles to be more readily recognized. Conventional IEM, in which virus reacts with antibodies in a fluid phase, resulting in aggregates of particles, is also of value, provided particles are not totally masked by excess antibody. IEM can also be used to measure antibody responses.

## Enzyme immuno-assays

Several research laboratories, particularly in the UK, USA and Japan, have developed assays for the detection of calicivirus antigens and to measure antibody responses to them. However, these tests rely on scarce reagents obtained from well-documented outbreaks or from human volunteer studies. Monoclonal and polyclonal antibodies to HuCVs and some SRSVs are being raised and assays should soon become available to diagnostic laboratories. Several strains of calicivirus, e.g. Norwalk, Hawaii, Toronto and Mexico, have been expressed in baculovirus and found to assemble as virus-like particles, which has enabled sensitive EIAs to be developed by research centres.

The ability to propagate astroviruses in CaCo2 and HT-29 cells has provided the potential to produce large quantities of antigen. EIAs have been developed, but the limited supply of typing sera and monoclonal antibody has restricted their use. A commercial assay for antigen is now available.

## Reverse transcription polymerase chain reaction

The success in obtaining the complete sequence of three caliciviruses (Norwalk and Southampton) in 1991 and Manchester in 1995 has enabled primers to be designed which are directed to the highly conserved 3D region of ORF1. Application of the technique is becoming more widespread for diagnosis of outbreaks of gastro-enteritis, but it is becoming increasingly apparent that a single set of primers will not detect all strains of HuCV. Sufficient genomic variability exists between strains to use sequence data for detailed epidemiological investigation of outbreaks

e.g. associating a particular source of oysters with an outbreak of gastro-enteritis.

RT–PCR has been applied for the diagnosis of astrovirus using primers directed to conserved regions within ORF2. Primers have been designed that are group specific and others that differentiate between the serotypes.

# EPIDEMIOLOGY

## Age distribution

Tests for antigen and sero-epidemiological surveys indicate that HuCVs and astroviruses have a worldwide distribution. All age groups can be affected, but outbreaks of morphologically typical HuCV and astrovirus infection most commonly involve infants, schoolchildren and the elderly. In contrast, SRSV outbreaks are more prevalent among adults and the elderly, although there are several reports of episodes in paediatric wards.

## Modes of transmission

The various routes of transmission are shown in Figure 56.6. Epidemiological studies can identify two characteristic epidemic curves for an outbreak. In one (Fig. 56.7), when most cases appear at about the same time, this usually results from a *point source*, e.g. contaminated food or water. In the other (Fig. 56.8), cases occur in smaller numbers over a longer period, often with short intervals between the occurrence of cases. This is characteristic of person-to-person spread.

## Faecal–oral route

Affected individuals may excrete large numbers of particles in their faeces and/or vomit ($>10^9$ particles per gram). Human volunteer studies indicate that stored viruses can remain viable for several years and that the infectious dose is 10–100 particles. It is therefore important to recognize that even apparently minor contamination of hands, work surfaces, taps, carpets, etc., can be a major source of infection. This is illustrated by the number of people who can become ill when food is contaminated by a single handler (Table 56.3).

## Respiratory route

There is strong epidemiological evidence that inhalation of aerosols of vomit or faecal material, from

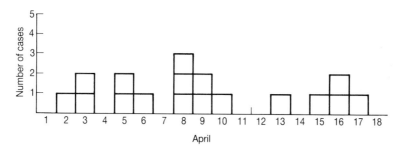

**Fig. 56.6** Routes of transmission of viruses associated with gastro-enteritis.

**Fig. 56.7** Distribution of cases of SRSV following a meal, indicative of a point source of infection.

**Fig. 56.8** Distribution of cases of astrovirus infection in a geriatric ward indicative of person-to-person spread.

| Table 56.3 | Food- and water-borne infections | | |
|---|---|---|---|
| Virus | Source | Origin | Attack rate (%) |
| SRSV | Asymptomatic food handler Salads | USA | 220/383 (57) |
| SRSV | Asymptomatic food handler Melon | UK | 239/280 (85) |
| SRSV | Caterers Cold foods | Japan | 835/3000 (46) |
| HuCV | Oysters | UK | 500/1700 (29) |
| SRSV | Oysters | Japan | 63/121 (52) |
| SRSV | Cockles and mussels | UK | >130/>300 |
| SRSV | Drinking water Secondary home contacts | USA | 495/647 (76) 719/1740 (41) |

bedlinen or nappies, can result in infection. At present, however, there is no evidence that virus replicates in the respiratory tract.

## Cold foods

Cold foods which undergo extensive handling during their preparation are a major source of outbreaks of SRSV infection. It is important to note that the foods involved, e.g. sandwiches, iced cakes, melons and salads, are not generally considered as potential causes of food poisoning. It is therefore likely that the true extent of the problem has escaped attention.

## Shellfish

Numerous outbreaks of gastro-enteritis due to caliciviruses and occasionally astroviruses have been caused by the consumption of *bivalve shellfish*, i.e. oysters, clams, mussels, cockles and scallops. The reason for the problem is that they are harvested from estuarine or coastal waters polluted with faecal material which is greatly concentrated by the filter-feeding bivalves. Methods to cleanse them prior to consumption, i.e. holding them in tanks of ultraviolet-irradiated, circulating filtered water, although successful in removing bacteria, are ineffective in freeing them of viruses. A further problem is that shellfish are frequently eaten raw or after minimal cooking.

## Water

Outbreaks of calici- and astrovirus infection associated with the consumption of untreated water, contaminated municipal drinking water or ice have been reported in the USA, UK and Australia. In the developing world where water is often untreated the problem is likely to be far greater. This is emphasized by epidemics of a calicivirus, hepatitis E, in many parts of the world.

## Asymptomatic excretors

Epidemiological investigation and volunteer trials have shown that asymptomatic excretion of caliciviruses and astroviruses is not uncommon. Such individuals may serve as an important reservoir of infection, particularly in situations such as hospitals or the catering industry.

## TREATMENT

At present there is no specific treatment for infections with these agents. Severe dehydration in infants or elderly debilitated patients should be managed in hospital with parenteral fluid replacement.

## CONTROL

### Control of food-borne outbreaks

The following guidelines for the management of an outbreak associated with food have been proposed in the UK by the Public Health Laboratory Service Working Party on Viral Gastro-enteritis:

1. Staff who develop or have had symptoms such as diarrhoea and/or vomiting should be excluded from work until 48 h after recovery.

2. If kitchen or adjacent areas have been fouled (e.g. by vomitus) then (a) the area should be thoroughly cleaned and disinfected with a 10 000 p.p.m. hypochlorite solution, and (b) all food to be eaten uncooked should be destroyed.

3. The importance of hygienic practices, particularly handwashing, should be reinforced.

4. High-risk foods such as bivalve shellfish should be excluded from the kitchen, and other foods which require much handling (e.g. salads and sandwiches) should be bought in or obtained from other branches if at all possible.

5. Unnecessary kitchen traffic should be stopped: the kitchen should not be used as a short-cut for other staff, particularly during the period of an outbreak.

### Management and prevention of hospital outbreaks

1. Ensure that both bacteriological and virological investigations are instigated at the same time.

2. Whenever possible, affected patients should be isolated and infected nursing, medical and support staff excluded from work.

3. All staff and patients on an affected ward should be screened as asymptomatic infections are not uncommon.

4. Particular attention should be paid to handwashing; 70–90% methanol or ethanol has been shown to be effective against astroviruses and rotaviruses even in the presence of faeces.

5. Bed-pan washers need to be examined to ensure they are working efficiently.

6. In some outbreaks it may be necessary to close wards to new admissions until all patients have stopped excreting virus and no new cases have occurred for a period of 72 h.

7. Staff movement from affected to unaffected wards should be restricted, group activities stopped and visits by children discouraged.

## RECOMMENDED READING

Bradley D, Japaridze A, Cook E H et al 1988 Aetiological agent of enterically transmitted non-A, non-B hepatitis. *Journal of General Virology* 69: 731–738

Carter M J, Cubitt W D 1995 Norwalk and related viruses. *Current Opinion in Infectious Disease* 8: 403–409

Cowden J M, Wall P G, Adak C, Evans H, le Baigue S, Ross D 1995 Outbreaks of foodborne infectious intestinal disease in England and Wales; 1992 and 1993. *Public Health Laboratory Service Communicable Disease Report* 5, review 8

Kapikian A Z (ed) 1994 *Viral Infections of the Gastrointestinal tract*, 2nd edn. Marcel Dekker, New York, pp 471–518, 549–579

Murphy F A, Fauquet C M, Bishop D H L et al 1995 Caliciviridae. In: *Virus Taxonomy. Sixth Report of the International Committee on Taxonomy of Viruses*. Springer-Verlag, New York, pp 359–367

Willcocks M M, Carter M J, Madeley C R 1992 Astroviruses. *Reviews in Medical Virology* 2: 97–106

# 57

# Coronaviruses

**Upper respiratory tract disease**

*E. O. Caul and J. M. Darville*

The relatively short history of the coronaviruses began in the early 1930s when an acute respiratory infection of domesticated chickens was shown to be caused by a virus now known as avian infectious bronchitis virus (IBV). Similarly, in the early 1950s, it was shown that colonies of mice maintained for laboratory research were endemically infected with a virus which in some circumstances caused outbreaks of fatal hepatitis. This virus was termed mouse hepatitis virus (MHV). A longer history, however, may be claimed for feline infectious peritonitis virus (FIPV), which has been associated by retrospective diagnosis with a case reported in the literature in 1912.

In the 1960s, research with human volunteers at the Common Cold Unit near Salisbury showed that colds could be induced by nasal washings that did not contain rhinoviruses. Subsequent in-vitro work using organ cultures revealed the presence of enveloped viruses in these washings. Electron microscopical studies demonstrated a unique morphology for these viruses, and comparative studies demonstrated a similarity to the previously described IBV and MHV. The term *coronavirus* was adopted for these agents in 1968, reflecting their morphology in the electron microscope after negative staining, and in 1975 the name *Coronaviridae* was accepted for the family. It is now evident that coronaviruses are widespread in nature, infect a range of hosts with variable tissue tropisms and are highly species specific. Although in humans they appear to be limited to infections of the respiratory and probably the enteric tracts, their involvement in systemic disease in other animals has over the years given rise to the suspicion that they may also cause more severe human disease. Unless such a link is established, however, it is likely that the human coronaviruses will remain relatively under-researched.

## PROPERTIES

### Morphology and structure

The most studied coronaviruses are IBV and MHV. The particles are pleomorphic and enveloped, varying between 75 and 160 nm in diameter, although this measurement has been found to be affected by the choice of negative stain used for electron microscopy. Widely spaced club-shaped surface projections or peplomers (composed of surface or S protein) of approximately 20 nm in length are seen in all species. These give the particles their characteristic *fringed* appearance, reminiscent of the solar corona, when negatively stained (Fig. 57.1). It is from this unique appearance that the name of the virus (Latin, *corona* = crown) is derived. There is some variation in the morphology and spacing of the peplomers. Bovine coronavirus (BCV) has a distinct inner fringe of short peplomers of haemagglutinin esterase (HE), as well as the outer fringe. This double fringe is also seen in other coronaviruses of the same antigenic group including human coronavirus (HCV) OC43.

The genome is encoded in non-segmented single-stranded positive-sense RNA of approximately 30 kilobases. In the virion this is complexed with nucleoprotein (N) in an extended helical nucleocapsid of 9–11 nm diameter. This is enclosed within a lipoprotein envelope in association with a transmembrane protein (M) to which the peplomers are attached. Coronaviruses also have a small membrane (sM) protein which is thought to have a role in assembly and/or budding. S protein is the major inducer of neutralizing antibody, although monoclonal antibodies raised against M protein can neutralize infectivity in the presence of complement. Antigenic variation is a feature of the S protein although the N protein is relatively conserved.

**Fig. 57.1** Particles of HCV serogroup 229E grown in human fibroblast cells and stained with 1.5% phosphotungstic acid. The bar represents 100 nm.

**Table 57.1** Antigenic relationships of mammalian coronaviruses

**Group 1**

Human coronavirus (HCV) 229E
Porcine transmissible gastro-enteritis virus (TGEV)
Canine coronavirus (CCV)
Feline infectious peritonitis virus (FIPV)
Porcine epidemic diarrhoea virus (PEDV)

**Group 2**

Human coronavirus (HCV) OC43
Rat coronavirus (RCV)
Rat sialodacro-adenitis virus (SDAV)
Porcine haemagglutinating encephalomyelitis virus (HEV)
Bovine coronavirus (BCV)
Mouse hepatitis virus (MHV)

**Unclassified**

Human enteric coronavirus (HECV)
Rabbit coronavirus (RbCV)
Mink coronavirus (MkCV)
Cheetah coronavirus (ChCV)

## Taxonomy

The family Coronaviridae contains the two genera *Coronavirus* and *Torovirus*. As yet there is little firm evidence to associate toroviruses with human disease. Arteriviruses, although distinct from coronaviruses in both morphology and genome size, have some genetic similarity, and it has been proposed to include them in the 'Coronavirus superfamily'.

Human coronavirus (HCV) is the only human species so far recognized, although human enteric coronavirus (HECV) is a likely second species. Also firmly recognized are coronaviruses of chickens (causing bronchitis), mice (hepatitis, gastro-enteritis and encephalitis), pigs (gastro-enteritis and encephalomyelitis), dogs, turkeys, cattle, horses (all gastro-enteritis), rats (pneumonia and swelling of salivary glands) and cats (peritonitis). In addition, coronavirus-like particles have been demonstrated in the faeces of cats, monkeys and rabbits both with enteritis and in health. In all probability they infect all or most higher animal species.

The confirmed species of coronavirus may readily be distinguished from each other by their limited host range. Serological studies of the N, M and S proteins (see below) have revealed antigenic relationships, allowing classification into two mammalian (Table 57.1) and two avian groups.

## Cultivation

Some avian and mammalian coronaviruses can be cultivated in fertile eggs or in cell culture with relative ease. The study of many coronaviruses, including HCV, has, however, been hampered by a relative difficulty in cultivation. The traditional method of cultivating HCV has been in fetal tracheal organ culture. However, HCV strains related to 229E may be isolated more readily in human diploid cells and strains related to OC43 may be adapted to grow in them after initial isolation in organ culture.

## REPLICATION

Coronaviruses attach to either protein or carbohydrate moieties of glycoprotein receptors on host cells via their S (and HE) proteins. After penetration an RNA-dependent RNA polymerase is translated from the genomic RNA before making the negative strand template for new genomic RNA. The viruses replicate in the cytoplasm with a growth cycle of 10–12 h. They bud not from the plasma membrane but from the Golgi apparatus (where the M protein localizes) into intracytoplasmic vesicles and leave the cell by fusion of these with the plasma membrane.

Viral infection may result in cell lysis but fusion of adjacent cells leading to the formation of *syncytia* can also occur and the virus may have a potential for persistence. The optimum temperature for the replication of HCV is 33°C, reflecting the usual habitat in the upper respiratory tract.

## CLINICAL FEATURES AND PATHOGENESIS

As well as being markedly species specific, coronaviruses show strong tissue tropism. They usually infect via the gut and/or respiratory tract. While some remain in these sites others can spread to specific organs. Different isolates of the same coronavirus type show different tropisms for the gut and respiratory tract. This tropism is determined by the S protein and by the type and distribution of receptors.

### Human coronavirus

The only significant condition known to follow HCV infection is upper respiratory tract disease and it is estimated that up to 30% of '*common colds*' are caused by coronaviruses. This figure is based on serological responses to OC43 and 229E antigens and could well be higher depending on the prevalence of unclassified human coronaviruses. Statistically, coronaviruses cause more coryza and discharge than do rhinoviruses, which in turn cause pharyngitis and coughing, more frequently than coronaviruses. However, individual cases cannot be attributed to either virus group on clinical grounds.

In some cases infection is mild or even subclinical. In contrast, there is some suspicion that coronaviruses may cause severe lower respiratory tract infection in the very young and the very old. However, although coronaviruses have been detected in such cases they have also been detected in control groups and so at present the association remains tentative. Coronavirus infections of the upper respiratory tract have, however, been linked in several studies with *wheezing attacks*, especially in asthmatic children.

Although the morbidity caused by HCV infection is trivial to the individual, it is economically important as illness is so widespread in the community that the virus is a major contributor to time lost from work and from academic studies.

The incubation period is from 2 to 4 days, and virus is detectable at the onset of symptoms and for 1–4 days thereafter. Symptoms outlast virus shedding and typically persist for a week, probably as a result of secondary bacterial infection.

After infection, humoral and local serological responses are detectable and cellular immune responses probably develop. These are presumed to be responsible for clearing the virus. Despite this, however, re-infection commonly occurs, and this can happen as little as 4 months after infection with the same serotype. Detectable antibody usually disappears after about 1 year.

There has been much conjecture about but no firm evidence for non-respiratory coronavirus infections in humans.

### Non-human coronaviruses

In other animals coronaviruses regularly infect and cause disease beyond the mucosal surfaces. In infected adult mice, for example, hepatitis is sometimes a consequence of reactivation.

In rats and mice, MHV strain JHM has been shown to cause demyelinating disease via an auto-immune mechanism. This is dependent on factors such as the maturity of the central nervous and immune systems. Inevitably perhaps, the coronaviruses too have been added to the list of agents, viral and otherwise, which have been implicated in the aetiology of human multiple sclerosis, none with any substantial supporting evidence.

Again, the cause of an encephalomyelitis in pigs has been shown to be a coronavirus, haemagglutinating encephalomyelitis virus (HEC). FIPV frequently infects populations of most species and all ages, and there is evidence for a carrier state. Although usually asymptomatic, the infection may cause severe peritonitis through antibody-dependent enhancement of infectivity and is usually fatal.

### Pathogenesis

It is presumed that the major pathogenic process, at least in human coronavirus infection, is the direct cytolysis of infected cells as a result of viral replication. However, the ciliostasis observed in organ culture may also be a contributory factor in vivo. Since HCV can cause disease on reinfection soon after primary infection, it cannot be excluded that humoral antibody or some other component of the immune system has some role in causing or aggravating acute disease, but no evidence for this exists. That coronaviruses have the potential to cause disease by immunopathological mechanisms is shown in the examples already given of central nervous system disease in mice and rats and of peritoneal disease in cats. There is no evidence for long-term carriage of HCVs.

## LABORATORY DIAGNOSIS

There is no clinical requirement for laboratory diagnosis since human respiratory tract infections with coronaviruses are known to be mild. At present, therefore, laboratory diagnosis has essentially research and epidemiological applications.

### Virus isolation

Members of the OC43 group of HCV will only grow on primary inoculation in *organ culture* (hence the designation). Virus growth may be detected by indirect means, such as passage to suckling mouse brain (resulting in fatal encephalitis and yielding a complement-fixing antigen from brain tissue) or by the demonstration of a haemagglutinin. Passage to diploid cell cultures may result in a cytopathic effect while infection of human volunteers may result in clinically apparent respiratory disease. Premature inhibition of ciliary motion in organ cultures, i.e. ciliostasis, can be seen and, furthermore, characteristic particles can be demonstrated by electron microscopy.

In contrast to the OC43 group, the 229E group can be cultivated directly in human diploid cells such as WI38 or human embryo kidney. The cytopathic effect, often described as 'tatty', resembles the non-specific degeneration of aged cultures with individual cells rounding and detaching from the cell monolayer. However, overlays such as agarose or methylcellulose may reveal the development of plaques by some strains while others produce syncytia.

### Serology

Antibodies to HCV have been detected by complement fixation, by haemagglutination inhibition (some strains) and by neutralization. The last is always a complex procedure and is especially so with these viruses. More recently, reliable enzyme-linked immunosorbent assay (ELISA) tests for detecting anti-HCV antibody have been developed. ELISA is now the preferred technique although its use is still limited to research and epidemiology. Antibody is a marker of past infection but, as reinfections are well documented, such antibody cannot be regarded as reflecting immunity.

### Rapid techniques

Although not yet of any practical value in monitoring HCV disease the methods developed for the rapid diagnosis of other agents have been applied to HCV. For example, ELISAs have been used to detect antigens in respiratory secretions. Since coronavirus antigens are associated with cell membranes the virus can be detected using techniques based on monoclonal antibody immunofluorescence, as are other respiratory viruses. Finally, reliable reverse-transcriptase polymerase chain reaction techniques for detecting coronavirus RNA have also been described.

## TREATMENT AND PREVENTION

The treatment of coronavirus infections, in common with most viral infections, remains *symptomatic* only. Indeed, since disease in humans is almost invariably mild, coronavirus infection ranks low on the list of candidates for specific antiviral chemotherapy. Although tribavirin has an in vitro effect against coronaviruses there is no record of this drug being used in vivo. Recombinant α-interferon has been used to prevent infection in volunteers in experimental studies. Effective vaccines have been produced to control some of the economically important coronavirus infections of animals.

## EPIDEMIOLOGY

Studies using both virus isolation and serology have shown that HCV infections occur wherever in the world they have been sought. Similarly, HCV activity can be widespread in the community and in widely separated areas. Rates of infection are similar in all age groups and there are no other factors, e.g. sex or socio-economic status, known to influence the frequency of infection. Given the above, coronaviruses behave in the same way as other human respiratory viruses.

Infection with HCV is markedly seasonal, with peaks of disease usually occurring late in winter or early spring. However, the exact timing of the peak can vary within the season, as it does with respiratory syncytial virus, and occasionally peaks of infection have been observed outside the usual season.

The two serogroups 229E and OC43 display an unusual periodicity. Each group becomes prevalent every 2–3 years with only sporadic isolates being made of the non-dominant type within the same community. However, the cycles do overlap so that in a single season 229E might predominate in one region and OC43 in another. This short-term cycling indicates that despite the diversity which exists within the OC43 serogroups at least, there are functionally few serotypes of HCV. Were it not for the ease with which reinfection occurs, this might be thought to indicate the feasibility of control by vaccination.

## Transmission

HCV infects the respiratory tract by the air-borne route, i.e. by the inhalation of droplets or aerosols generated by the coughs and sneezes of infected individuals. There is some evidence that fomites are a secondary factor in transmission.

## HUMAN ENTERIC CORONAVIRUS

In 1975 simultaneous reports of the discovery of coronavirus-like particles in human faeces by electron microscopy were made in Bristol, UK, and in southern India. It was at first suggested that these particles were derived from host cells or mycoplasmas.

However, it was soon shown that they could be propagated in human fetal intestinal organ cultures with cytoplasmic replication and 'budding' from the smooth endoplasmic reticulum, indistinguishable from that which occurs with HCV. More recently, unconfirmed reports have been made of the serial propagation of these agents in intestinal organ culture and of their detailed biochemical analysis. Although a causative association of *human enteric coronavirus* (HECV) with human enteric disease has yet to be proven, there is no doubt that coronaviruses are significant agents of *enteritis* in other animal species. Recent studies indicate the existence of two serotypes of HECV, one of which is reported to cross-react serologically with HCV strain OC43.

Other than the labour-intensive organ culture method described above, the only means of detecting HECV is by electron microscopy. The introduction of other techniques awaits the confirmation and upgrading of the virus as a pathogen.

HECV appears to be endemic throughout the world with a high prevalence in the developing countries, in which there may be some seasonal variation. In Western countries the prevalence is high in travellers from third-world countries and in low socio-economic groups and is markedly higher in male homosexuals than in the normal population. Although it has not been proved that HECV is spread by the enteric or faecal–oral route, there is strong circumstantial evidence that this is so; transmission by contaminated water may also be possible. The observed high prevalence among Western male homosexuals may be explained by oral–anal–genital contact.

## CONTROL

Given the economic impact of the common cold, HCV infections, like those with rhinoviruses, are obvious targets for control. However, the ease of reinfection suggests that the development of conventional vaccines would be an unrewarding approach, which might indeed create further problems through postulated immune-mediated pathogenic mechanisms. Nevertheless, in the veterinary field, effective vaccines have been developed to protect animals of economic importance from outbreaks of infection in which flocks or herds can be devastated. For example, both attenuated and inactivated vaccines are available to protect chickens from IBV, and live vaccines are used in sows to give their piglets lactogenic immunity to porcine transmissible gastro-enteritis virus. There is, however, a need for improved vaccines.

RECOMMENDED READING

Ashley C, Caul E O 1989 Human enteric coronaviruses. In: Farthing M J G (ed) *Viruses and the Gut* (*Proceedings of the Ninth BSG: SK & F International Workshop 1988*). Smith, Kline and French Laboratories, Welwyn Garden City, pp 91–95
Monto A S 1989 Coronaviruses. In: Evans A S (ed) *Viral Infections of Humans: Epidemiology and Control*, 3rd edn. Plenum Press, New York, pp 153–167
Resta S, Luby J P, Rosenfield C R, Seigel J D 1985 Isolation and propagation of a human enteric coronavirus. *Science* 229: 978–981

Siddell S G (ed) 1995 *The Coronaviridae*. Plenum Press, New York
Siddell S, Wege H, ter Muelen V 1983 The biology of coronaviruses. *Journal of General Virology* 64: 761–776
Sturman L S, Holmes K V 1983 The molecular biology of coronaviruses. *Advances in Virus Research* 28: 35–112
Tyrrell D A J, Alexander D J, Almeida J D et al 1978 Coronaviridae: second report. *Intervirology* 10: 321–328

# 58

## Rhabdoviruses

### Rabies

*S. Sutherland*

The hosts of viruses constituting the family Rhabdoviridae include mammals, reptiles, birds, fish, insects and plants. By definition, members of the family must be enveloped, single-stranded RNA viruses, with bullet-shaped or rod-shaped morphology. As with other virus families its members are unrelated serologically unless they form part of a distinct genus. About 80 viruses have vertebrate hosts with many found in invertebrates also. Most of these rhabdoviruses have not as yet been fully categorized, but two genera are known whose members have important roles in animal or human disease. The smaller genus, with which this chapter is concerned has been designated *Lyssavirus*, the name being derived from the Greek word for madness or frenzy. This genus has rabies virus as its prototype. The larger genus, named *Vesiculovirus*, whose members are associated with the disease vesicular stomatitis, is particularly prevalent among horses, cattle and pigs in the Americas.

Rabies has been recognized in humans and animals for many centuries, even before biblical times, as a distressing disease which develops rapidly into an acute encephalomyelitis, often frenzied initially, then subsiding into delirium, coma and death. A prominent feature in humans is *hydrophobia* – fear of water and inability to swallow it. Figure 58.1 shows part of a case report from Edinburgh dated 1747.

## DESCRIPTION

The genus *Lyssavirus* includes rabies virus and five other rabies-related viruses, all of which have been isolated mainly from various animal and insect species in Africa (Table 58.1).

Rabies virus typically is bullet shaped (Fig. 58.2) and measures $75 \times 180$ nm. Established as a transmissible agent by Pasteur, it was shown in 1931 by the collodion filtration method to be an ultra-

LI. *A Hiſtory of the* Rabies canina; *by Dr.* ANDREW PLUMMER *Profeſſor of Medicine in the Univerſity of* Edinburgh.

Publiſhed by a

## SOCIETY in *EDINBURGH.*

VOLUME V. PART II.

Printed by W. and T. RUDDIMANS, for Meſſrs. HAMILTON and BALFOUR, Bookſellers.

## M. DCC. XLVII.

A Young Gentleman, about ſeventeen Years of Age, who had been Apprentice to a Surgeon in the Country, and had come to *Edinburgh* for his Improvement, about the Beginning of *December* 1728, was bit by a Dog in the middle Finger of the right Hand, about the Middle of the Nail. At firſt he ſaid the Dog belonged to a Perſon of his Acquaintance; which Dog had no Symptoms of Madneſs at the Time: But afterwards he affirmed, that he was bit by a ſmall Dog, which he obſerved ſtraggling on the Streets, when he was endeavouring to catch him; and that he never knew what became of the Dog.

**Fig. 58.1** Rabies case report, Edinburgh 1747. (By courtesy of Dr. A. G. Dempster, University of Otago, New Zealand.)

microscopical particle, and was first visualized by electron microscopy in 1962. Its inner nucleoprotein core of single-stranded RNA enclosed in nucleoprotein

**Table 58.1**  Lyssaviruses

| Species | Serotype | Source | Occurrence |
|---|---|---|---|
| Rabies (prototype) | 1 | Carnivores, cattle, man, bats (warm-blooded animals) | World-wide |
| Lagos bat (rabies-like) | 2 | Fruit-eating bats, cats | West Africa |
| Mokola (rabies-like) | 3 | Shrews, man, cats, dogs, rodents | Africa |
| Duvenhage (rabies-like) | 4 | Man, bats (insectivorous) | South Africa, Europe |
| Kotonkan (rabies-like) | No type allotted | *Culicoides* (midges) | West Africa |
| Obodhiang (rabies-like) | No type allotted | Mosquitoes | East Africa |

**Fig. 58.2**  Rabies virus particle. Bar, 30 nm. (By courtesy of Dr Joan Crick, Animal Virus Research Institute, Pirbright, UK.)

The viral membrane or matrix (M) protein lies between the core and the outer lipoprotein envelope, which is itself fringed with projections (Fig. 58.3). Extraction of the outer envelope releases a glycoprotein (G) which can induce the formation of neutralizing antibody. Such antibody is serotype-more than group-specific and can have a protective effect if circulating in the blood in sufficient amount at, or even shortly after, the time of a biting incident by a rabid animal. Molecular analysis of the G protein in virulent and avirulent variants has detected an amino acid substitution at site 333, where, in the more pathogenic variant, arginine has replaced glutamine or isoleucine.

Rabies virus is rapidly inactivated at 60°C. It can remain viable for some days at 4°C, for longer periods when stored as infected brain tissue suspended in

(N) with helical symmetry provides the group antigen for the genus. This antigen may have a role in cell-mediated immunity. The RNA has a molecular weight of $4.5 \times 10^6$ and is of negative sense. The enzyme RNA-dependent RNA polymerase is essential for the initiation of replication, and is enclosed within the virion in association with the ribonucleoprotein core.

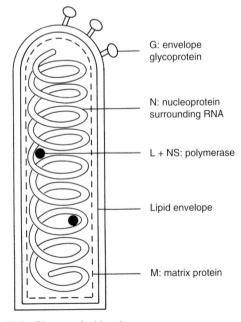

**Fig. 58.3**  Diagram of rabies virus.

G: envelope glycoprotein

N: nucleoprotein surrounding RNA

L + NS: polymerase

Lipid envelope

M: matrix protein

50% glycerol at 4°C and indefinitely when stored at or below −70°C or in a freeze-dried state. It is sensitive to lipid solvents, β-propiolactone, detergents and proteolytic enzymes.

## REPLICATION

Virus replication will occur in all warm-blooded animals, of which rabbits, guinea-pigs, rats and mice are useful for primary isolation. Growth also occurs in the chick or duck embryo and in a range of cell cultures, including baby hamster kidney and mouse neuroblastoma cells, human diploid lung fibroblasts, chick embryo fibroblasts and Vero monkey kidney cells, though with minimal cytopathic effects. The last three are among cells used in vaccine production.

Virus attaches via the glycoprotein of the envelope. In neural tissue virus attachment occurs at neuromuscular junctions via the acetylcholine receptors. However, while this may account for the localization and spread of the virus within the nervous tissue, there must be other receptors since the host cell range is broad and not confined to the central nervous system. Entry is by endocytosis; transcription of five messenger RNA species is catalysed by the virion RNA polymerase. The corresponding viral proteins are: N, the nucleoprotein; L and NS, together forming the polymerase; M, the internal membrane protein; and G, the protein which is glycosylated and inserted into the viral envelope (Fig. 58.3). Viral RNA is replicated on a positive-strand template by a viral polymerase. Only negative strands are enclosed in new virions. The M protein appears to be important in packaging the RNA and protein N and linking it to the envelope. Virions are formed by budding in association with the endoplasmic reticulum of the cell. The virus affects cell protein synthesis and the cell will die but, before this stage, it is possible to detect viral antigens by immunofluorescence or immunoprecipitation tests. Accumulation of cytoplasmic viral protein inclusions (*Negri bodies*) may be visible by light microscopy after appropriate staining. This has long been a useful diagnostic feature.

Newly recovered strains from animals are capable of killing laboratory animals such as mice within 10–20 days after intracerebral inoculation. The appearance of eosinophilic inclusions or Negri bodies, particularly in nerve cells of the hippocampus, brain stem or cerebellum, and specific rabies immunofluorescence confirm the diagnosis. Such strains, stemming from Pasteur, are called 'wild' or 'street' viruses. Serial animal passage may select out attenuated strains of lesser virulence called 'fixed' viruses. They are usually no longer able to multiply when injected extraneurally, but reversion to greater virulence is possible by the use of an alternative host.

## CLINICAL FEATURES AND PATHOGENESIS

Rabies may present as a predominantly encephalitic disease – *furious rabies* – or as a paralytic illness – *dumb rabies*. In humans, about two-thirds suffer the encephalitic form and die within 7 days, the rest initially present as paralytic then develop encephalitis, and death may not occur for 2–3 weeks. Survival is exceedingly rare.

The incubation period in humans, mostly pinpointed from the time of a bite, can be very variable. It may be less than a week after head and neck wounds, when the virus site of entry is close to the brain, or range up to several years. Recent molecular studies have identified cases with incubation periods of 4 and 6 years. On average it may range between 1 and 3 months; the duration is shorter in children than adults. Initial virus replication is considered to occur in the tissues at the point of entry, persisting there for 48–72 h. The virus then spreads to gain access to the nerves via the motor end plates. Once within the nerve fibres it is out of reach of any circulating antibody as it travels along the axons towards the central nervous system. To early manifestations of illness, fever, malaise and headache, may be added symptoms related to the wound site, e.g. tingling, pain, lumbar weakness and ascending paralysis after leg bites, and numbness, hyperaesthesia and pain with increasing shoulder weakness after hand or arm bites.

The prodromal symptoms include malaise, headache, fever, a profound sense of apprehension and feelings of irritation with paraesthesia at the wound sites. There are complaints of dry throat, cough and thirst, but patients will not drink. High fever, rigors, difficulty in swallowing and revulsion to water predominate, followed by bizarre behaviour, excitement, agitation, hallucinatory seizures, laryngeal spasms, choking and gagging, intermingled with lucid intervals. This state, the furious form of rabies, gradually subsides into delirium, convulsions, coma and death. Sometimes only the dumb form is seen, with symmetrical ascending paralysis followed by coma and death.

Clinically, the disease may resemble other types of acute encephalomyelitis although there will often be a history of exposure to, or an unprovoked attack by, a deranged animal. Tetanus with its severe spasms may confuse but it does not induce cerebrospinal fluid changes.

The predominantly neurological mode of spread has some experimental support, since section of the main nerve trunk proximal to the inoculation site can prolong the incubation period, as can the use of drugs which inhibit axonal flow such as colchicine. Experimentally pathogenicity has been related to the capacity of a strain to induce cell fusion in neuroblastoma cells.

Despite an inflammatory reaction from the developing encephalomyelitis accompanied by considerable virus multiplication, observable damage to the nerve cells in the brain appears minimal, though if survival is sufficiently prolonged, specific cytoplasmic eosinophilic inclusions (Negri bodies) will appear. Non-specific changes include a parenchymal microglial response and perivascular cuffing with lymphocyte and plasma cell infiltration in the grey matter of the brain stem and spinal cord. From the brain the virus spreads via efferent nerves to most body tissues, including salivary glands, with multiplication in the acinar cells and extrusion into the saliva; conjunctival cells with release into tears and exudates; the kidneys with excretion in the urine; and lactating glands and milk after pregnancy. Virus has also been found in the suprarenal glands, pancreas, myocardium and at the base of hair follicles, as in the neck. Study of saliva, corneal impression smears, conjunctival exudate or hair follicle biopsy from the nape of the neck, all by immunofluorescence, may provide an initial diagnosis.

## LABORATORY DIAGNOSIS

The history may be so characteristic that early laboratory confirmation of rabies, often a problem in itself, is not necessarily requested. Difficulties can arise when information about exposure to a rabid animal is not elicited, as shown in the USA where more than a fifth of deaths due to rabies are in this category. It is worth remembering that when any visits, particularly to known rabies endemic areas, have been made up to a year or more before a death which is ascribed to encephalitis, post-mortem examination of brain and cord tissue should include a search for rabies virus.

Because of risks from contact and handling, the British Advisory Committee on Dangerous Pathogens, in line with World Health Organization (WHO) safety recommendations, has classed rabies virus as a hazard group 4 pathogen on the basis that it can cause severe human disease and is dangerous for any person in contact, but effective prophylaxis is available. Regulations provide that high-risk diseases such as rabies and viral haemorrhagic fevers should be treated in secure isolation units, and the virological investigation of specimens from such patients is permitted only in specially designated laboratories. Similarly, for suspect rabid animals there is a designated veterinary laboratory. Stringent government regulations allow propagation of rabies virus only in designated category 4 laboratories.

Where rabies is endemic, wild animals or bats captured after biting incidents should be immediately sent for laboratory confirmation of rabies, but post-exposure treatment of persons bitten should not be delayed pending a laboratory diagnosis. Domesticated dogs and cats, particularly if previously vaccinated against rabies, may be observed in isolation for up to 10–14 days. If they survive for that time it is unlikely they were incubating rabies at the time of the incident but, if they succumb quickly, antirabies treatment of persons bitten should be started without waiting for laboratory confirmation. Britain, being free from indigenous rabies, usually offers vaccine only to persons bitten while abroad, but may make an exception for anyone bitten by a bat.

## Diagnostic methods

1. Identification of rabies antigen by specific immunofluorescence:
   a. Ante-mortem – in salivary, corneal or conjunctival smears or skin biopsy from the nape of the neck. Negative results, which are frequent, do not exclude rabies.
   b. Post-mortem – in impression smears of the cut surface of the salivary gland, hippocampus, brain stem or cerebellum.
2. Virus isolation:
   a. Ante-mortem – from saliva or cerebrospinal fluid.
   b. Post-mortem – from salivary gland or brain tissue extract by mouse intracerebral inoculation. Cell culture inoculation may be used but cytopathic changes are minimal and viral antigen must be looked for by specific immunofluorescence.
3. Histological examination of fixed brain tissues by staining or immunofluorescence, including a search for Negri inclusions.
4. Fluorescent tests or enzyme-linked immunosorbent assay (ELISA) on serum or cerebrospinal

fluid for evidence of specific antibody. This would not, however, be present until 7–10 days or more had elapsed since the onset of illness.

5. Amplification of DNA following reverse transcription of viral RNA is a research technique now in use. When combined with the use of restriction enzymes-species, specific variants can be identified allowing useful molecular epidemiology to trace the source of the virus in those cases without a history of exposure.

## IMMUNOPROPHYLAXIS

The risk of infection must first be assessed to take account of the type of exposure, the animal involved and whether rabies is known to be present in that species in the geographical area where the injury occurred. Since there is no effective antiviral, post-exposure prophylaxis must be started as soon as possible after the bite or other type of exposure. The WHO has recommended (1992) that this should comprise:

1. Thorough wound cleaning with 20% soap solution or a detergent.

2. Passive prophylaxis with antirabies immunoglobulin, preferably human, 20 IU/ml/kg body weight given half in and around the wound and half in the gluteal muscle.

3. Active immunization with inactivated whole virus cell culture grown vaccine, containing at least 2.5 IU/dose, given into the deltoid muscle. The complete course of post-exposure vaccination recommended in the UK comprises six intramuscular (IM) 1 ml doses on days 0, 3, 7, 14, 30 and 90. The WHO also approves two alternative schedules (a) the 2–1–1 regimen in which a 1 ml IM dose given into each deltoid muscle on day 0 is followed by one dose on days 7 and 21 and (b) an intradermal (ID) 2–2–2–0–1–1 regimen in which two doses of 0.1 ml are given on days 0, 3 and 7 and one dose of 0.1 ml on days 30 and 90. In individuals previously immunized against rabies, passive prophylaxis is not given but two booster doses are given on days 0 and 3.

## Vaccination

Vaccination after exposure to rabies was introduced by Pasteur in 1885 on the basis that a long incubation period should allow time for immunity to develop before the onset of symptoms. His vaccine was a crude extract of rabbit spinal cord containing virus 'fixed' as a result of serial passage. A well-publicized early success established the procedure, still in use despite various vicissitudes. Whether there was live virus in the original vaccine is uncertain, but increasing demand together with the use of larger animals such as sheep or goats for its preparation led to steps to inactivate residual virus without destroying antigenicity. A substance widely used was dilute phenol. A phenolized brain suspension formed the basis of the *Semple vaccine* used in the UK from 1919 until 1966. Its drawbacks included a variable but generally low potency, which necessitated a considerable number of daily, often painful, injections with an antibody response mainly of the IgM class. There was also the disadvantage that the amount of myelin in its nervous tissue content sensitized a proportion of those being immunized, estimated to range from 1 in 500 upwards, so that many went on to develop an allergic type of encephalomyelitis. When the risk of a possible exposure to a rabid animal was assessed as only marginal, it was a matter of debate whether the risk of rabies was greater than the risk of allergic encephalomyelitis.

A *suckling mouse brain vaccine* (SMBV) containing much less myelin and with a claimed five-fold reduction or more in the incidence of allergic encephalomyelitis was developed, and is widely used in Latin American countries. A non-neurogenic *duck embryo vaccine* (DEV) was used in the UK from 1966 to 1976. More recently, a purified version of DEV has shown increased potency, but this vaccine has been superseded by cell culture vaccines of which there are several types. Those available world-wide, though not necessarily used because of their high cost, include *diploid cell vaccine* (HDCV), *primary chick embryo cell vaccine* (PCECV) and *Vero cell vaccine* (PVRV). These have good immunogenicity and safety. HDVC is the only rabies vaccine licensed in the UK for both pre- and post-exposure prophylaxis. Severe reactions are rare after use, though up to 20% may report minor local effects, and a smaller proportion systemic, influenza-like or sensitization effects.

In the UK, stocks of vaccine and of human rabies immune globulin (HRIG) are held and distributed mainly through the Public Health Laboratory Service in England and Wales and from designated centres in Scotland and Northern Ireland.

Several vaccine types and modes of delivery have been used in animals. Those used in dogs and cats are given intramuscularly, and require boosting every 1–3 years depending on the vaccine type. Attempts have been made to control the infection in wild animals by the use of live attenuated vaccines delivered orally. By carefully selecting desirable baits, such as chicken heads for foxes, successful vaccination programmes have been carried out in several European countries.

Work continues on a number of recombinant and subunit vaccines and on alternative antibody preparations for use in humans.

## EPIDEMIOLOGY

During the period 1946–95 there were 19 human cases of rabies in the UK. All were infected in other countries, 18 the result of dog bites and one from cat scratches and bites. Of the 11 cases since 1975 none had received any post-exposure treatment. In Europe, between 1977 and 1994, 198 human cases were reported, of which 21 had been infected elsewhere. Russia and Romania have reported the majority (70) of the 104 European cases since 1989. World surveys of rabies report about 25 000 cases annually, but this is thought to be an underestimate.

Among animals the disease may spread via two intercommunicating pathways, urban and sylvatic. The *urban* mode, more immediately dangerous for humans, diffuses among domestic or scavenger dogs and cats, a situation prevailing in Third World countries. The *sylvatic* mode, as it affects small carnivores and mustelids, provides less opportunity for contact with humans. Its main focus in different regions may be confined to separate species, e.g. foxes in continental Europe, Canada and northern parts of the USA, racoons along the eastern seaboard, skunks in the mid-western states and coyotes in the southern states of the USA and the mongoose in the West Indies. Spread to other species or to humans, though a potential threat, appears unusual. Perpetuation of the disease comes particularly from salivary excretion of the virus during the early stages of illness combined with the biting tendencies of carnivores.

Dogs, and to a lesser extent cats, are the main sources of human infection so that control of such animals by surveillance, with elimination of strays and the initiation of vaccination programmes, as has occurred in the USA and many European countries has considerably reduced the incidence of human rabies in these countries. In other areas without the benefit of these programmes the incidence of both human and animal disease is much greater.

As well as the involvement of terrestrial animals there is widespread rabies infection in numerous species of bats. This was first noted in Brazil about 1916 when it was realized that both cattle and humans could develop rabies after being bitten by blood-sucking vampire bats. A similar situation was then found to exist in many Central and South American countries and also in the West Indies with considerable mortality in cattle. Some human and animal infections may have followed the eating of infected carcasses.

From 1953, reports, initially from the USA, have shown that many species of insectivorous and fruit-eating bats may also harbour rabies viruses with excretion and transfer of infection when they are sick. It is now believed that affected vampire bats, although thought to be mostly carriers, do ultimately succumb to the disease. Spread can readily occur in some bat colonies from the close contact among large numbers congregating together.

Most viruses isolated from bats in the Western hemisphere resemble the classic serotype 1 rabies virus, though in cross-protection and neutralization tests, as would be expected, minor antigenic differences are found. As dog rabies is brought under control in the USA and Europe a proportionate increase in bat rabies infections has been identified. Of 25 cases in the USA since 1980, 12 were bat variants even though a history of bat bites was obtained in only six. Bites by bats form the usual mode of transmission to humans, though in two reported fatal cases in the USA in 1956 and 1958 direct inhalation of virus while working in bat-infested caves in Texas led to the disease.

In continental Europe the fox provides the main animal reservoir, but rabies-like viruses have also been recovered in a small number of instances from some bat species in Germany since 1954. Infected bats have also been identified in the former Yugoslavia, Turkey, the former USSR, Poland, Finland, the Czech Republic, Denmark, Holland, France, Switzerland and Spain. No interchange of viruses between bats and animals such as foxes has so far been observed. The European bat viruses more closely resemble the serotype 4 Duvenhage virus from South Africa than the American bat viruses, which are serotype 1 rabies virus.

In the UK the system of 6 months' quarantine for imported canines and felines was introduced in 1886, together with measures for the muzzling of dogs. By 1902 this step had succeeded in freeing the country from rabies. The disease was reintroduced in 1918 via a dog brought back illegally from Europe. The disease was again eliminated from animals by 1922. Since that time the UK has been free from indigenous rabies despite two incidents in 1969 and

1970 when dogs released from quarantine developed rabies but, fortunately, there was no further spread. The quarantine barrier, still in force, has been extended to include most other imported animals with an additional proviso that quarantined dogs and cats must be injected, under veterinary supervision, with an acceptable animal rabies vaccine on entry to quarantine and again after 1 month. In Britain, foxes do not appear to have been involved, and laboratory studies of bat species have not shown the presence of rabies or rabies-like viruses so far. Whether the Channel Tunnel link with Europe will alter the situation remains to be seen.

## Transmission

Rabies virus does not penetrate intact skin and, if deposited on it from saliva, would become inactivated through such factors as temperature, time and the process of drying. The portal of entry from the infected saliva of a rabid animal is via abrasions or scratches on the skin, or mucous membranes exposed to saliva from licks, but more frequently via deep penetrating bite wounds. The amount of virus excreted in saliva is variable and bites through clothing by absorption of the saliva may reduce the amount so that not every person bitten by a rabid animal necessarily develops the disease. Uncommon routes include inhalation while in bat-infested caves, or from aerosols released during centrifugation of infected materials in the laboratory, or from ingestion of the flesh of rabid animals. High doses of virus would be necessary in such instances.

Despite the excretion of virus in the saliva and conjunctival exudates and occasional misguided attempts at mouth-to-mouth resuscitation, humans do not figure as spreaders of rabies. Transfer via infected corneal transplants has, however, been reported on at least four occasions.

## CONTROL

Because rabies has a world-wide distribution its complete elimination would need the eradication of infection from all susceptible animal species. First steps in this direction have been the use of vaccine-impregnated baits to reduce rabies in foxes in Europe and Canada and racoons in the USA. Since most human exposure has resulted from contact with infected dogs and cats, vaccination of domestic dogs and cats combined with *post-exposure* prophylaxis for those exposed in specific incidents to suspect rabid animals and *pre-exposure* for those who may come in contact with such animals in the course of their work has reduced the number of human cases in many countries.

Pre-exposure immunization requires two injections of 1 ml of vaccine, given into the deltoid muscle 4 weeks apart. A test for neutralizing antibody is advised 4 weeks later. A reinforcing dose is given at 12 months, followed by boosters every 2–3 years. A booster should be given after any potential exposure.

Clear signs of case reduction have come from the developed countries which have applied this scheme, and now the need is to extend the procedure to other, particularly enzootic, regions where dogs are the major reservoir of the virus. Past attempts to control wild-life rabies by such draconian measures as shooting and gassing have had short-lived effects. Species vary in their susceptibility to rabies and live vaccine strains that may be used for one species may be unsuitable for another. Extension to canine and other species may become feasible when suitable oral vaccine strains are identified. A number of vectors such as vaccinia, racoon poxvirus, fowlpox, canarypox and adenovirus have been used to express a recombinant rabies glycoprotein gene with successful induction of neutralizing antibody in a variety of animal species.

RECOMMENDED READING

Baer G M 1994 Rabies – an historical perspective. *Infectious Agents and Disease* 3: 168–180

Fishbein D B, Robinson L E 1993 Rabies. *New England Journal of Medicine* 329: 1632–1638

Porterfield J S 1989 *Viruses of Vertebrates*, 5th edn. Ballière Tindall, London, pp 214–229

Rupprecht C E, Dietzschold B, Koprowski H (eds) 1994 Lyssaviruses. *Current Topics in Microbiology and Immunology* 187

Smith J S 1989 Rabies virus epitopic variation: use in ecologic studies. *Advances in Virus Research* 36: 215–253

Smith J S, Fishbein D B, Rupprecht C E, Clark K 1991 Unexplained rabies in three immigrants in the United States. *New England Journal of Medicine* 324: 205–211

Winkler W G, Bogel K 1992 Control of rabies in wildlife. *Scientific American* June: 56–62

# 59

# Transmissible spongiform encephalopathies

**Scrapie; kuru; Creutzfeldt–Jakob disease**

*J. W. Ironside*

## INTRODUCTION

The transmissible spongiform encephalopathies are a unique group of fatal neurodegenerative disorders occurring in humans and animals which take their name from two major characteristics:

1. All are experimentally transmissible to a variety of animals. The precise nature of the transmissible agents involved is unknown, but they have a very small size (less than 30 µm) and possess physical and chemical properties which are quite distinct from those of conventional viruses and bacteria. One hypothesis concerning these agents suggests that they are composed entirely of protein, without any nucleic acid, for which the term *prion* (protein-aceous infectious particle) is used.

2. The disorders caused by these agents are characterized in all species by spongiform change in the central nervous system. This consists of numerous small vacuoles (10–200 µm) which are formed within neurones and in the neuropil of the grey matter, where they coalesce to form larger cystic cavities. This is accompanied by neuronal death and a reactive proliferation of astrocytes and microglia. Prion protein (PrP) accumulates within the central nervous system both as diffuse deposits and in the form of amyloid plaques. No evidence of a host immune reaction has ever been found in this group of diseases.

## SCRAPIE

The first animal spongiform encephalopathy to be described was *scrapie*, an endemic disorder of sheep and goats which has been present in Europe for at least two centuries. Affected animals become ataxic and wasted, and often rub or scrape the fleece off the sides of their bodies, hence the name. The first experimental transmission of scrapie from affected to healthy sheep by intraocular injection of spinal cord homogenate was reported in 1936. Scrapie can be transmitted from ewe to lamb, but there is no evidence to suggest that this occurs in utero. Natural transmission is thought to occur at parturition, or by scarification or via the oral (alimentary) route. The placenta from an infected ewe is one known source of infection which can allow contamination of the farm environment.

### The scrapie agent

The scrapie agent has been the subject of intense research and is by far the best-characterized of the transmissible spongiform encephalopathy agents. Although its precise nature is unknown, it is sub-viral in size and notoriously resistant to inactivation by many physical and chemical agents including heat, exposure to ionizing or ultraviolet radiation, DNAase, RNAase, formaldehyde and glutaraldehyde. The agent has been studied by experimental transmission following inoculation into mice and hamsters, in which around 20 strains of the scrapie agent have now been identified. These strains are defined on the basis of their incubation period and on the nature and distribution of the pathology in the brain when transmitted under identical conditions to genetically similar animals. Incubation periods range from 60 days to more than 2 years, which is close to the natural life span of mice and hamsters. The incubation period is influenced by the route of inoculation (intracerebral inoculation is the most efficient mode of infection, whereas oral or parenteral routes are less efficient), the dose of the injected inoculum and its infective titre. Host genetic factors also influence the incubation period (susceptibility) of these diseases and it has recently been recognized that the major host gene involved is the PrP gene.

Electron microscopical studies of extracts from scrapie-infected brain have revealed abnormal fibrillary structures named scrapie-associated fibrils which comprise a modified host glycoprotein, which is protease resistant (PrP$^{RES}$). Scrapie-associated fibrils were found to be closely associated with the presence of the transmissible agent in scrapie-infected brains; these structures do not occur in the brains of healthy animals. PrP$^{RES}$ is a truncated form of a host-encoded glycoprotein, the normal precursor of which is expressed in a variety of cells including neurones in the central nervous system, where it is thought to play a role in synaptic function. This protein has a molecular weight of 33–35 kDa and is highly conserved through a wide range of species, but its amino acid sequence varies from one species to another. This variation is thought to influence the species barrier, a factor which regulates the success of disease transmission from one species to another under experimental conditions. During the course of scrapie infection the normal glycoprotein undergoes subtle but unknown post-translational modifications to convert to PrP$^{RES}$, becomes relatively resistant to digestion with proteinase K and acquires the ability to form scrapie-associated fibrils, which accumulate in the brain. In the prion hypothesis, conversion of the normal glycoprotein to disease-associated PrP$^{RES}$ is thought to occur by direct interaction which sparks off a self-replicating catalytic conversion. This conversion has been replicated experimentally in a cell-free system, but it remains to be demonstrated that this biochemical change accounts for all the biological properties of the scrapie agent. Many of the physical and chemical features of the scrapie agent can be explained by the prion hypothesis. However, the mechanisms by which the various strains of scrapie agent have different effects in genetically identical mice are as yet unclear and some research groups continue to believe that a second molecule, not PrP, determines the strain of the infectious agent.

## Pathogenesis

Transmission of scrapie to experimental hamsters and mice can be achieved by inoculation of infected brain tissue into a number of sites in the body; the most rapid onset of disease in experimental animals occurs following intracerebral inoculation. With peripheral inoculation spread of infection appears to occur along sympathetic nerve fibres which connect via the splanchnic nerve complex to the spinal cord. Infection then spreads to the brain at a rate of around 1 mm/day, and there is evidence to support transport of the scrapie agent within neurones. The mechanisms through which spongiform change occurs in grey matter within the central nervous system are unknown, although dilatation of neuronal lysosomal, Golgi and endoplasmic reticulum structures has been suggested.

## Other animal transmissible spongiform encephalopathies

Scrapie-like diseases have been recorded in an increasing number of captive or domesticated animals (Table 59.1), the most significant of which in the UK is bovine spongiform encephalopathy (BSE), which was first identified in 1985 and spread rapidly throughout the cattle population to affect around

**Table 59.1**  Animal diseases caused by scrapie and related agents

| Disease | Occurrence | Hosts |
| --- | --- | --- |
| Scrapie | Common in many countries world-wide | Sheep and goats |
| Transmissible mink encephalopathy | Very rare, mostly in farms in the USA | Mink |
| Chronic wasting disease | Isolated foci in Colorado and Wyoming | Mule deer and elk |
| Bovine spongiform encephalopathy | Widespread epidemic in dairy cattle in the UK, smaller outbreaks in other countries | Domestic cattle |
| Unnamed spongiform encephalopathy | Small number of exotic ungulates in zoos | Nyala Gemsbok Greater kudu Arabian oryx Eland |
| Feline spongiform encephalopathy | Small numbers of domestic cats in the UK and a few large cats in zoos | Domestic cats Cheetah |

1% of all adult cattle in the UK in 1992. It appears that this epidemic resulted from oral ingestion of the scrapie agent via contaminated meat and bone meal in cattle feed; changes in the rendering processes by which these feeds were produced in the 1980s allowed the scrapie agent to persist as a contaminant. Recycling of contaminated cattle carcasses in the meat and bone meal subsequently fed to cattle appears to have fuelled the epidemic, but the incidence of the disease is now declining as a result of a ban on the use of bovine organs as foodstuffs for other animals. Experimental studies on BSE indicate that it represents a single agent strain. In addition to transmission to cattle, this strain of agent has also transmitted by foodstuff to domestic cats, large cats and exotic ungulates in zoos (Table 59.1). There has been much speculation as to whether BSE might be transmissible to humans via the food chain or by direct contact with contaminated foodstuffs or contaminated animal carcasses. However, there is at present no epidemiological evidence to suggest that this has yet occurred (see below).

## HUMAN DISEASES

Human transmissible spongiform encephalopathies were first described in the 1920s by *Creutzfeldt* and *Jakob*; the commonest form of this disease now bears their name. Three other related disorders have subsequently been identified; the next to be recognized was the *Gerstmann–Sträussler–Scheinker syndrome* (GSS), a familial disorder characterized clinically by cerebellar ataxia, described in 1936. In the 1950s another human spongiform encephalopathy, *kuru*, was described in the Fore tribe of New Guinea. The identification of PrP and sequencing of the human PrP gene on chromosome 20 have allowed con-

siderable advances in our understanding of human transmissible spongiform encephalopathies (Table 59.2). In 1986 a very rare inherited disorder, *fatal familial insomnia*, was described and although not recognized at first as a human spongiform encephalopathy, it was reclassified as one of this group of disorders in 1992 on the basis of a characteristic mutation in the human PrP gene and accumulation of PrP$^{RES}$ in the brain.

## Creutzfeldt–Jakob disease

Creutzfeldt–Jakob disease (CJD) occurs most commonly as a sporadic disorder, affecting around 1/million population/year in most recent epidemiological studies. CJD usually presents as a rapidly progressive dementia of less than 1 year's duration which is often accompanied by other neurological abnormalities including cerebellar dysfunction, pyramidal and extrapyramidal signs, cortical blindness and akinetic mutism. Many of these features evolve as the disease progresses, and electro-encephalography often shows characteristic diffuse periodic spike discharges. Middle-aged adults are most often affected, but the disease has also been described in teenagers and may occasionally present in the ninth decade. The disease is untreatable and invariably fatal; most patients survive for only 4–8 months after the onset of major symptoms. The cause of this disorder remains unknown; it might possibly reflect selective exposure to a ubiquitous agent, perhaps causing disease only in genetically susceptible individuals (see below), or a somatic mutation involving the PrP gene in a central nervous system neurone (Fig. 59.1). No specific occupational or dietary factors exist for CJD, and the distribution of CJD cases in the UK bears no relation to that of scrapie or BSE. The distribution of CJD on a world-wide basis is markedly different from that of scrapie, particularly in Australia, where scrapie has been eradicated for many decades, but CJD occurs as a sporadic disorder.

Around 10% of cases of CJD occur as inherited disorders; these are associated with mutations or insertions in the single open-reading frame of the human PrP gene on chromosome 20 (Fig. 59.1). In recent years, many new mutations and insertions have been identified in the PrP gene in familial human spongiform encephalopathies. A naturally occurring methionine/valine polymorphism at codon 129 in the PrP gene is of major influence in determining susceptibility to CJD. Around 50% of the normal population are heterozygous at this locus, but in both sporadic and iatrogenic CJD the instance of

**Table 59.2** Human spongiform encephalopathies classifed by aetiology

| | |
|---|---|
| Sporadic disorders | CJD (around 90% of all cases) |
| Inherited disorders | CJD (around 10% of all cases)<br>Gerstmann–Sträussler–<br>Scheinker syndrome<br>Fatal familial insomnia |
| Transmitted from human to human | Kuru<br>Iatrogenic CJD (less than 1% of all cases) |

CJD, Creutzfeldt–Jakob disease.

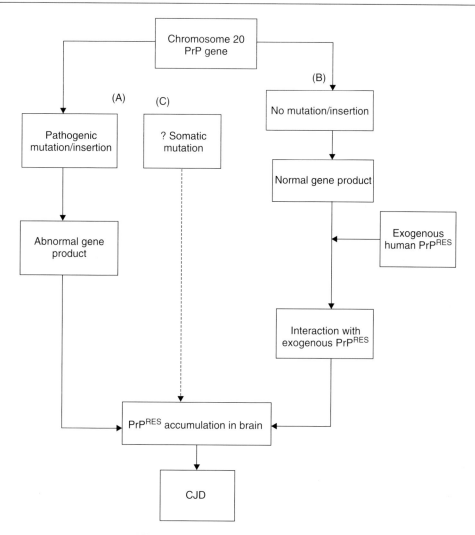

**Fig. 59.1** Postulated mechanisms of PrP$^{RES}$ accumulation in CJD. In A, an inherited PrP gene mutation results in familial CJD. In B, exogenous human PrP$^{RES}$ interacts with the normal host precursor protein, resulting in PrP$^{RES}$ accumulation. This mechanism is thought to operate in iatrogenic CJD. The cause of sporadic CJD is unknown, but proponents of the prion hypothesis have suggested that a somatic mutation in a neurone (C) might initiate the process of PrP$^{RES}$ accumulation in the brain. This 'rare event' might also explain the low incidence of sporadic CJD.

homozygosity is greatly increased (up to 90%). The mechanism for this influence on disease susceptibility is as yet unclear. CJD also occurs as an iatrogenic disorder following accidental transmission from one human to another (Fig. 59.1). Iatrogenic CJD was first described in 1974 in a corneal graft recipient. Since then, other examples of iatrogenic CJD have involved central inoculation of contaminated material from a human CJD victim to another patient, for example following the implantation of inadequately decontaminated intracerebral electrodes, or via human dura mater grafts. In the UK, the

commonest form of iatrogenic CJD occurs in recipients of human growth hormone derived from cadaveric pituitary glands, at an approximate incidence of 1/10 000 at-risk individuals with an average age at death of 25 years and incubation periods of up to 20 years. This variant of CJD is unusual in its clinical features, in which a cerebellar syndrome predominates with prominent ataxia, gait and visual disturbances; gross cerebellar atrophy and a predominant accumulation of PrP within the cerebellum are characteristic neuropathological features.

## Gerstmann–Straussler–Scheinker syndrome

GSS is the best known example of an inherited human transmissible spongiform encephalopathy. In this very rare disorder, which occurs as an autosomal dominant disease affecting middle-aged adults, cerebellar ataxia, nystagmus and gait abnormalities are prominent clinical features, with dementia occurring only towards the end of the illness. The neuropathology is characteristic, with enormous multicentric PrP amyloid plaques present throughout the central nervous system and a widespread loss of neurones which is particularly severe in the cerebellum and basal ganglia. However, these changes are not entirely specific; similar features may occur in both sporadic and other familial cases of CJD. GSS was the first human disease found to be associated with a mutation in the PrP gene; a codon 109 proline-to-leucine mutation was first identified in 1989 and has subsequently been found in several GSS families, including the original kindred described in 1936.

## Kuru

Kuru was a disease occurring in the Fore tribe of Papua New Guinea, apparently in association with practices related to ritualistic cannibalism. It still remains uncertain as to whether the brain was actually eaten, but it was handled after death by members of the tribe, particularly females and children, who went on to develop this disorder. The name *kuru* means shivering or trembling in the local dialect, which reflects the predominant clinical manifestations of a progressive cerebellar syndrome accompanied by dementia. The incubation period of the disease was variable, ranging from around 4 to 30 years. No evidence of mother-to-child transmission occurred in this disease, although its increasing prevalence made it the primary cause of death in most individuals within the tribes in the 1960s. The disease is now virtually extinct since cannibalistic practices have been abandoned.

## Fatal familial insomnia

Fatal familial insomnia is an extremely rare inherited disorder, characterized clinically by disturbances of sleep and autonomic function with relative intellectual preservation in middle age. This disorder is associated with a unique PrP genotype (codon 178 asparagine, 129 methionine/methionine), and neuro-

pathological changes which predominantly involve the thalamus. The relationship between the genotype, neuropathology and clinical features of this enigmatic disorder await further study.

## Neuropathology

The principal neuropathological features of human transmissible spongiform encephalopathies are spongiform change, neuronal loss, astrocytosis and amyloid plaque formation (Fig. 59.2). These were noted to resemble changes occurring in the brains of scrapie-affected sheep, and recognition of these similarities led to the first successful attempts to transmit kuru to experimental animals in 1966, followed by CJD in 1968, GSS in 1981 and fatal familial insomnia in 1995. In recent years, the enormous increase in our knowledge of the biochemistry and molecular biology of the transmissible agents responsible for this group of diseases has prompted a re-evaluation of their neuropathology and the study of PrP$^{RES}$ accumulation within the central nervous system. PrP$^{RES}$ deposition is confined to the central nervous system, and can occur in a variety of patterns including amyloid plaques, perivacuolar deposition around areas of spongiform change, perineuronal and axonal deposition. None of these patterns is entirely specific for any single disease category within the human transmissible spongiform encephalopathies. It is recommended that investigation of all suspected CJD cases by autopsy is performed. Only by examination of the central nervous system can the diagnosis of CJD be confirmed, placing a high priority on autopsy in suspected cases. The development of polyclonal and monoclonal antibodies to PrP has allowed the establishment of sophisticated diagnostic investigations on brain homogenates and sections from individuals thought to be suffering from CJD or a related disorder (Fig. 59.2).

## A new variant of CJD

The emergence of BSE as a new epidemic in cattle has clear potential implications for human disease, under the assumption that this disorder may be transmitted to humans through the food chain. Given the long incubation periods which are characteristic of human transmissible spongiform encephalopathies and their potential relationship to the BSE epidemic, a National CJD Surveillance Project was established for the UK in May 1990, based at the Western General Hospital, Edinburgh. In 1996, the CJD Surveillance Unit identified a new a                                                                              b

**Fig. 59.2** **a** Spongiform change in the cerebral cortex in a case of sporadic CJD consists of numerous small cyst-like spaces which tend to coalesce in the neuropil and around neurones (centre). Haematoxylin and eosin stain, ×200. **b** In this case of sporadic CJD, PrP accumulation in the cerebellum has occurred in the form of numerous plaques which stain intensely on immunocytochemistry for PrP. ×250.

variant form of CJD which so far has affected 14 patients in the UK and one in France. The age of onset is unusually young (mean = 26 y) with a prolonged illness of average duration of 14 months. The clinical features are unusual for CJD, with psychiatric and sensory symptoms at onset, followed by ataxia and myoclonus with dementia only in the final stages of the illness. The neuropathological features are relatively uniform and consist of massive accumulations of PrP$^{RES}$ throughout the brain, with the formation of multiple amyloid plaques (similar to those described in kuru) surrounded by spongiform change. Biochemical analysis of the PrP$^{RES}$ from these cases has shown a similar banding pattern in Western blot preparations to PrP$^{RES}$ from BSE in cattle and BSE in other species, including mouse, macaque monkey and cat. Sporadic CJD shows a different banding pattern relating to differential glycosylation of PrP$^{RES}$. Neuropathological studies of the macaque monkeys experimentally inoculated intracerebrally

with BSE showed similar changes to the new variant form of CJD with multiple amyloid plaques surrounded by spongiform change. These findings support the hypothesis that the new variant form of CJD is causally linked to BSE, but final proof will await the results of experimental strain typing studies in mice.

## CONCLUSION

A group of human and animal fatal neurodegenerative disorders are caused by unconventional transmissible agents which result in spongiform change, neuronal loss, reactive gliosis and amyloid plaque formation in the affected brain. Although the precise nature of the transmissible agents involved is not known, they are closely associated with an abnormal protein, PrP$^{RES}$, which accumulates within the brain in these disorders. PrP$^{RES}$ is derived from a larger precursor host glycoprotein which is normally expressed in neurones and is encoded by a gene on chromosome 20 in humans. Most examples of spongiform encephalopathies in humans occur as sporadic disorders, the underlying cause for which is unknown. A minority of cases occur as inherited disorders, which are invariably associated with mutations or insertions in the human PrP gene on chromosome 20. A large body of evidence exists to support the claim that susceptibility to both iatrogenic and sporadic human diseases is controlled by a naturally occurring polymorphism at codon 129 in the PrP gene; individuals who are homozygous at this locus

account for the large majority of CJD patients. A new variant form of CJD has been identified in the UK which appears to be causally linked to exposure to the BSE agent; final proof of this link awaits the result of strain typing studies and at present the magnitude of the risk to the UK population is uncertain. Extensive investigations on the nature of the infectious agent in these disorders has so far failed to reach any conclusion. However, the prion hypothesis, which states that the transmissible agent is composed entirely of PrP, has gained much favour at present since it appears to explain many of the transmissible and genetic aspects of these remarkable diseases.

## RECOMMENDED READING

Advisory Committee on Dangerous Pathogens 1994 *Precautions for Work with Human and Animal Transmissible Spongiform Encephalopathies*. HMSO, London

Allen I V (ed) 1993 Spongiform encephalopathies. *British Medical Bulletin* 49

Bastian F O (ed) 1991 *Creutzfeldt–Jakob Disease and Other Transmissible Human Spongiform Encephalopathies*. Mosby Yearbook, St Louis

Bradley R, Savey M, Marchant B (eds) 1991 *Sub-acute Spongiform Encephalopathies*. Kluwer, Amsterdam

Collinge J, Sidle K C L, Meads J et al 1996 Molecular analysis of prion strain variation and the aetiology of 'new variant' CJD. *Nature* 383: 685–690.

Prusiner S B, Collinge J, Powell J, Anderton B (eds) 1992 *Prion Diseases of Humans and Animals*. Ellis Horwood, Chichester

Will RG 1992 BSE and the spongiform encephalopathies. In: Kennard C (ed) *Recent Advances in Clinical Neurology*. Churchill Livingstone, Edinburgh vol 7, pp 115–127

Will R G, Ironside J W, Zeidler M et al 1996 A new variant of Creutzfeldt-Jakob disease in the UK. *Lancet* 347: 921–925

# Part 5
## FUNGAL PATHOGENS AND PARASITIC INFECTIONS

# 60

# Fungi

**Thrush; ringworm; subcutaneous and systemic mycoses**

*E. G. V. Evans*

Fungi constitute a large, diverse group of hetero-trophic organisms which exist as saprophytes, parasites or commensals, mostly in the soil and on decaying plant material. Fungi are eukaryotic, with a range of internal membrane systems, membrane-bound organelles, and a well-defined cell wall composed largely of polysaccharides and chitin. They vary considerably in size and form, but can be divided into two main groups: *moulds* and *yeasts*.

*Moulds*.   Moulds, also known as *filamentous* or *mycelial* fungi, are composed of branching filaments called *hyphae* which grow by apical extension, forming an interwoven mass, the *mycelium*; in most fungi the hyphae have regular cross-walls (*septa*) but in lower fungi these are usually absent (Fig. 60.1). In some higher fungi the hyphae may be compacted together to form a fungal tissue from which macroscopic structures such as mushrooms and toadstools are formed.

Moulds reproduce by means of *spores* which are produced, often in large numbers, by asexual cell division or as a result of sexual reproduction. Many fungi can produce more than one type of spore, depending on the growth conditions. The precise method of spore production and the type(s) of spore produced are unique to each individual fungal species. In laboratory cultures, moulds mainly produce asexual spores (Fig. 60.2).

*Yeasts*.   Yeasts are predominantly unicellular and oval or round in shape. Most reproduce by an asexual process called *budding* in which the cell develops a protuberance which enlarges and eventually separates from the parent cell. A few reproduce by fission. Some yeasts produce chains of elongated cells (*pseudomycelium*) that resemble the mycelium of moulds; some species also produce true mycelium (see Fig. 60.1).

*Dimorphic fungi*.   Fungi that can change their growth to either a mycelial or yeast phase, depending on the growth conditions, are called *dimorphic fungi*. Many of the fungi pathogenic for man are dimorphic.

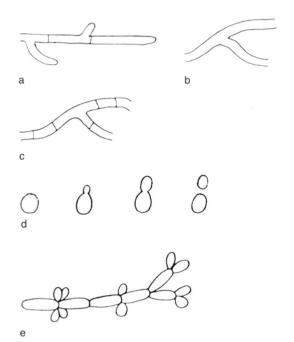

**Fig. 60.1**   Diagrammatic representation of vegetative forms of fungi: **a** hyphal tip with lateral branching; **b** aseptate (coenocytic) hypha; **c** septate hypha; **d** yeast cells showing stages in budding; **e** yeast pseudomycelium (pseudohypha). (From Evans E G V, Gentles J C 1985 *Essentials of Medical Mycology*. Churchill Livingstone, Edinburgh.)

*Identification*.   The identification of moulds is based on their macroscopic and microscopic morphology and, in particular, the type of spores they produce. Yeasts are primarily identified according to their ability to ferment sugars and to assimilate carbon and nitrogen compounds.

*Classification*.   The classification of fungi is based primarily on the method of sexual reproduction, although morphology and the method of asexual reproduction are also important. The kingdom Fungi, containing moulds and yeasts, is organized into four divisions or phyla, one of which is an artificial group

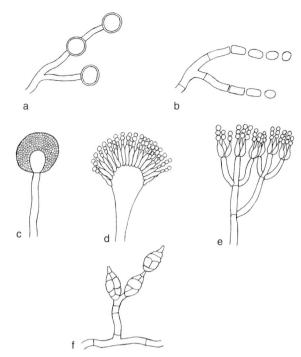

**Fig. 60.2** Types of asexual spores produced by moulds: **a** chlamydoconidia; **b** arthroconidia; **c** sporangium of *Mucor* species, containing sporangiospores; **d**, **e** sporing heads of *Aspergillus* and *Penicillium* species, respectively, with unicellular conidiospores; **f** multicelled conidia of *Alternaria* species.

which contains fungi with no known sexual phase. All the divisions contain fungi that are pathogenic for humans.

## FUNGAL DISEASES OF MAN

About 180 of the 250 000 known fungal species are known to cause disease (*mycosis*) in man and animals. Most are moulds, but there are number of pathogenic yeasts and many are dimorphic. Dimorphic fungi usually assume the mould form when growing as saprophytes in nature, and the yeast form when causing infection.

Some fungi, like the systemic pathogens *Histoplasma capsulatum* and *Coccidioides immitis* are able to establish infection in all exposed individuals. Others, such as *Candida* and *Aspergillus* species, are opportunists, which ordinarily cause disease only in a compromised host. In some mycoses the form and the severity of the infection depend on the degree of exposure to the fungus, the site and method of entry into the body, and the level of immunocompetence of the host. Occasionally, fatal toxic effects may occur after ingestion of poisonous toadstools or consumption of mouldy food that contains toxic secondary metabolites (*mycotoxins*). Allergic disease of the airways may result from inhalation of fungal spores.

Most fungal infections are caused by environmental saprophytes, but some yeasts are commensals of man and cause endogenous infections when there is some imbalance in the host. Only ringworm (dermatophyte) infections are truly contagious.

Certain fungal diseases are constrained to specific geographical regions, usually because the causal agents are saprophytes which are restricted in their distribution by soil and climatic conditions.

## Types of infection

### Superficial mycoses

Diseases of the skin, hair, nail and mucous membranes are the most common of all fungal infections and have a world-wide distribution.

**Ringworm.** This is a complex of diseases which affects the keratinous tissues of hair, nail and the horny layer of the skin; it is caused by a group of closely related mould fungi called *dermatophytes* which can colonize and digest keratin. Ringworm infections occur in both humans and animals.

**Yeast infections.** These affect the skin, nail and mucous membranes of the mouth and vagina, and are usually caused by *Candida* species, notably *C. albicans*, which are human commensals. Yeast infections are generally endogenous, but genital infections can be transmitted sexually. The yeast *Malassezia furfur*, a skin commensal, can cause an infection of the skin called *pityriasis versicolor*.

### Subcutaneous mycoses

Mycoses of the skin, subcutaneous tissues and bone, which show slow localized spread, occur mainly in the tropics and subtropics; they result from the inoculation of saprophytic fungi from soil or decaying vegetation into the subcutaneous tissue. The principal subcutaneous mycoses are mycetoma, chromomycosis and sporotrichosis.

### Systemic mycoses

Deep-seated fungal infections generally result from the inhalation of air-borne spores produced by moulds present as saprophytes in soil and on plant material. They are mostly caused by dimorphic fungi and occur mainly in the Americas. The principal diseases are coccidioidomycosis (caused by *C. immitis*), blastomycosis (*Blastomyces dermatitidis*), histoplasmosis (*H. capsulatum*) and paracocci-dioidomycosis (*Paracoccidioides brasiliensis*).

Systemic mycoses due to opportunistic pathogens such as *Aspergillus*, *Candida* and *Cryptococcus* species are more widespread. These infections are increasingly common in patients compromised by disease or drug treatment. In transplant patients, for example, they are among the most frequent causes of mortality due to infection.

## Incidence

The incidence of all the mycoses is related directly to factors which affect the degree of exposure to the causal fungi, e.g. living conditions, occupation and leisure activities. Ringworm of the foot (*athlete's foot*), with associated infections of the nails and groin, occurs most commonly in swimmers, sportsmen and industrial workers who use communal bathing facilities. Animal ringworm is an occupational hazard for farmers, veterinarians and others closely associated with animals. Field workers in warm climates who wear little protective clothing frequently contract subcutaneous infections following minor injuries from thorny vegetation. Systemic mycoses occur most frequently in workers in agriculture or the construction industry and following disturbance of soils containing the causal agents. The incidence of infections due to opportunistic pathogens has increased with developments in medical and surgical practice and with the increased number of immuno-compromised individuals, including those with the acquired immune deficiency syndrome (AIDS).

## Pathogenesis and immunity

Relatively little is known about the pathogenesis of fungal infections or the mechanisms of immunity to fungal disease, but it is clear that infection often arises due to deficiencies in the host rather than because of any inherent pathogenic properties of the fungus.

Antigenic variation on the surface of *Candida* cells may help the organism to avoid host defences. Furthermore, mannan, a cell wall polysaccharide of *Candida* species, and the capsular mucopolysaccharide of *Cryptococcus neoformans* have been shown to suppress cellular immunity. However, the importance of various fungal antigens in the disease process has yet to be elucidated fully; since anergy is a feature of serious disseminated mycotic disease, it is possible that some antigens, depending perhaps on their mode of presentation, may be inducing this anergic state.

## Clinical diagnosis

Superficial and subcutaneous mycoses often produce characteristic lesions which strongly suggest a fungal aetiology but they may also closely resemble and be confused with other diseases. Also, the appearance of lesions may be modified beyond recognition by previous therapy, e.g. with topical steroids.

The first indication that a patient may have a systemic mycosis is often their failure to respond to antibacterial antibiotics. Since early diagnosis considerably increases the chances of successful treatment, it is important that the possibility of fungal involvement should be considered from the outset, particularly in those known to be at risk of developing a fungal infection.

## Laboratory diagnosis

Laboratory diagnosis depends on recognition of the pathogen in tissue by microscopy, isolation of the causal fungus in culture, and the use of serological tests. It is important that the correct type of specimen, with adequate clinical data, is sent to the laboratory so that the appropriate investigations can be carried out. Information on factors such as travel or residence abroad, animal contacts and the occupation of the patient will enable the laboratory staff to direct their investigations towards a particular fungus or group of fungi when appropriate.

***Types of specimen.*** Skin scales, nail clippings and scrapings of the scalp which include hair stubs and skin scales are most suitable for the diagnosis of ringworm; these are collected into folded paper squares for transport to the laboratory. Swabs should be taken from suspected *Candida* infections of the mucous membranes and preferably sent to the laboratory in 'clear' transport medium. For sub-cutaneous infections the most suitable specimens are scrapings and crusts, aspirated pus and biopsies. In suspected systemic infection, specimens should be taken from as many sites as possible.

***Direct microscopy.*** Most specimens can be examined satisfactorily in wet mounts after partial digestion of the tissue with 10–20% potassium hydroxide. Gram films may also be used for the diagnosis of yeast infections of mucous membranes. Giemsa staining of smears is advised for detection of the yeast cells of *H. capsulatum* because of their small size. Fluorescent antibody staining can be used to demonstrate fungi in tissues and smears, but this requires specific antisera which are not widely available.

***Histology.*** Invasive procedures are required to obtain specimens for histological examination and, while sometimes necessary to provide firm evidence of invasive disease, such procedures are often impracticable on patients who are already seriously ill. Haematoxylin and eosin staining is seldom of value for demonstrating fungi in tissue, and specific fungal stains such as periodic acid–Schiff (PAS) and Grocott–Gomori methenamine–silver are widely used.

*Culture.* Most pathogenic fungi are easy to grow in culture. The agar media most commonly used are Sabouraud's glucose agar and 4% malt extract agar. These may be supplemented with chloramphenicol (50 mg/l) to minimize bacterial contamination and cycloheximide (500 mg/l) to reduce contamination with saprophytic fungi. Many fungal pathogens have an optimum growth temperature below 37°C. Consequently, cultures are incubated at 25–30°C and 37°C. With some of the dimorphic pathogens, the mould form develops at 22–27°C on Sabouraud's agar and enriched media such as brain-heart infusion or blood agar are used, with incubation at 37°C to promote growth of the yeast phase.

Many fungi develop relatively slowly, and cultures should be retained for at least 2–3 weeks and in some cases up to 6 weeks before being discarded; yeasts usually grow within 1–5 days. Moulds are identified by their macroscopic and microscopic morphology. Yeasts are identified by sugar fermentation and other biochemical tests, although commercial kits are available for the identification of medically important yeasts.

Culture may provide unequivocal evidence of fungal infection when established pathogens are isolated or when fungi are recovered from normally sterile sites. However, when commensals such as *Candida* species are isolated, results must be interpreted according to the quantity of the fungus isolated, the source and clinical evidence.

*Serology.* Serological tests for fungal antigens or specific antibodies are used mainly in the diagnosis of systemic fungal infections. Many tests lack sensitivity or specificity and their precise value varies from disease to disease.

The most common tests for fungal antibodies are: immunodiffusion (ID), countercurrent immuno-electrophoresis (CIE), whole cell agglutination (WCA), complement fixation (CF) and enzyme-linked immunosorbent assay (ELISA). For antigen detection, latex particle agglutination (LPA), ELISA and radio-immuno-assay (RIA) are used.

## Treatment of mycoses

There are relatively few therapeutically useful antifungal agents compared to the large number of anti-bacterial agents that are available (see Chs 5 and 65). This is due mainly to the fact that fungi and humans are both eukaryotes, and most substances that kill or inhibit fungal pathogens are also toxic to the host. Most antifungal agents exploit differences in the sterol composition of the fungal cell membrane.

Antifungal agents vary considerably in their spectrum of activity (see Table 5.5, p. 54). Primary or acquired resistance is not a major problem. About 12% of clinical isolates of yeasts are resistant to flucytosine, and resistance may also develop during therapy. More significantly, resistance to azole antifungals is increasing, and some yeast species (e.g. *Candida krusei*) are inherently resistant to some of the newer azoles such as fluconazole. Consequently, sensitivity testing is carried out for flucytosine and fluconazole and for any drugs failing to produce the expected therapeutic response.

Most antifungal agents are available only for topical use and relatively few can be administered systemically. Some such as itraconazole and terbinafine are usually administered orally; others like amphotericin B and miconazole are given parenterally because of poor absorption from the gastro-intestinal tract; flucytosine and fluconazole are available for oral or parenteral administration.

Combinations of antifungal agents may be useful in some systemic infections. A combination of amphotericin B and flucytosine, for example, allows amphotericin B, a toxic drug, to be used at a lower dose and reduces the likelihood of the emergence of resistance to flucytosine. Combinations of azole drugs and amphotericin B are seldom used therapeutically because they are antagonistic, at least in vitro.

Antifungal prophylaxis may be used for the prevention of opportunistic infections in patients undergoing transplants or cardiac surgery and those with haematological malignancies. Oral or topical antifungals are also used to prevent recurrent vaginal candidosis.

## SUPERFICIAL INFECTIONS

### Ringworm

Ringworm infections are common diseases of the stratum corneum of the skin, hair and nail; they are also referred to as *dermatophytosis* or *tinea*, a name which is qualified by the site affected, e.g. *tinea pedis* or *tinea capitis* for infections of the feet or scalp, respectively.

The infections are caused by about 20 species of dermatophyte fungi which are grouped into three genera, *Trichophyton*, *Microsporum* and *Epidermophyton* (Tables 60.1 and 60.2); some species are restricted to or are more common in certain parts of the world. Most ringworm infections in Europe are caused by *Trichophyton rubrum*, *T. mentagrophytes*, *T. tonsurans*, *T. verrucosum*, *Epidermophyton floccosum* and *Microsporum canis*. Some dermatophytes are primarily animal pathogens which may also infect humans (Table 60.2); a few species are saprophytes of keratinous material in soil, but these only occasionally infect humans and animals.

Ringworm infections are spread by direct or indirect contact with an infected individual or animal. The infective particle is usually a fragment of keratin containing viable fungus. Indirect transfer may occur via the floors of swimming pools and showers or on brushes, combs, towels and animal grooming implements. Dermatophytes can remain viable for long periods of time, and the interval between deposition and transfer may be considerable. Some abnormality of the epidermis, such as slight peeling or minor trauma, is probably necessary for the establishment of infection.

In the industrialized countries, ringworm of the scalp accounts for only a small proportion of infection, and is mostly caused by dermatophytes of animal origin, although *T. tonsurans* infections are on the increase in Europe. However, the use of communal bathing facilities has resulted in a considerable increase in the incidence of foot ringworm and associated nail and groin infections. These now constitute about 75% of all ringworm infections diagnosed in temperate zones. In developing countries, particularly in warm climates, scalp, body and groin infections predominate, with *T. rubrum* and *T. violaceum* among the most common causes.

There is no evidence of natural immunity to ringworm. Scalp ringworm is predominantly a disease of children, and foot ringworm a disease of adults, particularly adult males. Resistance to infection is partly determined by the production of inhibitory fatty acids and the rate of epithelial cell turnover, but the development of active T cell-mediated

**Table 60.1** Common dermatophyte pathogens of man

| Species | Common site(s) of infections | Main area of distribution |
|---|---|---|
| *Epidermophyton floccosum* | Groin, feet (nail)[a] | World-wide |
| *Microsporum audouinii* | Scalp (body) | Africa, America and Europe |
| *M. ferrugineum* | Scalp (body) | Africa, Balkans and Asia |
| *Trichophyton mentagrophytes* var. *interdigitale* | Feet, (nail, groin) | World-wide |
| *T. concentricum* | Body | South Pacific |
| *T. rubrum* | Feet, nail, groin, body | World-wide |
| *T. schoenleinii* | Scalp (body, nail) | Eurasia and North Africa |
| *T. soudanense* | Scalp (body) | Africa |
| *T. tonsurans* | Scalp body, (nail) | Europe and America |
| *T. violaceum* | Scalp body, (nail) | Africa and Eurasia |

[a]Parentheses indicate secondary sites of infection.

**Table 60.2** Common dermatophyte species of animals

| Species | Animals commonly affected | Main area of distribution |
|---|---|---|
| *Microsporum canis* | Cat, dog | World-wide |
| *M. distortum* | Cat, dog | Australasia, USA |
| *M. nanum* | Pig | World-wide |
| *M. persicolor* | Bank field voles | Europe |
| *Trichophyton mentagrophytes* var. *mentagrophytes* | Rodents (horse, cat, dog) | World-wide |
| *T. equinum* | Horse | World-wide |
| *T. erinacei* | Hedgehog | UK, New Zealand |
| *T. quinckeanum* | Mice | Europe, North America |
| *T. simii* | Monkey, chicken | India |
| *T. verrucosum* | Cattle | World-wide |

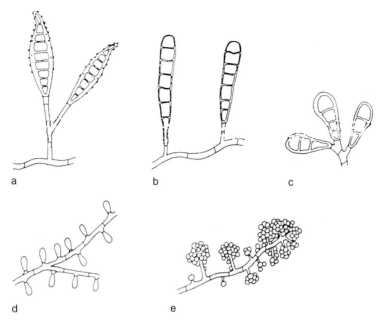

**Fig. 60.3** Dermatophyte spore forms: **a** macroconidia of *Microsporum* species; **b** macroconidia of *Trichophyton* species; **c** macroconidia of *Epidermophyton* species; **d** microconidia along sides of vegetative hyphae (*en thyrses*); **e** microconidia in grape-like bunches (*en grappe*). (From Evans E G V, Gentles J C 1985 *Essentials of Medical Mycology*. Churchill Livingstone, Edinburgh.)

immunity and, in follicular infections, phagocytosis by neutrophils, also play a part.

Dermatophytes invade keratin by enzymic digestion and mechanical pressure; the hyphae grow into newly differentiated keratin as it is formed, keeping pace with the keratin growth. In tissue the dermatophytes take the form of branching hyphae, which may eventually break up into arthroconidia, particularly in infected hair.

Many dermatophytes produce two types of asexual spore: *macroconidia* and *microconidia* (Fig. 60.3). Classification into the three genera *Trichophyton*, *Microsporum* and *Epidermophyton* is based on the morphology of the macroconidia, although the identification of species is also based on the shape and disposition of the microconidia and the macroscopic appearance of the colony. Biochemical tests can be used to differentiate some species.

## Pathogenesis

Ringworm lesions vary considerably according to the site of the infection and the species of fungus involved. Sometimes there is only dry scaling or hyperkeratosis, but more commonly there is irritation, erythema, oedema and some vesiculation. More inflammatory lesions with weeping vesicles, pustules and ulceration are usually caused by zoophilic species of dermatophyte.

In skin infections of the body, face and scalp, spreading annular lesions with a raised, inflammatory border are produced. Lesions in body folds, such as the groins, tend to spread outwards from the flexures. In foot ringworm, infection is often confined to the toe clefts, but it can spread to the sole; sometimes painful secondary bacterial infection occurs in the toe clefts. Infected nails become discoloured, thickened, raised and friable; most infections involve toenails and are due to *T. rubrum*.

In scalp infections there is scaling and hair loss, the extent of which depends on the causal fungus. Some zoophilic species give rise to a highly inflammatory, raised suppurating lesion called a *kerion*; kerions may also occur in the beard area of adults. It is important that scalp ringworm is recognized and treated promptly since it can lead to scarring and permanent hair loss.

In scalp infection the fungus invades the hair shaft and then the hyphae break up into chains of arthroconidia. In some species (e.g. *T. tonsurans* and *T. violaceum*) the arthroconidia are retained within the hair shaft (*endothrix* invasion), whereas in others (e.g. *Microsporum* species and *T. verrucosum*) they are produced in a sheath surrounding the hair shaft (*ectothrix* invasion) (Fig. 60.4). The pattern of hair

**Fig. 60.4** Diagrammatic representation of various forms of hair invasion by dermatophytes as seen in longitudinal and transverse sections of hair shaft: **a** ectothrix (e.g. *M. audouinii*, *M. canis* and *T. mentagrophytes*) with hyphae sparsely distributed within hair shaft and a sheath of arthroconidia on the outside; **b** endothrix (e.g. *T. tonsurans* and *T. violaceum*) with heavy arthroconidia formation completely filling hair shaft; **c** favus (*T. schoenleinii*) showing sparse hyphal growth and formation of air spaces. (From Evans E G V, Gentles J C 1985 *Essentials of Medical Mycology*. Churchill Livingstone, Edinburgh.)

invasion affects the clinical appearance of the lesion: in endothrix infection the hair breaks off at, or just below, the mouth of the follicle, which then becomes plugged with dirt and sebum to give what is described as *black dot* ringworm, but in ectothrix infection the hair usually breaks off 2–3 mm above the mouth of the follicle, leaving short stumps of hair. In the condition called *favus*, caused by *T. schoenleinii*, fungal growth within the hair is minimal and the hair remains intact but intense fungal growth within and around the hair follicle produces a waxy, honeycomb-like crust on the scalp.

Infections of the groins, hands and nails are nearly always secondary to infection of the feet and are usually caused by *T. rubrum*, *T. mentagrophytes* or *E. floccosum* (mixed infections can also occur).

Occasionally, patients with inflammatory ringworm infections develop a secondary rash known as an *id* reaction, which is thought to be an immunological reaction to fungal antigens. In patients with foot ringworm this takes the form of a vesicular eczema of the hands, whereas patients with scalp ringworm (especially kerion) develop a follicular rash usually on the trunk or limbs. None of these secondary lesions contains any viable fungus and they disappear spontaneously when the ringworm infection subsides.

## Laboratory diagnosis

Ringworm infections may be reliably diagnosed by direct microscopical examination and culture of skin, crusts, hair and nail.

***Collection of samples.*** The site should first be cleaned with surgical spirit, especially if greasy ointments or powders have been applied. Skin, hair and nail samples are best collected into folded squares of black paper, which can be fastened with a paper clip. The use of paper allows the specimen to dry out, which helps reduce bacterial contamination and provides conditions under which specimens can be stored for 12 months or more without loss in viability of the fungus.

Nail samples should be collected by taking clippings from any discoloured, dystrophic or brittle parts of the nail and by scraping material from underneath the nail. The sample should be taken from as far back as possible from the free edge of the nail.

Scales from skin lesions should be collected by scraping outwards with a blunt scalpel from the edges of the lesions where most viable fungus is likely to be. Specimens from the scalp should include hair stubs, the contents of plugged follicles and skin scales. Infected hairs are usually easy to pluck from the scalp with forceps. Cut hairs are unsatisfactory since the focus of infection is usually below or near the surface of the scalp.

***Wood's lamp.*** This is a source of long-wave ultraviolet light that can be used to detect fluorescence in infected hair. It is especially useful for the detection of inconspicuous scalp lesions, and to select infected hairs for laboratory investigation.

***Hairbrush sampling technique.*** Adequate material from minimal lesions may be obtained by brushing the scalp with a sterilized plastic hairbrush or scalp massage pad; this is then used to inoculate an appropriate culture medium by pressing the brush or pad spines into the agar.

***Processing of specimens.*** If there is insufficient material for both microscopy and culture, the sample should be used for culture, since this is generally more sensitive (except for nails).

The specimen should first be examined macroscopically; hair samples are examined under a Wood's lamp. Material from representative parts, and any fluorescent hairs, are divided up into 1–2 mm fragments with a sterile scalpel blade before microscopical examination and culture.

***Direct microscopy.*** Microscopy of wet mounts of keratinous material in potassium hydroxide is simple and reliable. The preparation should be allowed to stand for 15–20 min to allow digestion and 'clearing' of the keratin. Dermatophytes are seen in skin and nail as branching hyphae which often appear slightly greenish in colour and run across the outlines of the colourless host cells.

***Culture.*** Small fragments of keratinous material are planted or scattered on Sabouraud's glucose or 4% malt extract agar and incubated at 27–30°C for up to 3 weeks; room temperature is adequate but the dermatophytes grow more slowly. Only *T. verrucosum* grows well at 37°C.

Identification of dermatophytes is based on colonial appearance and colour, pigment production, and the micromorphology of any spores produced. Special tests exist for differentiating certain morphologically similar species. Thus, the ability of *T. mentagrophytes* to produce urease within 2–4 days distinguishes it from *T. rubrum*, and the ability to grow on rice grains distinguishes *M. canis* from *M. audouinii*.

## Treatment and prevention

Topical therapy is satisfactory for most dermatophyte infections of skin. However, oral antifungals are required to treat infections of the nail and scalp, and severe skin infections. Some chronic infections require prolonged oral and topical therapy.

Topical agents such as Whitfield's ointment and tolnaftate have been largely superseded by terbinafine and azole compounds. Oral griseofulvin is useful for scalp, skin and fingernail infections, but for toenail infections up to 18 months' treatment is required and the cure rate is only 30–40%. Terbinafine and itraconazole are gradually replacing griseofulvin for the treatment of all forms of ringworm since they give much better cure rates with shorter periods of treatment (e.g. 80–85% cure for toenails after 3 months' therapy) and lower relapse rates.

Relatively little has been done to control the spread of ringworm, although improved living conditions and standards of hygiene, and better diagnosis, have led to a reduction in the incidence of scalp ringworm. The prophylactic use of antifungal foot powder after bathing is beneficial in reducing the spread of infection among swimmers; the foot-baths containing antiseptic solutions which are commonplace in swimming pools are of no value and only serve to concentrate infected skin material in one area where everyone is expected to walk.

## Superficial candidosis

Superficial *Candida* infections may involve the mucous membranes of the mouth and vagina (*thrush*), the skin or nails. *Candida albicans* accounts for 80–90% of cases, but other species, notably *C. tropicalis*, *C. krusei*, *C. glabrata*, *C. parapsilosis*, *C. guilliermondii* and *C. lusitaniae* may occur.

*Candida* species, usually *C. albicans*, are found in small numbers in the mouth, gastro-intestinal tract, vagina and skin of about 20% of the normal population. The carriage rate tends to increase with age and is higher in the vagina during pregnancy. Commensal yeasts are more prevalent among hospital patients. Yeast overgrowth and infection occur when the normal microbial flora of the body is altered or when host resistance to infection is lowered by disease. Infection is most likely when several factors operate together to compound their effects, and in some cases deep-seated candidosis may result (see p. 574).

Immunity depends on a combination of non-specific and immunological defences. In superficial infections, non-specific factors include inhibitors in serum, such as unsaturated transferrin, and epithelial proliferation. Specific immunity largely depends on the appearance of sensitized T lymphocytes and phagocytes, particularly neutrophils.

On Sabouraud's glucose agar, *Candida* species grow predominantly in the yeast phase as round or oval cells, 3–8 μm in diameter. A mixture of yeast cells, pseudomycelium and true mycelium is found in vivo and under micro-aerophilic growth conditions on nutritionally poor media. *C. glabrata* does not form either mycelium or pseudomycelium.

## Pathogenesis

***Mucosal infections.*** These are the commonest forms of superficial candidosis; they are characterized by the development of discrete white patches on the mucosal surface which may eventually become confluent and form a curd-like pseudomembrane.

In oral candidosis, white flecks appear on the buccal mucosa and the hard palate, and although these are adherent, they can be removed; the surrounding mucosa is red and sore, and infection may spread to the tongue. Infection occurs most frequently in infancy and old age, or in severely immunocompromised patients, including those with AIDS. Other forms of oral candidosis occur: in those who wear dentures, lesions often appear in the occluded area under the denture, and in some individuals antibiotic therapy may result in a painful *Candida* infection of the tongue. Chronic oral candidosis may also occur with extensive leucoplakia and infection of the angles of the mouth (*angular cheilitis*).

In vaginal candidosis, typical white lesions on the epithelial surfaces of the vulva, vagina and cervix are accompanied by itching, soreness and a non-homogenous white discharge. Sometimes the mucosa simply appears inflamed and friable. The perivulval skin may become sore and small satellite pustules may appear around the perineum and natal cleft. Vaginal candidosis is common, especially during pregnancy; most women will have at least one episode during their lifetime and some suffer recurrent attacks.

Chronic, intractable oropharyngeal candidosis is common in AIDS patients and may extend to give oesophageal infection. The appearance of this infection is often the indicator of the transition from human immunodeficiency virus-positive status to true AIDS.

***Skin and nail infections.*** *Candida* infections of the skin almost invariably occur at moist sites such as the axillae, groins, perineum, submammary folds and occasionally the toe clefts. In infants, *Candida* species are frequently involved in napkin dermatitis. Infection of the finger webs, nail folds and nails is an occupational disease of housewives, nurses and barmaids, who frequently immerse their hands in water. Superficial infections occasionally occur on the penis after intercourse with females with vaginal thrush. The yeast may also infect the outer ear.

***Chronic mucocutaneous candidosis.*** This rare disease usually becomes apparent in childhood and takes the form of a persistent, sometimes granulomatous infection of the mouth, skin and nails. Those who develop this condition may have subtle defects in lymphocyte or neutrophil function.

## Laboratory diagnosis

Specimens of skin and nail are collected in the same way as for suspected ringworm. For infections of the mouth or vagina, scrapings taken with a blunt scalpel or a spatula from areas with erythema or white plaques are better than swabs, if the material is to be processed immediately. However, swabs are more convenient for transport to the laboratory, and they are better for collecting vaginal discharge. Swabs should be moistened with sterile water or saline before taking the sample, and sent to the laboratory in 'clear' transport medium.

In Gram-stained smears of mucous membrane samples the fungus is seen as budding Gram-positive yeast cells; mycelium is usually present except in the case of *C. glabrata*. Contrary to popular belief, the presence of *Candida* mycelium in clinical material does not confirm infection with the organism, particularly as it may have developed in the period between collection and processing.

*Candida* species grow well on Sabouraud's medium or on bacteriological media such as blood agar at 25–37°C, and typical yeast colonies appear within 1–2 days. *C. albicans* isolates can be identified by the germ tube test: the yeast is incubated at 37°C in serum for 1.5–2 h, and under these conditions *C. albicans* produces hyphae known as *germ tubes*. Other yeasts may be identified with one of the commercial kits, or by fermentation and assimilation tests. It is useful for culture results to be quantified, especially in the case of vulvovaginal samples, since this may help to distinguish between commensal carriage and infection.

## Treatment and prevention

Azoles have now largely superseded nystatin and amphotericin B for treating these infections. Most respond well to topical therapy. In addition to treating the *Candida* infection, it is important, if possible, to identify and correct any predisposing factor.

In oral candidosis, nystatin, amphotericin B and miconazole may be effective in lozenge or gel form. Vaginal candidosis can usually be treated successfully with a single application of an azole derivative or with oral therapy with fluconazole or itraconazole for 1 day. Intermittent prophylaxis with azole vaginal pessaries is of benefit in controlling recurrent vaginal candidosis.

Treatment of chronic paronychia involves a combination of antifungal therapy, nail care and avoidance of prolonged exposure to water by use of protective gloves; patients should dry their hands carefully after washing. Regular application of an azole lotion or an azole given orally is appropriate, but it may take several months to cure the condition; antifungal creams or ointments are less effective.

Oral therapy is essential for the treatment of intractable chronic *Candida* infections; treatment is given until remission is achieved, but in some patients (e.g. those with AIDS) relapse is common, and intermittent therapy may be required. Prolonged or intermittent therapy may lead to the development of resistance, as occasionally happens with fluconazole.

## Pityriasis versicolor

Pityriasis versicolor is a mild, chronic infection of the stratum corneum which produces a patchy discoloration of the skin caused by the lipophilic yeast *Malassezia furfur*.

*M. furfur* is a common member of the normal skin flora, and most infections are thought to be endogenous. Disease is probably related to host or environmental factors. It is very common in the tropics and is most prevalent in young adults.

*M. furfur* requires lipids for growth, and media containing Tween and lipid supplements are used. On skin and in conditions such as dandruff and seborrhoeic dermatitis (in which its precise role is uncertain), *M. furfur* is present as an oval or bottle-shaped yeast (2–3 × 4–5 μm), which characteristically produces buds on a broad base; in this form the organism is known as *Pityrosporum ovale*. In pityriasis versicolor the organism produces predominantly round yeast cells and short hyphae, the *P. orbiculare* form. All forms are Gram-positive. The optimum growth temperature is about 30°C, but in culture the colonial morphology and growth rate vary with the strain and the medium.

## Pathogenesis

Small, well-demarcated, non-inflammatory, scaling macules are usually present on the upper trunk or neck; they may appear hypo- or hyperpigmented, depending on the degree of pigmentation of the surrounding skin. The lesions tend to spread and coalesce, and occasionally spread to other sites.

## Laboratory diagnosis

The diagnosis can be confirmed reliably by direct microscopy of skin scales; culture is unnecessary. Clusters of characteristic round yeast cells (5–8 μm in diameter) are seen together with short, stout hyphae, which may be curved and occasionally branched.

## Treatment

Pityriasis versicolor responds well to topical therapy with 1% selenium sulphide or azoles in cream, lotion or shampoo. Oral azole therapy is sometimes used for recalcitrant or widespread infections. Relapse is common, particularly in hot climates.

## Other superficial infections

### Skin and nail

Certain non-dermatophyte moulds may cause infection of skin and nail. It is important that these are recognized since they are often resistant to the agents used to treat ringworm and superficial candidosis.

In the UK, about 5% of fungal nail infections are caused by non-dermatophyte moulds. *Scopulariopsis brevicaulis*, a ubiquitous soil saprophyte, is the most common, although other saprophytes such as *Fusarium*, *Aspergillus* and *Penicillium* species are also occasionally implicated. There is some debate as to whether these moulds are primary pathogens of nails; infection usually follows trauma and in many cases a dermatophyte is also present.

Two other moulds, *Scytalidium dimidiatum*, a pathogen of fruit trees, and *Scy. hyalinum*, a soil fungus, occasionally cause infection of nails and skin in the tropics. Scytalidium infections are diagnosed by microscopy and culture, as for ringworm infections. However, the moulds are both sensitive to cyclo-heximide and will not grow if this antibiotic is included in the medium.

Non-dermatophyte mould infections do not respond to existing antifungal agents. Attempts may be made to remove the nail with topical 40% urea paste.

**Tinea nigra.** This is a superficial, asymptomatic skin disease characterized by pigmented macules of variable size, usually on the palms and soles. It is caused by a black mould, *Exophiala werneckii*, and occurs mainly in the tropics. Tinea nigra is not contagious but is contracted by contact with the fungus in soil.

Diagnosis is made easily by recognition of the dark-coloured hyphal elements on micro-scopical examination of skin scrapings in potassium hydroxide. On Sabouraud's agar the fungus develops as grey, yeast-like colonies which gradually become more mycelial and darker coloured with age.

Tinea nigra responds well to treatment with keratolytic agents such as Whitfield's ointment.

### Hair

**White piedra.** This disease, caused by the yeast *Trichosporon beigelii*, results in soft, white, greyish or light-brown nodules on the hair shafts, mainly in the axillae. The hair often breaks at the point of infection, leaving hairs with a clubbed or swollen end. Shaving of the affected area is usually sufficient to effect a cure.

**Black piedra.** This condition, caused by *Piedraia hortae*, is characterized by the presence of black, hard nodules up to 1 mm in diameter, mainly on the hairs of the scalp. It occurs in humid, tropical climates. Crushing the nodules reveals the sexual reproductive phase, club-shaped asci, each with eight ascospores. Culture is unnecessary. Shaving to remove infected hairs is a satisfactory treatment.

## Otomycosis

About 10–20% of chronic ear infections are due to fungi, most commonly species of *Aspergillus*, notably *A. niger*. The fungi are easy to see in material from swabs or scrapings and grow readily in culture. Treatment with topical antifungals is usually successful, although relapse is common. Any concurrent bacterial infection or other underlying abnormality should also be treated.

## Mycotic keratitis

Fungal infections of the cornea are secondary to injury, bacterial infection and treatment with antibacterial agents and steroids. They are caused by common saprophytic moulds, in particular species of *Aspergillus* and *Fusarium*. Culture results should be interpreted with care since these fungi are also encountered as contaminants. Superficial swabs are of no value for laboratory investigation, and scrapings should be taken from the base or edge of the ulcer. The branched, septate hyphae may be rather sparse in potassium hydroxide mounts, and some of the material should also be stained with PAS or methenamine–silver techniques. Treatment is with topical antifungal agents, in particular natamycin.

# SUBCUTANEOUS INFECTIONS

## Mycetoma

Mycetoma is a chronic, granulomatous infection of the skin, subcutaneous tissues, fascia and bone, which most often affects the foot or the hand. It may be caused by one of a number of different actinomycetes (*actinomycetoma*) (see Ch. 21) or moulds (*eumycetoma*). The disease is most prevalent in tropical and subtropical regions of Africa, Asia and Central America. Infection follows traumatic inoculation of the organism into the subcutaneous tissue from soil or vegetable sources, usually on thorns or splinters. Consequently, the disease is most common in male agricultural workers, who acquire minor skin injuries.

A large number of organisms have been implicated, including species of *Madurella*, *Exophiala*, *Acremonium*, *Pseudallescheria*, *Actinomadura*, *Nocardia* and *Streptomyces*. Within host tissues the organisms develop to form compacted colonies (grains),
0.5–2 mm in diameter, whose colour depends on the organism responsible; for example, *Madurella* grains are black and *Actinomadura pelletieri* grains are red.

## Pathogenesis

Localized swollen lesions, which develop multiple draining sinuses, are usually found on the limbs, although infections occur on other parts of the body. There is often a long period between the initial infection and formation of the characteristic lesions; spread from the site of origin is unusual but may occur, particularly from the foot up the long bones of the leg (see Fig. 21.2, p. 224).

## Laboratory diagnosis

The presence of grains in pus collected from draining sinuses or in biopsy material is diagnostic. The grains are visible to the naked eye, and their colour may help to identify the causal agent. Grains should be crushed in potassium hydroxide and examined microscopically to differentiate between actinomycetoma and eumycetoma; material from actinomycetoma grains may be Gram stained to demonstrate the Gram-positive filaments. Samples should also be cultured, at both 25–30 and 37°C, on brain–heart infusion agar or blood agar for actinomycetes and on Sabouraud's agar (without cycloheximide) for fungi. The fungi that cause eumycetoma are all septate moulds which appear in culture within 1–4 weeks, but their identification requires expert knowledge. Serological tests for precipitins have been used to differentiate between eumycetoma and actinomycetoma and to identify specific causal agents, but their diagnostic value has yet to be confirmed and they are not in routine use.

## Treatment

The prognosis varies according to the causal agent, so it is important that its identity is established. Actinomycetoma responds well to rifampicin in combination with sulphonamides or co-trimoxazole, but an average of 9 months of therapy is required. In eumycetoma, chemotherapy is ineffective, and radical surgery is usually necessary. However, some of the newer antifungals have yet to be properly evaluated in this condition.

# Chromomycosis

This disease, also known as *chromoblastomycosis*, is a chronic, localized disease of the skin and subcutaneous tissues, characterized by crusted, warty lesions usually involving the limbs. The disease is mainly encountered in the tropics. The principal causes are *Fonsecaea pedrosoi*, *F. compacta*, *Phialophora verrucosa* and *Cladosporium carrionii*. Like mycetoma, the disease is seen most often among males in rural areas.

## Laboratory diagnosis

The dark-coloured fungal elements are relatively easy to see on microscopical examination of skin scrapings, crusts and pus. Culture on Sabouraud's agar at 25–30°C yields slow-growing, greenish grey to black, compact, folded colonies. Cultures should be incubated for 4–6 weeks. Specific identification of these closely related fungi is usually left to a reference laboratory. Serological tests are not used routinely.

## Treatment

Treatment is unsatisfactory, but itraconazole either alone or in combination with flucytosine may be useful. Early, solitary lesions may be excised.

## Phaeohyphomycosis

This is a general term given to non-specific solitary subcutaneous lesions caused by any black fungus. Diagnosis is often made at surgery, and treatment is by excision. These fungi may also cause opportunistic, deep-seated infections, such as brain abscesses, which require therapy with amphotericin B and flucytosine.

## Sporotrichosis

Sporotrichosis is a chronic, pyogenic granulomatous infection of the skin and subcutaneous tissues which may remain localized or show lymphatic spread. It is caused by *Sporothrix schenckii*, a saprophyte in nature. The disease occurs mainly in Central and South America, parts of the USA and Africa, and Australia; it is rare in Europe.

*S. schenckii* is a dimorphic fungus. In nature and in culture at 25–30°C, it develops as a mould with thin (1–2 µm) septate hyphae; spore-bearing hyphae carry clusters of oval spores. The yeast phase is formed in tissue and in culture at 37°C, and is composed of spherical or cigar-shaped cells (1–3 × 3–10 µm).

## Pathogenesis

Sporotrichosis most frequently presents as a nodular, ulcerating disease of the skin and subcutaneous tissues, with spread along local lymphatic channels. Typically, the primary lesion is on the hand with secondary lesions extending up the arm. The primary lesion may remain localized or disseminate to involve the bones, joints, lungs and, in rare cases, the central nervous system. Disseminated disease usually occurs in debilitated or immunosuppressed individuals.

## Laboratory diagnosis

Diagnosis is confirmed by isolation of the causative organism by culture of swabs from moist, ulcerated lesions or pus aspirated from subcutaneous nodules; biopsy specimens may be necessary in some cases. Direct microscopy is of little value since so few of the small *S. schenckii* yeast cells are present in diseased tissue. The mycelial phase develops within 7–10 days on Sabouraud's agar or blood agar at 25–30°C, and the yeast phase develops in 2 days at 37°C.

Identification depends on the micromorphology of the mould phase and conversion to the yeast phase at 37°C. An LPA test is of value for the diagnosis of the extracutaneous forms of sporotrichosis. The test has poor prognostic value since titres change little after successful therapy. A skin test with sporotrichin antigen is positive in almost all patients with cutaneous sporotrichosis.

## Treatment

For the cutaneous form, treatment with potassium iodide or itraconazole is satisfactory. In disseminated disease, intravenous amphotericin B is required.

## Rhinosporidiosis

This is a chronic, granulomatous disease which results in the production of large polyps or wart-like lesions in the nose or conjunctiva. More than 80% of reported cases have been from India and Sri Lanka, although the disease is also seen in South America.

Attempts to isolate the putative cause, *Rhinosporidium seeberi*, from clinical material have failed but the morphology suggests that it is related to aquatic fungi. Laboratory diagnosis depends on the demonstration of sporangia, which may be visible to the naked eye. It has been suggested that the condition is not due to an organism at all but results from the accumulation of polysaccharide material in the nasal passages and the host response to it. Treatment is by surgical excision.

## Other subcutaneous mycoses

Several other fungi, including *Loboa loboi*, *Basidiobolus haptosporus* and *Conidiobolus coronatus*, occasionally cause subcutaneous infections, usually in the tropics. Surgical excision is often curative in *L. loboi* infections; antifungal therapy may be of use for the other infections, but the newer drugs have not been properly evaluated.

# SYSTEMIC MYCOSES

## Coccidioidomycosis

Coccidioidomycosis is primarily an infection of the lungs caused by *Coccidioides immitis*, a dimorphic fungus found in the soil of semi-arid areas, mainly in the south-west USA and northern Mexico. Agricultural workers with a higher exposure risk and dark-skinned people are especially prone to the disease. In endemic regions over 90% of inhabitants may exhibit positive skin tests, and infection rates of 20% or higher have been recorded among newcomers to the areas in their 1st year of residence. Recovery from coccidioidomycosis usually confers lifetime immunity.

In culture and in soil, *C. immitis* grows as a mould, producing large numbers of barrel-shaped arthroconidia ($4 \times 6\,\mu m$ diameter), which are easily dispersed in wind currents. In the lungs the arthroconidia form spherules ($30–60\,\mu m$ in diameter) which contain numerous endospores ($2–5\,\mu m$ in diameter). Endospores are released by rupture of the spherule wall and develop to form new spherules in adjacent tissue or, following dissemination, in other organs of the body. In culture the mycelial colony is initially moist and white but changes within 5–12 days to become pale grey or brown.

### Pathogenesis

*C. immitis* usually causes an asymptomatic or self-limiting pulmonary illness, but a progressive and sometimes fatal secondary disease occasionally develops. Primary pulmonary coccidioidomycosis develops 7–28 days after infection. Skin rashes develop in up to 20% of those with the primary disease and indicate a good prognosis. In some cases primary infection may result in a chronic, cavitating, pulmonary infection which may resolve after several years, or may progress to the dis-seminated form. Localized subcutaneous infection

may result from direct inoculation of the fungus through the skin or may be secondary to pulmonary disease.

Disseminated infection occurs in about 1% of those who contract the primary pulmonary disease; it is more common in immunocompromised individuals, and in Filipinos, Black Americans and Native Americans. When dissemination occurs, it involves virtually every tissue of the body, including the central nervous system, skin and joints. The prognosis for disseminated coccidioidomycosis is generally poor, particularly in immunosuppressed individuals and those with meningeal involvement.

### Laboratory diagnosis

Microscopical examination of sputum, pus and biopsy material is helpful since the relatively large size and numbers of mature spherules present make their detection and identification comparatively straightforward. Material for culture should be inoculated on test-tube slopes of Sabouraud's agar and incubated at 25–30°C for at least 3 weeks. The fungus can be identified by its colonial morphology and the presence of numerous thick-walled arthroconidia formed in chains from alternate cells of the fine, septate hyphae.

The arthroconidia are highly infectious and are a serious danger to laboratory staff. Consequently, Petri dishes should *never* be used for isolation of the organism and all procedures should be carried out in a safety cabinet. Preparations for microscopy should be made only after wetting the colony to reduce spore dispersal.

Skin tests and serological tests are useful although cross-reactions may occur in patients with histo-plasmosis and blastomycosis. The tests use either coccidioidin, a culture filtrate antigen from the mycelial phase of *C. immitis*, or spherulin, an extract of the spherules. The skin test does not distinguish present from past infection and a negative skin test does not preclude infection with *C. immitis*.

Serological tests play an important part in diagnosis. The precipitin test is most useful for detection of early, primary infection or exacerbation of existing disease; precipitins appear 1–3 weeks after infection but are seldom detectable after 2–6 months, or in patients with disseminated coccidioidomycosis. The LPA test gives similar results to the precipitin test, but is not as specific. The CF test is most useful for detecting disseminated disease: CF antibodies appear 2–3 months after infection and persist until death or recovery.

## Treatment

Intravenous amphotericin B is indicated and concomitant intrathecal therapy is required in the meningeal form. Ketoconazole and itraconazole are also useful.

## Histoplasmosis

Histoplasmosis is ordinarily an asymptomatic or relatively mild, self-limiting pulmonary infection, although chronic or acute disseminated disease may also occur. The causative organism, *Histoplasma capsulatum*, is an intracellular parasite found in soil enriched with the droppings of birds and bats, and infection results from the inhalation of spores. The major endemic areas are the Mississippi and Ohio river valleys of the eastern USA, where the prevalence of infection may be as high as 95%. It also occurs in other parts of the USA and many other temperate and tropical areas.

*H. capsulatum* grows in soil and in culture at 25–30°C as a mould and as an intracellular yeast in animal tissues. The yeast phase cells (2–3 × 3–4 μm) can also be produced in vitro by culture at 37°C on blood agar or other enriched media containing cysteine. The mould colonies are fluffy, white or buff-brown; the mycelium is septate and two types of unicellular asexual spores are usually produced: large round, tuberculate macroconidia (8–14 μm in diameter) are most prominent and are diagnostic, but smaller broadly elliptical, smooth-walled microconidia (2–4 μm in diameter) are also present in primary isolates.

## Pathogenesis

Most infections are asymptomatic and are detected only when individuals develop a positive skin test reaction. Sometimes an acute influenza-like illness develops with fever and a non-productive cough. These infections are usually self-limiting, but patients are frequently left with discrete, calcified lesions in the lung.

A chronic form of histoplasmosis occurs mainly in adults; large cavities develop directly from primary lesions in the lung or by reactivation of old lesions. The clinical picture closely resembles tuberculosis; in some cases the infection may disseminate to give acute generalized disease.

Occasionally, patients develop an acute progressive form of the disease, with widespread infection of the reticulo-endothelial system and dissemination to other organs of the body. The rate of progression of the disease varies considerably, but generally the prognosis is poor. Disseminated infection occurs most often in old age and infancy, or in individuals with impaired immune responses.

## Laboratory diagnosis

Microscopy of smears of sputum or pus should be stained by the Wright or Giemsa procedure. Blood smears may be positive for *H. capsulatum*, especially in patients with AIDS. Liver or lung biopsies stained with PAS, or methenamine–silver may provide a rapid diagnosis of disseminated histoplasmosis in some patients. *H. capsulatum* is seen as small, oval yeast cells, typically packed within macrophages or monocytes.

Specimens should be cultured on Sabouraud's agar at 25–30°C to obtain the mycelial phase. Mycelial colonies develop within 1–4 weeks but cultures should be retained for 6 weeks. The fungus is identified by its colonial morphology and the presence of the characteristic macro- and microconidia. Culture at 37°C for the yeast phase is not used for primary isolation, but conversion from the mould to yeast phase is useful to confirm the identity of isolates. Mould cultures of *H. capsulatum* are a hazard to laboratory staff, and consequently test-tube slopes rather than Petri dishes should be used for isolation.

A histoplasmin skin test has been used, but a positive result does not differentiate between active and past infection, and false-positive reactions can occur in patients with other fungal infections; furthermore, skin testing induces humoral antibodies which complicate the interpretation of subsequent serodiagnostic tests.

Serological tests are useful, but cross-reactions can occur, mainly with *C. immitis*. CF, precipitin and LPA tests are commonly used in combination. The CF test, with histoplasmin or killed whole yeast cells as antigen, is positive in up to 96% of culturally proven cases. Generally, titres of 8 are regarded as presumptive evidence of infection, and titres of 32 or above indicate active disease. Low titres or negative results do not exclude infection. The precipitin test gives positive results in up to 85% of infected patients; there are few problems with cross-reactions but positive results should be confirmed by a CF test. The LPA test is useful for detection of acute histoplasmosis but is of less value than CF and precipitin tests.

Antibody tests fail to detect antibodies in up to 50% of immunosuppressed individuals although more sensitive techniques such as ELISA give improved results. Detection of *H. capsulatum* polysaccharide antigen in blood and urine by RIA is useful, but the test is not widely available.

## Treatment

Intravenous amphotericin B is the treatment of choice for disseminated histoplasmosis in immuno-compromised patients. Ketoconazole and itraconazole give good results in less ill cases.

## African histoplasmosis

This disease, caused by *Histoplasma duboisii*, is mainly restricted to the continent of Africa. It is primarily a disease of the cutaneous and subcutaneous tissues with little evidence of pulmonary involvement. *H. duboisii* is morphologically identical to *H. capsulatum* in its mycelial phase but differs in that the yeast phase, both in vivo and in vitro, has larger cells (12–15 µm in diameter); some consider *H. duboisii* to be a variety of *H. capsulatum*. Treatment is as for histoplasmosis.

## Blastomycosis

Blastomycosis is a chronic infection of the lungs which may spread to other tissues, particularly skin and bone. It is caused by *Blastomyces dermatitidis* and occurs mainly in the central and mid-western states of the USA and eastern Canada. The fungus has been isolated from the environment on only a few occasions, and its exact ecological niche has yet to be established. Infection results from inhalation of spores, and most infections appear to be contracted sporadically in cool, wet climatic conditions. The disease is seen most often among males in the 30–50 year age group. It is slowly progressive, and if left untreated has a poor prognosis. A subclinical pulmonary form, similar to that seen in cocci-dioidomycosis and histoplasmosis, probably exists.

*B. dermatitidis* is a dimorphic fungus. In culture at 25–30°C it grows as a mould with a septate mycelium. The colony varies in texture from floccose to smooth and from white to brown in colour. Asexual conidia are produced on lateral hyphal branches of variable length; the conidia range in size from 2 to 10 µm in diameter, and some may be dumb-bell shaped. In tissue and in culture at 37°C the fungus grows as a yeast (8–15 µm in diameter) which characteristically produces broad-based buds from a single pole on the mother cell.

## Pathogenesis

Primary pulmonary disease is usually relatively mild, but within a few weeks the disease may disseminate to other tissues. The chest radiograph can resemble that of tuberculosis or carcinoma. In disseminated infection the chronic pulmonary disease persists, and abscesses and granulomatous lesions are found in most organs and body tissues including bone. Disseminated blastomycosis has been described in immunosuppressed patients. Chronic cutaneous lesions occur in about 80% of patients with pulmonary infection; the characteristic secondary skin lesions are typically raised with a well-demarcated edge. It is from these skin lesions that the diagnosis is most often made. Primary cutaneous infection resulting from the introduction of the fungus to the skin is rare and produces a localized, self-limiting lesion.

## Laboratory diagnosis

Direct microscopy of pus, scrapings from skin lesions, or sputum usually shows thick-walled yeast cells (8–15 µm in diameter) which characteristically produce buds on a broad base (4–5 µm); the buds remaining attached until they are almost the size of the parent cell, often forming chains of three or four cells. In biopsy material the yeasts are best seen in sections stained with PAS or methenamine–silver.

*B. dermatitidis* will grow in culture on Sabouraud's agar or blood agar, but since it is sensitive to cycloheximide this must not be used in isolation media. The mycelial phase develops slowly at 25–30°C and cultures must be retained for 6 weeks. Test-tube slopes rather than Petri dishes are used for culture. Identification is usually confirmed by subculturing at 37°C to convert it to the yeast phase.

Most skin and serological tests are unreliable because of poor sensitivity and cross-reaction with histoplasmosis and coccidioidomycosis. However, an ELISA test has been developed that appears to be more than 90% specific.

## Treatment

Intravenous amphotericin B is used to treat all forms of blastomycosis and is the drug of choice in serious infection. Hydroxystilbamidine has been used in localized disease or when amphotericin B fails or proves too toxic. Oral ketoconazole or itraconazole are also effective and are now the drugs of choice in less serious, extra-central nervous system blastomycosis.

## Paracoccidioidomycosis

This is a chronic, granulomatous infection, caused by *Paracoccidioides brasiliensis*, which may involve the lungs, mucosa, skin and lymphatic system. The disease is fatal if untreated.

*P. brasiliensis* enters the body via the lungs; it grows as a saprophyte in nature but the precise reservoir is unknown. The disease occurs most frequently in humid mountain forests of South and Central America. Most infections are seen in rural workers 20–40 years of age.

*P. brasiliensis* grows in the mycelial phase in culture at 25–30°C, and in the yeast phase in tissue or at 37°C on brain–heart infusion or blood agar. The mould colonies are slow-growing with a variable colonial morphology, although most are white and velvety to floccose in texture with a pale brown reverse. Spore production is usually sparse and best seen in 8–10 week cultures. Asexual conidia may be produced but are not characteristic, and the identification of *P. brasiliensis* depends on its conversion from the mycelial to the yeast phase. The yeast phase consists of oval or globose cells 2–30 μm in diameter with small buds attached by a narrow neck, encircling the parent cell.

## Pathogenesis

The disease usually presents as an ulcerative, granulomatous infection of the oral and nasal mucosa and the adjacent skin. The lymphatic system, spleen, intestines, adrenals and liver are also often involved. Primary skin lesions are rare. There is evidence of prolonged latent infection before overt disease develops, and a mild, self-limiting pulmonary form probably exists.

## Laboratory diagnosis

Microscopy of sputum or pus, crusts and biopsies from granulomatous lesions usually reveals numerous yeast cells of *P. brasiliensis*. Yeasts showing the characteristic multipolar budding are diagnostic. Tissue sections should be stained with PAS or methenamine–silver. In culture the mycelial and yeast phases both develop slowly and cultures must be retained for 6 weeks. The mould phase can be isolated on Sabouraud's agar supplemented with yeast extract at 25–30°C, but colonies may take 15–25 days to appear. Blood agar (without cycloheximide) and incubation at 37°C are recommended for isolation of the yeast phase.

Skin tests for paracoccidioidomycosis are of limited diagnostic value because of poor sensitivity and cross-reactivity with other systemic mycoses. Serological tests are of value for diagnosis and for monitoring the response to therapy. Precipitin tests and CF tests, when used together, detect about 98% of infections. Cross-reactions are rare, particularly with the precipitin test.

## Treatment

Intravenous amphotericin B and sulphonamides have been used. Intravenous miconazole and oral ketoconazole or itraconazole also give good results. The choice of therapy depends on the site of infection and its severity; amphotericin B is the drug of choice for serious infections.

# Cryptococcosis

Cryptococcosis is most frequently recognized as a disease of the central nervous system, although the primary site of infection is the lungs. It occurs sporadically throughout the world but it is now seen most often in patients with AIDS.

There are four serotypes of the capsulate yeast *Cryptococcus neoformans* (A, B, C and D) which represent two varieties of the organism, namely, *C. neoformans* var. *neoformans* (A and D) and *C. neoformans* var. *gattii* (B and C). Most infections are caused by *C. neoformans* var. *neoformans*, which is commonly found in the excreta of wild and domesticated birds throughout the world. Pigeons carry *C. neoformans* in their crops, and counts of up to $5 \times 10^7$ cells/g of pigeon faeces have been found. The birds themselves do not appear to become infected, probably because of their high body temperature. *C. neoformans* var. *gattii* is associated with the flowers of *Eucalyptus camaldulensis* (red river gum tree), and the distribution of this tree coincides with the occurrence of infections due to *C. neoformans* var. *gattii*.

## Pathogenesis

Infection follows inhalation of the cells of *C. neoformans*, which, in nature, are thought to be small, allowing the organism to enter deep into the lung. The disease is more common in males than females. The meningeal form can occur in individuals who appear otherwise healthy, but occurs most frequently in patients with abnormalities of T lymphocyte function, including those with Hodgkin's disease, sarcoidosis, collagen disease and neoplasms. However, most cryptococcal infections are now seen in individuals with AIDS, 3–20% of whom develop cryptococcosis.

A mild, self-limiting pulmonary infection is believed to be the commonest form of cryptococcosis. In symptomatic pulmonary infection there are no clear diagnostic features. Lesions may take the form of small discrete nodules which may heal with a residual scar or may become enlarged, encapsulated and chronic (*cryptococcoma* form). An acute pneumonic type of disease has also been described.

Chronic meningitis or meningo-encephalitis develops insidiously with headaches and low-grade pyrexia, followed by changes in mental state, anorexia, visual disturbances and, eventually, coma. The disease may last from a few months to several years, but the outcome is always fatal unless it is treated. AIDS patients with cryptococcosis generally develop a chronic meningeal form with milder symptoms.

Although predominantly a disease of the central nervous system, lesions of the skin, mucosa, viscera and bones may also occur; in its disseminated form, the disease may resemble tuberculosis. Rarely, lesions of skin and bones may occur without any evidence of infection elsewhere.

### Laboratory diagnosis

*C. neoformans* is readily demonstrated in cerebrospinal fluid (CSF) or other material by direct microscopy, culture or serological tests for capsular antigen. The yeast load is generally higher in patients with AIDS. The cellular reaction and chemical changes in CSF usually resemble those seen in tuberculous meningitis. The yeast cells are round (4–10 µm in diameter) and are surrounded by a mucopolysaccharide capsule. The width of the capsule varies, and is greatest in vivo and on rich media in vitro.

In unstained, wet preparations of CSF mixed with a drop of India ink or nigrosin, the capsule of *C. neoformans* can be seen as a clear halo around the yeast cells. Capsulate yeasts are seen in the CSF of about 60% of patients with cryptococcosis, but the capsule may be difficult to visualize in some cases. Sputum, pus or brain tissue should be examined after digestion in potassium hydroxide, and here the capsulate yeasts are often delineated by the cellular debris. For examination of tissue sections it is best to use a specific fungal stain such as PAS; alcian blue and mucicarmine stain the capsular material, enabling the organisms to be differentiated from *H. capsulatum* and *B. dermatitidis*.

The yeast is easily cultured from CSF although large volumes or multiple samples may be required in some cases. On Sabouraud's agar (without cyclo-heximide) cultured at 25–30 and 37°C, colonies normally appear within 2–3 days, but cultures should be kept for 3 weeks. In culture, *C. neoformans* appears as creamy-white to yellow-brown colonies, which are mucoid in appearance in well-capsulated strains and dry in poorly encapsulated strains. The cells produce buds at any point on the cell surface but

mycelium or pseudomycelium is not normally produced. Preliminary identification depends on demonstration of the capsule, but this may be absent or difficult to see. *C. neoformans* is distinguished from other yeasts by its lack of fermentative ability, its ability to produce urease, to grow at 37°C and to assimilate inositol.

The most useful serological test is the LPA test for the detection of cryptococcal polysaccharide antigen. This test is highly sensitive and specific for the diagnosis of cryptococcal meningitis and disseminated forms of the disease and gives better results than microscopy and culture. With CSF samples the LPA test is positive in well over 90% of infected patients. In patients with AIDS, titres of over $1 \times 10^6$ may be detected. Antigen may also be detected by ELISA.

Tests for serum antibody (WCA) are positive in less than 50% of proven cases of cryptococcal meningitis, since antibodies are rapidly neutralized by the large amounts of capsular antigen released during evolution of the infection. Antibodies may subsequently reappear in patients after successful treatment. Consequently, the progress of the disease and the response to therapy can be monitored by using antigen and antibody tests in combination.

### Treatment

Intravenous amphotericin B in combination with flucytosine is the treatment of choice. Intrathecal amphotericin B may also be used in severe meningeal disease. Patients with AIDS commonly relapse after the initial course of therapy, and many react badly to the drugs. Fluconazole can be administered orally, and is useful if amphotericin B proves too toxic; it is also used as a maintenance therapy to control cryptococcosis in AIDS patients. Resistant strains of *C. neoformans* have emerged after prolonged therapy with fluconazole.

Individuals at risk of developing cryptococcosis should avoid contact with bird droppings.

## Aspergillosis

There are more than 100 species of *Aspergillus*, but only a few have been implicated in human disease: the most important are *Aspergillus fumigatus*, *A. niger*, *A. flavus*, *A. terreus* and *A. nidulans*. All are mycelial fungi with septate hyphae and distinctive sporing structures; the spore-bearing hypha (conidiophore) terminates in a swollen cell (vesicle) surrounded by one or two rows of cells (sterigmata) from which chains of asexual conidia are produced (see Fig. 60.2). *Aspergillus* spores are ubiquitous, and in winter months counts may reach 600 spores/m$^3$ of air in the UK. The fungus is particularly prevalent in decaying vegetation, such as mouldy hay, and counts as high as $2.1 \times 10^7$ spores/m$^3$ of air have been recorded inside farm buildings.

Aspergillosis most frequently affects the lungs, but infections at other sites such as the nasal sinuses and superficial tissues may also occur. Disease is usually caused by *A. fumigatus*. Inhalation of the spores may lead to colonization of existing lung cavities (*aspergilloma* form) or a hypersensitivity reaction (*allergic aspergillosis*). Rarely, *Aspergillus* species may cause invasive disease of the lung, and the fungus may disseminate to other organs; this form is seen in severely immunocompromised patients.

## Pathogenesis

***Allergic aspergillosis.*** Allergy to *Aspergillus* species is usually seen in atopic individuals with elevated IgE levels; about 10–20% of asthmatics react to *A. fumigatus*. Asthma with eosinophilia is a more chronic form, which manifests as episodes of lung consolidation and fleeting shadows on chest radiography; the fungus grows in the airways to produce plugs of fungal mycelium which may block off segments of lung tissue and which, when coughed up, are a diagnostic feature. Allergic alveolitis follows particularly heavy and repeated exposure to large numbers of spores. Breathlessness, fever and malaise appear some hours after exposure, and repeated attacks result in progressive lung damage. A form of the disease, *maltster's lung*, occurs in workers who handle barley on which *A. clavatus* has sporulated during the malting process.

***Aspergilloma.*** In this form of aspergillosis, also referred to as *fungus ball*, the fungus colonizes pre-existing (often tuberculous) cavities in the lung and forms a compact ball of mycelium, eventually surrounded by a dense fibrous wall. Aspergillomata are usually solitary. Patients are either asymptomatic or have only a moderate cough and sputum production. Occasional haemoptysis may occur, especially when the fungus is actively growing, and haemorrhage following invasion of a blood vessel is one of the complications of this condition. Surgical resection is most often used to treat this condition.

***Invasive aspergillosis.*** This form occurs in severely immunocompromised individuals who have a serious underlying illness. *A. fumigatus* is the species most frequently involved. The lung is the sole site of infection in 70% of patients, but dissemination to other organs often occurs. There is widespread destructive growth of *Aspergillus* species in lung tissue, and the fungus invades blood vessels, causing thrombosis; septic emboli may spread the infection to other organs, especially the kidneys, heart and brain. Invasive aspergillosis has a poor prognosis and is often diagnosed post mortem.

***Endocarditis.*** *Aspergillus* species may rarely cause endocarditis in immunosuppressed patients and those who have undergone open-heart surgery. The condition has a poor prognosis and successful therapy depends on a combination of antifungal treatment and surgical removal of infected tissue.

***Paranasal granuloma.*** *A. flavus* and *A. fumigatus* may colonize and invade the paranasal sinuses, and the infection may spread through the bone to the orbit of the eye and brain. This condition is seen most often in warm dry climates and is common in parts of the Sudan and northern India.

## Laboratory diagnosis

The value of the laboratory in diagnosis varies according to the clinical form of aspergillosis; the diagnosis of invasive disease is particularly difficult.

***Direct microscopy.*** In sputum the fungus appears as non-pigmented septate mycelium (3–5 μm in diameter) with characteristic dichotomous branching and an irregular outline; rarely the characteristic sporing heads of *Aspergillus* species are present.

In allergic aspergillosis there is usually abundant fungus in the sputum, and mycelial plugs may also be present. In aspergilloma, fungus may be difficult to find on microscopy. In invasive aspergillosis, microscopy is usually negative, and biopsy may be the only reliable method of making a definitive diagnosis, although this is a procedure many clinicians are reluctant to undertake because of the associated risk.

In tissue sections, *Aspergillus* species are best seen after staining with PAS or methenamine–silver.

***Culture.*** Aspergilli grow readily at 25–37°C on Sabouraud's agar without cycloheximide; colonies appear after incubation for 1–2 days. Isolates can be identified by their colonial appearance and micromorphology. The ability of *A. fumigatus* to grow well at 45°C can be used to help identify this species or to selectively isolate it.

Since aspergilli are among the commonest contaminants in the laboratory, quantification of the amount of fungus in sputum helps to confirm the relevance of a positive culture. Large quantities of fungus are usually recovered from the sputum of patients with allergic aspergillosis, but cultures from those with aspergilloma or invasive disease are commonly negative or yield only a few colonies. Blood cultures are negative in invasive disease.

***Skin tests.*** Skin tests with *A. fumigatus* antigen are useful for the diagnosis of allergic aspergillosis. All patients give an immediate type I reaction and 70% of those with pulmonary eosinophilia also give a delayed type III Arthus reaction.

***Serological tests.*** ID and CIE are widely used for the detection of precipitins in the diagnosis of all forms of aspergillosis, particularly aspergilloma and allergic bronchopulmonary aspergillosis.

Antigen detection has also been used successfully for diagnosis of invasive aspergillosis by techniques such as LPA, RIA and ELISA. However, currently available tests generally lack sensitivity and are best used along with other laboratory tests.

### Treatment

Allergic forms of aspergillosis are treated with corticosteroids. Aspergilloma is treated by surgical excision or sometimes with antifungal agents. In invasive aspergillosis, the treatment of choice is intravenous amphotericin B; itraconazole has given good results in some cases but has yet to be fully evaluated.

## Systemic candidosis

Systemic forms of candidosis may be localized, e.g. in the urinary tract, liver, heart valves (endocarditis), meninges or peritoneal cavity, or the infection may be widely disseminated and associated with a septicaemia (*candidaemia*). Deep-seated candidosis is difficult to diagnose and treat, and the prognosis is generally poor.

Systemic candidosis usually follows overgrowth of commensal yeasts in association with serious abnormality of the host. It is generally an iatrogenic infection encountered among certain groups of hospital patients who carry more yeasts in the mouth and gastro-intestinal tract than the normal population. Several factors predispose to yeast overgrowth (Table 60.3), but the highest numbers of yeasts occur in patients treated with antibiotics or steroids, in immunosuppressed patients, and after surgical procedures such as organ transplants or heart surgery.

Candidaemia is seen mainly in postoperative or immunosuppressed patients; in some patients it clears spontaneously, or disappears when contaminated intravenous catheters are removed. However, some patients with candidaemia, notably those treated with cytotoxic drugs or corticosteroids, develop generalized or localized deep-seated infection.

Common sites of involvement in disseminated infection include the kidney, liver, spleen, brain and

**Table 60.3** Factors associated with yeast overgrowth and candidosis

1. Natural receptive states (infancy, old age, pregnancy)
2. Changes in local bacterial flora (e.g. secondary to antibiotics)
3. Changes to epithelial surfaces (e.g. due to moisture, local occlusion, trauma)
4. T lymphocyte defects (primary or secondary to disease, e.g. AIDS or immunosuppression)
5. Neutropenia (primary or secondary to disease or immunosuppression)
6. Endocrine disease (e.g. diabetes mellitus)
7. Miscellaneous conditions (e.g. zinc or iron deficiency)

gastro-intestinal tract; pulmonary infections are rare. One common sign of deep-seated candidosis is the presence of white candidal lesions within the eye (*Candida* endophthalmitis). *Candida* endocarditis usually follows surgery for valve replacement, but also occurs in drug addicts and occasionally in patients on immunosuppressive therapy. Infection of the kidney is usually blood-borne and ascending infection is thought to be rare. Bladder infections are usually associated with the presence of an indwelling urinary catheter and the infection often clears when the catheter is removed.

*C. albicans* accounts for most cases of systemic candidosis but infections due to *C. tropicalis*, *C. lusitaniae*, *C. glabrata*, *C. krusei* and *C. parapsilosis* are increasingly implicated. For example, *C. parapsilosis* is responsible for about 25% of cases of yeast endocarditis, and *C. glabrata* is often involved in infections of the urinary tract. The mycological features of these organisms have been outlined in the section on superficial candidosis (see p. 563).

### Laboratory diagnosis

Diagnosis of deep-seated candidosis is difficult and many cases are revealed post-mortem. There are no distinctive clinical signs, unless endophthalmitis is present, although some patients develop a macular skin rash. Hepatosplenic candidosis has a characteristic computerized tomography (CT) scan appearance.

Laboratory diagnosis is complicated by the fact that *Candida* species may be present as commensals in the absence of infection. Isolation of *Candida* species from clinical material, except from sites that are normally sterile, is therefore of little significance. Similarly, candida antibodies can be detected in uninfected individuals because of their exposure to commensal yeasts, although a change in antibody titre may be of diagnostic significance. In suspected systemic candidosis, samples from as many sources as possible should be examined by direct microscopy and culture, and results should be interpreted in the light of clinical findings.

***Direct microscopy.*** Appropriate samples are examined microscopically in potassium hydroxide or after Gram staining. In tissue sections, the fungus is seen best if stained with PAS or methenamine–silver. Mycelium is often abundant but the presence of mycelium in sputum or urine does not confirm that the yeast is present as a pathogen.

***Culture.*** *Candida* species grow readily in culture at 37°C on common isolation media, such as Sabouraud's agar (see p. 564). Blood cultures provide the most reliable evidence of systemic infection, although repeated attempts to isolate the organism may be necessary. However, transient candidaemia is not uncommon, especially in patients with indwelling intravenous catheters. Isolation of the yeast from otherwise sterile sites provides reliable evidence for the diagnosis but cultures of urine, faeces and sputum are of value only if done quantitatively over a period of time. Cell counts of the yeast in urine in excess of $10^4$/ml are usually taken to indicate urinary tract infection, except in patients with indwelling urinary catheters.

Since *Candida* species multiply rapidly in clinical material it is important that specimens are processed as soon as possible after collection.

***Serological tests.*** Current tests lack specificity and sensitivity, and the results must be interpreted with care. The most widely used tests are ID and CIE for detection of precipitins to somatic extracts of *C. albicans* and *C. parapsilosis*. A positive test does not necessarily indicate infection since the antigens used are unable to differentiate antibodies formed during mucosal colonization from those produced during deep infection. Similarly, a negative antibody test does not necessarily rule out deep-seated candidosis in immunocompromised patients who are incapable of mounting an adequate antibody response; in such cases a more sensitive assay system such as ELISA gives better results. Antigen tests based on ELISA, RIA, passive haemagglutination (PHA) and LPA, to detect either cell wall mannan or cytoplasmic components, have been developed, and antigen detection is useful for serodiagnosis of some forms of systemic candidosis.

## Treatment

Intravenous amphotericin B in combination with flucytosine is the treatment of choice for most forms of systemic candidosis. Flucytosine is not used on its own due to problems of resistance. Fluconazole, ketoconazole and itraconazole have also been used successfully.

# Zygomycosis

Zygomycosis, also referred to as *mucormycosis* or *phycomycosis*, is a relatively rare, opportunistic infection caused by saprophytic moulds, notably species of *Rhizopus*, *Mucor* and *Absidia*. The fungi are characterized by having broad, aseptate mycelium, with large numbers of asexual spores inside a sporangium which develops at the end of an aerial hypha.

The best known form of the disease is rhinocerebral zygomycosis, a rapidly fulminating infection which is almost invariably associated with either acute diabetes mellitus, or with debilitating diseases such as leukaemia or lymphoma. There is extensive cellulitis with rapid tissue destruction, most commonly spreading from the nasal mucosa to the turbinate bone, paranasal sinuses, orbit and brain. Rhinocerebral zygomycosis is rapidly fatal if untreated and, although the prognosis of this infection has improved over recent years, most diagnoses are still made at necropsy.

Pulmonary and disseminated infections can occur in severely immunocompromised individuals. Primary cutaneous infections have also been reported, but these are extremely rare and usually occur in patients with severe burns. Subcutaneous forms of zygomycosis are less serious.

## Laboratory diagnosis

Recognition of the fungus in tissue by microscopy is considerably more reliable than culture, but material such as nasal discharge or sputum seldom contains much fungal material and examination of a biopsy is usually necessary for a firm diagnosis. Direct examination of curetted or biopsy material in potassium hydroxide may reveal the characteristic broad, aseptate, branched mycelium and sometimes distorted hyphae. However, they are seen much more clearly when stained with methenamine–silver; the hyphae of these fungi do not stain with PAS.

The fungi are readily isolated on Sabouraud's agar at 37°C but isolation of the causal agents is of little diagnostic significance in the absence of strong supporting clinical evidence of infection. There are no established serological tests for the diagnosis of zygomycosis.

## Treatment

Successful treatment depends on early diagnosis of the infection, allowing prompt therapy with intravenous amphotericin B and aggressive surgical intervention.

## Other opportunist fungi

*Penicillium marneffei* is a major pathogen of AIDS patients in South-East Asia. It causes serious disseminated disease and is dimorphic, forming yeast-like cells in infected tissues; these are often intracellular, resembling histoplasmosis. *P. marneffei* is associated with the bamboo rat (*Rhizomys sinensis*), and has been isolated from their burrows and internal organs.

Almost any fungus may invade a severely immuno-compromised host, and infections with many common fungi including *Fusarium* species, *Trichosporon beigelii* and *Pseudallescheria boydii* have been reported.

Diagnosis is made by culture of the causative organism from clinical specimens; serological tests play little part. Tissue sections are often not very helpful since the causal fungi either have no special features to enable identification, or they resemble other fungal pathogens.

Infections are usually treated speculatively, and sometimes successfully, with amphotericin B.

### RECOMMENDED READING

Clayton Y, Midgley G 1985 *Medical Mycology. Pocket Picture Guide Series.* Gower, London

Evans E G V, Gentles J C 1985 *Essentials of Medical Mycology.* Churchill Livingstone, Edinburgh

Evans E G V, Richardson M D (eds) 1989 *Medical Mycology. A Practical Approach.* Oxford University Press, Oxford

Kibbler C C, Mackenzie D W R, Odds F C (eds) 1996 *Principles and Practice of Clinical Mycology.* Wiley, Chichester

Kwon-Chung K J, Bennett J E 1992 *Medical Mycology.* Lea and Febiger, Philadelphia

Odds F C 1988 *Candida and Candidosis*, 2nd edn. Baillière Tindall, London

Richardson M D, Warnock D W 1993 *Fungal Infection: Diagnosis and Management.* Blackwell Scientific, Oxford

Warnock D W, Richardson M D (eds) 1991 *Fungal Infection in the Compromised Patient*, 2nd edn. Wiley, Chichester

|   |   |   |
|---|---|---|
| 1 | 2 | 3 |

**Plate 1**   Stages in the erythrocytic cycle of *Plasmodium vivax.*

**Plate 2**   Ring form trophozoites of *P. falciparum.*

**Plate 3**   Trophozoites of *P. falciparum.* Note peripheral location of the parasites (*appliqué* or *accolé* forms) and light stippling of the red cells (*Maurer's spots*).

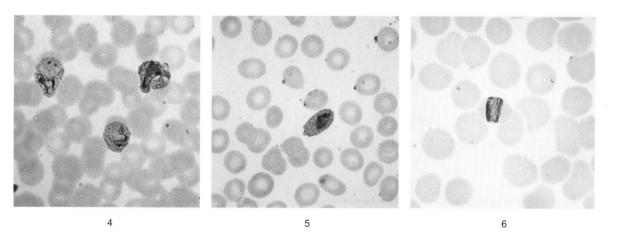

|   |   |   |
|---|---|---|
| 4 | 5 | 6 |

**Plate 4**   Amoeboid trophozoites of *P. vivax.* Note the marked enlargement of the parasitized red cells and the intense stippling (*Schüffner's dots*).

**Plate 5**   Trophozoite of *P. ovale.* Note the fimbriate, oval-shaped red cell and marked stippling (*James' stippling*).

**Plate 6**   Band-form trophozoite of *P. malariae.*

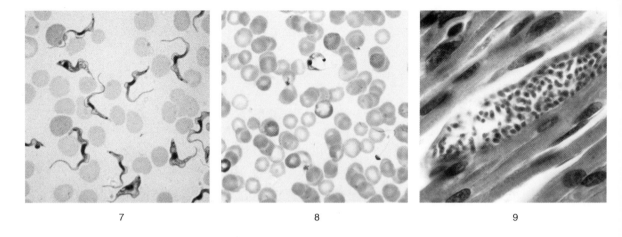

7                              8                              9

**Plate 7**   Trypomastigotes of *Trypanosoma brucei rhodesiense* in mouse blood.

**Plate 8**   Trypomastigote of *T. cruzi* in blood. Note the prominent kinetoplast and the 'C' shape adopted by the parasite.

**Plate 9**   Amastigotes of *T. cruzi* in heart muscle.

10                             11                             12

**Plate 10**   Amastigotes of *Leishmania tropica* in a ruptured macrophage from a cutaneous lesion (*Oriental sore*).

**Plate 11**   Promastigotes of *L. tropica* from laboratory culture in Novy, MacNeal and Nicolle's (NNN) medium.

**Plate 12**   Tachyzoites of *Toxoplasma gondii* in a macrophage (top left) and lying free (bottom right.)

2

# 61

# Protozoa

Malaria; toxoplasmosis; cryptosporidiosis; amoebic dysentery; sleeping sickness; Chagas' disease; leishmaniasis; giardiasis; trichomoniasis; pneumocystis pneumonia

## D. Greenwood

Infection with pathogenic protozoa exacts an enormous toll of human suffering, notably, but not exclusively, in the tropics. Numerically the most important of the life-threatening protozoan diseases is malaria, which is responsible for at least 1 million deaths a year, mostly in young children in tropical countries.

Pathogenic protozoan parasites are conveniently dealt with by placing them in four groups: *sporozoa*, *amoebae*, *flagellates* and a miscellaneous group of other protozoa that may cause human disease (Table 61.1).

## SPOROZOA

This group includes the malaria parasites and related coccidia, which exhibit a complex life cycle involving alternating cycles of asexual division (*schizogony*) and sexual development (*sporogony*). In malaria parasites, the sexual cycle takes place in the female anopheline mosquito (Fig. 61.1).

## Malaria parasites

### Description

Four species are encountered in human disease: *Plasmodium falciparum*, which is responsible for most fatalities; *P. vivax* and *P. ovale*, both of which cause *benign tertian malaria* (febrile episodes typically occurring at 48 h intervals); and *P. malariae*, which causes *quartan malaria* (febrile episodes typically occurring at 72 h intervals). The appearances of trophozoites of the four species as seen in Romanowsky-stained films of peripheral blood are illustrated in the colour plate section (facing p. 576).

***Life cycle.*** When an infected mosquito bites, *sporozoites* present in the salivary glands enter the bloodstream and are carried to the liver, where they

| **Table 61.1** | Principal protozoan pathogens of man | |
|---|---|---|
| Group | Species | Disease |
| Sporozoa | *Plasmodium falciparum* | Malignant tertian malaria |
| | *P. vivax* | Benign tertian malaria |
| | *P. ovale* | Benign tertian malaria |
| | *P. malariae* | Quartan malaria |
| | *Toxoplasma gondii* | Toxoplasmosis |
| | *Isospora belli* | Diarrhoea |
| | *Cryptosporidium parvum* | Diarrhoea |
| | *Cyclospora cayetanensis* | Diarrhoea |
| Amoebae | *Entamoeba histolytica* | Amoebic dysentery |
| | *Naegleria fowleri*[a] | Meningo-encephalitis |
| | *Acanthamoeba* spp.[a] | Keratitis |
| Flagellates | *Giardia lamblia* | Diarrhoea, malabsorption |
| | *Trichomonas vaginalis* | Vaginitis, urethritis |
| | *Trypanosoma brucei gambiense* | Sleeping sickness |
| | *T. brucei rhodesiense* | Sleeping sickness |
| | *T. cruzi* | Chagas' disease |
| | *Leishmania* spp. | See Table 61.4 |
| Others | *Babesia microti*[a] | Babesiosis |
| | *B. divergens*[a] | Babesiosis |
| | *Balantidium coli*[a] | Balantidial dysentery |
| | *Encephalitozoon cuniculi*[a] | Microsporidiosis |
| | *Enterocytozoon bieneusi*[a] | Microsporidiosis |
| | *Nosema connori*[a] | Microsporidiosis |
| | *Blastocystis hominis*[b] | Pathogenicity doubtful |
| | *Pneumocystis carinii*[b] | Pneumonia |

[a]These organisms are rarely encountered in human disease.
[b]Organisms of uncertain taxonomic status.

invade liver parenchyma cells. They undergo a process of multiple nuclear division, followed by cytoplasmic division (*schizogony*) and, when this is complete, the liver cell ruptures, releasing hundreds of individual

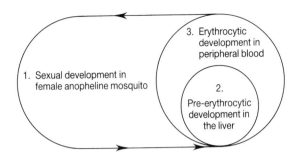

1. Sexual development in female anopheline mosquito

2. Pre-erythrocytic development in the liver

3. Erythrocytic development in peripheral blood

**Fig. 61.1** Schematic representation of the life cycle of malaria parasites.

parasites (*merozoites*) into the bloodstream. The merozoites penetrate red blood cells and adopt a typical 'signet-ring' morphology.

In the case of *P. vivax* and *P. ovale*, some parasites in the liver remain dormant (*hypnozoites*), and the cycle of pre-erythrocytic schizogony is completed only after a long delay. Such parasites are responsible for the relapses of tertian malaria that may occur up to 2 years after the initial infection.

In the bloodstream, the young ring forms (*trophozoites*) develop and start to undergo nuclear division (*erythrocytic schizogony*). Depending on the species, about 8–24 nuclei are produced before cytoplasmic division occurs, and the red cell ruptures to release the individual merozoites, which then infect fresh red blood cells.

Instead of entering the cycle of erythrocytic schizogony, some merozoites develop within red cells into male or female *gametocytes*. These do not develop further in the human host, but when the blood is ingested by the insect vector, the nuclear material and cytoplasm of the male gametocytes differentiate to produce several individual *gametes*, which give it the appearance of a flagellate body (*exflagellating male gametocyte*). The gametes become detached and penetrate the female gametocyte, which elongates into a zygotic form, the *ookinete*. This penetrates the mid-gut wall of the mosquito and settles on the body cavity side as an *oocyst*, which is yet another multiplicatory phase within which numerous *sporozoites* are formed. When mature, the oocyst ruptures, releasing the sporozoites into the body cavity, from where some find their way to the salivary glands.

*P. falciparum* differs from the other forms of malaria parasite in that developing erythrocytic schizonts form aggregates in the capillaries of the brain and other internal organs, so that only relatively young ring forms are found in peripheral blood.

The cycle of erythrocytic schizogony takes 48 h, except in the case of *P. malariae*, in which the cycle

occupies 72 h. Since febrile episodes occur shortly after red cell rupture, this explains the characteristic periodic fevers. However, with *P. falciparum*, the cycles of different broods of parasite do not become synchronized as they do in other forms of malaria, and typical tertian fevers are not usual in falciparum malaria.

## Laboratory diagnosis

Acute falciparum malaria is a medical emergency that demands immediate diagnosis and treatment. To establish the diagnosis, a drop of peripheral blood is spread on a glass slide. The smear should not be too thick; a useful criterion is that print should be just visible through it. The smear is allowed to dry thoroughly and stained by Field's method. This is an aqueous Romanowsky stain which stains the parasites very rapidly and haemolyses the red cells, so that the parasites are easy to detect despite the thickness of the film.

With experience, the species of malaria can usually be determined from a thick blood film, but some of the characteristic features used to establish the identity of the parasites (Table 61.2), such as the typical stippling of the red cell that accompanies infection with *P. vivax* or *P. ovale*, are better observed in a conventional thin blood film stained by one of the many modifications of Giemsa's or Leishman's stain. The water used to dilute the stain should be at pH 7.2 (not 6.8 as used for haematological purposes). Several other diagnostic tests have been devised, including an indirect immunofluorescence test, a simple fluorescent staining technique and DNA probes, but visualization of the parasites in Romanowsky-stained peripheral blood films remains the most reliable method.

## Treatment

For many years the standard treatment for acute malaria was chloroquine. However, resistance to that drug in *P. falciparum* (and, less commonly, in *P. vivax*) is now widespread and alternative agents often have to be used. The most reliable alternative to chloroquine is quinine (or quinidine), the traditional remedy that has been available for centuries in the form of cinchona bark. Some antibiotics, including tetracyclines and clindamycin, exhibit some anti-malarial activity and are used as an adjunct to quinine therapy.

Newer antimalarials include mefloquine and halofantrine. Although these compounds are active against chloroquine-resistant strains, resistance to

**Table 61.2** Differential characteristics of human malaria parasites as seen in Romanowsky-stained thin films of peripheral blood (see also colour plates 1–6)

| Species | Morphology of trophozoite | Morphology of red cell | Stippling of red cell | Morphology of gametocyte | No. of merozoites in mature schizont |
|---|---|---|---|---|---|
| P. falciparum | Ring forms only | Normal | Maurer's spots[a] | Crescentic | (16–24)[b] |
| P. vivax | Rings, becoming amoeboid during development | Enlarged | Schüffner's dots | Large, round | 16–24 |
| P. ovale | Rings, becoming compact during development | Slightly enlarged; sometimes oval with fimbriate edge | James's stippling[c] | Round | 8–12 |
| P. malariae | Rings, becoming compact, stretched across red cell | Normal or slightly shrunken | (Ziemann's dots)[d] | Small, round | 8–12 |

[a]Maurer's spots (or clefts) are relatively scanty and accompany more mature ring forms.
[b]Mature schizonts of P. falciparum are rarely seen in peripheral blood.
[c]James's stippling is similar to the intense stippling of Schüffner's dots.
[d]Ziemann's dots are rarely seen, except in intensely stained preparations.

them is already increasing in prevalence, and both drugs are associated with occasional problems of toxicity. Derivatives of artemisinin (a natural product from the plant *Artemisia annua*), including artemether and sodium artesunate, are being successfully used in some countries.

Treatment of acute malaria with chloroquine, quinine or other antimalarials will not eliminate exo-erythrocytic parasites in the liver. For this purpose the 8-aminoquinoline drug primaquine must be used. This agent carries the risk of precipitating haemolysis in individuals who are deficient in the enzyme glucose-6-phosphate dehydrogenase.

## Prophylaxis

Chloroquine and the antifolate drugs pyrimethamine (often combined with sulfadoxine or dapsone) and proguanil have been widely used for antimalarial prophylaxis, but the development of resistance to these agents has made it difficult to offer definitive advice to travellers, particularly those going to regions where *P. falciparum* is prevalent. One solution has been to suggest a combination of antifolate drugs, together with either chloroquine or mefloquine. Such cumbersome regimens invite lapses in compliance and increase the risk of side-effects, particularly if a sulphonamide is used; moreover, they are not completely protective. For these reasons some authorities recommend a simple prophylactic regimen such as daily proguanil, or weekly mefloquine, together with advice to bring any fever to medical attention. The combination of daily proguanil and weekly chloroquine is also widely recommended.

Whatever prophylactic advice is given, it should be combined with recommendations to avoid exposure to mosquito bites: wearing long clothing in the evening when the insects are most active; use of insect repellants; and sleeping under mosquito netting impregnated with insecticide.

Because parasites in the pre-erythrocytic stage of development escape the action of prophylactic drugs, prophylaxis should continue for at least 4 weeks after leaving a malarious area. This will effectively prevent the development of falciparum malaria, although long-term relapses of other types may occur up to 2 years after exposure.

## Other sporozoa

### Toxoplasma gondii

This is a coccidian parasite of the intestinal tract of the cat that is transmissible to many other mammals. Serological evidence suggests that human infection is common, presumably as a transient febrile illness or a subclinical attack, and of world-wide occurrence. Occasionally, more severe infection occurs: intra-uterine toxoplasmosis is an important cause of still-birth and congenital abnormality, and cerebral toxoplasmosis sometimes occurs in immunocompromised patients, such as those suffering from the acquired immune deficiency syndrome (AIDS).

Mature oocysts excreted by infected cats contain two sporocysts, within which *tachyzoites* develop. On ingestion the tachyzoites pass to the bloodstream and lymphatics to invade macrophages, in which they multiply (see colour plate 12). As the immune response develops, other cells are infected and tissue cysts containing slowly metabolizing *bradyzoites* are formed. Infection is acquired by ingestion of oocysts, or of tissue cysts in undercooked meat. Intra-uterine infection is acquired transplacentally.

It is not usually possible to demonstrate toxoplasmas in clinical material. Diagnosis of acute infection is made by demonstration of a rising titre of serum antibodies to *T. gondii*. The *Sabin–Feldman dye exclusion test* recognizes the ability of serum antibody to kill viable toxoplasmas. Other serological tests, including an enzyme-linked immunosorbent assay (ELISA), are available and have the advantage that they avoid the use of live toxoplasmas.

The combination of pyrimethamine and a sulphonamide is effective against active tachyzoites. Spiramycin is also effective and may be preferred during pregnancy. Clindamycin, azithromycin and, possibly, atovaquone, offer alternatives in patients with cerebral toxoplasmosis.

### Isospora belli

This coccidian parasite usually causes a mild, self-limiting diarrhoea, but it is occasionally associated with more severe infection, particularly in patients with AIDS. It is more common in areas of poor sanitation. Co-trimoxazole is usually effective if antimicrobial treatment is necessary.

### Cryptosporidium parvum

Cryptosporidia have long been known as animal parasites. One species, *Cryptosporidium parvum*, is now recognized as a common cause of diarrhoea in humans. Large numbers of oocysts are often present in faeces; they are partially acid-fast and can be demonstrated by modifications of the Ziehl–Neelsen method with carbol–fuchsin or auramine as the primary stain.

The infection usually responds to symptomatic treatment, with fluid replacement if necessary. In severely immunocompromised patients, cryptosporidia may cause a severe life-threatening diarrhoea for which the aminoglycoside, paromomycin, appears to offer some benefit.

### Cyclospora cayetanensis

Originally described as cyanobacterium-like or coccidian-like bodies, these parasites are now known to be typical coccidia. Unlike cryptosporidia to which they are related, cyclospora develop intracellularly in the gut mucosa. The immature oocysts are excreted in the faeces as round bodies about 10 μm in diameter, with a characteristic 'mulberry' appearance. They are more variably acid-fast than are cryptosporidia.

*Cyclospora cayetanensis* causes diarrhoea and is associated with poor sanitation. As with other coccidian parasites, infection is more severe in the immunocompromised, particularly those with AIDS. Mild infection is treated symptomatically, with rehydration if necessary. Co-trimoxazole appears to be effective in serious infection.

### Sarcocystis species

The animal parasites *Sarcocystis bovihominis* and *S. suihominis* occasionally invade the intestinal tract or muscle of humans. Infection is usually subclinical and discovered accidentally.

## AMOEBAE

### Entamoeba histolytica

This is the most important amoebic parasite of humans. The amoebae invade the colonic mucosa, producing characteristic ulcerative lesions and a profuse bloody diarrhoea (*amoebic dysentery*). Systemic infection may arise, leading to abscess formation in internal organs, notably the liver. Such disease may arise in the absence of frank dysentery.

### Laboratory diagnosis

In acute amoebiasis, blood-stained mucus, or colonic scrapings from ulcerated areas, are examined by direct microscopy. The material should be examined within 2 h of collection. *Entamoeba histolytica* may be recognized by its active movement pushing out finger-like pseudopodia and sometimes progressing across the microscope field. If mucosal invasion has occurred, the amoebae usually contain ingested red blood cells, but these may be absent if infection is confined to the gut lumen. The nucleus is not usually visible in unstained 'wet' preparations, but in fixed smears stained with haematoxylin, it is seen as a delicate ring of chromatin with a central karyosome (Fig. 61.2).

Typical amoebic trophozoites may also be seen in aspirates of liver abscess. The pus often has a distinctive red-brown 'anchovy sauce' appearance. Since the amoebae actively multiply in the walls of the abscess, the last few drops of pus drained from

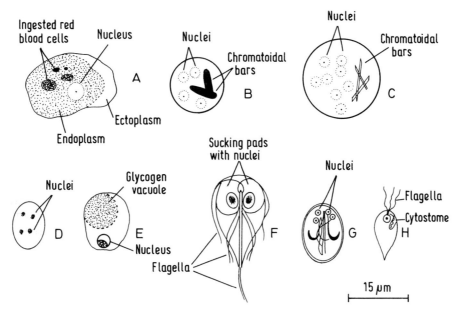

**Fig. 61.2** Diagrammatic representation of some intestinal parasites: **A** *Entamoeba histolytica*, trophozoite with ingested red blood cells; **B** *E. histolytica*, mature cyst; **C** *E. coli*, mature cyst; **D** *Endolimax nana*, mature cyst; **E** *Iodamoeba buetschlii*, mature cyst; **F** *Giardia lamblia*, trophozoite; **G** *G. lamblia*, mature cyst; **H** *Chilomastix mesnili*, trophozoite.

the lesion are most likely to yield recognizable forms of the parasite.

In the intestinal carrier state active amoebae are usually absent, but the encysted form, by which infection is spread, may be found. They are spherical, about 10–15 μm in diameter, and contain one to four of the nuclei typical of *Entamoeba* species: a circular ring with a central dot. Young, uninucleate cysts may also contain a large glycogen vacuole and, in fresh specimens, cysts of all stages of development may exhibit one or more thick, blunt-ended *chromatoidal bars* (Fig. 61.2).

Although demonstration of active amoebae or cysts is the best way to make a definitive diagnosis, serology is also sometimes helpful, particularly in systemic disease. Various immunodiagnostic tests have been described, but they are usually performed only in reference centres. Culture of *E. histolytica* is unhelpful as a diagnostic procedure.

### Treatment

Not all strains of *E. histolytica* are invasive and some (sometimes classified as *E. dispar*) never cause disease. Nevertheless, it is not possible readily to distinguish pathogenic from non-pathogenic strains in asymptomatic cyst excreters and, at least in areas of the world in which amoebiasis is uncommon, it is prudent to treat all excreters, particularly if they are food handlers. For this purpose, diloxanide furoate is often used.

Acute amoebiasis is usually effectively treated with metronidazole or tinidazole. Chloroquine is also useful in amoebic liver abscess. Older drugs, including emetine and dehydroemetine, are effective, but more toxic.

### Non-pathogenic intestinal amoebae

Although there are occasional reports of diarrhoea associated with other intestinal amoebae, notably *Dientamoeba fragilis* (an amoeba flagellate), most occur as commensals and are important only because of potential confusion with *E. histolytica*. The greatest opportunity for confusion arises with the other intestinal *Entamoeba* species, *E. hartmanni* and *E. coli* (Fig. 61.2). *E. hartmanni* is morphologically identical to *E. histolytica*, but is smaller and the trophozoite never contains ingested red blood cells. *E. coli* is somewhat larger than *E. histolytica*, particularly in the cyst form. The trophozoites are more sluggish than those of *E. histolytica*, and mature cysts contain up to eight nuclei; chromatoidal bars, if present, are fine and pointed, rather like slivers of broken glass.

The differential characteristics of these and other non-pathogenic intestinal amoebae are compared with those of *E. histolytica* in Table 61.3.

**Table 61.3** Differential characteristics of intestinal amoebae

| Species | Trophozoites | | Cysts | | | |
|---|---|---|---|---|---|---|
| | Size (μm) | Ingested red blood cells | Size (μm) | No. of nuclei[a] | Chromatoidal bars | Nuclear morphology[b] |
| *Entamoeba histolytica* | 10–40 | + | 10–15 | 4 | Solid, blunt-ended | Fine ring of chromatin with central karyosome |
| *E. hartmanni* | 4–10 | – | 6–10 | 4 | As above | As above |
| *E. coli* | 10–40 | – | 15–25 | 8 | Slender, pointed | As above, but karyosome may be eccentric |
| *E. gingivalis*[c] | 10–25 | – | No cyst stage | | | |
| *Iodamoeba bütschlii* | 10–20 | – | 10–15 | 1 | None | Chromatin massed at one end of ring |
| *Endolimax nana* | 5–12 | – | 5–8 | 4 | None | Small shadowy masses of chromatin |
| *Dientamoeba fragilis* | 5–10 | – | No cyst stage | | | Ring containing several chromatin granules |

[a]Refers to mature cyst.
[b]Refers to the trophozoite or cyst.
[c]*E. gingivalis* is a commensal of the mouth.

## Free-living amoebae

Environmental amoebae belonging to the genus *Naegleria* (usually *N. fowleri*) have occasionally been implicated in meningo-encephalitis. The outcome is ordinarily fatal, although amphotericin B has been successfully used. *Acanthamoeba* species occasionally cause keratitis, sometimes following use of contaminated cleaning fluids for soft contact lenses. Optimal antimicrobial chemotherapy remains to be defined, but topical propamidine in combination with neomycin or other agents has been used.

## FLAGELLATES

### *Giardia lamblia* (syn. *G. intestinalis*)

This intestinal parasite lives attached to the mucosal surface of the small intestine, notably in the duodenum. Vast numbers may be present, and their presence may lead to malabsorption of fat and a chronic bulky diarrhoea.

The trophozoite form is kite shaped, with two nucleated sucking pads, and four pairs of flagella (Fig. 61.2). Trophozoites may be found in duodenal aspirate, but examination of faeces usually reveals the cyst form by which the disease is transmitted. This is oval, about 10 × 8 μm, and contains up to

four nuclei as well as the remains of the skeletal structure of the trophozoite (Fig. 61.2).

Cysts of other, non-pathogenic, intestinal protozoa, including *Chilomastix mesnili*, *Enteromonas hominis* and *Retortamonas intestinalis*, may be mistaken for *G. lamblia*, but they are usually smaller and lack the regular oval shape and characteristic internal morphology. These non-pathogenic protozoa may also be found as trophozoites during microscopy of diarrhoeic faeces, but the most common intestinal flagellate is *Trichomonas hominis*, which is recognizable by its undulating membrane. There is no cyst form.

Giardiasis can be treated with 5-nitroimidazoles such as metronidazole, or, on the rare occasions when this fails (and re-infection is excluded), with mepacrine.

### *Trichomonas vaginalis*

*T. vaginalis* is a flagellate protozoon with four anterior flagella and one lateral flagellum which is attached to the surface of the parasite to form an undulating membrane. There is no cyst form; the parasite is transmitted by sexual intercourse.

As the name suggests, *T. vaginalis* is predominantly a vaginal parasite, although urethritis may occur in the male consorts of infected women. The organism is responsible for a mild vaginitis, with discharge, which ordinarily responds to treatment with metronidazole or tinidazole.

*T. vaginalis* is readily identified by its characteristic motility in untreated 'wet' films of vaginal discharge and can be cultivated in appropriate culture media.

## Trypanosomes

In contrast to the flagellates already described, trypanosomes have a complex life cycle involving an insect vector. The diseases that are caused in humans, African trypanosomiasis (*sleeping sickness*) and South American trypanosomiasis (*Chagas' disease*), are restricted in distribution according to the habitat of the insect host.

## African trypanosomiasis

African sleeping sickness is caused by trypanosomes that are subspecies of *Trypanosoma brucei*, an important aetiological agent of *nagana* in cattle in tropical Africa. The human parasites are: *T. brucei gambiense*, which occurs in west and central Africa, where it is transmitted by riverine tsetse flies, notably *Glossina palpalis*; and *T. brucei rhodesiense*, a parasite transmitted by *G. morsitans* in the savannah plains of east Africa, where cattle and wild antelope act as reservoirs of infection.

### Pathogenesis

Following the bite of an infected tsetse fly, a localized *trypanosomal chancre* may appear transiently, but invasion of the bloodstream rapidly occurs. The parasites multiply in blood, and at this stage there may be non-specific symptoms with occasional febrile episodes and some lymphadenitis. Swollen lymph glands in the posterior triangle of the neck (*Winterbottom's sign*) are often present in *T. brucei gambiense* infection. If untreated, the disease inexorably progresses to involve the central nervous system with the classic signs of sleeping sickness and, ultimately, death.

Infection with *T. brucei rhodesiense* tends to follow a more acute, fulminating course over a period of a few months, whereas *T. brucei gambiense* infection usually progresses slowly, sometimes over several years.

### Laboratory diagnosis

During the parasitaemic stage, scanty trypanosomes may be found in peripheral blood in unstained 'wet' mounts or in smears stained by the Giemsa or Leishman methods. Examination of lymph node exudate may be helpful. Once the disease has progressed to involve the central nervous system, examination of cerebrospinal fluid reveals a lymphocytic exudate, often with *morula cells* (plasma cells) and scanty motile trypanosomes.

The parasites have a characteristic morphology: they are elongated, about 20–30 μm in length, with a single anterior flagellum arising via an undulating membrane from a basal body situated near a posteriorly placed kinetoplast (Fig. 61.3 and colour plate 7).

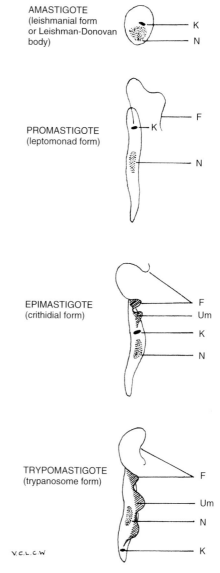

**Fig. 61.3** Forms which may be adopted by *Leishmania* and *Trypanosoma* spp. In parentheses are given the terms for the forms under the old nomenclature now superseded. F, flagellum; K, kinetoplast; N, nucleus; Um, undulating membrane.

In vitro cultivation is unreliable, but animal inoculation is sometimes useful, particularly with *T. brucei rhodesiense*, which infects laboratory mice more readily than *T. brucei gambiense*.

Various immunodiagnostic tests have been described, but they are not as reliable as direct microscopy in establishing a definitive diagnosis.

## Treatment

In the early, parasitaemic stage the infection is amenable to treatment with suramin or pentamidine, but if the disease has progressed to sleeping sickness, the trivalent arsenicals melarsoprol or tryparsamide are used. Less toxic alternatives are clearly required; encouraging results have been obtained with eflornithine in *T. brucei gambiense* infections, but, surprisingly, this drug is not effective in disease caused by *T. brucei rhodesiense*.

## South American trypanosomiasis

Chagas' disease, caused by *T. cruzi*, is quite different from African trypanosomiasis. The insect vectors are various species of reduviid bugs, often called *kissing bugs* because of their predilection for feeding round the mouths of sleeping individuals. The trypanosomes are not transmitted by the bite, but are present in the bug's faeces, which the unwitting sleeper rubs into the irritating bite wound. The trypanosomes enter the bloodstream, but do not multiply there; instead, they invade cells of the reticulo-endothelial system and muscle, where they lose their flagellum and associated undulating membrane and adopt a more rounded shape (Fig. 61.3). This morphological form is called an *amastigote*, and suggests a phylogenetic relationship with *Leishmania* species (see below). The amastigotes multiply in muscle and are liberated from ruptured cells as trypanosomal forms (*trypomastigotes*) to disseminate the infection and to provide the parasitaemia needed to infected fresh reduviid bugs when they next feed.

## Pathogenesis

Chagas' disease is a chronic condition, characterized by extensive cardiomyopathy, sometimes with gross distension of other organs (e.g. mega-oesophagus and megacolon). Death is usually from heart failure.

## Laboratory diagnosis

Trypomastigotes of *T. cruzi* may be seen in peripheral blood, but are often extremely scanty. They are shorter than those of the *T. brucei* group and have a characteristically large kinetoplast (colour plate 8). Unlike the African trypanosomes, *T. cruzi* can be grown in vitro in the rich blood agar medium also used to isolate leishmania (see below). Biopsy of skeletal muscle may be performed but is usually of little value. The appearance of amastigotes in heart muscle is shown in colour plate 9.

*T. cruzi* is infective to laboratory mice. Alternatively, a procedure known as *xenodiagnosis* may be used: uninfected reduviid bugs are allowed to feed on the patient, and after about 3–4 weeks the gut contents of the bug are examined for trypanosomes.

Immunofluorescence tests, ELISA and complement fixation tests may be used for presumptive serological diagnosis.

## Treatment

There is no reliable antimicrobial chemotherapy for Chagas' disease, but the nitrofuran derivative nifurtimox and the imidazole compound benznidazole have been used with modest success.

## *Leishmania* species

*Leishmania* species are intracellular parasites of the reticulo-endothelial system. They are related to trypanosomes, but exist in only two morphological forms: *amastigotes* (non-flagellate forms), which occur in the infected lesion; and *promastigotes* (flagellate forms that lack an undulating membrane), which occur in the insect vector, or in laboratory culture (Fig. 61.3 and colour plates 10 and 11).

The parasites are transmitted by sandflies (*Phlebotomus* or *Lutzomyia* species) in various parts of the world, including the Middle East, India, South America, the Mediterranean littoral and parts of Africa.

## Pathogenesis

Several distinct types of disease are recognized (Table 61.4), although they are caused by morphologically identical parasites. The taxonomic relationships between the various forms have still not been entirely clarified. *Cutaneous leishmaniasis (oriental sore)* is the least troublesome, causing a boil-like swelling on the face or other exposed part of the body. The central part of the lesion may become secondarily infected with bacteria, but the leishmania organisms reside in the raised, indurated edge of the lesion. The sore usually heals spontaneously, leaving a scar, but with some species a more severe *disseminated cutaneous*

**Table 61.4** *Leishmania* species involved in human disease

| Species | Form of disease | Common names | Main geographical distribution |
|---------|-----------------|--------------|-------------------------------|
| *Leishmania tropica* | Cutaneous | Oriental sore, Baghdad boil, Delhi boil, etc. | Middle East, central Asia |
| *L. major* | Cutaneous | | Africa, Indian subcontinent, central Asia |
| *L. aethiopica* | Cutaneous, DCL | | Ethiopia, Kenya |
| *L. donovani* | Visceral | Kala azar, Dum-dum fever | Middle East, Africa, Indian subcontinent, |
| *L. infantum*[a] | Visceral | | Mediterranean coast, Middle East, China |
| *L. chagasi* | Visceral | | Tropical South America |
| *L. mexicana* complex | Cutaneous, DCL | Chiclero's ulcer | Central America, Amazon basin |
| *L. braziliensis* complex | Mucocutaneous | Espundia | Tropical South America |
| *L. peruviana* | Cutaneous | Uta | Western Peru |

DCL, disseminated cutaneous leishmaniasis.
[a]*L. infantum* may be a subspecies of *L. donovani*.

leishmaniasis may occur. Parasites of the *Leishmania mexicana* complex may cause a destructive lesion of the outer ear (*Chiclero's ulcer*).

In *mucocutaneous leishmaniasis (espundia)*, which is associated with the *L. braziliensis* complex, disfiguring lesions of the mouth and nose may be caused. However, the most serious form of leishmaniasis is *visceral leishmaniasis (kala azar)*, which is a life-threatening disease involving the whole of the reticulo-endothelial system. A late complication of kala azar, *post-kala azar dermal leishmaniasis*, may be confused with leprosy or other skin conditions.

### Laboratory diagnosis

In the cutaneous or mucocutaneous form of the disease, typical intracellular amastigotes may be recognized in Giemsa-stained smears of material obtained from tissues at the margin of the lesion (see colour plate 10). Free amastigotes are commonly seen because of rupture of the macrophage host cell. Material should also be cultured in Novy, MacNeal and Nicolle's (NNN) medium or a modification thereof. This is a rabbit blood agar containing antibiotic to prevent bacterial contamination and a buffered salt overlay solution in which the parasites grow as promastigotes (see colour plate 11). Incubation is maintained for up to 3 weeks at room temperature (*not* 37°C).

In kala azar, spleen puncture is the most reliable method of diagnosis, but sternal marrow aspirate is safer and is usually preferred. Smears and cultures are made and examined as for cutaneous leishmaniasis.

Various serological tests have been designed. A haemagglutination test and an indirect fluorescent

antibody test have been successfully used in the diagnosis of kala azar, but demonstration of the parasite by microscopy or culture is preferable whenever possible.

### Treatment

The pentavalent antimony compounds sodium stibo-gluconate and meglumine antimoniate offer the most reliable therapy for leishmaniasis. Paromomycin (aminosidine), antifungal azoles and amphotericin B (preferably in the liposomal formulation) are also used.

## OTHER PATHOGENIC PROTOZOA

### *Babesia* species

These are predominantly animal parasites related to the piroplasmas that cause theileriasis in wild and domestic animals in many parts of the world.

Babesiae are transmitted by arthropod vectors, usually ixodid ticks, and human infection is uncommon. European cases have mostly been in patients whose resistance was impaired by lack of a functioning spleen; the causative parasite was usually *Babesia divergens*. In contrast, babesiosis caused by *B. microti* has been reported in otherwise healthy persons in parts of the east coast of North America.

Babesiae are intracellular parasites living within red blood cells; they superficially resemble young ring forms of plasmodia. The disease in immunocompetent individuals is usually self-limiting, so that specific treatment is not required. Optimal treatment for more serious cases has not been properly defined, but the combination of quinine with clindamycin has been successfully used.

## Balantidium coli

*Balantidium coli* is the only representative of the ciliates to exhibit pathogenicity to humans. It is a common parasite of the pig, and human infections have usually been traced to contact with these animals. The infective form is a large (about 50 μm in diameter), thick-walled cyst. The trophozoite inhabits the lumen of the gut and may attack the colonic mucosa in much the same way as *E. histolytica*, to cause balantidial dysentery. Many highly motile ciliate trophozoites are readily seen in untreated 'wet' films of diarrhoeic faeces.

Treatment has not been fully defined, but tetracyclines and metronidazole are said to be effective.

## Microsporidia

These animal parasites are represented by several genera, including *Encephalitozoon*, *Enterocytozoon* and *Nosema*, which have, on rare occasions, been implicated in opportunistic infections of immuno-compromised patients, especially those with AIDS. Infections of the eye, meninges and other organs have been reported. Albendazole may be useful in treatment, but is not always curative.

## ORGANISMS OF UNCERTAIN TAXONOMIC STATUS

### Blastocystis hominis

This organism, formerly thought to be a yeast, is probably a form of amoeba. It is commonly found in faeces. Any pathogenic role is the subject of dispute, but it has been associated with diarrhoea in the absence of other known pathogens. Metronidazole is said to be useful if true infection is suspected.

### Pneumocystis carinii

There is evidence that this organism may be a fungus, but its morphology, behaviour and response to anti-microbial agents are more typical of a protozoon. It was originally described as a cause of atypical pneumonia in malnourished infants, but is now more widely recognized as a common cause of pneumonia in patients with AIDS.

Diagnosis depends on the identification of typical octonucleate 'cysts' in material obtained from the lung, since serology is unreliable. Simple expectorated sputum commonly fails to reveal evidence of the organism, and broncho-alveolar lavage or biopsy may be needed to establish the diagnosis.

The organisms are sensitive to co-trimoxazole, which is the treatment of choice, but patients with AIDS may suffer unacceptable side-effects to the high doses used. In such patients, pentamidine has been widely used. This drug is most effective when given by the intravenous route, but to minimize the risks of toxic side-effects it is sometimes instilled into the lungs by nebulizer. Several alternative drugs are used in patients who do not respond to standard therapy; these include trimetrexate, atovaquone and eflornithine.

### RECOMMENDED READING

Bradley D J, Warhurst D C 1995 Malaria prophylaxis: guidelines for travellers from Britain. *British Medical Journal* 310: 709–714

Cook G C (ed) 1996 *Manson's Tropical Diseases*, 20th edn. W B Saunders, London

Fleck S L, Moody A H 1988 *Diagnostic Techniques in Medical Parasitology*. Wright, London

Goodgame R W 1996 Understanding intestinal spore-forming protozoa: cryptosporidia, microsporidia, isospora, and cyclospora. *Annals of Internal Medicine* 124: 429–441

Maegraith B 1989 *Adams and Maegraith's Clinical Tropical Diseases*, 9th edn. Blackwell, Oxford

Peters W, Gilles H M 1995 *A Colour Atlas of Tropical Medicine and Parasitology*, 4th edn. Wolfe, London

World Health Organization 1991 *Basic Laboratory Methods in Medical Parasitology*. WHO, Geneva

World Health Organization 1990 *Practical Chemotherapy of Malaria. Technical Reports Series*, No 805. WHO, Geneva

# 62

# Helminths

**Intestinal worm infections; filariasis; schistosomiasis; hydatid disease**

*D. Greenwood*

---

Medical helminthology is concerned with the study of parasitic worms. These creatures are responsible for an enormous burden of infection throughout the world and, although few helminth infections are life-threatening, their impact on human health is incalculable. Most helminths have no independent existence outside the host and are therefore truly parasitic. Since they rely on the host for sustenance, it is not in their interest to cause the host harm; consequently they do not usually exhibit great virulence and are characterized more by the novel methods that they have evolved to prevent rejection by the host defences. The pathogenic manifestations of helminthic disease, which can nonetheless be considerable, are ordinarily due to physical factors related to the location of the worms, their life-style or their size (see Ch. 13).

There are two major groups of helminths: *nematodes*, or roundworms, and *platyhelminths*, or flatworms. Flatworms are, in their turn, represented by two classes: *trematodes* (flukes) and *cestodes* (tapeworms).

## NEMATODES

The principal nematode parasites of humans are conveniently considered under two headings: intestinal nematodes and tissue nematodes.

## Intestinal nematodes

Infection with intestinal roundworms (Table 62.1) is generally associated with conditions of poor hygiene. Such infections are extremely common, particularly throughout the tropics and subtropics, although a number are also found in temperate regions.

### Ascaris lumbricoides

This is the common roundworm which probably infects over a 1000 million people in the world. The adults are large and fleshy, rather like a garden worm, and as with many nematodes (other than the hookworm group), the smaller male can be recognized by his characteristically crooked tail. The eggs (ova) are produced in huge numbers; they are thick walled, bile stained and typically exhibit a corrugated albuminous coat (Fig. 62.1a). In the absence of a male worm, the female will produce infertile eggs, which tend to be more elongated and irregular than the fertile variety (Fig. 62.1b).

**Table 62.1** Principal intestinal helminths of man

| Species | Common name | Relevant examination |
|---|---|---|
| *Ancylostoma duodenale* | Hookworm | Stool concentration (ova) |
| *Ascaris lumbricoides* | Common roundworm | Stool concentration (ova) |
| *Enterobius vermicularis* | Threadworm | Peri-anal swab (ova), adult worms on stool |
| *Necator americanus* | Hookworm | Stool concentration (ova) |
| *Strongyloides stercoralis* | – | Stool concentration (larvae) or culture |
| *Toxocara canis*[a] | Dog roundworm | Serology |
| *Trichostrongylus* spp. | Hookworm | Stool concentration (ova) |
| *Trichuris trichiura* | Whipworm | Stool concentration (ova) |

[a] Not an intestinal parasite of man; causes visceral larva migrans (see text).

**Fig. 62.1**    Eggs of intestinal helminths: **a** *Ascaris lumbricoides* (fertile eggs); **b** *A. lumbricoides* (infertile egg); **c** *Trichuris trichiura*; **d** hookworm.

e                      f

**Fig. 62.1** (Cont'd)   **e** *Strongyloides stercoralis* (larva); **f** *Enterobius vermicularis*.

In warm, moist conditions, infective larvae develop within fertile eggs, but do not hatch. Such eggs can survive for long periods in soil. If ingested, the eggs hatch in the duodenum and the larvae penetrate the gut mucosa to reach the bloodstream. They are carried to the pulmonary circulation, where they gain access to the lung and undergo two moults before migrating via the trachea to the intestinal tract. Having completed their round-trip, they mature in the gut lumen and live for several years.

*Ascaris lumbricoides* is a well-adapted parasite that is not usually pathogenic in the ordinary sense. However, pneumonic symptoms may accompany the migratory phase and the adult worms may invade the biliary and pancreatic ducts. Moreover, heavy infection with these large worms can cause intestinal obstruction. Allergy is also sometimes a problem.

The dog ascarid, *Toxocara canis*, may accidentally infect humans. Larvae hatch in the small intestine and penetrate the gut wall, but they are unable to complete their migratory phase. Instead, they find their way to remote parts of the body, a condition known as *visceral larva migrans*. Occasionally the larvae reach the eye and cause serious retinal lesions. Larvae of several other roundworms, including *Angiostrongylus*, *Gnathostoma* and *Anisakis* species, are occasionally implicated in visceral larva migrans in some parts of the world.

## Trichuris trichiura

This is the common whipworm, often found together with ascaris. The adults live with the head (the 'whip' end of the worm) embedded in the colonic mucosa. Each female lays thousands of characteristic 'tea-tray' eggs (Fig. 62.1c) every day. Like those of ascaris, they develop infective larvae in warm, moist conditions, but the ova do not hatch outside the body. However, after ingestion and hatching, there is no migratory phase and adult worms develop directly in the large intestine.

Infection is usually trivial, though massive infections can cause rectal prolapse in young children, and a form of dysentery is described.

## Hookworm

The two human hookworms, *Ancylostoma duodenale* and *Necator americanus*, are widely distributed throughout the tropics and subtropics. The two species produce indistinguishable thin-walled eggs (Fig. 62.1d) which hatch in soil. The larvae undergo several moults before infective larvae are produced. These are capable of penetrating unbroken skin, and in this way they gain access to the bloodstream to begin a migratory phase similar to that of ascaris. When they reach the gut they attach by their mouthparts to the mucosa of the small intestine.

Hookworms ingest blood and, moreover, move from site to site in the gut mucosa, leaving behind small bleeding lesions. These two facts are responsible for the chief pathological manifestation of heavy infection with hookworms: iron deficiency anaemia.

Larvae of animal hookworms, notably the dog hookworm, *A. caninum*, may penetrate human skin, but do not migrate further. They do, however, cause irritation by wandering locally through subcutaneous tissue to cause *cutaneous larva migrans*.

## Trichostrongylus *species*

Various species of *Trichostrongylus* have been associated with human disease, particularly in the Middle East. The eggs are similar to those of hookworm, but are more elongated.

## *Strongyloides stercoralis*

This parasite is also related to the hookworms, but differs in several important respects. There is a distinct free-living phase in the life cycle, during which males and females reproduce. Human infections arise after penetration of infective larvae through skin and there is a migratory phase involving the lungs. However, human infection appears to be restricted to female worms, which reproduce parthenogenetically after attaching to the gut mucosa. Eggs contain fully developed larvae when laid, and these hatch within the intestinal lumen so that larvae, not eggs, are found in faecal samples (Fig. 62.1e). Infection can persist for many years, probably because some larvae can develop sufficiently within the body to initiate a fresh cycle of development and cause auto-infection.

Symptoms are usually benign, but in debilitated individuals larvae may be activated to penetrate the gut wall and invade other organs, a serious condition known as *hyperinfection*.

## *Enterobius vermicularis*

This is the common threadworm, which infects children throughout the world. It has the simplest life cycle of all intestinal worms. Adults live in the large intestine and are occasionally found in the appendix. Mature, gravid females crawl through the anus at night and lay their eggs in the perianal area. The eggs are characteristically flattened on one side (Fig. 62.1f) and usually contain fully developed larvae. Ingestion of these eggs initiates a fresh infection. Symptoms are restricted to itching (*pruritus ani*) associated with the deposition of eggs.

Since eggs are not discharged by the worm into faeces, faecal examination is not appropriate in the laboratory diagnosis of threadworm infection. The diagnosis is established by finding the characteristic threadworms on the surface of formed stools, or by examination of swabs (or Sellotape impressions) of unwashed peri-anal skin for the characteristic ova.

## *Treatment of intestinal nematode infections*

In endemic areas, the need to treat intestinal worm infections has to be balanced against the severity of symptoms (if any), the inevitability of reinfection, and the use of scarce medical resources. In the industrially developed world, where the infections are less common and mostly imported, a more liberal approach to treatment can be adopted.

The range of options is listed in Table 62.2. Most effective (and expensive) are the benzimidazole derivatives, especially albendazole and mebendazole.

---

**Table 62.2**  Spectrum of activity of drugs used in the treatment of intestinal helminthiasis

| Drug | Ancylostoma duodenale | Necator americanus | Ascaris lumbricoides | Strongyloides stercoralis | Trichuris trichiura | Enterobius vermicularis |
|---|---|---|---|---|---|---|
| Tetrachloroethylene | + | +++ | – | – | – | – |
| Piperazine | – | – | +++ | – | – | +++ |
| Bephenium | +++ | + | + | – | – | – |
| Levamisole | ++ | ++ | +++ | – | – | – |
| Pyrantel pamoate | ++ | ++ | +++ | + | ++ | +++ |
| Thiabendazole | ++ | ++ | +++ | ++ | – | ++ |
| Mebendazole | ++ | ++ | +++ | + | ++ | +++ |
| Albendazole | +++ | ++ | +++ | ++ | ++ | +++ |

From Greenwood D (ed) 1995 *Antimicrobial Chemotherapy*, 3rd edn. Oxford University Press, Oxford.
+++, highly effective; +, poorly effective; –, no useful activity.

## Tissue nematodes

This group includes the filarial worms, the Guinea worm (*Dracunculus medinensis*) and *Trichinella spiralis* (Table 62.3).

Filarial worms have a complex life cycle involving developmental stages in an insect vector. They vary considerably in their pathogenic effects, but some are responsible for disabling diseases that have a major impact on communities living in endemic areas.

### Wuchereria bancrofti

This filarial worm is transmitted by the bite of various species of mosquito throughout the tropical belt of the world. It is believed that over 100 million people are infected. The larvae invade the lymphatics, usually of the lower limbs, where they develop into adult worms. Presence of the adult worms causes lymphatic blockage and gross lymphoedema, which sometimes leads to the bizarre deformities associated with bancroftian filariasis, *elephantiasis*.

Embryonic forms (*microfilariae*) are liberated into the bloodstream. They retain the elastic egg membrane as a sheath, which covers the whole larva (Fig. 62.2a). Microfilariae remain in the pulmonary circulation during the day, emerging into the peripheral circulation only at night, to coincide with the biting habits of the insect vector. The physiological basis of this nocturnal periodicity is not understood, but it can be reversed by altering sleep patterns in, for example, night-shift workers. Moreover, strains of *Wuchereria bancrofti* encountered in some Pacific islands do not exhibit a nocturnal periodicity. Aside from these exceptions, blood for examination for *W. bancrofti* must be taken during the night, optimally between midnight and 2 a.m.

### Loa loa

This worm is restricted in distribution to central and western parts of tropical Africa, where it is transmitted by the mango fly (*Chrysops* species). The adult worms live in subcutaneous tissue and wander round the body, provoking localized reactions known as *Calabar swellings* and sometimes migrating across the front of the eye.

The sheathed microfilariae of *Loa loa* (Fig. 62.2b) exhibit diurnal periodicity, so that, unlike those of *W. bancrofti*, they appear in peripheral blood only during the day.

### Brugia malayi

This parasite is probably related to *W. bancrofti*. It is transmitted by mosquitoes in parts of India, the Far East and South-East Asia. Adult worms inhabit the lymphatics and, like *W. bancrofti*, can cause elephantiasis. Microfilaraemia usually shows a nocturnal periodicity.

### Onchocerca volvulus

This filarial worm is common in parts of tropical Africa and Central America. It is transmitted by *Simulium damnosum*, and related species of blackfly, which breed in vegetation on the banks of rivers. Adult worms develop in subcutaneous and connective tissue, and often become encapsulated in nodules which form on bony parts of the body, such as the hip, elbow and (particularly in central America) the head. The microfilariae are not found in blood, but live in the superficial layers of the skin causing itching and, in heavy, chronic infections, gross thickening of the skin. The eye is commonly invaded by microfilariae, which may cause corneal

| Table 62.3 | Principal tissue nematodes of man | | |
|---|---|---|---|
| Species | Intermediate host | Geographical distribution | Relevant examination |
| *Wuchereria bancrofti* | Mosquitoes | Tropical belt | Night blood |
| *Loa loa* | *Chrysops* spp. | West and Central Africa | Day blood |
| *Brugia malayi* | Mosquitoes | South-East Asia | Night blood |
| *Mansonella perstans* | *Culicoides* spp. | Tropical Africa, South America | Blood |
| *M. ozzardi* | *Culicoides* spp. | West Indies, South America | Blood |
| *Onchocerca volvulus* | *Simulium* spp. | Tropical Africa, Central America | Skin shavings |
| *M. streptocerca* | *Culicoides* spp. | West and Central Africa | Skin shavings |
| *Dracunculus medinensis* | Water fleas | Africa, Indian subcontinent | Adult worm when mature |
| *Trichinella spiralis* | None[a] | World-wide | Muscle biopsy, serology |

[a] Pork forms the chief reservoir.

**Fig. 62.2** Sheathed microfilariae of **a** *Wuchereria bancrofti* and **b** *Loa loa*; **c** tail of microfilaria of *W. bancrofti* showing tip devoid of somatic nuclei; **d** tail of microfilaria of *L. loa* showing nuclei extending to tip of tail.

and retinal lesions that lead to blindness. Because of the association of the vector with rivers, the condition is known as *river blindness*.

If nodules are present, diagnosis can be made by finding macroscopic worms within an excised nodule. Otherwise, superficial slivers of skin, taken from calves, buttocks and shoulders, are suspended in a drop of saline and examined microscopically for motile microfilariae.

## Mansonella species

*Mansonella perstans* (formerly *Acanthocheilonema perstans* or *Dipetalonema perstans*) is widespread throughout tropical Africa and parts of South America; the related *M. ozzardi* is restricted to parts of the West Indies and South America. They are transmitted by biting midges (*Culicoides* species). The unsheathed microfilariae appear in the bloodstream, and exhibit no periodicity. They are generally regarded as being non-pathogenic.

*M. streptocerca* (formerly *A. streptocerca*) causes skin infections similar to those of *O. volvulus*, although the symptoms are usually milder. It is restricted to parts of western and central Africa.

## Differential characteristics of microfilariae

The microfilariae of filarial worms can be differentiated in stained preparations of clinical material by various criteria, the most useful of which are the presence or absence of a sheath and the disposition of the somatic nuclei in the tip of the tail (Table 62.4 and Fig. 62.2c and d). Giemsa stain is suitable for the demonstration of somatic nuclei, but hot (60°C) haematoxylin is necessary to stain the sheath.

## Treatment of filariasis

Diethylcarbamazine (DEC) has been used for many years for the treatment of all forms of filariasis. It effectively kills microfilariae, but is not reliably lethal to adult worms. It is relatively non-toxic, but death of the microfilariae is often accompanied by a severe allergic reaction (*Mazzotti reaction*), especially in onchocerciasis. Suramin kills the adult worms, but is much more toxic than DEC.

The treatment of onchocerciasis has been revolutionized by use of the veterinary anthelminthic *ivermectin*. This drug appears to be highly effective in a single oral dose and is less likely than DEC to elicit a severe reaction. The infection can be controlled in endemic areas by administering ivermectin at 6-monthly or yearly intervals. Ivermectin also appears effective in other forms of filariasis. Since it exhibits activity against some intestinal nematodes, including *A. lumbricoides*, these may be incidentally expelled during treatment.

## Dracunculus medinensis

This is the *Guinea worm*. The infective larvae develop within water fleas of the genus *Cyclops*, and human infection is normally acquired through infected drinking water. The larvae penetrate the gut mucosa and grow to maturity in connective tissue, usually of the lower limbs. The male is small and insignificant, but the female may reach a length of 1 m. After fertilization, the female worm incubates the larvae to maturity and, when ready to give birth, emerges to the skin surface to provoke an intensely irritating blister. When the sufferer immerses the blister in water, the uterus of the female worm bursts, liberating up to 1 million larvae, which are ingested by water fleas to continue the cycle.

---

**Table 62.4** Differential features of human microfilariae

| Species | Site in human host | Periodicity | Sheath | Nuclei in tip of tail | Length (μm) |
|---|---|---|---|---|---|
| *Wuchereria bancrofti* | Blood | Nocturnal[a] | Present | Absent | 250–300 |
| *Loa loa* | Blood | Diurnal | Present | Present | 250–300 |
| *Brugia malayi* | Blood | (Nocturnal)[b] | Present | Present[c] | 200–250 |
| *Mansonella perstans* | Blood | Non-periodic | Absent | Present | 150–200 |
| *M. ozzardi* | Blood | Non-periodic | Absent | Absent | 180–220 |
| *Onchocerca volvulus* | Skin | Non-periodic | Absent | Absent | 250–300 |
| *M. streptocerca* | Skin | Non-periodic | Absent | Present | 180–240 |

[a] Subperiodic forms occur in the Pacific Islands.
[b] Partial nocturnal periodicity.
[c] Two small, well-separated nuclei in the tip of the tail.

Attempts can be made to wind out the dead worm over several days, but breakage of the worm often occurs, and pyogenic cocci may be carried into the tissues to cause a cellulitis. Prevention is the best approach, and campaigns for the provision of safe water are having an impact on the prevalence of this disease, with the eventual aim of complete eradication.

### Trichinella spiralis

Unlike most parasitic worms, *Trichinella spiralis* has an extremely wide host range. Humans are infected accidentally, usually by eating undercooked pork products, although other meat, including bear and walrus meat, has been incriminated. The infected larvae lie dormant in skeletal muscle (Fig. 62.3) and are released when the meat is digested. Male and female worms develop to maturity attached to the mucosa of the small intestine. The female is viviparous, producing numerous larvae during a life-span of only a few weeks. The larvae penetrate the gut wall and migrate to skeletal muscle, where they enter the quiescent phase. Most of the symptoms of trichinosis, which can be very severe, even life-threatening, are associated with the migration of larvae.

Mebendazole is said to be effective against the adult worms and the larvae, but treatment is unsatisfactory. Symptoms usually develop only during the invasive stage, and measures to control the sequelae of invasion are more important than anthelminthic therapy.

## TREMATODES

The flukes (Table 62.5) are a diverse group of worms that share a similar life cycle involving a snail intermediate host and, often, a second intermediate host that provides the vehicle for the transmission of infection. Most flukes have a restricted geographical distribution that reflects the habitat of the appropriate type of snail.

Most trematodes are hermaphrodite, but the most important human flukes, the schistosomes, are differentiated into separate sexes.

### Life cycle

When excreted from the body, the eggs often contain a fully developed ciliated organism called a *miracidium*, although in some species immature eggs are produced which require a period of development before the miracidium is formed. In water, the miracidium escapes, either through a lid-like *operculum*

**Fig. 62.3** Larvae of *Trichinella spiralis* in muscle.

**Table 62.5** Principal trematode parasites of man

| Species | Common name | Intermediate host First[a] | Intermediate host Second | Geographical distribution | Relevant examination |
|---|---|---|---|---|---|
| *Clonorchis sinensis* | Chinese liver fluke | *Bithynia* sp. | Freshwater fish | Far East | Stool concentration |
| *Fasciola hepatica* | Sheep liver fluke | *Lymnaea* sp. | Vegetation | World-wide | Stool concentration, serology |
| *Fasciolopsis buski* | Giant intestinal fluke | *Segmentina* sp. etc. | Water chestnut | Far East | Stool concentration |
| *Paragonimus westermani* | Lung fluke | *Semisulcospira* sp. | Crabs and crayfish | Chiefly Far East | Sputum |
| *Schistosoma mansoni* | Bilharzia | *Biomphalaria* sp. | None (water) | Africa, West Indies, South America | Stool concentration, rectal biopsy |
| *S. haematobium* | Bilharzia | *Bulinus* sp. | None (water) | Africa | Terminal urine (midday) |
| *S. japonicum* | Bilharzia | *Oncomelania* sp. | None (water) | Far East | Stool concentration, rectal biopsy |

[a] The first intermediate host is a snail in each case.

in the egg shell, or (in the case of the schistosomes) by osmotic rupture of the egg. The miracidium penetrates the appropriate species of snail and undergoes several stages of asexual reproduction before emerging as a free-swimming body called a *cercaria*. The cercariae encyst in the muscle of fish (*Clonorchis sinensis*), crabs and crayfish (*Paragonimus westermani*), water chestnuts (*Fasciolopsis buski*) or vegetation (*Fasciola hepatica*), and humans become infected by ingesting the metacercarial form. In the case of *Schistosoma* species, the cercariae remain in water and penetrate unbroken skin to gain access to the body.

## Clonorchis sinensis (syn. *Opisthorchis sinensis*)

This is the Chinese liver fluke. Infection is acquired from uncooked freshwater fish, notably carp. The metacercariae excyst in the small intestine and pass into the bile ducts, where they mature. Typical small, flask-shaped eggs with a prominent operculum (Fig. 62.4a) are excreted in large numbers into the faeces.

Infection is commonly asymptomatic, but fibrosis of the bile ducts with impairment of liver function may occur in heavy, chronic infections. As with most fluke infections, praziquantel is emerging as the drug of choice for treatment.

A closely related fluke, *Opisthorchis felineus*, which is a parasite of the cat, has been associated with human disease in parts of eastern Europe.

## Fasciola hepatica

This is the cosmopolitan liver fluke of sheep. Human infections have usually been associated with eating wild watercress from infected sheep pastures. The adult worm is larger than *C. sinensis*, and lighter infections can cause biliary fibrosis and obstructive jaundice. The large, immature eggs with an indistinct operculum (Fig. 62.4b) may be found in faeces, but are usually scanty.

Unlike other trematode infections, fascioliasis does not reliably respond to praziquantel, and treatment with the veterinary anthelminthic triclabendazole, or the more toxic chlorophenol derivative bithionol, may be required.

## Paragonimus westermani

This is the lung fluke, which is found in parts of the Far East. Closely related species have occasionally been implicated in human disease in parts of Africa and South America. Human infection follows ingestion of raw, infected muscle of freshwater crabs and crayfish. The metacercariae penetrate through the gut wall and diaphragm to reach the lung, where they develop to maturity. Occasionally the larvae find their way to the brain. Pulmonary infection usually provokes the production of sputum, in which the characteristic large eggs (Fig. 62.4c) can be found, often associated with flecks of altered blood. Praziquantel is used for treatment.

**Fig. 62.4**   Eggs of trematodes: **a** *Clonorchis sinensis*; **b** *Fasciola hepatica*; **c** *Paragonimus westermani*; **d** *Schistosoma mansoni*.

e

f

**Fig. 62.4** (*Cont'd*)  **e** *S. haematobium*; **f** *S. japonicum*.

## Intestinal flukes

Several genera of intestinal flukes cause human infection, particularly in the Far East. *Fasciolopsis buski* is found in restricted foci in China and South-East Asia. Infection is often acquired by the habit of opening water chestnuts with the teeth. The adult flukes live attached to the wall of the small intestine, and produce a large number of eggs which resemble those of *F. hepatica*.

Other intestinal flukes include *Gastrodiscoides hominis*, *Heterophyes heterophyes*, *Metagonimus yokogawai* and various species of *Echinostoma*. Infection is usually asymptomatic unless the worm burden is large. Such evidence as exists suggests that praziquantel is effective in these cases.

## *Schistosoma* species

The schistosomes, or *blood flukes*, also known as *bilharzia* after the discoverer, Theodor Bilharz, are the most important of the pathogenic trematodes. At least 200 million people are infected, principally in Africa, where *Schistosoma mansoni* and *S. haematobium* are widespread. *S. mansoni* is also found in parts of the West Indies and South America; *S. japonicum* and the related *S. mekongi* are restricted to the Far East.

Human infection follows exposure to cercaria in water that harbours infected snails. The cercariae penetrate the skin, often causing a transient dermatitis, called *swimmer's itch*. Once in the bloodstream, the schistosomula migrate to the liver, where they develop into mature male and female worms. The integument of the mature male worm is adapted in the form of two long flaps, the *gynaecophoral canal*, in which the female is held. The mature worms migrate to the small veins of the rectum (*S. mansoni*, *S. japonicum* and *S. mekongi*) or the bladder (*S. haematobium*). Eggs, which contain a fully developed miracidium, are passed through the rectal mucosa onto the surface of colonic faeces or through the bladder wall into the urine.

The ova of *S. mansoni* possess a characteristic lateral spine, while *S. haematobium* has a terminal spine (Fig. 62.4d and e). Terminal-spined eggs found in faeces usually belong to another species that may infect humans, *S. intercalatum*. The more rounded eggs of *S. japonicum* and *S. mekongi* do not have a prominent spine, but may exhibit a rudimentary nipple-like appendage (Fig. 62.4f).

### Pathogenesis

The adult worms adopt the subterfuge of coating themselves with host antigens to evade attack by host defences and, in themselves, the adults are innocuous. Most of the serious manifestations of schistosomiasis are associated with the deposition of eggs, with the formation of granulomata and fibrotic lesions of the liver, bladder or other organs. Such effects may herald malignant changes. Heavy infection with *S. mansoni* may give rise to *schistosomal dysentery*, while *S. haematobium* infections are commonly accompanied by a marked haematuria.

## Laboratory diagnosis

Ova of rectal schistosomes can be sought on the surface of formed faeces. Blood-stained mucus should be examined, if present. Alternatively, microscopical examination of snips of rectal mucosa teased out in a drop of saline on a microscope slide may reveal viable or calcified eggs.

For the diagnosis of infection with *S. haematobium*, the last few drops of urine at the end of micturition (*terminal urine*) are most likely to be rich in ova. Excretion is said to be maximal around midday.

To test for viability of the eggs after treatment, ova can either be hatched in water (the motile miracidia can be seen with the help of a hand-lens) or the eggs can be examined microscopically for the characteristic flickering movement of excretory 'flame-cells'.

Various serodiagnostic tests, including enzyme-linked immunosorbent assay (ELISA), are available, but are no substitute for demonstration of the ova. Antigen detection methods have also been developed and are becoming available.

## Treatment

Sodium antimony tartrate was used for many years, but is difficult to administer and highly toxic. Several other antischistosomal drugs, including niridazole, metriphonate and oxamniquine, were subsequently introduced, but none exhibits a complete antischistosomal spectrum (Table 62.6).

Praziquantel is effective against all the human schistosomes and is now established as the drug of choice; because of its lack of toxicity and simplicity in administration it has been used in control programmes in addition to molluscicides and water purification.

## CESTODES

The most common species of tapeworm to be involved in human infection are listed in Table 62.7.

## *Taenia* species

*Taenia saginata*, the *beef tapeworm*, is much more prevalent than the related *T. solium*, the *pork tapeworm*. Both have a relatively simple life cycle, alternating between humans and the intermediate host. Human infection is acquired by eating raw or undercooked beef or pork containing the encysted larval stage, the *cysticercus*. The larvae hatch in the small intestine, and attach to the mucosal surface by four suckers on the head (*scolex*) of the worm. The scolex of *T. solium* additionally carries a crown of hooklets. The worm grows backwards from the head, first producing immature segments (*proglottids*) which continue to develop as they become more distant from the head. When sexually mature, the proglottids, which exhibit both male and female characteristics, cross-fertilize one another, and eggs start to be produced in the uterine canal. This becomes grossly distended as more eggs are produced, so that the fully gravid segments at the end of the worm become nothing more than bags full of eggs. The complete chain of segments is known as a *strobila*, and may measure 10 m or more.

**Table 62.6** Spectrum of activity of drugs used in the treatment of schistosomiasis

| Drug | Schistosoma mansoni | S. haematobium | S. japonicum |
|------|---------------------|----------------|--------------|
| Sodium antimony tartrate | +++ | ++ | ++ |
| Niridazole | + | +++ | + |
| Metriphonate | – | +++ | – |
| Oxamniquine | +++ | – | – |
| Praziquantel | +++ | +++ | +++ |

From Greenwood D (ed) 1995 *Antimicrobial Chemotherapy*, 3rd edn. Oxford University Press, Oxford.
+++, highly effective; +, poorly effective; – no useful activity.

**Table 62.7** Principal cestode parasites of man

| Species | Common name | Intermediate host | Relevant examination |
|---------|-------------|-------------------|---------------------|
| *Taenia saginata* | Beef tapeworm | Cattle | } Mature segments on stool |
| *T. solium* | Pork tapeworm | Pig | |
| *Diphyllobothrium latum* | Fish tapeworm | *Cyclops* spp./fish | Mature segments on stool |
| *Hymenolepis nana* | Dwarf tapeworm | None | Ova in stool |
| *Echinococcus granulosus*[a] | Hydatid worm | Sheep, man | Ova in stool; Radiology; serology |

[a] Dog tapeworm; man is one of the intermediate hosts.

Eggs are not laid. They are retained within the proglottids which become detached from the end of the worm and are passed with the faeces. Animals become infected by ingesting the eggs from pastures which are contaminated with inadequately treated sewage or, possibly, by birds that scavenge in untreated sewage.

Considering the size of the worm, infection is usually remarkably asymptomatic. However, in the case of *T. solium*, eggs may hatch in the human host and form cysticerci. When these lodge in the brain, they may cause a serious epileptiform disease, *cerebral cysticercosis*.

### Laboratory diagnosis

Taenia infection is usually diagnosed by finding the typical segments in faeces. Since eggs are not laid, faecal examination for ova is inappropriate. *T. saginata* can usually be differentiated from *T. solium* if the segment is pressed between two microscope slides and examined macroscopically. In the case of *T. saginata*, numerous branchings of the central uterine canal are evident, whereas there are usually far fewer branchings with *T. solium* (Fig. 62.5a and b). The eggs (Fig. 62.6a) are thick walled and contain an *oncosphere* with six hooklets. The eggs of *T. saginata* and *T. solium* are indistinguishable.

### Treatment

Tapeworm infection was treated traditionally (and often successfully) with an extract of the rhizome of male fern (*Dryopteris filix-mas*). This has now been abandoned in favour of niclosamide or praziquantel.

### Diphyllobothrium latum

This is the *fish tapeworm*, which is prevalent in lakeland areas where fish is eaten raw. The life cycle is reminiscent of that of the trematodes. The mature adult worm, which may attain a length of 10 m, lays numerous operculate eggs which eventually develop a ciliated body called a *coracidium*. This hatches in water and is ingested by the water flea (*Cyclops* species). After a period of development, the larva awaits ingestion by a freshwater fish in which it invades the muscle as an infective *plerocercoid larva* or *sparganum*.

Human infection is usually asymptomatic, although a form of pernicious anaemia caused by competition for dietary vitamin $B_{12}$ has been described.

The characteristic immature eggs with an indistinct operculum (Fig. 62.6b) are usually present in large numbers in faeces. Occasionally, a length of the worm may break off and be passed in the stool.

Niclosamide or praziquantel are used for treatment.

### Hymenolepis nana

In contrast to the enormous length of *Taenia* species and *D. latum*, *Hymenolepis nana* is only 2–4 cm long, and is consequently known as the *dwarf tapeworm*. It has a very simple life cycle with no known intermediate host. The characteristic 'poached egg' ova (Fig. 62.6c) are directly infective, and it is surprising ·that infection is not more common.

Infection is usually asymptomatic; heavy infections can be treated with praziquantel or niclosamide.

A slightly larger species, *H. diminuta*, is occasionally found in humans. This is a parasite of small rodents, and is transmitted by their fleas.

### Echinococcus granulosus

This is the tapeworm of the dog and other canine species and, unusually, humans are an intermediate host. It is a very small worm consisting usually of just four segments and measuring only a few millimetres in length. Sheep are the usual intermediate hosts. Other animals, including humans, may become infected, especially in sheep-farming areas, where the cycle of transmission is maintained between sheep and dogs.

a

b

**Fig. 62.5**    Segments of **a** *Taenia saginata* and **b** *T. solium*. The uterine canal has been injected with India ink to show the branchings.

After ingestion of the eggs, which resemble those of *Taenia* species, larvae hatch in the small intestine, penetrate the gut mucosa and are carried by the bloodstream to various organs (commonly the liver), where they are filtered out by the capillaries. The larva starts to grow, eventually forming a cystic cavity, the *hydatid cyst*. The inner wall of the cyst contains the *germinal layer*, from which develop *brood capsules* that bud off and fall into the cyst cavity. Within these brood capsules new scolices develop, and some of these may initiate the formation of daughter cysts within the main cavity.

The young cyst may die and calcify, but it often continues to grow inexorably, eventually seriously compromising the function of the organ in which it is situated.

In certain parts of the world, notably the arctic regions of North America and Siberia, infection with a related canine tapeworm, *E. multilocularis*, is encountered. The hydatid cyst infiltrates the surrounding tissue, making it difficult to remove surgically.

### Laboratory diagnosis

The diagnosis is usually made on clinical and radiological evidence. Examination of the cyst fluid (*hydatid sand*) reveals the typical invaginated scolices (Fig. 62.7), but diagnostic puncture of cysts is not recommended because of the risk of spillage (see below).

Immunodiagnostic tests can be used. ELISA is the preferred method, but complement fixation,

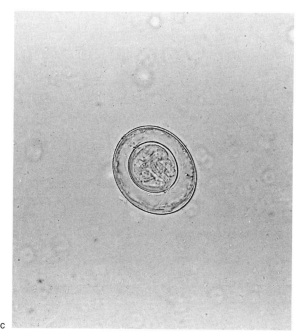

**Fig. 62.6**   Eggs of cestodes: **a** *Taenia* species; **b** *Diphyllobothrium latum*; **c** *Hymenolepis nana*.

indirect agglutination and latex agglutination tests are also available. A skin test with antigen derived from hydatid fluid (*Casoni test*) was formerly employed, but is not reliably specific.

## Treatment

Cysts of *E. granulosus* can often be removed surgically, but accidental spillage of viable scolices into body cavities may cause an anaphylactic reaction and,

**Fig. 62.7** Scolices of *Echinococcus granulosus* from hydatid cyst.

moreover, is likely to lead to the development of fresh cysts. For this reason the hydatid cyst is first injected with a scolicidal agent, such as chlorhexidine or hydrogen peroxide.

The relative impermeability of the cyst militates against successful chemotherapy, but some success has been obtained with benzimidazole derivatives, notably albendazole, and with praziquantel.

## RECOMMENDED READING

Cook G C (ed) 1996 *Manson's Tropical Diseases*, 20th edn. W B Saunders, London

Fleck S L, Moody A H 1988 *Diagnostic Techniques in Medical Parasitology*. Wright, London

Maegraith B 1989 *Adams and Maegraith's Clinical Tropical Diseases*, 9th edn. Blackwell, Oxford

Muller R 1975 *Worms and Disease: A Manual of Medical Helminthology*. Heinemann, London

Peters W, Gilles H M 1995 *A Colour Atlas of Tropical Medicine and Parasitology*, 4th edn. Wolfe, London

World Health Organization 1991 *Basic Laboratory Methods in Medical Parasitology*. WHO, Geneva

# Part 6
## DIAGNOSIS, TREATMENT AND CONTROL OF INFECTION

# 63
## Infective syndromes

*R. C. B. Slack*

Throughout this book, infections have been dealt with as appropriate according to the micro-organisms involved. In this chapter, the study of infection is considered by syndromes associated with the major organs in order to emphasize the variety of microbes that may attack different body systems. The subject is presented in broad outline, and the reader should refer back to earlier chapters for a more extensive account of specific themes.

In infectious diseases, as in other branches of clinical practice, a diagnosis may be obvious and require little investigation, e.g. a case of chickenpox during an epidemic, or may only be established after laboratory and radiological examination, as

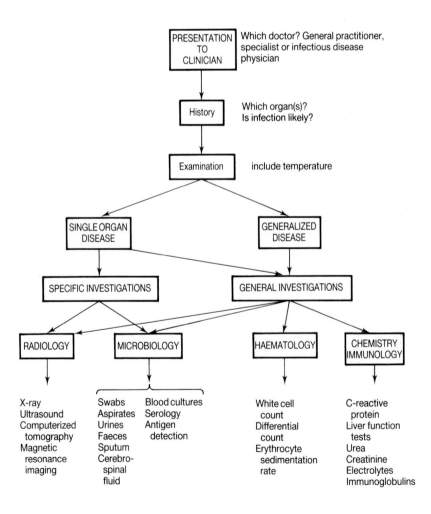

**Fig. 63.1** Flow diagram for the diagnosis of infection.

with a patient with pyrexia of unknown origin (PUO). Figure 63.1 shows a flow chart of a rational approach to diagnosis and management of a patient with infection. In practice, treatment is often started before isolating and identifying the pathogen and in many viral conditions the exact cause can only be determined during convalescence, either by serological tests or after prolonged growth in tissue culture. The availability of rapid methods of diagnosis and new chemotherapeutic agents has made the study of infectious disease even more important.

## SPECIFIC SYNDROMES

### Upper respiratory tract

The upper respiratory tract is frequently the site of general and localized infections. Indeed, this group

of ailments is amongst the most common presenting to domiciliary practice. It is the primary site of infection for most viral diseases which are spread by sneezing, coughing or direct contact with materials contaminated by respiratory secretions. Although the majority of such symptoms are viral in origin, secondary bacterial infection may often follow, particularly in the very young and malnourished. Resident bacteria in the upper respiratory tract such as *Haemophilus influenzae*, *Streptococcus pyogenes* and *Str. pneumoniae* are the most common causes. Figure 63.2 shows the anatomical sites of respiratory infection and the appropriate specimens which may be taken for microbiology.

### Sore throat

Bacterial acute tonsillitis or pharyngitis is commonly due to *Str. pyogenes* (group A), and a few are caused

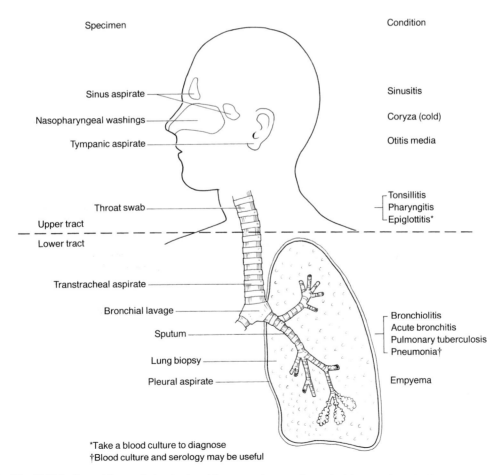

**Fig. 63.2** Microbial infections of the respiratory tract and the appropriate specimens for laboratory investigation.

by groups C and G. Viruses are even more common causes of sore throats, especially the milder, non-exudative forms. However, it is important to make a definitive diagnosis of streptococcal pharyngitis for two reasons:

1. *Str. pyogenes* remains sensitive to penicillin, which should be used for treatment.

2. Group A β-haemolytic streptococci, if untreated, may give rise to septic complications such as a peritonsillar abscess, or to immune-complex disease (glomerulonephritis, rheumatic fever).

On the other hand, since *Str. pyogenes* may account for only 20% of patients presenting with typical symptoms, many courses of antibiotics would be prescribed unnecessarily if all suspected cases were treated. Even in experienced hands it is difficult to predict on clinical grounds alone which cases are streptococcal. This has led to three approaches:

1. Treat all children with a penicillin, or erythromycin if allergic. Adults are treated if the throat looks very inflamed or if there is pus on the tonsils.

2. Swabs are taken for culture of streptococci and antibiotics are started as above but stopped if *Str. pyogenes* is not found.

3. Swabs are taken for rapid diagnosis (by antigen detection) and penicillin commenced only if the throat swab is positive.

There are pros and cons to each method. One drawback to early use of antibiotics is that the patient may react to the drug. If ampicillin is used, there is a strong chance of a skin reaction if the sore throat is the harbinger of glandular fever. In defence of the antibiotic lobby, there is no doubt that complications of streptococcal disease are seen far less commonly when there is access to medical service and pharmacies. However, these improvements have occurred in concert with better housing and social conditions.

There is little need to make a virological diagnosis as specific therapy is not available. However, epidemiological studies of patients with throat symptoms have revealed how common and varied are the viruses in the respiratory tract.

In the severely ill child with toxaemia and a membrane, diphtheria must be considered and treatment should not await laboratory confirmation. Moreover, the laboratory needs to do special tests to isolate and identify *Corynebacterium diphtheriae*, and communication (by telephone, if possible) between the clinician and laboratory is essential. Other corynebacteria such as *C. ulcerans* and *Arcanobacterium haemolyticum* may rarely cause

ulcerated sore throats. In the sexually active, gonococcal pharyngitis should not be missed and again the laboratory needs to be told as they will use special selective media for *Neisseria gonorrhoeae*.

## Common cold (coryza)

This common complaint, characterized by a nasal discharge (acute rhinitis) which is usually watery with scanty cells, afflicts humans of all ages who congregate together. Since there are many types of rhinoviruses, coronaviruses, adenoviruses, etc., and since immunity may be short lived, individuals in a crowded environment, such as at school and university or travelling on public transport, may suffer three or four clinical infections a year. Most of these do not seek medical help knowing that there is little to offer. This is a condition for which many 'alternative' remedies are tried from garlic to peppermint and vitamin supplements.

Bacterial superinfection with pneumococci and *H. influenzae* can occur in the nasopharynx but is only symptomatic when the sinuses or middle ear are involved. Pharyngitis and, occasionally, tracheobronchitis may occur with a cold or develop in more susceptible individuals. Respiratory syncytial virus (RSV) may cause upper respiratory symptoms in children and adults but in those contracting the virus for the first time (usually infants under 1 year of age) acute bronchiolitis is common.

## Sinusitis and otitis media

Direct extension of a viral or bacterial infection from the nasopharynx into frontal and maxillary sinuses in adults and into the middle ear in children is not uncommon. Obtaining adequate material for microbiology is difficult and requires the expertise of ear, nose and throat specialists. In most cases of acute sinusitis or otitis media the microbial cause is not found. It is assumed that severe pain and discharge of pus from the nose or ear is suggestive of bacterial infection and antibiotics are usually given to cover streptococci (mainly *Str. pneumoniae*) and *H. influenzae*. In adults with recurrent or chronic sinusitis, anaerobes (peptostreptococci or bacteroides) are often found in sinus washings.

## Lower respiratory tract

### Epiglottitis

Although situated in the upper part of the respiratory tract, *epiglottitis* behaves like a serious systemic infection which requires urgent admission to hospital and treatment. The diagnosis should be made clinically in a toxic child (usually under 5 years old) with respiratory obstruction and stridor. The most useful investigation is blood culture, which invariably grows *H. influenzae* type b unless antibiotics have been given. The epiglottis, which is swollen and cherry-red in appearance, should only be examined by skilled paediatricians prepared for a respiratory arrest. A lateral radiograph shows a soft tissue swelling in the throat.

## Laryngotracheobronchitis

In adults, some viral infections cause acute laryngitis with voice loss or tracheitis with a dry cough. Respiratory tract infection in children is usually generalized and presents as *croup*. This may lead to respiratory obstruction and, as with haemophilus epiglottitis, urgent admission to hospital is necessary. The condition may be caused by a variety of respiratory viruses, with para-influenza, adeno- and enteroviruses the most common. RSV can also cause croup, but more commonly this virus attacks infants in the first few months of life. In the UK there are winter epidemics of *acute bronchiolitis* due to RSV. This clinical syndrome starts as a cold which is followed by wheezing. In older children, asthmatic attacks are often precipitated by viral respiratory infections.

## Whooping cough

Pertussis may be confused with croup, and, as special specimens need to be taken, the laboratory must be informed. A pernasal swab in special transport medium is required, and *Bordetella pertussis* will only grow on enriched culture media in conditions of high humidity.

## Acute bronchitis

Acute exacerbations of chronic obstructive airways disease (COAD) is the commonest adult lower respiratory infection. It is invariably due to pneumococci, non-encapsulated haemophili, or both. Sometimes, acute bronchitis follows a viral infection. Although often examined, expectorated sputum from ambulatory patients with COAD is almost always a waste of effort.

Cystic fibrosis patients have frequent exacerbations and, in those situations, sputum examination is valuable because the causative bacteria (*Staphylococcus aureus*, *H. influenzae* and *Pseudomonas aeruginosa*)

may show variable antimicrobial resistance and appropriate therapy is essential.

## Acute pneumonias

It is sometimes possible on clinical and radiological grounds to distinguish between *lobar pneumonia* (pneumococcal), *bronchopneumonia* (staphylococcal and klebsiellal) and '*atypical*' *pneumonias* (mycoplasmal and chlamydial). This division is of importance in guiding primary treatment, but should not give the clinician a blinkered view in investigation as some cases will invariably not follow a textbook! Expectorated sputum is often poorly collected and may not yield the pathogen. Blood cultures should always be taken from pneumonia patients but may not yield an organism, especially if antibiotics have been started. *Antigen detection* in urine or sputum by fluorescent antibodies, immuno-electrophoresis, latex agglutination or enzyme-linked immunosorbent assay (ELISA) is a useful method for rapid diagnosis but may lack sensitivity. New amplified DNA detection methods are likely to improve diagnostic accuracy in respiratory infections. At present most cases of 'atypical' pneumonia are diagnosed by obtaining acute and convalescent sera and finding a significant titre or a rising titre of antibodies. *Legionnaires' disease* may be diagnosed by culture of *Legionella pneumophila* from sputum or a biopsy, but this has too low a sensitivity and treatment must often be given on the grounds of serological evidence or clinical suspicion.

## Chronic chest disease

Tuberculosis must always be considered in any patient with fever, cough and weight loss. Again, a request for examination for mycobacteria must be included on the request card.

In the immunocompromised, various opportunist pathogens may give rise to respiratory infection. *Pneumocystis carinii* is demonstrated by fluorescent antibody staining of bronchial lavage. Fungal infections are diagnosed by growth of the pathogen or by serology. Special investigations are required for all these situations and unless the diagnosis is considered the laboratory cannot assist the clinician.

# Gastro-intestinal infection

Acute diarrhoea with or without vomiting is a common complaint. Microbial causes, either by multiplication in the intestine or from the effects of preformed toxin, are the most important reasons for

**Table 63.1** Common microbial causes of infectious intestinal disease

| | |
|---|---|
| Viruses | Rotavirus |
| | Astrovirus |
| | Calicivirus |
| Bacteria | *Salmonella* spp. |
| | *Campylobacter* spp. |
| | *Shigella* spp. |
| | *Escherichia coli* (ETEC, EIEC, EPEC, EHEC) |
| | *Vibrio cholerae* |
| | *V. parahaemolyticus* |
| | *Yersinia enterocolitica* |
| Protozoa | *Cryptosporidium parvum* |
| | *Entamoeba histolytica* |
| | *Giardia lamblia* |

ETEC, enterotoxigenic *Esch. coli*; EIEC, entero-invasive *Esch. coli*; EPEC, enteropathogenic *Esch. coli*; EHEC, enterohaemorrhagic *Esch. coli*.

acute gastro-intestinal upset in an otherwise healthy individual. The cause of inflammatory bowel disease such as ulcerative colitis has not been established. A patient may present similarly but usually the natural history and chronicity of the condition make the distinction obvious.

Although many new causes of bowel infection have been discovered in the past 15 years the majority of food-related and short-lived episodes do not yield a microbial cause. In part this is due to the wide range of viruses, bacteria and protozoa which may be sought (Table 63.1). A search for all causes involves extensive and expensive laboratory effort, and this is often considered unnecessary for a condition which is usually self-limiting and relatively harmless.

Toxin-mediated disease of microbial origin ranges in severity from relatively trivial episodes of food poisoning caused by enterotoxin-producing strains of *Staph. aureus*, *Clostridium perfringens* and *Bacillus cereus*, to the life-threatening systemic disease (*botulism*) caused by *Cl. botulinum*, and the severe *pseudomembranous colitis* caused by *Cl. difficile*, which occasionally follows depletion of the gut flora by antibiotic treatment. There are, in addition, many non-microbial causes of food poisoning, such as that due to the ingestion of certain toadstools, undercooked red kidney beans or various types of fish (*ciguatera toxin*, *scombrotoxin*); most notorious is the puffer fish which, during part of its reproductive cycle, produces a neurotoxin that is responsible for more than 100 deaths a year in Japan, where the delicacy *fugu* is enjoyed.

It may be possible on clinical grounds to distinguish between patients with dysentery, in which bloody diarrhoea and mucus are found, and those with watery diarrhoea, due to the toxic effects of the pathogen on the small intestinal mucosa, leading to accumulation of fluid in the bowel. Some conditions such as staphylococcal food poisoning and some viral illnesses present largely with vomiting. A specific cause is also suspected if there is a history of foreign travel, if the case forms part of an outbreak which is food or water associated, or if the individual has a relevant food history.

*Travellers' diarrhoea* encompasses many clinical and microbial causes but the commonest organisms implicated are enterotoxigenic strains of *Escherichia coli* (ETEC). However, a host of microbes must be considered. Some, such as salmonellae, are found world-wide; others, such as vibrios, have a more limited distribution.

More chronic intestinal infections contracted in warmer climates usually do not present with diarrhoea but with vague abdominal symptoms. Many helminths and protozoa are found on screening faeces for other pathogens.

## Urinary tract infections

The diagnosis of urinary tract infection cannot be made without bacteriological examination of the urine because many patients with the frequency-dysuria syndrome have sterile urine and, conversely, asymptomatic bacteriuria is a common condition. Infection is most commonly caused by members of the Enterobacteriaceae (Table 63.2), but there are great variations in antimicrobial susceptibility and control of chemotherapy requires laboratory examination. Occasionally, *Mycobacterium tuberculosis* invades the kidney and appropriate tests must be carried out if this is suspected.

Infection in the urinary tract may be confined to particular anatomical sites, e.g. urethritis or renal abscess. Alternatively, the urine may become infected

**Table 63.2** Common causes of urinary tract infection (approximate percentages)

| Organism | Domiciliary | Hospital |
|---|---|---|
| *Escherichia coli* | 70–80 | 50 |
| *Proteus mirabilis* | 10 | 1–5 |
| *Klebsiella* spp. | 1–5 | 5–10 |
| *Staphylococcus saprophyticus* | 10–15 | 0 |
| *Staph. epidermidis* | 1–5 | 10–20 |
| Enterococci | 1–5 | 10–20 |
| Other coliforms | <1 | 5–10 |
| *Pseudomonas aeruginosa* | 1–2 | 5–10 |

and, in cases of obstruction or reflux, bacteria may ascend from the bladder to give rise to kidney infections. *Urethritis* is really a genital infection and is most commonly due to sexually transmitted organisms such as chlamydiae or *N. gonorrhoeae*. Confirmation depends on obtaining, by swabbing or scraping, a sample of urethral discharge for microscopy and culture. *Metastatic abscesses* in the kidney and *perinephric abscesses* cannot usually be diagnosed by urine examination, although pyuria may be present. Specific radiological or surgical exploration is necessary, as with any localized infection.

Throughout most of their life-span women suffer far more attacks of urinary tract infection than men. In young adult women who become sexually active, frequency and dysuria are common reasons to seek medical attention. Only about one-half of these yield an organism in 'significant' numbers, usually defined as above $10^7$ organisms per litre. The commonest cause by far is *Esch. coli* (Table 63.2), some strains of which possess specific uropathogenic determinants. It has been suggested that many of the culture-negative infections are due to coliforms which are present in small numbers in urine. Infection of the urine is common and may be asymptomatic in many elderly patients.

## Infections of the central nervous system

### Meningitis

Meningeal irritation may occur in association with other acute infections (*meningism*) or with non-infective conditions such as subarachnoid haemorrhage. In the early stages of meningococcal disease, signs of meningitis may be absent yet examination of the cerebrospinal fluid (CSF) yields *N. meningitidis*. Thus, CSF and blood cultures should be examined from all suspected cases. There are contra-indications to performing a lumbar puncture in any patient with raised intracranial pressure because of the danger of herniation through the foramen magnum (*coning*). Thus, lumbar puncture should only be carried out in hospital. In fulminating disease, especially if it is meningococcal, it is prudent to give penicillin as soon as the diagnosis is suspected and before admission. This has led to a greatly reduced yield by culture of suspected cases. Antigen and DNA detection have become increasingly important in confirming the diagnosis.

It is often possible to consider the likely pathogen on clinical and epidemiological grounds. *H. influenzae* type b occurs almost always in infants from 6 to 24 months of age. *Str. pneumoniae* is seen generally in

| Table 63.3 | Causes of aseptic meningitis |
|---|---|
| Viruses | Enteroviruses (echo-, polio-, coxsackie-viruses) Mumps (including post-immunization) Herpes (herpes simplex and varicella–zoster) Arboviruses |
| Spiral bacteria | Syphilis (*Treponema pallidum*) Leptospira (*Leptospira canicola*) |
| Other bacteria | Partially treated with antibiotics Tuberculous (*Mycobacterium tuberculosis*) Brain abscess |
| Fungi | *Cryptococcus neoformans* |
| Protozoa | *Acanthamoeba, Naegleria Toxoplasma gondii* |
| Non-infective | Lymphomata, leukaemias Metastatic and primary neoplasms Collagen-vascular diseases |

the very young and the elderly. *Meningococcal meningitis* is characteristically a disease of children and young adults. In the neonate, coliforms (mainly *Esch. coli* K1), *Listeria monocytogenes*, group B streptococci and pneumococci may be found. In infants a few months old, salmonella meningitis is an important condition in some warm-climate countries.

If no readily cultivated organism is found, but the CSF shows an increase in cells, the syndrome of *aseptic meningitis* is present. Table 63.3 shows some of the causes of this condition. If the symptoms are short in duration, viruses are most likely. If the child has been unwell for more than 1 week, *tuberculous meningitis* must be considered. This is one of the most difficult and important microbiological diagnoses to make.

In the immunocompromised, listeria meningitis may be seen in the adult and *Cryptococcus neoformans* in all age groups but particularly those with human immunodeficiency virus (HIV) infection. Central nervous system disease in patients with acquired immune deficiency syndrome (AIDS) is a very complicated differential diagnosis (Table 63.4).

### Cerebral infections

*Encephalitis* may extend into the meninges with signs and CSF findings of an aseptic meningitis. Many viral infections may, however, only infect the brain cortex and clinical symptoms may be vague: loss of consciousness, fits, localized paralysis. This can also occur in toxaemia, cerebral malaria, electrolyte disturbances or vascular accidents.

**Table 63.4** Causes of neurological damage in HIV-infected patients

| Direct HIV infection | Subacute encephalomyelitis (AIDS–dementia complex) |
|---|---|
| Opportunist infections | |
|    Viruses | Cytomegalovirus |
| | Herpes simplex |
| | Varicella–zoster |
| | Papovavirus |
|    Bacteria | *Treponema pallidum* (syphilis) |
|    Fungi | *Cryptococcus neoformans* |
|    Protozoa | *Toxoplasma gondii* |
| Malignancy | |
|    Primary | Brain lymphoma |
|    Secondary | Kaposi's sarcoma |
| | Systemic lymphoma |

In western Europe, herpes simplex or varicella–zoster viruses are the most common causes of encephalitis but in many parts of the world arboviruses such as Japanese B encephalitis virus are important.

*Abscesses* in the brain or subdural space may arise from haematogenous spread during bacteraemia or by direct extension, either through the cribriform plate from the nasopharynx or from sinuses or the middle ear. They may be clinically silent or present as a space-occupying lesion accompanied by fever and systemic upset. Skilled radiological scanning by computerized axial tomography (CAT) or magnetic resonance imaging (MRI), if available, and early neurosurgical intervention will reduce complications and, if appropriate systemic antibiotics are given for a prolonged period, the success rate is nowadays good.

## Skin and soft-tissue infections

Human skin acts as an excellent barrier to infection. Some parasites, such as hookworm larvae and schistosome cercariae can penetrate skin to initiate infection. This may also be true of some bacteria, notably *Treponema pallidum*, although in primary syphilis the spirochaete probably enters through minute abrasions which are present even in healthy skin. Primary skin infection such as *impetigo* is due to *Staph. aureus* or *Str. pyogenes*, or both, gaining access to abrasions, usually in children. This may occur in association with ectoparasite infestation, in particular, scabies. *Dermatophyte* fungi are specialized to grow well in keratinized tissue.

*Skin lesions* are a feature of some virus infections, such as warts, herpes simplex and molluscum contagiosum. In other virus diseases, including rubella, measles, chickenpox (and, before its eradication, smallpox) a characteristic rash follows the viraemic phase of the illness. *Wound infections* may be accidental or postoperative and many organisms can cause sepsis. Even after surgery many wounds are infected with the endogenous flora of the patient. Swabs, or preferably pus, obtained directly from the wound or abscess, are adequate to find the causative organisms. *Anaerobic* sepsis most commonly occurs following amputations or in contaminated traumatic wounds, particularly if the blood supply has been compromised or the bowel perforated. In classic *gas gangrene*, bubbles of gas may be felt in the wound and surrounding tissues and the muscle and fascia have a black necrotic appearance. Less florid examples of anaerobes causing extensive cellulitis are more commonly seen and the laboratory should be requested to look carefully for anaerobes in all situations where deep wounds may be contaminated with endogenous flora.

## Genital tract infections

In the male, acute urethritis is a common condition which is usually due to a sexually transmitted microbe such as *N. gonorrhoeae*, *Chlamydia trachomatis* or *Ureaplasma urealyticum*. If untreated these organisms can cause prostatitis or epididymitis, and gonorrhoea may produce unpleasant consequences such as urethral stricture or sterility. Genital ulcers in both sexes may be due to herpes simplex virus, syphilis or chancroid (*H. ducreyi*).

The more complicated female reproductive organs are subjected to many more infections with a greater scope for sequelae. Vaginitis may present as vaginal discharge or irritation and often these are due to infections that are not always exogenously acquired. *Trichomonas vaginalis* is the most common sexually acquired microbe, although both *N. gonorrhoeae* and chlamydia may also present as discharge. Thrush due to *Candida* species is especially common in pregnancy and in diabetics. It is usually an endogenous condition due to disturbances in the normal commensal flora. Another cause of vaginal discharge, but usually without inflammatory cells and irritation, is associated with an alteration of local pH with proliferation of *Gardnerella vaginalis* and anaerobic spiral bacteria, now termed *Mobiluncus* species. The alkaline conditions and characteristic amines found in *bacterial vaginosis* allow a diagnosis to be easily made on examination of the patient.

This condition, which used to be called non-specific vaginitis, is a common condition in sexually active women, although probably not a venereal disease in the usual sense.

The endocervical canal is the site of infection with *N. gonorrhoeae* and *C. trachomatis* in the sexually mature woman. During parturition both organisms may be passed to the baby's eyes to give rise to *ophthalmia neonatorum*. The cervix may also be infected with human papillomavirus (HPV), and this is associated with a high risk of cervical cancer. HPV commonly causes warts on the external genitalia, perianally as well as in the vagina and cervix. Herpes, chancroid and syphilis may cause ulcers in parts of the genital tract which are not visible without a speculum.

Ascending genital infection due to gonococci or chlamydia is a common sequela. In cases of *acute gonococcal salpingitis* there is usually fever and pelvic pain. On vaginal examination, there is referred lower abdominal pain on moving the cervix (*cervical excitation*) and tenderness in the iliac fossa on abdominal palpation. Signs and symptoms in cases due to *C. trachomatis* are much less pronounced, and some women develop chronic *pelvic inflammatory disease* (PID) without having suffered a recognizable acute episode. PID, although most often initiated by these two common sexually transmitted pathogens, is usually a polymicrobial infection, in which endogenous commensals, particularly anaerobes, play an important role.

Infection may progress outside the fallopian tubes to give rise to *pelvic abscesses*, especially in the pouch of Douglas, and peritonitis. Spread across the peritoneal cavity may give rise to *perihepatitis*, which was first described in gonorrhoea as the Fitz-Hugh–Curtis syndrome, but also occurs in chlamydial disease.

## Eye infections

Various microbes may cause acute conjunctivitis. Ophthalmia neonatorum may be due to gonococci or chlamydia. In the newborn, *Staph. aureus* is commonly found in 'sticky eyes', either as a primary cause of conjunctivitis or after infection with another pathogen. In older infants and children, *H. influenzae* and *Str. pneumoniae* are common. Chlamydiae give rise to *trachoma*, the commonest cause of blindness in the world, and to a milder form of inclusion blennorrhoea in sexually active individuals.

Primary viral conjunctivitis often occurs in epidemics when certain types of adenovirus are implicated. This is usually a mild condition with few sequelae compared with the keratitis due to herpes simplex virus or in shingles when the ophthalmic division of the trigeminal nerve is infected with varicella–zoster virus.

Corneal damage due to fungi as well as herpesviruses is seen in immunosuppressed patients, and keratitis caused by free-living amoebae (*Acanthamoeba* species), though rare, is becoming more common, particularly in wearers of contact lenses.

Penetrating injuries of the eye and ophthalmic surgery may introduce a wide range of bacteria and fungi into the chambers of the eye which may give rise to *hypopyon* (pus in the eye). This condition requires prompt surgical drainage and instillation of appropriate antibiotics such as gentamicin. *Ps. aeruginosa* and *Proteus* species are among the more common organisms isolated.

Infections of the back of the eye (choroidoretinitis) are seen in many diverse infectious diseases (see Table 63.5).

**Table 63.5** Causes of choroidoretinitis

| | |
|---|---|
| Viruses | Cytomegalovirus, rubella |
| Bacteria | *Treponema pallidum* |
| Protozoa | *Toxoplasma gondii* |
| Helminths | *Toxocara canis, Onchocerca volvulus* |

# SYSTEMIC AND GENERAL SYNDROMES

## Pyrexia of unknown origin

PUO may be defined as a significant fever (greater than 38°C) for a few days without an obvious cause, i.e. no apparent infection of an organ or system. In the classic studies of PUO only patients with persistent fever for at least 3 weeks were included. These chronic cases are often due to non-infective causes such as malignancy (especially lymphomata) or auto-immune and connective tissue diseases (such as systemic lupus erythematosus).

In determining an infective aetiology some of the most important questions to be asked of the patient are:

1. Have you been abroad recently?
2. What is your occupation (especially, is animal contact involved)?
3. What immunizations have you had – in particular have you had BCG?
4. Have you or your family ever had tuberculosis?
5. Are you taking or have you recently had any drugs (especially antibiotics)?

## Character of fever

The individual with suspected PUO should be admitted to hospital so that measurements can be made regularly by skilled staff. Rarely, malingerers may be found out and drug reactions discovered by controlling intake. Rhythmical fevers such as the quartan fever (every 72 h) of *Plasmodium malariae* or undulant fever of *Brucella melitensis* may be rarely found and point to the aetiology. More commonly, fevers are intermittent with rises at the end of the day and falls after rigors or extensive sweating.

The degree of temperature depends also on the host response as well as the pyrogens produced by microbes. Generally, the older the patient the less able they are to mount a pyrexia. Many elderly patients with septicaemia may have normal or subnormal temperatures whereas infants can have fevers of 40°C and febrile convulsions with otherwise mild respiratory viral infections.

## Endocarditis

Infections of the tissue of the heart usually involve damaged valves, either post-rheumatic fever or with atheroma. Another important group of patients are those who have had heart surgery, in particular prosthetic valve replacements. In addition, intravenous drug addicts or patients who have had indwelling vascular devices are liable to bacteraemia and, occasionally, endocarditis may follow. The most common causative organisms are listed in Table 63.6.

## Septicaemia

It is not clinically useful to distinguish between *bacteraemia*, organisms isolated from the bloodstream, *septicaemia*, which is a clinical syndrome, and *endotoxaemia*, which is circulating bacterial endotoxin. The spectrum of clinical disease ranges from hypotensive shock and disseminated intravascular coagulation (DIC) with a high mortality, to transient bacteraemia, which may occur in healthy individuals during dental manipulations.

The vascular compartment is sterile and usually intact. Microbes gain entry from breakages of blood vessels adjacent to skin or mucosal surfaces or by phagocytic cells carrying organisms into capillaries or the lymphatic system. Active multiplication within the bloodstream probably only occurs terminally, but in many cases of septicaemia there are high numbers of bacteria recovered from blood cultures, which often only sample 10 ml at a time. This occurs from a heavily contaminated site such as an indwelling urinary catheter which releases bacteria into veins on movement. Septic shock may be due to Gram-negative lipids (endotoxins) or Gram-positive toxins (e.g. staphylococcal enterotoxin), which are usually proteins. The end result of both is to initiate a cascade of events involving cytokines, especially tumour necrosis factor and interleukin-2, vascular mediators and platelets, which combined lead to DIC and hypotension. This process becomes irreversible and produces failure of all major organs. Patients die from a variety of terminal events which make up the syndrome of *septic shock*. The main microbial causes are listed with approximate frequency in Table 63.7.

---

**Table 63.6** Common causes of infective endocarditis (approximate percentages)

| Organism | Non-operative | IVDA/surgery |
|---|---|---|
| Viridans group of streptococci | 70 | 35 |
| Enterococci | 5 | 3 |
| Other streptococci (group G, F) | 10 | <1 |
| *Staphylococcus epidermidis* | 10 | 25 |
| *Staph. aureus* | 5 | 25 |
| Gram-positive rods (diphtheroids) | <1 | 5 |
| *Haemophilus* spp. and other fastidious Gram-negative organisms[a] | <1[b] | <1 |
| Gram-negative bacilli (coliforms, *Pseudomonas* spp.) | 0 | 5 |
| *Coxiella burnetii* (Q fever) | <1[b] | 0 |
| *Chlamydia psittaci* | <1 | 0 |
| Fungi (*Candida* spp.) | <1 | 2 |

IVDA, intravenous drug abusers.
[a] *Neisseria, Brucella, Cardiobacterium, Streptobacillus* spp.
[b] These are rough UK figures; in some parts of the Middle East, brucellae and Q fever cause significant numbers of infective endocarditides.

**Table 63.7**  Major causes of septicaemia (approximate percentages)

| Organism | Community acquired | Hospital acquired | Sources and comments |
|---|---|---|---|
| *Escherichia coli* | 35 | 30 | UTI (catheters), biliary tract |
| Other enterobacteria | 5 | 10 | UTI, chest |
| *Pseudomonas* spp. | 5 | 5 | UTI, immunocompromised |
| Other Gram-negative rods | 2 | 5 | Ventilator pneumonia |
| *Neisseria meningitidis* | 3 | 0 | Characteristic skin rash |
| *Staphylococcus aureus* | 30 | 25 | Vascular, postoperative |
| *Staph. epidermidis* | <1 | 20 | Vascular devices |
| *Streptococcus pneumoniae* | 10 | 0 | Pneumonia |
| *Str. pyogenes* | 5 | 2 | Skin, soft tissue |
| Other Gram-positive cocci | 2 | 0 | Skin |
| *Listeria monocytogenes* | <1 | 0 | Bowel, foods |
| *Clostridium* spp. | <1 | 0 | Bowel, gangrenous wounds |
| *Bacteroides* spp. | 3 | 1 | Bowel, pelvis, wounds |
| Mixed infection | 10 | 7 | Bowel, intensive care |

Data from Dr P. Ispahani, Nottingham Public Health Laboratory UK.
UTI, urinary tract infection.

Clinical features may occasionally suggest the aetiological agent, e.g. the characteristic purpuric rash of meningococcal disease and the black lesions (*ecthyma gangrenosum*) seen on the skin of compromised patients with pseudomonas septicaemia, but in the majority of bacteraemias the agent can only be determined after blood culture. Sometimes, prior antibiotic therapy may render cultures negative and new methods of antigen detection or gene probes may be useful. Non-specific investigations such as those shown in Figure 63.1 may offer some help that the cause of the illness is infective. C-reactive protein (CRP), an acute-phase protein which is often greatly elevated in the serum during bacterial infections, may be the most useful of these but, as with peripheral leucocyte counts, there are a significant number of errant results.

## Imported fevers

An important group of patients with fever are those who have recently returned from abroad. In whichever country a doctor may practise, travellers with unfamiliar disease will be encountered. A knowledge of medical geography is useful but conditions vary greatly within one country and with time. Up-to-date information is held, often on computer, by communicable disease centres and tropical disease hospitals and schools. The World Health Organization and the Centers for Disease Control, Atlanta, USA, publish international notification data and maps. Undoubtedly, the most important condition to diagnose is malaria due to *Plasmodium falciparum*, which may be rapidly fatal without appropriate treatment in the non-immune subject. The wide distribution of drug resistance in *P. falciparum* has led to difficulties in giving adequate prophylaxis and in treating an acute attack. Other common febrile illnesses which are imported into northern countries are typhoid and paratyphoid. These do not usually present with diarrhoea so the possibility of an enteric fever may not be considered. It is also obvious, but sometimes overlooked, that the fever may not be related to the travel history and that the cause is a microbe which could have been caught at home.

## Imported infections

Table 63.8 lists some of the more common causes of infectious diseases imported from tropical countries into temperate regions where the diseases are not normally transmitted. There are three groups of patients which are considered separately, but the separation of diseases and microbes is not exclusive:

1. Short-term travellers or *tourists* who usually visit major cities or special holiday areas and stay in good accommodation and have minimal contact with the indigenous population.
2. Long-term visitors who may be engaged in lengthy overland trips or be working abroad as *expatriates*.
3. *Immigrants* who were brought up abroad and visit or have residence in the host country: also settled immigrants who pay short-term visits to their country of origin.

Individuals who travel abroad vary in their risk behaviour and their exposure to potential pathogens.

**Table 63.8** Some important infective conditions imported to temperate regions from the tropics

| Causative organism | Tourists[a] | Expatriates[a] | Immigrants[a] |
|---|---|---|---|
| Viruses | Hepatitis A<br>Influenza | HIV<br>Yellow fever<br>(Other arboviruses) | Hepatitis B<br>Haemorrhagic fever |
| Rickettsiae and chlamydiae | Tick typhus | Q fever | Trachoma |
| Bacteria | Typhoid<br>Toxigenic *Escherichia coli* | Brucellosis<br>Shigellosis | Tuberculosis, leprosy<br>Cholera |
| Protozoa | Cryptosporidiosis<br>Falciparum malaria<br>Cutaneous leishmaniasis | Giardiasis<br>Malaria (all)<br>Schistosomiasis | Amoebiasis<br>Vivax malaria<br>Kala azar (visceral leishmaniasis) |
| Helminths | — | Tapeworm<br>Stronglyloidiasis<br>Filariasis | Roundworm<br>Hookworm |
| Ectoparasites<br>(ticks, mites and insects) | — | Myiasis<br>Jigger flea | Scabies |
| Fungi | — | Dermatophytosis<br>Histoplasmosis | Mycetoma |

[a] These categories are not mutually exclusive.

Generally, advice given by travel operators, tourist offices, embassies and medical sources has greatly improved in the past few years. Companies sending out expatriate workers tend to look after their staff well. Nevertheless, many tourists (up to 50% in some studies) have episodes of travellers' diarrhoea, which in some cases results in admission to hospital. The major groups who are missed in preventative programmes are overland travellers and immigrants returning to their homeland, often with young families who have never been exposed to the infectious risks of their parents' home. Immigrants returning for visits to malarious areas seldom take prophylactic advice, believing themselves to be immune, but protective immunity wanes with prolonged absence.

## Cryptogenic infections

Some of the commonly encountered sites of infection which may give rise to fever, and must be considered in the differential diagnosis of PUO, are listed in Table 63.9.

**Table 63.9** Some common sites of infection in PUO

| | |
|---|---|
| Abdomen | Subphrenic abscess<br>Appendix abscess<br>Ileal tuberculosis<br>Pelvic abscess |
| Liver and biliary tract | Intrahepatic abscess<br>Empyema of gallbladder<br>Ascending cholangitis<br>Cholecystitis<br>Viral hepatitis |
| Kidney and urinary tract | Perinephric abscess<br>Renal tuberculosis<br>Pyelonephritis (especially children) |
| Bones | Vertebral osteomyelitis<br>Tuberculosis<br>Prosthetic infections |
| Cardiovascular | Endocarditis<br>Graft infections |
| Respiratory | Tuberculosis<br>Empyema and lung abscess |
| Nervous system | Cryptococcal or tuberculous meningitis<br>Brain or spinal abscess |

## RECOMMENDED READING

Christie A B 1987 *Infectious Diseases: Epidemiology and Clinical Practice*, 4th edn. Churchill Livingstone, Edinburgh, vols 1 and 2

Emond R T D, Rowland H A K 1987 *A Colour Atlas of Infectious Diseases*, 2nd edn. Wolfe, London

Grist N R, Ho-Yen D O, Walker E, Williams G R 1993 *Diseases of Infection*, 2nd edn. Oxford University Press, Oxford

Lambert H P, Farrar W E 1982 *Infectious Diseases Illustrated*. Pergamon, Oxford

Mandell G L, Bennett J E, Dolin R 1995 *Principles and Practice of Infectious Diseases*, 4th edn. Churchill Livingstone, New York

Shanson D C 1989 *Microbiology in Clinical Practice*, 3rd edn. Wright, London

Weatherall D J, Ledingham J G G, Warrek D A 1996 *Oxford Textbook of Medicine*, 3rd edn. Oxford University Press, Oxford

# 64

# Diagnostic procedures

*R. C. B. Slack*

The role of the laboratory in assisting clinicians in the diagnosis of infection is illustrated in the specimen flow diagram shown in Figure 64.1. The choice of specimen depends on following the principles outlined in Chapter 63. The microbiology laboratory

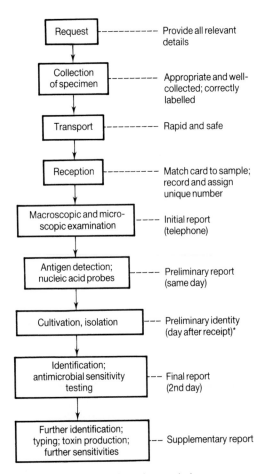

* viruses, fungi and some bacteria may take longer

**Fig. 64.1** Steps in the isolation and identification of pathogens from an infected patient.

requires enough information on the request card accompanying the specimen to use the optimal methods necessary for identification of potential pathogens in particular infective syndromes. At the most basic level, it is obvious that when a swab is received in the laboratory, it is necessary to know if it comes from the throat or the vagina! But additional information is also essential: is the patient being investigated for pharyngitis or diphtheria; for vaginal discharge or septic abortion? Furthermore, the specimen must be obtained with care and transported to the laboratory without delay in an appropriate manner. The value of the result is in direct proportion to the attention given to these details, as well as to the skill and efficiency of the laboratory. For further details of laboratory methods, including specimen containers and culture media used, the reader is encouraged to consult the companion volume *Practical Medical Microbiology* listed in the recommended reading section.

## COLLECTION OF SPECIMENS

Samples for microbiological examination need to be carefully collected, if possible without contamination with commensals or from external sources. Some points to remember with specimens from individual sources are shown in Table 64.1. It is essential to use sterile containers which are leak-proof and able to withstand transportation through the post if necessary. It is more convenient for both the clinician and microbiologist if the laboratory provides request cards, containers and an efficient transport system. There is a need for staff to be aware of safety regulations and for all parties to understand who has responsibility for each step of the process and how to minimize handling by untrained people. Special precautions required for 'high-risk' specimens need to be defined by the laboratory and hospital manage-

**Table 64.1** Some important points to remember in the collection of specimens for microbiological examination

**Respiratory secretions**

| | |
|---|---|
| Nasal swab (anterior) | Only for carriage of staphylococci and streptococci |
| Nasopharyngeal swab | For pertussis and meningococci |
| External ear swab | Wide range of microbes including fungi |
| Myringotomy and sinus samples | As for abscesses – including anaerobes |
| Throat (pharyngeal) swab | Specify if only for streptococci; mention if diphtheria possible; use special transport media for virology |
| Saliva | Used for antibody detection; otherwise discard |
| Laryngeal swab | Specify if for mycobacteria |
| Expectorated sputum | Often poorly collected; specify mycobacteria, legionellae, pneumocystis |
| Transtracheal aspirate, bronchoscopy specimens, lung biopsy | Specify likely diagnosis; ask for specific tests |
| Pleural fluid | Treat as pus; always look for mycobacteria |

**Gastro-intestinal specimens**

| | |
|---|---|
| Vomitus | Only for virology |
| Gastric washings | For mycobacteria (particularly in children) |
| Gastric biopsy | For *Helicobacter pylori* |
| Duodenal/jejunal aspirates | Protozoa (*Giardia lamblia*, microsporidia, etc.) |
| Liver aspirates | As for pus (anaerobes); consider amoebae |
| Spleen puncture | For *Leishmania* spp. |
| Rectal biopsy | Schistosomiasis |
| Rectal swab | Only for gonococci and chlamydia |
| Colonic biopsy | Histopathological diagnosis of amoebiasis, pseudomembranous colitis (*Clostridium difficile*) |
| Colonic scrapings | Protozoa; amoebic trophozoites (deliver to laboratory immediately) |
| Faeces | Specify possible diagnosis; ask for clostridial toxins, parasite examination if suspected |
| Peri-anal swab | For eggs of threadworm |

**Urine**

| | |
|---|---|
| Mid-stream (MSU) | Suitable for most patients |
| Clean catch | Infants and elderly – increased contamination |
| Suprapubic aspirate | Infants and neonates |
| Ureteric/bladder washout | To localize infection |
| Prostatic massage | Collect samples before, during and at end of micturition |
| Terminal urine | Schistosome ova |
| Complete early morning or 24 h urine | Mycobacteria (tubercle) |

**Central nervous system**

| | |
|---|---|
| Cerebrospinal fluid by spinal tap | For meningitis collect sample for protein and glucose – test blood sugar simultaneously, specify virology, fungi or syphilis serology |
| Ventricular tap | Specify if through an indwelling shunt or catheter |
| Brain abscess | As for pus (include anaerobes) |

**Table 64.1** (cont'd)

| | |
|---|---|
| **Skin and soft tissue** | |
| Skin scraping/nail clipping | Dermatophyte fungi |
| Skin swab | Rarely valuable without pus |
| Skin snips | Onchocerciasis – seek advice |
| Vesicle fluid | Suitable for electron microscopy for viruses |
| Wound swab | Obtain pus if possible; record site |
| Pus, tissues, aspirates | Describe site and any relevant operative details |
| **Genital** | |
| Urethral swab | Pus for gonococci, scrape for chlamydia |
| Vaginal swab (adult) | Only for candida, trichomonas and bacterial vaginosis |
| Vaginal swab (prepubertal) | State age; caution required if abuse possible |
| Cervical swab | Separate media for chlamydia |
| Ulcer scrape | Immediate dark-ground microscopy; separate media for virology or chancroid |
| Uterine secretions | Specify puerperium or post-abortion |
| Pelvic aspirates | As for pus |
| Laparoscopy specimens | Include chlamydia specimen |
| **Eye** | |
| Conjunctival swab | Separate virology; scrape for chlamydia |
| Aspirates | As for pus |
| **Blood** | |
| Culture | Strict aseptic technique; take large sample in special media before antibiotics |
| Bone marrow | Valuable for leishmania, mycobacteria, brucella |
| Film | Malaria (thick and thin), filaria, borrelia, trypanosomes |
| Whole blood | Filaria (day or night samples as appropriate) |
| Serum antigen | Rapid diagnosis of many microbial diseases (e.g. hepatitis B) |
| Serum antibody | Retrospective diagnosis of common viral diseases, syphilis and other selected infections; need rising titre or specific IgM |

ment. Storage of clinical material must be separate from food and drugs and this may necessitate provision of additional refrigerator space and transport facilities.

## Food and water

The examination of non-clinical specimens is beyond the scope of this book and readers are referred to appropriate reading. However, an outbreak of gastro-intestinal disease inevitably leads to the question of identifying the source. When disease is due to pre-formed toxins, as with staphylococcal food poisoning, faecal examination is unhelpful, and the diagnosis can only be made by testing the food. Frequently, the offending item has been discarded and the

examination of food and water related to specific patients is often unrewarding. Routine sampling of water sources and potentially contaminated food such as poultry at various critical points of production is essential in maintaining good public health.

## TRANSPORT

Many microbes may perish on transit from the host's body to a laboratory incubator. Some contaminants, especially coliforms, may overgrow the pathogen and so mask its presence. These two constraints make it essential that any material for cultivation of microbes is transported as quickly as possible to the labora-

**Table 64.2**  Types of transport medium

| Type of organism | Medium | Comments |
|---|---|---|
| Bacteria | Stuart's semi-solid agar | Contains charcoal to inactivate toxic material |
| Anaerobic bacteria | Various systems, including gassed-out tubes and anaerobic bags | Not widely used, but essential for some strict anaerobes |
| Viruses | Buffered salts solution containing serum | Contains antibiotics to control bacteria and fungi |
| Chlamydiae | Similar to viral transport medium, but without agents that inhibit chlamydiae | Chlamydial antigen media contain detergent to lyse infected cells |
| Protozoa, helminths | Merthiolate–iodine–formalin | Kills active protozoa, but preserves cysts and ova in a form suitable for concentration and microscopy |

tory in a manner expected to protect the viability of any pathogens. Such problems may be minimized by the use of antigen or gene probe detection because of the relative stability of the chemical structures identified.

The ideal situation is to bring the patient to the laboratory for specimen collection or take the laboratory to the clinic. Both approaches are used for special purposes but are obviously inconvenient for many patients and inappropriate and costly for complicated techniques such as virus isolation which need specialized (and safe) facilities.

To overcome any drawbacks due to delay in reaching the microbiology department the following methods may be used:

1. *Transport media* (Table 64.2).
2. *Boric acid.* The addition of boric acid to urine at a concentration of 1.8% (v/w) will stop bacterial multiplication but lower concentrations are ineffective and higher ones may kill the pathogen.
3. *Dip slides.* These provide a convenient way of inoculating urines at the clinic. They comprise small plastic spoons or strips holding a thin layer of agar which is dipped into the urine and then put in a screw-topped bottle for transport. The agar adsorbs a fixed volume of urine and, after incubation, colony counts of bacteria give a semi-quantitative estimation of numbers.
4. *Refrigeration.* Storage at 4°C before processing will prevent multiplication of most bacteria. However, delicate microbes such as neisseriae may not survive whereas certain organisms, notably listeriae, flourish at low temperatures.
5. *Freezing.* Temperatures of −70°C or below which can be achieved in liquid nitrogen or special deep freezes will preserve many microbes, providing they are protected by a stabilizing fluid such as serum or glycerol.

## RECEPTION

The importance of good documentation cannot be overstressed. No matter how well the specimen was taken, transported and processed in the laboratory, the end result depends on communication between people. The clinician making the request must give complete details on the request card and specimen to reduce errors. Staff receiving specimens in the laboratory must match them with the cards and record them into a book or computer. This is usually done by assigning a unique number to each specimen and labelling both the specimen and the request. When parts of the specimen are separated from the original bottle, e.g. after centrifugation of serum, the laboratory number becomes the only recognizable identification. Transcription errors are especially important for requests for human immunodeficiency virus (HIV) or syphilis serology, which may have disastrous consequences and medicolegal implications if wrong results are given. Transcription mistakes in laboratories are far more common than is supposed: studies in chemical pathology departments have shown a significant number of 'errors' amounting to 5% of the total samples.

## EXAMINATION

Looking at clinical material with the naked eye or hand-lens should be part of the examination of a patient at the bed-side. Sadly, many doctors delegate this to nurses or to the laboratory staff. Many unnecessary laboratory tests could be avoided if unsuitable specimens were rejected on the ward or in the general practitioner's surgery. These would include: crystal-clear urine from patients with 'cystitis'; well-formed stools from patients with 'diarrhoea'; and mouth washings or saliva from patients with respiratory symptoms. It was once common practice to carry out certain basic investigations in ward side-rooms, and kits offering 'near-patient testing' are becoming available. However, there are cogent arguments against bedside pathology, including issues of safety, time, competence and quality control.

## Microscopy

Microscopy is an important part of the examination of many specimens. For bacteriology, the Gram and Ziehl–Neelsen stains are usually sufficient, but for the demonstration of fungi or parasites special stains or concentration techniques may be required. 'Wet' mounts, i.e. unstained preparations of fluid material, are widely used in looking at cells in urine, cerebrospinal fluid, faeces and vaginal secretions. None of these procedures takes more than 5 or 10 min and all are inexpensive in reagent costs and capital equipment. They are therefore ideal rapid methods and new diagnostic techniques have to be judged against microscopy. An initial report, such as 'Gram-negative diplococci and pus cells seen' from meningitic cerebrospinal fluid, can be issued within minutes of receiving the specimen and will aid the clinician in confirming the diagnosis and starting appropriate antibiotics.

Similarly, a rapid diagnosis of falciparium malaria can be life-saving. Indeed, suspected pyogenic meningitis and falciparum malaria are among the few conditions for which it is clearly justifiable to call upon emergency laboratory services outside normal working hours.

Electron microscopy requires more elaborate preparation than does light microscopy and it is therefore much slower. It is, however, valuable in the relatively rapid diagnosis of certain viral infections, including viral diarrhoea. The non-specific nature of electron microscopy gives it the advantage over virus-specific techniques in that any type of viral agent, if present in sufficient numbers, may be recognized.

## Non-culture methods

There are many situations where isolation of microbes in vitro or in tissue culture is impossible or is insufficiently sensitive to make a microbiological diagnosis. Some microbes are so fastidious or slow-growing that useful information cannot be given to clinicians. The isolation of many viruses requires laborious tissue

culture methods that are too slow to influence patient management. Microscopy is usually of low sensitivity, e.g. the threshold of detection of acid-fast bacilli in sputum is about $10^5$ microbes per millilitre. Microscopy also has low specificity; for example, Gram staining of faeces would yield millions of Gram-negative rods, but it is not possible to recognize those that are pathogenic by this means.

To overcome these deficiencies probes have been developed which combine a part that reacts with a specific microbial structure and a part that will produce a signal (colour, fluorescence or radio-activity) after the reaction. Many microbes are detectable in this way. Antibodies labelled with fluorescent molecules are widely used in diagnostic virology, e.g. for respiratory secretions to find respiratory syncytial virus. Enzyme-linked antibodies are available as enzyme-linked immunosorbent assay (ELISA) kits for chlamydia detection, and many other *immunoprobes* are commercially produced or under investigation. The explosion in molecular biology has led to the widespread availability of DNA and RNA probes, which have changed from complicated research techniques requiring radio-isotopes to relatively simple methods that can be carried out with minimal expertise. Use of the *polymerase chain reaction* (see p. 68) has greatly increased the sensitivity of nucleic acid probes. Provided a unique sequence of nucleotides is used, the method is highly specific. Nonetheless, as the new technology becomes more commonplace traditional methods will not discarded. More likely it will complement them.

One of the chief advantages of probes – their specificity – is also one of their major disadvantages. For example, in the investigation of diarrhoea, it would be impossibly laborious to have to use a separate probe for each of the possible microbial causes. Furthermore, use of probes leaves little scope for detection of the unexpected and hampers the discovery of previously unsuspected aetiological agents of disease.

## Serology

In situations in which microbial isolation is impossible and probes are unavailable, evidence of infection may be obtained by finding a rise in antibody titre or the presence of specific IgM. Serology is still the most common method of diagnosing the causes of 'atypical' pneumonia (mycoplasmal pneumonia, psittacosis, Legionnaires' disease), syphilis, brucellosis and many viral infections, including HIV. It is preferable to take a blood sample early in the illness (the *acute serum*) and another 10–14 days after the onset (the *convalescent serum*); a four-fold or greater rise in antibody titre in the second specimen is diagnostic of acute infection.

## Isolation of micro-organisms

The basis of the study of medical microbiology was laid over a century ago by the isolation of microbes in pure culture outside the host animal. The methods used by the fathers of bacteriology have been adapted, simplified and, in some cases, automated for the modern diagnostic laboratory. The principles remain the same: use sterile equipment and media (with cell lines if necessary) and add clinical material. After incubation at 37°C, for a variable time, from a few hours for enterobacteria to weeks for mycobacteria and some viruses and fungi, a visible effect will be produced. This might be colonies growing on agar or a cytopathic effect (CPE) in tissue culture. The skill of microbiology is in identifying the microbes responsible for the effect.

There are limits to the methods that can be used in a routine hospital laboratory to isolate microbes. The choice of media used is dictated by the specimen and by the clinical condition of the patient. For example, in some areas of the world there is little point in looking for *Corynebacterium diphtheriae* in every throat swab, so that the specific media needed are not routinely used. It is therefore incumbent on the doctor to make sure that the laboratory is alerted to look for diphtheria bacilli in any suspicious case. Similarly, clinicians need to know which microbes are routinely sought from particular specimens so that they can make a special request if they suspect the unusual.

'New' causes of illness are often found and new methods of investigating old diseases regularly appear on the market. It is a difficult decision for the laboratory manager to assess at what point a 'new' pathogen becomes sufficiently important to be routinely sought, or to balance the advantages of new (and expensive) technology against cheap and well-tried techniques.

## Identification

The full identification of each microbe isolated in a clinical laboratory is uneconomic and unnecessary. Short-cuts must be made in order to satisfy the clinical demand of a final report which the doctor can understand and which is available in time to influence management of the patient. In practice, most laboratories use simple and incomplete methods of identification, depending on the level of useful information required. Typing of isolates is for epidemiological or other special reasons, and this is usually done in national reference centres.

Examples of the extent of identification are shown in Table 64.3. This shows that the same organism may not be identified even to the genus level, or it may have extensive genetic investigation depending on the reason for the request. In a cost-conscious climate you get what you pay for and what the service thinks you need!

## Antimicrobial sensitivity testing

One advantage of good bacterial identification is that it helps greatly in choosing antibiotics and in some situations in-vitro tests of susceptibility are unnecessary. However, the widespread occurrence of bacterial resistance, even in genera such as *Neisseria* and *Haemophilus* in which sensitivity to β-lactam antibiotics was previously assumed, has meant that tests are often performed on all significant clinical isolates of bacteria. The relevance of information generated in the extremely artificial conditions of the laboratory is discussed in Chapter 65.

As there are technical problems in carrying out sensitivity tests at the same time as the primary culture, the report will be delayed for at least 24 h

**Table 64.3** Examples of bacterial identification in medical laboratories

| Reason for request | Extent of identification | |
|---|---|---|
| | Example 1 | Example 2 |
| Test of sterility | Bacteria present | |
| Initial blood culture report | Gram-negative rod | Gram-positive cocci |
| Urine examination | 'Coliforms' | Staphylococci |
| Wound swab | *Escherichia coli* | *Staphylococcus aureus* |
| Outbreak epidemiology | *Esch. coli* O157 | *Staph. aureus* phage type 80/81 |
| Pathogenicity tests | *Esch. coli* O157 Vero toxin-producing | *Staph. aureus* enterotoxin A-positive |

after isolation of the pathogen. Tests of slow-growing bacteria such as mycobacteria take much longer and tests involving fungi, viruses and protozoa are not ordinarily available. In general, all patients with acute symptoms will receive treatment before the report returns to the doctor so that the result will merely confirm that correct treatment had been chosen. Sometimes, the laboratory report will allow speculative antimicrobial therapy to be modified, e.g. by allowing one or more drugs in a precautionary mixture to be discontinued.

A frequent difficulty facing microbiologists is which, out of a rapidly increasing number of agents, should be tested and, of those tested, which should be reported. Most laboratories test a few representative compounds from among the many penicillins, cephalosporins, aminoglycosides, tetracyclines, quinolones, etc., and restrict those reported to the clinician to two or three agents selected for their appropriateness in the particular infection. In this way, institutional antibiotic policies are reinforced and the impact of the promotional activities of pharmaceutical companies is lessened. If the primary agents are unsatisfactory for any reason, a telephone call to the laboratory will establish what other agents have been tested, or what further tests may be useful.

## REPORTS OF RESULTS

Just as it is important to obtain as accurate a result as possible, so it is vital to transfer the information rapidly to the user of the laboratory in a form that is easily intelligible. Laboratory workers need to tailor their reports to suit their customers and to recognize their needs. Trained microbiologists are used to the vagaries of microbial taxonomy and the profusion of antibiotics with similar names, but physicians and surgeons are easily confused by laboratory jargon and changes in nomenclature. On the other hand, clinicians rightly expect laboratory reports to be explicit and helpful. As in so many spheres of health care, a spirit of mutual respect and cooperation is in the best interests of the patient, and this is most likely to happen if microbiologists regularly visit the wards and if clinicians are encouraged to discuss problems with laboratory staff.

In these days of computers and facsimile machines it is attractive to use the latest technology to transfer results, but the personal touch is essential, particularly for important results such as positive blood or cerebrospinal fluid cultures. Clinicians dealing with

difficult problems enjoy the reassurance that the laboratory has found the cause of a patient's illness and advice on management is generally well received. Seeing the problem for oneself and discussing it with the responsible doctors is the ideal. The telephone is a satisfactory substitute in many cases and is far preferable to a report form printed by a computer and arriving after the crisis is over. It behoves us all to communicate better and faster.

## NOTIFICATION OF INFECTIOUS DISEASES

In addition to making a clinical diagnosis and treating the individual there is a need with some infectious diseases to determine the source and prevent further spread. In some countries there are public health laws specifying the method of reporting these. The list of *notifiable diseases* in England and Wales is shown in Table 64.4. This reporting system requires a clinical diagnosis, although laboratory confirmation may be sought separately. In England and Wales each health district has a consultant responsible for communicable disease control, who is usually the 'proper officer' for the local government authority. Notifications are sent by this officer to the Office of National Statistics (ONS) and the Communicable Disease Surveillance Centre (CDSC).

There is also an obligation, which in some circumstances may be statutory, for laboratories to report isolates of certain pathogens to central authorities for surveillance purposes. In an outbreak, or

| Table 64.4   List of notifiable diseases in England and Wales | |
|---|---|
| Acute encephalitis | Ophthalmia neonatorum |
| Acute poliomyelitis | Paratyphoid fever |
| Anthrax | Plague |
| Cholera | Rabies |
| Diphtheria | Relapsing fever |
| Dysentery (amoebic or bacillary) | Rubella |
| | Scarlet fever |
| Food poisoning | Smallpox |
| Leprosy | Tetanus |
| Leptospirosis | Tuberculosis |
| Malaria | Typhoid fever |
| Measles | Typhus |
| Meningitis | Viral haemorrhagic fever |
| Meningococcal septicaemia (without meningitis) | Viral hepatitis |
| | Whooping cough |
| Mumps | Yellow fever |

where the pathogen is highly infectious, it is essential for the head of the laboratory to inform both the clinician looking after the patient and local communicable disease control staff. In this way a coordinated approach can be made to prevent further spread of infection.

---

## RECOMMENDED READING

Baron E J, Finegold S M 1990 *Bailey and Scott's Diagnostic Microbiology*. C V Mosby, St Louis

Collee J G, Fraser A G, Marmion B P, Simmons A 1996 *Practical Medical Microbiology*, 14th edn. Churchill Livingstone, Edinburgh

Johnson F B 1990 Transport of viral specimens. *Clinical Microbiology Reviews* 3: 120–131

Murray P R, Baron E J, Pfaller M A, Tenover F C, Yolken R H 1995 *Manual of Clinical Microbiology*, 6th edn. American Society for Microbiology, Washington, DC

Tyrrell D A J, Phillips I, Goodwin C S, Blowers R 1979 *Microbial Disease: The Use of the Laboratory in Diagnosis, Therapy and Control*. Edward Arnold, London

# 65

# Strategy of antimicrobial chemotherapy

*R. C. B. Slack*

In the previous chapter the work of the laboratory in assisting doctors in making a definitive microbiological diagnosis was described and summarized in Figure 64.1. Ideally, management of an infection should involve these stages plus choice of an appropriate antimicrobial agent (if necessary) and follow-up tests of cure. Chapter 5 listed the different classes of antimicrobial agents from which the doctor may prescribe. The objectives of an antibiotic strategy are to implement clinical guidelines which cover the treatment of an individual patient and policies based on these which will have a maximum public health effect. These include cost-effectiveness and limiting the spread of antibiotic resistance.

or the presence of a foreign body. In the latter situation it is more important to send specimens to the laboratory and start empirical therapy to cover likely pathogens.

2. The organisms causing many common clinical syndromes have predictable antibiotic sensitivities allowing a rational choice to be made.

3. The results of laboratory tests may lead to modification or withdrawal of chemotherapy.

Although 'best guess' or empirical therapy is commenced before the results of laboratory tests are available, it is wrong to argue that this approach is incorrect since early administration of an antimicrobial is sometimes life-saving.

## CHOICE OF TREATMENT

Infections are so common in general practice that it is not practical for each patient to be fully investigated and a rational choice of antimicrobial agent made on the results. Because many have a viral aetiology and most respond rapidly to simple symptomatic relief, the choice is not which agent to use but whether to prescribe at all. Many patients who make the effort to see a doctor expect drug treatment. Although the time taken to educate the public and convince the individual is often longer than that needed to write a prescription, it is important that prescribers do not yield to pressure if antibiotics are not indicated. Figure 65.1 shows a flow diagram of choice of antibiotics which is applicable to many common conditions. There are three main points in the diagram:

1. Patients may be categorized on clinical grounds into those with mild, moderate or severe infection and also into those who were previously healthy or have underlying disease which may affect their response to therapy, for example impaired immunity

## LABORATORY MONITORING

### Susceptibility tests

As well as providing routine tests of sensitivity on individual isolates, the laboratory should provide a general picture of the prevalence of different pathogens occurring in the local population and their pattern of resistance. Different lists should be prepared and regularly circulated to general practitioners, hospital consultants and specialized units. The methods used and limitations of susceptibility testing are outlined in Chapter 5. Sometimes individual patients will need to be monitored for the efficacy of treatment and to determine if failure has occurred due to acquired resistance or replacement with a more resistant organism. This is especially important in the assessment of new agents in clinical trials.

### Antibiotic assay

Rapid methods are now available to determine the amount of antibiotic in serum and other body fluids during treatment. These assays can be used to monitor

*Choice based on predictable sensitivity or local resistance patterns.
Broken line indicates a course of action that will depend on circumstances

**Fig. 65.1**    General strategy of antimicrobial chemotherapy.

the adequacy of dosage or to avoid possible toxic effects of overdosage.

In practice, it is necessary to carry out such assays only in a small minority of patients in hospital: those who are seriously ill with infections such as endocarditis; those receiving potentially toxic agents, such as aminoglycosides and vancomycin; and those who may be compromised with regard to absorption or excretion of the drug.

The interpretation of the results of antibiotic assays may be difficult if the patient is receiving multiple antibiotics. In such cases, the power of the body fluid to inhibit or kill the infecting organism in vitro may be a more useful measurement of adequate dosage; for example, in bacterial endocarditis, the patient's serum should kill the causative organism at a dilution of 1 in 4 or more.

It is important to know the relationship of the sample being assayed to the time of dosage: maximum or *peak* levels are usually measured in serum 0.5–1 h following a dose; minimum or *trough* levels are from a sample taken shortly before the next dose.

Assays should always be carried out in close collaboration with the microbiologist to ensure the correct timing of samples and to avoid errors of interpretation.

## Assay of urine

Urine samples may be screened for antibacterial activity. This can be of value in determining patient compliance with treatment and also in interpreting the culture result in relation to possible inhibition by residual antibiotic.

## Clinical correlation of laboratory tests

The epithet *sensitive* or *resistant* is a clinical description; in laboratory tests it is usual to select a concentration of the agent which is known to be easily attained in serum, other body fluids or tissue after normal recommended dosage. Organisms susceptible to this, or lower concentrations, are regarded as sensitive; those failing to grow are resistant. The correlation between this interpretation and clinical results is generally good, but not perfect. Discrepancies may be due to a failure to attain adequate concentrations at the site of infection, resulting in clinical failure. However, there are many factors on which the outcome of the host–parasite relationship in infection depends, and it would be surprising if a complete correlation between in vitro tests and the results of chemotherapy was observed. The best correlation occurs with penicillin treatment of acute gonorrhoea in males where outcome is easy to assess and single-dose therapy is standard.

## PREDICTABLE SENSITIVITY

Once the identity of an infecting organism is known, the sensitivity pattern is often predictable with a fair degree of accuracy. Not surprisingly, however, the susceptibility of common pathogens may change with time. Thus, predictable sensitivity of micro-organisms, while useful, is a changing concept and will have local variations, so that the advice of local microbiologists should be sought.

### Organisms with predictable sensitivity patterns

*Streptococcus pyogenes* is a good example of an organism that has retained a sensitivity pattern that has changed little in 50 years. Thus, penicillin is always the drug of choice for the treatment of haemolytic streptococcal infections. Other β-lactam

antibiotics are also uniformly active against *Str. pyogenes*. Erythromycin is an alternative if the patient cannot be given penicillin because of allergy, but an increasing number of strains in some areas show some resistance to this antibiotic in vitro.

Until recently, most strains of *Str. pneumoniae* were highly sensitive to penicillin. An increasing number of penicillin-resistant pneumococci are now found in cases of invasive disease in some institutions, and are posing a major problem world-wide.

Reproducible patterns of sensitivity to antimicrobial drugs can be shown for many other groups of bacteria and offer a useful guide to the choice of chemotherapy (Table 65.1). However, exceptions to these patterns occur and resistant variants may become prevalent in some localities, particularly under the pressure of intensive antibiotic usage.

In the same way that organisms may exhibit predictable sensitivity to some agents, they may be predictably resistant. Some examples are shown in Table 65.2.

## ORGANISMS OF VARIABLE SENSITIVITY

Many groups of pathogenic bacteria, notably staphylococci and enterobacteria, vary unpredictably in their sensitivity to antimicrobial drugs. With these organisms there is a greater need to carry out sensitivity tests on individual isolates.

### Staphylococci

Staphylococci, including coagulase-negative strains, show great variability in susceptibility, and this can

**Table 65.1** Examples of organisms and antimicrobial agents for which susceptibility is *usually* predictable

| Organism | Antimicrobial agents normally active |
|---|---|
| Streptococci | Penicillin, erythromycin, vancomycin |
| Enterococci | Ampicillin, vancomycin |
| Anaerobic cocci | Penicillin, erythromycin, metronidazole |
| Staphylococci | Flucloxacillin, clindamycin, fusidic acid, gentamicin, vancomycin |
| *Haemophilus influenzae* | Co-amoxiclav, tetracycline, cefotaxime, erythromycin |
| *Escherichia coli* } *Proteus mirabilis* } | Gentamicin, cefotaxime, co-amoxiclav, ciprofloxacin |
| *Pseudomonas aeruginosa* | Gentamicin, ceftazidime, azlocillin, ciprofloxacin, imipenem |
| *Bacteroides fragilis* | Metronidazole, cefoxitin, co-amoxiclav |
| Rickettsiae } Chlamydiae } | Tetracyclines, macrolides, rifampicin |
| Mycoplasmas | Tetracyclines, erythromycin |
| *Candida albicans* | Nystatin, amphotericin B, miconazole |
| Herpes simplex virus | Acyclovir |

**Table 65.2** Examples of organisms and antimicrobial agents for which resistance is usually predictable

| Organism | Antimicrobial agents not normally active |
|---|---|
| Streptococci } Enterococci } | Aminoglycosides, nalidixic acid, aztreonam |
| Staphylococci | Most penicillins[a], nalidixic acid, aztreonam |
| *Escherichia coli* | Penicillin, vancomycin, erythromycin, metronidazole |
| *Klebsiella* spp. | Most penicillins, erythromycin, metronidazole |
| *Pseudomonas aeruginosa* | Most penicillins and cephalosporins, erythromycin, metronidazole |
| Anaerobes | Aminoglycosides, aztreonam, nalidixic acid, fluoroquinolones |

[a]Except methicillin and isoxazolylpenicillins.

severely limit choice of antibiotics. Four main kinds of staphylococci may be encountered:

1. *Penicillin-sensitive strains.* Before the widespread use of penicillin in the 1940s, most *Staphylococcus aureus* isolates were sensitive. Usually these strains are susceptible to other antistaphylococcal agents (macrolides, aminoglycosides and fusidic acid). Penicillin-sensitive strains now account for about 10% of isolates.

2. *β-lactamase-producing strains.* Staphylococcal penicillinase confers resistance to all penicillins except methicillin, the isoxazolyl group (cloxacillin etc.) and nafcillin. These strains usually retain susceptibility to cephalosporins. Most *Staph. aureus* and *Staph. epidermidis* strains found in clinical practice belong to this group.

3. *Methicillin-resistant strains (MRSA).* Methicillin, the first penicillinase-stable penicillin, is used as the test compound to identify these strains in the laboratory. Strains of *Staph. aureus* resistant to methicillin are also resistant to virtually all β-lactam agents. MRSA have epidemiological significance as a group and have been isolated from hospital outbreaks in different countries. Many of these epidemic strains are multi-resistant, exhibiting resistance to aminoglycosides, macrolides and other antistaphylococcal agents including the topical compound, mupirocin, which has been used to eradicate the organism from carriers of MRSA. Vancomycin or teicoplanin may be the only agents available for treatment.

4. *Other antibiotic-resistant strains.* Multiple resistance to antistaphylococcal antibiotics may be seen in strains which are methicillin-sensitive. They are found in similar situations to MRSA, namely hospital units with severely debilitated patients and problems with cross-infection. Such resistance patterns are more common in coagulase-negative staphylococci.

## Enterobacteria

*Escherichia coli* includes many strains of variable sensitivity, but among the general population in the UK most strains (about 60%) are sensitive to ampicillin and amoxycillin and an even higher proportion are sensitive to cephalosporins, co-amoxiclav (the combination of amoxycillin and clavulanic acid) and trimethoprim.

Variable sensitivity is also a feature of other enterobacteria. Multi-resistant typhoid is a particular problem in many countries where the disease is endemic. If there is doubt about the clinical response, or the sensitivity of the strain, laboratory tests should be carried out.

## Other organisms

Several pathogens which were formerly reliably sensitive to standard agents, including neisseriae, *Haemophilus influenzae*, pneumococci, enterococci, mycobacteria and *Plasmodium falciparum* are now commonly resistant to first-line therapy. In some cases, options for treatment of infection with these organisms have become severely constrained.

# ANTIBIOTIC POLICIES AND THE CONTROL OF RESISTANCE

The benefits of the use of antibiotics, not only in medicine but also in animal husbandry, must be taken into account in considering the merits of restrictive policies undertaken to control antibiotic resistance.

There is, without doubt, a problem of resistance among many commonly occurring micro-organisms. Indeed, difficulties are already being experienced with infections highly refractory to therapy with available agents. However, most of the problems of resistance occur among patients susceptible to colonization by resistant strains within closed communities such as hospitals. This is most marked in areas of intensive care, where large amounts of antibiotics are used in highly susceptible patients with low immunity to infection. In the general community, multiple resistance to antibiotics is presently not a major problem, but the spread of MRSA out of hospitals into nursing and residential homes may herald a change in this situation.

Accordingly, attention should be directed to those hospital units in which the problem of resistance is significant and which may be the most important source of spread to the general community. As resistance in bacteria has many of the features of an epidemic disease, the application of classic rules for the prevention of infection may prevent the spread of antibiotic-resistant organisms from such units.

## Restrictive policies

The use of antibiotics by general practitioners and clinicians is influenced by the prescribing habits of other medical colleagues and by the promotional efforts of the pharmaceutical companies. Thus, an ordered and systematic use of antimicrobial drugs might be of benefit in the general strategy of chemotherapy. Since the use of antibiotics acts as a powerful selective factor in the emergence and spread of resistant micro-organisms, restriction of use should have the opposite effect and reduce the proportion of resistant organisms in a community. The acceptance of this thesis has encouraged restrictive policies involving temporary bans on the use of certain antibiotics. Such policies may also lead to a reduced chance of prescription error and some cost benefits.

## Rotational policies

Periodic changes of antibiotics used in treatment might also help to avoid the emergence of resistant strains by altering the selective pressures and discouraging opportunistic pathogens such as *Pseudomonas* and *Acinetobacter* species. Such a rotational policy might help to retain the therapeutic value of antibiotics over a longer period. The availability of a large range of clinically useful antibacterial substances (Table 65.3) makes this kind of policy more practicable.

## PROPHYLACTIC USE OF ANTIBIOTICS

The unnecessary prophylactic use of antibiotics should be discouraged since this may result in increased selection of resistant variants or super-infection with resistant flora. However, there are several circumstances in which chemoprophylaxis is clearly beneficial.

A widely accepted use of antimicrobial agents for the prevention of infection is in patients who have suffered from rheumatic fever, or are thought otherwise to be at risk of rheumatic carditis to prevent further streptococcal infection. Among other indications for chemoprophylaxis are the use of peri-operative antibiotics in patients undergoing joint replacement to reduce the chance of potentially disastrous infection. Similarly, patients undergoing lower bowel resection receive peri-operative treatment with combinations of agents intended to suppress the lower bowel flora. The clinical and laboratory evidence for the

**Table 65.3** Main groups of antibiotics available for clinical use

| Antibacterial agent | Route of administration | | Antibacterial spectrum[a] | | Some indications for therapy |
|---|---|---|---|---|---|
| Phenoxymethylpenicillin | O | | + | | Streptococcal infections |
| Benzylpenicillin | | P | + | | Community-acquired pneumonias/meningitis |
| Ampicillin } Amoxycillin | O | P | + | − | Respiratory, hepatic, biliary infections |
| Flucloxacillin | O | P | + | | Staphylococcal infections |
| Co-amoxiclav | O | P | + | − | Infections due to β-lactamase-producing organisms |
| Imipenem | | P | + | − | Serious infections with mixed organisms |
| Cephalosporins | O | P | + | − | Respiratory and urinary infections; staphylococcal infections |
| Aminoglycosides | | P | | − | Gram-negative coliform infections; endocarditis (with penicillin) pseudomonas infections |
| Macrolides | O | P | + | | Streptococcal and staphylococcal infections and those due to legionellae, campylobacters, chlamydiae and coxiellae |
| Tetracyclines | O | P | + | − | Respiratory infections and those due to chlamydiae, mycoplasmas and rickettsiae |
| Chloramphenicol | O | P | + | − | Serious infections due to *Haemophilus influenzae*, salmonellae and rickettsiae |
| Fusidic acid | O | T | + | − | Staphylococcal infections |
| Glycopeptides | O | P | + | | Resistant staphylococcal infections; *Clostridium difficile* enteritis |
| Trimethoprim } Co-trimoxazole | O | P | + | − | Urinary and respiratory infections; salmonellosis |
| Imidazoles | O | P | + | − | Anaerobic infections |
| Sulphonamides | O | T | + | − | Intestinal and eye infections |
| Fluoroquinolones | O | P | | − | Urinary infections; pseudomonal infections; salmonellosis |

O, oral; P, parenteral; T, topical; +, mainly active against Gram-positive bacteria; −, mainly active against Gram-negative bacteria.
[a]See also Table 5.1, p. 45.

benefit of these kinds of prophylaxis is now well established.

Chemoprophylaxis is also justified in preventing pneumococcal infection in splenectomized patients and pneumocystis pneumonia in people with human immunodeficiency virus (HIV). In healthy individuals who are close contacts of infectious diseases such as meningococcal meningitis, short courses of antibiotics are justified to prevent acquisition of the organism or eradicate carrier status. Travellers to regions in which malaria is endemic should take antimalarial prophylaxis.

## HOST FACTORS INFLUENCING RESPONSE

In most individuals with normal immune systems an antimicrobial drug assists in a more rapid recovery from infection, but the choice of agent is often not critical providing it has some effect on the causative organisms. In very serious infections or when the patient is at a disadvantage because of impaired or absent immunity, the role of the antibiotic becomes more important and more care should be taken in its selection, dosage and administration.

### Problems of toxicity

The final choice of the most appropriate antimicrobial drug may be influenced by the history and responses of the patient. Known hypersensitivity to a drug such as penicillin means that neither this antibiotic nor other penicillins can be safely given and alternatives must be used. Side-effects such as nausea, vomiting, diarrhoea or pruritis may be severe enough to warrant a change in treatment. Some antibiotics have potentially serious side-effects, such as the ototoxicity of the aminoglycosides, and care must be taken to avoid these by laboratory monitoring of drug levels, since such toxicity is usually dose related. Intercurrent disease may require modification of the dosage of certain antibiotics because of specific organ deficiency, e.g. liver failure or impaired renal function. Ototoxicity of the aminoglycosides must always be borne in mind in patients who have poor renal function.

### Failure to reach the site of infection

The absorption of oral antibiotics varies widely from patient to patient and, if poor, may be a cause of treatment failure. Alternatively, infection may be localized within a large collection of pus or at an anatomical site that is penetrated by antibiotics with difficulty. Obstruction to the flow of body fluids may likewise militate against success; this is important in infections of the urinary tract, biliary system and the central nervous system. In some of these cases more radical interference may be indicated to relieve the obstruction.

### Alteration of normal flora

Antibiotic therapy may upset the patient's microflora and result not only in the selection of resistant strains of commensals, such as staphylococci on the skin, or *Esch. coli* in the intestinal tract, but also colonization with species not normally present. This can lead to antibiotic-induced infection, such as candidosis. Diarrhoea is frequently associated with antibiotic therapy, and reflects disturbance of the normal bowel flora. In a few patients the clinical condition can be severe and proceed to pseudo-membranous colitis associated with the toxins of *Clostridium difficile* (see Ch. 23).

### Intravenous administration

When antibiotics are given intravenously, they should normally be administered directly into the vein and not added to other infusion fluids; otherwise adequate blood levels of the drug may not be attained owing to excretion outpacing administration. There is also the possibility of incompatibility between the antibiotic and the contents of the fluid. In all cases, the manufacturer's instructions and recommendations about the administration of the drug should be closely followed.

## COMBINATIONS OF ANTIBIOTICS

The clinical benefits of the use of combinations of antibacterial agents tend to be exaggerated. The combination of two or more agents has been long accepted in the treatment of tuberculosis, so limiting the selection of mutants resistant to the individual components. The use of β-lactam antibiotics with an aminoglycoside in the treatment of streptococcal endocarditis is also accepted, since the mixture is more bactericidal than the individual components.

A combination of a β-lactam antibiotic with a β-lactamase inhibitor may prevent destruction of the antibiotic. Thus, the enzyme inhibitor clavulanic acid in combination with amoxycillin (co-amoxiclav) restores the activity of the antibiotic against many β-lactamase-producing bacteria.

Potentiation of the antibacterial effect by combinations is referred to as *synergy*; some combinations exhibit a lesser effect than the individual components, and this is called *antagonism*. These interactions are generally displayed in vitro, and it is difficult to establish evidence of advantages or disadvantages in the patient. Thus, the combination of trimethoprim and sulphamethoxazole (co-trimoxazole) can be shown to be synergistic in the test-tube, but it has been difficult to demonstrate any clinical benefit, and trimethoprim is now often used on its own to avoid the chance of toxic reactions to sulphonamides.

## ANTIVIRAL THERAPY

Relatively few agents have yet found a place in the prophylaxis or treatment of viral infections (see Table 5.6, p. 54).

Acyclovir is the most widely used agent at present, and is prescribed for the treatment of herpes simplex and herpes zoster. This drug can be given orally, but in severely ill patients it is administered intravenously, for example in treating herpes encephalitis. Acyclovir is also used in the prophylaxis and treatment of varicella, particularly in immunocompromised patients. The related compound ganciclovir is available for the treatment of cytomegalovirus infection, but is associated with considerable toxicity.

Amantadine is active against influenza A virus, but not against influenza B virus. This drug, and the related rimantadine, have been chiefly used for the prophylaxis of influenza.

Tribavirin (ribavirin) is useful in the treatment of respiratory syncytial virus infections in children and some haemorrhagic fever viruses, such as Lassa fever virus.

Zidovudine (azidothymidine) is an inhibitor of HIV and is used in the management of patients with acquired immune deficiency syndrome (AIDS). There are a number of new anti-retroviral agents (see Ch. 5 and 9).

## ANTIFUNGAL THERAPY

Superficial fungal infections are very common. Systematic fungal disease is relatively rare in the UK, except in patients who are immunosuppressed or otherwise compromised. There are few effective antifungal agents that can be used systemically (see Table 5.5, p. 54) and some have considerable toxicity.

For many years the chemotherapy of superficial fungal infections depended on preparations of benzoic, salicylic or undecanoic acid. More effective is griseofulvin, given orally, sometimes over long periods, for the treatment of dermatophytoses; the new allylamine, terbinafine, seems to be at least as effective in these conditions. Nystatin and other polyenes are used for the topical treatment of superficial candidosis (thrush). Imidazoles such as clotrimazole are also used in the treatment of vaginal yeast infections.

Amphotericin B is used parenterally for the treatment of systemic candidosis, cryptococccal infections and aspergillosis. Flucytosine is also active against yeasts and has been used in combination with amphotericin B. Amphotericin B is toxic and treatment has to be carefully monitored to obtain the most satisfactory clinical results. New formulations of the drug appear to be safer.

Ketoconazole, and triazoles such as itraconazole and fluconazole, also have a fairly wide range of antifungal activity, and are being used more widely in the treatment of systemic fungal disease because of their relative lack of toxicity, although resistance may be a problem.

## CHEMOTHERAPY OF SYSTEMIC INFECTIONS

### Serious generalized infection

Patients with serious and often overwhelming generalized infection include those with *bacterial shock syndrome* and others with the symptomatology of acute infection without localizing signs. These syndromes may be related to post-operative infection, to instrumentation, or to the aggravation of a previously mild infection (e.g. extension of a middle ear infection to the brain). Generalized infection may also follow a reduction in the natural resistance of the patient. Such a situation may arise in renal failure, immune deficiency states, in blood dyscrasias and in neoplastic disease. Specific measures used in the treatment of these diseases may further reduce resistance to infection and the clinical features characteristic of infection may be muted or absent.

Appropriate specimens should be submitted to the laboratory before treatment is begun, in an effort to isolate the causative organisms. However, these patients may require immediate treatment and often there will be little indication of the nature of the infecting organism; more than one species may be involved, especially when the source of the infection is within the abdomen. Empirical chemotherapy must therefore cover Gram-positive cocci, Gram-negative bacilli and anaerobes such as bacteroides. A combination of amoxycillin, an aminoglycoside and metronidazole is suitable. Co-amoxiclav improves the spectrum of amoxycillin and allows omission of the metronidazole. Alternatively, an expanded-spectrum cephalosporin such as cefotaxime can be used. Therapy may be subsequently changed according to the results of laboratory tests. If the patient fails to respond after treatment for 3 days, the use of alternative agents should be considered.

In some patients in intensive care, and in the immunocompromised, the possibility of systematic fungal infection or activation of dormant viruses, such as cytomegalovirus, must be considered.

It must always be remembered that bacterial toxins are unaffected by antibacterial therapy. Supportive treatment will include correction of fluid and electrolyte imbalance and appropriate treatment of any coexisting organ failure. In future, immunotherapy such as the use of anti-endotoxin preparations may find a place in treatment.

## Infective endocarditis

Whenever possible, treatment of endocarditis should be related to the results of sensitivity tests made on the organism isolated from the blood. Formerly, viridans streptococci were the most common isolates and penicillin was the drug of choice. Viridans streptococci are now isolated from only about one-third of patients and the organisms from the remainder are usually relatively resistant to penicillin. In a proportion of cases believed to be infective on clinical evidence, no organism can be isolated and treatment must be empirical.

It seems to be important to kill all the organisms growing in heart valve tissue since the normal body defences find it difficult to penetrate this site to assist the antibiotic. Bactericidal therapy with a penicillin in combination with an aminoglycoside is usually indicated. It is sometimes helpful to carry out bactericidal tests against the causative organism and it may also be useful to monitor the progress of the patient by assays of the bactericidal activity of the serum against the causative organism.

After operations for the replacement of heart valves it may be difficult to isolate an organism and there may be doubt as to whether or not infection has become superimposed. The risk of withholding treatment, however, is so great that empirical

treatment may be indicated, and as staphylococcal infection may occur in such circumstances, it is best to include an antistaphylococcal antibiotic.

For the prevention of bacterial endocarditis in patients at risk following dental extraction, 3 g of amoxycillin, given orally 1 h before surgery, is recommended.

Rare causes of infective endocarditis in which blood cultures are negative include infections with *Coxiella burnetii* or certain chlamydiae. The diagnosis of these conditions depends largely upon serological evidence as it is difficult to isolate the organisms. An aetiological diagnosis is important, as treatment with an appropriate antibiotic, usually tetracycline, may be life-saving.

## Urinary tract infections

### Uncomplicated cystitis

Uncomplicated urinary infections and asymptomatic bacteriuria are common in adolescent and adult women seen in general practice and maternity clinics. Most infections are due to *Esch. coli*, and most are sensitive to a wide range of drugs. In most cases eradication of the organism is achieved after a short course of therapy with an oral agent such as trimethoprim. The remainder will often respond to a second course of treatment, but if the bacteriuria still persists, fuller urological investigation is required since failure of treatment is more usually related to an abnormality of the urinary system than to resistance of the organism.

Recurrence of bacteria within weeks of a short course of treatment is quite common, and patients should have their urine bacteriologically examined 3–7 days after the cessation of any antibacterial treatment and again after 1 month.

### Infections following catheterization

Infection of the urinary tract sometimes occurs after instrumentation such as catheterization or cystoscopy; it is almost unavoidable if indwelling catheters are used. Often the strains causing these infections are derived from the hospital environment, and include resistant strains of Gram-negative bacilli, sometimes in mixed culture. Frequently, the patient is not greatly inconvenienced by such infection, and chemotherapy is not indicated in most areas. If therapy is required, elimination of the organisms can be difficult, particularly if there is residual pathology or a degree of urinary obstruction. Sensitivity tests must be carried out to assist in the choice of therapy. The most useful agents are cephalosporins, trimethoprim and ciprofloxacin; for more serious or refractory cases, in which there is the hazard of systemic spread of the infection, parenteral treatment with an aminoglycoside or an expanded-spectrum cephalosporin must be considered.

### Recurrent infection

In chronic pyelonephritis and recurrent bacteriuria it may be important to control infection by continuous treatment with antibiotics such as trimethoprim. Unfortunately, some patients may become reinfected with resistant species so that alternative drugs must be used. Thus, long-term therapy may require periodic bacteriological reassessment and sensitivity tests on the flora isolated to indicate when changes in therapy are required.

### Prostatitis

Prostatitis is common in men over a wide age range and it is often difficult to obtain categorical evidence of bacterial infection; examination of seminal fluid, prostatic secretions and urine specimens may help. Treatment with trimethoprim, ciprofloxacin or erythromycin is sometimes beneficial as these drugs penetrate well into the prostate, but short-term use is rarely curative. Prophylaxis during prostatectomy is now well established; cephalosporins such as cephradine or cefotaxine have been used for this purpose.

## Respiratory infections

Respiratory tract infections are extremely common, and, although many are primary virus infections, those that are more severe and prolonged usually indicate secondary bacterial invasion. Laboratory diagnosis of these conditions is important since effective treatment depends on use of an antibiotic specifically active against the causative organisms.

### Upper respiratory tract infections

A number of bacteria may be associated with sore throat, pharyngitis and sinusitis, including *Str. pyogenes*, *Str. pneumoniae*, *H. influenzae* and Vincent's organisms. The most important infections from the point of view of the development of sequelae are those due to *Str. pyogenes*, for which the treatment of choice is penicillin given for at least 7 days to ensure eradication of the organism. All the other important bacterial pathogens will also respond to this treatment, with the exception of *H. influenzae*, for which treatment with amoxycillin, tetracycline, co-trimoxazole or erythromycin is appropriate.

If for some reason a penicillin cannot be prescribed, the antibiotic of choice is erythromycin or co-trimoxazole. Ampicillin and amoxycillin should be avoided if there is any likelihood of glandular fever because these antibiotics tend to cause a rash and prolong the disease. Tetracyclines should be avoided in young children because of the risk of discoloration of developing teeth.

### Lower respiratory tract infections

Lobar pneumonia is most frequently caused by pneumococci and penicillin is the drug of choice; erythromycin or cefotaxime are good alternatives. Infections due to klebsiellae or other organisms will require treatment with antibiotics according to the results of sensitivity tests; cefotaxime or cefuroxime are usually effective if laboratory confirmation is not available. Other coliform bacilli are rarely involved in pulmonary infections although they often colonize the upper respiratory tract; they seldom require specific treatment.

Among atypical pneumonias, mycoplasma infections respond best to a tetracycline or erythromycin; and legionella infections to erythromycin, alone or combined with rifampicin.

Bronchopneumonia is most frequently associated with pneumococci or haemophilus, so that amoxycillin, tetracycline or trimethoprim should be effective. More rarely, bronchopneumonia is caused by *Staph. aureus* and flucloxacillin, fusidic acid or clindamycin is urgently required for treatment.

Acute exacerbations of chronic bronchitis are almost invariably associated with either *Str. pneumoniae* or *H. influenzae*. Amoxycillin, tetracycline or trimethoprim is usually effective.

In bronchiectasis, lung abscess or cystic fibrosis, antimicrobial treatment should be prescribed according to laboratory culture and sensitivity test results. Combinations of antibiotics may be effective in some of these patients. In pulmonary tuberculosis, combination treatment, usually with rifampicin, isoniazid and pyrazinamide, is mandatory.

## Meningitis

A Gram film and cell count of cerebrospinal fluid (CSF) will usually differentiate viral from bacterial meningitis. If bacteria cannot be seen, initial treatment is with cefotaxime or ceftriaxone. This choice ensures adequate treatment of infections with Gram-negative bacilli (most common in neonates) and of infections with *Neisseria meningitidis*, *H. influenzae* and *Str. pneumoniae*, which are the most common causes of meningitis in young children. Care must be taken to differentiate *Listeria monocytogenes* infection, as this organism is less sensitive to penicillin and cefotaxime; a combination of amoxycillin and gentamicin is usually used.

When the causative organism is isolated, therapy may be altered to penicillin for meningococcal or pneumococcal infections. *Pseudomonas aeruginosa* meningitis may occasionally occur as a nosocomial infection and should be treated with full doses of gentamicin plus a β-lactam agent such as azlocillin. It is rarely necessary to give intrathecal antibiotics.

Where there is increased CSF pressure, as in spina bifida, shunts are inserted to facilitate the circulation of fluid. These often become contaminated, usually with staphylococci, probably derived from the skin. Antistaphylococcal antibiotics are used to control the growth of the infecting organism in anticipation of replacement of the prosthesis.

## Intestinal infections

Mild bacillary dysentery, salmonella food poisoning and other forms of bacterial diarrhoea do not ordinarily require chemotherapy. Indeed, such therapy may make intestinal carriage more likely and increase the risk of the selection of antibiotic-resistant strains. The most important treatment is correction of fluid balance.

Patients with invasive infection (e.g. typhoid and paratyphoid fever) and those with severe bacillary dysentery or cholera may warrant treatment (see appropriate chapters).

Many intestinal infections are due to viruses, for which there is presently no specific chemotherapy. Cryptosporidiosis is now being diagnosed more frequently, but is usually self-limiting except in the immunocompromised. Infection with other protozoa, such as *Giardia lamblia* or *Entamoeba histolytica*, requires treatment with metronidazole.

Spread of infection from the bowel may give rise to serious infections and associated toxaemia. If subphrenic, retrocolic or pelvic abscesses form, drainage is the most important aspect of treatment, but antibiotics can assist recovery of the patient. Cephalosporins or an aminoglyoside plus ampicillin are useful in empirical treatment, and metronidazole should be added if bacteroides is likely to be present. Acute peritonitis after non-specific inflammation of the bowel, such as appendicitis, is usually effectively treated with amoxycillin (with or without clavulanate) or cefotaxime combined with metronidazole.

## Liver infections

Bacterial infections of the liver and portal pyaemia are best treated with large doses of cefuroxime, cefotaxime, or an antibiotic chosen on the basis of laboratory findings (e.g. ampicillin against enterococci). Liver abscesses occur most frequently by spread via the portal tract of intestinal Gram-negative bacilli, or to retrograde spread in the biliary passages of streptococci (especially *Str. milleri*) and anaerobes from the gall bladder. Ampicillin is selectively concentrated in the bile, and is often useful in treatment of cholecystitis. Amoebic abscess requires prompt and specific treatment with metronidazole, and its possibility should always be kept in mind, particularly in a patient who has been abroad.

Infection caused by the hepatitis viruses B and C is treated by α-interferon with variable success.

## Bone and joint infections

Most infections of bones and joints are due to *Staph. aureus*. Large doses of flucloxacillin should be given in combination with either fusidic acid or clindamycin.

Penicillin in prolonged high dosage is the drug of choice for streptococcal arthritis. Where other organisms, such as *H. influenzae*, neisseriae or Gram-negative rods are involved, specifically directed therapy is required.

## Genital tract infections

Venereal infections such as syphilis and gonorrhoea are traditionally treated with penicillin, but a proportion of isolates of gonococci are now resistant to this agent, in which case ceftriaxone, co-amoxiclav or ciprofloxacin should be used.

Non-specific infections of the genital tract are common in women; aerobic and anaerobic bacteria, *Candida* species or *Trichomonas vaginalis*, may be involved. Frequently, an abnormal flora is isolated in the absence of an inflammatory exudate, and it may be difficult to decide on the necessity for chemotherapy. Bacterial vaginosis is such a clinical syndrome associated with *Mobiluncus* spp. which responds to metronidazole or amoxycillin. Vaginal candidiasis is usually treated topically with nystatin or an antifungal imidazole. In trichomoniasis, metronidazole is indicated.

More serious pelvic infection in women is often associated with chlamydiae, and tetracycline or erythromycin is the drug of choice. Anaerobic bacteria may be involved, and metronidazole or co-amoxiclav may be prescribed.

## Surgical wound infections

Most surgical infections are caused by the patient's own organisms, but some arise exogenously, often by cross-infection. In orthopaedic units, most exogenous infections are due to staphylococci, but in gastro-intestinal units, Gram-negative bacilli and anaerobes are more common. The situation may change from time to time as a result of ecological movements in the microbial flora within the unit, associated with selective pressures of antibiotic use.

Specimens from infected lesions should always be sent to the laboratory, since the identity of the isolate may have epidemiological significance as well as being of importance in the management of the patient. The microbiologist should always be informed of any therapy as this may affect the interpretation of bacteriological tests.

## Superficial infections

Skin and soft-tissue infections are common in general practice. Most are of bacterial origin, although some have a fungal or viral aetiology.

Common lesions such as boils, carbuncles, impetigo and infected wounds are associated with *Staph. aureus* and *Str. pyogenes*. Systemic treatment with appropriate antibiotics may be indicated in some patients, but topical treatment is often effective. The use of antibiotics commonly prescribed for systemic infections should be avoided in favour of topical antiseptics or topical antibiotics such as mupirocin.

RECOMMENDED READING

Christie A B 1987 *Infectious Diseases*, 4th edn. Churchill Livingstone, Edinburgh
Greenwood D (ed) 1995 *Antimicrobial Chemotherapy*, 3rd edn. Oxford University Press, Oxford
Kucers A, Bennett N Mck 1987 *The Use of Antibiotics*, 4th edn. Heinemann, London

Lambert H P, O'Grady F, Finch R G, Greenwood D (eds) 1997 *Antibiotic and Chemotherapy*, 7th edn. Churchill Livingstone, Edinburgh
Mandell G L, Douglas R G, Dolin R (eds) 1995 *Principles and Practice of Infectious Disease*, 4th edn. Churchill Livingstone, New York

# 66

# Epidemiology and control of community infections

*D. Reid*

When you can measure what you are speaking about and express it in numbers, you know something about it; when you cannot express it in numbers, your knowledge is of a meagre and unsatisfactory kind.

William Thomson, Lord Kelvin
(*Popular Lectures and Addresses*, 1891)

Good surveillance does not necessarily mean the making of right decisions but it reduces the chances of wrong ones.

Alexander Langmuir, 1963

Once is happenstance, twice is coincidence, the third time it's enemy action.

Ian Fleming
(*Goldfinger*, Jonathan Cape, 1959)

Attempts to observe and record diseases in order to devise means of determining their cause and control have a long history. Hippocrates (460–361 BC) 'the father of medical science' and Herodotus (484–425 BC) 'the father of history' both related environmental factors to health. Hippocrates when writing of the occurrence of diseases distinguished between the 'steady state', the 'endemic state' and the abrupt change in incidence, the 'epidemic'.

Probably the first public health measures based on case reports of infectious diseases taken by a European government occurred in 1348 when the Republic of Venice excluded ships with affected people on board in order to control outbreaks of pneumonic plague (the *black death*). Fifty years later, again in Venice, the concept of *quarantine* was introduced when ships from plague-stricken areas had to stay outside the harbours for 40 days (*quaranta giorni*).

Also because of the fear of a plague epidemic, the first of the *Bills of Mortality*, in which causes of death were recorded, was published in London in 1532. In 1662 John Graunt (1620–74) in his book *Natural and Political Observations Made Upon the Bills of Mortality* was the first to count the number of persons dying in London from specific illnesses and to advocate the value of obtaining numerical data on a population in order to study the causes of disease (Table 66.1). In 1837 the office of the Registrar General was established to develop the work started

**Table 66.1** Selection of causes of death in London taken from the Bills of Mortality, 1632

| Causes of death | Numbers |
|---|---|
| Chrisomes[a] and infancy | 2268 |
| Consumption[b] | 1797 |
| Fever | 1108 |
| Aged | 628 |
| Smallpox | 531 |
| Teeth | 470 |
| Abortive and stillborn | 445 |
| Bloody flux[c], scouring[d] and flux | 348 |
| Dropsy[e] and swelling | 267 |
| Convulsions | 241 |
| Childbed | 171 |
| Measles | 80 |
| Ague[f] | 43 |
| King's evil[g] | 38 |

[a]A child who died during the 1st month of life or a child who died unbaptized. [b]Usually pulmonary tuberculosis.
[c]Dysentery.
[d]Diarrhoea.
[e]Oedema.
[f]Malaria.
[g]Tuberculosis of the skin.

by John Graunt; the English physician William Farr (1807–83) added reports to those of the Registrar General which dealt with infectious diseases, occupational diseases, accidents or hazardous work conditions.

The importance of keen observation of disease in order to deduce the likely cause has been demonstrated on many occasions. In 1849, 34 years before the identification of *Vibrio cholerae* by Robert Koch (1843–1910), John Snow (1813–58), a London physician, proved by epidemiological observation that cholera is mainly spread by drinking infected water and not through the air in the form of miasmas as was commonly thought at the time. Similarly, William Budd (1811–80), a general practitioner from Devon, showed in 1873 how typhoid was caused,

635

even though it was not until 1885 that *Salmonella typhi* was first isolated in the laboratory. More recently, William Pickles (1885–1969), a general practitioner in Wensleydale, Yorkshire, was able to elucidate many of the epidemiological characteristics of hepatitis and other infections well before microbiological advances were to confirm his observations.

From these beginnings the surveillance of infection has assumed national and international proportions. In the UK, information on microbial disease is collated in England and Wales by the Communicable Disease Surveillance Centre (CDSC) at the Central Public Health Laboratory, London, and in Scotland by the Scottish Centre for Infection and Environmental Health (SCIEH) at Ruchill Hospital, Glasgow. The Royal College of General Practitioners also undertakes regular recording of disease voluntarily reported by various practices. Elsewhere, national surveillance is carried out in different countries (e.g. at the Centers for Disease Control (CDC) in Atlanta, USA). On a world-wide basis the World Health Organization (WHO) provides important liaison and support. This international co-operation is vital as 'germs do not recognize boundaries'.

The most outstanding achievement of international surveillance was the development of a programme for smallpox eradication. The multidisciplinary approach adopted by the WHO, in which programmes were community based with measurable goals and constant monitoring, resulted in the last endemic case being recorded in October 1977; smallpox was officially declared eradicated in December 1979.

## EPIDEMIOLOGY: DEFINITIONS AND PRINCIPLES

Epidemiology is usually defined as *the study of the nature, distribution, causation, mode of transfer, prevention and control of disease.* It has also been regarded as 'the natural history of disease' or as 'the human face of ecology'. Closely linked with the study of epidemiology is the concept of surveillance, which is the most effective infection control technique available. Surveillance is defined as: *the epidemiological study of a disease as a dynamic process involving the ecology of the infectious agent, the host, the reservoirs, the vectors as well as the complex mechanisms concerned in the spread of infection and the extent to which this spread will occur.* The three main elements of surveillance of infection are:

1. The systematic collection of pertinent data

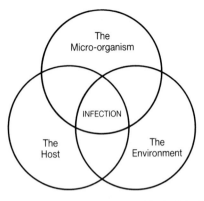

**Fig. 66.1**  The three main factors involved in the infectious process.

2. The orderly consolidation and evaluation of the data
3. The prompt dissemination of the findings, especially to those who can take appropriate action.

Surveillance provides for the recognition of acute problems requiring immediate local, national or international action, and for the assessment of specific problems by revealing trends or facilitating forecasts. It also provides a rational basis for planning and implementing efficient control measures and for their evaluation and continuing assessment. Although particularly appropriate to the study of infectious diseases, epidemiological principles are also used to elucidate the causes of non-communicable diseases.

The infectious process is a dynamic state involving three main factors: the micro-organism, the host and the environment (Fig. 66.1).

## The micro-organism

Since few micro-organisms are harmful to humans the concept of *virulence* (i.e. the degree of pathogenicity of an infectious agent indicated by fatality rates and/or its ability to invade and damage the tissues of the host) must be recognized. The degree of virulence depends on *invasiveness* (i.e. the capacity of the organism to spread widely through the body) and *toxigenicity* (i.e. the toxin-producing property of the organism) (see Ch. 8). A second variable is the *dosage* of the organism, and this is closely related to the virulence. A small number of organisms of high virulence is usually sufficient to cause disease in a susceptible person, whereas if the organism is of low virulence it often fails to cause disease. A third variable is the *portal of entry*. Many organisms have a predilection for a particular tissue or organ. For example, the causal organism of typhoid fever, *Salmonella* Typhi, usually causes typhoid only when it enters the human body through the mouth in food or water.

## The host

The reaction of the host to a micro-organism will depend on the ability to resist infection. The individual may not possess sufficient resistance against a particular pathogenic agent to prevent contraction of infection when exposed to the organism. Alternatively, the individual may possess specific protective antibodies or cellular immunity as a result of previous infection or immunization. However, immunity is relative and may be overwhelmed by an excessive dose of the infectious agent or if the person is infected via an unusual portal of entry; it may also be impaired by immunosuppressive drug therapy, concurrent disease, or the ageing process.

### Herd immunity

Herd immunity is an important element in the balance between the host population and the micro-organism and represents the degree to which the community is susceptible or not to an infectious disease as a result of members of the population having acquired active immunity from either previous infection or prophylactic immunization (see Ch. 68). Herd immunity can be measured:

1. *Indirectly* from the age distribution and incidence pattern of the disease if the disease is clinically distinct and reasonably common. This is an insensitive and inadequate method for those infections which manifest themselves subclinically.

2. *Directly* from assessments of immunity in defined population groups by antibody surveys (sero-epidemiology) or skin tests; these may show 'immunity gaps' and provide an early warning of susceptibility in the population. Although it may be difficult to interpret the data in absolute terms of immunity and susceptibility, the observations can be standardized and reveal trends and differences between various defined population groups in place and time.

The decision whether to introduce herd immunity artificially by immunization against a particular disease will depend on several epidemiological principles:

1. The disease must carry a substantial risk
2. The risk of contracting the disease must be considerable
3. The vaccine must be effective
4. The vaccine must be safe.

The effectiveness and safety of immunization programmes are monitored by observing the expected and actual effects of such programmes on disease transmission patterns in the community by appropriate epidemiological techniques.

## The environment

The environment plays a major role in the causation, spread and control of infection. In the UK, the virtual disappearance of relapsing fever, plague and cholera, the rarity of indigenous typhoid fever and the relative infrequency of tuberculosis and bacillary dysentery are all indications of the improvements which have taken place in environmental conditions. The decrease in overcrowding and infestation together with the demand for cleaner water supplies and better sanitation have been of paramount importance in producing these dramatic advances. This is well illustrated in the case of tuberculosis, which was declining before the availability of chemotherapy and mass BCG vaccination in countries where socio-economic conditions were improving (Fig. 66.2). Paradoxically, better living conditions may unexpectedly create new problems; for example, poliovirus infection, previously experienced mainly in early childhood, is usually postponed in more favoured communities to older ages when paralysis is a more likely complication unless there is an adequate immunization programme.

## THE SPREAD OF INFECTION

Infection spreads in well-defined epidemiological patterns. A knowledge of these will lead to an understanding of the best methods of control, or even eradication, and enables an estimate to be made of the likelihood of this happening.

## Infection spread directly from one person to another

Among this group can be included such highly infectious diseases as measles. Infection is passed directly from a person with the disease to a susceptible contact. Diseases in this category are usually clinically apparent and healthy carriers are not a feature. When it is possible to diminish the number of susceptibles in the target population then eradication becomes feasible, as has happened with smallpox.

**Fig. 66.2**    Notifications of tuberculosis in England, Wales and Scotland, 1915–95.

## Infection in which healthy carriers are involved

Because apparently healthy individuals may harbour the bacilli responsible for such diseases as typhoid, paratyphoid and diphtheria, often for long periods after having acquired the infection, it is possible for such infections to be transmitted to others and the source remains undetected.

## Infection in which persons harbour the organism before the onset of clinical illness

Organisms such as *Streptococcus pneumoniae* may not cause the person any harm until an event such as a skull fracture allows for the transfer of the bacterium from the middle ear to the cerebrospinal space where it can cause a potentially lethal meningitis.

## Infection derived from animal sources

Diseases derived from animals, such as leptospirosis, Q fever, anthrax, rabies and brucellosis are known as *zoonoses*. These diseases are spread by direct contact with the animal concerned or indirectly by such means as the ingestion of infected milk, contact with infected bone products, etc.

## Infections derived from environmental sources

The spread of legionellae from cooling towers and air conditioning units to cause Legionnaires' disease is an example of illness derived from an infected environment. By dealing appropriately with the infected source the population is protected.

## OUTBREAKS OF INFECTION

The crowding together of humans (or for that matter animals, fish or birds) provides the necessary conditions to allow micro-organisms to multiply and spread. When humans led nomadic lives there was less opportunity for outbreaks to occur; the main opportunities came when large numbers gathered for a pilgrimage or had other reasons for a meeting. These clusterings facilitated the spread of infection, resulting in outbreaks; the subsequent dispersal of the group enabled the causative organism to be carried elsewhere.

The threat of outbreaks in overcrowded and difficult conditions is particularly well illustrated in military history; on many occasions the germ has been as important in determining the outcome of a campaign as the sword or gun. The typhoid bacillus caused severe effects during both the American Civil War (1861–65) and the Boer War (1899–1902). The use of typhoid vaccine in the latter years of the First World War meant that the main impact of typhoid in this war subsided after 1916. Similarly, typhus was rife in the Civil War in Britain (1642–49), when both the Parliamentary and the Royalist armies were affected. The pandemic of influenza in 1918–19, in which about 700 million people were affected with approximately 22 million deaths, was a scourge of military camps and affected many servicemen returning home from the First World War.

# Nomenclature of outbreaks

The term *outbreak* is often confused with other epidemiological terms used to enumerate infection:

1. *Sporadic case*: a person whose illness is not apparently connected with similar illnesses in another person.

2. *Outbreak*: the occurrence of cases of a disease associated in time or location among a group of persons. A *household outbreak* involves two or more persons resident in the same private household and not apparently connected with any other case or outbreak. A *general outbreak* involves two or more persons who are not confined to one private household.

3. *Epidemic*: the large-scale temporary increase in the occurrence of a disease in a community or region which is clearly in excess of normal expectancy.

4. *Pandemic*: the occurrence of a disease which is clearly in excess of normal expectancy and is spread over a whole geographical area, usually crossing national boundaries.

# Types of outbreak

There are three main patterns of outbreak which may be revealed by the construction of graphs of occurrence of cases over time:

1. *The explosive outbreak*. This is characterized by the occurrence of a large proportion of cases in a relatively short period of time (Fig. 66.3); there is a sharp rise and fall in the number of infected persons, since the usual cause of such an event is a common source which infects the people concerned. This type of outbreak is also frequently termed *a common source outbreak* or a *point source outbreak*. This pattern of infection is often discovered when water or food becomes contaminated, although other vehicles of infection can also be responsible for this type of outbreak.

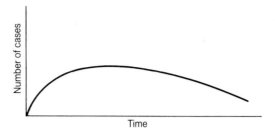

**Fig. 66.4** Epidemic curve apparent when there is person-to-person spread of infection.

**Fig. 66.5** Epidemic curve apparent when there is person-to-person spread subsequent to a common source outbreak.

2. *Person-to-person spread*. Outbreaks caused by infections which are spread from person to person have a more protracted course taking longer than explosive outbreaks to build up and to subside.

An infective agent may be passed from person to person by a variety of routes. Diseases such as dysentery, hepatitis type A and gastro-enteritis which are usually spread by the faecal–oral route often follow this pattern of spread (Fig. 66.4).

3. *Explosive outbreaks with subsequent person-to-person spread*. This pattern is often apparent when there is contamination of a common water or food source and the initial cases subsequently infect their contacts. Thus, the pattern of the outbreak is a combination of that seen with an explosive outbreak, but followed by a slower decline (Fig. 66.5).

# Analysis of outbreaks

The investigation of an outbreak should be approached in a logical and methodical way. The cause may be elucidated by determining details of the *persons* involved, the *place* where they had been and the *time* when they became ill.

The fundamental pieces of information which should be sought whenever an outbreak occurs are as follows:

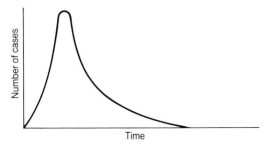

**Fig. 66.3** Epidemic curve apparent when there is an explosive (common or point source) outbreak.

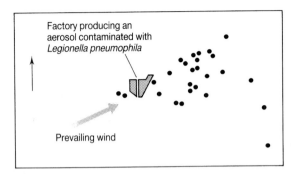

**Fig. 66.6** Occurrence of Legionnaires' disease in persons living downwind from a factory with an evaporative condenser contaminated with *Legionella pneumophila*.

1. *WHO gets infected?* What is their age? For example, if a possible food-borne outbreak mainly affects children, could the source be milk or ice-cream?

2. *WHERE were those who became infected?* Where have they recently been? For example, in a hospital outbreak were they all in the same surgical ward? Could a member of the operating staff be a carrier of a pathogen? In a community outbreak of Legionnaires' disease were those affected living downwind from a contaminated source of infection? (See Fig. 66.6.)

3. *WHEN did the infection occur?* By knowing the incubation period of the infection it may be possible to trace back to an event which was attended by all those affected.

4. *WHAT was the common factor?* For example, in a food poisoning episode, the ingestion of an article of food by most of those affected but not by those unaffected may be a vital piece of evidence.

5. *HOW did those involved become infected?* For example, abscess formation among recently immunized persons might be due to contaminated vaccine.

6. *WHY did the infection occur?* For example, the reheating of meat is often the cause of a *Clostridium perfringens* food poisoning outbreak.

## Investigation of outbreaks

In the investigation of outbreaks it is important to have a standardized approach to the various steps involved. Such an approach might have the following as a basis:

1. *Verify the diagnosis.* It is always prudent to confirm that the clinical history is compatible with the diagnosis. Occasional 'pseudo-epidemics' can occur, sometimes resulting from contamination of specimens.

2. *Establish the existence of an outbreak.* The increased interest of an investigator or a change in the mechanism of reporting can sometimes result in an increase in the number of reports of illness. It is important to check the previous level of investigation of a clinical entity or alteration in laboratory methods.

3. *Establish the extent of an outbreak.* Often the number of cases notified is only a proportion of the total number of those affected. It is necessary to seek out the additional cases or vital information may be lost.

4. *Identify common characteristics or experiences of the affected persons.* An individual history from each confirmed or suspected case is required in order to detect any common factor among those affected (e.g. eating the same item of food).

5. *Investigate the source and vehicle of infection.* In addition to ascertaining the general characteristics of the material suspected as being the source or vehicle of infection, appropriate laboratory investigation will often have to be done. Good co-operation with the laboratory staff is vitally important.

6. *Analyse the findings.* The data should be analysed by the various epidemiological criteria, especially persons, time and place. Denominators should be obtained in order to calculate attack rates.

7. *Construct a hypothesis.* On the basis of the evidence a hypothesis should be constructed concerning the origin of the outbreak. This may be confirmed by laboratory findings but action to control the outbreak may be needed in advance of such findings.

## Control of outbreaks

The investigation of an outbreak should be carried out as swiftly as possible so that adequate control measures can be started without delay. Knowledge of the *source of infection*, the *route of transmission* and the *persons at risk* should allow appropriate action to be taken in order to achieve success.

### Sources of infection

These may be:

1. Human cases or carriers
2. Animal cases or carriers
3. The environment.

If the initial cases have readily identifiable clinical features (e.g. measles) then control is often easier as it is much more likely that the index case will be located. On the other hand, it is more difficult to control diseases in which apparently healthy carriers are responsible, as it is necessary to search for an infected person who may be asymptomatic.

It may be important to isolate the case or carrier, and possibly to institute appropriate treatment, until the patient is no longer infectious. The degree of isolation will depend on the type of disease as not all infections require strict isolation. For example, a patient with a highly infectious disease may require very strict isolation whereas the salmonella excreter will usually need only to cease food handling activities and observe a high standard of personal hygiene until free from infection. In contrast to 'isolation' the term 'quarantine' applies to restrictions on the healthy contacts of an infectious disease.

If an animal reservoir is responsible, action has to be directed at ensuring that the source of infection is eradicated, withdrawn from consumption, or rendered harmless (e.g. by the pasteurization of milk or the adequate cooking of meat).

When the environment is the source of an outbreak the control measures required will depend on the nature of infection and the mode of spread. In recent years, water-borne spread of Legionnaires' disease (e.g. from shower heads, air-conditioning systems, or droplet spread from cooling towers) has become increasingly recognized (Fig. 66.7). Environmental measures, such as the use of biocides, can destroy the causative legionellae at their source and so prevent further cases.

The hospital setting is particularly dangerous since the presence of compromised patients can result in tragic consequences. Moreover, the increasing use of invasive techniques and the appearance of antibiotic-resistant strains of micro-organisms further compound the problem. In a survey of hospital patients in England and Wales 9% of all patients acquired infection while in hospital. The early detection of infection by effective surveillance, the emphasis on the cleanest possible environment and awareness among the staff of potential problems are among the measures that need to be stressed in order to control infection among hospital patients (see Ch. 67).

## Route of transmission

Infection may be spread by:

1. Direct or indirect contact
2. Air-borne transmission
3. Percutaneous transmission
4. Food- and water-borne transmission
5. Insect-borne transmission
6. Transplacental transmission.

There are various ways in which the routes of transmission occurring during an outbreak may be blocked by measures appropriate to the route involved: effective handwashing; disinfection or disposal, if necessary, of the patient's belongings; and strict adherence to high standards of personal hygiene by the *contacts* of a case are important measures. When the disease is air-borne, overcrowding should be avoided and, where appropriate, dormitory or ward beds should be well spaced out. The acquired immune deficiency syndrome (AIDS) is a good example of a disease which can be spread *percutaneously* via contaminated needles as well as by other routes. *Food* and *water* should be as free as possible from infection as these are major causes of outbreaks. To deal with *insect-borne transmission*, eradication policies and repellents should be considered. The *transplacental* route is important in the spread of diseases such as hepatitis B.

## Persons at risk

Where indicated and feasible, susceptible persons at risk should be protected as soon as possible. Among the measures available, the following may need to be considered:

1. Immunization
2. Chemoprophylaxis for close contacts.

Immunity against several infectious diseases can be obtained either by active or passive immunization (see Ch. 68). Examples of rapid effective protection of communities by active immunization are the 'ring vaccination' policy used to protect close contacts of

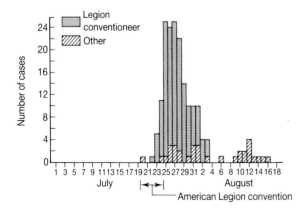

**Fig. 66.7** Legionnaires' disease among those associated with a convention in a hotel in Philadelphia (July to August 1976): an example of an explosive outbreak.

poliomyelitis and so stop more widespread dissemination of poliovirus, and the early (within 72 h of exposure) administration of measles vaccine to close contacts in an institution. Passive immunization, usually by means of human normal immunoglobulin or human specific immunoglobulin, gives rapid protection to contacts of hepatitis A and some other infections, although protection is short lived. Chemoprophylaxis is effective in the protection of close contacts of meningococcal infections and diphtheria.

## MATHEMATICAL MODELS

Mathematical modelling techniques attempt to define by use of relatively simple estimates and assumptions, the conditions governing transmission of communicable agents. Details of the multiplication and growth rates of micro-organisms and the spread of infection under natural or experimental conditions need to be known. Measurable factors include: the number of infective persons or sources of introduction of infection; the proportion of susceptible persons in a community at risk; the duration of immunity; the introduction of new susceptibles; the removal rate of infective persons (by isolation, immunity or death); and the response to vaccines and chemotherapeutic agents. Mathematical models can be used to predict institutional outbreaks and epidemics. This approach has been used to forecast the number of cases of AIDS that are likely to occur, the effect of control measures such as immunization or the number of cases over time.

## ASSOCIATION AND CAUSATION OF INFECTION

A problem commonly encountered by microbiologists and epidemiologists is the attribution of an infectious disease to a particular micro-organism. How do we determine if the relationship is one of causation or merely a chance association? Koch addressed this when he formulated his 'postulates' in 1891. These state that:

1. The organism must always be found in the given disease
2. The organism must be isolated in pure culture
3. The organism must reproduce the given disease after inoculation of a pure culture into a susceptible animal

4. The organism must be recoverable from the animal so inoculated.

For many organisms pathogenic to man it is not possible to fulfil all of Koch's postulates; moreover, they are not applicable to the study of the transmission of infection within a population. For this purpose it is more appropriate to consider the following factors, suggested by the medical statistician Bradford Hill, in order to establish whether a disease is caused by a particular infectious agent:

1. *Strength.* What is the strength of the association? During the cholera epidemic in London in 1854 John Snow compared the death rates among persons drinking the sewage-polluted drinking water of the Southwark and Vauxhall Company and those receiving the purer water of the Lambeth Company; he discovered that the rate in the former was 14 times higher (Table 66.2). This strength of association allowed Snow to consider that polluted water was a cause of cholera, although at that time the causative organism itself had not been identified.

2. *Consistency.* Similar observations, made by different people at different times in different places, add confidence to a conclusion that causation is likely.

3. *Specificity.* If the association is limited to a specific group of persons, with a specific type of illness, who have all been subjected to the same specific infection, then a cause and effect relationship can be more strongly suspected.

4. *Temporality.* This can be of especial importance when persons in particular occupations become infected (e.g. leptospirosis in fishworkers). The history of working in a particular environment *before* infection rather than vice versa is particularly relevant.

5. *Biological gradient.* If a dose–response curve is apparent then the evidence for causation is much stronger.

6. *Plausibility.* Is the possibility biologically plausible? The likelihood of veterinary surgeons becoming

**Table 66.2** Deaths in London during the cholera epidemic of 1854 according to source of water supply

| Water source | Number of houses supplied | Deaths |
|---|---|---|
| Southwark and Vauxhall Company (polluted) | 10 000 | 71 |
| Lambeth Company (non-polluted) | 10 000 | 5 |

ill with a zoonotic infection from affected cattle which they have recently been treating seems biologically plausible.

7. *Coherence.* If all the evidence is coherent (e.g. if the same micro-organism is isolated from the index case, the vehicle of transmission and from the victims) this is strong support for causation.

8. *Experiment.* Is the frequency of infection reduced if certain preventative measures are taken? The beneficial effects of the pasteurization of milk to diminish the number of cases of milk-borne salmonellosis is presumptive evidence of a zoonotic relationship.

9. *Analogy.* Has there been similar evidence in the past? The known capacity of the rubella virus to cause congenital abnormalities in the infants of infected mothers makes it easier to accept the possibility of other viruses causing similar problems if maternal infection occurs.

## CONCLUSION

Because of the multifactorial causation of infection it is usually necessary to study the epidemiology of infection in a *multidisciplinary* manner. The microbiologist, the clinician, the epidemiologist, the infection control nurse, the veterinarian, the environmental health officer, and other appropriate personnel, must all be involved; the extent of the involvement will depend on the nature of the infection. Success will depend on the expertise and co-operation of these members of the team.

## RECOMMENDED READING

Anderson R M, May R M 1991 *Infectious Diseases of Humans: Dynamics and Control.* Oxford University Press, Oxford

Benenson A S (ed) 1995 *Control of Communicable Diseases in Man*, 16th edn. American Public Health Association, Washington, DC

Campbell D M, Paixao M T, Reid D 1988 Influenza and the 'spotter' general practitioner. *Journal of the Royal College of General Practitioners* 38: 418–421

Eylenbosch W J, Noah N D 1988 *Surveillance in Health and Disease.* Oxford University Press, Oxford

Giesecke J 1994 *Modern Infectious Disease Epidemiology.* Edward Arnold, London

Grist N R, Ho Yen D O, Walker E, Williams G R 1993 *Diseases of Infection*, 2nd edn. Oxford University Press, Oxford

Last J M (ed) 1983 *A Dictionary of Epidemiology.* Oxford University Press, Oxford

Mims C A 1982 *The Pathogenesis of Infectious Disease*, 2nd edn. Academic Press, London

Noah N D, Reid D 1979 Sources of data on infectious diseases in England, Wales and Scotland. *Journal of Infection* 1: 259–298

Reid D, Grist N R, Pinkerton I W 1986 *Infections in Current Medical Practice.* Butterworth, London

Pickles W N 1939 *Epidemiology in Country Practice.* Wright, Bristol (re-issued 1972 by the Devonshire Press, Torquay)

Tyrrell D A J 1982 *The Abolition of Infection. Hope or Illusion? Rock Carling Fellowship Lecture.* Nuffield Provincial Hospitals Trust, London

Velimirovic B, Greco D, Grist N R, Mollaret H, Piergentili P, Zampieri A 1984 *Infectious Disease in Europe. A Fresh Look.* World Health Organization Regional Office for Europe, Copenhagen

# 67

# Hospital infection

*R. A. Simpson*

Historically, hospitals have a notorious reputation for infection. The hazards of puerperal sepsis and the horrors of septic infection in the pre-Listerian era have been well documented; admission to hospital in the mid-19th century was associated with the fear of gangrene and death.

Since that time, surgical and medical techniques have developed dramatically, basic standards of building and hygiene have greatly improved, and the identification and treatment of most infecting micro-organisms have become possible. Despite such changes, infection acquired in hospitals remains a major cause of morbidity and mortality, leading directly or indirectly to an enormous increase in the cost of hospital care and to the emergence of new health hazards for the community. Advances in biomedical technology and therapeutics are producing greater numbers of highly susceptible patients requiring treatment in hospitals, and this is aggravated by the occurrence of transferable resistance to antibiotics in pathogenic bacteria and the emergence of new pathogens transmitted by a variety of routes.

## CLASSIFICATION

In determining the extent of hospital infection, the following categories should be considered:

1. Infections contracted and developing outside hospitals which require admission of the patient (e.g. pneumonia).
2. Infections contracted outside hospital which become clinically apparent when the patient is in hospital (e.g. measles).
3. Infections contracted and developing within hospital (e.g. postoperative wound infection).
4. Infections contracted in hospital but not becoming clinically apparent until after the patient has been discharged (e.g. breast abscess).

5. Infections contracted by hospital staff as a consequence of their work, whether or not this involves direct contact with patients (e.g. hepatitis B).

On average, 5–10% of all hospital patients will develop an infection as a result of their stay in hospital. Urinary, respiratory and wound infections are the most common.

## FACTORS THAT INFLUENCE INFECTION

Hospital infection, also known as *nosocomial infection*, may be exogenous or endogenous in origin. The exogenous source may be another person in the hospital (*cross-infection*) or a contaminated item of equipment or building service (*environmental infection*). A high proportion of clinically apparent hospital infections are endogenous (*self-infection*), the infecting organism being derived from the patient's own skin, gastro-intestinal or upper respiratory flora.

Most infections acquired in hospital are caused by micro-organisms that are commonly present in the general population, in whom they cause disease less often and usually in a milder form than in hospital patients. Thus, contact with micro-organisms is seldom the sole or main event predisposing to infection. Various risk factors, alone or in combination, influence the frequency and nature of hospital infection.

### Susceptibility to infection

Natural resistance to infection is lower in infants and the elderly, who often constitute the majority of hospital patients. Pre-existing disease, such as diabetes, or other conditions for which the patient was admitted to hospital and the medical or surgical treatment, including immunosuppressive drugs, radiotherapy or splenectomy, may also reduce the patient's natural resistance to disease. Moreover, the natural defence mechanisms of the body surfaces may be bypassed either by injury or by procedures such as surgery, insertion of an indwelling catheter, tracheostomy, or ventilatory support.

## CONTACT WITH OTHER PATIENTS AND STAFF

In common with any larger institution or workplace, the patients and staff of a hospital share many facilities in close or crowded conditions. Outbreaks of diarrhoeal and food-borne disease may be traced to a common source via the hospital water or food supplies. The specific role of hospitals in admitting infected patients or carriers for treatment or isolation clearly serves as a potential source of infection for others. Patients with comparable susceptibility to infection tend to be concentrated in the same area, e.g. in neonatal units, burns units or urological wards, where infected and non-infected patients may be cared for by the same staff, thus creating numerous opportunities for the spread of micro-organisms by direct contact.

### Inanimate reservoirs of infection

Equipment and materials in use in hospitals often become contaminated with micro-organisms which may subsequently be transferred to susceptible body sites on patients. Gram-positive cocci, derived from the body flora of the hospital population, are found in the air, dust and on surfaces where they may survive along with fungal and bacterial spores of environmental origin. Gram-negative aerobic bacilli are common in moist situations and in fluids, where they often survive for long periods, and may even multiply in the presence of minimal nutrients. Awareness of the common reservoirs of environmental and contaminating hospital micro-organisms provides the basis for maintaining standards of hygiene (cleaning, disinfection, sterilization) throughout the hospital.

### Role of antibiotic treatment

At least 30% of hospital patients receive antibiotics, and this exerts strong selective pressures on the microbial flora. Sensitive species or strains of micro-organisms which normally maintain a protective function on the skin and other mucosal surfaces, tend to be eliminated, whereas those that are more resistant survive and become endemic in the hospital population. This may restrict the range of agents available for treatment and may lead to the transmission of plasmid-mediated antibiotic resistance into strains that show increased virulence, survival and spread within the hospital.

## MICRO-ORGANISMS CAUSING HOSPITAL INFECTION

The most important micro-organisms responsible for hospital infection are listed in Table 67.1.

The explosive outbreaks of *Staphylococcus aureus* infection that were often seen in surgical wards and maternity units up to the mid-1970s demonstrate the infectious potential of strains exhibiting particular virulence and colonizing capabilities. When combined with resistance to antibiotics, as subsequently occurred in epidemic or pandemic strains characterized by resistance to methicillin (MRSA), the challenge for outbreak control is even more daunting. In contrast, other strains of MRSA persisting in some UK hospitals appear better able to colonize patients or staff than to produce systemic disease. This illustrates the adaptation and evolutionary changes possible within common hospital bacteria revealed by careful epidemiological typing and observation. The changing patterns may be related to particular events and infection control measures, so that lessons can be learnt for future control and prevention.

**Table 67.1** Commonly occurring micro-organisms in hospital infection

| | |
|---|---|
| Urinary tract infections | *Escherichia coli*<br>*Klebsiella, Serratia, Proteus* spp.<br>*Pseudomonas aeruginosa*<br>*Enterococcus* spp.<br>*Candida albicans* |
| Respiratory infections | *Haemophilus influenzae*<br>*Streptococcus pneumoniae*<br>*Staphylococcus aureus*<br>Enterobacteriaceae<br>Respiratory viruses |
| Wounds and skin sepsis | *Staph. aureus*<br>*Esch. coli*<br>*Proteus* spp.<br>Anaerobes<br>*Enterococcus* spp.<br>Coagulase-negative staphylococci |
| Gastro-intestinal infections | *Salmonella* spp.<br>*Shigella sonnei*<br>Viruses |

With the advent of more elaborate surgery and intensive care, combined with the use of broad-spectrum antibiotics and immunosuppressive drugs, the Gram-negative bacteria have risen in importance. Many Gram-negative bacilli such as *Pseudomonas aeruginosa* are *opportunists* capable of causing infection in compromised patients. Such organisms may be found in the patient's own flora, or in damp environmental sites, including patient equipment and medicaments. They may exhibit natural resistance to many antibiotics and antiseptics and the ability to colonize traumatized skin such as burns and bedsores.

In recent years, groups of micro-organisms which formerly played no recognized part in hospital infection have emerged. These include the coagulase-negative staphylococci present in normal skin flora. Viral or fungal infection, particularly of the immunocompromised patient, has become more important. *Legionella pneumophila*, disseminated from environmental sources such as cooling towers, causes sporadic cases or outbreaks of respiratory infection in the hospital community. Awareness of the risks of blood-borne viruses, including hepatitis B, human immunodeficiency virus (HIV) and cytomegalovirus has increased in patients and in staff.

## ROUTES OF TRANSMISSION

The hospital offers many opportunities for the ex-change of microbes, many of which are harmless and a normal part of the balance between man and his environment. For there to be a significant risk of infection, several factors, including the right susceptible host and the appropriate inoculum of infecting micro-organism, must be linked via an appropriate route of transmission. Understanding of the sources and transmission routes of hospital infection enables efforts to be concentrated in more effective preventive measures.

Common routes of transmission for different micro-organisms are shown in Table 67.2.

## Air-borne transmission

Infections may be spread by air-borne transmission from the respiratory tract (talking, coughing, sneezing), from the skin by natural shedding of skin scales, during wound dressing or bed making and by aerosols from equipment such as respiratory apparatus and air-conditioning plants. Infectious agents may be dispersed as small particles or droplets over long distances (Fig. 67.1). Staphylococci survive well on mucosal secretions, skin scales and dried pus and may be redistributed in the air after initial settlement during periods of increased activity (Fig. 67.2). Gram-negative bacilli do not generally survive desiccation in air, and this route of transmission is therefore limited to conditions of high humidity such as ventilatory equipment.

**Table 67.2** Hospital infection: sources and spread

| Route | Source | Examples of disease |
|---|---|---|
| **1. Aerial (from persons)** | | |
| Droplets | Mouth | Measles, tuberculosis, pneumonia |
| | Nose | Staphylococcal sepsis |
| Skin scales | Skin exudate, infected lesion | Staphylococcal and streptococcal sepsis |
| **2. Aerial (from inanimate sources)** | | |
| Particles | Respiratory equipment | Gram-negative respiratory infection |
| | Air-conditioning plant | Legionnaires' disease, fungal infections |
| **3. Contact (from persons)** | | |
| Direct spread | Respiratory secretions | Staphylococcal and streptococcal sepsis |
| Indirect via equipment | Faeces, urine, skin and wound exudate | Enterobacterial diarrhoea, *Pseudomonas aeruginosa* sepsis |
| **4. Contact (environmental source)** | | |
| | Equipment, food, medicaments, fluids | Enterobacterial sepsis (*Klebsiella/Serratia/Enterobacter* spp.) *Ps. aeruginosa* and other pseudomonads |
| **5. Inoculation** | Sharp injury, blood products | Hepatitis B, HIV |

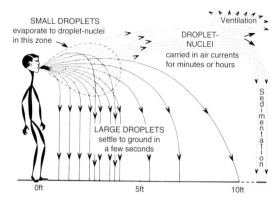

**Fig. 67.1** Spread of respiratory infections by droplets and droplet nuclei.

**Fig. 67.2** Infection of the air with dust particles derived from nasal and oral secretions contaminating hands, handkerchief, clothing and surrounding surfaces: **A**, hand soiled with secretions from lips or nose-picking; **B**, clothing contaminated by hand; **C**, soiled handkerchief; **D**, infected dust from handkerchief; **E**, dust from clothing (e.g. from near handkerchief pocket); **F**, infected dust raised after settling on floor.

## Contact spread

The most common routes of transmission for hospital infection are by *direct* contact spread from person to person or by *indirect* contact spread via contaminated hands or equipment. Faeces, urine or pus as well as contaminated dust particles or fluids may be carried on thermometers, bed-pans, bed-linen, cutlery or other shared items. Hands and, to a lesser extent,

clothing of hospital staff serve as vectors of Gram-negative and Gram-positive infection around a busy theatre or ward. Procedures involving contact with mucosal surfaces, e.g. insertion of a urinary catheter, may introduce micro-organisms from the contaminated hands of the operator or from the patient's own urethral flora into the normally sterile bladder. Similarly, intravenous fluids and topical medicaments have direct contact with vulnerable sites for infection.

Food-borne infection may originate in the hospital kitchen, or in special diets, infant feeds, kitchen or commercial supplies. Deteriorating hygiene standards may support the proliferation of flies, cockroaches and other insects or rodents which damage stored products and act as carriers of microbes. Of special note is the accidental transmission of predominantly blood-borne infections such as hepatitis B by needlestick or contaminated 'sharp' injury.

## Self-infection and cross-infection

The interaction between different sources of infection may be illustrated by the example of a patient undergoing lower bowel surgery. *Self-infection* may occur due to transfer into the wound of staphylococci (or occasionally streptococci) carried in the patient's nose and distributed over the skin, or of coliform bacilli and anaerobes released from the bowel during surgery. Alternatively, *cross-infection* may result from staphylococci or coliform bacilli derived from other patients or healthy staff carriers: the organisms may be transferred into the wound *during operation* through the surgeon's punctured gloves or moistened gown, on imperfectly sterilized surgical instruments and materials, or by air-borne theatre dust; or *post-operatively* in the ward from contaminated bed-linen, by air-borne ward dust or in consequence of a faulty wound dressing technique.

Of all the possible routes, by far the most likely in this example is self-infection from the patient's own bowel flora and it is therefore against this route that most specific preventive measures in colorectal surgery are directed. Understanding of possible sources of infection and the methods available to block transmission to susceptible sites forms the basis of hospital infection control.

The site and extent of infection and the time it was first recognized after the date of operation often help to establish whether cross-infection occurred during operation or postoperatively in the ward: clustering of cases according to a common surgical team or location in the ward may suggest a common source and may be the first firm indication of an outbreak of hospital infection.

Cross-infection from other patients or from staff carriers is especially dangerous because the causal organisms are often strains that have been selected in the hospital population for high infectivity and resistance to antibiotics. They are, however, potentially preventable by the practice of basic hygienic precautions.

Soon after admission to hospital, individuals commonly become contaminated with the 'hospital flora'. This has been shown with *Staph. aureus* in studies of patients before and during hospital treatment. Patients who need to stay longer in hospital, e.g. those requiring intensive care or the elderly, are less able to withstand infection and the risks of hospital infection are greater.

## PREVENTION AND CONTROL

### The infection control policy

The establishment of an effective infection control organization is the responsibility of good management of any hospital. There will normally be two parts:

1. An *infection control committee*, meeting regularly to formulate and update policy for the whole hospital on matters having implications for infection control and to manage outbreaks of nosocomial infection.

2. A team of workers, headed by the *infection control doctor* (usually the microbiologist), to take day-to-day responsibility for this policy.

The functions of the *infection control team* include surveillance and control of infection and monitoring of hygiene practices, advising the infection control committee on matters of policy relating to the prevention of infection and the education of all staff in the microbiologically safe performance of procedures. The *infection control nurse* is a key member of this team. Close working links between the microbiology laboratory, infection control nurse and the different clinical specialties and support services (including sterile services, laundry, pharmacy and engineering) are important to establish and maintain the infection control policy, and to ensure that it is rationally based and that the recommended procedures are practicable. Some of the control measures in which the infection control team should be involved are shown in Figure 67.3.

### Sterilization

The provision of sterile instruments, dressings and fluids is of fundamental importance in hospital

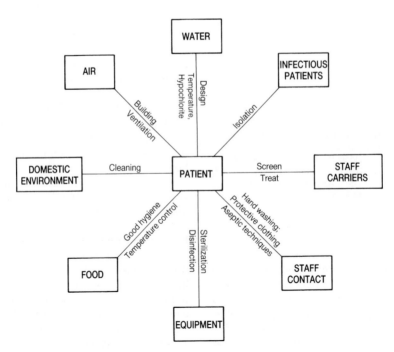

**Fig. 67.3** Control measures to reduce exogenous hospital-acquired infection.

practice. By the end of the 19th century, heat processing of instruments, dressings, surgical gloves, face-masks and theatre clothing began to supersede the phenol antiseptic soaks of the Lister era. Sterilization in autoclaves and hot-air ovens became accepted hospital practice. The development of automatic, high-vacuum sterilizers for processing wrapped goods facilitated the provision of a centralized service of sterile supply to wards, complementing the existing theatre service. The availability of a wide range of prepacked single-use items (syringes, needles, catheters and drainage bags) sterilized commercially by γ irradiation or ethylene oxide has further improved aseptic procedures and removed the need for reprocessing items that are difficult to clean and therefore impossible to sterilize.

Most fluids for topical use or intravenous administration are now prepared commercially or in regional units where standards of quality control and efficiency for bulk processes are more readily achieved than in individual hospital pharmacies.

## Aseptic techniques

The provision of sterile equipment will not prevent the spread of infection if there is carelessness in its use. Wherever possible, *no-touch* techniques must be used, coupled with strict personal hygiene on the part of the operator. These routines are rigidly laid down in operating theatre practice and may be modified as required for other procedures such as wound dressing and insertion of intravenous catheters.

## Cleaning and disinfection

The general hospital environment can be kept in good order by attention to basic cleaning, waste disposal and laundry. The use of chemical disinfectants for walls, floors and furniture is necessary only in special instances, such as spillages of body fluids from patients with blood-borne virus infections. Ward equipment such as bed-pan washer/disinfectors and dishwashers should be monitored to ensure reliable performance, and cleaning materials such as mop-heads and cloths should be heat disinfected and stored dry after use. Precleaning of contaminated instruments and equipment, preferably by means of an automatic washing process with an ultrasonicator, is an essential step before disinfection or sterilization.

## Skin disinfection and antiseptics

The ease of acquisition and transfer of transient hospital contaminants, particularly Gram-negative bacilli on the hands of staff, is an important factor in the spread of hospital infection. Thorough hand-washing after any procedure involving nursing care or close contact with the patient is essential. Gloves may be worn for many dirty contact procedures, such as emptying a urinary drainage bag or bed-pan, although it should not be forgotten that the gloved hand may also become colonized by transient hospital flora.

Procedures for pre-operative disinfection of the patient's skin and for surgical scrubs are mandatory within the operating theatre. The use of antiseptics for irrigation of the wound site at operation or for other mucosal surfaces such as the bladder after urological surgery in catheterized patients or the peritoneum during dialysis may also be beneficial. Dilute 'in-use' solutions of antiseptics may readily become colonized with Gram-negative bacteria and should be replaced regularly. Ideally, *single-use* preparations should be used. Restriction should be placed on the indiscriminate use of antiseptics and disinfectants by means of a *disinfectant policy* agreed by pharmacists, microbiologists and key users, such as theatre staff.

## Prophylactic antibiotics

Widespread and haphazard use of antibiotics hastens the emergence of antibiotic-resistant bacteria and increases both the incidence of toxic side-effects and the cost of treatment. However, rational antibiotic prophylaxis plays an important role in infection control. Specific indications include peri-operative prophylaxis in gastro-intestinal and gynaecological surgery directed predominantly against anaerobic infection and for patients known to have bacteriuria at the time of urological surgery or instrumentation, directed against the urine isolate. An *antibiotic policy* which limits the choice of broad-spectrum agents is important both for prophylaxis and treatment (see Ch. 65).

## Protective clothing

Different activities within the hospital require different degrees of protection to staff and patients. In operating theatres the wearing of sterile gowns, gloves, headgear and face-masks minimizes the shedding of micro-organisms. The properties of fabrics available for theatre use have improved, and now include close-weave ventile fabrics that are comfortable to wear and allow evaporation of moisture. 'Total protection' of the operating site may be considered for certain high-risk clean surgery such as hip replacements, during which the surgical team may wear exhaust-ventilated suits and operate under conditions of ultraclean laminar airflow.

For many ward procedures in which there may be soiling, or for simple *barrier nursing* of patients with communicable diseases, plastic aprons and gloves are used. Gloves, face-masks and goggles are also indicated for specific procedures when blood contact is likely through splashes or aerosols, such as dental procedures.

## Isolation

The isolation policy should list facilities and procedures needed to prevent the spread of specific infections to other patients (*source isolation*) and to protect susceptible or immunocompromised patients (*protective isolation*). Effective isolation demands a highly disciplined approach by all staff to ensure that none of the barriers to transmission (air-borne, direct and indirect contact) are breached. Multi-bedded rooms may be used, and even wards converted during hospital outbreaks, but the simplest solution wherever possible is to use single rooms.

'Cubicle' isolation, by which the patient is nursed alone in a room separated by a door and corridor from other patients, confers a substantial measure of protection. Preferably, each isolation room has its own toilet and washing facility. Clean, filtered air is supplied to the room, which should be at negative pressure (*exhaust ventilated*) to the corridor for source isolation or at positive pressure (*pressure ventilated*) to the corridor for protective isolation. If, however, there is a small airlock vestibule separating the room from the outer corridor, then exhaust ventilation of the airlock will give effective isolation for either situation. The vestibule or lobby should contain a washbasin and include space for gowning and equipment.

In some critical situations such as bone marrow transplant units, where air-borne contamination with environmental fungal spores is a problem, the efficiency of air filtration may be increased and laminar airflow maintained as a barrier around the patient. Stringent isolation, such as a plastic tent or 'Trexler' isolator, is required only for patients with highly contagious infections, such as those due to Lassa, Marburg and Ebola viruses, who are nursed in a *high-security isolation unit*.

## Hospital building and design

The routine maintenance of the hospital building is important, ensuring that surfaces wherever possible are smooth, impervious and easy to clean. Major rebuilding works on or near the hospital site may generate dust containing fungal and bacterial spores with implications for specialized units serving immunocompromised patients. Close communications with the works department and hospital administration are necessary to co-ordinate any protective action. When a new hospital or modification of existing building is planned, the infection control team should be closely involved in discussing the plans. In many countries, guidance on new building design exists to minimize potential hospital-acquired infection. Areas requiring special attention include operating theatres, kitchens, acute wards, laboratories and air-conditioning systems. The risk of Legionnaires' disease is reduced by installing water supplies that circulate below 20°C for the cold and above 60°C for the hot circuit.

## Equipment

Any object or item of equipment for clinical use should be assessed to determine the appropriate method, frequency and site of decontamination. Wherever possible, heat processes are preferred, although this may be precluded for certain thermolabile items such as fibre-optic endoscopes (see Ch. 7).

## Personnel

An occupational health service in hospitals should screen staff pre-employment and offer appropriate immunization. Hepatitis B vaccine should be given to those at special risk, such as those working in renal dialysis units and dental practice. All staff (including medical students) should receive general health protection. The notification and screening of staff with specific infections such as diarrhoeal disease or following needlestick injury should be understood within the infection control policy.

## Monitoring

Routine microbiological monitoring of the environment is of little benefit, although monitoring of the physical performance of air-conditioning plants and machinery used for disinfection and sterilization is important. In the event of an outbreak of hospital infection, more specific monitoring targeted at the known or likely causative micro-organism should be considered.

Microbiological screening of staff or patients is not undertaken routinely, but it may be needed for specific purposes, such as before cardiac surgery, to eliminate *Staph. aureus* from carriage sites which may otherwise cause self-infection, or for detection of staff carriers in critical areas such as dialysis units (hepatitis B).

## Surveillance and the role of the laboratory

The detection and characterization of hospital infection incidents or outbreaks rely on laboratory data that alert the infection control team to unusual clusters of infection, or to the sporadic appearance of organisms that may present a particular infection risk or management problem. Bacterial typing schemes and antibiograms (see Ch. 3) are very important in this regard. Regular visits to the wards are also important to record data on infected patients for whom specimens have not been received and to respond to problems as they occur. Such visits also serve to provide opportunities for practical teaching, which is another important element of the infection control team's responsibility.

## EFFICACY OF INFECTION CONTROL

There is acceptable proof of efficacy for only a few infection control measures. These include sterilization, handwashing, closed-drainage systems for urinary catheters, intravenous catheter care, peri-operative antibiotic prophylaxis for contaminated wounds and techniques for the care of equipment used in respiratory therapy. Isolation techniques are assumed to be reasonable as suggested by experience or inference. Measures which are now considered to be ineffective include the chemical disinfection of floors, walls, sinks and routine environmental monitoring.

Effective surveillance and action by the infection control team have been shown to reduce infection rates. One important role of the team is to monitor compliance with practices known to be effective and to eliminate the many rituals or less effective practices which may even increase the incidence or cost of cross-infection. As further advances occur in medical care and limited health care resources are spread across hospital and community needs, innovations in infection control will need to be evaluated for efficacy and cost-effectiveness. With this understanding it is possible that hospital infection can be controlled and largely prevented. The dictum of Florence Nightingale, made over a century ago, that 'the very first requirement in a hospital is that it should do the sick no harm', remains the goal.

### RECOMMENDED READING

Ayliffe G A J, Collins B J, Taylor L J 1990 *Hospital Acquired Infection*, 2nd edn. Wright, Bristol

Ayliffe G A J, Lowbury E J L, Geddes A M, Williams J D 1992 *Control of Hospital Infection*, 3rd edn. Chapman and Hall, London

British Medical Association 1989 *A Code of Practice for Sterilisation of Instruments and Control of Cross Infection*. Edward Arnold, London

Maurer I M 1985 *Hospital Hygiene*, 3rd edn. Edward Arnold, London

Report 1995 *Hospital Infection Control. Guidance on the Control of Infection in Hospitals*. Department of Health and Public Health Laboratory Service, London

Wenzel R P (ed) 1987 *Prevention and Control of Hospital Infection*. Williams and Wilkins, Baltimore

# 68

# Prophylactic immunization

*J. G. Collee*

Prophylactic immunization is only one of the measures that may be used for the control of infectious diseases. Its cost and efficacy must be assessed against other forms of defence such as: environmental sanitation; safe sewage disposal; a secure water supply; food hygiene; clean air and adequate ventilation; good animal husbandry with effective quarantine arrangements where necessary; insect vector control; and improved nutrition.

Other aspects of community defence against infection include: the surveillance of infectious diseases; early detection; prompt and adequate treatment; and isolation facilities, when appropriate, with proper measures to control cross-infection and transmission (Table 68.1). A detailed knowledge of the epidemiology of infections, and of the correct use of antimicrobial drugs and immunological products for therapy or prophylaxis, is crucial.

Much of the morbidity and mortality of infection is still either not assuredly preventable by immunization or presents great difficulties. For example, many of the diarrhoeal diseases and respiratory infections that take a heavy toll of life and health among young children in poor and overcrowded communities are not amenable to control by specific vaccines. Nor are the common bacterial infections associated with haemolytic streptococci, staphylococci and coliform bacilli, or many virus infections. However, some spectacular successes can be claimed, and encouraging efforts are being made to extend the range of success.

## RATIONALE OF IMMUNIZATION

The objective is to produce, without harm to the recipient, a degree of resistance sufficient to prevent a clinical attack of the natural infection. The degree of resistance conferred may not protect against an overwhelming challenge, and other control measures must operate in concert with any immunization policy, as discussed above.

## PASSIVE IMMUNIZATION

### Homologous and heterologous sera

*Artificial passive immunization* is used in clinical practice when it is considered necessary to protect a patient at short notice and for a limited period. Antibodies, which may be antitoxic, antibacterial or antiviral, in preparations of human or animal serum are injected to give temporary protection. Human preparations are referred to as *homologous*, and are much less likely to give rise to the adverse reactions occasionally associated with the injection of animal (*heterologous*) sera. An additional advantage of homologous antisera is that, although they do not confer durable protection, their effect may persist for 3–6 months, whereas the protection afforded by a heterologous serum is likely to last for only a few weeks.

**Table 68.1** Approaches to the prevention of infectious disease: an indication of priorities

- Preventive engineering: water, sewage, ventilation, food production and food processing
- Surveillance and diagnostic awareness
- Prompt management: recognition, treatment, isolation and contact tracing where necessary
- Improvement and maintenance of good socio-economic conditions: housing, nutrition, education, medical and social care
- Increased resistance to infection by appropriate active immunization policies and in some special circumstances by passive immunization

## Equine antitoxins

Antiserum raised in the horse against diphtheria toxin (*equine diphtheria antitoxin*) is available for the prophylaxis and treatment of diphtheria. A similar heterologous antiserum is available for emergency use in cases of suspected botulism and to protect those thought to be at risk. Equine tetanus antitoxin is still used in some countries, but it should be abandoned in favour of human tetanus immunoglobulin (see Ch. 23, p. 240). It is most important to give an intended recipient of equine serum a prior test dose to exclude hypersensitive subjects who may have been sensitized by a previous dose of equine serum.

## Pooled immunoglobulins

Protective levels of antibody to a range of diseases are present in pooled normal human serum. *Human normal immunoglobulin* (HNIG) is available in the UK and elsewhere for the short-term prophylaxis of hepatitis A in contacts or travellers who intend to visit countries where hepatitis A is common (but note that active immunization against hepatitis A is now an alternative for frequent adult travellers to areas where hepatitis A is relatively common). HNIG also protects an immunocompromised child temporarily against measles if given promptly after contact with a case. However, HNIG does not give reliable post-exposure protection against mumps or rubella.

## Specific immunoglobulins

Preparations of specific immunoglobulins are available in the UK for passive immunization against tetanus (human tetanus immunoglobulin; HTIG), Hepatitis B (HBIG), rabies (HRIG), varicella–zoster (ZIG) and vaccinia (AVIG).

## ACTIVE IMMUNIZATION

## Types of vaccine

### Toxoids

If the signs and symptoms of a disease can be attributed essentially to the effects of a single toxin, a modified form of the toxin that preserves its antigenicity but has lost its toxicity (a *toxoid*) provides the key to successful active immunization against the disease. This has been spectacularly successful with tetanus and diphtheria.

### Inactivated vaccines

If the disease is not mediated by a single toxin, it may be possible to stimulate the production of protective antibodies by using the killed (inactivated) organisms. This is done as a routine with vaccines against pertussis (whooping cough), typhoid and influenza. There is also an inactivated polio vaccine.

### Attenuated live vaccines

In some cases, the inactivation procedure to make a killed vaccine destroys or modifies the protective antigenicity (*immunogenicity*) of the organisms. Hence, another approach is to use suspensions of living organisms that are reduced in their virulence (*attenuated*) but still immunogenic. This strategy has yielded: mumps, measles and rubella vaccines (now combined); the live-virus polio vaccine; and yellow fever vaccine.

Sometimes it is possible to use a related organism with shared antigens. Thus, the vaccinia virus vaccine was used to eradicate smallpox, and a bovine tubercle bacillus was modified by Calmette and Guérin to make bacille Calmette–Guérin (BCG) which protects humans against tuberculosis.

### Special procedures

Some vaccines, such as influenza (virus) vaccine, can be refined by a process that removes unwanted protein and other reactive material but retains the important protective antigens. Some others must be conjugated to proteins to render them immunogenic. Some vaccines, such as hepatitis B vaccine, can be bio-engineered. There is much current interest in the possibility of developing *subunit vaccines* consisting of purified fragments of the major immunogenic components of micro-organisms, particularly viruses.

## Immune response

Antibodies against the agents of some bacterial and viral infections may be present in the mother's blood and be passively acquired by the baby. This gives some protection to the infant at a time when it is poorly equipped to produce specific antibodies, but it may interfere to a varying extent with the infant's capacity to respond to the stimulus of injected or ingested vaccines in the very early months of life. Although the capacity of the infant to produce specific antibody to injected antigens is poorly developed in the first few months of life, this problem can often be resolved by the use of *adjuvants*. Thus, effective responses are produced to powerful antigens such as alum-adsorbed toxoids. Pertussis whole-cell vaccines have an adjuvant effect of their own, so the combination of adsorbed toxoids and whole-cell pertussis vaccine (the triple diphtheria, tetanus, and pertussis vaccine) is an effective immunizing complex that can be given at 2, 3 and 4 months of age to cover the period when the lethal potential of pertussis is greatest (see Ch. 33). The tissues of the newborn respond effectively to BCG vaccine because the protection here is cell mediated. The use of a high-potency measles vaccine at 6 months of age is likely to be exploited in countries where measles kills or severely injures the very young.

When a good specific antibody response is being sought to a toxoid or a killed antigen, the usual procedure is to give three doses of the antigen at spaced intervals. The first or 'priming' dose evokes a low level of antibody after a latent period of about 2 weeks, but the second dose elicits a much greater (secondary) antibody response, and this is further boosted by the third dose. The efficacy of injected antigen preparations can be enhanced by slow-release agents such as mineral carriers which have adjuvant effects. With most antigens, the response is better if the first two doses are separated by an interval of a month or two. A third dose is generally recommended at some time thereafter, and further booster doses may be given to maintain immunity.

## Duration of immunity

After an effective course of active immunization, a protective amount of antibody may persist in the blood for some years and a subsequent booster injection may maintain protection for a further decade. Much depends upon circumstances that will vary for different vaccines and different groups of people. The duration of active protection cannot be absolutely equated with the presence of demonstrable antibody because factors such as the sensitivity of the test and the actual protective role of the antibody detected have to be taken into consideration.

## Age of commencement of active immunization

This must take account of the immaturity of the antibody-forming system in the very early months (see above) and the infectious challenges that a child may encounter early in life and in later years. The start of any immunization programme must be adjusted to the known epidemiology of the diseases that are prevalent in the country in which it is to be instituted, and it must also be related to any serious infective challenges that may be imported from time to time. Poliomyelitis is a good example of a disease that has been largely eradicated from many communities; however, the disease is quick to strike back if the immunization shield is lowered.

## CONTROLLED STUDIES OF PROPHYLACTIC VACCINES

Combined field and laboratory studies aim to provide confidence in the efficacy of vaccines. A field trial can show only whether or not the actual preparation of vaccine used was successful under the circumstances prevailing at the time. Accordingly, trials require very sophisticated design and much care in their execution. They are very expensive. In order to satisfy the requirement for reproducibility, the method of preparation of the vaccine must be meticulously described and controlled. Much work continues to define and to refine laboratory tests for the protectiveness of a particular vaccine that might be correlated with its efficacy in field trials. The laboratory test that gives results most closely corresponding to the protective value in the field trials may then be adopted as the test for standardizing future batches of vaccine.

Manufacturers of vaccines for commercial use are required in the UK and in many other countries to satisfy certain standards relating to the purity, safety, potency and stability of their products. In addition, the World Health Organization has established internationally agreed requirements. At the national level, a system for continuing surveillance of the efficacy of prophylactic vaccines with continuing notification of any suspected adverse reactions is essential.

## CONTRA-INDICATIONS TO THE USE OF VACCINES

The delivery of an important immunization programme should not be unwisely prejudiced by catch-all statements that take a legalistic view of theoretical hazards and thus err on the side of opting out. The risk of opting out of an immunization schedule should be clearly appreciated.

It is difficult to make valid generalizations about contra-indications to vaccination, but there are some useful general principles: do not give a vaccine to a patient with an acute illness, but do be sure that the postponed immunization is subsequently given. Do not give a live vaccine to a pregnant woman, unless there is a clear balance of risk in favour of vaccination; in general, avoid giving any vaccine in the first trimester of pregnancy. Do not give live vaccines to patients receiving immunosuppressive drugs or irradiation, or to patients suffering from malignant conditions of the reticulo-endothelial system – delay until after successful therapy when they are in remission.

Experience with human immunodeficiency virus (HIV) antibody-positive patients with or without the signs and symptoms of the acquired immune deficiency syndrome (AIDS) indicates so far that measles, mumps, rubella and polio (live virus) vaccines can be given, but that BCG vaccine should not be given. Inactivated vaccines are not contra-indicated.

## Hazards of immunization

Possible adverse reactions to active immunization with an injected preparation generally range from mild or moderate pain at the site of injection, to fever and malaise for a day or two after. Anaphylactic reactions are very rare; as they may be fatal, doctors and nurses should be aware of the possibility and should be prepared for such an emergency by carrying drugs and equipment for resuscitation (a 'shock box') to all immunization sessions. No death of a child attributed to an anaphylactic reaction to an active immunizing agent was notified in the UK in the decade 1979–89. This is reassuring, but it is also a challenge to maintain our collective and individual vigilance.

During the first few years of life when many vaccines are given, children tend to have various health problems that include occasional febrile convulsions and may, sadly, include an unexplained cot death or other tragedy. It is inevitable that some of these events will coincide with the period shortly after a vaccine was given to a child and the possibility of a causal relationship will be entertained. The probability of such a link certainly deserves to be considered, but it is most important to bear in mind that the issue is emotive and that ill-balanced or ill-informed adverse publicity can do irreparable harm to an immunization programme. For example, annual notifications of whooping cough in England and Wales dropped from more than 100 000 in the early 1950s to some tens of thousands in the late 1950s as the vaccine gained ground. By the early 1970s (and after modification of the vaccine to take account of a possible deficiency in its protective cover), whooping cough was largely controlled in the UK with about 75% of children

immunized. In the late 1970s, after some ill-informed adverse publicity, acceptance rates for the vaccine fell steeply to 30% or lower, and the uptake of other vaccines was also affected. Epidemics of whooping cough followed in the UK in 1978 and 1982 with tens of thousands of children affected. It should be remembered that the morbidity associated with whooping cough is still very considerable, and very young children still die of the disease or are severely injured by it (see Ch. 33). Deaths attributable to whooping cough averaged seven per year in the 5 years from 1976 to 1981. In the UK epidemic of 1978–80, 0.02% of notified cases died.

As a result of efforts to restore confidence in pertussis vaccine, uptake figures increased in the 1980s and the disease again began to be brought under control. Preliminary results of tests with new (acellular) pertussis vaccines indicate that these are safe and probably more effective.

Children who are most vulnerable are likely to be least protected. Pertussis, polio and measles spread most effectively when living conditions are over-crowded and unhygienic. To some extent, these diseases depend upon population density for their spread. Some underprivileged groups in a community are in very real danger when the average rate of vaccine uptake falls, because they often represent the extreme end of the fall in vaccine cover.

In view of the stringency of the regulations that control the quality and efficacy of vaccines, the probability of error lies more with the vaccinator than with the producer. There is a special obligation to ensure that a vaccine is properly stored, properly reconstituted (if relevant) and properly administered (Table 68.2). The appropriate instructions and local protocols should be followed in detail. *An injectable vaccine must be given with a sterile syringe and needle, and a separate sterile syringe and needle must be used for each injection.*

## Site of injection

This will vary with the vaccine to be given. Specific instructions should be followed. In general, and

---

**Table 68.2** Safety considerations

- Use a separate sterile syringe and needle
- Avoid errors: check the vial personally
- Consider the patient's history: note pregnancy and various contra-indications
- Keep careful records

with the exception of BCG, injectable vaccines are given by intramuscular or deep subcutaneous injection. The anterolateral aspect of the thigh or upper arm is the preferred site for infants. Some doctors and nurses use the upper outer quadrant of the buttock, but fat in this area may interfere with the efficacy of the vaccine.

## HERD IMMUNITY

When most of the people in a community are immune to a particular infection that is spread from person to person, the natural transmission of the infection is effectively inhibited. Thus, if almost all children in a residential school have been immunized against measles, the school is most unlikely to have an outbreak of measles; even the few children who have not been immunized will enjoy a measure of protection afforded by the general herd immunity in that they will not be challenged within the school. This will only apply so long as the school population is largely composed of immune pupils and a non-immune pupil does not encounter a visitor who is infected with measles. If there is an influx of non-immunes, the level of herd immunity will fall and the general protection will be lost. When the pupils go into other communities at holiday times, the non-immune individuals are liable to get measles at their first contact with an infective case.

For herd immunity to operate well in a community or a country, vaccine uptake rates must exceed 90%. For some highly transmissible infections such as measles, uptake rates above 95% are the target. Bear in mind that herd immunity operates only for infections transmitted from person to person. Tetanus is not transmitted in this way; a non-immune person is fully vulnerable to tetanus even if he or she is surrounded by fully immunized colleagues in a closed community (Fig. 68.1).

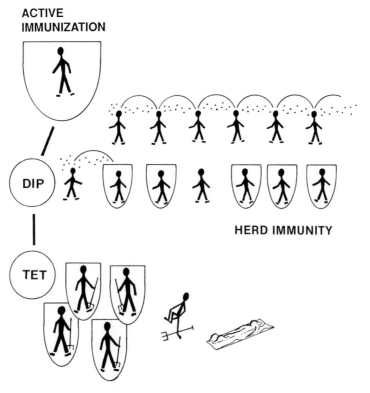

**ACTIVE IMMUNIZATION**

DIP

**HERD IMMUNITY**

TET

**Fig. 68.1** If almost all of the members of a community receive active immunization against a disease that is normally transmitted from person to person, the resulting herd immunity confers some advantage even upon an occasional non-immune member because rapid transmission of the disease through the community is prevented. This is true for diphtheria, but not for tetanus, which is not dependent on person-to-person spread.

# IMMUNIZATION PROGRAMMES

An immunization campaign carried out without provision for its continuation as a routine procedure will not give satisfactory results unless complete eradication of the disease is achieved. Thus, in planning immunization schedules, consideration must be given to ensuring that the general public is receptive and understands the policy. It is essential to secure the trust and co-operation of parents who have to bring their children to the doctor or clinic for a series of inoculations and who will undoubtedly seek reassurance that the benefits are considerable and the risks negligible. Parental consent must be obtained for each immunization.

In the planning and execution of a programme, immunological points that merit special attention are:

1. The use of combined antigens and the simultaneous administration of killed and live vaccines
2. The incorporation of adjuvants in killed vaccines and toxoids
3. The age of commencement
4. The dosage and spacing of antigens.

# IMMUNIZATION SCHEDULES

The provision of a programme of active immunization to a community should be governed by considerations of need, efficacy, safety and ease of administration. An overriding consideration is the cost and the availability of skilled manpower. Circumstances vary widely in different countries, and priorities vary.

In the UK, it is generally agreed that protection of the susceptible population against diphtheria, whooping cough and tetanus (with a triple vaccine), *Haemophilus influenzae* type b (with an inactivated conjugated Hib vaccine), poliomyelitis (with a live vaccine), and mumps, measles and rubella (with a combined live vaccine) merit priority in the very early years of life. BCG vaccine is offered to tuberculin-negative children at 10–14 years and in some high-risk populations neonatally. In the UK it is now recommended that the DTP triple vaccine with the Hib vaccine and oral polio vaccine are started early, at 2 months, with further doses at 3 months and 4 months (Table 68.3). This secures earlier protection against pertussis in the months when the disease is most dangerous to the young child.

**Table 68.3**  Schedule of immunization for children in the UK: a model for countries with adequate public health services

| Age | Vaccine | Notes |
|---|---|---|
| During year 1 | Diphtheria<br>Tetanus<br>Pertussis | DTP triple vaccine: start at 2 months; second dose at 3 months and third dose at 4 months by intramuscular or deep subcutaneous injection |
| | Hib vaccine | Give at the same times as the DTP injections |
| | Oral polio vaccine | Give at the same times as the DTP injections |
| During year 2 | Measles<br>Mumps<br>Rubella | MMR vaccine: give one injection of the combined live vaccine at age 12–18 months |
| At 4–5 years | Diphtheria<br>Tetanus<br>MMR[a] | Booster |
| | Oral polio vaccine | Booster |
| At 10–14 years | Rubella[b]<br>BCG vaccine[b] | For girls if they have not received MMR vaccine<br>For tuberculin-negative children |
| At 15–18 years | Tetanus/low-dose diphtheria<br>Oral polio | Booster<br>Booster |

[a] To be introduced in the UK.
[b] Allow an interval of at least 3 weeks between rubella and BCG.

## NOTES ON SOME VACCINES IN COMMON USE

### Adsorbed tetanus toxoid

The preparation in routine use in the UK is adsorbed onto an aluminium salt; it is is more effective and less reactive than simple toxoid. It is a component of the triple DTP vaccine. A course of three injections given at intervals of about 6 weeks and 6 months immunizes for at least 5 years. A booster dose at school entry then protects for 10 years, and booster doses can be given thereafter at intervals of 10 years. Prevention of tetanus should be considered in relation to the management of wounds (see Ch. 23, p. 239).

### Diphtheria toxoid

The adsorbed preparation used in the UK and incorporated into the triple DTP vaccine contains aluminium phosphate and affords good protection which is boosted at school entry age. This preparation is not used for adults; a dilute adsorbed diphtheria vaccine preparation is used for people who are more than 10 years old and is now incorporated with tetanus toxoid for school leavers. Active immunization of adults against diphtheria is not practised in the UK as a routine, unless there is a potentially high occupational risk of encountering the organism in laboratory or clinical work, or unless a person has been in contact with a case of diphtheria or travelling to an endemic area and protection is deemed necessary. A course of erythromycin gives further protection to a close contact, and this has replaced the use of diphtheria antitoxin in contacts. The falling level of immunity to diphtheria among adults in communities that regard themselves as having good preventive medical services gives some cause for concern and calls for continuing vigilance particularly because of large outbreaks in eastern Europe.

The Schick test (see Ch. 18, p. 192) can be used to check the immunity of those recruited to work where there is an occupational hazard of diphtheria.

### Pertussis vaccine

The vaccines in general use are whole-cell preparations of killed *Bordetella pertussis*. Acellular vaccines containing antigenic components of the organism have been developed and are being assessed for their protective potency; results so far are very promising. The protection afforded by the whole-cell vaccines is generally acknowledged to be considerable, but the acellular vaccines seem to be more effective. Three injections are given at intervals of 1 month or more. Whole-cell pertussis vaccine is a component of the DTP triple vaccine, and it has the added advantage of being an adjuvant in that combination.

Adverse reactions that may be associated with pertussis vaccine include soreness at the site of injection, irritability and pyrexia. Other reactions such as persistent screaming, shock, vomiting and convulsions have been reported, but the association with pertussis vaccine is not invariably clear. Sometimes an association with a different vaccine is claimed, and sometimes there is no history of recent vaccination. Thus, while there may be a causal association, in some cases there seems to be a considerable chance that the association is casual and not attributable to the vaccine. Particular attention has been paid to a possible association of convulsions and encephalopathy and cerebral damage. It should be noted that unexplained convulsions occur in young children, especially during the period when the immunization programme is set, and that such an incident may occur by chance shortly after a vaccine has been given. Moreover, the age at which certain cases of cerebral damage begin to be apparent coincides with this age range. Accordingly, we are quite uncertain if there is a risk of permanent brain damage associated with whole-cell pertussis vaccine; if there is, it must be very small and it must be greatly outweighed by the known risk of neurological and other damage that may be life-threatening when the natural disease occurs. It is hoped that acellular pertussis vaccines which are much less likely to cause reactions will resolve the problem.

### *Haemophilus influenzae* type b (Hib) vaccine

Invasive encapsulated strains of *H. influenzae*, almost always of serotype b, are associated with meningitis, bacteraemia, epiglottitis and other serious infections particularly affecting young children. The risks of severe morbidity and mortality are highest in children in the age range 3–18 months. Hib conjugate vaccines containing the capsular polysaccharide linked to a protein are immunogenic. The Hib vaccines used in the UK are given as deep subcutaneous or intramuscular injections; three doses of 0.5 ml are injected at intervals of 1 month. The preparation now in use is combined in the DTP vaccine. Children in the age range 1–4 years who have not received Hib vaccine can be protected by a single dose of Hib vaccine. Routine immunization of older children or adults with Hib vaccine is not generally recommended.

## Poliomyelitis vaccines

The control of poliomyelitis is one of the great success stories of active immunization, and the world-wide eradication of poliomyelitis by the year 2000 is a goal of the World Health Organization. The Salk vaccine came first; this is a killed mixture of the three types of poliovirus (1, 2 and 3). A course of three injections is given at appropriate intervals.

The polio vaccine favoured in the UK and many other countries is the live attenuated form developed by Sabin. This is a mixture of the three types, and it is given orally on three occasions, usually at the same time as the triple DTP vaccine is given in the early months. Note that the oral polio vaccine (OPV) is not given by injection. As it is a live preparation, the vaccine must be stored and held according to the manufacturer's instructions and not allowed to become inactivated in a bottle on the desk. OPV colonizes the gut and gives rise to local and humoral antibodies. The faeces contain live virus for some time, and poliomyelitis caused by a vaccine strain is a rare, but recognized hazard. Any non-immune contact in the household should be advised to be immunized at the same time, but difficulties in arranging this should not delay the primary job of getting the baby immunized. It is important to advise on the hygienic handling of the baby's nappies during the period of excretion of the virus (and at any other time, for that matter!).

## Measles, mumps and rubella (MMR) vaccine

This is a mixture of live attenuated strains of these three viruses in freeze-dried form; it has to be stored at 2–8°C (not frozen), reconstituted according to the manufacturer's instructions and used promptly. One injection of the mixture is given in the 2nd year of life in the UK schedule, and there are proposals to give a second dose in the 5th year.

The measles component may give rise to fever or malaise and sometimes a rash about a week after inoculation. The mumps component may cause some parotid swelling seen about 3 weeks after inoculation. Very occasional cases of mumps vaccine-associated meningo-encephalitis are being reported; these also occur at 3 weeks and follow a generally benign course, but there may be confusion with other non-benign syndromes in this age group. The rubella component is not usually associated with reactions in this age group, though temporary malaise, mild fever and arthralgia occurring about the 9th day after vaccination have been noted in some older recipients of rubella vaccine.

It is hoped that the incorporation of two doses of MMR vaccine in the UK schedule will eradicate measles, mumps and rubella in this country. Much depends upon an adequate uptake of the vaccine, as these diseases are highly transmissible. Meanwhile, a dose of rubella vaccine alone will be offered to girls aged 10–14 years who have not received the booster dose of MMR vaccine, and rubella vaccine is offered to all seronegative women of child-bearing age and to seronegative professional attendants who might come into contact with pregnant women at clinics, etc. Although rubella vaccine is not thought to be teratogenic, any woman of child-bearing age who is given the vaccine should avoid pregnancy for a month.

## BCG

The attenuated strain of bovine tubercle bacillus known as bacille Calmette–Guérin (BCG) produces cross-immunity to human tuberculosis and has significantly contributed to the control of the disease in many countries. An intradermal injection of the live attenuated vaccine is given on the lateral aspect of the arm at the level of the deltoid insertion, but not higher, or on the upper lateral surface of the thigh. Instruction on the reconstitution of the freeze-dried vaccine, the dosage and the detailed technique of giving a truly intradermal injection should be most carefully observed. With the exception of newborn children, any recipient of BCG vaccination should have been tested for hypersensitivity to tuberculin and found to be negative. Tuberculin tests include the *Mantoux test*, in which diluted tuberculin is injected intradermally, and the *Heaf test*, which is done with a multiple puncture apparatus (see Ch. 19). Be sure to appreciate the difference between the tuberculin test and a BCG vaccination; and note that attention to detail in the sterilization of the Heaf apparatus is of crucial importance.

## Hepatitis B vaccine

For the protection of groups of people considered to be at special risk of acquiring hepatitis B, a bio-engineered vaccine is now in common use. A course of three intramuscular injections is given (not into the buttock) at intervals of 1 and 5 months; thus, it takes 6 months to complete the course, and this is of practical importance. Protective antibody responses are generally achieved in about 90% of those given the vaccine with a range of responses from weak to

| Table 68.4 | Vaccines for active immunization of people at special risk |
|---|---|
| Anthrax | Pneumococcal infection* |
| Cholera | Q fever |
| Hepatitis A | Rabies |
| Hepatitis B | Smallpox (vaccinia vaccine) |
| Influenza* | Typhoid* |
| Japanese B encephalitis | Typhus |
| Meningococcal infection | Varicella–zoster* |
| Plague | Yellow fever |

The asterisk indicates that there are some problems (see text).

strong, but there is a worrying minority of non-responders (10–15% in the over-40 years age group). Antibody responses should be checked 3–4 months after completion of a course, and it may be prudent to give poor responders or non-responders a booster dose or a repeat course. Non-response rates are particularly worrying among patients on maintenance haemodialysis. In the general population, the protection afforded to responders is thought to last for about 5 years, when a booster dose of vaccine may be given. Established policy must await further experience with hepatitis vaccines, which in many countries are being given universally as part of the routine schedule.

## Other vaccines

Various vaccines are available for the protection of special groups of people or for individuals in special circumstances (Table 68.4). The reader is referred to the appropriate chapters for more detailed consideration of such topics as: the prevention of tetanus in wounded patients; the indications for pneumococcal vaccine; the management of rabies; the control of Q fever; the protection of those at special risk from hepatitis B; and the protection of HIV antibody-positive individuals and patients with AIDS.

## PROTECTING THE TRAVELLER

An intending traveller to another country should seek advice in advance about the prevailing diseases and the precautions that should be taken. Advice on immunization is unlikely to be of much help if the traveller unwisely runs the risk of drinking raw water or eating uncooked salads and vegetables in a country where sanitation is inadequate and water supplies are insecure.

In advising travellers about exotic diseases, do not forget that diseases now uncommon in countries with developed medical services may still be common in countries that lack such services. Thus, a booster dose of poliomyelitis vaccine may be appropriate, for example. If work in a hospital or health clinic is envisaged, include the risk of diphtheria in your list. Do not forget that tetanus is still a major killer on a global scale. Remember that tuberculosis is still common in some countries. If the traveller is going to Central Africa or Central America, bear in mind the need for protection against yellow fever. Other vaccines that may be indicated include those that will afford some protection against typhoid. Some of the special vaccines listed in Table 68.4 may also merit inclusion, especially if the traveller's activities when abroad are likely to expose him or her to the relevant diseases.

Active immunization against hepatitis A can be offered to frequent travellers to areas where hepatitis A is relatively common or to those intending to stay for more than 3 months in these areas. Passive protection against hepatitis A for some months is conferred by the injection of human normal immuno-globulin (HNIG, see p. 653) and this is still the preferred option for a short-term traveller to an endemic area. Give the injection shortly before your patient sets off, but not so late that the patient still has sore buttocks while in transit.

An effective malaria vaccine has been sought for many years, but none is yet available. Consequently, it is essential to ensure that any traveller to (or through) a malarious zone is adequately protected by relevant advice and by the proper prophylactic drugs (see Ch. 61).

## UNRESOLVED PROBLEMS

Nothing is perfect (see Table 68.5). Some vaccines are more imperfect than others, and some circumstances pose special problems. The influenza virus

| Table 68.5 | Properties of an ideal vaccine |
|---|---|

- Promotes effective immunity
- Confers lifelong protection
- Safe (no side-effects)
- Stable
- Cheap
- Seen to be good and effective (protected from adverse publicity by regular appraisal and informed comment)

has shifts and drifts in its antigenic pattern, so vaccines must be frequently updated. Then decisions have to be made on the patients who merit this special protection. As these include many old people and many patients with respiratory or cardiovascular impairment, the decisions are quite difficult.

Cholera vaccines have had a chequered record with very little evidence of real efficacy for the traveller, who is much better protected by a basic knowledge of hygiene. Some new developments with oral vaccines are a little more promising.

Acute purulent (bacterial) meningitis is a dramatic clinical problem. A vaccine that affords some protection against groups A and C of the meningococcus is available, but a group B vaccine is not available at the time of writing (1996) and group B strains are more common in many areas.

We are still quite unclear about the place of pneumococcal vaccine (see Ch. 17). A vaccine produced against 23 types of pneumococci is recommended, particularly for the protection of patients who do not have a spleen or are about to be splenectomized in the course of therapy. It is also suggested that the vaccine may be of use, sometimes with additional penicillin prophylaxis, for the protection of various groups of patients against pneumococcal infections.

Typhoid vaccine is associated with reactions of pyrexia and malaise attributable to the lipopolysaccharide endotoxin content of the presently available preparation. An attenuated strain, Ty21a, has been developed with a built-in metabolic error which is the basis for the live vaccine given by the oral route.

Several vaccines have been developed against various herpesviruses including herpes simplex, varicella–zoster and Epstein–Barr viruses. There have been many difficulties, but a live attenuated varicella vaccine has been developed.

A vaccine effective against HIV is being urgently sought in the fight against AIDS. There have been many disappointments, and we are still hoping.

## RECOMMENDED READING

Anonymous. Immunological products and vaccines. In: *British National Formulary*. British Medical Association and Royal Pharmaceutical Society of Great Britain, London (revised at intervals of about 6 months)

Department of Health, Welsh Office, Scottish Home and Health Department 1995 *Health Information for Overseas Travel*. HMSO, London

Department of Health, Welsh Office, Scottish Home and Health Department, DHSS (Northern Ireland) 1996 *Immunisation against Infectious Disease*. HMSO, London

Mackett M, Williamson J D 1995 *Human Vaccines and Vaccination*. Bios Scientific Publications, Oxford

Nicholl A, Rudd P (eds) 1989 *British Paediatric Association Manual on Infections and Immunizations in Children*. Oxford University Press, Oxford

Reid D, Grist N R 1987 Tetanus immunization. *Update* 34: 149–156

Root R K, Warren K S, Griffiss J M, Sande M A 1989 *Immunization*. Churchill Livingstone, New York

The health authorities of some countries issue useful booklets with guidelines appropriate to the local conditions.

# Index